BASIC HANDBOOK

OF

Child Psychiatry

VOLUME TWO

BASIC HANDBOOK OF
Child Psychiatry

Joseph D. Noshpitz / *Editor-in-Chief*

VOLUME TWO

Disturbances in Development

JOSEPH D. NOSHPITZ

EDITOR

Basic Books, Inc., Publishers / New York

To all those

who strive to ease the pain

and better the lives of troubled children

these books are dedicated

Library of Congress Cataloging in Publication Data
Main entry under title:

Basic handbook of child psychiatry.

Includes bibliographies and indexes.
CONTENTS: v. 1. Development.—v. 2. Disturbances
in development.—
1. Child psychiatry. I. Noshpitz, Joseph D.
RJ499.B33   618.9′28′9   78–7082
ISBN 0–465–00590–X

Copyright © 1979 by Basic Books, Inc.
Printed in the United States of America
DESIGNED BY VINCENT TORRE
10 9 8 7 6 5 4 3 2 1

CONTENTS

PART A / Etiology

PART B / Nosology

PART C / Syndromes

CONTRIBUTORS

STEVEN LURIA ABLON, M.D.
Assistant Professor of Psychiatry, Harvard Medical School, Boston; Director of Child Psychiatry Training, Cambridge-Somerville Mental Health and Retardation Center, Cambridge, Massachusetts.

PAUL L. ADAMS, M.D.
Professor of Psychiatry, University of Louisville, Louisville, Kentucky.

THOMAS F. ANDERS, M.D.
Associate Professor of Psychiatry and Pediatrics and Director of Child Psychiatry, Stanford University School of Medicine, Stanford, California.

ADRIAN LEE BAL, PHARM.D.
Resident of Clinical Pharmacy, Long Beach Memorial Hospital, Long Beach, California.

RONALD M. BENSON, M.D.
Clinical Associate Professor, Department of Psychiatry, University of Michigan; Director, Youth Outpatient Program, Children's Psychiatric Hospital, Ann Arbor, Michigan.

SIDNEY BERMAN, M.D.
Clinical Professor of Psychiatry, George Washington University School of Medicine; Senior Advisory Staff, Children's Hospital, Washington, D.C.

DENNIS P. CANTWELL, M.D.
Director of Training in Child Psychiatry, University of California School of Medicine, Los Angeles, California.

MORTON CHETHIK, M.S.W.
Associate Professor, Department of Psychiatry, University of Michigan, Ann Arbor, Michigan.

JOHN C. COOLIDGE, M.D.
Senior Staff Psychiatrist, Judge Baker Guidance Center, Roxbury; Assistant Clinical Professor in Child Psychiatry, Harvard Medical School, Boston, Massachusetts.

LEON CYTRYN, M.D.
Clinical Professor of Psychiatry and Behavioral Sciences, and of Child Health and Development, George Washington University, School of Medicine, Washington, D.C.; Staff Psychiatrist, Unit on Childhood Mental Illness, National Institute of Mental Health, Bethesda, Maryland.

CHRISTINA C. DUBLIN
Former Research Social Worker, Children's Hospital National Medical Center, Washington, D.C.

LEON EISENBERG, M.D.
Maude and Lillian Presley Professor of Psychiatry, Harvard Medical School; Senior Associate in Psychiatry, Children's Hospital Medical Center, Boston, Massachusetts.

MILTON ENGEL, M.D.
Clinical Professor of Child Psychiatry, Georgetown University School of Medicine; Child Psychiatrist, Saxe Therapeutic School, Washington, D.C.

SHERMAN C. FEINSTEIN, M.D.
Clinical Professor, Pritzker School of Medicine, Michael Reese Hospital, University of Chicago, Chicago, Illinois.

STUART M. FINCH, M.D.
Lecturer, University of Arizona College of Medicine, Tucson, Arizona.

BARBARA FISH, M.D.
Professor of Psychiatry, Division of Child Psychiatry and Mental Retardation, University of California, Los Angeles; Associate Member, Mental Retardation Research Center, Los Angeles, California.

Contributors

SUSAN M. FISHER, M.D.
Assistant Clinical Professor, Department of Psychiatry, Tufts Medical School; Clinical Instructor, Harvard Medical School, Boston, Massachusetts.

ELLEN D. FREEMAN, M.D.
Assistant Clinical Professor of Psychiatry, Cornell University Medical Center, New York, New York.

RICHARD GALDSTON, M.D.
Assistant Clinical Professor of Psychiatry, Harvard Medical School, Boston, Massachusetts.

JOSEPH M. GREEN, M.D.
Professor of Psychiatry; Director, Division of Child and Adolescent Psychiatry, University of Wisconsin School of Medicine, Madison, Wisconsin.

RICHARD GREEN, M.D.
Professor, Departments of Psychiatry, Behavioral Science, and Psychology, State University of New York, Stony Brook, New York.

STANLEY I. GREENSPAN, M.D.
Supervising and Teaching Staff, Children's Hospital and Medical School, George Washington University, Washington, D.C.; Chief of Clinical Research, Mental Health Study Center, National Institute of Mental Health, Adelphi, Maryland.

JAMES G. KAVANAUGH, JR., M.D.
Assistant Professor of Psychiatry and Pediatrics, Division of Child and Adolescent Psychiatry, University of Virginia Medical Center, Charlottesville, Virginia.

EDWIN S. KESSLER, M.D.
Clinical Professor of Psychiatry and Director, Children's Psychiatric Services, Georgetown University Medical Center, Washington, D.C.

VIKI LABRECQUE, PH.D.
Director of Psychological Services, Kellogg Psychiatric Hospital, Corona, California.

MAURICE W. LAUFER, M.D.
Professor of Psychiatry and Human Behavior, Brown University Program in Medicine, Providence; President and Physician-in-Chief, Emma Pendleton Bradley Hospital, Riverside, Rhode Island.

PAUL C. LAYBOURNE, JR., M.D.
Professor of Psychiatry and Family Practice; Associate Professor of Pediatrics; Director, Division of Child Psychiatry, University of Kansas Medical Center, Kansas City, Kansas.

MELVIN LEWIS, M.D.
Professor of Pediatrics and Psychiatry, Yale Child Study Center, New Haven, Connecticut.

DAVID LOOFF, M.D.
Private Practice, Adolescent and Child Psychiatry, Lexington, Kentucky.

REGINALD S. LOURIE, M.D., MED.SCD.
Professor Emeritus, Child Health and Development, Department of Psychiatry and Behavioral Sciences, George Washington University, Washington, D.C.; Senior Research Scientist, National Institute of Mental Health, Bethesda, Maryland.

ALEXANDER R. LUCAS, M.D.
Head, Section of Child and Adolescent Psychiatry, Mayo Clinic; Professor in Psychiatry, Mayo Medical School, Rochester, Minnesota.

JOHN E. MACK, M.D.
Professor of Psychiatry, Harvard Medical School, The Cambridge Hospital, Cambridge, Massachusetts.

DONALD H. MCKNEW, JR., M.D.
Clinical Assistant Professor of Psychiatry and Behavioral Science, and of Child Health and Development, George Washington University School of Medicine, Washington, D.C.; Staff Psychiatrist, Unit on Childhood Mental Illness, Adult Psychiatry Branch, National Institute of Mental Health, Bethesda, Maryland.

ÅKE MATTSSON, M.D.
Professor of Psychiatry and Attending Physician at New York University Medical Center; Attending Physician, Bellvue Hospital; Director of Child and Adolescent Division, New York University Medical Center, New York, New York.

J. GARY MAY, M.D.
Director, Adolescent Inpatient Services, Department of Psychiatry, University of Colorado Medical Center; Child Psychiatry Consultant, Denver Public Schools, Denver, Colorado.

JOHN E. MEEKS, M.D.
Medical Director, Child and Adolescent Services, The Psychiatric Institute of Washington, Washington, D.C.

DEREK MILLER, M.D.
Chief, Adolescent Program, Institute of Psychiatry, Northwestern University, Evanston, Illinois.

FRANCIS K. MILLICAN, M.D.
Associate Clinical Professor of Psychiatry, Georgetown University School of Medicine;

Faculty Associate, Department of Psychiatry, Children's Hospital National Medical Center, Washington, D.C.

HUMBERTO NAGERA, M.D.
Professor and Director, Child Analytic Study Program and Chief, Youth Services, Children's Psychiatric Hospital, University of Michigan Medical Center, Ann Arbor, Michigan.

JOSEPH D. NOSHPITZ, M.D.
Professor of Psychiatry, George Washington University; Professor of Psychiatry and Director of Education and Training, Department of Psychiatry, Children's Hospital National Medical Center, Washington, D.C.

ROBERT A. NOVER, M.D.
Clinical Assistant Professor of Psychiatry and Behavioral Sciences and Child Health and Development, George Washington University, Washington, D.C.; Section Chief in Child Psychiatry, Mental Health Study Center, National Institute of Mental Health, Adelphi, Maryland.

KARL FREDERICK NYSTROM, M.D.
Clinical Instructor of Psychiatry, University of Southern California School of Medicine, Los Angeles, California.

JOHN B. REINHART, M.D.
Professor, Pediatrics and Child Psychiatry, University of Pittsburgh, School of Medicine; Director, Division of Behavioral Sciences, Children's Hospital of Pittsburgh, Pittsburgh, Pennsylvania.

EDWARD R. RITVO, M.D.
Professor, Division of Mental Retardation and Child Psychiatry, University of California School of Medicine, Los Angeles, California.

CAROLYN B. ROBINOWITZ, M.D.
Deputy Medical Director and Director, Office of Education, American Psychiatric Association, Washington, D.C.

CLYDE L. ROUSEY, PH.D.
Private Practice, Topeka, Kansas.

TARANATH SHETTY, M.D.
Clinical Assistant Professor of Pediatrics, Brown University Program of Medicine; Director, Division of Pediatric Neurology, Rhode Island Hospital, Providence, Rhode Island.

LARRY B. SILVER, M.D.
Professor of Psychiatry and Pediatrics, Chief, Section of Child and Adolescent Psychiatry, Rutgers Medical School, New Brunswick, New Jersey.

RAYMOND SOBEL, M.D.
Professor Emeritus, Department of Psychiatry, Dartmouth Medical School, Hanover, New Hampshire.

JOHN A. SOURS, M.D.
Private practice; Clinical Assistant Professor of Psychiatry, Columbia Psychoanalytic Center for Training and Research, College of Physicians and Surgeons, Columbia University, New York, New York.

ROBERT J. STOLLER, M.D.
Professor of Psychiatry, University of California at Los Angeles School of Medicine, Los Angeles, California.

GEORGE TARJAN, M.D.
Professor of Psychiatry, University of California at Los Angeles School of Medicine; Director of the Mental Retardation and Child Psychiatry Division, Neuropsychiatric Institute, University of California School of Medicine, Los Angeles, California.

JOSEPH D. TEICHER, M.D.
Professor of Psychiatry, University of Southern California School of Medicine; Director, Los Angeles Child Guidance Clinic, Los Angeles, California.

JOHN S. WERRY, M.D.
Professor and Head of the Department of Psychiatry, University of Auckland, New Zealand.

HENRY H. WORK, M.D.
Deputy Medical Director for Professional Affairs, American Psychiatric Association; Clinical Professor of Child Psychiatry, George Washington University and Georgetown University, Washington, D.C.

JOAN J. ZILBACH, M.D.
Director, Family Therapy and Research Program, Judge Baker Guidance Center, Roxbury; Senior Consultant, Child/Family Program, Boston Veterans Administration Hospital and Tufts Medical School, Boston, Massachusetts.

PREFACE

Child psychiatry is now in its seventieth year. It has passed through an early phase of clinic practice, a later period of intense concern with inpatient care, and, most recently, a move into the universities. In the course of this evolution child psychiatry has advanced from a set of unique skills and techniques to an ever more complex scientific endeavor. It involves a basic science dimension, a wide array of specialized practices, and an increasingly intricate universe of research. Along with these have come an extensive literature, now international in scope, and an ever-widening impact on the culture generally and on medicine and psychiatry in particular.

So rapidly has this growth proceeded that it has heretofore been difficult to find any single work that embraced the full complexity of the development of child psychiatry. The emphasis of most authors has been on specialized aspects of the field; only a few have attempted more comprehensive efforts in the form of textbooks, and some of these have tended to be rather brief surveys of major topics. As a result, teachers and residents in the many training programs and individual practitioners in the communities have long felt the need for an additional book—comprehensive in its scope—in which the array of topics would be sufficiently exhaustive and in which the study of each area would be examined in enough depth to satisfy student, scholar, and practitioner alike. It was the pressure to fill this need that brought forth the idea of the *Basic Handbook of Child Psychiatry*. The same sense of urgency led the more than 250 contributors and the six editors to commit time, energy, and industry to the accomplishment of this task. And it was in response to these pressures that the authors, editors, and publisher worked together for six years to produce these volumes. If their undertaking succeeds in its intent, the *Handbook* should provide a primary reference source for many of the questions and needs that arise within the discipline. It is with this hope that the *Basic Handbook* is presented.

The arrangement of materials in these volumes speaks for something of the logic of the discipline of child psychiatry. To begin with there is an account of the first basic science of the field, a detailing of *child development*. This is followed by a series of brief descriptions (the sort of statements that can be read quickly in connection with individual clinical cases) of different *varieties of child development*. Next comes a recounting of one of the major subdisciplines of child psychiatry, the *nature of assessment*, a section written in large part by Dr. Richard L. Cohen. These three topics comprise Volume I. The second volume is given over to the second basic science of child psychiatry, that of *child psychopathology*. Included here are studies of etiology and nosology and an account of the more important syndromes. Volume III follows, and treats another great subdiscipline, the field of *therapeutics*. The final volume, Volume IV, covers the field of *prevention* and contains a series of studies on the impact of current cultural issues on children and child psychiatry.

It should be noted that the *Handbook* is calculatedly eclectic. It is written by the working child psychiatrist as well as by the researcher and by other mental health professionals; a variety of views and opinions are therefore presented. Differences will be found among theories of development, techniques of assessment, modes of psychopathology, and approaches to treatment. No one will agree with them all—the editors certainly do not. Nonetheless they are all serious positions that demand respect if not accord. Such is the state of the art.

Grants from the Commonwealth Fund, the Maurice Falk Medical Fund, and the Grove Foundation supported the development of these volumes, and the funds are gratefully acknowledged.

Early on, Ginger Bausch lent the use of the offices of the American Academy of Child Psychiatry in Washington as a mailing address and a site to store *Handbook* materials, and Jeanne DeJarnette took on the coordination of the *Handbook* as an after-hours job. She acted as guardian angel, financial manager and factotum, kept track of documents, typed correspondence, maintained files, saw that people were informed about what was happening, and, all in all, made the enterprise work. Three years after it began, the central effort shifted from her capable hands to the secretarial staff of the Department of Child Psychiatry at the Children's Hospital National Medical Center. The Chairman of the Department was at that time Jerry Wiener, who gave a full measure of support to the demanding effort that the host of accumulated documents required. Later, Dr. James Egan took over the chairmanship and continued the pattern of unstinting support. Within the department, Mrs. Shirley Wells, ably backed up by Mrs. Penny Nolton, carried the brunt of the responsibilities, and it was she who brought the work to its final form. The sheer time involved was prodigious.

While this was going on in Washington, parallel efforts were being exerted in Pittsburgh by Dr. Cohen and his staff; in Ann Arbor by Dr. Harrison and his people; in Seattle and then in Davis, California, by Dr. Berlin and his associates; in Irvine by Dr. Call and his associates; and in San Antonio by Dr. Larry Stone, his wife Marnette, and others who worked with him. Indeed, when one ponders the amount of university assistance offered to the many authors, as well as the intensive and extensive efforts made by their staffs, it is no small contribution that the *Handbook* received from the academic world in its largest sense. The work entailed a truly massive effort, and it is impossible to list the names of the many, many people who helped it come to fruition.

For the publisher, the *Handbook* was shepherded through its labyrinthine way by the tireless efforts of Herb Reich, Behavioral Science Editor of Basic Books. This involved visits back and forth between Washington, D.C., and New York, endless attention to detail, and a sort of total immersion in the fullness of the effort needed to turn the mass of documents into a printable manuscript. Among the highly skilled staff at Basic Books who labored long hours over the thousands of pages that comprised the manuscript were Pamela Dailey and Debra Manette. They copy edited the text, cleaned up bibliographies, queried areas of uncertainty, and saw to it that scholarly rigor and clarity of expression prevailed throughout. Maureen Bischoff as project director coordinated the publication work, and all played vital roles in the final outcome.

One final point remains. The original manuscript grew to such excessive proportions that it became necessary to cut out, cut down, and shorten materials. This distressing process was initiated by the publisher and then carried by the several editors, who trimmed and tightened until a shorter, more compact work emerged. In the course of editing, a number of papers were eliminated and several others were shortened. It caused both publisher and editors considerable pain to perform this task, yet it was vital to the actual production of the work. Both the editors and the publisher hope that the outcome will justify the surgery.

JOSEPH D. NOSHPITZ
Washington, D.C.
February 15, 1979

BASIC HANDBOOK

OF

Child Psychiatry

VOLUME TWO

PART A
Etiology

1 / The Psychodynamic Aspects of Behavior

Sidney Berman

In the material that follows, various aspects of the behavior of children and adolescents will be considered from a psychodynamic point of view, especially as they relate to psychoanalytic concepts of development. Basic to this approach is the crucial assumption that all behavior emanates from the organic matrix of the central nervous system. A second assumption is that the mind is active in an understandable and predictable way; the term psychodynamics refers to the laws of such mental action. This mental activity follows certain lines of development and organization; metaphorically, these functions are ascribed to a psychic apparatus. This psychic apparatus operates in keeping with a number of integrating principles. The nature of the psychic apparatus, of its functions, and of its conscious and unconscious organization can be ascertained by psychological methods of investigation. These involve: the reconstruction of childhood experience through adult psychoanalysis, direct observation by means of child psychoanalysis, psychoanalytic research, and longitudinal developmental studies. An additional rich source of information arises from myths, folklore, and fairy tales. Thus, meaning can be ascribed to unconscious and conscious mental activity as represented by thoughts, emotions, and actions.

Introduction

The behavior of children and adolescents is tempered by their fantasy life. This is by no means self evident; often it is misunderstood. This occurs for two reasons. The first is the fact that all adults experience an amnesia for their own childhood and adolescence; as a result, they find much of the behavior of children to be incomprehensible. The second is the tendency of children to communicate with adults either symbolically or in a cryptic language which the adults often do not understand.

During the formative years, personality characteristics are determined in great measure by the psychodynamic functions of the mind; their investigation and study therefore become essential for the understanding of both normal and abnormal psychological development. These insights are not easy to come by. In the early months of life, before children have developed verbal language, their highly personal responses are only inferentially understood. Even to begin to grasp such meanings requires a kind of emotional contagion based on empathy in the adult.[25] After nonverbal and verbal communication has developed, children will still try to conceal any mental activity which they feel is reprehensible or embarrassing, and they will censor their thoughts and experiences.

In turn, adults tend to consider the expressions and actions of children in conventional terms, such as cute, intelligent, silly, dull, cruel, sensitive, and the like. They also tend to treat the behavior of children as transitory phenomena and not very significant. They feel that children's minds may be molded by various techniques of behavior modification, by the use of reward and punishment, or by learning techniques. In particular, the child's unconscious mental activity is treated as inconsequential. Nevertheless, these various dynamic occurrences and experiences and their mental representations are the ultimate determinants of the personality characteristics of the growing child. The theory of psychodynamics endeavors to give a plausible account of these mental phenomena.

The Mental Apparatus and the Psychodynamic Process

Freud[31] formulated the idea that in every individual there is a coherent organization of mental processes. In order to understand more thoroughly the dynamic relationships within the mind and to describe them more clearly, Freud conceptualized the mind as a mental apparatus differentiated into an id, an ego, and a superego.

For an understanding of psychodynamics, psychoanalysis uses this "structured" model of the psychic apparatus. Although this theory of psychoanalysis is gone into in greater detail elsewhere, a brief statement is in order here.

Developmentally, the id precedes the ego and superego. It is unconscious, and at birth it becomes differentiated from the totally undifferentiated psychic apparatus. It is the mental expression of the instincts or drives from which it derives its energy, and it seeks to obtain satisfaction for these drives. These drives, libidinal and aggressive, are associated with hunger, tactile sensation (which may be the forerunner of closeness), urethral and anal experience, genital gratification, and the avoidance of physical pain. Simple as they seem, with the emergence of the other mental functions, they find expression as remarkably intricate patterns of psychic activity. According to the model, these drives are unconscious, but press toward conscious expression. As they move toward consciousness, they achieve psychodynamic signifi-

cance. Where there is insufficient gratification of the basic requirements for physical and psychological survival, psychic development becomes undermined. When this occurs early, it leads to serious psychodynamic pathology. For example, from birth on, a child with minimal cerebral dysfunction may suffer from inordinate hyperactivity. This impairs the mother's capacity to hold him and, ultimately, to help him achieve impulse control. It evokes frustration and anger in those about him, and he develops paranoid fantasies and fantasies of power to compensate for these deficits. As a way of trying to control his inner disorganization, he often plays compulsively with inanimate objects, repetitiously attempting to master his movement and action.

The id tensions compel the child or adolescent to seek satisfaction, that is, to engage in some kind of behavior which permits a discharge of his tension. He is hungry, he wants to eat now. However, forces both from within and without may demand modulation, inhibition or postponement of the fulfillment of the gratification. He must wait till mealtime, he must wait till grace. The nature of the response will be determined by an inner regulatory agency which operates to delay, detour, or even frustrate the child. This frustration may be total. Thus, certain foods might be forbidden, or he may have to wait until his sense of reality deems gratification appropriate. This regulatory agency is referred to as the ego.

The ego is conceptualized as having functions which emerge with the development of perception. As the child's visual and auditory processing becomes more mature, it also undergoes sequential development, beginning with his capacity to discriminate between his mother and himself. Hartmann[41] defined the attributes of the ego as possessing developmental qualities. The ego apparatuses such as perception, mobility, language, intelligence, reasoning and the like were described as emerging autonomously; around them the other ego functions develop. Their characteristics are constitutionally determined, and they provide the somatic and mental basis for ego functions.

Initially the action of the ego is to mediate between the demands of the id and of reality. As regards the id, the ego endeavors to control its drives, deciding whether they shall be satisfied immediately, postponed until they can be gratified under more favorable circumstances, or suppressed completely. The ego also performs the tasks of adapting to or modifying the external world in order to try to have the psychic needs gratified. Gradually, as a result of the long period of dependence upon the parents, a portion of the ego incorporates the parental expectations. It achieves a certain coherence and autonomy and begins to function both as conscience and ideals. This new organization is called the superego. In effect, the ego takes in a series of internal restraints which are the expression of parental demands, prohibitions, and sanctions. In time these extend to include family traditions and customs, social influences, and cultural values. The ensuing psychic structure, the superego, also undergoes developmental changes. From its archaic precursors in infancy and early childhood (the scary, devouring witch mother), it achieves a concise organization in latency (where it has learned guilt and fair play) and it continues to change during adolescence and into adulthood. This component of the mental apparatus becomes a formidable factor in treatment; it may make the young child or adolescent very reluctant to talk about many conflicted feelings, especially those involving the parents, especially parental disapproval.

Vulnerability

Every child is born potentially vulnerable.[2, 24, 62] Helpless and totally dependent in the beginning of life, the child is dependent upon the physical and psychological environment created by his mother during pregnancy and for many months thereafter. The genetic endowment given the child by both parents will play an important role in determining his maturational qualities and psychological potentials. Beyond this, the quality of the life experienced by the child in his family, and the psychological interactions between them, will be the proving ground for his subsequent development. What occurs in this setting during the first six years of life will determine how the functions of the mental apparatus will evolve, how the child will cope with social expectations, and how he will be influenced by the traditional forces operating in his culture.

The mind's capacity to combine such elements as perception, memory, thought, and action into a dynamic synthetic process is an amazing phenomenon. The capacity to bring all these functions together belongs to the synthetic function of the ego. But this is a complex, hazardous process, subject to many dangers.

Some of the major factors which may expose a child to mental dysfunction are as follows:

1. Biologic disorders such as hereditary and constitutional deficits, neurological and other physical disabilities, paranatal infections, physical trauma at birth, anoxia, and prematurity. Any of these may severely impair the underlying structures and the associated ego functions of the child's mental apparatus.[75] This is due to two factors. One is the distortion of stimuli and data that the child receives both from within and from without; this influences the development of the child's image of his body. The mental manifestations are often the most sensitive evidence of such pathology which may range from the most obvious to the elusive and indefinite. The other is the bewilderment and frustration experienced by the caretakers of such a child in attempting to respond to the child's nurturance needs. These children often have the most violent fantasies, frequently with a paranoid theme. This is one way in which they attempt to cope with their physical deficit and their aggression; the fantasies serve as a defense against their helplessness. Paradoxically, they are distrustful of those close to them, believing that they can be hurt by them. Yet, in their struggle to achieve stability, they express a hunger for affection.

Other physical disabilities such as a loss of hearing or sight, hypersensitivity to tactile stimuli, loss of a limb, defective impulse control, learning disability or other developmental anomalies invariably impair the ego apparatuses (as defined by Hartmann[41]) and thus disturb the functions of the ego. These children are certainly different from other children, and they require special therapeutic and educational programs to help them adapt to their handicap and to their problems with family and social relationships. They feel damaged, evil, insecure, and vulnerable to life's normal demands, and they protect themselves by the use of such mental mechanisms as denial and projection, along with paranoid or grandiose fantasies.[59]

2. The world of infancy and childhood fantasy possesses its own psychic reality. Children cannot express their feelings of fear, pain, disappointment, sadness, or anger effectively and appropriately; instead, they respond with fantasy as a way of coping with their tormented mental content. Due to the power of their own impulses or their anticipation of retribution by the forces of reality, they experience fear and, presently, anxiety may arise. The fantasy they then elaborate becomes a means of defense against this anxiety, a means of inhibiting or controlling instinctual conflict. More than that, however, it is an expression of reparative wishes.

It is true that fantasy is an active presence in

the minds of all children, normal or neurotic. In some children, however, there is a difference. There seems to be a special sensitivity to these early experiences, which exists on a constitutional basis. The child can seize on this fantasy as a mental representation of the conflict. This becomes an enduring presence in his life, with significant after-effects.[43] The most common pathological fantasies are associated with unresolved sibling rivalry, severe castration anxiety and separation anxiety; under such conditions, primitive magical thinking dominates the child's construction of his inner and outer world.

Where there has been an accentuation of pleasurable experiences, it may become difficult for the child to relinquish them. The opposite is also true; a frustration may lead to a sequence of disappointments. Even in the face of the most favorable environment, certain vulnerable children may respond with pathological fantasies and associated symptom formation.

Fantasy represents an attempt at the fulfillment of a wish; it may be conscious or unconscious. An example of a conscious fantasy could be the desire to kill a sibling as a rival for mother's love. The same theme may be expressed unconsciously in the form of severe passive dependent behavior where the child insists on remaining home due to a school phobia. Another child may avoid physical games because he has compared his penis to the size of his father's genitals and developed the fantasy of being inadequate and anatomically damaged. Or, he may fantasize that his sister has lost a penis and thus fear injury in his play with other boys. For some children, these distortions of reality and the accompanying disturbances of affect and reasoning lead to intense conflict and create serious adaptational problems.

3. In the course of development, as children move from one stage of development to another, internal stresses are inevitable. As a result, it is impossible for the child to escape maturational and developmental conflict. However, these developmental crises may be mild or severe.[29] Although most such reactions are circumscribed and transitory, some continue to be nodal points for subsequent serious psychopathology. Thus, developmental crises occur at those transitional points where a new phase of growth emerges and begins to dominate the life of the child. These phases are regulated by a maturational sequence according to which these new functions unfold and are integrated into the psychic structure. One after another, the child must master the oral, anal-urethral, phallic and genital libidinal drives. He

must cope with these in the early phases of development, integrate and control them in the latency phase, and ultimately consolidate these not altogether coherent sets of mastery functions during adolescence.

Many children are ambivalent about moving from one phase to another; for a period of time they feel impelled to resist change. The reasons for these constitutional differences are insufficiently known, yet the observable phenomena demonstrate the primitive ways in which children respond to the demand for change. For example, some infants may engage in a severe hunger strike when they have to relinquish the breast or the bottle. At the next phase of development, there are children who tenaciously hold on to their own way of disposing of feces and urine and fight any attempt on the part of the parents to train them. Others are reluctant to undergo separation and individuation and cling to the blanket with a death grip. There are children who are frightened by genital arousal and fear genital injury; they react with nightmares, or elaborate fantasies of immense power, or experience a desire to be of the opposite sex. In latency, there are children who hold on to the prelatency fantasies and find it very difficult to master the tasks of socialization. In adolescence, genital arousal may create severe transitory disturbances of development, with feelings of panic and fantasies of impending disaster. The psychodynamic factors which are at work here will find expression in the fantasies cherished by these children at the point of crisis.

4. Children are particularly vulnerable to pathological environmental influences. This is true whether these influences arise within the family or are visited upon the child by environmental deprivation. Retrospective studies of adults and children show in glaring relief that deprivations, frustrations, and trauma during early childhood are significantly related to psychiatric illness and deviant character formations.[3]

The resultant psychodynamic disorganization invariably has a devastating impact upon a child's psychic growth. As an example, a child from a violent slum area often suffers from somatic complaints, and his inner life (ordinarily revealed to no one) is burdened by oral, anal, and phallic conflict. One such youngster was filled with repressed hostility, had fantasies of starring in horror films and wished nothing bad would happen to him. He drew people with large heads and weak, small bodies and spoke of protecting himself by learning karate. Another child whose father had abandoned the family yearned for his father's return. His inner world was one of great sadness. In yet another case, a child, from birth onward, was subject to multiple surrogate parents. The mother abandoned him in order to pursue her own interests, and the father was uninterested in his son. This youngster peopled his inner world with many monsters, he was concerned with things getting blasted off, and he expressed grandiose and demanding fantasies. Although he wanted his mother very much, he feared she would punish or reject him if he asked too much of her. Another child whose father died reacted with severe depression, felt his world would explode and be completely shattered, and felt weird and overwhelmed. His sadness and rage at abandonment were somatized as stomach pains and insomnia; he could no longer go to school; and he wanted only to curl up and isolate himself.

Among large populations it is possible to find people who have had similar experiences but who function adequately. As a result, such experiences are not always predictors of later psychopathology. At the same time, it is fallacious to minimize such traumata or to assume that they are not necessarily detrimental. In fact, normality as a defense is one way of surviving such serious conflict, and this is an intrinsic quality of the multiple functions of the mental apparatus. Acceptable behavior may occur just as well for neurotic reasons as for healthy, adaptive reasons. A child traumatized by blind neglect or one hurt by the death of parents may get along beautifully with people. Because of his fantasized fear of rejection or abandonment, he may cope by presenting a "noble image." A sexually molested child who is physically aroused by a seductive adult or a child brutalized by a sadistic adult may also, to all intents and purposes, appear normal. In his personal adult sexual life, however, he may yet relive the conflict with sad consequences.

Principles of Defense and Adaptation

Defense is a general term used to describe the response of the ego when it seeks to protect itself against anxiety caused by real or fantasied danger. From a psychoanalytic point of view, it is important to distinguish between a defense and a defense mechanism.[66] Defense refers to the behavior, affects or ideas which are evoked for defensive purposes. The content of the defense (be it behavior, affect, or idea), although usually unconscious, can be rendered conscious by psychoanalytic work. The defense mechanism, on the other hand, is a theoretical abstraction which describes how such behaviors, affects, and ideas work to protect, that is, how they modify an unwanted discharge of an impulse. Although one tends to refer to the content of the mental activity as synonymous with the way in which it comes about, the differentiation between defense and defense mechanisms is parallel to the distinction between content and process; to draw this distinction heightens the observer's sensitivity to the meaning of a child's behavior, the way he feels, or how he thinks, which results in the use of a defense.

Bibring[13] listed thirty-nine defenses, demonstrating the versatility of the human mind to respond to conflict. Of more significance to the child therapist, however, is the fact that particular defenses appear at specific phases of development. They are, in fact, among the emerging or developmental functions of the ego. Thus, the earliest defenses are primary identification, splitting, introjection, projection and incorporation; those which develop later include identification with the aggressor, displacement, and isolation; and so on up.

Anxiety arises as a function of the ego; it appears when there is a movement toward consciousness of some mental content associated with a real or imagined danger, or with a fear of punishment. Before it erupts into full awareness there is a flash of anxiety. It is a normal response and has a signal function. In effect, it alerts the ego to initiate unconscious defensive operations in order to ward off the painful conscious awareness of the wish, desire, or fear. These dangers are experienced in childhood with enormous intensity. At first they are conscious; later on they are repressed and rendered unconscious. They are usually associated with (1) loss of or separation from the one who cares for and loves the child, (2) the loved ones' anger or disapproval, (3) fear of damage to the genitals (referred to as castration anxiety), and (4) a bad conscience based upon the child's disapproval of himself. (This appears only after the formation of the internal censorship system, the superego). In the formative years of infancy and childhood, these conflicts emerge in sequential order, and regularly overlap one another.

As the child matures physically, the ego grows in a parallel way. Gradually there emerges an ever more elaborate system of means for coping with conflict. One aspect of this process is the patterning of psychic action referred to previously as the defense mechanisms. These are devices which the ego uses to cope with and to survive otherwise unbearable situations. In the normal course of events, some of these defenses are phase specific, that is, they tend to occur with greater frequency at certain periods of the child's development and then, inconspicuously, disappear. Others remain operative throughout life.

All mental processes produce movement, change, and transformation in one or another aspect of psychic life. However, mental mechanisms denote relatively durable and circumscribed responses which serve to inhibit, avert, or modulate troublesome impulses. Thus, by preventing their direct discharge, the defense mechanism keeps the child out of trouble, i.e. it facilitates adaptation. Children are largely body oriented in relation to the world and limited in their ability to distinguish whether stimuli are coming from within or from without. Their ideas about themselves and others, are inconsistent, diffuse, and concretistic. The mental mechanisms reflect this state of affairs and have all the characteristics of magical thinking. Ideas, feelings, and acts which are painful can disappear, be denied, made into the opposite, attributed to something or someone else, avoided, and the like. As these defenses are erected, the children's lives become more tolerable. They can now compromise their wishes with reality.

Another set of ego functions are also related to adaptation, and these functions too undergo development along a continuum. They consist of memory, speech, control of motor impulses, reality testing, judgment, learning, and reason. These functions of the ego perform the task of integrating the internal needs with the demands both of the outside world and of the superego.[41] Again, this is part of the process defined as adaptation. As the child grows, reality thinking comes to govern behavior. In effect, this demands a renunciation of primitive desires created by the drives. Based upon the child's knowledge of reality, it speaks for postponement of pleasure now in order to achieve later gratification. Obviously, the effort to maintain the mental apparatus in effective balance places a considerable demand upon the child's developing ego functions.

Undue stress may arise at any point along the developmental continuum. This can impair the important ego functions which make for adaptation. Inevitably, such stress carries with it the experience of psychic pain. Because of his distress, the child can no longer use his skills, his talents,

his intellect, his memory, or his other healthy ego equipment. The defense mechanisms may then become the major means for coping with conflict, either temporarily or over an extended period of time. When this occurs, it is indicative of serious psychic functional impairment. Precipitating factors such as lack of protection against dangerous aggression, severe disappointments, feelings of abandonment, feelings of mortification, fears of body injury, or self-destructive impulses may impair the adaptive functions of the ego and mobilize pathological defensive responses. Defense mechanisms can be employed to control drives completely in a rigid manner, or they can be too infantile or too precocious for the child's age. There may also be excessive use of a particular defense. The problem may be due to the strength of the drives, the ineffectiveness or severity of the superego, or the weakness of the ego. As an example, a girl of five had been vivacious, exhibitionistic and enjoyed feminine clothing. At some point, however, she became withdrawn, reserved, no longer played with other little girls, and preferred to wear pants. A study of the case reveals that she reacted in this way when her brother was born. For her, this constituted a narcissistic mortification which evoked the mechanisms of reversal isolation and constriction as primary defenses. At the appearance of the little boy, she felt betrayed by her father. She sought to deal with the sibling rivalry by turning to her mother. This was no minor reaction. At the age of eighteen years, she continued to remain close to her mother. More than that, she continued to rely on isolation and inhibition as her primary defenses. These markedly restricted her intellectual, emotional, and volitional activities. Asceticism had replaced a normal developmental process.

Anna Freud[30] made a classic contribution to the understanding of the mechanisms of defense. She studied the various defensive operations of the ego and related them to the source of anxiety and danger. Among the mental mechanisms most commonly noted are repression, projection, introjection, denial, regression, reaction formation, isolation, undoing, identification with the aggressor, turning against the self, displacement, identification, sublimation, and a specific one ascribed to adolescence, alienation. They do not occur in individual form, although one or more may dominate personality function. In addition to their presence in various combinations, one observes an admixture with other ego functions. Bibring[13] presents a glossary of defenses which include not only the specifically described unconscious mechanisms, but also a wide range of complex functional responses of a defensive nature.

REPRESSION

This is the only defense mechanism which is elementary or irreducible. Its function is the total elimination of a given intrapsychic conflict from conscious awareness. Thus, all dangerous thoughts, knowledge, and feelings, external and internal, may be kept completely out of awareness. What becomes repressed is the memory of undesirable instinctual demands. Sometimes repression is not effective against unbearable thoughts and feelings; in such instances they may reappear in disguised form. Thus, when a child's oedipal rage toward father threatens to boil over, it may be displaced onto an authoritarian teacher.

A frequent example of repression as a defense is the statement that nothing is remembered about infancy and early childhood, that the earliest memory is seldom before six. As a defense, repression becomes pathological when it leads to a crippling of the instinctual life and restricts the natural expansion of ego functions. Brenner[16] discusses in detail the development of the concept of repression in Freud's writings from a historical and theoretical perspective.

Freud[34] attributed the repression of sexual wishes and memories to certain sequences in the development of psychic functioning. At the end of each different phase of development, a certain amount of repression occurs. This serves to free the ego of the conflicts of that phase and prepares it to master the tasks of the next stage. As an example, the events prior to the age of six undergo an "infantile amnesia." In effect, the child no longer remembers his oedipal struggles. This liberates the ego, which now redirects the drive energy to master the broader tasks associated with the processes of socialization and learning. The same appears to hold true for subsequent phases of development; many adolescents can no longer accurately recall significant events from their latency. It is the nature and degree of repression that determines its developmental utility, or pathology. In hysterical conditions, on the other hand, repression is excessive. Thus the various kinds of dissociation (such as fugue or multiple personality or psychic amnesia) are examples of undue resort to this mechanism.

PROJECTION

This mechanism of defense occurs early in the lives of all children. It permits the child unconsciously to externalize undesired feelings. It thus provides a sort of "easy way out" by allowing the child to rid himself of uncomfortable thoughts and feelings, especially hostile ones. In general, these are feelings which would otherwise create overwhelming anxiety. It may be dramatically observed in the so-called eight-month anxiety of young children who cry when they see a stranger. Paradoxically, this begins with the child's yearning for a kind, tender, protective response from his parents. Since this cannot always be forthcoming, some degree of frustration is inevitable. In turn, this evokes intense feelings of anger or hatred toward the caretaker. These, however, cannot be long endured; basically the child yearns for love, and these negative emotions threaten the child's sense of security. Therefore, the hatred is projected onto a person, thing, or symbol removed from the parents. This, then assumes the quality of an alleged persecutor. Later on these feelings are projected onto the witch or the monster. A certain amount of projection is universal. Adolescents may project their internal conflicted and warded off dependency needs onto the school or society; these are accused of confining them or not doing enough for them. However, when it serves as the major defense in a child's life, it becomes a matter of grave concern, for it then has a paranoid quality indicating serious maladjustment.

INTROJECTION

From retrospective studies, this mechanism of defense seems to appear in infancy. It represents the process of perceiving and treating that which is in fact outside as though it were inside one's self. Thus, for the infant, the loved and hated external caretaker is symbolically taken into the self. How the child experiences being held, fed and bathed creates in him the feeling of "good enough mothering" or "bad mothering." In the course of the nursery experience, the psychological attributes of the mother are figuratively ingested; this aspect of the psychological relationship is referred to as incorporation. What the child takes in by this process is determined by the quality of the mothering. This concept is used to explain primitive forms of psychopathology, such as the failure to thrive syndrome in which the infant's refusing or vomiting food is a way of repudiating the painful relationship with the mothering person. A later derivative of this conflict may take the form of psychogenic vomiting; the child is literally trying to vomit up the introjected other. This same mechanism plays an important role in depression. Here, the child may feel rage and hatred toward his mother which he cannot allow himself to experience consciously. He then directs these unacceptable feelings onto the incorporated mother within and thus, in effect, onto himself. This may lead to his being accident prone[68] or even suicidal.

DENIAL

This defense mechanism occurs very early. It is used by the child to ward off some painful aspect of reality or to ward off a painful internal perception. In effect, the child disavows what he sees or fears; he turns off reality. For him, the undesired experience no longer exists. Like projection, it may be used to lessen guilt, avoid shame, and deny the fear of seeming loss of body parts or persons. A child from an environmentally impoverished background called both her aunt and grandmother "mama" but always called her actual mother, with whom she lived, by her first name. This persisted in spite of her mother's attempts at correction. Children deny acts to avoid punishment or the withdrawal of love. They may also deny sexual differences and insist on being neuter or of the opposite sex as a way of coping with castration anxiety. This particular defense mechanism is ubiquitous and serves throughout life as a means of avoiding anxiety. When relied on to excess, it makes for major disturbances in one's appreciation of reality.

FIXATION AND REGRESSION

A child or adolescent may encounter a wish or a fear that stems from his current developmental conflicts and that feels too threatening to face. He may then take flight by turning back to acts, thoughts, or feelings which belonged to an earlier phase of development. In effect, in order to avoid intense anxiety or guilt which cannot be mastered, the ego stages a retreat. Such a developmental retreat is termed regression. It may be caused by transitory stress, neurotic and psychotic processes, bodily illness, toxic drugs, and/or stressful life experiences.

Transitory regression occurs under normal conditions when a child or adolescent is experiencing envy over a new baby, a desire for a past gratification, a reluctance to respond to the demands of reality, or alterations of body functions due to fatigue, illness, or injury. Thus a child of four may temporarily want to take the bottle or breast away from the newly arrived sibling. When he is engaged in other pleasurable activities, he may have "accidents." When fatigued, fretful for attention, or ill, he may suck his thumb or return to a transitional object such as a blanket. Usually the feelings of shame or guilt and the desire for approval and acceptance are strong enough to motivate the child to return to age appropriate behavior.

Another normal manifestation of regression occurs when a child passes from one developmental phase to another. The thrust of maturational change and the accompanying advance place stress upon the child; his very progress requires him to give up the hard won achievements and pleasures of one period of growth for another. The ensuing psychic and physical imbalance invariably evokes transient regression as a defense. In other words, older patterns of behavior may be used temporarily to support efforts both to master and to change it. These reactions are brief, circumscribed, and reversible. They are regressive responses which are actually in the service of growth, that is, they benefit the ego by providing support in mastering the immediate developmental crisis.

These regressive phenomena are commonly observed at each phase of body change and psychological progression; they demonstrate the enormous psychological significance of all the body's erotogenic zones. Their integration into the formation of the body image and their impact on psychic development are obvious. There is a complex interaction which occurs between the child and his parents in taming these functions. The natural and appropriate response of weaning at the optimum time creates in some infants a fretfulness, irritability and anguish which may last for several days. Such babies refuse to accept milk in any way other than the one which has satisfied their need. The psychic pain may cause a regression to a stage of total helplessness, a need to be held and responded to. Rebellion at the demands for toilet training may cause a child to continue to soil secretly for an extended period of time. Preoccupation with genital autostimulation and concern with sexual anatomy may be expressed by food fads and separation anxiety. The demands of education and socialization may evoke regression in the form of difficulty arising in the morning, dawdling and loss of personal belongings. In prepuberty and early adolescence, the phenomenon may be expressed in the form of exhibitionism and various forms of anal and oral symbolic behavior, such as defiance, obstinancy, messiness, changes in food habits, burping, and the like. Such transitional events in moving from one phase to another occasionally create anxious concern in parents; they require that the child psychiatrist be able to discern between behavior that is transitory and that which represents a significant arrest of psychic development.

Pathological regression such as that noted in the psychoses and neuroses, in sexual deviance, and in disturbed behavior presaging character disorder always merit alarmed concern. When the regressive behavior becomes striking in its consistency, intensity, and persistence, and the disturbed ideas and fantasies defensively dominate the mental life of the child, they indicate a serious disruption of psychic development. Severe regression to earlier levels may be expressed by such symptoms as encopresis, enuresis, night terrors, school phobia (related to separation anxiety), depression in the prepubertal and pubertal periods, and other severe manifestations. Every regression activates primary process thinking, that is, primitive, irrational types of wishful thought, and revives old defenses and earlier ego patterns of dealing with reality. The child turns to earlier modes of defense; he returns psychologically to periods in the past when a solution to the conflict was attempted through magical thinking and other primitive mechanisms. These are described as points of fixation. In psychoanalytic parlance, fixation refers to the unusual concentration of the psychic energy of a drive upon a given object or fantasy or aspect of the self. This overcharge of psychic energy may be a conscious or unconscious attachment to an idea, image, fantasy, symbol, or concept. The preoccupation with unresolved conflict then remains operational and is never fully abandoned. If it is extremely severe, it will cause an arrest of development. However, it usually does not interfere with psychic development until an episode of severe stress occurs later in life. Then, regression may occur as a defense. When this happens, the emotional interest attaches to an object or mode of gratification on which the patient was fixated earlier in life. An example of this is the case of a boy who had formed an intense attachment to the mother in the oedipal phase of development. In latency he made a reasonable adjustment in school because of his superior intellectual ability. During this time he maintained an indirect involvement with his mother, watching television in her bed and using her shower. However, when adolescence was reached, he was paralyzed by the emergence of his genital drives; he regressed to the point of infantile fixation by wanting to remain home and be cared for by her.

REACTION FORMATION

This defense mechanism is evoked when the child experiences tender love or adequate care from his parents, coupled with stern injunctions about behavior. In the face of this he experiences conflict; his drives tell him one thing, his parents another. He begins to fear that his drives are too intense and may overwhelm him. In a similar way, the indoctrination of severe and punitive religious values may also cause the child to fear his impulses. The child therefore makes a decision: the expression of the desired impulse is turned exactly into its opposite. The decision is soon repressed, yet it continues (automatically) to influence the child's behavior. For example, anger at the mother for bearing a new infant may be expressed by the child becoming oversolicitous about her health, while his rage at the baby is expressed by repeated declarations of affection. Adolescent asceticism is a striking example of the use of virtue as a defense against sexual impulses. This defense mechanism will not be observed in predelinquent children, children whose parents neglect them, or where the parents are ambivalent in the treatment of their children. Although the appearance of this mechanism may be transient, it may persist in the form of a character trait, especially in obsessional children.

ISOLATION

As a rule, thoughts come to mind with a certain emotional quality attached to them. By dint of this mechanism, however, the ideas are split from the feelings and the feelings repressed. Isolation thus deprives the thought of its motivational force. As a result, action is thwarted and guilt avoided; the thought exists, but has little power. This mechanism of defense occurs with the formation of the superego. Normally an act requires the existence of both thought and feeling, that is, a conviction which justifies the act. However, in this case the thought exists without any intense emotion and without the child doing anything about it. A child may express the thought that he could kill his sibling, but he refrains from acting. He may also think of shouting obscenities, but remains silent.

Another child may think of plunging a knife into someone but this thought, too, is "just an idea," and quickly recedes from awareness. Under certain circumstances, these emotion-denuded thoughts can become recurrent and oppressive; when this happens, the child suffers from an obsessional neurosis and is severely handicapped.

UNDOING

With this mechanism, a magical gesture annuls a forbidden act or thought. It is commonly seen in children and takes the form of crossing fingers or legs to nullify a thought, or going back around a tree in the opposite direction to ward off a possible evil fate. In a child with an obsessive-compulsive neurosis, such an act may have to be repeated several times in order to atone for some forbidden mental activity. As an example, a child may have to wash his hands repeatedly, or avoid touching a wall in order to extinguish the guilt about masturbation or about murderous impulses. Another child may become accident prone as atonement for chronic anger at his mother. Or another child may be obsessed with coprophagia or coprophilia in order to ward off the fear of losing a part of his body, whether it be feces or genitalia. The anxiety can be undone by looking, smelling, or defecating frequently, thereby providing reassurance that the loss is not permanent.

TURNING AGAINST THE SELF

The manifestations of this defense can be most dramatic. Either the aggressive or libidinal drives may be turned in their aim against the originator of the impulse. A melodramatic form of this phenomenon frequently occurs in the psychiatric treatment of children; a child whose mind is filled with violent aggression symbolically kills off the dolls which represent his family and then takes a toy gun and shoots himself dead. In other words, the child has turned sadism into masochism as he directs the hostile aggression at himself. A child in a rage may also beat himself rather severely. In a milder form, it may be a seemingly meaningless self-reproach. In its most intense form, it may lead to suicide because the child feels bitter anger at a loved one, and the bursting hostile rage overwhelms the ego. The destructive impulse is caused either by the child fearing his own sadism as a dangerous internal enemy that can destroy him, or by the child destroying an internal object as a revenge against that loved one. This mechanism of defense is closely related to introjection and

identification. Here, the attributes of the parents are internalized in the form of the superego; this determines the child's self-esteem. The working of this mechanism gives a clue to the strength of the drives or the severity of the superego.

DISPLACEMENT

This mental activity permits the child symbolically to exchange one part of the body for another, or one person for another. It may be used to obtain indirect gratification of a repressed desire for erotic bodily sensations, especially masturbatory impulses. Instead of manipulating the genitals, the displacement may be to stroking the hair and touching the nose, or to rhythmic movements of other parts of the body. (This is commonly noted in the body movements of children during the oedipal and early adolescent phases). It may also be used to allay fears of injury to the body, especially the genital area. In such instances it is expressed as pain in the extremities or fear of injury to the limbs or nose. The child may, then, avoid any kind of athletic activities.

Displacement also may be from one object to another, either as a substitute object of gratification or as a substitute for the expression of repressed hostile feelings. The hatred a child feels toward his parent may be directed instead toward teachers or toward a sibling; either one thereupon becomes the innocent victim of the displaced anger. Affection also may be directed toward others as a means of gratifying what is felt as prohibited love.

Displacement redirects not only a prohibited idea toward a substitute, but also the effect related to that idea. Thus it reinforces the conviction that the mental activity is not associated with the original object.

IDENTIFICATION

This is perhaps the most important of all the mental mechanisms which facilitate the adjustment of the growing child. It may have prominent and significant preconscious and conscious components, but the motives which power it are always unconscious. When it operates, in certain aspects, the child unconsciously becomes the same as his parents or others. In effect he internalizes one or more aspects of their behavior. These internal "presences" then exert a regulatory influence upon the child's behavior; in effect the child treats absent people as though they were still present, argues with them, submits to them, defies them, or placates them. In extreme cases he may attack them (himself), or try to run away from them (the marvelous initial burst of freedom some runaways describe). This process emerges as a normal aspect of development, and its nature and complexity depend upon many variables. These include the genetic and conceptual level the child has attained, the people about him with whom he can identify, the host of factors that facilitate or impede specific identifications at given times, and the like. Schafer[65] provides a comprehensive study of this phenomenon.

In its more mature form, this mechanism of defense becomes operational during approximately the third year of life; it begins with the work of separation and individuation. These early identifications coalesce with the products of other defense mechanisms to form the matrix which eventually becomes structured as the superego.

Prior to three years of age, important primitive psychological experiences occur which exercise a crucial if subtle influence on the child's development. These are referred to as primary identifications. They take place around experiences which are primarily related to biological stimuli (tactile, auditory, visual, visceral and kinesthetic), and generally speaking, they are aroused in the emotional climate in which the mother administers to the child's needs. They represent the mother's earliest caretaking functions as the infant experienced them—and they become internalized. These many caretaking events provide rhythmicity and constancy which are of great importance to the infant's viability. At first these attributes of the mother are internalized as various forms of introjection. Gradually, as differentiation occurs, the child begins to imitate; he imitates the mother primarily, but this extends to others who are important to him. These experiences precede the process of identification, and if all has gone well, they create in the child a state of stability described as basic trust.[7]

In time, as the child becomes less dependent and more autonomous, it is important that he establish inner controls in relation to internal and external stimuli. The process of identification provides this regulatory function. As a result of its operation, the child becomes like the parents as he takes in their attitudes about body functions, speech, sexual identity, aggression, and moral values. In normal development, the child is provided with three important support functions. First, by internalizing the various qualities of the parents, the child can be separated from them and still be able to adjust on his own to that which he

experiences in the external world. Also, by dint of responding to parental expectations, he wins their regard. This enhances his feeling of being loved as well as secure. In time, the child begins to construct an inner image of how he is supposed to be. This is formed in part of parental expectations; the child aspires to live up to these "standards." Such an internal presence is called the ego-ideal. Finally, the child protects himself from any angry feelings he may have toward his parents from time to time by idealization; that is, he overestimates them and thereby retains them as loved objects in spite of his anger.

On the other hand, when parents are cruel, inconsistent, seductive, or antisocial, faulty object relations ensue. Fearing a cruel parent, a child may express the hostility he feels by displacing it onto other children in an irrational manner. He does to the other children what has been done to him; he is thus the ally of the parent and not the victim. This is referred to as identification with the aggressor. A child raised by a puritanical, depressed mother may take in her endless denunciations of his natural appetites in the form of severe archaic superego identifications. Now he has an inner voice to condemn and devalue him. Presently this results in a childhood depression. All too often, children identify with their parents' antisocial characteristics and engage in serious delinquency. Such a child is described as suffering from sociopathy. The impact on the child of parental seduction or rejection may also result in pathological identifications. An example of this would be a boy who identifies himself with his mother in order to save himself from a fantasied fear of castration; or the girl who struggles against identification with her mother due to her disappointment at not having a penis. The boy in such a case can become effeminate, and the girl may defensively identify with her father and become a tomboy. In general, when the identification is with a loved person, separation becomes more tolerable. When, instead, it is with a person who exploits the relationship for whatever reason, the identification leads to serious pathology.

SUBLIMATION

This refers to mental activity which results in highly valued achievements. In general, the sexual and aggressive drives must be defended against by the ego. If the defense is not altogether successful, this creates anxiety. Under optimal circumstances, however, the defense works well. These drives are then deflected from instinctual aims and find expression in ways which are socially and culturally valued. There is a harmony among the mental institutions—the drives, the ego, and the superego—which results in outstanding achievement in art, science, and religion. This, then, is hardly a "mechanism" in the usual sense, in that the drives undergo desexualization and deaggressivization. That is, the psychic energy is channeled into socially acceptable or "sublimated" forms of mental activity. They are not inhibited or blocked and forced to seek gratification through defensive patterns which restrict ego functions. Examples of sublimation of drives may be noted in the talented, creative, and artistic accomplishments of some children in art and science. Such expressions are free from inhibition, a sense of compliance or a burden of discontent. This highly complex form of mental activity in which the ego ideal plays a significnt role in supporting the nondefensive functions of the ego is discussed in detail by Hartmann[42] in "Notes on the Theory of Sublimation."

ALIENATION

This defense mechanism is activated in adolescence when a specific need arises to place psychological and physical distance between the adolescent and his parent. Its function is to modify incompatible ideas related to the sexual and aggressive drives and to the superego; its goal is to master the sexual drive and direct it toward nonincestuous object relationships.[11] The adolescent must relinquish his libidinal ties to and dependency upon his parents no matter how compatible this relationship has formerly been. He must struggle to free himself from the identifications of childhood as represented in the superego in order to master and integrate the sexual drives into the body schemata and then direct them toward new objects which are nonincestuous. During this transitional phase, the ego uses the power of the intense sexual and aggressive drives in order to modify the superego; in effect the youth attacks his own conscience. By doing so, however, he achieves mastery of the drives and separation and individuation from the parents. This mental mechanism is manifested overtly by behavior in which the adolescent becomes alienated from, but not totally removed from, his parents. The process by which the influence of the superego is modified is in the service of instinct regulation and is referred to as alienation. New behavior, attitudes, feelings, thoughts, and body posture emerge, reflecting new external and internal rela-

tionships. Where the superego is too severe, the ego may fail in its efforts to bring about change; instead ti falls victim to the rigid and unmodifiable superego. This can result in severe pathology. Depending on the degree of failure and the rest of the youngster's resources, this may take form variously as depression, reactive schizophrenia, neuroses, passive-dependent character formation, or asceticism. On the other hand, if the superego is seductive or corrupt, the process of alienation may result in a chaotic and frenetic hunger for new pathological object relationships and a tendency to resort to drugs to tame the drives. Normally, once adulthood is reached and the psychic changes are consolidated, this particular mechanism disappears.

Additional Psychodynamic Factors
Basic to Health and Illness

IDENTITY

This broad and generally used concept is not free of ambiguities. Erikson[23] has written about this extensively from a psychosocial point of view. From a psychoanalytic perspective, identity refers to the experience of the "self" as a distinct coherent entity. It involves the person's wishes, thoughts and memories, and his own distinctive appearance. Whereas the concept of personality refers to what others perceive of an individual's behavior and physical appearance, identity refers to the individual's self-awareness, the way he perceives himself combined with his sense of how he is seen by others. Identity formation is not confined to any specific phase; it is an ongoing life-long process. Over time, it produces an enduring schema representing how the person consciously and unconsciously perceives himself. Erikson[22] describes identity as self-realization based upon a specific configuration. It is established gradually by successive ego synthesis and resynthesis integrating "the constitutional given, idiosyncratic libidinal needs, favored capacities, significant identifications, effective defenses, successful sublimations and consistent roles."

To know how a child sees himself provides the child psychiatrist with critical understanding of the child's mental development. Identity focuses upon the psychological and social factors which determine for the child who he is and what is his relationship to the world in which he lives. A striking example of the disruption of this process is observed in some adopted children who are told early in life that they are adopted.[81] A vulnerable group undergoes a disorganization of the process of identity formation and has difficulty in establishing a permanent sense of self. They wonder, "Who am I, what is my real name, who are my parents?" They are never content, never sure of where they belong. In general, children may grow to adulthood seeing themselves as loved or rejected, omniscient and powerful, or injured and vulnerable, belonging or estranged, male or female, and the like. Halloween offers a fascinating opportunity for ascertaining a child's self-image; in this, he demonstrates in fantasy and attire how he sees himself. If observed over time, it reveals the ever changing nature of the process of identity.

During infancy, as the child receives nurturance from the mother, identity formation begins. When circumstances are favorable, a relationship of reciprocal satisfaction develops between mother and child. For the child, this creates an internal feeling of confidence and an external feeling of trust.[7, 70] In parallel with his good physical experiences, the child also takes into himself psychologically the good emotional relationship to the mother. By the same token, a significant disturbance of this relationship may leave the child psychologically impaired, an impairment that may range in form from psychosis to character disorder. Whatever else ensues, one outcome common to all children subjected to early emotional deprivation is a debilitating chronic depression, a fragmentation of the concept of self, a discontent with the self-perception.[48]

Early life experiences are the bases upon which later identifications are structured. These identifications are in turn determined by the quality of the relationships the child experiences with the adults in his life, especially his parents. Out of this matrix emerge adaptive patterns which represent a compromise between the quest to satisfy inner needs and the demands of reality. Although these patterns of behavior are initially conscious, they recede into the partially or the totally unconscious and form the child's self-image. In theoretical terms, during infancy and childhood, the child constructs a composite self-image. This consists of his body image, the psychic representations of his inner state, and the mental representations of objects or persons of great significance to him. These mental representations play a vital role in developing the child's conception of himself. Body image development, identity formation and ego development continue to interact with one another at each developmental stage. The outcome of this process determines the child's growing awareness of his own self and his sense of his body; ultimately these form the child's "self-image" and his sense of identity.

For a child or adolescent to experience a relative sense of well-being, both psychologically and socially, among other things he must feel comfortable about his own body. In addition he must possess an inner feeling of closeness to and acceptance from those who mean so much to him.

Glaring examples of a disturbance of this process are all too common. They can be observed in predelinquent children who see themselves as oppressed, persecuted, and who turn on their world, bitter and vengeful. Other children may show serious disturbances in assuming appropriate male and female roles. Their underlying fantasies support their conflict over gender identity. A most dramatic example of a disturbance of identity may be observed in adolescents who suffer from acute identity diffusion. In general, this is a mental state in which there is an inability to experience oneself as having continuity and sameness within the process of developmental change. As part of such a state, there is a loss of capacity for work, including academic work, an inability to concentrate, a feeling of being adrift in time, a yearning for intimacy based upon dependency needs, and an oppositionalism to the demands of reality. In its most extreme form, the adolescent sees himself as barren, despicable, evil, and abandoned; he wants only to be dead.

Estrangement from parents tends to create a sense of a loss of identity, an inability to assume prescribed personal and social roles. This is especially so during adolescence. This is the moment when the identifications of childhood, which are so essential for security, must be disavowed. When this separation is harsh and severe, the response to family and society becomes scornful, snobbish, and hostile. Adolescents choose what Erikson describes as a negative identity, that is, roles and values which the parents and the community see as undesirable or dangerous. The adolescent feels that it is better to follow a deviant path through adolescence than to lose one's sense of self by being an automaton run by the parents and society. The quest for an identity may be expressed through intense narcissistic interest in others with similar conflicts; such a pattern is seen in delinquent gangs, drug-oriented groups, various religious cults, communes, homosexual communities, and the like. No longer can ambitious, controlling, or insensitive parents direct the life of the adolescent; the influence of the superego is renounced. An adolescent following such a pattern often is not influenced by psychotherapy; the behavior has become egosyntonic, that is, compatible with the ethical standards of the self or peers. Indeed, the feeling of belonging to a deviant or variant group becomes necessary as a defense against the disorganization experienced during the adolescent process of ultimate separation and individuation.

Disturbances of Parenting

OBJECT LOSS

The term object loss has been used to describe the loss of a parent by death,[37] divorce,[20, 77] separation and abandonment,[63, 71] and hospitalization.[67] Whatever its origin, it produces a profound influence upon the child's mental development.[63] Separation from, abandonment by, or death of the loved object tends to arrest ego development at the level achieved at the time of the loss. It may also result in regression to an earlier stage of development in expressing a wished-for relationship with the lost object.[59] The child may also experience a loss when the parent is present but rejects him, or the parent is chronically depressed or psychotic. Additionally, the fantasy life of the child may be organized around the feeling of parental loss because of the birth of a sibling or because of fantasies associated with adoption. The resentment, hostility, and feelings of loss may be internalized; ultimately they may lead to a state of depression which has nothing to do with external object relations. On the other hand, the rage at loss may be externalized by means of projection and then, for example, a teacher or the principal of a school may become a target for the hostility of a boy who has experienced intense anger at the loss of his father by death. With a new baby a child will usually express anger at the younger sibling rather than toward the mother for having the baby. A certain group of adopted children turn against their adoptive parents, to help ward off the rage they feel toward their natural parents for abandoning them; they may then idealize the unknown biologic parents in fantasy and even search for them. The most common pattern is to deny the meaning of the loss in order to avoid the pain of mourning and perpetuate the fantasy that the relationship continues. The absence of a parent during normal development creates a serious developmental deficit, with fantasies of reunion, either in harmony or in conflict. Although such ruminations shield the child from the persistent aspects of grief, it always leaves a serious void in the development of healthy relationships to others.

CHRONIC EMOTIONAL DEPRIVATION

This dreadful and severe form of childhood deprivation is noted especially among the children of families living in poverty, and is also referred to as social or environmental deprivation. However, it can occur at any level of society. These children are alleged to be resourceful in surviving the deprivation, neglect, and, often, terror in the social setting in which they are raised; in fact, however, they react with feelings of passivity, helplessness and hopelessness, and they exhibit strong dependency wishes. Some respond by turning their helplessness into aggression or by identifying with an aggressor. Although chronic depression and apathy are common forms of psychological sequelae, there are, in addition, a wide range of pathological syndromes such as psychoses, neuroses, psychosomatic reactions, and character disorders. Moreover, in an atmosphere of psychological impoverishment, abandonment, and violence, intellectual development also becomes impaired.[19, 55, 61]

Regardless of the specific behavior they manifest, examination of these children shows them to be chronically depressed, as are their mothers. During their earliest years these children have often experienced multiple object relationships devoid of any security. Their fantasies are filled with violence, yearnings to be cared for, distrust, and magical solutions. They also demonstrate confusion about their sexual identity. In their drawings of a person they exhibit strong oral needs, helplessness, an immature body ego, and confusion about sexual differences.

OVERSTIMULATION AND FLOODING

Overstimulation of a child may occur as the result of one of three factors: stimuli from without which may overwhelm the stimulus barrier of the ego, stimuli arising from within which may be so intense that the ego can't bring them under control, and defects of the ego or immaturity of the ego which will leave the ego incapable of dealing either with increased tension or even normal tension by the usual methods.

Overstimulation may occur at any point in time

along the developmental continuum and severely impair the growth of the ego. The earlier the ego is subjected to overstimulation, the more serious the resulting ego defects. At birth, before object relations develop, the external stimuli are defended against by what Freud[33] called a stimulus barrier (the *Reizschutz*). However, there is no protection against stimuli arising from within. A good example of flooding by internal stimuli is noted in children suffering from minimal brain dysfunction. Here the nature of their ego defects makes them helpless to master their drives; they then succumb to hyperactivity which the mother is unable to relieve. Atypical children also suffer from serious ego defects which leave them vulnerable to inner and outer stimuli.[10, 80] Flooding may also be caused by maternal neglect and rejection. When the baby is overcome by hunger, a need for soothing, or a need for changing, the mother must serve as a supplementary barrier against the noxious stimuli; when she does not, ego development is disturbed.[73] More than that, the mother may herself strongly overstimulate the infant, thus preventing the natural emergence of mastery with the associated growth in ego functions. Later, this may make it especially difficult for the child to separate from the mother.[14] Such sequences can be the preconditions for serious pathology, such as psychoses, homosexuality, borderline states, antisocial character disorder, learning disabilities, excessive eating tendencies, and the like.

During the anal stage of development, maternal overstimulation can take the form of administering frequent enemas, or excessive wiping, cleaning, douching, and bathing. These experiences may create fantasies of terror and annihilation or seductive pleasure, depending upon the emotional climate in which they are carried out.

In the phallic-oedipal period, overstimulation may involve physical and/or psychological trauma. Some children are subjected to overstimulation of the genitalia, seduction, constant fondling, or exposure to the primal scene as a form of violence. A violent father may batter the child physically and overwhelm his defenses psychologically. The child will identify with the father in order to survive and pay the inevitable price of impaired development. Such overstimulation creates conditions that deprive the child of the ability to discharge tension appropriately; this brings about premature arousal and intense anxiety beyond the child's powers of control or coping. The ego is "flooded" with anxiety before it has developed the capacity to master and integrate such stimuli in an effective manner.

Adolescence offers a classic example of overstimulation from within; his drives may indeed overwhelm the adolescent. Parental overstimulation, too, covertly or overtly, may overwhelm and paralyze the child's capacity to separate and find his own identity.

REPETITIOUS SEPARATIONS

There are fathers who spend long hours at work, mothers who for various reasons seek full-time employment, parents who go out almost every evening in the week or take frequent vacations away from their children, and divorced parents who date frequently and have many preoccupying encounters with different people. The frequent absence of a parent from the home and the introduction of a bewildering number of other adults into the home cannot enhance a child's feeling of security and relatedness. For optimal development, children require reasonably stable dual parenting, a stimulating psychological climate, and a continuing, unbroken relationship with the parents. Those children who are exposed to repetitive separation often ward off the resulting depression and the hostility by denial, projection and displacement, as they search frantically for a replacement of the unavailable object. Such children commonly idealize the unavailable parents in order to deny their nonavailability and to avoid the frightening feelings of hostility. When they are young, children may protest such parental activities, but as they grow older, they learn to endure the situation. As a result of these experiences, their object relations become fragile. These children frequently show intense anxiety and restlessness as an expression of their depression. Defective impulse-control is present along with unstable peer group relationships and a strong identification with the longed-for parent.

INSUFFICIENT, INCONSISTENT AND
OVERINDULGENT PARENTING

In general, parenting requires an adequate response to the phase specific needs of the child. The nature of this nurturing response has a powerful influence upon the child's development. If it is insufficient, inconsistent or excessive, there will be a derailment of this highly sensitive and complex process.

As has been demonstrated by Spitz, Provence, A. Freud, Mahler and many others, insufficient parenting at any level of development will interfere with drive organization and ego growth. It will cause children to experience intense frustration to which, in turn, they may react with detachment, inordinate demands for satisfaction, or a frantic search for gratification through action or through fantasy. These children are overwhelmed by feelings of depression; their every moment is tinged with helplessness, emptiness, and powerlessness. Their fantasies often have demoniacal features, and they experience volcanic aggressive feelings which they strive desperately to control. Their pathological object relationships distort their patterns of identification; this predisposes them to psychoses, borderline states, the formation of disordered, oral dependent character structuring, or the syndrome of environmental deprivation. Some children desperately seek substitute oral gratification, putting any material objects in their mouth for relief which may result in pica or lead poisoning.[56]

Inconsistent parenting also disorganizes the normal development of the child. Fenichel[27] demonstrated that the alternation of extreme parental permissiveness with extreme hostility resulted in a person incapable of introjecting any consistent parental images; because of this there was an inability to develop a normally functioning superego. It seems safe to say that any factors which interfere with consistent handling of drives will impair ego development. Before the age of three, the child is particularly vulnerable to such experiences as separation, a lack of interest, or a lack of patience on the part of the mother in feeding, weaning and training for cleanliness. Such a relationship with gratification at one moment and lack or excessive delay of gratification on the other may lead to a disturbance of ego development. The stronger the child's instinctual drives, and the greater the inconsistency, the more severe the final picture. Up until the time when separation-individuation is completed (somewhere about three to four years), the child is particularly likely to respond to inconsistent instinctual gratification by a form of development which may lead to delinquent behavior.[12, 35] This results from a weakening of ego functions in the regulation of impulses. Such children become vulnerable to pathological castration anxiety and oedipal conflict. The instinctual drive seeks gratification through pregenital activity such as by the loss of impulse control and delinquent behavior. This embarks the child on a course which must ultimately interfere with the socialization process. The behavior of such children represents the chronic hostile desire for both revenge upon and gratification from the inconsistent mother. Szurk[76] pointed out that a parent may selectively encourage antisocial behavior and Johnson[44] described how these parents could influence certain circumscribed areas of behavior in their children by creating "superego lacunae."

Excessive gratification can be experienced at any given level of development. It will result either in a reluctance to give up the pleasurable experience or in a fear of being overwhelmed by impulses which are beyond the child's control. When parents overindulge their children, they do so because of their own unresolved emotional problems. In effect, they unconsciously exploit the children as an expression of their own narcissistic needs, repressed hostility, guilt feelings, sibling rivalry, and the like. As compared to deprivation, very little study has been accorded this type of parent-child interaction.

Overindulgence has the quality of overstimulation; the infant or child is not given the opportunity to master instinctual tension normally as it arises with each phase of development. Ideally, at each level, the child should have the opportunity to master the discharge of his drives with the cooperation of the parents who teach him limits and define what are and what are not appropriate means for the gratification of his impulses.

During the oral phase, overindulgence may cause the child to develop a false optimism and a deep-rooted conviction that everything should go well for him. Some children respond with an intense need for direct oral gratification expressed in such symptom-formation as obesity.[18] Or, they may respond with the formation of a passive dependent character employing oral activity or its derivatives to bind aroused impulses, whatever their cause.[69] Levy[51] described this phenomenon as "maternal overprotection" and elaborated on its complications.

During the anal-urethral developmental phase, the mother may overstimulate the child by the use of enemas, by wiping the child excessively each time the child urinates or defecates, and by responding intensely with glee or disgust at having the child constantly clean. Where they don't fight back, such children are condemned to inactivity and passivity in the mastery of these functions by masochistically submitting to the mother's control. This may then be carried over into the school; if the child's performance is not appreciated by the teacher, he will defy her, or refuse to produce for her. The lowering of self-esteem under such circumstances creates unconscious, self-inflicted suffering and chronic discontent. What emerges is the state of moral masochism.[17] There can be bitter complaints about the teacher because she does not respond to his performance in a way similar to that of his mother. There is the fantasy that he will be rewarded for clean living, clean thinking, and his unusual productivity. Often these children show an aversion to certain foods as a symbol of their inability to handle their anal impulses. They thus force the mother to give them food which is symbolically acceptable.

During the phallic-oedipal phase, many mothers, and at times, fathers, overindulge or overstimulate the "little man" or "little woman" who represents some aspect of their own oedipal conflicts. In Western culture, this takes the form of sleeping in the same bed, taking showers together, parading nude in an exhibitionistic manner, overstimulating the child's genitalia, touching him provocatively, and the like. These serve to excite the child, arouse fantasies of special status, or evoke fears of physical or psychological vulnerability. This type of excessive stimulation may also cause the child to dramatize a false excitement in which he complies in order to alleviate castration anxiety or in order to evoke further overstimulation. Ultimately, this too will interfere with the normal process of socialization.

In general, excessive satisfactions and overindulgence make children unable to bear the normal frustrations which less spoiled children learn to tolerate.[27] Divorce and separation as well as conflicts between parents tend to cause parents to displace their indulgences or frustrations onto their children. Children in such a dilemma are either being spoiled or neglected; as a result, they are all too likely to suffer from pathological narcissism, that is, either feeling a special exaggerated self-interest or a painful, brooding self-preoccupation, or both.

FOSTERING PATHOLOGICAL IDENTIFICATIONS

Whatever its character, the child's identification with his parents is essential for his psychological survival. Unfortunately, as this process proceeds, whatever psychopathological attributes the parents possess will necessarily become part of his way of life.

Identification with the person whom the child fears may be lost or whom he has lost, may lead to a denial of the loss. Rochlin[64] refers to this phenomenon as a loss complex. Where this is the case, in the face of the object loss, regression takes place. In order to preserve the relationship, the child returns to the point where the identification with the object was fixed. Invariably this brings about an arrest of development of certain ego functions and an impairment of other object relations. Aside from identification, in order to preserve the lost object, the child may also express the pain of loss by withdrawal, regression and other symptoms of depression. Thus one child may evoke a noble image of himself so as to attain from others eternal approval and love. Another child may identify with the mother and mourn the loss of his father through her. He may then withdraw, show irritability, tearfulness, and self-hatred, and feel helpless. There may also be the direct identification with the lost parent; one boy became withdrawn and depressed like his father who was this way for two years before committing suicide. The child's fantasies included a reunion with his father in heaven in which he would meet this parent on a cloud.

Identification with a seductive mother may be used to protect the child from castration anxiety and object loss. The child will have a false sense of power based upon his identification with his powerful mother. Such children harbor a grandiose illusion of oneness with her and a reluctance to relinquish this relationship.

Delinquent children often identify with their parents. They carry out antisocial acts in response to an unconscious directive from the parent with whom they have identified.[45] The delinquent behavior thus becomes a means of establishing a reunion, through the act, with the parent from whom the child feels separated.

Identification with the aggressor always plays havoc with a child's ability to live with other children. This costly mental mechanism permits the child to survive the fear of the parent in a situation which threatens his very existence. It also arouses in the child a strong sense of power as a defense against feeling powerless. Such children forgive themselves too easily for their pathological behavior just as their parents approve of and defend their behavior since it also represents their own unrealized fantasies.[30]

Some boys engage in transvestitism by identifying with both the mother and father, thus having what the woman has without being castrated.[40, 68] The wearing of clothing appropriate to the opposite sex assures the child that through fantasy, the desire to be like both mother and father, female and male, can be achieved without damage to his body. Also, some boys assume the effeminate traits of their mothers; they adopt her mannerisms and the pitch of her voice. By thus identifying with the mother, they deny that they can be castrated. The young man becomes a sex object like his mother and looks for another young man to love him as he wished his mother would, free from castration fear. In this way he identifies with his mother and has the homosexual object identity with himself. This identification is either out of the fear of the aggressor or attachment to the seducer. During childhood, in fantasy and in drawings, these children express their wish to be effeminate. They show a powerful reluctance to separate from the mother and manifest as well a considerable fear of injury to the body.

Because of severe early deprivation and frustration, certain children suffer from what Erikson[23] describes as a loss of a sense of identity. Although it may be observed more frequently among children subjected to cultural deprivation, it also may be observed in young children caught in the web of divorce, death, or abandonment by a parent. Such children lack a sense of relatedness and continuity in their lives. Although they feel dreadful isolation and loneliness, they sometimes express themselves with unexpected naughtiness and provocative behavior. The child may also struggle against identification with the parent. This may cause him to deny the importance of this relationship, the pain of separation, and the hostility felt toward the parent. Such a child struggles to deny oral, libidinal, and sadistic impulses in relation to that parent; however, he may express these feelings in dramatic play with dolls in a treatment setting. He is unable to use the mother or father as a real external object as a basis for developing a stable sense of self and for relating to the world of reality.[39]

Children who suffer from schizophrenia demonstrate severely disturbed early object relationships and difficulty in differentiating between themselves and the external world. Their problem is not one of identification; rather it is one in which the ego actively uses separation for defensive purposes. The central problem for these children is a prolonged pathological autism-symbiosis conflict, and fusion with the mother is experienced as engulfment and annihilation. Such children shut out the human object world and show a preoccupation with repetitive, apparently purposeless behavior.[21, 54] An unusual phenomenon, however, is noted in children with borderline states. Such children show an overlapping of oral, anal, and phallic-oedipal conflict. Albeit seemingly neurotic, they may present good impulse control at one moment and then as the result of internal conflict or a disturbance in communication with the therapist, quickly switch to the most bizarre, im-

pulsive, and primitive behavior. This appears to be an identification with parents who have given highly charged, inconsistent care to the child in the autistic-symbiotic level of development.[53]

Precocity

The study of precocity, either psychological or physical, has been sporadic and fragmented in spite of the fact that there is a consensus that this can create painful problems for many children.

The premature development of ego functions, especially memory, or of the libidinal or aggressive drives, may result in serious maladaptive behavior. Learning and maturation normally occur along balanced developmental lines. However, a child born with precocious mental endowment, i.e., one who demonstrates early intellectual prowess, an unusual memory, and a rich fantasy life may have difficulty in structuring stable parental identifications because he is offered inordinate narcissistic gratification. Such children tend to be treated as special, with very little consideration given to their emotional and social needs. People relate to them with great interest and even with awe, thereby evoking in them a false evaluation of reality. Adulation by parents and the gratification such children receive from their exhibitionism restrict their emotional maturity and natural peer group experiences. This self-containment may result in pathological development in adolescence or later as their interests move into narrower channels and more specialized pursuits.[50] With the impairment of reality testing, with defective internalization of stable object relations, and without normal environmental stimulation they dry up. Many children with extraordinarily high intellectual development ultimately succumb to academic failure. In these highly gifted children, unusual intelligence serves only to weaken their adaptation to reality in that it obviated the necessity to learn to function cooperatively with others. The omniscience they fantasize in the oedipal period and the accompanying desire for adulation, coupled with their strong dependency needs, ill prepares them for the disciplined academic tasks required either at high school or at college. As one youngster put it, "when it got hard and was not fun, I didn't like it." Responsibilities which demand delay of gratification burden them with displeasure and may even lead to boredom or depression.

In some of these children, their precocity favors

a selective hypertrophy of certain ego functions which bind their libidinal and aggressive drives. Thus a child may become a whiz at mathematics, science, writing, art, music, chess, or drawing caricatures, thereby evoking admiration. However, the intrapsychic needs of the child flow continuously into the activity; in effect it becomes the receptacle for the sexual and aggressive drives. Thus, one major source of pleasure may be tapped through exhibitionism. In clinical cases, this marked investment in one activity represents a defense against anxiety connected with separation from an admiring parent and defense against the pain of the loss of the oedipal object.

Another, and most serious type of precocious development, occurs when a child has a surplus of aggressive energy on a hereditary basis.[1] This creates an imbalance between the ego and the drives. Early in life this kind of child shows signs of serious impairment of object relations. It is impossible for him to develop part and total object relationships which will bring about a balance between the internal and external environment. Fantasies of power, fears of being overwhelmed, and vulnerability to impulsivity usually result in delayed superego development. As a result there is an inability to establish latency as a developmental phase.

Precocious physical maturation also creates serious developmental stress. Throughout childhood the body image plays an important role in how the child feels about himself. This body image is built upon stimuli arising from within the body and from the reactions of other people to the child's physical attributes. Precocious physical growth, especially with the onset of puberty, will cause a child a great deal of stress. This physical upheaval subjects the child to an imbalance of psychic functions to which he often reacts with great discontent. The internal overstimulation and precocious changes in the structure of the body image result in an inability of the ego to neutralize the drives; this leaves the child disorganized, vulnerable to impulsivity and unable to study. Since adults and peers also tend to relate to such children as if they are older, this increases their discomfort and feeling of estrangement. They feel unacceptable, passively negativistic, restrained, sad, and unsure. When the tension becomes unbearable, the child may suddenly decompensate with chaotic, impulsive behavior, thus demonstrating that all control has been lost over the mental and physical functions.

Finally, precocious intellectual development combined with delayed physical maturation, especially in puberty, may result in depression, painful self-consciousness, shame, and outbursts of anger (often referred to as narcissistic rage). This precocious intellectual endowment unfortunately is used for defensive purposes rather than for healthy narcissistic satisfaction.

Traumatic Life Events

Far too many children are cruelly neglected, physically and psychologically, so that their development is marred for life. Often enough, the cruelty and deprivation which a parent has experienced during his own infancy and childhood will be inflicted on his children. This malignant phenomenon clearly demonstrates how conflicts arising during infancy and childhood remain active in adulthood and are repeated with the next generation of innocent victims. This consideration is basic to any study of the epidemiology of abnormal behavior and illustrates the importance of the integration of motherliness and fatherliness into early life.[4, 74]

The child-caring functions of a parent do not depend solely upon his ability and willingness to care for the child. The child's capacity to respond to care is another important ingredient. As an example, congenital or other physical or acquired disabilities may impair the child's response and may presently provoke a parent to emotional and material neglect. Child-abusing parents in particular will tend to see such a child as "bad" or "out to get me upset," and may react with yelling, violent slapping, severe beating, or burning the child. There can be a convergence of parental problems so that passive masochistic mothers will maintain homes in which their alcoholic or violent-tempered husbands victimize and abuse their children.

Certain infants, subject to such neglect, fail to thrive physically and mentally. They demonstrate poor eating patterns and withdrawal or fretful behavior.[26, 28, 38] Later they may show a breakdown of eating and toilet functions, delayed speech, and bizarre behavior. Older children often react with restlessness, hostility, distrust, poor impulse control, fantasies of violent interpersonal relationships, and dreams and stories concerned with gruesome monsters, violence, helplessness, and the desire for power. Many repress these grim experiences, act out their conflicts within a turbulent sexual life, and ultimately reactivate these conflicts of childhood with their own children.

Spitz[72] observed that the loss of the mother in the second half of the first year of life created a major life crisis for children. It led to a psychological syndrome of depressive nature which he called anaclytic depression. These children present a picture of weepiness, withdrawal, expressionless eyes and a harassed facial expression. They refuse to eat and display loss of weight and, at times, insomnia. All show a susceptibility to colds or eczema and a gradual decline in their development quotient. In some, this syndrome followed a catastrophic course ending in the death of the infant. This same phenomenon may occur even when the mother is present if she subjects the infant to psychological and material deprivation due to her own depression or her rejection of the child.[52] From a psychodynamic point of view, the infant reacts by withdrawing from the mother; in effect, the mother is lost as a libidinal object. The malevolent aspect of the mother as the "bad" object is introjected, following which the infant projects the distrust onto others who seek to care for him. Not every person can reverse this process, for the infant responds favorably only to those who possess certain psychological qualities which modify the projection system.[7, 47]

Whenever divorce occurs, it precipitates an acute crisis in all the involved children, since it prevents the child from working through the normal triadic relationships which are necessary to attain ultimate separation and individuation as an adult. The fantasies of these children represent the intrapsychic response to the crisis. They are of great variety and depend upon the child's relationship to both parents. For some children it may represent the victorious affirmation of an oedipal victory. For others, it might reactivate a negative Oedipus complex in which the parent of the opposite sex is seen as malevolent. It is not unusual for these children to exploit the permissiveness of one parent and to use it in the service of expressing hostility against the natural authority of the other. New adult relationships established by either parent may be reacted to with fear of the loss of that parent or with a feeling of betrayal. Fantasies of romantically bringing about the restitution of the marriage may also influence the behavior of the child. Again, if either spouse remarries, this may aggravate the child's oedipal conflicts and create serious family crises.[78]

Any premature removal of the child from his mother, from his father, or from the child's familiar envoronment will plunge him into a developmental crisis. The child's reaction depends on many variables, such as the nature of the relationship to the mother or father, the length of the separation, the age of the child, and the stage of drive and ego development. The response to separation as described by Bowlby[15] goes through three phases: protest, despair, and detachment. Situations such as prolonged hospitalization of the child or the mother, premature consignment of a child to camp or boarding school, prolonged absence of a parent from the home (such as occurs during an extended holiday), or parental death incline the children toward a state of chronic affective and cognitive disorganization and discontent.

Rochlin[64] stated that rather than coping with the management of his grief and working it through, the child deals with his pain by fixation or regression. In the course of this, he returns to the point where the identification with the lost object was fixed in order to preserve the relationship with the lost object. The mental life of the child may be directed toward a desire for reunion with the absent parent and burdened by sadness and anger at his loss. This preoccupation with such wishes for restitution may last for months; even though it gradually undergoes repression, the loss complex continues to be expressed as various derivatives of grief and anger. Since no child can survive in an object-less state, mechanisms of defense such as repression, denial, and substitution gradually take over. However, the attachment cathexis to the lost object is so strong that it is never relinquished, as is the sense of loss and unfulfillment.

Seduction and Molestation

Seduction occurs when a child is prematurely overstimulated sexually. The ego becomes bound to the seducer as a pathological object who restricts the child's normal psychological development. The seducer invites the child's participation by exhibitionism, such as provocative nudity, or by physical arousal through erotic caresses, mutual bathing, masturbation, fellatio, or sexual intercourse. In molestation, the child is forced to engage in a sexual act, either as a voyeur or as a physical participant.

It is not uncommon for a parent to be psychotic

or to suffer from a defective superego which allows the drives to be inappropriately gratified by using the child as a sexual object. Such a parent may be demanding, controlling, and seductive in order to arouse the child's participation. The child becomes trapped in the excitement of the experience and overwhelmed by arousal; he joins the behavior in a state of helpless dependency along with the fear of rejection. Beres[8] describes the role of parental influences in such a disturbed parent-child relationship; such a parent has an especially adverse effect on the child's superego formation by offering the child the model of uncontrolled sexual activities. The child may in turn experience profound unhappiness, remorse, distress, and apathy; he relies on his dependence upon the parent to protect him against the fear of loss of parental love. Also, the fear of the control exerted by the parent is managed by denial and projection; the child feels threatened by the outside world and expresses an inordinate need to remain close to the parent. Seduction, whether physical or psychological, usually results in a fixation of psychosexual development. Ultimately, this will impair the child's capacity to achieve a non-incestuous object relationship. Furthermore, since children normally have powerful oedipal fantasies and wishes which stimulate and arouse excitement, they are vulnerable to any advances made by adults who activate these fantasies. Although they may submit masochistically to the seducer and show no overt anxiety, it has been shown that parental restraint and aggressive control over the child may precipitate somatic complaints, neurotic or psychotic symptoms.[5] Molestation, whether heterosexual or homosexual, always carries with it the danger of precipitating a traumatic neurosis or premature arousal with subsequent chronic guilt or shame. The excitement may cause a primitive leap forward in libidinal development with severe pathological consequences.[46]

Chronic Scapegoating

A child may be assigned the role of family scapegoat. For reasons which are unconscious, the parent who dominates the household selects a particular child for this fate. At times, the children selected for this purpose recognize the parent's irrationality; however they try desperately to accommodate to the parent's disturbed behavior in order to continue to receive this parent's love. All too often, parents seek treatment for such a scapegoat child only to be surprised to find that he had been sacrificed in order to contain their own conflict. It then comes as a surprise that treatment is recommended for them instead of for the child. In such a situation, the child becomes the victim of a sado-masochistic relationship existing between the parents.

Although one child usually serves as scapegoat, on occasion more than one child is victimized. Who is selected and how he is treated depend upon the psychological and social problems which impinge on the parents and on their own unresolved childhood conflicts. Either the sex of the child, the birth order in the family, or the child's appearance may determine the selection process. Both parents may become intensely involved in the child's difficulties and in this way avoid the problems which exist between them. All too often, this is observed when a child suffers from a chronic illness, such as fibrosis cystica or minimal brain dysfunction. It is used as the excuse for a father to abandon the family when his problem actually is related to the marital conflict. The child also may be used to continue the parents' conflict after a divorce.

In his attempt to establish a secure object relationship, such a child becomes a psychological yo-yo. Although he may appear compliant to the unconscious directives of the parent, the child is overwhelmed by a feeling of disorganization, hostility, and vulnerability to his own impulses. Some children isolate their feelings and develop a façade of passivity and resignation. Other children displace the conflict onto the social situation with outbursts of hostility and delinquent behavior. At home they display irritability, hostility towards other siblings, withdrawal, defiance or tearfulness, and the like, as an expression of their feelings of futility. An assessment of their intrapsychic organization reveals their helplessness, dependency, depression, confusion about their sexual identity, the wish to be nurtured, and the most intense hostile fantasies.

Scapegoating is a defensive function which supports and maintains the operation of the family by isolating the problem in the child and denying its serious nature. The child becomes the sacrificial victim whose development is seriously impaired. This is reflected in his adjustment to the home, the school, and the community and is caused by defective identifications and a disorganization of superego formation.[6]

Chronic Devaluation

Certain parents have a need to select a child to be stupid, subjecting the child to chronic devaluation, destructive criticism, or overprotection; this stifles the child's assertiveness and phase specific mastery of the external world.[9] The child may represent certain unacceptable attributes of the parent, or of others to whom the parent was related in childhood. Often these children were unwanted or conceived for irrational reasons.

Devaluation (which may be expressed in the form of overprotection) intensifies the child's feelings of vulnerability and helplessness; the child is made to feel he can't do anything for himself. Such children feel hopeless; they can never do anything right. They have a defective self-image and an intense ambivalence toward the parent, along with the need to comply with the parent's directives. The impact of this type of care is devastating, and the developmental deficit often remains in the form of a character disorder in which the victim feels a lack of self-esteem and an absence of self-confidence. Intense affect hunger and anxiety occur in the presence of any tasks which require separation and individuation. Sado-masochistic fantasies and dreams represent the malevolent influences to which the child has been subjected. Passivity and chronic despair, with an accompanying impairment of intellectual, social, psychological, and sexual development reflect the severe constraints on ego functions. In some children the mental inertia is so powerful that it severely constricts intellectual and social development and denies the child any satisfactions from life. Loneliness may become their lifestyle, and television, the haven for their fantasy life as they live in the shadow of the oppressive parent.

Cultural Deprivation

This is a concept which creates strong differences of opinion about its nature and powerful resistances as to the choice of any interventional strategies. This phenomenon nevertheless has a crippling effect upon the psychological development of a child and ill prepares him to cope with survival in this society. This syndrome is bred by differences in cultural values and by transcultural conflict; it finds expression in poverty, racism, violence, malnutrition, child abuse, one-parent homes, and a vulnerable dependence upon a welfare program. Each generation of children so reared continues to grow at a high level of risk, and their children are, in general, assured the same fate.

These children are cared for or loved in a most inconsistent, fragmented and chaotic environment. They often have multiple parent surrogates with many caretakers coming in and out of their lives, so that it is difficult for them to achieve the object constancy so necessary for internal stability. As already mentioned in connection with the work of Spitz, Provence, Meers and others, adverse environmental stimulation has a disruptive effect on the child's psychological development, his relationships to others, and his intellectual development. In their early years, these children appear compliant, and it may seem from their behavior that their experiences have had no ill effects. However, their aggression is not bound to stable object love, and the course of their lives did not nurture an inner calm. When their feelings are explored, they express a yearning for tender care which, however, is tempered by distrust, along with violent fantasies of rage and revenge. Their adaptations may help them survive the culture in which they were reared, but they do not help them to transcend these experiences. When they start school, a serious deficit already exists in the quality of their early object relationships. This prevents them from establishing the object constancy required for the steady work of learning. The unconscious mental structures are bound to unfulfilled dependency needs, hostile fantasies, helplessness, and an inability to establish a positive identification with the teacher. Inevitably, learning becomes burdensome. The people available to them as models for identification are unable to give these children a feeling of stability and confidence in a climate of security. Chaos and, at times, violence force upon them a response of apathetic or depressive behavior, defensive passivity, and dependence based upon fear. When these children reach adolescence, for many of them it becomes a specially vulnerable period. The ego lacks the ability to master the sexual and aggressive drives effectively; superego formation is defective and the adults and peer groups they know offer them no support. With the absence of such necessary organizers of behavior, adolescence ill prepares too many of these adolescents for the psychological tasks of adulthood.

Family Romance and Family Secrets

Family romance refers to a sense of disillusionment with one's real parents and the need to search for them in fantasy as though they were lost objects. This is an extremely common fantasy in the lives of children; they think of themselves as adopted or as having somehow been assigned to different parents at birth; usually this involves the dream of having been born to parents of higher status. It often takes the form of a daydream and occupies very little attention mentally. This fantasy usually occurs in latency and preadolescence; it is a late displacement from oedipal fantasies. It is seen more frequently in children who are adopted and where a relatively undisturbed preoedipal development was followed by traumatic experiences in the oedipal phase. Knowing of their adoption, these children construct the family romance in their search for the idealized lost parents. The forerunner of the fantasy lies in the preoedipal period when the child's feelings of omnipotence are projected as powerful fantasies. In the oedipal phase, it is experienced as a search for an ideal parent figure in the person of a neighbor or relative. In latency it may be expressed as daydreams of glory and adventure. A common fantasy is the child as superman, of divine birth and looked up to by everyone. The family romance fantasy is born out of the need to deny the primal scene, to negate the relationship of the child to the parents, to avoid castration anxiety, and to evade the acceptance of the oedipal relationships.[32, 49]

In adolescence, a derivative of the family romance fantasy may manifest itself in the form of a repudiation of the family of origin. One becomes reborn as a member of a new family in a cult or a movement. Thus the feeling of hostility or contempt toward the parents may be extremely intense; this helps to wean the adolescent away from the oedipal attachments to his family[36] and turns him from the temptation to restructure once again the fictitious happy family of childhood.

Family secrets also operate as irritating nuclei in the psychic functions of a child. The defense required to encapsulate the family secret usually paralyzes the child's normal assertiveness and spontaneity. The family secret may be constructed by parents for various reasons such as concealing a death by suicide, the hospitalization of a retarded or psychotic family member, an imprisonment of a member of the family, alcoholism, child abuse, sexual abuse, and the like. The need for secrecy is usually for the protection of the parents and the avoidance of shame or censorship. Such children may be rendered depressed, passive, reluctant to play with peers, and lack the aggressivity required to master educational tasks.

Folie à Deux

Although infrequently observed, this phenomenon occurs when a child is under close supervision of a parent who is psychotic, hysterical, or fanatically religious. The child takes on the characteristics of this adult, sharing the same delusional ideas. It also may occur when a child assumes a similar delusional system as a sibling. The process has more of the features of imitation than those of identification, for if such a child is separated from the aberrant behavior of the other person, the distorted thinking is gradually relinquished. A variant of this is seen in children of divorced parents where a child will take on all of the bitterness and recrimination one parent holds against another. As one listens to the child, it is noted that there is a remarkable similarity in the complaints and criticism expressed by the one parent or the other. Another variant is observed when a child, because of the extreme closeness to the parent (particularly the mother), assumes all of the physical complaints of this parent. In treatment, this type of child tends to disengage quickly from the influence his parent has over his mental functions.

Coping and Adaptation

The concept of normality has limited usefulness in appraising what constitutes mental health and what constitutes psychiatric risk.

Unusual behavior is not necessarily abnormal and frequently encountered behavior is not necessarily normal. Transitory regressive states are essential in supporting the child's development, whereas compliance due to a reaction formation which controls hostile aggression may severely restrict the child's developmental capacities. Also, behavior which is considered normal in one subculture of this society is considered abnormal in another. The concept of "normality" is not that of a static process; it more closely approximates coping and adaptation. The more balanced or "healthier" the defenses, the better the coping abilities.[58] When the ego is not impaired, early in life, by severe conflict associated with struggles to gratify basic psychological and physical needs, its capacity to adapt to the internal and external environment is so much the greater.[79]

The inherent coping and adapting tendencies are expressed by the child's innate urge to master each developmental phase, to reach appropriate drive satisfaction, to render experiences free from anxiety, to assimilate and mitigate new experiences and to develop stabilizing object relations. In discussing the adult, Hartmann[41] states that "the degree of adaptiveness can only be determined with reference to environmental situations" whether it is "average expectable" or "average not expectable." However, for the child, in view of the fluid nature of his development, a more precise method of assessment is required in order to determine whether psychodynamic operations are progressive or regressive.

This, A. Freud[29] formulated in her procedure for the assessment of normality and pathology in childhood along development lines. This sensitive instrument for scrutinizing and assessing a child's development provides a vehicle for evaluating each one of the dynamic factors considered in this chapter within the broader framework of ego psychology; as they relate to pathological mental processes, to the environmentally expectable behavior, and to prevention.[24, 57]

Psychodynamic concepts derive from empirical observations and are constructs used for the purpose of clarifying and better understanding observed behavior. These activities of the mind operate upon the principle of psychic determinism, that is, they are complex mental processes which do not occur at random or by chance. Although various mental operations have been teased out of a highly complex child psychoanalytic psychology and child development, they stand in their own right as nuclear issues related to the stress which all children must bear, whether, for example, internally in the form of superego prohibitions, or externally, as it applies to object relationships, separation, loss, cultural deprivation, and the like.

None of these are the result of one all-pervasive motive; they are usually the outcome of many conflicting forces. Any shift within the constellation of conflicting forces can result in a radically different behavior, a phenomenon which is relevant to the treatment of pathological behavior. Psychodynamics defines the fluidity of these forces and their relationship to each other.

REFERENCES

1. ALPERT, A., NEUBAUER, P. B., and WEIL, A. P., "Unusual Variations in Drive Endowment," in Eissler, R. S., et al. (Eds.), *The Psychoanalytic Study of the Child*, vol. 11, pp. 125–163, International Universities Press, New York, 1956.

2. ANTHONY, E. J., "Introduction. The Syndrome of the Psychologically Vulnerable Child," in Anthony, E. J., and Koupernik, C. (Eds.), *The Child and His Family: Children at Psychiatric Risk*, pp. 3–10, John Wiley, New York, 1974.

3. ———, and KOUPERNIK, C. (Eds.), *The Child and His Family: Children at Psychiatric Risk*, John Wiley, New York, 1974.

4. ———, and BENEDEK, T. F., *Parenthood: Its Psychology and Psychopathology*, Little, Brown, Boston, 1970.

5. BARRY, N. J., and JOHNSON, A. M., "The Incest Barrier," *The Psychoanalytic Quarterly*, 27:485–500, 1958.

6. BELL, N. W., and VOGEL, E. F., "The Emotionally Disturbed Child as The Family Scapegoat," in Handel, G. (Ed.), *The Psychosocial Interior of the Family*, pp. 424–442, Aldine, Chicago, 1960.

7. BENEDEK, T. F., "Towards the Biology of the Depressive Constellation," *Journal of the American Psychoanalytic Association*, 4:389–427, 1956.

8. BERES, D., "Vicissitudes of Superego Functions and Superego Precursors in Childhood," in Eissler, R. S., et al. (Eds.), *The Psychoanalytic Study of the Child*, vol. 13, pp. 324–351, International Universities Press, New York, 1958.

9. BERGER, M., and KENNEDY, H., "Psuedobackwardness in Children: Maternal Attitudes as an Etiological Factor," in Eissler, R. S., et al. (Eds.), *The Psychoanalytic Study of the Child*, vol. 30, pp. 279–306, International Universities Press, New York, 1975.

10. BERGMAN, P., and ESCALONA, S. K., "Unusual Sensitivities in Very Young Children," in Eissler, R. S., et al. (Eds.), *The Psychoanalytic Study of the Child*, vol. 3/4, pp. 333–352, International Universities Press, New York, 1949.

11. BERMAN, S., "Alienation: An Essential Process of the Psychology of Adolescence," *Journal of the American Academy of Child Psychiatry*, 9:233–250, 1970.

12. ———, "Antisocial Character Disorder: Its Etiology and Relationship to Delinquency," *American Journal of Orthopsychiatry*, 29:612–621, 1959.

13. BIBRING, G. L., et al., "A Study of Psychological Processes in Pregnancy and of the Earliest Mother-Child Relationship," in Eissler, R. S., et al. (Eds.), *The Psychoanalytic Study of the Child*, vol. 16, pp. 9–72, International Universities Press, New York, 1961.

14. BOYER, L. B., "On Maternal Overstimulation and Ego Deficits," in Eissler, R. S., et al. (Eds.), *The Psychoanalytic Study of the Child*, vol. 2, pp. 236–256, International Universities Press, New York, 1956.

15. BOWLBY, J., *Attachment and Loss*, vol. 1, Basic Books, New York, 1969.

16. BRENNER, C., "The Nature and Development of the Concept of Repression in Freud's Writings," in Eissler,

R. S., et al. (Eds.), *The Psychoanalytic Study of the Child*, vol. 12, pp. 19–46, International Universities Press, New York, 1957.

17. BROMBERG, H., "Stimulus Response Cycle and the Masochistic Ego," *Journal of the American Psychoanalytic Association*, 7:277–297, 1959.

18. BRUCH, H., "Transformation of Oral Impulses in Eating Disorders: A Conceptual Approach," *Psychiatric Quarterly*, 35:458–481, 1961.

19. CHESS, S., "Disadvantages of the Disadvantaged Child," *American Journal of Orthopsychiatry*, 39:4–6, 1969.

20. DESPERT, J. L., *Children of Divorce*, Doubleday, Garden City, N.Y., 1962.

21. EKSTEIN, R., and WALLERSTEIN, J., "Observations on the Psychology of Borderline and Psychotic Children: Report From a Current Psychotherapy Research Project at Southard School," in Eissler, R. S., et al. (Eds.), *The Psychoanalytic Study of the Child*, vol. 9, pp. 344–369, International Universities Press, New York, 1954.

22. ERIKSON, E. H., "The Problem of Identity," *Journal of the American Psychoanalytic Association*, 4:56–121, 1956.

23. ———, *Childhood and Society*, W. W. Norton, 1950.

24. ESCALONA, S., "Intervention Programs for Children of Psychiatric Risk; The Contribution of Child Psychiatry and Child Developmental Theory," in Anthony, E. J., and Koupernik, C. (Eds.), *The Child and His Family: Children at Psychiatric Risk*, pp. 33–46, John Wiley, New York, 1974.

25. ———, "Emotional Development in the First Year of Life," in Senn, M. J. (Ed.), *Problems of Infancy and Childhood*, pp. 11–90, Josiah Macy Foundation, New York, 1953.

26. EVANS, S. L., REINHART, J. B., and SUCCOP, R. A., "Failure to Thrive: A Study of 45 Children and Their Families," *Journal of the American Academy of Child Psychiatry*, 11:458–466, 1972.

27. FENICHEL, O., *The Psychoanalytic Theory of Neurosis*, W. W. Norton, New York, 1945.

28. FISCHHOFF, J., "Failure to Thrive and Maternal Deprivation," in Anthony, E. J. (Ed.), *Explorations in Child Psychiatry*, pp. 213–225, Plenium Press, New York, 1975.

29. FREUD, A., *Normality and Pathology in Childhood*, International Universities Press, New York, 1965.

30. ———, *The Ego and the Mechanisms of Defense*, International Universities Press, New York, 1946.

31. FREUD, S., "The Ego and the Id," in *The Standard Edition of the Complete Psychological Works of Sigmund Freud* (hereafter: *The Standard Edition*), vol. 19, pp. 12–66, Hogarth Press, London, 1961.

32. ———, "Family Romances," *The Standard Edition*, vol. 9, pp. 237–241, Hogarth Press, London, 1959.

33. ———, "Beyond the Pleasure Principle," *The Standard Edition*, vol. 18, pp. 7–64, Hogarth Press, London, 1955.

34. ———, "The Interpretation of Dreams," *The Standard Edition*, vols. 4 and 5, Hogarth Press, London, 1953.

35. FRIEDLANDER, K., "Latent Delinquency and Ego Development," in Eissler, K. R. (Ed.), *Searchlights on Delinquency*, pp. 205–215, International Universities Press, New York, 1949.

36. FROSCH, J., "Transference Derivatives of the Family Romance," *Journal of the American Psychoanalytic Association*, 7:508–522, 1959.

37. FURMAN, R. A., "Death and the Young Child: Some Preliminary Considerations," in Eissler, R. S., et al. (Eds.), *The Psychoanalytic Study of the Child*, vol. 19, pp. 321–333, International Universities Press, New York, 1964.

38. GREEN, A. H., "A Psychodynamic Approach to the Study and Treatment of Child Abusing Parents," *Journal of the American Academy of Child Psychiatry*, 15:414–429, 1976.

39. GREENSON, R. Q., "The Struggle Against Identification," *Journal of the American Psychoanalytic Association*, 2:200–217, 1954.

40. HARRISON, S. I., "Reared in the Wrong Sex," *Journal of the American Academy of Child Psychiatry*, 9:44–102, 1970.

41. HARTMANN, H., *Ego Psychology and the Problem of Adaptation*, Translated by David Rapaport, International Universities Press, New York, 1958.

42. ———, "Notes on the Theory of Sublimation," in Eissler, R. S., et al. (Eds.), *The Psychoanalytic Study of the Child*, vol. 10, pp. 25–28, International Universities Press, New York, 1955.

43. ISAACS, S., *Developments in Psycho-Analyses*, Hogarth Press, London, 1952.

44. JOHNSON, A. M., "Sanctions for Superego Lacunae of Adolescents," in Eissler, K. R. (Ed.), *Searchlights on Delinquency*, pp.225–245, International Universities Press, New York, 1949.

45. ———, and SZUREK, S. A., "The Genesis of Antisocial Acting Out in Children and Adults," *Psychoanalytic Quarterly*, 21:323–343, 1952.

46. KATAN, A., "Children Who Were Raped," in Eissler, R. S., et al. (Eds.), *The Psychoanalytic Study of the Child*, vol. 28, pp. 208–224, International Universities Press, New York, 1973.

47. KLEIN, M., et al., *Developments in Psychoanalysis*, Hogarth Press, London, 1952.

48. KRAMER, P., "On Discovering One's Identity," in Eissler, R. S., et al. (Eds.), *The Psychoanalytic Study of the Child*, vol. 10, pp. 58–74, International Universities Press, New York, 1955.

49. KRIS, E., "The Personal Myth," *The Selected Papers of Ernst Kris*, pp. 272–300, Yale University Press, New Haven, 1975.

50. ———, "The Recovery of Childhood Memories in Psychoanalyses," in Eissler, R. S., et al. (Eds), *The Psychoanalytic Study of the Child*, vol. 11, pp. 54–88, International Universities Press, New York, 1956.

51. LEVY, D. M., *Maternal Overprotection*, Columbia University Press, New York, 1943.

52. LOURIE, R. S., "Experience with Therapy of Psychosomatic Problems in Infants," in Hoch, P. H., and Zubin, J. (Eds.), *Psychopathology of Childhood*, pp. 254–266, Grune & Stratton, New York, 1955.

53. MAHLER, M. S., *On Human Symbiosis and the Vicissitudes of Individuation: Infantile Psychosis*, vol. 1, International Universities Press, New York, 1968.

54. ———, "On Child Psychosis and Schizophrenia: Autistic and Symbiotic Infantile Psychosis," in Eissler, R. S., et al. (Eds.), *The Psychoanalytic Study of the Child*, vol. 7, pp. 286–305, International Universities Press, New York, 1952.

55. MEERS, D. R., "Contributions of a Ghetto Culture to Symptom Formation," in Eissler, R. S., et al. (Eds.), *The Psychoanalytic Study of the Child*, vol. 25, pp. 209–230, International Universities Press, New York, 1970.

56. MILLICAN, F. K., and LOURIE, R. S., "The Child with Pica and His Family," in Anthony, E. J., and Koupernik, C. (Eds.), *The Child and His Family*, pp. 333–348, John Wiley, New York, 1970.

57. NOSHPITZ, J. D., "Toward a National Policy for Children," *Journal of the American Academy of Child Psychiatry*, 13:385–401, 1974.

58. OFFER, D., and SABSHIN, M., *Normality*, Basic Books, New York, 1974.

59. Panel Report, Tourkow, L., reporter. "Psychic Consequences of Loss and Replacement of Body Parts," *Journal of the American Psychoanalytic Association*, 22:170–181, 1974.

60. Panel Report, Levin, S., reporter, "Depression and Object Loss," *Journal of the American Psychoanalytic Association*, 14:142–153, 1966.

61. PAVENSTEDT, E., "A Comparison of the Child-rearing Environment of Upper-lower and Very Low-lower

Class Families," *American Journal of Orthopsychiatry,* 35:89–98, 1965.

62. PROVENCE, S., "Some Relationships Between Activity and Vulnerability in the Early Years," in Anthony, E. J., and Koupernik, C. (Eds.), *The Child and His Family: Children at Psychiatric Risk,* pp. 157–166, John Wiley, New York, 1974.

63. ——, and LIPTON, R. C., *Infants in Institutions,* International Universities Press, New York, 1962.

64. ROCHLIN, G., "The Loss Complex: A Contribution to the Etiology of Depression," *Journal of the American Psychoanalytic Association,* 7:299–316, 1959.

65. SCHAFER, R., *Aspects of Internalization,* International Universities Press, New York, 1968.

66. SIEGAL, R. S., "What are Defense Mechanisms," *Journal of the American Psychoanalytic Association, 17:* 785–807, 1969.

67. SOLNIT, A. J., "A Study of Object Loss in Infancy," in Eissler, R. S., et al. (Eds.), *The Psychoanalytic Study of the Child,* vol. 25, pp. 257–271, International Universities Press, New York, 1970.

68. SPERLING, M., *The Major Neuroses and Behavior Disorders in Children,* Jason Aronson, New York, 1974.

69. SPITZ, R. A., "The Derailment of Dialogue: Stimulus Overload, Action Cycles and the Completion Gradient," *Journal of the American Psychoanalytic Association, 12:*752–775, 1964.

70. ——, *No and Yes: On the Genesis of Human Communication,* International Universities Press, New York, 1957.

71. ——, "Anaclitic Depression," in Eissler, R. S., et al. (Eds.), *The Psychoanalytic Study of the Child,* vol. 2, pp. 313–342, International Universities Press, New York, 1946.

72. ——, "Hospitalism. An Inquiry into the Genesis of Psychiatric Conditions in Early Childhood," in Eissler,

R. S., et al. (Eds.), *The Psychoanalytic Study of the Child,* vol. 1, pp. 64–70, International Universities Press, New York, 1945.

73. ——, and WOLF, K. M., "Autoerotism. Some Empirical Findings and Hypotheses on Three of its Manifestations in the First Year of Life," in Eissler, R. S., et al. (Eds.), *The Psychoanalytic Study of the Child,* vols. 3/4, pp. 85–120, International Universities Press, New York, 1949.

74. STEELE, B., "Parental Abuse of Infants and Small Children," in Anthony, E. J., and Benedek, T. (Eds.), *Parenthood,* pp. 449–477, Little, Brown, Boston, 1970.

75. STONE, L. J., SMITH, H. T., and MURPHY, L. B., (Eds.), *The Competent Infant: Research and Commentary,* Basic Books, New York, 1973.

76. SZUREK, S. A., "Genesis of Psychopathic Personality Trends," *Psychiatry,* 5:1–6, 1942.

77. WALLERSTEIN, J. S., and KELLY, J. B., "The Effects of Parental Divorce: The Adolescent Experience," in Anthony, E. J., and Koupernik, C. (Eds.), *The Child in His Family: Children at Psychiatric Risk,* John Wiley, New York, 1974.

78. ——, and KELLY, J. B., "The Effects of Parental Divorce: Experiences of the Preschool Child," *Journal of the American Academy of Child Psychiatry,* 14:600–616, 1975.

79. WEINSHEL, E. M., "The Ego in Health and Normality," *Journal of the American Psychoanalytic Association, 18:*682–735, 1970.

80. WEIL, A. P., "Certain Severe Disturbances of Ego Development in Childhood," in Eissler, R. S., et al. (Eds.), *The Psychoanalytic Study of the Child,* vol. 8, pp. 271–287, International Universities Press, New York, 1953.

81. WIEDER, H., "On Being Told of Adoption," *Psychoanalytic Quarterly,* 46:1–22, 1977.

2 / Constitutional-Organic Factors in Etiology

Dennis P. Cantwell and George Tarjan

Although child psychiatrists recognize that both normal and abnormal human behavior results from the interplay between the constitutional organic matrix of the child and environmental factors, many tend to overlook the importance of the matrix in this interaction. When one does consider the ways that the relationship between the somatic structure of a child and his behavior has been conceived, three traditional schools of thought can be recognized: the "hard," "soft," and "intermediate."[6, 37, 111, 123]

From the viewpoint of the "hard" school some brain lesion is seen as directly producing a behavior disorder. This may either be a specific "brain damage syndrome"[110] or a number of different clinical pictures depending on the sight or the type of the lesion.[123]

The "soft" school considers the organic structure to play only a minor role in the genesis of a child's behavior. Environmental aspects are seen to be of primary and overriding importance.[13, 123]

The "intermediate school" takes the stance that there are certain primary organic deficits which are the result of structural or functional abnormalities of the brain. However these organic deficits do not directly lead to certain types of behavior. Rather, specific behavioral syndromes in children with such deficits are determined by the reaction of the individual child to both his environment and to his primary deficit.

These three viewpoints have recently been elegantly expanded upon by Sameroff and Chandler.[97] They have described the three different models for evaluating the relative role of constitutional and environmental factors in the genesis of children's behavior as: a "main effect model," an "interactional model," and a "transactional model."

The main effect model states that irrespective of any environmental circumstances some type of defect in the organic matrix of any child will produce a deviant child.

A "strict" interactional model should enable one to predict a child's behavioral picture from the known combination of only two factors: the child's organic-constitutional makeup and his psychosocial environment. While this type of interactional model has been shown to hold up better than the main effect model in predicting behavior, by itself it is inadequate for several reasons. Sameroff and Chandler point out that neither the child's constitutional-organic makeup nor his environment are necessarily constant over time. Moreover, they note that the changes in both the constitutional makeup and the environment of the child are not independent of each other. Rather they change as a function of their mutual influence on each other. Sameroff and Chandler therefore propose moving from a static interactional model to a dynamic theory of developmental transaction—a transactional model.

This transactional model stresses that the child plays an active role in molding and shaping his environment just as the environment plays an active role in molding and shaping the child. Thus, the child is actively engaged in attempts to organize and structure his environment and environmental variables modify to a large degree *both* the child's organic-constitutional makeup and his reaction to the environment at any one time.[83]

The present authors believe that this transactional model offers the best perspective for viewing the interplay of constitutional and environmental factors in the production of normal and abnormal behavior in children. This chapter will review what is presently known about the role that the constitutional factors of the child play in this transaction.

Constitutional Factors and Behavior in Children—General Principles

This section will review recent research which supports the following general statements:

1. The Lockean idea that the newborn baby comes into this world as a tabula rasa merely to be written on, or a lump of clay merely to be molded by his parents is now known to be false. The constitutional matrix of the newborn child has a degree of complexity and organization that is only now beginning to be fully appreciated. Moreover, newborn babies are not mere passive recipients of attention from adults. The process of interaction between a newborn child and his environment is a complex one with very young children taking an active part in initiating and maintaining the interaction between themselves and adults.
2. There are great differences in the capabilities of individual children right from the time of birth.
3. There are multiple determinants of these individual differences in children.
4. These individual differences in children lead indirectly to differences in their behavior as a result of interaction with certain environmental experiences.

The Constitutional Complexity of the Newborn

There is a good deal of evidence now that the auditory and language capabilities of very young children are much greater than what was previously thought. Studying young children both in the home and at the laboratory, Friedlander has demonstrated not only that newborns can hear, but that they can discriminate well between different types of sound. During the first few months of life, the baby's ability to make fine auditory discriminations undergoes a marked and rapid development.[41] Friedlander's studies have utilized "Playtest" equipment: a machine containing a pre-programed selection of two channel tapes. The two tapes contain conversations with marked differences in degree of redundancy and in type of intonation: one conversation being highly redundant, the other being of very low redundancy; one conversation carried on with flat intonation, the other with bright intonation. The baby can operate switches which control a loud speaker and a stereotape player by differentially sucking on a nipple-like part of the apparatus. In the first few months of life the babies differentially select and respond to differences in flat and bright intonation and between conversation of high redundancy and low redundancy. While this does not mean that they can understand these differences, they definitely can distinguish them.

Other researchers have shown that infants as young as two months of age can *direct* conversation with an adult. Trevarthen and his colleagues at the University of Edinburgh[115] sought to test when infants developed behaviors indicating that they perceive people differently from objects. They filmed babies on a once-a-week basis from the time of birth until they were six months old, filming them either in a situation with the mother chatting to them or with a small toy suspended in front of them. In every instance the babies demonstrated elaborate activity that was specific to communicating with the mother which did not occur when only the suspended object was there. Movements of the hands and the voice and facial expressions were the behaviors most notably different in the two situations. Trevarthan hypothesizes that the young infant "communicates" with persons and "does" with objects. With objects the babies demonstrate such behaviors as: visually exploring and tracking, trying to grasp the object, trying to kick or step on it, or trying to put it in the mouth. With their mothers chatting to them, however, infants as young as two months old demonstrate "pre-speech" activity. This type of activity occurs in the context in which speech usually occurs, and the movement of the lips and the tongue make it look like a rudimentary form of speech. Even when sounds weren't made, a specific pattern of breathing was noted with this pre-speech activity. Distinctive movements of the hands were also associated with these pre-speech behaviors. Trevarthen feels these are developmentally related to the gestures of adults when they are engaged in eager and graphic conversation. He concludes that the foundation for interpersonal communication between human beings is present at birth and is remarkably useful even by eight weeks or age when cognitive processes are just beginning.

Other researchers have also looked at very young babies' reactions to sound by noting changes in muscle activity, heart rate, and breathing. Newborn babies have been shown to be very sensitive to different types of sounds. They respond to patterns, (square wave) tones, and to the human voice much more readily than they respond to pure (sine wave) tones.[21]

Moreover, for both square wave tones and sine wave tones, infants respond much more to frequencies within the range of the human voice. It has also been shown that babies seem to lose interest with repeated presentations of a given tone. When a tone of a different frequency is presented or when the same tone is presented at a different amplitude the baby will produce a renewed response.[21]

There is also evidence that the visual capabilities of young children are much greater than previously thought. Fantz and other researchers[38, 39] have provided evidence showing that young infants also show very reliable preferences for visual forms and patterns. Infants have the capacity for pattern vision and pattern selectivity, and a preference for patterns in individual children is evident from the time of birth. Within the first few days of life, babies will look for much longer periods of time at black and white patterns, such as a set of stripes as narrow as an eighth of an inch apart, than they will look at an unpatterned gray patch of equal brightness. In a similar vein they will look for longer periods of time at line drawings of a face with black lines drawn on white background than they will at simply three black dots on a white background. As with auditory stimuli, infants seem to lose interest when the same visual pattern is presented repeatedly. They will look away and spend less and less time looking at the same visual pattern. However, they become interested once again when a new pattern is presented to them.[21]

More than just pattern recognition has been investigated by Bower and his colleagues.[14] He has presented different stimuli to infants which project the same retinal image size. The stimuli have been either a solid object in three dimension, a two-dimensional representation of the object by photograph, or two three-dimensional objects varied in size and distance from the baby's eyes. Bower's work has conclusively shown that by as early as the second week of life infants reach for the *actual* three-dimensional object rather than for the photograph of the same object. This evidence thus suggests that the newborn baby even from the earliest days after birth may experience a three-dimensional world.

Finally, there is evidence that very young children can use both visual and auditory input to classify information. A series of elegant studies by Carpenter has shown how very young infants respond differently to a stranger's face and voice than to a mother's face and voice.[21] Carpenter first asked whether newborns could respond to *any* differences between three-dimensional facial forms. Her first study presented to each baby for a fixed time the mother's face, a model of a face, and an abstract facial form. In this experiment the infants discriminated between the three-dimensional forms very distinctly. By two weeks of age the infants looked reliably *longer* at both artificial faces than at their mother's face. Since these were black infants and the models were white, Carpenter assessed the possibility that the darker faces of the black mothers provided less distinct contrast to the background thus explaining the rather unexpected results.

Carpenter controlled for this with a new sample of Caucasian infants. Again three faces were shown, but this time the mothers faces were Caucasian and of equivalent brightness to the model face. A black model was also added to the study. However, this new sample of infants also looked at the Caucasian and black models more frequently than they looked at their mother's face.

At each age from one week of age to eight weeks of age the amount of time spent looking at the mother when she was stationary was virtually the same for both samples of infants. When the faces were moved rather than stationary they all attracted more attention, but even with this the mother was looked at *less* frequently than the models. There was not a statistical difference in the amount of time spent looking at the Caucasian or black models. Thus stimulus brightness was not the basis of differential response of the infants.

Carpenter then hypothesized that the turning away from the mother's face may have been due to the fact that although the mother's face was more familiar than either of the facial models that the stationary experimental setup meant that the *familiar face* was presented in an *unfamiliar setting*. She hypothesized that the turning away from the mother rather than from the model could be looked upon as visual withdrawal from something that seemed incongruous to the infant. If this were true, one would expect the infants to turn away less and less the more closely the experimental condition conformed to the usual setting in which the mother's face was seen.

To test this proposition she examined infants from the age of two weeks through seven weeks and measured their responses to the following situations: the mother's face alone, the mother's face plus the mother's voice, the mother's face with a stranger's voice, and a stranger's face with the mother's voice. By as early as two weeks of age the infants discriminated well between all

four of these situations. They made the most discrimination between the mother's face and a stranger's face. Infants looked for longer periods of time at the mother's face than they did the stranger's face regardless of whose voice was combined with the face. Each face was looked at longer if it was accompanied by a voice, but the mother's face without voice attracted much more attention than the stranger's face did with either a strange voice or the mother's voice. The infants turned away most when the faces and voices were mismatched. Thus, this group of infants was capable of detecting differences between two live female faces and two live voices during the very earliest weeks of life.

Since the infants turned away more when the face had a mismatched voice, this suggested that voices were also used by the infants as a discriminating cue. This further suggests that associations between a familiar face and a familiar voice have already been learned by the earliest weeks of life.

In summary, Carpenter's studies indicate that babies in the earliest weeks of life pay more attention to a mother's stationary face than to a live stranger's stationary face. They pay less attention to a mother's stationary face than to an artificial face. When a more familiar situation is created by combining a voice with a face, the infants looked even longer when the mother's face was combined with the mother's voice. But they turned away from the most unfamiliar situation: when the mother's voice was combined with a stranger's face. This suggests that from the earliest weeks of life the sensory inputs a child receives undergo a process of multiple categorizations. Moreover, infants at this very early age may be able to respond to more than just *immediate* sensory events. Carpenter's findings seem to indicate that they are also able to screen environmental input with reference to information stored from everyday experience and that more than one category may be used in classifying such information. That is, the infants may discriminate between inanimate and animate objects, discriminate between auditory and visual cues and so forth.

This view is supported by the work of investigators such as Freedman[40] and Wolff.[127] They have shown that the infant smiles from the time of birth when there does not appear to be any external stimulus which gives rise to the smile. However the onset of social smiling is more closely related to the age taken from the point of conception than the age taken from the point of birth. This suggests that smiling is innate and that a maturational factor is involved. In systematic studies Wolff found that smiling could be elicited by a variety of noises by the first week of life. During the third week of life the first clear indication of a social smile appears when a human voice is the best elicitor. In the fourth week, the best elicitor is not an auditory stimulus, but a visual one—that of eye to eye contact.

Finally, Rudolf Schaffer's studies of newborn's sleeping and eating habits seem to reveal endogenous patterns governing these aspects of behavior.[102] Studies of the sleep patterns of infants indicate two essential characteristics: spontaneity and periodicity. The responses from a newborn infant can not be explained in terms of environmental stimuli alone. Spontaneous changes that take place tend to occur in definite rhythm. The sleep/wake cycles of infants are of much shorter duration than those of adults. Kleitman and others[56] have demonstrated that within the first year of life a shift occurs in the distribution of sleeping and waking towards the diurnal pattern of the adult. However in infants with demonstrable injury to the CNS, the cyclical nature of this activity may be impaired or entirely absent. This is an indication that endogenous regulating devices exist within the central nervous system, even in the very young infant, and that these regulating devices can be disrupted by early injury to the CNS.

The characteristics of spontaneity and periodicity are also evident in the infant's sucking behavior.[102] Sucking is not just a reflex action to a certain type of stimulus. It regularly occurs spontaneously, particularly in certain types of arousal states. On the other hand it may be impossible to elicit sucking at all, even with contact with the nipple. Sucking responses in infants show the characteristics of a high frequency rhythm, being organized on a burst/pause pattern. The number of sucks per burst range from about five to twenty, and periods between the bursts vary between four and fifteen seconds. There is a definite pattern underlying this response cycle that is primarily regulated by endogenous mechanisms. And, just as for the sleep/wake cycle, it has been demonstrated that in some infants with CNS injury the burst/pause rhythm of sucking shows marked irregularity.[102]

In summary, the research just outlined indicates that the somatic matrix of the newborn child has a degree of complexity, organization, and endogenous regulation that is only now being appreciated and that has yet to be fully elucidated.

Individual Differences in Constitutional Factors

Given that the newborn infant comes into the world as a complex organization, are the "constitutional givens" for each separate child the same or are there individual differences in these capabilities? Recent research provides evidence that in fact not only are newborns capable individuals from the moment of birth, but that there are great differences in capabilities between individual children.

The studies of Rudolph Schaffer, mentioned earlier in connection with the sucking behavior of infants, indicated marked individual differences in the burst/pause patterns of infants. These individual differences were also found to have consistency over a short term period of time.[102] Korner[59, 60] has also studied the mouthing behavior of newborn infants ranging in age from forty-five to eighty-eight hours of birth. Through the use of videotapes Korner demonstrated marked degrees of individual differences in the frequencies of mouthing and sucking behavior and hand/face and hand/mouth contact between newborn infants. She also looked at startle behavior of the infants during sleep, a behavior that was common to all of the newborns. Again there were major individual differences in the pattern of startle response between these infants. Some infants demonstrated long intervals between startle responses while others would startle several times in rapid succession.

Bridger and Birns[16] have found very consistent individual differences in the heart rate changes in response to babies being touched and in the infants' responses to various attempts at being pacified following stressful stimuli. In their studies of two- to five-day old babies they found very stable individual differences in cardiac responses to tactile stimulation. Moreover, when they rank-ordered the babies in terms of their behavioral responses to a standard stimulus, consistent individual differences in the intensity of the response of the babies were observed.

A large literature on infant conditioning has also arisen in the last several years. Investigators such as Lipsitt[63] and Brackbill and Fitzgerald[15] have emphasized that the normal human infant shows an exceptional ability for differential respondent conditioning and discrimination learning. Marked individual differences between infants have been found on almost all measures of conditioning that have been employed.[77]

The NIMH study[25] on twins provides dramatic evidence that even genetically identical monozygotic twins may be born with very different constitutional capabilities. Differences in such areas as: ability to attend, to remain calm, and to adapt physiologically were large between the genetically identical monozygotic twins. Eight sets of monozygotic and two sets of dizygotic twins were followed from the time of diagnosis of twin pregnancy to the age of five years to assess the different levels of functioning. Of interest in the present discussion is the assessment of the congenital endowment of the twins during the first week of life. A rating scale was devised called the First Week Evaluation Scale (FES) which consists of six variables that can be rated on a five point scale with one indicating very poor functioning and five indicating excellent functioning. The six variables rated on the FES include: general health, attention, vigor, physiological function and adaptation, calmness, and neurological performance. In the NIMH study of twins the mean FES score for the twins was twenty-two, with a range from a low of eighteen to a high of thirty. The mean intra-pair difference between the twins in FES scores was six. This is a strong indication of *nongenetic* determinants of very early *congential differences* in constitutional endowments since these were all genetically identical individuals. These ratings of the infants agreed quite strongly with the type of ratings used by Thomas[112] which will be described next.

would be conceptualized as a formal characteristic of a child's behavior that is present with a variety of contents of behavior. Thomas and his colleagues have used the word "temperament" to describe these formal characteristics. Thomas[112] recorded observations in the first months of life of a selected group of children in New York. Half of the infants were less than two and a half months of age at the time that they were studied. From their parental reports they were able to isolate nine temperamental characteristics. These were labeled as follows:

1. Activity level—High, Medium, Low
2. Rhythmicity—Regular, Variable, Irregular
3. Approach-Withdrawal—Approach, Variable, Withdrawal
4. Adaptability—Adaptive, Variable, Nonadaptive
5. Threshold of Responsiveness—High, Medium, Low
6. Intensity of Reaction—Intense, Variable, Mild
7. Quality of Mood—Positive, Variable, Negative
8. Distractibility—Yes (Distractible), Variable, No (Nondistractible)
9. Attention Span and Persistence—Yes (Persistent), Variable, No (Nonpersistent)

The longitudinal stability of the temperamental characteristics of these children has been demonstrated up to at least the age of five years.

In summary, the research reviewed in these first sections indicates that the newborn human infant comes into the world with many capacities as well as with certain individual biases in the way that it will use these capacities to interact with his environment.

The New York Longitudinal Study

The New York Longitudinal Study of Thomas, Chess, and their colleagues[112] is probably the best known study of individual differences in children and their relationship to later abnormal and normal behavior. These investigators proposed a distinction between the *content* of behavior and the *formal characteristics* of a behavior. The contents of behavior are the "what" of the behavior. These include such behaviors as crying, playing, exploring, and many others. However, the formal characteristics of the behaviors are the "how" of the behaviors. That is, a child may *persist* in crying despite attempts to pacify him and persist in playing and exploring. Persistence in this instance

Individual Differences in the Constitutional Matrix in Children— Possible Sources

Given that the research just summarized (and other studies not mentioned here) has demonstrated the variety of individual behavioral and physiological differences between infants at a very early age, what can be considered the source of these individual differences? These have been nicely summarized by Berger and Passingham[8] into four possible areas: (1) nonheritable prenatal and postnatal factors, (2) possible differences in rates of brain growth, (3) sex-linked factors, and (4) genetic factors.

1. PRE- AND POSTNATAL FACTORS

Children in utero and in the early stages of life are constantly exposed to a variety of somatic stimuli which may produce varying degrees of change. There are major methodological problems when one attempts to do research on prenatal and postnatal determinants of differences in characteristics of children.[52] However, among the various factors that seem to be known to place the fetus at risk include: parity of the mother, age of the mother, socioeconomic status, ethnic group membership, physique, cigarette smoking, prenatal and postnatal infections of the central nervous system, nutritional state of the mother, drugs given to the mother during pregnancy, interuterine hypoxia and low birth weight.[8, 11, 82]

Since the newborn infant has such a degree of structural and behavior complexity and since our methods for assessing the structural and functional integrity of the young infant are so relatively crude, we can not be more specific about all of the factors that may promote the individual differences which are already present in the neonatal period. It is obvious that there are also certain influences that may be operating that have escaped detection up to now.

2. DIFFERENCES IN RATES OF BRAIN GROWTH

Dobbing and Sands[34] have presented evidence that two major growth spurts take place during the time of gestation and early infancy. The first spurt takes place in the fifteenth to twentieth week of pregnancy and the second growth spurt begins in the twenty-fifth week of pregnancy and lasts well into the second year after birth. When one considers the extent of variability of such measurements as head circumference for the same chronological age, it seems reasonable to hypothesize that the rate of brain growth is not uniform for all individuals. Rather it is much more likely that different central nervous system subsystems develop at different rates in different individuals. Moreover, it is likely that individual differences observed in neonates and in infancy are to some degree a function of this differential rate of brain growth.

3. SEX DIFFERENCES

Theories of child development have paid little attention to sex differences, but recent research evidence indicates that the physical and physiological consequences of a child's sex are evident at birth and throughout the life span. Hutt[51] has pointed out that there are three related characteristics which seem to be inherent in development of males. First, males are more vulnerable and more at risk for a variety of disorders. Second, males are characterized by a greater phenotypic variability. Third, despite the fact that sexual differentiation occurs earlier in males, males are slower in their development.

In considering her first point, it is notable that the ratio of male to female births is about 1.25 to 1 and more male than female fetuses are aborted. Not only are male infants more susceptible to perinatal and postnatal complications, but it seems that throughout their life span males are more at risk for the occurrence of most developmental disorders such as childhood psychosis, learning disabilities, language retardation, mental retardation, and behavioral disturbances.

The greater phenotypic variability of males means that characters which are distributed continuously throughout the population occur more commonly in males at the extreme ends. For example, both very high and very low IQs are more frequently found among men, although the average male/female intelligence difference is negligible.

The fact that males are generally slower in their development means that girls tend to be physically more mature than boys even though boys are generally larger and stronger. The greater maturity of girls is on the order of several weeks at birth, as much as one year by the time that both sexes enter school, and two years by the time of puberty.[86]

On a developmental level girls sit, crawl, and walk at an earlier age; they acquire language earlier and develop proficiency in intellectual skills before boys. It is felt that this accelerated development in girls is under the control of female hormones. Hutt[51] argues that if boys do have longer periods of development that means that "periods of risk" or "critical periods" are also extended in males. This would allow stress influences of all types a longer time to operate in males. Rutter has shown that there are in fact major sex differences in response to family stress.[88] In an epidemiologic study using a "high risk population" defined in terms of children having at least one parent with a mental illness, Rutter[90] found that these children in families with one mentally ill parent showed more behavioral disturbances than a control group of children. Three variables seemed to be related to which children in this high risk group became behaviorally deviant and which did not. These included: separation experiences, temperamental attributes, and the sex of the child. For the purpose of our present discussion only the sex differences will be considered here.

Boys in this high risk group were found to be much more susceptible to the effects of family discord created in the families of mentally ill parents than were girls. This sex difference applied whether or not the children were raised in broken or unbroken homes as long as discord was present. When stresses associated with short term admissions into foster care were examined in a similar study the same sex difference was found to apply. That is, more boys than girls were found to become behaviorally deviant due to the stress of a short term admission into foster care. These short term admissions were often a result of family discord. Rutter is quick to point out, though, that other studies have shown that not all psychological stresses are associated with greater vulnerability in males. Girls seem to be just as likely as boys to suffer from the effects of long term institutional care.[128, 132]

Another high risk population for psychiatric disorder, children with organic brain pathology, were studied in a similar epidemiologic investigation on the Isle of Wight.[93] Girls were just as likely as boys to suffer psychologic disorder in this high risk population.

A Swedish study by Bergman,[9] who investigated both boys and girls between the ages of ten and thirteen years who had missed long periods of school due to illness or who had experienced some family discord, also revealed major sex differences. In this longitudinal study of the intellectual performance of over a thousand children the psychological stresses just mentioned depressed the boys intellectual skills much more than those of the girls, particularly nonverbal skills. Girls experiencing the same stresses seemed to remain relatively unimpaired.

Hutt's studies[51] of 200 nursery school children have shown that from a very early age boys and girls began to develop different life styles. The boys were found to be more energetic, more exploratory, and more "thing oriented." Girls were found to be more affiliative, and "person oriented." They were also more easily inhibited by novelty or uncertainty. Boys were much more aggressive, physically and verbally, than girls and they also elicited aggression more frequently.

Some studies have suggested that most of these features of early sex differences are under the control of the male hormone. Studies of genetic females who have been exposed to androgens in utero reveal that they develop tomboyish behavior; that is, showing a preference for physical activities and boys' toys while having little interest in child care or in marriage.[69]

Boys who are exposed to excess androgen in utero are found to be even more aggressive than their brothers who did not experience such hormonal exposure. Conversely, genetic males who become phenotypic females due to ineffectiveness or absence of sex hormones show predominantly female interests, and boys who had been exposed in utero to female hormones show reduced levels of aggression, more characteristic of female behavior. These data indicate that there are certain sex differences in predisposition, sensory capacity, and behavior which to some degree are under a measure of genetic control.

However, to a large extent, males and females develop different life styles because of the reinforcement they receive for these various differences that occur early in their lives. Thus fathers are likely to reinforce aggression in boys (who are already predisposed to be more aggressive) and to not reinforce aggressive behavior in girls (who are already inclined to be less aggressive). Similarly, doll play and other "feminine type" behavior would not be likely to receive reinforcement in a male child, but would in a female child. Evidence that such differential reinforcement occurs in the very earliest months of life is available. Moss, for example, studied newborn infants over a three-month period of life and their interaction with their mothers. Male newborn infants cried more and did less sleeping than female newborn infants, but what was most notable was that these behaviors had different effects on the mother depending on the sex of the infant.[73]

4. GENETIC FACTORS

While it is generally agreed that genetic differences to a great degree underlie the behavioral and physiological differences between individuals, genetic sources of behavioral differences between human beings has not been explored as extensively as they should be.[35]

Some indication of genetic control of sexual differences in behavior were mentioned previously. Some other important contributions in this area will be briefly reviewed here.

Freedman[40] studied social responses of infants to an adult using groups of twins who were seen at frequent intervals in the first year of life. Each twin's behavior was filmed separately and the films were scored separately by separate groups of raters using an infant behavior profile developed by Bayley. Freedman concluded that independent ratings demonstrated that identical twins were significantly more alike than fraternal twins in both quality and quantity of social behavior. These social behaviors included the development of a positive social orientation, including smiling and the emergence of fear of strangers. Identical twins are much more alike in: the time, the quality and quantity of smiling; vocalizing and attending to the mother and to the experimenter. Even with substantial differences in birth weight the identical twins were much more alike than the fraternal twins in these early social behaviors. Concordance in the timing and intensity of fear of strangers was noted in identical pairs while the appearance and the duration of fear of strangers varied markedly in fraternal pairs.

The Louisville Longitudinal Twin study has reported similar findings. Vandenberg[116] has shown that identical twins show fewer within pair differences in developmental status than do fraternal twins. The fluctuations in status on these various parameters also are under a large degree of genetic control so that if one member of a twin pair scores lower on one occasion than he did on a previous occasion, his twin is much more likely to show a similarly lowered score if they are identical than if they are fraternal twins.

The temperamental characteristics described by Thomas and his colleagues[112] have also been shown to have a substantial hereditary component. As part of the overall New York Longitudinal study eight pairs of twins including three monozygotic pairs and five dizygotic pairs and twenty-six pairs of sibs were studied.[95] At the time of analysis all of the children were at least two years of age. If any of the temperamental characteristics rated could be considered to have a largely genetic basis then the monozygotic pairs of twins should have been more alike than the dizygotic pairs, the dizygotic pairs would be no more alike than sibs, and no large difference should be found within monozygotic pairs. All of these conditions were met with most of the temperamental characteristics rated by Thomas and his colleagues. The strongest evidence for a genetic component was present for the temperamental characteristics of activity, approach-withdrawal, and adaptability. Intensity, threshold, and mood appeared to have a genetic basis in only one of the three years of analyses done. Regularity did not appear to be genetically determined by any of the analyses. Evidence for genetic influence was stronger in the first year for all of the temperamental characteristics than in either of the two subsequent years of study.

To say that these temperamental characteristics have a strong genetic component does not mean that they are unchangeable or immutable. Both the studies of Thomas and others have indicated that environmental influences do in fact modify these temperamental characteristics to a large degree.[83]

Individual Differences in the Constitutional Matrix of Children and Their Relationship to Differences in Behavior

The evidence reviewed in the previous three sections is consistent with the following:

1. Each individual child comes into the world as a complex organization with many capabilities and capacities.
2. There are large individual differences, right from the time of infancy, between children with regard to these capabilities and capacities.
3. There are many possible determinants for these individual differences.

This section will attempt to review the evidence concerning how enduring these individual differences in the constitutional makeup of children are and whether they in fact lead to large differences in behavior, both normal and abnormal. Finally, some consideration of the mechanisms by which these constitutional differences lead to differences in behavior will be considered.

The evidence that will be reviewed, in the authors opinion, indicates that constitutional differences in children are associated with the development of later problem behavior. Of more interest to the child psychiatrist is not the *association* between these constitutional differences and differences in behavior but in the *mechanism* by which individual differences may either *predispose* an individual child or *protect* an individual child from development of psychiatric disorder. A full exploration of these mechanisms requires further research, but the work reviewed here will indicate that at least several mechanisms may be operating.[83]

First, these individual differences in children probably lead to differences in their response to stressful situations and in the ability of a child to accommodate to the situations and overcome hazards. Secondly, temperamental attributes of a child will certainly play a role in shaping his life experience. Thirdly, the temperamental attributes of a child will determine the child's perception of his environment and influence what is an "effective" environment for them. And lastly, temperamental differences in children have as one of their main effects the structuring of how other people respond to them. That is, these individual differences may predispose children to develop psychiatric disorder, at least in part, because they lead people to treat the child differently than they treat other children.

With regard to the questions of how enduring the individual differences in the constitutional makeup of children are and their connection with later life behavior of the child, some information from the NIMH twin study mentioned previously is relevant.[25] The First Week Evaluation Scale (FES) would give a rating of thirty to a perfectly endowed newborn. As mentioned in the longitudinal study of ten sets of twins, the FES scores ranged from a high of thirty to a low of eighteen. In a follow-up study each of these children was re-evaluated at the age of three and one half years in a research nursery school. In the nursery school setting, observation and rating were made of the following items: the child's general behavior, his play, his relationship to his mother, his reaction to the teacher, and his reaction to strangers.

What emerged from these ratings was a picture of each child's general competence at age three and a half in the nursery school setting. When one looked back at the first week evaluation scale scores, it was found that the FES scores correlated highly with the child's competence in the nursery school setting. What was found was that those toddlers at age three and a half who in a nursery school setting had more thematic play, more mature speech, and more originality in their behavior were those with the highest scores on the FES. While those toddlers in the nursery school setting at age three and a half were more fearful and more distractible than were those with the lower scores.

As part of the follow-up study each child was also visited at home by a psychologist. In this home setting, psychological interview ratings were made of the following items: the child's attention, his speech, his originality, distractibility, social relatedness, and other aspects of social competence. These ratings in the home setting

correlated well with the measures in the nursery school setting.

As with the nursery school measures, those children on the home measures who emerged as the more competent and socially mature children were those with the highest FES scores.

Finally, the mothers of the children were given the Vineland Social Maturity Scale and the Childhood Personality Scale developed by Dibble and Cohen.[32] Both of these measures, the Vineland and the Childhood Personality Scale, had high correlations with measures obtained in the nursery school setting and with the psychological interview obtained in the home setting with the child.

The overall picture then, that emerges from these observations, is that there are characteristics, measurable in the first week of life, which are highly predictive of competence and social-emotional maturity at age three and one half. This is true whether the measures at three and a half are taken in the home setting, the school setting, or are based on parental reports.

With regard to stability of temperamental characteristics, Rutter has recently critically reviewed the Berkeley Growth Study and the New York Longitudinal Study.[89] He attempted to assess the evidence from these two studies as to how well we are able to predict a child's later psychological development from measures taken some time during infancy.

The Berkeley study is hampered in that it relies entirely on observations made during testing situations of the children. Different types of ratings were made at different ages. Before the age of three years, seven point bipolar scales were used which measure such factors as the child's response to persons, his activity level, the speed of his movements, his degree of responsiveness, the amount of positive behavior exhibited by the child, the child's excitability, and his mood. After the age of three years and before the age of nine years ratings were made of the child's friendliness, his cooperation, his attentiveness and his facility. Certain other ratings were made after the age of nine years in addition to those made between the ages of three and nine. The overall findings indicated that ratings made in infancy bore little relationship to ratings made in later childhood. However, ratings made when the child was four years of age or older showed greater stability over time. Only the rating of activity made in early infancy seemed to predict at all the behavior in later childhood.

Rutter's conclusion[89] was that the Berkeley

Growth Study offered no support for the hypothesis that one would reliably predict the social and emotional development of children at later ages based on ratings made in infancy. One other defect of the Berkeley Growth Study was that there were no systematic psychiatric evaluations made of the children. Thus, the possibility of meaningfully classifying the behavior disturbances shown by the children at later ages and of correlating them with the longitudinal data obtained earlier was eliminated.

The methodology of the New York Longitudinal Study eliminated some of the defects of the Berkeley Growth Study. The behavioral development of 136 children was followed from the earliest months of infancy onward and data have been analyzed up to the middle childhood period. The data were gathered prospectively at sequential age levels on the nature of each child's individual characteristics of functioning: in the home, in the school, and in standardized test situations. Measures of parental attitudes and child care practices and evaluations of special environmental events in the life of the child and the child's reactions to them were also obtained. Data collection was obtained by several means including: interviews with the parents and teachers, direct observation of the children; and psychological testing was done at the ages of three years, six years, and at sometime during the middle childhood period. Psychiatric evaluation was done of each child who presented with clinically significant symptomatology. Special testing and neurological evaluations were also done when they were needed. Reliability and validity of various measures were checked and found to be satisfactory. The earliest reports from the New York Study[113] emphasized the continuity in the behavioral development of the child over time. However later reports[93, 112] indicated that the correlations between ratings of the nine temperamental attributes made during the first year of life and those made of the same attributes at five years of life are negligible. Rutter[95] concludes that it is unlikely from the currently available findings of the New York Longitudinal Study that a strong relationship will be found between measures of temperament in later childhood and the ratings of temperament made in early infancy.

However, this conclusion applies only to predictions within the *normal* range of behavioral development. When one considers predictions of abnormal personality development and the development of psychiatric disorder, the story is somewhat different. Certain temperamental characteristics in infancy were significantly associated with the later development of behavioral disorders in children. No significant prediction could be made on the basis of the first year's ratings, but significant differences were apparent in the ratings made at the second year of life.

Forty-two of the 136 children developed a degree of behavioral disturbance significant enough to be brought to clinical psychiatric attention. Two types of analyses were undertaken to examine the relationship between temperamental characteristics and the development of behavior disorder. First, comparisons were made between the group of 42 children with clinically significant behavior disorders and the remainder of the 136 children in the group (who did not have clinically significant behavior disorders). This type of comparison enabled the investigators to tease out the temperamental differences between the two groups. The categories of temperament that seemed to predict the later development of behavioral disturbance were: low regularity, high intensity, and low adaptability.

A second and different type of analysis involved the isolation of temperamental patterns or clusters. This type of analysis revealed three groups of children with similar clusters of temperamental patterns. The names given to the children characterized by these temperamental clusters were: (1) "difficult children," (2) "easy children," and (3) "slow to warm up children."

Difficult children were characterized by the following temperamental pattern: irregularity of biological function, negative withdrawal responses to new stimuli, difficulty in adapting to change, frequent negative mood, and high intensity of reactions. Only 10 percent of the entire sample of the New York Longitudinal Study were categorized as difficult children. Yet 25 percent of the children who later developed behavior disorders had this temperamental cluster.

The temperamental pattern which characterized the easy child included: regularity, positive approach responses to new stimuli, ease in adaptability to changes, preponderance of positive mood, and mild to moderate intensity of reactions. The great majority of those labeled as easy children did not develop a behavior disorder, and they contributed only a small number of cases to those who developed a clinically significant behavior disorder.

The slow to warm up children early in life had appeared to be slow in adapting, showed low intensity of reaction, low activity level, and would initially withdraw from situations. They are quite different from the difficult children, however, in that their withdrawal from new situations is done quietly rather than loudly. They do not have the irregularity of functions, frequent negative mood, and intense reactions that the difficult children have.

In summary, this section briefly reviews the evidence that there are certain constitutional characteristics present from an early age which do seem to predispose children to the development of behavioral and psychiatric disorders in later life.

Mechanisms of Development

This next section will discuss the possible mechanisms by which behavior disorders develop as a result of these constitutional differences in children.

The first possibility to be considered is that these individual differences in children may lead to differences in their ability to accommodate to certain stressful situations and to overcome the hazards of everyday life.

A study by Graham, Rutter, and George[45] gives strong support to this possibility. Their study was designed to test whether the findings of the New York Longitudinal Study could be replicated on a different population of children. The population chosen was a population at "high risk" for the development of psychiatric disorder because one of the parents had a mental illness.[29, 90] The sample consisted of all of the families containing a child under the age of fifteen years living in the old London Borough of Camberwell in which one parent had been referred to a psychiatric clinic for some type of mental disorder. Children in these families with a mentally disordered parent were compared with a control group matched for age, sex, and school class neither of whose parents had a mental disorder. As expected, the children of the mentally ill parents did show more behavioral deviance than the control children.

For the purposes of the study in question only the children between the ages of three years and seven years, eleven months were considered. Temperamental characteristics were rated by the use of a standardized interview and were similar to those in the New York Longitudinal Study. Temperamental characteristics rated included: negative mood, low intensity, high intensity, high activity, low activity, low regularity, low malleability, low

fastidiousness, and withdrawal from people. It was found that children who developed a behavior disorder one year after the time they initially were evaluated were characterized in their temperamental pattern by high irregularity in their sleep and eating patterns, low malleability, and low fastidiousness. Comparing the mean temperamental characteristic scores for the psychiatrically disordered and normal groups at two points in time a year apart, shows that the child most likely to develop a behavior disorder is characterized by the following.

At the time of initial evaluation, the children who later developed behavior disorders showed more intensity of emotional expression and were more tolerant of dirt and messiness (i.e., they were low in fastidiousness). A year later, those who had developed a behavior disorder were the ones who at the beginning of the study were characterized as having significantly more negative mood and were considered to be less regular in their biological functions. The temperamental characteristics identified by Graham et al.[45] as being associated with the development of behavior disorder in this high risk population are similar to those obtained in a much different population by Thomas, Chess and Birch.[112] (The Thomas population was a middle-class professional group whereas the London population[45] was a predominantly working class group.)

The temperamental characteristics that predicted the later development of psychiatric disorder in the New York Longitudinal Study were low regularity, high intensity, and low adaptability. In the London study the temperamental characteristics that were mainly associated with the later development of behavior disorders were low regularity, low malleability and low fastidiousness. The London workers use of malleability is similar to the use of adaptability by the New York workers. (Thomas et al. did not assess the temperamental characteristic of fastidiousness.)[45, 112]

Graham et al.[45] then went on to discuss a number of possible explanations as to *why* these particular temperamental characteristics were associated with the later development of behavior disorder. Four mechanisms were considered as likely possibly causes. These four mechanisms were:

1. The possibility that disturbed parents may produce children with temperamental characteristics that predispose the children to the development of psychiatric disorder.
2. The possibility that certain temperamental characteristics may lead to psychiatric disorders in

the child, which psychiatric disorder in turn produces disturbed relationships in the family.

3. The possibility that certain temperamental characteristics and disturbed family relationships may act independently to produce a psychiatric disorder in the child.
4. The possibility that the temperamental characteristics themselves do not lead directly to psychiatric disorder in the child, but rather certain clusters of temperamental characteristics make the child more vulnerable to the adverse effects of certain environmental stresses, particularly discord in the family.

The possibility that psychiatrically disturbed parents produce children with temperamental characteristics that lead to psychiatric disorders was considered to be unlikely because the association between disturbed family relationships and temperamental characteristics was not very strong. One would have to hypothesize a much stronger relationship between the two to propose that the primary association is between some type of disturbed family relationship and development of certain types of temperamental characteristics in the child.

The second possibility was considered to be equally unlikely because the data indicated that the disturbed family relationships *preceded* the development of the behavior disorder in the child.

The third possibility, i.e., both disturbed family relationships and certain temperamental characteristics acted independently to produce psychiatric disorder was also considered to be unlikely because of the positive association between the temperamental characteristics and the disturbed family relationships. Thus, it was concluded that the fourth possibility was the most likely explanation. That is, that particular temperamental characteristics made an individual child more vulnerable to whatever adverse effects appeared in his environment, particularly those of family discord.

Although it is clear that certain temperamental characteristics may influence a particular child's threshold for stress, it is also likely that temperamental characteristics probably have a lot to do with shaping a child's life experiences. A child who is timid, passive, and withdraws from new situations is likely to have very different life experiences than the active, extroverted child, who will create a whole different universe of experiences for himself.[83]

The timid passive child may never find himself in many social situations which are commonly met by the active, outgoing, exploratory child. Thus his relationships with his peers and with other significant people in his environment are likely to be quite different, both in quantity and quality. To the extent that life experiences, peer relationships, and other human relationships play a role in the development of psychopathology in childhood, it can be seen then that this is another way in which temperamental characteristics may affect the development of psychopathology in children.

As a corollary to this it is likely that not only will the constitutional characteristics of the child shape his life experiences, but they will also determine to some extent the way the child perceives the world about him. Thus, a child's temperamental characteristics will influence what is an "effective" environment for him.[92]

When considering environmental influences on children, it is important to distinguish between what is an "objective" and what is an "effective" environment for the child. As is pointed out by Rutter and Sussenwein,[92] if intelligent, highly verbal parents keep talking to a child who is hard of hearing, they are providing a richly stimulating language environment from the "objective" point of view. However to the child who can not hear, the "effective" environment they are producing is a very poor and potentially harmful one. There is evidence that children not only differ in their threshold to sensory stimuli, but that these differences vary according to the stage of maturation. Thus these individual constitutional differences do play a role in determining what is an effective environment for the individual child and consequently help determine the impact of environmental influences of all types on the child.

However, it is the authors' feeling that the major mechanism by which temperamental characteristics exert their effect on the development of behavior disorders in children is in terms of the response that these temperamental characteristics *elicit* from significant others in the child's environment.

Child development and child psychiatric research for many years has tacitly assumed a unidirectional impact of parent-child interaction. It is only in recent years that parent-child interaction has been looked upon as a bi-directional phenomenon. Several different types of studies have shown that children do in fact have an important influence on their parents and that many of the behaviors of parents and significant others in the child's environment are not spontaneously emitted but are elicited by many of the child's own characteristics and behaviors. In two seminal papers, Bell[4, 5] has reinterpreted the literature on the "direction of effects" in studies of socialization of children. He began by noting that data from several classic studies do not fit with a "one way model" of parental determination of child behavior. Bell's own studies using a parent attitude scale have shown that scores on these scales were consistently found to be higher in mothers of children with congenital defects than in mothers of children without any such defects. The limitation in coping ability of the mothers associated with the congenital defect of their children could best explain the altered parental attitudes of these two groups of parents.

Levy[62] found that "maternal greeting" behavior, that is, the way nursing mothers responded to their babies was related more to the state of the infant when it was brought to the mother than to the mother's "maternal attitude." Yarrow[130] found that the behavior of a foster mother varied according to the behavior of the child that was assigned to her at different times. The most dramatic case was of extreme differences in maternal care shown by the same foster mother toward two infants of the same age and sex assigned to her at the same time. It was clear that certain individual characteristics of the two infants evoked very different behavior from the same mother which could not be explained on the basis of a "general maternal attitude" or general set of "maternal behaviors."

Bell then summarized the rather strong research evidence supporting the hypothesis that there are congenital determinants of such childhood traits and behaviors as: human assertiveness, sensorimotor capability, and sociability. Variations in these traits and behaviors are very likely to differentially affect parents in their response to individual children. Parents do not have fixed techniques for socializing children, but rather they have a repertoire of behaviors which they use to accomplish different objectives. Bell divides these into two major types: "upper limit control behaviors" and "lower limit control behaviors." Upper limit control behavior is used to reduce and redirect behavior of the child which exceeds parental standards. Lower limit behaviors are used to stimulate the child's behavior which is below parental standards. Thus Bell views parental control behavior as being homeostatic relative to the child's behavior and that parental behavior in all cases needs to be rated with reference to the stimulation of the child. Bell concludes that there is a good deal of evidence to believe that there are congenital contributors to child behaviors which activate different aspects of the social repertoire of parents, which effect a level of parental response within certain response hierarchies, and which differentially reinforce certain parental behaviors once they have been elicited.

Thus there are good reasons to believe that a child's constitutional characteristics are likely to be important factors in modifying the effects of his interactions with his parents and significant others in his environment.

However the most important question is not whether such characteristics *might* exert an influence on the behavior of significant others in the child's environment, but *do* actually do so and *are* they actually important in the etiology of childhood psychiatric disorder?

Evidence that they are important is provided most dramatically by the New York Longitudinal Study and also by the Graham, Rutter and George study mentioned previously. Thus in the London study certain temperamental characteristics in the children were associated with the development of psychiatric disorder. These characteristics were low regularity, low malleability, and low fastidiousness. However, these temperamental features did not lead *directly* to psychiatric disorder in the child, rather they seemed to make the child more vulnerable to the stress of discord within the family setting.

However it is important to note that the children with these adverse temperamental characteristics, those that were shown to be associated with behavior disorders, did not come from different types of families than those children without adverse temperamental characteristics. That is, they were no more likely to come from homes that were unhappy, homes that were full of discord, than other children. However, *within* these families which had great deal of disharmony, those children with the adverse temperamental characteristics were more likely to be singled out as the target of parental criticism. It was as if the parents took out their frustrations on these irregular, nonmalleable, difficult children who acted as the focus for their parents irritability.[83]

Similarly in the New York Longitudinal Study, it was the physiologically irregular, nonadaptive, intense child with predominance of negative mood who was the one most likely to develop a behavior disorder late in life. But these temperamental characteristics did not lead *directly* to the development of behavior disorder as there were many children with these temperamental characteristics who did not develop a clinically significant psychiatric problem.

Thomas and his colleagues in several publications[23, 24, 112, 113] have given numerous examples of children with similar temperamental characteristics from early infancy, one developing a behavior disturbance, the other not doing so. They have been able to tease out environmental aspects which combined with these temperamental characteristics to produce a behavioral disorder in one child while a child with the same temperamental characteristics exposed to a different environment did not develop any behavioral disorder.

Thus a key issue in the development of behavior disorders in the children with adverse temperamental characteristics is the attitude and practices of parents, teachers, and significant others in the child's environment. In the view of Thomas et al. one of the most important factors leading to normal development appeared to be the existence of a consonance or "goodness of fit" between the child's individual characteristics and the demands and expectations of both intra- and extra-familial environments.[112]

All of what has been said thus far in this chapter has been summarized nicely by Rutter.[85]

1. The infant and even the neonate is a complex, organized being who both reacts to the environment and acts on the environment. He is not the passive creature he was once thought to be.
2. There are many behavioral and physiological differences between babies even at birth. Human individuality is present from the outset.
3. To a very important extent they are shaped by genetic and other biological influences.
4. To some extent these individual differences persist as the children grow older, although of course, they are also modified to a considerable degree by the child's life experiences.
5. These individual differences help determine how people respond to the child.
6. To some extent the individual child's temperamental attributes determine what is an effective environment for him.
7. Differences in temperamental attributes will also determine to some extent what are a child's life experiences.
8. Finally, the child's adaptability, the ease with which he accommodates to changing circumstances and modifies his behavior in response to different needs will influence his susceptibility to stress.

Brain Damage and Brain Dysfunction as Etiologic Factors in the Psychiatric Disorders of Childhood

In beginning a discussion of brain damage and brain dysfunction as etiologic factors in the psychiatric disorders of childhood one must first consider the problem of terminology and of methodology.

When one critically reviews the literature concerning the relationship between "brain damage" and "brain dysfunction" and the development of behavior problems in childhood, it is quickly evident that there is a confusion in terminology. "Brain damage" in its literal sense should only be used to describe a condition in which there is definitely a *structural change* in the brain. "Brain dysfunction" should be used when there is an *abnormal functioning* of the brain (such as an abnormal electrical discharge). Abnormal functioning may occur with or without evidence of an abnormality of the organic brain structure. However these terms are often used interchangeably.[123]

Secondly, if one is to infer a causal relationship between brain damage and dysfunction and behavior disorder one is faced with the problem of measuring both brain damage or dysfunction and behavior disorder. However there is almost negligible recognition given in the literature to the methodological difficulties of such measurement. Currently there are four possible techniques to make a diagnosis of brain damage and/or dysfunction in common use: a history from the parents, review of medical records, physical and neurological examinations, and laboratory studies.

HISTORY FROM THE PARENTS

The history from the parents is the most used, yet least useful and most inaccurate technique. There are several reasons why this is so. First, the information given by the parents is often inaccurate. Authors such as Chess et al.[24] and Wenar[119] have shown that developmental histories are extremely unreliable. Most of the important details of pregnancy, delivery, and neonatal status are not recalled by mothers. For example, Minde and his colleagues found that when one used histories of the parents *only*, prenatal and perinatal factors seemed to be associated with hyperactivity in children. However, when they went back to the actual medical records, the association between the perinatal factors and the behavioral syndrome of hyperactivity disappeared.[68]

MEDICAL RECORDS

This would seem to indicate that the use of medical records would be an improvement over taking a history from the parents. However, when medical records are used, information in such records are seldom systematically recorded. Thus, the critical data necessary to make a positive diagnosis of brain damage are often missing. Moreover, we can not make a one-to-one relationship between a history of perinatal complications and actual damage to the brain, since we do not know that events which are *potentially* traumatic *actually* do lead to some type of brain damage in every case. And further, we do not know what percentage of those potentially traumatic events that *do* lead to actual brain damage, also lead to some type of behavioral abnormality in the child.

PHYSICAL AND NEUROLOGICAL EXAMINATIONS

The third set of major techniques used to diagnose brain damage in children is represented by the standard physical and neurological examinations. These examinations are very accurate in detecting major degrees of brain damage, where a lesion impinges on a nonsilent area of the brain and gives rise to specific signs (such as the Babinski reflex).[123] However, these "hard" signs are prevalent in only a minority of children with psychiatric problems. Thus the concept of equivocal or "soft" neurological signs has been advocated as evidence of "minor" or "minimal" brain damage in behaviorally disordered children. Unfortunately, most of this literature presents data collected by examinations which were not standardized and for which there are no normative values.[123]

Moreover, the term "soft neurological signs" has been used in at least two different ways: to describe signs which are "soft" with regard to the reliability of their being found and to describe signs which are "soft" with regard to their neurological significance.[93] In short, although children with psychiatric problems *may* often show soft neurological signs, the significance of these findings is not clear, and they certainly cannot be used as an indication of brain damage—minimal or major.

LABORATORY STUDIES

The fourth major technique currently used to diagnose brain damage in children is some form of laboratory test or battery of tests. The two most common tests seem to be the electroencephalogram and certain psychological tests.

Abnormalities in the EEG may be more common in children with psychiatric problems than in the general population, but in one controlled study by Werry et al.[125] abnormal EEGs were found more frequently in neurotic children than they were in hyperactive children—this despite the fact that the hyperactive child is supposed to be a "minimally brain damaged" child, while the neurotic child has a behavior disorder based on some internalized conflict. Moreover, studies that use the EEG generally do not point out that there is often a lack of agreement between readers of the EEG on both the criteria of abnormality and on the neurological significance of the abnormality.[123]

The situation is similar (but worse) when one looks at psychological tests as indicators of brain damage. Reviews by Graham and Berman,[44] Herbert,[50] Meyer,[66] and Yates[131] have clearly shown that the validity of using any psychological test or combination of tests to make a diagnosis of brain damage in children is unestablished. The reasons for this have been reviewed by Yule[93] and Herbert.[50]

First, the validation of the tests of brain damage in children have been faulty vis-a-vis their clinical application. They have been validated on their ability to differentiate between children with no brain damage and normal intelligence and children with brain damage and below normal intelligence. But in clinical practice they are used to try to determine the presence of brain damage in children without hard neurological abnormalities who present only with deviant behavior.

Secondly, even the standardization studies comparing the results between brain damaged children and children without brain damage have had to rely on a neurological diagnosis to delineate the brain damage group. When the neurological diagnosis has limited validity, then the results of the psychological tests will also tend to be ambiguous.

Lastly, the concept of a "psychological test of brain damage" implies both that brain damage leads to a uniform psychological picture in children, and that the psychological effects of brain damage are qualitatively different from those found in normal children. Both of these premises are false.

The current state of the art in making a diagnosis of brain damage or brain dysfunction in children has been nicely summarized by Werry.[123] He states:

The diagnosis of brain damage or brain dysfunction, unless gross, depends on a group of medical, historical and psychological measures most of which are of low or untested reliability, which discriminate poorly between normal and brain damaged populations, and which apparently measure a variety of unrelated functions instead of a homogenous variable "brain damage." Under the circumstances, the diagnosis of brain damage or dysfunction in the majority of children with behavior disorders is no more than an enlightened guess. [p. 83]

Finally, even when a diagnosis of brain damage can be firmly established in a child with a behavior disorder, there is generally no way of definitely proving, in an individual case, that it is a cause rather than a correlate of the behavior disorder.

Where then does that leave us with the concept of brain damage and brain dysfunction and their relationship to behavior disorders in children and adolescents? This is the problem that will be considered next in this chapter.

We will begin with a consideration of brain damage (i.e., an abnormality of the anatomical structure of the brain), and brain dysfunction (i.e., an abnormality of brain function) and their relationship to childhood behavior disorders. The questions that we will ask are the following:

1. Is there an increased prevalence rate of psychiatric disorder in children with brain damage and brain dysfunction?
2. Is there an increased prevalance rate of brain damage and brain dysfunction in children presenting with psychiatric disorders?
3. Is there a specific type of psychiatric disorder that occurs in children with brain damage or brain dysfunction?
4. Is there an association of psychiatric disorder with certain specific etiologic types of brain damage or brain dysfunction in children?
5. What are the mitigating factors that either predispose a child with brain damage or brain dysfunction to develop a psychiatric disorder or protect him from doing so?
6. What are the mechanisms for the development of psychiatric disorder in children with brain damage or brain dysfunction?

While this area requires much more in the way of careful research and many questions remain unanswered, the recent work of Rutter and his colleagues,[93] Shaffer,[105] and Werry[123] have done much to clarify the issues. Much of what follows is a summary of their work. As we attempt to answer these six questions we will try, wherever possible, to make a distinction between the role of brain damage versus brain dysfunction. Since the terms are so often confused in the literature a clear distinction will not always be possible.

Is There an Increased Prevalence Rate For Psychiatric Disorder in Children With Brain Damage?

Werry[123] has recently reviewed the literature in which a patient population of children with brain damage was selected and an attempt was made to determine the prevalence of psychiatric disorder in the selected population. He reviewed both retrospective and prospective studies in which the types of *both suspected* and *proven* brain damage included pre- and perinatal complications, prematurity, encephalitis, epilepsy, cerebral palsy, and head injury. His conclusion, after reviewing this massive literature, was that the better methodologically designed studies using properly matched control groups failed to show a significantly increased frequency of childhood psychiatric disorder in populations of children with brain damage. Most of the studies reviewed by Werry would more properly be considered as studies of children with brain dysfunction rather than actual damage.

Rutter has similarly reviewed the literature for cerebral palsy, epilepsy, and organic brain disorders other than cerebral palsy.[93] With regard to cerebral palsy, there is a very large literature on behavioral characteristics of cerebral palsied children, most of which result from anecdotal, uncontrolled studies, and thus no positive conclusions can be drawn regarding the prevalence or types of behavior disorders in this population. Likewise, Rutter points out that although there is a large literature on the behavioral and psychiatric disorders of epileptic children, the great majority of the studies are likewise unsystematic and do not allow for a definite conclusion that the rate of psychiatric disorder in epileptic children is significantly higher than the rate of psychiatric disorder in the general population of children. Finally, Rutter came to essentially the same conclusion when considering psychiatric consequences of organic brain diseases other than cerebral palsy. That is, that the rate of psychiatric disorder in these children compared with children in the general population is unknown.

Rutter and his colleagues then went on to provide us with a definitive answer to our first question by their extensive epidemiologic studies on the Isle of Wight. They selected as their population all children born between March 1, 1950 and August 31, 1960 who suffered from any type of "neuro-epileptic disorder" which was chronic, which was currently present at the time of their assessment of the child, and which was associated with a persistent or recurrent handicap. Cases were excluded in which a diagnosis of brain dysfunction had to be made on the basis of *only* soft signs or on the presence of some type of behavioral or cognitive abnormality, which may or may not have signified actual damage to the brain. Thus, theirs is a study of truly "brain damaged" children.

By a series of screening procedures, a number

of children were collected who might have possible neuro-epileptic disorders. Parents and teachers were sent questionnaires about these children and on the basis of all the information garnered from all of the selection procedures and from both of the questionnaires, Rutter and his colleagues decided whether to include each individual child in an intensive phase of the study. Valid and reliable means of assessing the neurological state of each of the children as well as the psychiatric state of each of the children were developed as part of the study and are described in detail.

Two hundred and sixty-two children were picked up during the screening phase of the study to be included in the intensive phase of the study. When all of the information was available and a final diagnosis was made, there were a total of 186 children with definite neuro-epileptic disorder. The diagnositic breakdown of this group was as follows: 64 had uncomplicated epilepsy; 40 had severe intellectual retardation; 35 had cerebral palsy; 20 had some other brain disorder; 19 had a lesion below the brain stem; 15 were blind; 14 were deaf; 9 had a developmental language disorder; and 2 had a spinal defect but no other associated neurologic problem. There was some overlap between these diagnostic groups.

The definition of psychiatric disorder used by Rutter and his colleagues was an operational one: "abnormality of behavior, emotions, or relationships which was sufficiently marked and sufficiently prolonged to cause handicap to the child himself and/or distress or disturbance in the family of community and which was continuing up to the time of the assessment."[93] Six main diagnostic categories of psychiatric disorder were used: neurotic, conduct, mixed-conduct and neurotic, the hyperkinetic syndrome, childhood psychosis, and other. Comparisons of the prevalence rate of psychiatric disorder were made between various groups of the Isle of Wight children. These groups included:

1. The general population—all 3,300 children who were ten and eleven years old at the time of study and were still living on the Isle of Wight. Only limited information was available on these children, including group achievement tests of verbal and nonverbal intelligence, teacher and parent behavior rating scales, and certain demographic information on the family such as social class and family size.

2. A random control group—A random control group of nine and ten year old children was selected for a more detailed comparison with the neuro-epileptic children. They were studied in the same intensive way as the neuro-epileptic children.

3. Neurologic disorders—The neuro-epileptic group was divided into four groups for comparison: (a) children with uncomplicated epilepsy, (b) children without epilepsy but who did have a definite structural anatomical abnormality which was above the level of the brain stem, (c) children with epilepsy who also had a definite anatomical lesion above the level of the brain stem, and (d) children who had a lesion below the level of the brain stem.

4. All blind and deaf children.

5. Children with a chronic physical disorder without neurological manifestations. These were children ten and eleven years old at the time of the study who had conditions such as asthma, diabetes, and heart disease. Extensive psychiatric study of this group was also performed.

6. Children with psychiatric disorder.

All children age ten and eleven years old living on the Isle of Wight at the time of the study in 1965 were also assessed for the presence of psychiatric disorder in the general population of children. A two-stage procedure for identifying psychiatric disorder in these groups was also performed similarly to that performed for the selection for the neuro-epileptic children. They were selected for intensive psychiatric study on the basis of high scores on a teacher and parent questionnaire, or because they belong to certain administrative groups, i.e., those who had received psychiatric help during the previous year. The intensive individual psychiatric examination of the groups included a psychiatric interview (of demonstrated relability and validity) with the child, an interview (of likewise demonstrated reliability and validity) with the parent, and the Rutter Teacher Rating Scale. Diagnosis of psychiatric disorder was an over-all clinical judgment based on all the information obtained.

Results of this very carefully controlled study indicate that the answer to our first question is a definite yes: 6.8 percent of the ten and eleven year old children living on the Isle of Wight were found to have a clinically significant psychiatric disorder. (When children not attending school because of significant mental retardation were excluded, this rate drops to 6.6 percent.)

Those children who had chronic physical disorders not involving the brain (such as asthma, diabetes, etc.) had a rate of psychiatric disorder of 11.6 percent. This is almost twice as high as the general population. Because of small numbers, reliable comparisons could not be made relating psychiatric diagnosis to a particular physical condition.

Psychiatric disorder was found in 16.6 percent of the blind children, 15.4 percent of the deaf children, 13.3 percent of children with lesions at or below the level of the brain stem. The evidence is quite clear that psychiatric disorder is significantly high in children with a variety of physical disorders that do *not* directly involve the brain.

What is even more striking in this study is the very high rate of psychiatric disorder occurring in children with definite brain disorders. This figure was 34.3 percent, a rate some five times as great as that in the general population and three times as great as those children with chronic physical disorders that do not involve abnormality of the brain structure. Children with uncomplicated epilepsy had a prevalence rate for psychiatric disorder of 28.6 percent while children with epilepsy who had definite abnormalities above the level of the brain stem had a rate of psychiatric disorder of 58.3 percent. Children who had lesions above the brain stem, but did not suffer from epileptic disorder, had a rate of 37.5 percent.

The major findings of this study relevant to our first question then are that there is definitely an increased prevalence of psychiatric disorder in children with demonstrable physical abnormality of the brain. And there is likewise a definitely increased prevalence of psychiatric disorder in children with at least one form of abnormal brain functioning without a demonstrable physical abnormality of the brain (uncomplicated epilepsy).

rotic disorders, conduct disorders, and children with special symptom reactions.

In considering this literature Werry concluded that when psychiatrically disturbed children are considered as a group, they *probably do* have increased frequency of soft neurological signs and EEG abnormalities, and *may* have an increased incidence of pre- and perinatal complications. However, as we have pointed out, the relationship between pre- and perinatal complications and actual damage to the brain is a tenuous one, and the relationship between brain damage or dysfunction and soft neurological signs and/or abnormal EEGs is even more tenuous.

A more direct answer to our second question again comes from the Isle of Wight Study of Rutter and his colleagues.[93] They found that less than 5 percent of the ten- and eleven-year-old children who had clinically significant psychiatric disorders also had detectable pathological disorders of the brain. The total prevalence on the island of children with pathological disorders of the brain was 6.4 per thousand. (This is a minimal figure since it does not include children with uncomplicated epilepsy, language delay, clumsiness, and other conditions which may be due to structural brain pathology but which cannot be picked up by our current techniques.) In any event, these figures do indicate that in a large scale, carefully controlled, epidemiologic study only a minority of children with clinically significant psychiatric problems have demonstrable evidence of brain damage. However, the figures also indicate that compared to the general population of children those with psychiatric disorder do have an increased prevalence rate for structural abnormality of the brain. Thus based on the best available data, the answer to both our first two questions seems to be an unqualified "yes."

Is There an Increased Prevalence Rate of Brain Damage or Brain Dysfunction in Children Presenting With Psychiatric Disorders?

Werry has also reviewed this voluminous literature in which children are selected on the basis of having some type of psychiatric disorder and an attempt is made to determine how many have some form of brain damage or dysfunction.[123] Werry's review covered studies of general psychiatric populations and populations of children with specific behavioral syndromes such as the hyperkinetic syndrome, childhood psychosis, neu-

Is There a Specific Type of Psychiatric Disorder That Occurs in Children With Brain Damage?

This question can be looked at in two ways— *first* by taking a population of brain damaged children and seeing if a specific type of psychiatric disorder is likely to result or if several specific types are more likely to result than others. Werry concluded, after reviewing the studies of psychiatric disorder in populations of brain damaged children, that when psychiatric disorder is associated with brain damage in children it can take *any* form.[123] The hyperkinetic syndrome—hyperactivity, distractibility, excitability, and impulsive behavior—which is often thought to be characteristic of brain damage in children[3] turns out to be one of the *least common* outcomes.[123]

The Isle of Wight Study[93] clearly shows that there is *no* specific behavior syndrome that occurs in children with known brain damage. Neurotic and antisocial disorders were the most common psychiatric disorders seen in children of the general population on the Isle of Wight. These were likewise the most common disorders seen in children with uncomplicated epilepsy and in children with lesions above the brain stem. One child of 111 in the general population psychiatrically disordered group was considered to have the hyperkinetic syndrome; one of 18 of the children with uncomplicated epilepsy, and 3 of the 16 with lesions above the brain stem had the hyperkinetic syndrome. The only child with infantile psychosis was in the group with lesions above the brain stem. Thus psychiatric diagnoses varied little among the psychiatrically disordered group with known brain damage compared to the larger group of psychiatrically disordered children in the general population. Rutter also looked at items of behavior that are often thought to be associated with brain damage such as restlessness, fidgetiness, poor concentration, irritability, and fighting. While both teachers and parents reported these symptoms higher in the brain disordered group and in the uncomplicated epileptic group than they did in the general population, they were *equally common* in children *without any neurologic abnormality* who had neurotic and antisocial behavior disorders. The same held true when these items of behavior were looked at based on the psychiatric interview with the child.

This same type of analysis was carried out for "motor behavior" items, "neurotic" items, "antisocial" behavior, "relationship" items, and "developmental and other" items of behavior. A summary of these analyses indicates that there were very few features of either behavior, emotions, or relationships which are absolutely characteristic of organic brain disorder. Thus the results of the best controlled study support the contention that there is *not* a specific type of psychiatric disorder that occurs in children with brain damage.

Secondly, this question can be looked at from a slightly different standpoint. When one asks if there are certain psychiatric conditions that are more likely to be associated with brain damage, the answer is a probable "yes," the clearest evidence being for infantile autism. A large number of autistic children have been shown to have clear evidence of brain damage, although no specific type of brain damage has been found. However, even when the majority of children have been found to have some type of organic dysfunction, there is a sizeable minority of cases where no evidence of damage to the central nervous system can be found.*

From Werry's review[123] it can be tentatively concluded that evidence suggestive of brain damage or brain dysfunction is more likely to be found in children with the hyperkinetic syndrome than in children with conduct disorders or neurotic problems. And children with conduct disorders are probably more likely to have such evidence than neurotic children. This last conclusion, however, is by no means definitely established since really proper comparative studies taking into account factors such as social class, family discord, etc., have not been done.

Finally, it should be noted that children with levels of intellectual retardation at the moderate level and below are likely to have evidence of organic brain dysfunction.[93]

Is There an Association of Psychiatric Disorder With Certain Specific Types of Brain Damage or Brain Dysfunction in Children?

Numerous attempts have been made to relate specific types of psychiatric disorder in children to specific etiological conditions producing brain damage or dysfunction. A number of these have been recently reviewed by Shaffer.[105] For example, in the area of chromosomal abnormalities, much has been written about the XYY syndrome and its association with antisocial behavior disorders. As recently pointed out by Kessler[55] the validity of this association is far from proven. Kessler has shown that the possible increased rate of institutionalization for XYY males is more likely due to their environmental and social backgrounds than to the presence of an extra Y chromosome. The extra Y chromosome cannot be considered a

---

* See references 22, 48, 58, 91, 105.

causal role for whatever behavioral problems they show because associated and environmental variables have not been controlled for.

Likewise there is abundant literature regarding the "characteristic personality" of Down's syndrome—children who are felt to be more musical, outgoing and friendly than other retarded children. A careful review of this literature suggests that this stereotype does not hold up under careful scrutiny.[87] The same can be said about the so-called "epileptic personality."[114]

While there are studies showing that certain children with metabolic disorders such as PKU and galactosemia may have high rates of psychiatric disorder if they are untreated, there is no evidence from comparative studies of children matched for chronological and mental age that there is any specific type of psychiatric disorder associated with these metabolic abnormalities.

In short, a review of what available evidence there is suggests that there is not an association of psychiatric disorder with certain specific etiological types of brain damage in children. What evidence there is is probably more related to the *site* of the damage than it is to the specific etiological agent causing the damage.

This then leads us to the next question.

What Are the Mitigating Factors That Either Predispose a Child With Brain Damage to Develop a Psychiatric Disorder or Protect Him from Doing So?

Although children with brain damage and brain dysfunction do seem to have a higher risk for the development of psychiatric disorder than children in the general population, not every brain damaged child develops a psychiatric disorder. Thus, there must be mitigating factors, other than the brain damage itself, which either predispose a child with brain damage to develop a psychiatric disorder or to protect him from doing so. The following factors have been considered to possibly be important in this regard: (1) the etiologic type of the brain lesion, (2) the site of the lesion in the brain, (3) the amount of damage to the brain, (4) the age of the child at the time of the injury

to the brain, (5) presence of associated intellectual retardation, (6) presence of associated abnormal physiological brain function, (7) the sex of the child, and (8) environmental variables.[93, 105, 123] We will consider each of these in turn.

ETIOLOGIC AGENT CAUSING THE BRAIN DAMAGE

As noted, there have been attempts to relate specific types of psychiatric disorder to specific etiological types of brain damage. The best available evidence suggests that specific etiological agents, including pre- and perinatal abnormalities, metabolic disease, infection, epilepsy, chronic metabolic abnormalities, and structural damage due to trauma do not give rise to specific types of psychiatric disorder. Moreover, there is no good evidence from systematic comparative studies to suggest that independent of other variables any one specific type of brain damage or brain dysfunction is more likely to lead to a psychiatric disorder than any other type.

SITE OF THE LESION IN THE BRAIN

There are studies in adults[64] showing that a psychiatric disorder occurs most commonly after trauma to the left temporal, left parietal, and either frontal areas of the brain. Apparently there are no comparable studies in children.[93] There does seem to be a good deal of evidence that psychiatric disorder does occur more commonly in children with a temporal lobe epilepsy.[1, 74, 76, 93] However, Shaffer[105] points out that one cannot conclude from these studies that it is the *actual locus* of the lesion that leads to the high frequency of concomitant behavior disorder. He feels that even in focal epilepsy in children the presence of a psychiatric disorder may relate more to a generalized disturbance of cortical activity rather than to the specific site of the lesion. Many authors, including Rimland,[81] Laufer and Denhoff,[61] and Eisenberg,[37] have presented theoretical reasons why the site of the lesion should influence whether or not a child develops a psychiatric disorder and possibly even what type of psychiatric disorder the child should develop (such as the hyperkinetic syndrome or infantile autism). However, this remains a theoretical question at the present time but does seem to be a fruitful area for investigative work.

EXTENT OF THE BRAIN DAMAGE

Theoretically it makes sense to presuppose that the development of a behavior disorder would be influenced by the extent of damage to the brain. Rutter[93] has reviewed this literature and points out that it is fairly well established in adults that following head injury psychiatric disorder is more likely to develop when the wound penetration and total amount of brain tissue destroyed are greater. However, there is apparently no comparable data available to make the same statement about the development of psychiatric disorder in children and its relationship to the amount of brain damage. This again would be a very fruitful area for research.

THE AGE OF THE CHILD AT THE TIME OF THE INJURY TO THE BRAIN

Considering the relation between the development of psychiatric disorder and the age at which brain injury occurs, two competing influences must be considered. The younger the child, the more immature the brain, and the younger the child, the more rapidly brain growth is occurring. Rutter has pointed out that organs are most susceptible to being damaged both when they are immature and when the growth is most rapid.[83, 93] However, the brain is also at its most plastic stage of development when it is immature and there is evidence that this plasticity of functional representation may mitigate to some degree the effects of damage to the brain at an early age. There is a rather large literature which suggests that the age at the time of injury does affect later disturbances of language development and of other forms of cognitive development.[93, 105] There is at least a suggestion from the work of Black et al.[12] that psychiatric disorders develop more commonly after head injury in children than they do in adults and the type of symptoms experienced are different in childhood than they are in adults.[105]

However, there is as yet no systematic study of the relationships between age at the time of brain injury and the subsequent development of psychiatric disorder comparable to those existing for cognitive deficits.[93]

THE PRESENCE OF ASSOCIATED INTELLECTUAL RETARDATION

Many epidemiological studies have shown that deviant behavior in children is considerably commoner in intellectually retarded children than in children of normal IQ.[94] In the Isle of Wight Study more than 25 percent of the children with an IQ below 70 were considered psychiatrically ill on the basis of parental questionnaires—three times the rating in the control group. On the basis of the teacher questionnaire more than 40 percent were considered to exhibit signs of psychiatric disorder. When severe intellectual retardation was concerned (i.e., child with IQ below 50) half of these children were felt to demonstrate psychiatric disorder compared to 6.6 percent in the general population.

Thus it is quite clear from the best available epidemiologic study on this topic and from other investigations that psychiatric disorder is significantly more common in children with an IQ of 70. The mechanisms of this relationship are not entirely clear and probably more than one mechanism is operating. Of interest to us at the present time is whether or not in brain damaged children psychiatric disorder is more common in children with IQ below 70 than IQ above 70; i.e., does the association of psychiatric disorder with low IQ hold up in populations of children with brain damage? The Isle of Wight Study again offers us a definite "yes" in answer to this question. As noted in the Isle of Wight Study 34 percent of the children with a neuro-epileptic condition were found to have a psychiatric disorder. This association held true after controlling for IQ, age, sex, and severity of the physical handicap. It was difficult to determine the presence of brain damage conclusively in the Isle of Wight Study as it is in all studies, and thus comparisons of the rate of psychiatric disorder in intellectually retarded children with and without brain damage are difficult. However, it was found that psychiatric disorders were more common in intellectually retarded children who had definite or possible neurological abnormalities than in retarded children without neurological abnormalities. Looked at the other way around, an IQ of 85 or less was more than twice as common in epileptic children who had a psychiatric disorder compared to epileptic children who were free of psychiatric disorder. In children with brain disorder low IQ was also strongly associated with psychiatric disorder. Eighty-three percent of those with psychiatric disorder had an IQ of 85 or less compared to only 40 percent of the brain disordered children who did not demonstrate psychiatric abnormality. Thus one can conclude that the association of psychiatric disorder in brain damaged children might be due to associated intellectual retardation in a significant number of cases.

Rutter[93] has pointed out that in adults psychiatric disorder occurs more commonly after a trauma to the head when epilepsy develops after the trauma.[64]

Also psychiatric disorder seems to occur more commonly after lesions to the temporal lobe where epileptic seizures develop as a result of that lesion.[10] Moreover, there are numerous reports of an improvement in psychiatric disorder following temporal lobectomy for an active temporal lobe focus.[27, 46] Rutter has also pointed out that among mentally retarded children, behavioral abnormalities are more frequent among those with epileptic seizures or other types of *active* brain disturbance than among children with a *loss* of brain function.[93] It is safe to conclude then that *active* brain malfunction causing an interfering effect upon the remaining intact nervous system is much more likely to lead to psychiatric disorder than a *loss* of brain function.

SEX OF THE CHILD

Psychiatric disorder in childhood seems to be commoner in boys than it is in girls, both from the study of child guidance clinic populations and from epidemiologic studies of total populations.[94]

The reasons for this excess of psychiatric disorder in males are probably multiple but are not known conclusively at this time. Therefore, it is interesting that in Rutter's epidemiologic study, psychiatric disorder in brain damaged children was as common in girls as it was in boys. Evidently, several factors must play a role in causing the greater prevalance of psychiatric disorder in boys. Whatever they are, however, this suggests that they are overcome by the process of damage to the brain.

What Are the Mechanisms for the Development of Psychiatric Disorder in Those Children With Brain Damage or Brain Dysfunction?

In considering the mechanisms by which brain damage or brain dysfunction may lead to psychiatric disorders, two broad classes will be considered: direct and indirect. We will examine whether the psychiatric disorder produced in brain damaged children is a direct result of damage to the brain or whether the brain damage interacts with environmental variables, such as: familial variables, academic failure, social attitudes of others to the child, distorted social perceptions of the child, and the effect of drugs.[93, 105, 123]

Is psychiatric disorder in children with brain damage due to a direct effect or an indirect effect of the CNS damage or dysfunction? As we have seen from the above discussion, brain damage per se does not lead to universal "brain damage behavioral syndrome" in children. We have also seen that there is no direct evidence that either the site of the lesion, the amount of brain damage, the etiological type of lesion, or the age of the child at the time of injury have been conclusively shown to be related to the prevalence or type of psychiatric disorder in children. This would indicate then that when psychiatric disorder does develop in a brain damaged child, other variables play a large role.

However, there are biologic factors which did seem to be more frequently associated with the development of psychiatric disorder in Rutter's study on the Isle of Wight. None of the children in the Isle of Wight Study, who had a strictly unilateral brain disorder, were found to have a psychiatric problem. Strabismus and language disorder were also significantly more frequent in those brain damaged children with a psychiatric disorder than in the brain damaged children without a psychiatric disorder. Nearly twice as many chlidren with a psychiatric disorder had epileptic seizures. This suggests that to some extent there are biological factors which play a role in the likelihood of development of psychiatric disorder in brain damaged children. But the authors feel that there is much greater evidence for a transactional effect between presence of brain damage and certain other factors which lead to the development of psychiatric disorder in children.

What are the factors which interact with brain damage in children to heighten the likelihood of development of psychiatric disorder? We will consider in order: familial variables, educational retardation, the social attitude of others, and distorted social perceptions of the child.

The familial variables to be considered include: psychiatric illness in family members and other family pathology, broken homes, social disadvantage, and family attitudes toward the handicap of the child.

In an early study, Grunberg[47] showed that epileptic children with a behavior disorder came from more deviant families than those without psychiatric problems. They compared fifty-three epileptic children with conduct disorders to fifty-three children without conduct disorders. Three broad categories of possible etiologic factors for the behavior disorders were considered: organic, genetic, and social. There were no significant differences between the two groups on any of the organic factors looked at. Thirty of the fifty-three children with conduct disorder had a family history of psychiatric disorder as opposed to sixteen in the group without a conduct disorder. A family history of psychopathy was the most significant finding. However, the greatest differences between the two groups were in the social and environmental factors, particularly in those factors having to do with "maternal attitude" and "breaks and changes" in the child's environment. Thirty-four mothers in the group of children with conduct disorder were felt to have a disturbed attitude toward the child, as opposed to ten in the nonconduct disorder group. A disturbed paternal attitude was found in seventeen of the fifty-three children with conduct disorder as opposed to six without. The conduct disorder group also came from families in which there was greater marital discord, greater number of breaks and changes in their environment, and from family settings in which the children were more likely to be deprived of normal social opportunities. The authors then went on to compare thirty-five of these epileptic children with conduct disorder to thirty-five nonepileptic children with the same type of behavior problem. They were able to find the same adverse social and environmental factors in both groups.

Likewise Harrington and Letemendia[49] showed that children with head injuries who had a psychiatric referral had greater family pathology than those who were not referred to a psychiatrist. They examined the records of children seen between the years of 1947 and 1955 at the Children's Department of the Maudsley Hospital. They looked for a history of head injury in this group. They then examined the records of children admitted after head injury to the emergency service of the University College London and the Hospital in Birmingham between the years 1946 and 1955. All of the children were then personally examined in this investigation and one parent of each was interviewed. There were thirty-one cases from the Maudsley Hospital population, a psychiatric clinic population and thirty-two from

the "surgical clinics" population. In looking at the psychiatric status of both groups at the time of follow-up, eighteen of the surgical clinic group were asymptomatic as opposed to none of the psychiatric clinic group. This would be expected since they were taken from a psychiatric clinic population. The psychiatric clinic group also showed more severe and varied psychiatric symptoms than did the surgical clinic group. Eighteen of the group in the psychiatric clinic population were felt to have come from disturbed families. Twelve were felt to have a moderate degree of home disturbance and in six there was a severe disturbance. In eight of these families there was a history of overt psychiatric disorder in one or both parents. In contrast, only ten of the surgical clinic group were felt to have any disturbance in family background, nine of a moderate degree, one of a severe degree. One or both parents were receiving psychiatric treatment in five out of the thirty-two families in the surgical clinic group.

Finally, the authors noted that if one used the presence and extent of a fracture, the duration of unconsciousness, and the severity of neurological sequelae as criteria of severity of head injury, then the children followed up from the surgical clinic had more severe head injuries. And if one assumed that the head injuries were the *major* factor producing subsequent psychiatric problems, one would expect that the surgical group would have shown an equal or greater amount of behavior disorders than the psychiatric clinic group. However, this was not found. The authors concluded that many of these psychiatric symptoms were not *directly* attributable to the head injury alone, but were products of other factors. As in the Grunberg and Pond study,[47] family background seemed to be the major factor, for both genetic and environmental reasons.

In Rutter's Isle of Wight Study the incidence of family pathology, such as maternal depression or "malaise," and family quarrels was the same in the families with brain damaged children as among children with other forms of physical handicap that did not involve the central nervous system. However, the rate of psychiatric disorder in children with damage to the central nervous system was considerably higher, so that family pathology can not solely account for the development of psychiatric disorder in these children. However, 39 percent of the epileptic children with a psychiatric problem had a mother who had had a "nervous breakdown." This was compared to only 12 percent of the children with epilepsy who had no psychiatric disorder. The incidence of maternal malaise was 67 percent in the psychiatrically disordered epileptic population versus 26 percent in the mothers of the epileptic population without a psychiatric problem. Both of these differences were statistically significant at the 5 percent level. It is known that children being raised in families with psychiatric disorder in the family or with high rates of family pathology and discord are at risk for the development of psychiatric problems.[90] It seems that brain damaged children growing up in such families are even more at risk, and this family pathology is one of the mechanisms by which the vulnerable brain damaged child develops a psychiatric problem.

However, broken homes were not significantly more common in epileptic children with a psychiatric problem than in epileptic children without a psychiatric problem. Finally, among the uncomplicated epileptic children, psychiatric problems were significantly less common in children whose fathers had a nonmanual occupation. The meaning of this association with social class is not easily interpretable. And no association between social class and psychiatric problems was found in the Isle of Wight Study in either the general population or in the group of children with neurological problems other than epilepsy. In fact, none of the social factors which were investigated in the Isle of Wight Study showed any association between psychiatric disorder among the brain damaged children with conditions other than epilepsy. The father's occupation, the family size, whether or not the mother worked outside the home, degree of overcrowding in the home, all were unrelated to the development of psychiatric problems in the brain damaged group.

Also in contrast to the group of children with uncomplicated epilepsy, there was no significant increase of psychiatric disorder in the mothers of the children with psychiatric disorder. However, again in contrast to the epileptic group, broken homes were significantly more common in the brain damaged children with psychiatric problems than brain damaged children without a psychiatric problem. Thus, certain familial and social factors have been found to be associated with the development of psychiatric problems in children with brain damage and brain dysfunction. This area requires much further research.

One familial variable, the family's attitude toward the handicap in the brain damaged child, is likely to play a role in development of psychiatric problems. Little evidence is available on this point, but it seems likely that prejudice in the parents against such disorders as epilepsy may lead to the treatment of the child as "deformed" in some way and lead to the development of psychiatric disorder. Assessing such attitudes is difficult and makes research in this area necessarily extremely complex.

The next variable to be considered is academic retardation. Many epidemiological studies have indicated that underachievement in all academic subjects is associated with behavioral disturbance in children.[84]

The type of academic retardation most associated with psychiatric disorder is reading retardation, but it does appear that underachievement in other academic subjects is also associated with behavioral disturbance. The behavioral disturbance is most likely to be a "conduct" disorder rather than an "emotional" disorder. However, there is a tendency toward an increased rate of all types of psychiatric disorder in children with reading retardation.

Is one of the mechanisms of behavior disorder occurring in brain damaged children also the presence of academic retardation? In the Isle of Wight Study on epileptic children, three times as many children with psychiatric disorders had specific reading retardation at least two years below the expected, on the basis of the child's age and IQ as compared with the epileptic children without psychiatric disorder. In the children with brain disorder and psychiatric disorder, three times as many (64 percent) had a severe degree of specific retardation compared to the group without psychiatric disorder. Thus it may be that in brain damaged children one of the mechanisms for development of behavior disorder may be through academic failure.

Some authors such as Cruickshank[28] feel that a contributing factor to the development of psychiatric disorder in brain damaged child is the social attitudes of others toward their handicap. While this seems plausible at first glance, hard evidence to support this view is lacking. While social rejection certainly may adversely affect the child's social and emotional adjustment, as a practical matter it is difficult to assess if the child is rejected *because* he demonstrates odd or abnormal behavior or because he shows some type of physical deformity. In the Isle of Wight Study, for example, children were much more likely to be rejected by others because they manifested a psychiatric problem rather than because they were physically handicapped in some way. Moreover, psychiatric disorder was much more common in children *with* demonstrable brain damage who were also deformed and disabled than in children *without* central nervous system injury who were deformed and disabled because of orthopedic or muscular handicaps.

A view that has more evidence to support it is that brain injury in some children leads the child to have a distortion in social perception. This distortion in social perception may then affect the child's pattern of social interactions, producing a psychiatric problem. One study by Gallagher[42] on retarded children, comparing those who were brain injured and those who were not brain injured, showed that the brain injured group demonstrated characteristics such as impulsive behavior and inability to defer gratification which generated negative feelings from the environment towards them. These negative feelings then led to deviant behavior on the part of the child.

Finally, Seidel et al.[104] considered a number of these variables together. They reported a detailed psychiatric study of all crippled children between the ages of five and fifteen years who were listed on the local authority lists of handicapped children in three boroughs in the city of London. All of the children had normal intelligence (defined as a tested IQ of 70 or more). Thirty-three of the children were found to have a neurological disorder above the level of the brain stem. They were compared to forty-two children who had a neurological disorder below the brain stem. There were no significant differences between the two groups in age, sex, social class, overcrowding in the home, and whether or not the child came from a broken home. The diagnosis of psychiatric disorder was made from interviews with teachers, teacher's questionnaires, interviews with the parents and interviews with the child. Based on all available information, 24 percent of the group with lesions above the brain stem showed a psychiatric disorder with substantial social impairment. Only 12 percent of the group with neurological disorder below the brain stem had a similar degree of psychiatric disorder. Types of psychiatric disorder in the two groups were similar. Thus, among crippled children of normal intelligence, psychiatric disorder was shown to be twice as common when the neurological condition involved disease or damage to the brain.

The two groups also differed in mean IQ and in reading achievement. The mean IQ of the brain damaged group was 90.7; the mean IQ of those with a peripheral lesion was 100.8. Fifty-two percent of the brain damaged group were found to be significantly backward in reading, as opposed to 15 percent of those with a peripheral lesion. This difference between the two groups with respect to reading disability held true even after the effects of IQ were parceled out. There was no association in this brain damaged group between IQ and social class.

The authors then looked at the following factors in relation to the presence of psychiatric disorder: the degree of physical handicap, cognitive factors and schooling, and psychosocial factors. Somewhat surprisingly, psychiatric disorder was not associated with severity of physical handicap. In fact, it occurred significantly less often in those with severe physical incapacity as judged from the parental interview. This latter finding was unexplainable in terms of age of the child, sex of the child, type of lesion, IQ, presence of reading disability, or social class. The authors hypothesize that this finding might be due to the fact that children with a severe physical handicap had adjusted better to the fact that they would not be able to participate normally in society, whereas those with a mild handicap might continue to strive to do so and be continually frustrated.

There was not a significant association between low IQ and the presence of psychiatric disorder. Likewise the psychiatric disorder was not associated significantly with the presence of severe reading difficulties.

It was in the psychosocial factors that the greatest differences were found between the psychiatrically disordered group and the nonpsychiatric group. Psychiatric disorder was significantly associated with: an overcrowded household, a broken home, coming from a family in which there was marital discord, and the presence of psychiatric disorder in the mother.

The authors concluded then that although the presence of brain damage clearly increased the risk of development of psychiatric disorder, the psychiatric disorder was not directly caused by the brain damage, but developed as a result of a combination of increased biological susceptibility and certain psychosocial factors. Those psychosocial factors which were important in the genesis of the psychiatric order in the brain damaged group are the same psychosocial factors important in the genesis of psychiatric disorder in nonhandicapped children.

SUMMARY

In this section we have attempted to review the association between brain damage and brain dysfunction and the development of psychiatric disorder in children. Particularly, we have attempted to answer six specific questions based on a critical review of the available literature. This review allows us to conclude that there is an increased prevalence rate of psychiatric disorder in children with brain damage and brain dysfunction. And likewise there does seem to be an increased prevalence rate of brain damage and brain dysfunction in children presenting with psychiatric disorders. However, there does not appear to be any specific type of psychiatric disorder that is uniquely and specifically associated with brain damage in children. Nor does there seem to be an association of psychiatric disorder with specific certain etiologic types of brain damage. Finally, we considered mitigating factors that predispose the child with brain damage or brain dysfunction to develop a psychiatric disorder and have considered some possible mechanisms for the development of psychiatric disorder in children with brain damage or brain dysfunction.

A Model for the Investigation of the Psychiatric Disorders of Childhood

In this section the authors will present a six stage model which has been found useful for studying the interactive effects of organic and environmental factors in the etiology, natural history, and treatment responses of the psychiatric disorders of childhood. In using this model an investigator begins with an index population of children with a defined clinical problem and carries out studies that can be grouped under six "stages" of investigation. These six stages are as follows:

1. *Clinical Description:* A careful clinical description of the behavior problem the child presents with is the starting point for investigative work in this model. Obtaining this requires detailed, systematic, yet flexible questioning of the parents; obtaining reliable information from the school; and performing a reliable and valid diagnostic interview with the child. It also requires taking into account age appropriateness of behaviors, sex of the child, race, social class, and other factors that may affect the clinical picture.

2. *Physical and Neurologic Factors:* A systematic physical and pediatric neurologic examination should be performed and the results recorded in a standardized fashion. Special attention should be given to the evaluation of neuro-developmental abnormalities. It is important to inquire systematically about events in the history suggesting possible CNS involvement.

3. *Laboratory Studies:* Included here are the results of all types of laboratory investigations: blood, urine, spinal fluid, EEG, neurophysiological, etc. Valid, reliable psychometric studies can also be considered as laboratory investigations in this context.

4. *Family Studies:* Included in this stage are two different types of investigations: (a) Family Illness Studies: studies of the prevalence and types of psychiatric disorders in the close relatives of a clinically defined index group of child patients, and (b) Family Interaction Studies: studies of the relationships and interactions occurring between the members of a family.

5. *Longitudinal Natural History Studies:* Prospective and retrospective follow-up studies of an index population of children to trace the course and outcome of their disorder help determine whether the original group formed a homogeneous diagnostic category. They also provide a standard against which to judge the effectiveness of various forms of treatment.

6. *Treatment Studies:* At our present level of knowledge, marked differences in response to adequate trials of the same treatment, such as between complete recovery and marked deterioration, can be considered as evidence that the original group of children did not form a homogeneous group. Thus differential treatment response can also be used to subdivide the original index population of patients.

APPLICATION OF THE MODEL TO THE
HYPERKINETIC SYNDROME

Clinical Description: The cardinal symptoms of the hyperkinetic syndrome seems to be those of hyperactivity, impulsivity, distractibility and excitability.[18] There are a number of associated symptoms that also frequently occur. These include: learning disabilities, antisocial behavior, and depression and low self-esteem.

In selecting a population of children who chronically manifest this symptom pattern both in the home and school settings, investigators surely will begin with a heterogeous group of children. Some attempts can be made at making the population more homogeneous by such steps as limiting index group to (a) white boys between six and nine years of age; (b) currently attending school; and (c) with a full scale IQ of 85 or above on the Wechsler Intelligence Scale for Children. The population remaining after application of these inclusion and exclusion criteria will still be a rather heterogeneous one. Thus various subgroups of the original population should be formed when studies in the other five stages of the model are carried out with this index population. Some possible subgroups based on constitutional-organic factors will be discussed under each stage of the model.

Physical and Neurological Findings: The physical examination is usually normal in hyperkinetic children. In a minority of children defects of vision or hearing may be picked up[109] as well as abnormalities of speech.

One group of investigators[117] has reported a high incidence of minor physical anomalies in hyperkinetic children such as: epicanthus, widely spaced eyes, curved fifth finger, adherent earlobes, etc. The findings were more consistent for boys than for girls. These authors have suggested that the same factors operating in the first week of pregnancy led to both the congenital anomalies and the hyperkinetic behavior.

In a study of seventy-six hyperkinetic boys, Rapoport[79] not only confirmed the increased incidence of minor physical anomalies, but in this population the presence of these anomalies was associated with: severity of hyperactivity; a history of hyperactivity in the father; a history of early obstetrical difficulty in the mother; and higher than normal mean plasma dopamine-β hydroxylase activity. These findings suggest that those hyperkinetic children with minor physical anomalies may form a distinct subgroup of the total population of hyperkinetic children and that the physical examination early in life may identify children who are "at risk" for developing the syndrome.

There is agreement that certain neurological signs are more frequent among hyperkinetic children.[125] However, most studies have methodological deficiencies such as absence of proper control groups and failure to use a reliable, standardized neurological examination.[103, 125] The most common findings are those minor neurological abnormalities usually described as "soft signs" in the neurological literature.[7, 107, 123] While there has been a tendency to infer brain pathology from these signs,[54, 67] the evidence for doing so is lacking.[93, 123]

Only one study has compared carefully matched hyperkinetic, neurotic, and normal groups of children using a standardized neurological examination of demonstrated reliability.[125] The hyperkinetic children did have an excess of minor neurologic abnormalities indicative of sensorimotor incoordination. However, the hyperkinetic group did not have an excess of major neurologic abnormalities, of EEG abnormalities, or histories suggestive of trauma to the brain. The source and significance of these minor neurologic abnormalities thus remains obscure.[93] Their value in the diagnosis of the hyperkinetic syndrome is questionable since only about one half of behaviorally defined hyperkinetic children have even "soft" neurologic signs.[67, 98] However, there is some evidence that those with such signs are distinguished from those with no such neurological signs by a greater likelihood of response to stimulant drug treatment,[67, 98] suggesting that this may be a meaningful subgroup.

Laboratory Studies: Laboratory findings are generally more reliable, precise, and reproducible than are clinical descriptions. If some measure could be found that was consistently associated with the hyperkinetic syndrome, it would permit a more refined classification and possible subdivision of the syndrome. Some relevant laboratory studies are summarized below.

Electroencephalographic and Neurophysiologic Studies: Electroencephalographic findings are quite variable. Studies have reported 35 to 50 percent of hyperkinetic children have abnormal EEGs[98, 123] with an increase in slow wave activity being the most common finding. There are no EEG abnormalities specific to the syndrome, and there is even some question whether hyperkinetic children have a greater number of EEG abnormalities than carefully matched normal and nonhyperkinetic emotionally disturbed children.[36, 78, 123]

Neurophysiologic studies have been limited in scope and number and have reached different conclusions. Laufer and Denhoff[61] found hyperkinetic children to have a significantly lower mean EEG photo-metrazol threshold than non-hyperkinetic emotionally disturbed controls. The threshold was raised to normal levels by amphetamine. Satterfield[99] found that hyperkinetic children had lower skin conductance levels, larger amplitude, and slower recoveries of evoked cortical responses than normal children. These measures together with high amplitude EEG and high energy in the lower frequency (0–8 Hz) band of the resting EEG also distinguished hyperkinetic children who responded best to stimulant drug treatment from those who obtained a poor response. These authors interpreted their results to suggest that those hyperkinetic children who respond best to stimulant drug treatment have low CNS arousal.[99] Other auditory evoked potential studies[17] and studies using electronic pupillography[57] have also suggested low CNS arousal in hyperkinetic children who respond best to stimulant medication. However, studies of alpha rhythms[106, 133] have suggested the opposite conclusion—that hyperkinetic children who respond best to stimulants have high CNS arousal. Differing patient populations and diagnostic criteria, and differing experimental stimulus conditions make the results of these studies difficult to compare.

At present there is no neurophysiologic parameter that can be said to reliably distinguish hyperkinetic from normal or other emotionally disturbed children nor among subgroups of hyperkinetic children. However, this appears to be a fruitful area for future research.

Metabolic, Biochemical, and Chromosomal Studies: Disorders of monoamine metabolism in hyperkinetic children have been proposed by several authors but experimental evidence to support such abnormalities is sparse. Dextroamphetamine is thought to be ten times as potent as its isomer levoamphetamine in inhibiting catecholamine uptake by norepinephrine terminals in the brain. The two isomers are of approximately equal potency in inhibiting catecholamine uptake by dopamine neurons.[108] Thus the differential effect of the two isomers on the behavior of hyperkinetic children[2] offers indirect evidence that in some hyperkinetic children the disorder is mediated by dopaminergic systems and in others by norepinephrinergic systems.

More direct studies of a possible metabolic abnormality have been limited. Wender et al.[122] failed to detect any differences in the metabolites of serotonin, norepinephrine or dopamine in the urine of children with "minimal brain dysfunction" compared to a group of normal children. The study population was very heterogeneous however. Wender[121] did find very low concentrations of serotonin in the blood platelets of three children with "minimal brain dysfunction," all of whom were from the same family. In the rest of the study population the platelet serotonin levels were normal or in the borderline range. Coleman[26] demonstrated low platelet serotonin concentrations in 88 percent of twenty-five children with the hyperkinetic syndrome. The two most hyperactive children in the group were studied in a research ward. Interestingly, the serotonin concentration rose toward the normal range and the hyperactivity of the children lessened during the hospital stay. When both children returned home, the serotonin values dropped to prehospitalization levels and hyperactivity increased. Urinary monoamine metabolites in both of these children remained within normal limits during their hospital stay.

Rapoport[80] in contrast did find an inverse relationship between the degree of hyperactive behavior and urinary norepinephrine excretion within a group of hyperkinetic boys, but the mean twenty-four-hour urinary catecholamine excretion did not differentiate the hyperkinetic group from a normal comparison group. In addition, there was an inverse relationship between response of the hyperactivity to dextroamphetamine and urinary norepinephrine levels.

All of these studies are suggestive of a possible disorder of monoamine metabolism in the hyperkinetic syndrome. However, urinary and platelet data only imperfectly reflect brain monamine metabolism. Since direct measurement of central nervous system monoamine metabolism is not a possibility, the measurement of monoamine levels and turnover in cerebrospinal fluid, as has been done in adults with affective disorders,[43] might offer a more fruitful approach. More rigorous diagnostic criteria and control of factors such as diet, stress, and adrenal steroid levels are called for in future studies.[120]

The only reported chromosome study of hyperkinetic children failed to find any evidence of sex chromsome aneuploidy or other chromosome abnormality.[118] In view of the evidence for a possible genetically determined subgroup of hyperkinetic children, chromosomal studies may bear repeating in families with multiple cases of the hyperkinetic syndrome. These "multiplex families" would seem to be the most likely population to study if one is to find any type of metabolic, biochemical, or chromosomal abnormality specific for the syndrome.

Familial-Genetic Studies: Two studies of biologic parents of hyperkinetic children have revealed increased prevalence rates for alcoholism, sociopathy, and hysteria.[20, 72] One of these studies also reported a high prevalence rate of these same psychiatric disorders in the biologic second-degree relatives of hyperkinetic children.[20] In both studies it was noted that the hyperkinetic syndrome also occurred more often in the biologic first and second degree relatives of hyperkinetic children than in the relatives of control children. Moreover, a significant number of these "grown up" hyperkinetic children were found to be psychiatrically ill as adults with alcoholism, sociopathy, and hysteria. These findings suggest that the three adult psychiatric disorders—alcoholism, sociopathy, and hysteria—bear some familial relationship to the hyperkinetic syndrome. They also suggest that the hyperkinetic syndrome may be a familial disorder passed from generation to generation, but they do not explain whether the mechanism of transmission is genetic or environmental.

Two recent studies of the *nonbiologic* relatives of *adopted* hyperkinetic children revealed no increased prevalence rates for psychiatric illness or the hyperkinetic syndrome.[19, 71] These data are strongly suggestive of a genetic component operating in the syndrome. Safer[96] has reported that 50 percent of full sibs of children with "minimal brain dysfunction" gave histories suggesting the presence of the hyperkinetic syndrome. This type of history was present in only 14 percent of half sibs. These data also suggest that genetic factors may be important in the syndrome.

Twin studies of the hyperkinetic syndrome have been limited. Lopez[65] found a 100 percent concordance rate for the hyperkinetic syndrome in four monozygotic (MZ) twin pairs, while only one of six dizygotic twin (DZ) pairs was concordant for the syndrome. However, sex differences between the MZ and DZ twin pairs cloud the interpretation of the data.[75]

A larger study of ninety-three sets of same sexed twins has been reported by Willerman[126] who used a parent rating scale as a measure of hyperactivity. The heritability estimate was 0.82 for the males 0.58 for the females and 0.77 for males and females combined, suggesting a substantial genetic component to activity level. Willerman then arbitrarily defined children with scores on the parent rating in the top 20 percent as "hyperactive." There were eight MZ and sixteen DZ twin pairs with activity scores in this range. The heritability estimate for this group was 0.71. These results, too, are consistent with the notion that genetic factors play an important role in the hyperkinetic syndrome.

The mechanism of the possible genetic transmission can only be hypothesized at present. A single gene autosomal transmission is unlikely due to the excess of males with the condition.[124] Sex-linked transmission is equally unlikely due to the high degree of apparent transmission from father to son.[20, 72] The high percentage of parents manifesting the syndrome all but rules out a simple recessive trait, while the skipping of generations makes simple dominant transmission unlikely unless one invokes "reduced penetrance." Morrison[70] used Slater's method of analysis of ancestral cases to attempt to differentiate between polygenic transmission and dominant transmission with reduced penetrance. His preliminary evidence favors polygenic transmission.

The preceding brief review summarizes some of the pertinent findings regarding organic-constitutional factors in the hyperkinetic syndrome. How helpful are these studies in determining possible etiologically different subgroups of the syndrome, in predicting natural history, and in helping to predict response to various forms of treatment?

Natural History of the Hyperkinetic Syndrome: A number of prospective and retrospective studies paint the following picture of the hyperkinetic child in adolescence. Hyperactivity per se seems to diminish with age but the children are still more restless, excitable, impulsive, and distractible than their peers. Attentional and concentration difficulties remain as major problems. Chronic, severe underachievement in school in almost all academic areas is a characteristic finding. Low self-esteem, poor self-image, depression, and a sense of failure are common. Antisocial behavior occurs in up to one quarter, and 10-15 percent have had actual police contact or court referral. There are no published prospective studies of hyperkinetic children followed into adulthood. However, retrospective studies and other data indicate that hyperkinetic children are at risk for the development of significant psychopathology in adulthood, including alcoholism, hysteria, antisocial personality, and possibly other syndromes.[19, 129]

The mechanism of the association between hyperkinesis in childhood and antisocial behavior in later life is unknown at present. Since the percentage of hyperkinetic children who develop significant antisocial symptomatology increases with the age of the children, it could be hypothesized that the antisocial behavior develops as a reaction to the primary symptoms that define the syndrome. Children who are unable to succeed in the academic setting, who are unable to develop satisfactory peer relationships, and who find rejection at home and at school are likely prospects to act out and rebel against the values of society.

However, the familial-genetic studies previously described which suggest a genetic relationship between sociopathy and hyperkinesis, support another hypothesis; that is, that "antisocial hyperkinetic" children form an etiologically distinct subgroup of the hyperkinetic syndrome. There are other lines of evidence that tend to support such a view. Recent research on waking autonomic functions and EEG patterns in sociopathic adults suggest that many have the same underlying neurophysiologic abnormality that has been discovered in hyperkinetic children: lower levels of basal resting physiological activation than age matched normals.[31]

One way of studying this possibilty is by dividing hyperkinetic children into a family history positive (FH+) group and a family history negative (FH−) group. If the "low central nervous system arousal" subgroup of hyperkinetic children discovered in neurophysiological testing were also found to be the FH+ group and could be shown on follow up to develop significant antisocial behavior, this would suggest that "antisocial hyperkinetic" children are a meaningful, etiologically distinct subgroup. It would also suggest that in this group, there may be a genetically transmitted neurophysiological abnormality that leads to hyperkinesis in childhood and sociopathy in adulthood.

There is also some suggestive biochemical evidence that among hyperkinetic children antisocial, aggressive behaviors may be mediated by dopamine while the symptoms of hyperactivity may be mediated by norepenephrine.[2]

This evidence tends to indicate a possible biochemical difference between "antisocial hyperkinetic children" and those without antisocial behavior.

Finally, some authors have found antisocial hyperkinetic children to be very resistant to the psychopharmacologic agents so successful with non-antisocial hyperkinetic children.[53] Thus there is evidence from neurophysiologic studies, from biochemical studies, and from drug treatment studies that antisocial hyperkinetic children may be a meaningful, etiologically distinct subgroup of the total population of children with this syndrome. The evidence also suggests that in this subgroup one of the main etiologic factors is some type of constitutional abnormality.

The evidence from the physical and neurologic studies indicating a distinct subgroup of hyperkinetic children identified by the presence of minor physical anomalies also suggests a constitutional basis for a certain subgroup of children with this syndrome. None of these children have been followed long enough to tell if they form a distinct subgroup at outcome. But it is noteworthy that there is also a suggestion that the minor physical anomalies may also be associated with a biochemical abnormality in the monoamine system, adding further evidence to the very strong likelihood that in some children with this disorder, an abnormality of monoamine metabolism is one of the major etiologic factors.

Treatment Studies: A complete discussion of the treatment of the hyperkinetic child is beyond the scope of this chapter and is discussed elsewhere in this work. For the purpose of this discussion we will consider only response to stimulant drug treatment.

It is a well-established fact that a significant percentage of behaviorally defined hyperkinetic children do have a positive, short-term dramatic response to central nervous system stimulant medication. What effect do organic-constitutional factors play in this drug response? In one study some 70 percent of behaviorally defined hyperkinetic children have shown a favorable response to methylphenidate, while approximately 20 percent deteriorated following stimulant treatment.[100] These investigators have shown that those children who are most likely to respond to stimulant treatment are neurophysiologically and neurologically different from those with a poor response, as previously reviewed.[100, 101] At the present level of knowledge it is reasonable to assume that these two groups of children may have different conditions with similar clinical pictures. If this is so, one could expect these two groups to differ in many other areas of the model.

For example, beginning with a population of children with a clinical picture of the hyperkinetic syndrome, we find that one group shows a positive response to stimulant medication while another group shows a negative response. When we compare these two groups, the "responders" and the "nonresponders," we find they differ in a number of other parameters. The responders show: laboratory evidence of low central nervous system arousal, more abnormal EEGs, and a greater number of minor abnormalities on neurological examination. Thus, those in this group begin to look as though they have their disorder on a neurodevelopmental basis. One might then go back and take a closer look at the clinical picture of the two groups using techniques such as cluster analysis to see if differences can be found in the behavioral picture. A family study of the two groups may yield different familial patterns of illness and follow-up studies should reveal a different natural history for the two groups if they do in fact have different disorders.

Likewise, with the same population of hyperkinetic children, one might divide up the group with the negative family history on a number of parameters in this model. We might compare the behavioral pictures of the two groups or look at a variety of laboratory measures. Since the family studies offer tentative evidence for a possible genetically determined subgroup of hyperkinetic children, it is reasonable to assume that one might find metabolic, biochemical, or chromosomal differences between the FH+ and the FH− groups.

Summary

In the concluding section of this chapter the authors have presented a six stage model they have found useful for studying the effect of organic-constitutional factors in the etiology, natural history, and treatment of psychiatric disorders of childhood. We have also applied this model to one specific psychiatric disorder, the hyperkinetic syndrome. We believe that our review indicates that the continued application of this model to the same index population leads to increasingly refined diagnostic criteria and ultimately to more homogeneous subgroups of the original index patient population. These homogeneous patient populations provide the best starting point for studies of etiology and treatment. The role of organic-constitutional factors (as well as dynamic factors, family relationships, and sociological factors) in the etiology of any condition is more easily elucidated when the patient population under study is as diagnostically "pure" as possible. Likewise, response to any treatment modality be it psychotherapy, pharmacotherapy, behavior therapy, or some other modality is best evaluated in a homogenous patient population.

REFERENCES

1. AIRD, R. B., and YAMAMOTO, T., "Behaviour Disorders of Childhood," *Revue d'Electroencephalographie et de Neurophysiologie Clinique, 21:*148, 1966.
2. ARNOLD, L., et al., "Levoamphetamine and Dextroamphetamine: Differential Effect on Aggression and Hyperkinesis in Children and Dogs," *American Journal of Psychiatry, 130:*165, 1973.
3. BAKWIN, H., "Cerebral Damage and Behaviour Disorders in Children," *Journal of Pediatrics, 34:*371, 1949.
4. BELL, R. Q., "Stimulus Control of Parent or Caretaker Behavior by Offspring," *Developmental Psychology, 4:*63, 1971.
5. ———, "A Reinterpretation of the Direction of Effects in Studies of Socialization," *Psychological Review, 75:*81, 1968.
6. BENDER, L., *Psychopathology of Children with Organic Brain Diseases*, Charles C Thomas, Springfield, Ill, 1959.
7. ———, *Psychopathology of Children with Organic Brain Disorders*, Charles C Thomas, Springfield, Ill., 1956.
8. BERGER, M., and PASSINGHAM, R. E., "Early Experience and Other Environmental Factors: An Overview," in Eysenck, H. J. (Ed.), *Handbook of Abnormal Psychology*, 2nd ed., pp. 604, Pitman Medical, London, 1973.
9. BERGMAN, L., cited in Hutt, (ref. 51).
10. BINGLEY, T., "Mental Symptoms in Temporal Lobe Epilepsy and Temporal Lobe Gliomas," *Acta Psychiatrica Scandinavica*, vol. 33, Suppl. 120, 1958.
11. BIRCH, H. G., "Health and Education of Socially Disadvantaged Children," *Developmental Medicine and Child Neurology, 10:*580, 1968.
12. BLACK, P., et al., "The Post-Traumatic Syndrome in Children," in Walker, A. E., Caveness, W. F., and Critchley, M. (Eds.), *The Late Effects of Head Injury*, Charles C Thomas, Springfield, Ill., 1969.
13. BLAU, A., "The Psychiatric Approach to Posttraumatic and Postencephalitic Syndromes," in McIntosh, R. (Ed.), *Neurology and Psychiatry in Childhood*, Proceedings of the Association for Research in Nervous and Mental Diseases, vol. 34, p. 404, Williams & Wilkins, Baltimore, 1954.
14. BOWER, et al., cited in Carpenter, (ref. 21).
15. BRACKBILL, Y., and FITZGERALD, H. E., "Development of the Sensory Analyzers During Infancy," in Lipsitt, L. P., and Reese, H. W. (Eds.), *Advances in Child Development and Behavior*, p. 173, Academic Press, New York, 1969.
16. BRIDGER, W. H., and BIRNS, B., "Experience and Temperament in Human Neonates," in Newton, R., and Levine, S. (Eds), *Early Experience and Behavior*, Charles C Thomas, Springfield, Ill., 1968.
17. CALLOWAY, E., Personal communication, 1973.
18. CANTWELL, D. P., *The Hyperactive Child: Diagnosis, Management, and Current Research*, Spectrum Publications, New York, 1975.
19. ———, "Genetic Studies of Hyperactive Children: Psychiatric Illness in Biologic and Adopting Parents," in Fieve, R., Rosenthal, D., and Brill, H. (Eds.), *Genetic Research in Psychiatry*, p. 273, Johns Hopkins University Press, Baltimore, Md., 1975.
20. ———, "Psychiatric Illness in Families of Hyperactive Children," *Archives of General Psychiatry, 27:*414, 1972.
21. CARPENTER, G., "Mother's Face and The Newborn," *New Scientist, 61:*742, 1974.
22. CHESS, S., KORN, S. J., and FERNANDEZ, B., *Psychiatric Disorders of Children with Rubella*, Butterworth, London, 1971.
23. CHESS, S., THOMAS, A., and BIRCH, H. G., "Behavior Problems Revisited: Findings of an Anterospective Study, in Chess, S., and Thomas, S. (Eds.), *Annual Progress in Child Psychiatry and Child Development*, p. 335, Brunner-Mazel, New York, 1968.
24. ———, et al., "Interaction of Temperament and Environment in the Production of Behavioral Disturbances in Children," *American Journal of Psychiatry, 120:*142, 1963.
25. COHEN, D. J., et al., "Personality Development in Twins: Competence in the Newborn and Preschool Periods," *Journal of the American Academy of Child Psychiatry, 11:*625, 1972.
26. COLEMAN, M., "Serotonin Concentrations in Whole Blood of Hyperactive Children," *Journal of Pediatrics, 78:*985, 1971.
27. CRANDALL, P. H., "Postoperative Management and Criteria for Evaluation," in Purpura, D. P., Penray, J. K., and Walter, R. D. (Eds.), *Advances in Neurology*, vol. 8, p. 265, Raven Press, New York, 1975.
28. CRUICKSHANK, W. M., and RICE, H. V., *Cerebral Palsy: Its Individual and Community Problems*, Syracuse University Press, Syracuse, N.Y., 1965.
29. CUNNINGHAM, L., et al. "Studies of Adoptees from Psychiatrically Disturbed Biological Parents: Psychiatric Conditions in Childhood and Adolescence," *British Journal of Psychiatry, 126:*534, 1975.
30. DE HIRSCH, K., "Early Language Development and Minimal Brain Dysfunction," *Annals of the New York Academy of Sciences, 205:*158, 1973.

31. DE LA PENA, A., "The Habitually Aggressive Individual," *Progress Report to the National Institute of Mental Health*, 1973.

32. DIBBLE, E., and COHEN, D. J., "Companion Instruments for Measuring Children's Competence and Parental Style," *Archieves of General Psychiatry*, 30:805, 1974.

33. DOBBING, J., "Vulnerable Periods in Developing Brain," in Davison, A. N., and Dobbing, J. (Eds.), *Applied Neurochemistry*, Blackwell, Oxford, 1968.

34. ———, and SANDS, J., "The Timing of Neuroloblast Multiplication in Developing Human Brain," *Nature, 226:* 639, 1970.

35. DOBZHANSKY, T., "On Types, Genotypes, and the Genetic Diversity in Populations," in Spuhler, J. N. (Ed.), *Genetic Diversity and Human Behavior*, Aldine, Chicago, 1967.

36. EEG-OLOFSSON, O., "The Development of the Electroencephalogram in Normal Children and Adolescents from the Age of 1 through 21 years," *Acta Paediatrica Scandinavica, 208,* 1970.

37. EISENBERG, L., "Psychiatric Implications of Brain Damage in Children," *Psychiatric Quarterly*, 31:72, 1957.

38. FANTZ, R. L., "Visual Perception and Experience in Early Infancy: A Look at the Hidden Side of Behavior Development," in Stevenson, R. W., Hess, E. H., and Rhinegold, H. L. (Eds.), *Early Behavior*, John Wiley, New York, 1967.

39. ———, and NEVIS, S., "Pattern Preferences and Perceptual-Cognitive Development in Early Infancy," *Merrill-Palmer Quarterly*, 13:77, 1967.

40. FREEDMAN, D., "Hereditary Control of Early Social Behaviour," in Foss, B. M. (Ed.), *Determinants in Infant Behaviour II.*, Methuen, London, 1965.

41. FRIEDLANDER, B. Z., "Receptive Language Development in Infancy: Issues and Problems," *Merrill-Palmer Quarterly*, 16:7, 1970.

42. GALLAGHER, J. J., *A Comparison of Birth Injured and Non-Birth-Injured Mentally Retarded Children on Several Psychological Variables*, Monographs of the Society for Research in Child Development, vol. 22, 1957.

43. GOODWIN, F., and BUNNEY, W., "A Psychobiological Approach to Affective Illness," *Psychiatric Annals*, 3:19, 1973.

44. GRAHAM, F. K., and BERMAN, P. W., "Current Status of Behavior Tests for Brain Damage in Infants and Preschool Children," *American Journal of Orthopsychiatry*, 31:713, 1961.

45. GRAHAM, P., RUTTER, M., and GEORGE, S., "Temperamental Characteristics as Predictors of Behavior Disorders in Children," *American Journal of Orthopsychiatry*, 43:328, 1973.

46. GRIFFITH, H., and DAVIDSON, M., "Long-Term Changes in Intellect and Behavior After Hemispherectomy," *Journal of Neurology, Neurosurgery and Psychiatry*, 29:571, 1966.

47. GRUNBERG, F., and POND, D. A., "Conduct Disorders in Epileptic Children," *Journal of Neurology, Neurosurgery and Psychiatry*, 20:65, 1957.

48. HACKNEY, I. M., et al., "Phenylketonuria, Mental Development, Behavior and Termination of Low Phenylalanine Diet," *Journal of Pediatrics*, 72:646, 1968.

49. HARRINGTON, J. A., and LETEMENDIA, F. J. J., "Persistent Psychiatric Disorders After Head Injuries in Children," *Journal of Mental Science, 104:*205, 1958.

50. HERBERT, M., "The Concept and Testing of Brain Damage in Children: A Review," *Journal of Child Psychology and Psychiatry*, 5:197, 1964.

51. HUTT, C., "Sex: What's the Difference?," *New Scientist, 62:*405, 1974.

52. JOFFE, J. M., *Prenatal Determinants of Behavior*, Pergamon, Oxford, 1969.

53. KATZ, S., et al., "Clinical Pharmacological Management of Hyperkinetic Children," *International Journal of Mental Health, 4:*157, 1975.

54. KENNARD, M., "Value of Equivocal Signs in Neurologic Diagnosis," *Neurology, 10:*753, 1960.

55. KESSLER, S., "Extra Chromosomes and Criminality," in Fieve, R. R., Rosenthal, D., and Brill, H. (Eds.), *Genetic Research in Psychiatry*, p. 65, Johns Hopkins University Press, Baltimore, 1975.

56. KLEITMAN, N., et al., cited in Schaffer, 1974; (ref. 102).

57. KNOPP, W., et al., "Predicting Amphetamine Response in Hyperkinetic Children by Electronic Pupilography," *Pharmakopsychiatrie, 6:*158, 1973.

58. KOLVIN, I., "Psychoses in Childhood—A Comparative Study," in Rutter, M. (Ed.), *Infantile Autism: Concepts, Characteristics and Treatment*, Churchill, London, 1971.

59. KORNER, A. F., "Neonatal Startles, Smiles, Erections, and Reflex Sucks as Related to State, Sex and Individuality," *Child Development, 40:*1039, 1969.

60. ———, CHUCK, B., and DONTCHOS, S., "Organismic Determinants of Spontaneous Oral Behavior in Neonates," *Child Development, 39:*1145, 1968.

61. LAUFER, M. W., and DENHOFF, E., "Hyperkinetic Behavior Syndrome in Children," *Journal of Pediatrics, 50:*463, 1957.

62. LEVY, D. M., *Behavioral Analysis: Analysis of Clinical Observations of Behavior as Applied to Mother-Newborn Relationships*, Charles C Thomas, Springfield, Ill., 1958.

63. LIPSITT, L. P., "Learning Capacities of the Human Infant," in Robinson, R. J. (Ed.), *Brain and Early Behaviour*, Academic Press, London, 1969.

64. LISHMAN, W. A., "Brain Damage in Relation to Psychiatric Disability After Head Injury," *British Journal of Psychiatry, 114:*373, 1968.

65. LOPEZ, R. E., "Hyperactivity in Twins," *Canadian Psychiatric Association Journal, 10:*421, 1965.

66. MEYER, V., "Critique of Psychological Approaches to Brain Damage," *Journal of Mental Science, 103:*80, 1957.

67. MILLICHAP, J., "Drugs in Management of Minimal Brain Dysfunction," *Annals of the New York Academy of Sciences, 205:*321, 1973.

68. MINDE, K., WEBB, G., and SYKES, D., "Studies on the Hyperactive Child VI: Prenatal and Paranatal Factors Associated with Hyperactivity," *Developmental Medicine and Child Neurology, 10:*355, 1968.

69. MONEY, J., and EHRHARDT, A., *Man and Woman, Boy and Girl*, Johns Hopkins University Press, Baltimore, 1973.

70. MORRISON, J. R., "Bilateral Inheritance as Evidence for Polygenicity in the Hyperactive Child Syndrome," *Journal of Nervous and Mental Disease, 158:*226, 1974.

71. ———, and STEWART, M. A., "The Psychiatric Status of the Legal Families of Adopted Hyperactive Children," *Archives of General Psychiatry*, 28:888, 1973.

72. ———, and STEWART, M. A., "A Family Study of the Hyperactive Child Syndrome," *Biological Psychiatry*, 3:189, 1971.

73. MOSS, H. A., "Sex, Age and State of Determinants of Mother-Infant Interaction," *Merrill-Palmer Quarterly*, 13:19, 1967.

74. NUFFIELD, E. J., "Neurophysiology and Behavour Disorders in Epileptic Children," *Journal of Mental Science, 107:*438, 1961.

75. OMENN, G. S., "Genetic Issues in the Syndrome of Minimal Brain Dysfunction," *Seminars in Psychiatry, 5:*5, 1973.

76. OUNSTED, C., LINDSAY, J., and NORMAN, R., "Biological Factors in Temporal Lobe Epilepsy," *Clinics in Developmental Medicine*, No. 22, SIMP/Heinemann Medical, London, 1966.

77. PAPOUSEK, H., "Genetics and Child Development," in Spuhler, J. N. (Ed.), *Genetic Diversity and Human Behavior*, Aldine, Chicage, 1967.

78. PETERSEN, I., EEG-OLOFSSON, O., and SELLDEN, U.,

"Paroxysmal Activity in EEG of Normal Children," in Kellaway, P., and Petersen, I. (Eds.), *Clinical Electroencephalography of Children*, p. 167, Grune & Stratton, New York, 1968.

79. RAPOPORT, J., QUINN, P., and LAMPRECHT, F., "Minor Physical Anomalies and Plasma Dopamine-Beta-Hydroxylase Activity in Hyperactive Boys," *American Journal of Psychiatry, 131:*386, 1974.

80. RAPOPORT, J., et al., "Urinary Noradrenaline and Playroom Behaviour in Hyperactive Boys," *Lancet, 2:*1141, 1970.

81. RIMLAND, B., *Infantile Autism*, Appleton-Century-Crofts, New York, 1964.

82. RUSSELL, J. K., and THOMPSON, A. M., "Fetal Complications and the Selection of High-Risk Cases," *British Journal of Hospital Medicine, 3:*594, 1970.

83. RUTTER, M., "Individual Differences," in Rutter, M., and Hersov, L. (Eds.), *Child Psychiatry: Modern Approaches*, Blackwell Scientific Publications, London, 1977.

84. ———, "A Child's Life," *New Scientist, 62:*763, 1974.

85. ———, "One-Day Symposium on the Child and Family," Sponsored by the Association of Child Psychology and Psychiatry, 1972.

86. ———, "Normal Psychosexual Development," *Journal of Child Psychology and Psychiatry, 11:*259, 1971.

87. ———, "Psychiatry," in Wortis, J. (Ed.), *Mental Retardation*, vol. 3, Grune & Stratton, New York, 1971.

88. ———, "Sex Differences in Children's Responses to Family Stress," in Anthony, E. J., and Koupernik, C. (Eds.), *The Child in His Family*, John Wiley, London, 1970.

89. ———, "Psychological Development: Predictions from Infancy," *Journal of Child Psychology and Psychiatry, 11:*49, 1970.

90. ———, *Children of Sick Parents: An Environmental and Psychiatric Study*, Maudsley Monograph No. 16, Oxford University Press, London, 1966.

91. ———, and LOCKYER, L., "A Five-to-Fifteen-Year Follow Up Study of Infantile Psychosis. I. Description of Sample," *British Journal of Psychiatry, 113:*1169, 1967.

92. ———, and SUSSENWEIN, F., "A Developmental and Behavioral Approach to the Treatment of Preschool Autistic Children," *Journal of Autism and Childhood Schizophrenia, 1:*376, 1971.

93. ———, GRAHAM, P., and YULE, W., *A Neuropsychiatric Study in Childhood*, Lippincott, Philadelphia, 1970.

94. ———, TIZARD, J., and WHITMORE, K., *Education, Health and Behavior: Psychological and Medical Study of Childhood Development*, John Wiley, New York, 1970.

95. ———, KORN, S., and BIRCH, H. G., "Genetic and Environmental Factors in the Development of 'Primary Reaction Patterns,'" *British Journal of Social and Clinical Psychology, 2:*161, 1963.

96. SAFER, D. J., "A Familial Factor in Minimal Brain Dysfunction," *Behavioral Genetics, 3:*175, 1973.

97. SAMEROFF, A. J., and CHANDLER, M. J., "Reproductive Risk and the Continuum of Caretaking Casualty," in Horowitz, F. D., et al. (Eds.), *Review of Child Development Research*, vol. 4, p. 187, University of Chicago Press, Chicago, 1975.

98. SATTERFIELD, J., "EEG Issues in Children with Minimal Brain Dysfunction," *Seminars in Psychiatry, 5:*35, 1973.

99. ———, CANTWELL, D. P., and SATTERFIELD, B. T., "The Pathophysiology of the Hyperkinetic Syndrome," *Archives of General Psychiatry, 31:*839, 1974.

100. ———, et al., "Response to Stimulant Drug Treatment in Hyperactive Children: Prediction from EEG and Neurological Findings," *Journal of Autism and Childhood Schizophrenia, 3:*36, 1973.

101. ———, et al., "Physiological Studies of the Hyperkinetic Child: I," *American Journal of Psychiatry, 128:*1418, 1972.

102. SCHAFFER, R., "Behavioral Synchrony in Infancy," *New Scientist, 62:*16, 1974.

103. SCHAIN, R., *Neurology of Childhood Learning Disorder*, Williams and Wilkins, Baltimore, 1972.

104. SEIDEL, U. P., CHADWICK, O. F. D., and RUTTER, M., "Psychological Disorders in Crippled Children. A Comparative Study of Children With and Without Brain Damage," *Developmental Medicine and Child Neurology, 17:*563, 1975.

105. SHAFFER, D., "Psychiatric Aspects of Brain Injury in Childhood: A Review," *Developmental Medicine and Child Neurology, 15:*211, 1973.

106. SHETTY, J., "Alpha Rhythms in the Hyperkinetic Child," *Nature, 234:*476, 1971.

107. SILVER, A., "Postural and Righting Responses in Children," *Journal of Pediatrics, 41:*493, 1952.

108. SNYDER, S., et al., "The Role of Brain Dopamine in Behavioral Regulation and the Actions of Psychotropic Drugs," *American Journal of Psychiatry, 27:*199, 1970.

109. STEWART, M., et al., "The Hyperactive Child Syndrome," *American Journal of Orthopsychiatry, 36:*861, 1966.

110. STRAUSS, A., and LEHTINEN, L., *Psychopathology and Education of the Brain-Injured Child*, Grune & Stratton, New York, 1947.

111. TEUBER, H., "The Premorbid Personality and Reaction to Brain Damage," *American Journal of Orthopsychiatry, 30:*322, 1960.

112. THOMAS, A., CHESS, S., and BIRCH, H. G., *Temperament and Behavior Disorders in Children*, New York University Press, New York, 1968.

113. ———, et al., "Individuality in Responses of Children to Similar Environmental Situations," *American Journal of Psychiatry, 117:*9, 1961.

114. TIZARD, B., "The Personality of Epileptics: A Discussion of the Evidence," *Psychological Bulletin, 59:*196, 1962.

115. TREVARTHEN, C., "Conversations With a Two-Month-Old," *New Scientist, 62:*230, 1974.

116. VANDENBERG, S. G., "Hereditary Factors in Normal Personality Traits," *Research Report from the Louisville Twin Study Child Development Unit*, Department of Pediatrics, University of Louisville, Louisville, Ky., 1966.

117. WALDROP, M., and HALVERSON, C., "Minor Physical Anomalies and Hyperactive Behavior in Young Children," in Hellmuch, J. (Ed.), *The Exceptional Infant*, Brunner-Mazel, New York, 1971.

118. WARREN, R. J., et al., "The Hyperactive Child Syndrome: Normal Chromosome Findings," *Archives of General Psychiatry, 24:*161, 1971.

119. WENAR, C., "The Reliability of Developmental Histories: Summary and Evaluation of Evidence," *Psychosomatic Medicine, 25:*505, 1963.

120. WENDER, P. H., *Minimal Brain Dysfunction in Children*, Wiley-Interscience, New York, 1971.

121. ———, "Platelet Serotonin Level in Children With 'Minimal Brain Dysfunction,'" *Lancet, 2:*1012, 1969.

122. ———, et al., "Urinary Monoamine Metabolites in Children With Minimal Brain Dysfunction," *American Journal of Psychiatry, 127:*1411, 1971.

123. WERRY, J. S., "Organic Factors in Childhood Psychopathology," in Quay, H., and Werry, J. (Eds.), *Psychopathological Disorders of Childhood*, p. 83, John Wiley, New York, 1972.

124. ———, "Developmental Hyperactivity," *Pediatric Clinics of North America, 15:*581, 1968.

125. ———, et al., "Studies on the Hyperactive Child. VII. Neurological Status Compared With Neurotic and Normal Children," *American Journal of Orthopsychiatry, 42:*441, 1972.

126. WILLERMAN, L., "Activity Level and Hyperactivity in Twins," *Child Development, 44:*288, 1973.

127. WOLFF, P., "Observations on the Early Development of Smiling," in Foss, B. M. (Ed.), *Determinants of Infant Behaviour II.*, Methuen, London, 1963.

128. WOLKIND, S., and RUTTER, M., "Children Who Have Been 'In Care'—An Epidemiological Study," *Journal of Child Psychology and Psychiatry, 14:97,* 1973

129. WOOD, D. R., REIMHERR, F. W., and WENDER, P. H., "Diagnosis and Treatment of Minimal Brain Dysfunction in Adults: A Preliminary Report," *Archives of General Psychiatry, 33:1453,* 1976.

130. YARROW, L. J., "Research in Dimensions of Early Maternal Care," *Merrill-Palmer Quarterly, 9:101,* 1963.

131. YATES, A. J., "The Validity of Some Psychological Tests of Brain Damage," *Psychological Bulletin, 51:359,* 1954.

132. YULE, W., and RAYNES, N. W., "Behavioral Characteristics of Children in Residential Care," *Journal of Child Psychology and Psychiatry, 13:249,* 1972.

133. ZAHN, T., et al., "Minimal Brain Dysfunction, Stimulant Drugs, and Autonomic Nervous System Activity," *Archives of General Psychiatry, 32:381,* 1975.

3 / Family Development and Familial Factors in Etiology

Joan J. Zilbach

Introduction

To the small child, the family ways and the parents' ways are *the* way of life and *the* way for people to interact with one another . . . The family influences are so pervasive and transpire so naturally that it has required the comparison of family patterns in divergent societies and, more recently, the study of the effects of serious family pathology to realize how greatly the individual is shaped by the family mold and how greatly the continuity of the society depends on the nature of its families . . . The family forms the first imprint upon the still unformed child and the most pervasive and consistent influence that establishes patterns that later forces can modify but never alter completely.

Theodore Lidz
The Family and Human Adaptation

The family is the basic biosocial unit, a unity of interacting personalities,[26] that surrounds and encompasses children from birth to death. Since we are always part of or from a family, we know it well, in one sense, since it is omnipresent, but little, in another sense, due to its complexities. Some degree of distance or separation is necessary for objective observation, description, and understanding. The complexities of understanding the family are due to difficulty in achieving the necessary distance for pursuing investigation and further knowledge. The importance of the early years of life and, in recent years, even the first few weeks of life on the later development of the individual child is commonplace knowledge. In this chapter the influence of the surrounding family will be the center of attention, rather than the individual child.

There is a wide range of factors that generate and maintain psychopathology, and some familial factors contributing to disturbances of development in children and adolescents will be discussed here. First, certain characteristics of the family and normal family development will be summarized. The familial factors will be related to the description of family development.

GENERAL HISTORICAL ORIENTATION

The idea of development had entered the world and was touching other fields than biology; thinking in terms of growth and change was becoming a familiar habit of the age.

Milton Millhauser
Just Before Darwin

In the 1800s biology underwent an important conceptual change, from the use of static or mechanistic models to developmental concepts under the influence of Darwin. Freud was strongly influenced by these trends: his early writings in the 1890s,[42] which were based primarily on mechanistic models, progressed to a developmental framework.[48]

From Freud's early writings with an emphasis

on external traumatic events such as seduction, there was a shift inwards, with subsequent delineation of intrapsychic development and the emergence of an intricate series of psychosexual stages. Attention was focused almost entirely on the development of the individual child, but over the years attention broadened and included the child within the family, and even more recently the entire family of the child.

In 1905 Freud drew attention to the family of his famous patient Dora by stating:

It follows from the nature of the facts which form the material of psychoanalysis that we are obliged to pay as much attention in our case histories to the purely human and social circumstances of our patients as to the somatic data and the symptoms of the disorder. Above all, our interest will be directed toward their *family circumstances*—and not only, as will be seen later, for the purpose of inquiring into their heredity. (p. 18)[47]

In this case Freud did not direct much attention specifically to "the family circumstances". A few years later, however, in another famous early case, Freud did not treat the childhood phobic disorder himself. Instead, the work was done through a family member: the father in "Little Hans."

. . . It is true that I laid down the general lines of treatment, and that on one single occasion, when I had a conversation with the boy, I took a direct share in it; but the treatment itself was carried out by the child's father . . . (p. 5)[45]

This might be considered as the first case of family treatment! In "Little Hans,"[45] the actions and statements of the parents were further utilized to understand the development of the child's phobic illness, and the actual family circumstances were considered in some detail.

In the course of individual development, Freud also noted that a child has a different estimate of his parents at different periods in his life. However, several concurrent changes occur simultaneously. A child's "estimate" of parents' change is a function of his own development, but, some of these altered estimates result from the real changes the parents undergo as a function both of their own individual development as adults, and also, as a function of changes in the family as a unit. The changes in the entire family in the course of development over time will be described in the next section on family development. The family life cycle and basic family functions will be useful as a framework for understanding some familial factors which are important in the development of psychopathological conditions of childhood and adolescence.

Family Development

It remains for us to enumerate the various factors, internal and external that interfere with *development*, and to indicate the place in the mechanism on which the disturbance arising from each of them impinges. The factors that we shall enumerate can evidently not be of equal importance, and we must be prepared for difficulties in assigning an appropriate value to each.

Sigmund Freud
"Three Essays on the Theory of Sexuality"

The development of an instinct and some factors that may interfere or obstruct normal development was the central concern of Freud's *Three Essays on the Theory of Sexuality*.[48] In more recent years, the usefulness of a developmental approach in the understanding of individual or general human problems has been well accepted. In clinical or mental health fields, however, the developmental approach has, so far, been mostly confined to the understanding of individuals. In this section the development of the family as a unit moving through a family life cycle sequence will be described. (The term "development" refers to an orderly sequence of changes occurring over time: the progression or unfolding of one expectable stage of organization or function from a previous stage.) A sequence of stages in the family life cycle can be identified. Separate members of the family may be at widely varying points in individual psychological development, but the family unit or family group will be in *one* particular phase of the family life cycle. Family development is a complicated process that involves a number of individuals and many psychological and social forces. Clinicians usually acknowledge that a patient or child is a member of a family, but they do not directly consider the entire family as such, except in passing or in fragments. Even then it is the individual's stage of development, symptoms, inhibitions, prognosis, etc. which are described. But, in this section we are discussing the stages of development that the child's family may be in, may be looking forward to, and may have passed through.

The Family

In this chapter, the term family is defined as a small group, composed of two or more individuals. It refers to a group living in a household, "under the same roof." For clinical purposes this "household" definition has empirical advantages as the most general conception of the group in most frequent interaction. (This definition is similar to that used in some sociological family research and by the census bureau).[28] The family as a unit is a special type of small, natural group, and its development is a separate process distinguishable from the development of the individuals within the family.[29, 59, 115, 117]

The developmental patterns, progressions, etc. of the family life cycle may seem more complicated than those of individual family members. And yet, the development of the family as a whole may be intuitively perceived and recognized in frequent general statements: "We (family X) can do that now . . . We're in that stage . . . They do things like that . . . They are that kind of family . . ."

The Family Life Cycle

In general, families undergo a pre-family, gestational or courtship phase which precedes the early or initial phase (Stage I); then middle years of subsequent growth and development (Stages II through V), later years (Stage VI and VII), and an end. The sequences of the middle years may vary, but all stages will appear in the course of unimpeded family development. Some universal, "normal" characteristics will be described here. Developmental arrests and other pathological aspects of family development and its effects on the child may then be identified more clearly. These will be described in later sections.

In family development the phases in the family life cycle are:

Gestational: Courtship—Engagement or other alternative, introductory variant. This prehistory will affect, in many ways, the early days of the family.[95]

Early:

Stage I   The beginning of the family is at the point of marriage and/or the establishment of a common household by two people; from independence to interdependence.

Stage II   The arrival and subsequent inclusion of the first child represents the beginning of the second phase in family life—the incorporation of a dependent member; from interdependence to dependence.

Middle:

Stage III The exit of the first child from the immediate world of the family to the larger world by entrance into school or other extrafamilial environment such as daycare center; from dependence to beginning separations and partial independence.

Stage IV   The entrance of the last child of the family into the larger community; continuing expansion of partial separations.

Stage V   The exit of the first child from the family by the establishment of an independent household which may include marriage or other establishment of this independent entity; from partial separations to first independence.

Late:

Stage VI   The exit of the last child from the family. This has been termed the "shrunken family" or empty nest. This may include the beginning of grandparenthood; continuing expansion of independence.

Stage VII The later years include the death of one spouse and continue up to the point of the death of the other partner.

Basic Family Functions

The establishment, continuance, and maintenance of the family as a unit involve certain needs and tasks which have been entitled, *basic family functions*.[117] Most family functions have their origin in the first stage of family development and continue on through all later stages. In later stages there are necessary changes in these functions and, also, additional ones may be added. Inadequate development, distortion, or omission may occur in some or many of these basic family functions. This can take place in the first stage of family development or later. Patterns of maldevelopment are complicated and have important implications for disturbance in childhood and adolescence.

The importance of basic family functions is that they are the tasks that must be carried out by any new or distinctive social unit in order to attain a modicum of stability around fundamental social requirements. These functions form the substrate of a family, which then continue through all stages of family development. As has been mentioned, for several of these functions the earliest phase of family development is most crucial and also perhaps most vulnerable to maldevelopment. The first four family functions can be considered as a unit since they are primary functions of a family. (By primary, I mean that a family cannot exist without the establishment of these functions. They must be established in some fashion.) These are the tasks that have been described generally by some authors in the family field as "nurturance."[29, 76] In this publication they have been specified in accord with the way they are actually carried out within a family.

The first primary group are: (1) Housing-Shelter, (2) Supplies-Food, (3) Finances-Employment, and (4) Family Health. The second group of family functions has been broadly entitled socialization or enculturation.[49, 76, 91] This group includes provision of education, transmission of values, and other related functions.

Survival Processes

SHELTER-HOUSING

Shelter-housing is an important psychosocial function of the family. Every family establishes their space at the onset of family life. The boundaries of this space should be distinct and strong. The establishment of these family boundaries commonly is regarded as primarily an economic issue and, therefore, is disregarded by clinicians. As an example: frequently a new family moves in with the parents of one spouse and this is attributed only to economic pressures. But underlying family psychological issues such as difficulties in separating from parents may be the most powerful and persuasive force for this household union.

There are a variety of arrangements that can adequately establish this basic family function. Whatever the arrangement, there are basic qualities that must be fulfilled. Ideally these include: (a) adequate size, based on number in the family unit; (b) adequate basic structure so that c and d become possible; (c) facilities for food preparation; and (d) provision for other essentials such as heat, light, water, and bathroom facilities. Other qualities such as neighborhood are not so critical but may contain potentials for satisfactory family-community relations or for later difficulties. This aspect, positive or negative outcome, is also integrally connected with the development of socialization processes in the second group of basic family functions.

Although social, cultural, economic, and psychological factors will determine the conception of "adequacy" for each of these housing-shelter requirements, once these are defined and choices made, the actual physical arrangements determine many subsequent features of family behavior and interaction. An expanded or extended household arrangement, i.e., nonindependent, can provide adequately for the family function of housing as when two or more individuals become part of a larger household. (This joining and extension of a parental household, may be susceptible to later difficulties, but, such an outcome cannot be assumed without actual evaluation of maldevelopment.) In certain foreign cultures a new room is built onto the existing house for the newlyweds. In the societies in which an expanded household arrangement is frequent, there are fairly rigid social arrangements maintaining boundaries to the relationships betwen people that might otherwise lead to irresolvable conflict. The strength of physical boundaries will be undermined in families where social boundaries are indistinct.

SUPPLIES-FOOD

Beyond basic nutritional and preference requirements, it is clear that the significance of supplies—food in its association with family and household has many psychological implications. The arrangements for purchase, cooking, serving, and cleaning are based on fundamental psychological issues of reciprocity, of giving, and receiving that are of general importance in family life. (The well-known primary needs of an infant are warmth, shelter, and food. The first two family functions bear a striking similarity to those of an infant but are being described in relation to the family as a unit.)

The basic qualities for fulfillment of family needs are: (a) a consistent supply of nutriment over an extended period of time, (b) a quantity of nurture consistent with the size of the family, and (c) adequate quality and kind of food supplies for each given stage of family life. Such common requirements as (d) meeting minimal nutritional needs and (e) edibility also must be noted because in some severely disturbed families these basic requirements will not be met. Some of these needs may vary, but their stable fulfillment is a universal and continuing necessity for families.

FINANCES-EMPLOYMENT

In family life this set of psychoeconomic tasks subserves the first two family functions, which have just been described. It provides the source, in a money economy, for the purchase and provision of housing-shelter and supplies-food. This function includes: (a) provision and (b) management of finances-employment. Provision may be acquired by employment but there is a great variation in the spectrum of arrangements for gaining money for the family. Employment is distinguished from finances in order to describe these functions in a more universal way. There are many families for whom money comes from sources other than employment, such as from parents and/or siblings, from agencies (particularly public ones), or from other sources such as trusts. In this age of early marriages (see Stage I) a variety of arrangements are common, particularly in marriages of college students.

The management or handling of finances is also part of this basic family function. There are many variations, from a common family fund to separate budgets for different family members (especially husband and wife and, in later phases of family development, the older children). A common family fund carries a different affective tone with it into other areas of family functioning than separate or independent funds. It is also important to note that, since the area of finances-employment is so basic to the family's household functioning, priority in earnings and explicit or implicit rights of distribution lead to many other influences on family and household arrangements.

The basic family arrangement for handling money and its impact on family life are generally recognized. From the early days of family life when the arrangement is established, to the middle stages of family development when rearrangements will impinge particularly on the adolescent, there are many opportunities for maldevelopment. Part of the normal dramatic struggle for independence on the part of the adolescent will take place in this arena, i.e., over allowances, budgets and other expenditures of teenage requirements. The conflicts over establishment of independence by the adolescent may be expressed in all areas of family functioning, but those that have not been satisfactorily established will more often lead to difficulty.

FAMILY HEALTH

This complex function is the family equivalent of public health. This family function is divided into two subcategories: (a) maintenance of mini-mal physical and emotional health, and (b) recognition of health problems, both acute and chronic. The establishment and maintenance of minimal health levels is dependent, to some extent, on the adequacy of the three previously described basic family functions. But indicators of adequate health must be noted independently.

Acute and chronic health problems have different patterns and require the use of different facilities. The needs of acutely ill persons are distinguishable from the on-going and special needs of the disabled or from the chronic health problems of members who may be part of the family from the beginning or who join the family at later stages in the family life cycle.

The differentiation of these categories is important in estimating the adequacy of this function in a particular family. In acute conditions the outcome should be the disappearance of the problem and discontinuance of use of facilities. With chronic health needs, the opposite pattern is most effective and adaptive. Recognition of long-term needs should be followed by the continued use of indicated facilities.

Maintenance of family health is an important basic function. In its earliest phase this may be primarily provided on a continuing, individual basis as a holdover from the earlier, or gestational, pre-family years. This pattern becomes a more interlocking and familial one as the variety of health needs increase in the course of the family life cycle. The recognition of and equilibrium within family functioning, around both special physical abilities and disabilities, is not only a necessary basis for effective individual and family performance, but carries with it a host of emotional connotations that are significant in creating a familial sense of reciprocity and appreciation.

Appreciation of the importance of the care of individual bodies is well recognized, but the state of the "family body," the family collective whole, is also important. This is necessary to the development of a "family sense" or a "family atmosphere," or is, at least, an important ingredient of this atmosphere. Every family, as a unit, develops a health standard and ways of maintaining that standard, and there are many ways of maintaining the "family body." This standard of the "family body" may be set at a low level and foster a poor and unhealthy family atmosphere. Some families may expend an inordinate amount of their finances on family health, etc. in an attempt to be "super-healthy" with a "super-family body."

Socialization and Enculturation Processes: Extra-Familial Basic Family Functions

Much of the work on the family as an enculturating agent has been done in related fields.[91]

There is a second group of family functions which, though they have their origins early in the family life cycle, emerge as central in later phases (beyond Stage II). The first group of four family functions that have just been described are primarily oriented inward and between family members. These intrafamilial functions potentially create and enhance closeness and intimacy between family subgroups (for example, husband-wife or parent-child). The second group of family functions is oriented outward to the community and other extrafamilial institutions such as school. These functions create and enhance bonds outside the family and foster expansion of the family into the community and larger society.

SOCIALIZATION

The socialization functions of the family include: (a) the transmission of values and other educative mechanisms within the family, and (b) the development of extra-familial patterns including leisure, recreation, and others. Socialization is an interactive process which begins in the home through family member-to-member interactions, in multiple daily experiences of being together. Family members, including siblings, have important socializing functions as models (positive or negative) and as auxiliary teachers in the educative processes in the family.

Transmission of Values: Early feeding experiences, play within the family with siblings and peers, household chores, homework, and, eventually extrafamilial experiences are all areas of access for transmission of values around core issues, e.g., autonomy and independence. The amount of autonomy and independence is initially granted and slowly increased by parents according to their standards. As the family progresses through its life cycle, siblings add to these influences. In varying ways, in later stages members integrate the values of their family with outside influences such as peer and neighborhood groups. The family is, however, the first, continuing, and powerful influence in the transmission of values. The transmission of deviant values by parents,

impinging particularly upon the adolescent and contributing to maldevelopment, has been recognized in the production of antisocial behavior and delinquency.

Development of Extrafamilial Relationships: The family as a unit develops patterns of relationships with the "outside world" of relatives, friends, and the community. Patterns of leisure and recreation are established as a family function beginning in the early years of the family life cycle and continuing through all stages. Provision for education and patterns of association with these institutions are also part of this function. The function and extent to which these relationships are carried out on an individual or familial basis vary markedly by social class and cultural patterns.[49] This is a large and significant topic in its own right and full discussion is beyond the scope of this chapter.

DEVELOPMENT OF BASIC FAMILY FUNCTIONS

From the beginning of the family, basic family functions may manifest flexibility or rigidity and progressive or static characteristics; thus, they may continue progressing and changing or remain relatively unaltered during all stages of family development. But, there is no simple relationship between the establishment of effective methods of dealing with these issues at any one stage of development and the adaptability of the approach to new problems and issues posed by changes in the family situation. Thus, patterns may be established satisfactorily, for the earliest periods of family organization and then continue to function on that same level, remaining fixed and inflexible. On the other hand, the patterns may appear quite inadequate during the first stages of development and yet prove adaptable and increasingly, or varyingly, effective during subsequent developmental family phases. Moreover, the pattern of provision for basic family functions may not be uniform; there may be difficulties in only one or two or in all of these functions that emerge in the early stages of family development.

In summary, at the onset of family life, basic family functions may indicate progressive characteristics and continue as such, enabling the adaptive family to successfully manage all stages of the family life cycle. Or a pattern of satisfactory functioning in an early period of family life may become inelastic and nonprogressive and thus cause difficulty in the next or later periods. And another pattern, inelasticity or difficulties in development, may start only in the later phases of family development. The difficulties may be in one, two, or all of the basic family functions. The next section will deal with specific stages of the family life cycle and include some clinical examples of maldevelopment at each stage of family functioning (emphasis will be placed on the effects on the children in each of these stages of the family life cycle).

Stages of the Family Life Cycle

EARLY PHASES

Stage I: Each stage in family development involves all family members. And each one of the basic family functions will have its origin at this stage of family development.

A family starts with the establishment of a common household by two or more individuals, after marriage or otherwise. A family, as a household, may start with three persons, for example, with the addition, from the onset, of an inlaw, or a child from a previous marriage, or another relative. In many instances the marital couple is incorporated into an already existing larger family structure. However, even in a family with a pre-existing extended household pattern, the conjugal unit has basic tasks that must be accomplished as a unit, partially independent of other household members. When two pre-existing households join together after divorce, the new parental unit must again initiate basic family functions. The form and timing of the task resolution in the basic family functions are modified according to the particular kind of family and household structure.

This stage in the family life cycle is one of joining together and mutual establishment of the basic family functions. For individual family members, there is a progression from being dependent on their original family (to some extent varying according to age) to the establishment of interdependence.

In Stage I, the establishment of the relationship of the newly formed couple, the marital pair, is critical. Interdependence in fundamental interpersonal features, including the establishment of sexuality in marriage, the development of affectional ties, and the overt and covert authority patterns, are of utmost importance in creating the initial family environment. Moreover, the form and effectiveness of these relationships, although primarily a matter for the marital pair, have considerable significance for the development of cohesion and unity in the entire family. The specialized issues and development of the marital unit are beyond the confines of this chapter.[96]

The arrangement of financial support is a primary task of Stage I, since the other basic family functions depend upon this one. There are many alternatives, from total family support of both members of the marital pair (by one or both in-laws), to work by one or both members of the pair and various admixtures. The working through of interdependent financial arrangements must be accomplished, either with or without emotional complications.

The basic family function of provision of family finances-employment is often recognized as a source of stress in early stages of the family life cycle. It is common for families or individuals to recall, "Oh, since the beginning, we've always had trouble with money." However, even when not spontaneously or initially presented, direct scrutiny of the other two functions, supplies-food, and shelter-housing, will reveal interesting and significant material.

The family task of providing shelter-housing is a necessity in Stage I. This establishes the psychophysical boundaries of the family. At this early stage there are many variations in the establishment and accouterments of family space. But the fundamental characteristics described earlier can be discerned in all of these arrangements. If any of these characteristics seem vague, assumed, and unplanned, then it is likely that adequate establishment of this function has not occurred. For example, there are young unmarried couples who automatically assume that "they" will join the household of parents after the birth of an unplanned baby. This may lead to vagueness in the housing arrangements after the birth of the baby. When this kind of extended household is established without planning, discussion, and resolution, there will be considerable strain on all members of the family. This may also occur at later stages in the family life cycle with unplanned, unresolved family expansions.

The third family function of supplies-food at this early stage has been extensively described in the earlier section on basic family functions.

The basic family function of health ("the family body") has its origin in this early stage of family life. Acute health needs can continue to be provided primarily on an individual basis. However, if there are chronic health needs or disabilities in any of the family members this function

68

must be established on a more familial basis. This latter family situation is a fairly common cause of strain during the first stage of family development.

Stage II: The next stage of family development is signaled by the entrance into the family of its first dependent member, usually the first child. The birth of the first additional member of the family and the infant's dependent state have been the subject of much study. However, little attention has been devoted to the impact of this child on family organization and functioning. During this second family stage, the first three basic family functions of housing-shelter, supplies-food, and finances-employment must undergo many changes and considerable reorganization for satisfactory family development. In family terms, the entrance of the dependent infant heralds the beginning of being depended upon for the adult members of the family.

Housing must undergo many changes to accomodate new needs, such as the rhythm and sleeping patterns of an infant and the need for physical separation of the infant from adults. Supplies-food must change not only in amount, but also in kind, and the adaptability of the family in handling divergent food needs is tested. This family function of food has been described didactically, that is, in terms of the mother-infant relationship, and has omitted the influence of other important family members. The importance of the mother-child unit is obvious, but, the balance may be impaired by the functioning of the other members in relation to the dyad. If the functioning of the mother-child dyad assumes overwhelming importance, then family functioning, with integration of the total family, will be impaired. In this and later phases, the inclusion in all functions of family members at appropriate levels of intensity insures further development.

Maldevelopment has been recognized, e.g., the intensity of the schizophrenic dyad of mother-child has been described in relation to many family functions, including food and emotional supplies. If one looks, however, at other family functions beyond food into shelter-housing, particularly, other impairments may be seen, e.g., the schizophrenic mother may not separate the child from her in ways other than food. The bedroom-sleeping arrangements often remain close and undifferentiated for many years. The mothers of schizophrenic patients, after hospitalization of a child, are well known for their loyalty and persistence. They continue for decades, as their children become chronic patients, with uninterrupted

ties, bringing Sunday dinner every week after the hospital meal is served.[101]

Finances-employment also require readjustments in Stage II. These may have to undergo a necessary expansion in the amount of income, or readjustment and redistribution of available resources.

During this phase, the fourth function of maintenance of family health must become a family function. The health characteristics of the parents and the child are no longer individual matters. Each member affects the other in a complex and interlocking fashion.

The second group of family functions: Socialization and other family functions affecting child rearing emerge clearly at this stage of family functioning. Many of the significant socialization experiences of the infant/child/adolescent begin in the family.

The educative process of toilet training, for example, is markedly influenced by family structure. The attitude and experience of the proud first child who has "taught" the second child reflects this educative function. Similarly, oedipal experiences are modified by the number and sex of siblings with whom this experience may be enacted.

In Stage II of family development, the marital couple must make many changes. Indeed, in many societies, the husband and wife are hardly viewed as a family unit until they have a child. Among some subgroups in Western society a sharp distinction is made between "a couple" and "a family." In later stages of family development, the addition of more members adds to the importance of socialization, especially, as childrearing family functions become paramount. But, the necessary reorganization of previously existing functions, prior interactions and prior relationships, must not be overlooked. Additional children introduce further elements into family development and a much wider potential range of interactions and relationships. But they do not require the initial and basic transition to a new stage of developmental functioning as does the birth and introduction into the family of a dependent member (as occurs in the first part of Stage II).

An illustrative clinical example: An infant was brought for a diagnostic evaluation of "developmental retardation." Lengthy infections had been treated with unsatisfactory results and the pediatrician also noted lags in several areas of motoric development. The family consisted of a young artist and his student wife. This couple had been married for several years and had functioned at a satisfactory level in Stage I. They lived in an art studio and the wife worked to support the family, pursuing her studies on a part-time basis. Thus, the tasks of Stage I were accomplished; supplies-food, shelter-housing, and finances-employment were satisfactory up to the birth of the first baby. Within a few weeks, the wife returned quickly to work, as planned previously, since she provided the stable income. The marital couple had agreed that the father would do the major portion of early child rearing. Family development had proceeded with no difficulties in the resolution of the basic family tasks of Stage I: the studio provided adequate housing for the couple, food was arranged according to their needs, and the wife's work provided finances adequate for the needs of this marital pair. However, the inclusion of a dependent member, the baby, resulted in increased demands in all of these areas. Due to increased financial need, there was a demand on the artist father to sell his work which previously was not an issue. He was not automatically willing to do this. Superficially, the provision of food and housing for themselves and the baby might have been adequate in amount. But, pursuit of these areas revealed that the father often lost track of time and heard nothing when involved in his artistic pursuits. The father, though willing and agreeable, had not made any readjustments. When lost in his work, medication, food, and the cries of the baby went neglected. Food, housing, and financial arrangements had been agreed to by both of them and the baby was planned—she wanted to "produce also" and he had agreed that this was important. These unsatisfactory family patterns, illustrating difficulties of adjustment in the early phases of Stage II, were revealed not spontaneously, but through specific family developmental inquiries. More adequate arrangements for baby care were arranged, the infections improved and the development of the infant proceeded in a satisfactory fashion. The question of 'developmental retardation' was thus resolved. In addition, the father was able to adjust and offer his art for sale, and the mother was able to decrease her out of home jobs. Thus, in the area of finances, food, and other child rearing responsibilities, some readjustments took place.

It might be tempting to concentrate on understanding the individual intrapsychic state of the artist and his creativity, or his wife, or likewise, the intrapsychic development of the infant. But, this would not have been sufficient. The inflexibility of the family in meeting the new demands was not primarily an individual psychological matter, nor was it explained by the "symbolic meaning" of the baby to the wife or marital pair. The couple had developed effective basic family functions in Stage I, but not in Stage II. There was no direct intrapsychic intervention, treatment pursued family developmental blocks and a positive family outcome ensued. The interconnections and interweavings of the family as a unit and its component parts were crucial to successful treatment.

MIDDLE PHASES OF THE FAMILY LIFE CYCLE

Stage III: The entrance of the first child into the larger community, school or other institution,
which is a partial exit from the family, is the next landmark in family development. At this stage, the family function of socialization must take a big step to include the provision of education and other forms of transfer of information from one generation to the next. Education has distinctive characteristics that are important and may be vulnerable in some families. These characteristics include: (1) regular attendance at school is a minimal requirement; (2) steady, consistent, and appropriate grade progression is expected; and (3) special needs, such as retardation must be provided for by the family's use of appropriate facilities. If basic family functions are operating precariously, steady attendance of the child at school may be jeopardized. The additional needs of the school age child, getting dressed, breakfasted, and transported may be too great, and the child may frequently stay home. Frequent or prolonged absences from school have been discussed as a developmental issue of mother-child separation and vice versa. A more general separation problem may exist for the family as a unit (see later case example). The attitudes towards schooling of other important members of an extended household, including those of the maid or nurse in upper class socioeconomic families, may be crucial and are often overlooked.

The entrance of the child into the larger community necessitates a major change in the extrafamilial relationships of the child. Peer relations begin to assume great importance, and there are social and emotional pulls away from the family with the development of independence and social initiative on the part of the child. The patterns of peer relations vary from the street orientation of working class neighborhoods, to groups of children running in and out of many houses as in suburban communities, to the more structured schedules and activities of other, more urban, neighborhoods.

The movement of the child away from the home, both in the form of finding new authority figures in school and in the form of establishing new social and emotional relationships with other children in the school and in the community, has many implications for family development. On the one hand, it adds a new dimension to family patterns, in the sense that the child now also has an "extra-familial" life and this may provide a further (and often a first) link of the family to the local residential community. This link frequently involves the parent in a wider range of social relationships. This trend necessitates developmental changes within the household itself that may include making physical and psychological room for child visitors, accepting the absence of a child during his play with other children, and overall, a different conception of the family's relationships with the wider world. This is a serious problem for those families who are unable to accept either new authorities in the child's life or new emotional relationships that may lessen the intensity of ties to the parents.

The addition of other children into the family does not affect the fundamental nature of the various family functions, but rather tests their expandability, their flexibility or rigidity, and their basic effectiveness.

Stage IV: The next junction point is marked by the entrance of the *last* child into the larger community, which makes a significant difference in the family. As the last child expands the range of his social and emotional ties beyond the family, basic family functions must change and may seem to narrow as the parents begin to take a new position in family organization. But it is not in any sense a return to the early years of marriage, since the family remains as critical a base for functioning as ever, although it spills beyond the confines of the immediate household more freely. Actually some family functions will increase as the family base must expand and be flexible, as dependent members, particularly adolescent members, struggle to develop:

A middle class family with two children worried about the older adolescent daughter who was referred by a school counselor for school difficulties. Initially, this family indicated no other problems, and stated that they were otherwise comfortable, both financially and socially. Further discussion revealed that the mother had always worked and the father, who contributed "when he could" was, at that time, in one of his longest and most consistent working periods. In the course of diagnostic family sessions, the older daughter expressed some strong feelings of general deprivation, and the issue of *food* was specifically pursued. The girl indicated that she "never had breakfast." This was not an individually determined adolescent whim. There was often *no* food in the house. The mother bought food sporadically, and, since she was never up or awake in the morning, breakfast food was usually omitted from the to-be-purchased list. The mother's working hours determined this pattern, and the father had arranged his life accordingly. The daughter's general feelings of deprivation were derived, in part, from nonadequate provision of kinds, amount and consistency of supply of food in this middle-class household. This was determined primarily by the mother's sporadic pattern of buying food, and supplemented only by the father when he was *not* working. The issue of food revealed a pattern originating in the early days of this family. In Stage I, the mother never cooked, the father was free to eat many meals out and without any children, and when

the children were young, the pattern was adequate. Arrangements were made for feeding dependent infants but the reorganization in later stages was inadequate. Superficially, *housing* seemed adequate, but further questioning revealed that the apartment, furniture, etc. had been chosen at the start of marriage and had never changed or altered to meet later needs, or enlarged in any fashion. There were still only *two* chairs at the small kitchen table of this family that now had four members.

Shelter-housing had adequately established boundaries in the first years of family life, but had remained inflexible and unchanged over the middle stages of family development. In these middle years of family life, family members were rarely all at home at the same time. Intimacy, closeness, and communication dwindled. Isolation and alienation beyond expression of adolescent independence, were evident. Thus, supplies-food and shelter-housing were continuously inadequate in middle years of family development, and finances had a long history of sporadic difficulty. The emergence of both children into adolescence, with increased emotional and financial demands, tipped the precarious equilibrium in the family. The early information on basic family functions was crucial in understanding both the referral of one family member and current difficulties which affected all members but went unnoticed in the family.

The maintenance of generational boundaries becomes particularly important in middle stages of family development. The increasing expansion of the family functions of socialization in these middle periods will be affected by maintenance or blurring of boundaries. In this critical stage, there are many challenges to generational boundaries as the children move toward establishing a life separate from their parental family. This concept has usually been specified only in relation to the marital pair. The importance of banding-together, or *generational-alliance*, of the adolescent children is crucial. Splitting and blurring of these boundaries by the alignment of one child member with either parent can be a source of difficulty. These alignments can be observed changing in the course of development when an increase in the strength of the bonding occurs between the adolescent members. This may not be peaceful, but it is important in the progress of a family. Blurring of boundaries can destroy the meaning of differentiation of parenthood and childhood. The development and maintenance of sex-linked roles is aided by clear generational alliances and boundaries:

In Family C, with two late adolescent members, there was a long history of psychiatric difficulties in all members. They were referred for family sessions as the oldest daughter was attempting to finish college. Severe anxiety hampered her performance and her individual therapist wondered if family interaction contributed to the intensity and persistence of her symptoms.

In family interviews unswerving, strong father-son and mother-daughter alliances were clear. When either adolescent expressed anxiety, it was abetted by the opposite alliance. There was little if any sympathy or help given by either sibling to the other. In the course of family treatment the existing alliances were revealed and the altercations temporarily worsened. Gradually mother and father began to battle and then sister and brother. The therapist noted the new strength and change in the alliances. The identified patient turned directly to her brother and with tears said, "Now we are really sister and brother."

The generational alliances were established during the course of family treatment. The battles waxed and waned but there was a positive intensification of relationships in their new alliances.

Stage V: The exit of the first child (not necessarily the oldest child) from the family by marriage or other establishment of an independent household is the next milestone. There had been a widespread impression that the family as a functional entity began to diminish its activities with this event in urban, industrial societies, particularly in the United States. It is now clear that this is far from the case. Some functions may begin, e.g., grandparenthood, and there is a striking continuity in ties at all class levels and for many ethnic groups, between parents and the new nuclear families developed by their married children. This so-called "shrunken" stage of family development rapidly enlarges as the kind and frequency of grandparent-grandchildren interactions and other activities are noted. As in previous stages earlier family developmental patterns affect the organization and quality of these relationships.

Stage VI: This is signaled by the exit of the last child from the nuclear family. The role of grandparents has been mentioned in Stage V. Ideally, the grandparents' function should encompass the entire family with provision for varying needs. Problems are common in this function: There are grandparents who can deal comfortably with babies, and who, in their own nuclear family, dealt adequately with Stages I and II, but who had many difficulties in Stage III through VI. These may be recapitulated in their relationships to grandchildren. Conversely, there are grandparents who were incapable of dealing effectively with later stages of development in their own nuclear family, but whose growing perspective is an asset

during these stages in the development of their married children's families. That is, the family developmental issues of increasing independence may be helped by the active presence or intervention, in other ways, of grandparents. The relationships, at a familial level, between parent/child and grandparent/grandchild have been only minimally included in family developmental investigations.[9, 19]

The middle Stages III through VI of family development have been described separately for purposes of clarity. Ideally, they would be intermingled as they occur in a variety of sequences.

Scapegoating: In these middle stages of family development one child may become the main carrier and indicator of difficulties. This maneuver is an attempt to keep the family together and manage the tensions within the family. It is dysfunctional not only for the scapegoated member but for the entire family group. This is illustrated in the following case:

Family A came for help, self-referred, when they felt an "open and complete break" with their younger son was about to occur. They stated that "their trouble" was the behavior of this son, and it soon became clear that he was an indicator and carrier of difficulties in the middle stages of family development.

The family consisted of a father, mother, and two sons. The oldest was in his mid-twenties and the youngest in his mid-teens. The early years of this family were satisfactory in all areas. However, when the oldest son reached late adolescence he attempted to leave home in order to attend college, developed school difficulties, and somatic symptoms. On this basis he left college, returned home, and though about to marry at the point of referral, he was not planning to leave the family. After the first son returned home, the family again did well until the second son entered mid-adolescence. At this point, he attempted some preliminary moves away from the family and his behavior became more and more unbearable to the other family members. This had been the source of increasing strain and tension. A state of virtually complete noncommunication existed in this troubled family. There was no talk with the younger son and the parents feared an "open break." The oldest son, in a family session, said: "I went through a similar stage at the same time. There were arguments all the time—but the degree was different. I would leave the table after an argument—he (the younger brother) leaves the house." Father, mother, and older brother all attributed to the youngest son an attitude of "not caring" which was also intolerable to them. The youngest son's (Son B) attempts at "going out" had been completely banned, and eventually he resorted to leaving secretly via the window. Upon discovery, severe measures were taken. The mother described asking Son B where he was going and receiving no answer, she felt it was clear that B did not love her.

Father referred to any independence by Son B as being "cut off," in contrast to "under my support" which he clearly indicated was what he and the other family members preferred and required. Son A emphasized this family attitude, adding, "I've been afraid to say anything—I'll sound just like a third parent. Why can't he do what I did? How come I gave in and you won't?" The father's adolescence was described proudly and not seen as a source of any problems in this family: "I was never a child—I didn't date. I did a lot of reading and once a week I took my sister out to a movie." After this, father went into his father's business, and soon after, briefly dating only mother, they were married. The two generations lived in the same house as was still true at the time of referral.

Son B's adolescent behavior was felt by the family as a threat. This behavior was challenged as "not caring." The family response was one of increasing isolation and noncommunication. The issue of separation and independence had not been resolved in the previous generation. And, in this generation, the oldest son had made a brief attempt to go away to college and had returned. Now, under the impact of adolescence in the younger son, the family was encountering graver difficulties.

The issues of caring and independence were disentangled in the course of family sessions: Son B stated: "(Now) I feel comfortable about things. I want to go away to school not to get rid of my family, but to try independence." This became acceptable to all family members.

As a result, the learning difficulties and downward path, in which Son B had become increasingly nonfunctional in school, was reversed. In the family sessions, Son B had been brought into active interchange with other family members rather than remaining an outcast which was, at the same time, an indicator of the family difficulties and also intolerable to the family as a unit. This reinclusion of Son B was in a family role appropriate to Stage VI. He could not return as a totally dependent submissive member but there was family acceptance of him as an independent member, though still part of the family. Partial separation had been achieved.

Stage V, the exit of the first child from the family by marriage, was also a problem, as evidenced by Son A in the process of attempting this task. Some evidence of trouble appeared as he described altercations with his fiancée over the same issues as with his mother. There was little or no discussion of this soon-to-be marital pair leaving the family to establish an independent household; rather the establishment of a common household

was assumed. These difficulties were not apparent in the referral but did arise in family sessions. This aspect of family sessions and others, illustrate preventive work that may occur with family members other than the identified "troubled" referral member.

One common childhood disturbance is school phobia, when a child, physically healthy, is unable to attend school. Somatic symptoms, particularly morning stomach-aches and vomiting, are frequent symptoms. This has been described as a separation problem of a child in his interrelationship with mother, with the vicissitudes of aggression and hostility utilized as explanation of the difficulties. However, the family intertwinings are exemplified in the following case example:

An 11 year old child was referred by a school for "school phobia." Though the parents stated that the other children were normal, a family diagnostic interview was requested, and all family members were seen. The oldest son, twenty-one, returned from the army after brief unsatisfactory service. He was "staying home and doing nothing," pursuing no employment or schooling. No one in the family was particularly concerned with his state of "hanging around the house." The next sibling, a fifteen-year-old girl, was described as "sick." She was often out of school for long periods of time, with a vague and questionable diagnosis of rheumatic fever. This diagnosis had never been substantiated, her vague signs and symptoms were not questioned by the parents or other family members, and she remained home. The identified patient was often at home with "school phobia" detected by a guidance counselor. The youngest child, age seven, also spent a considerable amount of time out of school "with colds." This was acceptable to the family because, "All children are mostly sick in the early years of school." Mother, unable to drive, was very dependent upon father for any activity or errand outside the house. Father took care of them all. His job allowed him considerable "free time" which he spent at home performing many functions for family members who were "always around." The "troubled child" was identified as such, not within the family, but by the school authorities as a "problem."

This child was the only one of the younger children without marked somatic symptoms, so that his stay outside of school was not acceptable to the extrafamilial community. It is to be noted that the referral occurred after the exit of the last child into the larger community to school and at the point of an unsatisfactory attempt by the oldest child to stray from the family into the army. Thus, separation problems are prominent in all family members. In this family, the resolution of partial, exploratory, and other forms of separation were apparently absent, diminished or otherwise unsatisfactory.

Stage VII:

> Death be not proud
> Thy hand gave not this blow . . .
> And teach this hymn, aver with joy,
> The grave no conquest gets,
> Death has no sting.
>
> John Donne
"Elegy"

> Such wilt thou be to mee, who must
> Like th' other foot, obliquely runne;
> Thy firmness draws my circle just,
> And makes me end, where I begunne.
>
> John Donne
"A Valediction: Forbidding Mourning"

. . . We may not linger on this final stage of the family life cycle, the poets say.

During this stage of the last years in family life there are many changes, decreases, and diminishments, but often there are remarkable unnoticed enhancements and progressions. Some families experience a downward course to nothingness, with extremes of complication and pain, but this is not the only pattern for late family life.

Many joinings and separations have occurred during the family life cycle—from independence to interdependence, then dependence and partial separations. At this stage there are the final separations. Death may have been part of family life at earlier times, but the death of the second spouse marks the end of this stage in family development. The new families of their children will be in various stages of family development at this time and will resolve in their own way the death of their original family.

During this stage of later years in family life, the parental coalition undergoes many changes. The couple's function as parents diminishes sometimes to nothing, but, in a more successful traversal of this stage, new ways are discovered. Some families experience resolution of issues and integration only in this phase of family development. Reversal of independence to dependence may occur after the death of one parent, but is not limited to the parents. It is difficult to conceptualize and accept this phase, after the death of the second parent, but it is an end for this particular family unit.

Other Aspects of Family Development

MOTOR ACTIVITY

Every family, in the course of the family life cycle, develops an identifiable level of motor activity. The family motoric level is particularly observable in certain situations. For example, looking down on a beach where many family groups can be scanned, the differences in the activity level of each family group can be seen. They range over a spectrum, and those at the ends, the very active and the very inactive, will be noticed easily and most prominently. In early stages of family development, particularly Stages I and II, a relatively inactive motor level is harmonious with the development of the young family. But for persistently inactive families, varying amounts of strain may enter in the middle stages, as increasing numbers of children enter the larger community. At these middle stages, the extremely inactive or inflexible family will also experience difficulties from the requirements of various extrafamilial institutions. As the family moves towards the later stages, particularly the late stages of family development, the level of motor activity again can decrease.

AFFECTIVE TONE

There is a range of affective expression available to most family groups. However, a particularly striking or predominant affective tone is characteristic of some families. For example, in the anonymous atmosphere of the clinic waiting room when several families are present, the affective tone of an entire family may be observed more easily than in the therapy room with only one family. A family may be noisy, sad, even occasionally joyous, and they may be consistently characterized in this manner. This is not a reflection of the inner state of all individual family members. Here, as with the motoric level, the situations in which this can be observed are those in which other characteristics of the family are submerged and, again, extremes will be most noticeable. In the middle ranges, a wide and changing range of affective expression will be utilized. When a particularly dominant affective tone is present, there is a constriction or exaggeration of available affect range. Sad families are rather easy to identify. In these families the positive and happy affects are relatively absent. There are other predominant affective tones, such as cranky families, sharp families, bitter families, and others. The stresses of any period of family development may precipitate such a pattern. Certain affective tones may also be more characteristic for one period than for others. An inability to describe or identify affects, other than an extremely limited range, has been observed in delinquent families.[86] Individual deviations from a predominant family affective tone may be regarded as peculiar by the family.

COMMUNICATION PATTERNS

Verbal and nonverbal communications are basic instruments of family life. Normal communication patterns vary with the stage of the family life cycle. The verbal/nonverbal distribution changes in the course of family development. In Stage I, there will usually be an increasing amount of verbal and nonverbal communication as the marital pair struggles with the initial tasks. In Stage II, there must be a change in distribution, a progression that increases the nonverbal communication as the first dependent nonverbal infant joins the family. Families that do not establish these simple lines will carry deficiencies on into the next stages. For example, in the middle stages, the marked decrease in verbal communication that was experienced in Family A with two adolescent sons, described earlier, was a pattern of regression. There were changes in the course of treatment that allowed progression and an appropriate increase in verbal communication.

Difficulties in Communication Patterns: Communication gaps, monopolies, or communication exclusions of individual family members may occur throughout all family stages. For example, Family D:

A mother brought an adolescent boy for treatment because of "obnoxious behavior." The entire family was seen in family diagnostic sessions. It became quickly apparent that all verbal communication progressed through the mother who openly said, "I speak for everybody." The family pattern, in many areas, along with verbal communication was one of "mother-doing." The request for treatment, was precipitated by an adolescent surge against this pattern of "mother-doing" which included a monopoly of verbal communication with the external world by the mother. The boy's "obnoxious behavior" was a primitive and nonverbal expression of revolt against the family pattern. This boy had been silent in two previous years of individual treatment. This could then be understood not as "resistance" but rather as part of the family pattern. Out of the mother's range, where she could no longer do the speaking, all members of this family were insecure, incompetent, and inefficient. In family sessions she spoke first, and they all usually agreed.

In Stages I and II this had been tolerable for family members as primitive nurturance and care. But beginning in Stage II there were notably increasing difficulties with such a pattern. In the middle stages, and particularly for the adolescent as part of individual as well as family development, there was a necessary movement away from the family, and difficulties with the parent-dominated communication pattern came into ascendance. The "obnoxious behavior" increased as "speaking up" in the family was intolerable to the mother and other family members.

Double Bind: The concept of "the double bind" message, i.e., the simultaneous transmission of contradictory messages[12, 13] is a pattern of communication in families that has been emphasized in the literature. This concept has been described as an important component of families with a schizophrenic member and was originally described in these family units. It is, however, of more general interest, both as a mechanism of family interchange and often serves as a focus of intervention in a family.[88]

The term, double bind, is often used loosely for contradictory statements. The original definition clarifies a "double-bind" communication and requires that all characteristics must be present:

The general characteristics of this (double bind) situation are the following: 1) When the individual is involved in an intense relationship; that is, a relationship in which he feels it is vitally important that he discriminate accurately what sort of message is being communicated so that he may respond appropriately. 2) And, the individual is caught in a situation in which the other person in the relationship is expressing two orders of message and one of these denies the other. 3) And, the individual is unable to comment on the messages being expressed to correct his discrimination of what order of message to respond to, i.e., he cannot make a metacommunicative statement. (p. 374)[110]

The necessity to respond is crucial. An interested bystander noting contradictions will not experience a double-bind message and conflict. The changing patterns of communication in the course of the family life cycle have been mentioned. A prevalence of double bind messages can occur in any period of family development. In schizophrenic families, these messages seem to occur early and occupy a good portion of the communications within these families. The form of these messages and their impact will vary depending on the development of the verbal/nonverbal communication patterns within the family. Nonverbal "double-binding" contradictory communications also are important in family communication patterns and have been less stressed in the literature. The nonverbal double-bind messages start with the vulnerable infant. The progression of these nonverbal double-bind patterns to verbal double-bind patterns occurs in families with schizophrenics and others. Double-bind messages can also occur with a mixture of nonverbal to verbal interchanges in families delivering contradictory messages. No, as a verbal message and yes, nonverbally, is one type of contradiction. "Do as I say, not what I do." is a frequent message.

FAMILY HOMEOSTASIS

The concept of "family homeostasis" is derived from communication theory; family interaction, particularly communication, is viewed as a closed information system in which variations in input and behavior are fed back in order to correct the system's response:

The term *family homeostasis* is chosen from the concepts of Claude Bernard, and Cannon because it implies the relative constancy of the internal environment, a constancy, however, which is maintained by the continuous interplay of dynamic forces. (p. 79)[65]

The concept of family homeostasis implies a series of alterations in family functions, initially set off by a major internal or external change resulting in a return to a *previous* form of stability. This is an "error-activated" model in which, after an "input," the system adjusts and returns to a previously set level.

In a previous section, we have described the family life cycle, in which family relationships and interactions are in a state of continuing change over time and movement to new functional or dysfunctional levels of family development. The family is stable at any one moment or short time period, and the principle or homeostasis operates within this moment. Over longer time intervals the family is in developmental motion. Emphasis may be placed on consistency and stability, and this is often implicit and explicit when the term "system" is used. Over any small period of time a family's actions are undoubtedly patterned and the concept of family homeostasis can be applied usefully. Family interaction research has been limited to such moments and there has been relatively little exploration of interactional changes that occur over time in family development.

Disturbances in Family

Separation Processes

Separation-individuation, as a family process, occurs all through the family life cycle stages. Extreme inhibition or other, less severe, lack of progression of the separation-individuation process is a source of difficulty for all family members. In a society that places a premium on individuality, individual competence, and initiative, the focus on "fitting together" as a major component of family equilibrium leads to an inflexibility in family patterns, in which there is little accomodation to divergent needs of individuals, or in the developmental framework, little ability to shift adaptive patterns in response to changing contexts of family life.

PSEUDO-MUTUALITY

Pseudo-mutuality is a concept that frequently appears in the family literature. As Lidz says, "In describing pseudo-mutuality, we are emphasizing a predominant absorption in fitting together, at the expense of differentiation of the identities of the persons in the relations."[77]

A strong emphasis on "fitting together" may be an indication of difficulty in family development that will inhibit both family development and the development of its individual members. The middles stages of family development are particularly vulnerable to family separation problems. Pseudo-mutuality, in an extreme form, may include psychological merging of various individual family members with each other, particularly in the mother-child dyad. Pseudo-mutuality has been reported primarily in families with schizophrenic members, but can be seen in families with other problems.

ENMESHMENT

Enmeshment is another term for difficulties with family separation-individuation. It has not been defined precisely but has been utilized descriptively in clinical work with a variety of families.[83] Interesting clinical examples of enmeshment in the LaSalle and other delinquent families appeared in an early publication.[85]

Enmeshment implies more differentiation than the merging and "fitting-together" of pseudo-mutuality. The development of the family and its boundaries are wider and more extensive. Partial separations are acceptable but tangles and complications are prominent in enmeshed families.

Family Identity and Family Myth

Family identity, family flavor, and family atmosphere are characteristics difficult to define, that do exist, accompany each family, and seem to be part of its uniqueness. Sometimes a particular characteristic of a family is useful for definition, e.g., sports, in certain families, the "Hockey Howes" or the "Skiing Corcorans." In these families, all members participate actively, competitively, and have been trained extensively by their parents. Or, the family of Alexander Calder, in which three generations have been sculptors, and where this activity has certainly permeated and created the family identity. In less illustrious families, this quality is more difficult to define and yet plays an important role in family life. Family identity may change over time in the course of family development, but certain aspects of it start early, perhaps in previous generations, and continue throughout the life of the family. Fisher and Mendel[35] analyzed Rorschach data and TAT's in two or three generations of the same family. A "family flavor" appeared in their data that persisted over three generations. In more pathological families, the "shadow of an ancestor" has been described with an accompanying myth of inevitable illness.[101]

A family myth may have important prospective functions, particularly for the children present. This may strengthen and accentuate certain characteristics which are to be pursued in the lives of children within a family. When this family myth is strong and pervasive, the effect on a particular child may be very strong. It is what the child or children are to "become," and many, if not all, family members, have been influenced in this direction. The Kennedy family and their political lives are a known, easily recognized example. A family myth or myths that are additive and changeable in the course of family life are more useful for progressive and expansive development of family members.[99]

Summary: Family Development

A family developmental framework enables the seemingly inchoate continuing set of family influences to become organized and useful. These influences are not static or constant, but become predictable. The path of family development, in the course of its life cycle, can thus be traced with delineation of patterns of progression, or distortions and deficiencies. Dynamic growth changes in individual family members are contained within the family group in a sequence of family developmental stages. Certain developmental tasks have been specified as *basic family functions*. The normal development of the family requires the satisfactory resolution of these tasks, with progression and expansion in the course of family development.

PARENTAL-COALITION: THE MARITAL PAIR

Within a framework of family development, the "parental-coalition" or marital pair can be understood in full dynamic development, beginning in Stage I of family development, but with precursors in the courtship and engagement phase.[93, 96] Examined in Stage I, the couple will contain potential for progression or the precursors of later developmental problems. This parental coalition, once initially established, changes as development proceeds to meet new family issues, interactions, and relationships and at each stage of family development will have a specific range of characteristics. Of particular importance are the ways in which the parental coalition is maintained in response to new family demands and expectations at different stages, and how it is affected by differences in individual parent reaction to these changes. Thus, the birth of a new baby (Stage II) can be experienced quite differently by both parents without fundamentally disrupting a relatively flexible form of parental coalition. But, the same pattern of individual difference in response can make serious incursions on a parental coalition predicated on a rigid conception of husband-wife relationships. In a similar way, the emergence of adolescent children in the family (Stages III–V), representing a new focus of power and demand in the family, can be a basis for expanding the range and conception of the coalition between the parents, or conversely, it can threaten the entire arrangement by the development of new coalitions between one parent and an adolescent child. Flexibility and progression are as important in the parental coalition, the marital pair, as in the development of the family as a unit in the course of the family life cycle. Children are particularly vulnerable to maldevelopment, lack of progression, or other disturbances in family development.

The early stages of the family life cycle and its developmental tasks are important for understanding the contribution of family factors to disturbances of childhood and adolescence. Some families have difficulty from the outset and, in each stage of the family life cycle, experience difficulty with ensuing impairment and deviations in development.

Psychopathological Disturbances in Family Functioning

It was unpleasant coming home to have an illness.

T. S. Eliot
"The Family Reunion"

Of all the family variables, it is discord, quarrelling, unhappiness and disruption which are most consistently associated with disorder in the child.

Michael Rutter
*The Child in His Family**

INTRODUCTION

Family development, the family life cycle, and basic family functions, described in previous sections, establish a framework and baseline for discussion of some family factors affecting disturbances in childhood and adolescence. These disturbances can occur (1) at certain points in family development, and/or (2) in basic family functions with disturbances in one, many, or all of these family factors. Impairments in the normal family developmental sequence that has just been described will affect all members of the family. However, at each stage of this life cycle, children are particularly susceptible to lack of family developmental progression, fixation, or retrogression. Extreme pathological situations have revealed important clues and produced germinal work, such as the early work on infants in institutions deprived of human and, particularly, family contact. These infants, suffering from "hospitalism," brought attention to the importance of general stimulation which is usually provided by families.[106, 107] The emphasis in this early research was on the lack or absence of home, or family stimulation, as, "Even the most destitute of homes offers more mental stimulation than the usual hospital ward."[107] In another institution, weaning and subsequent loss of contact between the infants with mother occurred at three months. Stimulation was reduced to a very minimal amount. There was a subsequent rapid fall in IQ, which started at this age in these infants.

The effect of lack of human contact or other forms of early neglect occurs outside institutions, in families, and can be detected in "failure to thrive," marasmus and other similar states. Spitz elaborated a series of conditions in the first year

* From his article "Sex Differences in Children's Responses to Family Stress."

of life, in which maternal deprivation and stimulation were regarded as important etiological factors. These ranged from coma in the newborn to hypermotility (excessive rocking).[105] The symptoms of children with "failure to thrive," still within their families, bear a striking resemblance to those of "hospitalism." In these severe conditions the disturbance in basic family functions involving supplies-food may reach the extreme of survival as when child homicide is caused by starvation.

The psychosocial environment, including stimulation, primarily by mother, is part of a general family atmosphere and may range from weak, minimal, and neglectful to strong, overstimulation, and battering. There are many forms of psychosocial disturbances in which significant, if not causative, factors lie within the family. In pediatrics and public health, there are symptom groups in which strong "social," interpersonal causes within the family have been identified;[90] these "illnesses" include failure to thrive, accidents and ingestions, child abuse and neglect, pica and poisoning with lead based paint, rumination, excessive bottle feeding (often with iron-deficiency anemia as a consequence), "idiopathic" feeding disorders without demonstrable organic cause, "habit" disorders, learning disability, hyperactivity, and bronchial asthma. The particular vulnerability of the young child to family stress and neglect is emphasized in this list. Maltreatment may cause reversible and irreversible damage to intellectual development as indicated by the fall in IQ and in other developmental areas. These syndromes of maltreatment can be understood and classified by utilization of a family developmental framework, in which distortions and omissions in family development are determined.

The discussion of the battered child has broadened from a narrow definition in 1962[72] to the more general concern with child abuse and neglect. In these families with gross difficulties in nurturance (food-supplies), therapeutic endeavors have also noted strengths[71] which may be in family functions other than nurturance. There has been identification of "battered children" where disturbances have existed in families for at least two generations.[51, 71, 89, 90] Battering, severe neglect, and abuse occur in many forms, some as physical beatings with detectable bruises, but also with hidden bruises and/or with sexual molestations.

Severe psychopathological conditions illustrate clearly the effect of disturbed family functions. Family factors have been described in (1) schizo-

78

phrenia, (2) delinquency, and (3) in a group with pan-phasic disturbances, the *multi-problem* or *chronic* problem families.

FAMILY FACTORS IN FAMILIES WITH SCHIZOPHRENIC MEMBERS

The bonds of love and hate that exist in every family occur in an extreme form and with exaggerated intensity in the families of schizophrenics. Distortions of these bonds of love-hate are present in all members of a schizophrenic family. The need for early, partial, and continuing separation is established at the moment of birth and goes on through the life of every child and member of a family. In disturbed families, often with schizophrenic members, separations or differences are experienced as destructive and are accompanied by extremes of hate and violence. These difficulties and lack of separation have been termed symbiosis, particularly in the mother-child relationship. But, all members are affected, and this is not simply separation anxiety. A mother in such a family said, "We are all peaceful. She likes peace even if I have to *kill* someone to get it—a more normal happy kid (with her brothers and sisters) would have been hard to find." She was describing her family, and the "normal happy kid" was the schizophrenic daughter prior to hospitalization.

In the early 1960s, several groups of researchers pursued their interests in understanding the families of schizophrenics.*

Peculiarities, deficiencies, distortions, and other difficulties can be seen in these families in many areas of family functioning, starting early in the family life cycle. Laing[73] included some longitudinal histories of families along with description of disordered family processes which were entitled "mystification." Much of this work has emphasized communication patterns as basic mechanisms of disturbance in family life. As these researchers ventured beyond the inner world of the schizophrenic patient to their families, communication patterns were described in the mother-child dyad, and then extended to at least three members of the family.[110]

The "double-bind" mechanism, an initial mechanism noted in these families, provide incongruent conflicting levels of communications to which the child or other family member *must* respond, and then each response is labeled as wrong. This double-bind pattern of communications, among others, is an example of family factors which will

* See references 5, 11, 12, 21, 37, 50, 54, 63, 66, 67, 77, 78, 79, 80, 81, 99, 110, 113, 114.

influence particularly, child members of a family. The cognitive development of the child is seriously interfered with when any response that he must make, to many messages, is labeled as wrong. There will be difficulties in the development of learning sequences in the young child who must then maneuver between two wrong messages. The outcome will be seen in disturbances of thought processes and other integrative functions. Pseudomutuality, scapegoating, sick-role reinforcement and mystification are additional mechanisms that were identified in these families.*

PSEUDOMUTUALITY

Pseudomutuality, originally described in families with a schizophrenic member, is a description of an engulfing family atmosphere with implicit and explicit rules about communications and other expressions.[113] There is a complete or almost complete dismissal of divergences. There are dire consequences to openly recognizing divergences or pursuing individuation-separation issues within the family. The communication system will include massive use of double-bind messages in the service of obliterating and dismissing divergences.

MYSTIFICATION

Mystification has been used as a descriptive unifying concept in work in families with schizophrenic members. Stress for the parents in these families is not so much the loss of self in the merging and fusion of symbiotic relationships, but the development of any specificity or particular identity. Any personalization, realization, autonomy, or spontaneity is seen and identified as illness. The total mystification process will include many contradictory attributions, inconsistencies, and multiple disagreements. Family members cannot tell the difference from these statements about "what was and what was not."[73]

"Masking" is another mechanism that has been identified in these families. This is a particular form of mystification. The family agrees that something does not exist, or if it does, then don't ask about it. This may be done through lies or other kinds of pretenses. For example:

In Family X an adolescent had experienced serious difficulties including expulsion from school due to bizarre behavior. Whenever outside visitors came, the family pretended that this member was still in school. During these visits, the adolescent member automatically went to the basement so that his pres-

* See references 17, 34, 78, 104, 113.

ence was not apparent and the family could tell their stories more easily. Other family members agreed that this arrangement was "beneficial" and age-appropriate since in the basement this member was "free" to think his own seemingly idiosyncratic thoughts, which at times, approximated reality but a considerable portion were in disagreement with family statements. The adolescent experienced not being in school, but the family had many ways of stating the opposite.

The frequent occurrence of such mutually contradictory experiences is "training in irrationality"; this may be provided many times a day in family life.[78] Ordinary logic will not suffice, and paralogical thinking becomes necessary in the explanations of such experiences. Amorphous and fragmented styles of communication also have been noted.[114]

Pervasive and enduring difficulties for both parents and children, throughout formative years influence the functioning of all family members. The failure of integration in schizophrenic members of a family, some researchers ascribe to the faulty integration of the family as a unit.[77] Bizarre family patterns can be noted at times in normal and less disturbed families. But, it is likely that when communication and other difficulties predominate, then these factors will have a particularly serious influence on integrative functions in its members, and in some, schizophrenia is seen.

FAMILY FACTORS IN DELINQUENCY

We can understand children telling lies, when in doing so, they are imitating the lies told by grownup people, parents.
"Infantile Mental Life: Two Lies Told by Children"
Sigmund Freud

Psychopathy is probably the best documented form of intrafamilial learning of abnormal behavior. Young psychopaths often act out overt and covert wishes of parents who themselves may not misbehave grossly.
Adelaide Johnson and S. A. Azurek
*Psychoanalytic Quarterly**

We frequently see parents who describe the child's delinquent behavior with pleasure . . . the normal parent neither anticipates impending disaster nor dismisses monetary or other transgressions as trivial . . . the apparent mystery of adolescent homicides can be quickly dissipated if adequate background material is available . . . we could hardly believe the material given by this well-dressed, intelligent, attractive woman (mother) . . . she described wanting to "mutilate, stab, slice her throat, in relation to her daughter."
Mary Griffin, Adelaide Johnson, and Edward Litin
American Journal of Orthopsychiatry†

* From their article "The Genesis of Antisocial Acting Out in Children and Adults."
† From their article "Specific Factors Determining Anti-Social Acting Out."

The influence of family, particularly parents, is evident in the above quotations. Communication by direct transmission, of delinquent messages from parent to child is frequent and often obvious:

Two young sisters were apprehended and referred for evaluation after repeated shoplifting episodes; these included many handbags and other small items. The family consisted of mother and two daughters. Father had deserted immediately after the birth of the second child. The second pregnancy was complicated and an unexpected hysterectomy was performed. Mother described her feelings of emptiness following the hysterectomy and in subsequent early years of their family life. Her mood brightened as she described recent years. She said enthusiastically with eyes sparkling, "I told the girls to bring their bags, their gifts, back to me." She remembered telling the girls that she had wanted a larger family and how much she enjoyed them as infants. There was an oft-repeated family joke: "We—mother—need a baby to feel better." Early in adolescence the older sister became pregnant and presented this "new gift" to mother. The baby was eagerly received and mother reared the baby as if it were her own. The biological mother became "Sis" and grandmother was "Mom." Shoplifting was continued by the younger sister who, at that time, was not yet able to provide babies. The messages in this family were direct, from mother, and received and acted upon by the daughters as subsequently reported in treatment sessions.

The delinquent activities in this family were persistent, unavoidably connected with mother, and inevitable. The younger daughter also became pregnant in early adolescence. In this two generational one parent family, the ties were close. Delinquent patterns and messages were easily recognizable, strong and difficult to change.

PARENTAL COALITION: ROLE REVERSAL
IN DELINQUENCY AND INCEST

Parents serve as guides, educators, and models for offspring. Though individuals, as parents they function as a coalition, dividing roles and tasks in which they support one another.
Theodore Lidz
The Family and Human Adaptation

Family separation-individuation processes have been described in previous sections. The parental coalition is central in this process, with the development of mutual dependency between parents an integral component of the coalition. Weakness, blurring, distorted dependencies, or more complete lack of appropriate coalition in any stage of family development will have particularly negative effects upon the children. When there is weakness in the parental coalition, the child may become the bridge and spend considerable energy in closing the gap. Or, the child may become the villain, and the gap be attributed to the presence of the child in an overly strong alliance with one or the other of the parents. This is recognizable as a scapegoating maneuver.

Distorted development of coalitions is seen in role reversals. In these reversals generational boundaries become blurred: (a) One parent may use a child to fulfill the needs and position that the other parent would be in if strong generational boundaries existed; (b) The parents may rival for a child to be placed incorrectly within the generational boundary; (c) Boundaries may be distorted and the generational boundary weakened by strong mother-son or father-daughter relationships; (d) One parent may act like a child rather than a spouse, transgressing the generational boundaries completely.

When generational boundaries are weak and role reversal has occurred, there may be strong sexual wishes on the part of one parent for the child of the other sex. The maintenance of these gender linked roles within strong generational boundaries is important in aiding and diminishing incestuous tendencies particularly in adolescence. This is a function of the family as a system and not of one parent.

INCEST

Incest, the universal crime, violates a taboo that is as forceful among primitives as among sophisticated moderns. It is behavior that disrupts or destroys the social intimacy and sexual distance upon which family unity depends. . . . These processes of personality development could be traced back to early and later family influences. The two extremes of family organizations which influence the attitudes of the incest offenders pertained either to their inability to deflect their sexual desires to members outside the family, or to their inability to become and remain sensitized to family sex constraints. (p. 93)[111]

The strong, universal taboo against incest has prevented extensive examination of the family aspect of this problem. The mother's role in permitting, aiding, or even abetting a father-daughter incestuous relationship has, in the past, been said to have been embedded in the unconscious and it is! Or, father-dominance has been utilized as an explanation.[111] Interviews with family members indicate that overt actions within the entire family will show compliance,[70] if not actual provocation of incestuous relations and, within the parental coalition, role reversals:

In incest Family A:
Mother would fight with the husband and then immediately rush upstairs to the apartment of maternal grandmother. Father's sexual relations with the daughter, during her latency years, occurred only during these upstairs "absences" of mother. When she became adolescent, father discovered her engaging in sexual activity with young men, angrily took her home to mother, and complained about her sexual involvement with these "other boys." The daughter, upset and angry, told her mother for the first time about the long incestuous relationship with father. Early history revealed many areas of role reversal. Throughout her childhood, daughter rather than mother, had made father's daily lunches and taken care of all the younger siblings, in addition to the ongoing sexual relationship with father.

The parental coalition in this instance was weak and the daughter had taken over a major portion of the maternal roles with compliance and encouragement by the mother. The role reversal included not only the sexual relationship, but other basic family functions, particularly the nurturance and socialization of the other siblings. The maintenance of the role reversal was strengthened by all family members including siblings who benefited by the nurturance supplied by the sister-mother. The behavior of some of these incestuous girls, after being taken away from their families, while living in group homes, has been described as "regressed." Regression or becoming childlike in a new family may occur because they have been given permission to behave like a baby, in a situation that will provide nurturance for themselves.

In incest Family B:
From the outset, mother and father experienced many kinds of strain in their relationship, which over the years became overtly distant. Mother ousted father from their bed and when he went to sleep in another room, she would put her daughter in bed with the father. When asked about these actions, she said she felt "sorry" for him and took the daughter to him. Thus, early on in family life, daughter functioned in the place of mother, and these maneuvers maintained within bounds the family structure and tension levels within this household.

Incest is one of many familial mechanisms, including role reversals, that attempt to mitigate the strains between mother and father. Individual sexual difficulties or perversions are part of the intrapsychic paternal structure and function within a complementary family equilibrium. Incestuous girls may experience sexual relations as warm and giving, perhaps restituting for the nurturance and care that they themselves are providing within the family. Often, there are limitations and deficiencies in other basic family functions, including a more general inadequacy of supplies and nurturance. And, at times of severe family crisis and disequilibrium, extrusion of the incestuous child may be utilized as one means of attempting to reduce the strains and multiple needs of the family members.

This discussion of incest has not specifically mentioned the many forms of incestuous behavior, i.e., father-daughter, mother-son, brother-sister combinations. Particular distortions in family relationships occur in each of these incestuous patterns. However, it is not the intent of this chapter to focus incest, but rather to use it as an example of the influence of family factors on sexual development and sexual relationships within the family.

CHRONIC PROBLEM FAMILIES

There is another group of severely disturbed families that illustrate difficulties starting early in the family cycle, in all or almost all of the basic family functions, that have been entitled *multi-problem or chronic problem families*.[92, 93, 116] Delinquency, incest, and schizophrenia may co-exist in these families. The disturbances are broad, panphasic during the family life cycle and affect many basic family functions. These families and their difficulties should be considered as an entity, rather than as examples of individual varieties of pathology or disturbance. Multi-problem families have been described generally as poor, deprived, and disturbed, and, when examined as a unit, the chaos and disorganization begin to form patterns of insufficient or distorted development of basic family functions through the family life cycle:

Mrs. J. sat slumped in the midst of a dilapidated filthy apartment with her feet up on a soiled hassock, one of the few pieces of family furniture, uttering constant, mostly monosyllabic contradictory commands to her adolescent daughter. Mr. J. sat motionless and quiet. Past family history indicated that from the outset *food* had never been consistently available, but this was noted only by teachers when the children were hungry in school. The adolescent daughter lit the fire and did all the cooking for the entire family. Housing-shelter was grossly inadequate in a small wooden, unrepaired, private house. The family had experienced many relocations as agencies had placed them in more adequate surroundings in housing projects. The family had been evicted from these apartments due to complaints made about them for inadequate care and damage done by the unsupervised younger children to the apartment and outer premises of the project. Finances had been a long and constant problem with sporadic employment of any family members including the father. However, even when the funds were supplied by public agencies, the income was variable. Mother's reports to the welfare agency managed to cause funds to be reduced until the needs of the family would be evident in a periodic crisis and then there would be budget increase.

Finances-income from public agencies, and less from employment, went up and down according to the interactions of mother and others with employment and welfare agencies. As the children grew older, there were involvements and difficulties with many community agencies, schools, and courts. The earlier family life, in the grandparent generation, also indicated insufficiencies and severe deprivations.

This example is from a "poor family" in which economic circumstances are intermingled with severe deficits in all spheres of family functioning in at least two generations. These involve housing, food, finances, and health. At each junction in the family life cycle severe developmental difficulties cause the addition of more public and other service agencies, as these families attempt to deal with their needs.[85, 92, 116] This is a brief summary of one of these families. The profile of difficulties varies, including, in some families, an emphasis on one area such as health with medical emergencies, chronic disabilities, and multiple psychosomatic illnesses, or in another family, emphasis on a variety of antisocial behaviors. Thus, if all family members are included in an evaluation, difficulties will be detected in many more members and with more impeded functions than were originally presented to any one agency or clinician.

PSYCHOSOMATIC AND OTHER CHILDHOOD ILLNESSES: ANOREXIA NERVOSA AND EATING DISORDERS

The transactional patterns within a family with an anorexic son are reconstructed, from psychotherapeutic sessions and family conferences, to illustrate the occurrence of serious (familial) disturbances under the facade of seemingly normal functioning (p. 307).[24]

Family factors and disorder in the family scene have been described in childhood eating disorders. As in other areas, early studies on obesity concentrated on the individual child, then the mother-child dyad and, recently, the family environment. It is curious how often the presence of gross disturbances of food supply and other distortions of nurturant functions, including bizarre food rituals, are overlooked.[25]

Case example: Three massively overweight members of a family were admitted in succession to an inpatient diet program. They all did well as in-patients but regained to previous levels and beyond upon return to family life, though all stated that they were continuing on the program. A family interview revealed the father also was massively obese. After recognition occurred of family compliance with intricate patterns of stress and hostility intermingled with gross overeating, one member was able to begin weight reduction within the family. At this time, he recalled the detailed discussions with the nutritionist on the in-patient service. The amount and patterns of eating had not been available to him for accurate description until some disentanglement from the family had taken place.

Immediate life-saving endeavors in the treatment of anorexia nervosa necessarily concentrate on the individual sick patient. The families of anorexia nervosa patients often insist upon their "normality" and present an outward appearance of a well-educated, rather average, aspiring family. There is an intense hostile struggle over food after the onset of symptomatology. Knowledge of early family history and development is limited, though it has become an area of recent research interest. There is consensus among several authors that the early family situation is distorted and further investigation is underway to distinguish among families with particular disorders in their members.[10]

Feeding requires the active participation of another family member from shortly after birth. Later the family atmosphere around the dinner table or wherever eating occurs, may range from "being actively hit in the gut" to an atmosphere of implacable steely rigidity. In the eating disorders, the struggle around this function has been ascertained but differentiation awaits further research. In recent studies, physiological and biochemical determinations were made in the course of family interviews, so that members' responses to family stress could be physiologically measured and documented. Behavioral events, stressful interactions, among family members were measured in the bloodstream of other family members as they happened.[83]

In families with psychosomatic illness, interesting shifts occur when all family members are included in therapeutic sessions. In a family with one asthmatic child and one with obesity, as the concern changed to obesity, the asthmatic child's symptoms markedly diminished. The influence of the family on development of psychosomatic illness in the child has been related to three factors: (1) a particular type of family organization and functioning; (2) involvement of the child or children in parental conflict, and (3) physiological vulnerability. The latter is still somewhat vague and unspecified.[24]

These families are characterized by enmeshment, overprotectiveness, rigidity, and a lack of conflict resolution. The physiological vulnerability of the child seems to be a necessary but not sufficient component of psychosomatic illness. (p. 242–243)[83]

TREATMENT IMPLICATIONS

Some illustrative family factors in child and adolescent disturbances have been described. Examples and clinical descriptions have referred to family sessions, family treatment, or other kinds of family observations. Freud, in the historic Dora case[47] referred to the importance of "family circumstances," and in "Little Hans,"[45] the actions and statements of both parents, but particularly the father, were utilized to understand and treat the phobic illness.

As early as 1936 in her classic monograph on ego psychology, Anna Freud[41] indicated the need for direct therapeutic alliance with "external forces" . . . in the form of "those responsible for the child's upbringing."

Nevertheless, a little child is not a being of unbridled instinct nor, in ordinary circumstances, is it aware of the pressure of instinctual anxiety within it. In the external world, i.e., in the educational influences brought to bear upon it, its feeble ego had a powerful ally against its instinctual life. The situation does not arise in which it has to measure its own puny strength against the very much stronger instinctual impulses, to which, if left to itself, it must inevitably succumb. We hardly leave it time to become aware of its own wishes or to estimate its own strength or weakness in relation to its instincts. Its attitude towards the ego is simply dictated to it by the promises and threats of other people, that is to say, by the hope of love and the expectation of punishment.

Under such external influence little children, in the course of a few years, acquire a very considerable capacity for controlling their instinctual life, but it is impossible to determine how much of this achievement is to be attributed to their ego and how much to direct pressure by external forces. (pp. 154–155)[41]

These "external forces" of the parents were considered important and became an integral part of psychoanalytic therapy of children, though defined as "education."

Family therapy as a distinct clinical area of interest, therapeutic practice, and research is relatively recent in origin. In the 1950s there was considerable direct interest in research and treatment of the family.* New forms of therapeutic intervention progressed from an individual sick patient and his mother to the family as an entire unit and have provided extensive data on family processes and family intervention. In 1961 Bell published a monograph entitled *Family Group Therapy*,[16] and by 1964 a summary text of conjoint family therapy had appeared.[100] Since that time there has been a steady burgeoning of this literature.†

---

* See references 13, 22, 27, 54, 64, 69, 77, 82, 110, 113.
† See references 1, 3, 14, 15, 33, 36, 60, 83, 94, 115, 118, 119.

Therapeutic work with families has been done in conjunction with descriptive research. Direct observation of families (entitled "deroofing") has investigated the families of psychotic patients including their off-spring and verified earlier impressions of serious developmental effects on these children.[8, 97, 98]

The details of family therapeutic endeavors are beyond the scope of this chapter. This chapter has presented a family orientation and developmental framework beyond the individual child to all members of the family, in which some family factors have been described. Family therapy as a research endeavor has played an important role in elucidating the structure of family dynamics, and thus has facilitated further understanding of family influences in the development of child and adolescent disturbances.

Summary and Conclusion

The family is the basic psychosocial unit into which children are born and in which they develop. That process continues with the creation of another family and the cycle repeats itself.

The family as a "unity of interacting personalities" has been described through a progression of developmental stages. This process of change, with joinings and separations occurring over the life span of a family, has been a recurring theme within this chapter. The *epigenetic* model,[32, 33] in which each phase of a development is based on the accomplishment of and successful progression through the preceding phase, has been a second principle underlying this material. The developmental framework has been explicated in relation to the family as it impinges on the development of child members. Concurrent development by family members as a unit and interaction among family members have been stressed rather than intrapsychic development. Interpersonal and inter-experiential observation of the whole family is an important method of family research and treatment. Dynamic changes over time, largely responsive to life cycle changes which affect whole families, have been defined and described as a sequence of stages in family development.

Some fundamental characteristics of the family have been emphasized. The changing patterns of basic family functions including nurturance, dependence, and socialization, have been traced. Tasks during stages of family development, the changes in these tasks, and the changing character of the same task have been specified as basic family functions. The normal development of a family requires the satisfactory and effective resolution of these tasks. In the process, families undergo progressive changes and alterations or, in pathological instances, reveal an inability to change basic patterns of family functioning in response to new demands.

The basic family functions previously described are strong influences on each child. In the life of any particular child, some family factors and certain periods in the family life cycle may be particularly influenced in the development of childhood disturbances. These have been discussed in schizophrenia, delinquency, incest, and psychosomatic illnesses including anorexia nervosa and psychogenic obesity. The need for early, partial, and continuing struggles with separations is established at the moment of birth and continues through the life of a child and of every member of a family. Even very young infants, living primarily in the parental bedroom who continue to be close, and may become almost part of mother, also may experience adequate separation, if this is accomplished by the family unit as a whole. Later, in individual and family development, oedipal resolution in each family member may be affected by the lack of adequate boundaries and/or instability or partial separations.

Distortion in familial communication patterns such as predominant use of double bind messages, enmeshments, and other mechanisms have been described in severely disturbed families. These mechanisms are present in the daily lives of less disturbed families but not to such an extent as to interfere with developmental sequences necessary for satisfactory family progression. The predominant use of such mechanisms inhibits the adequate maintenance of generational boundaries in the course of the family individuation-separation process.

Such factors operating within the family life cycle have been shown to be a strong and continuing influence on individual child members of a family. Examples of families in family therapy have been utilized to exemplify these influences on the development of psychopathological conditions.

REFERENCES

1. ACKERMAN, N. W., *Treating the Troubled Family*, Basic Books, New York, 1966.
2. ——, *Psychodynamics of Family Life*, Basic Books, New York, 1958.
3. ——, BEATMAN, F. L., and SHERMAN, S. N. (Eds.), *Exploring the Base for Family Therapy*, Family Service Association of America, New York, 1961.
4. ACKERMAN, N. W., PAPP, P., and PROSKY, P., "Childhood Disorders and Interlocking Pathology in Family Relationships," in Anthony, E. J., and Koupernik, C. (Eds.), *The Child in His Family. The International Yearbook for Child Psychiatry and Allied Disciplines*, vol. 1, pp. 241–267, John Wiley, New York, 1970.
5. ALANEN, U., "Some Thoughts on Schizophrenia and Ego Development in the Light of Family Investigations," *Archives of General Psychiatry*, 3:650–656, 1960.
6. ALBERTI, B., "Della Famiglia," in Anthony, E. J., and Koupernik, C. (Eds.), *The Child in His Family. The International Yearbook for Child Psychiatry and Allied Disciplines*, vol. 1, John Wiley, New York, 1970.
7. ANTHONY, E. J., "The Influence of Maternal Psychosis on Children-Folie à Deux," in *Parenthood: Its Psychology and Psychopathology*, pp. 571–599, Little, Brown, Boston, 1970.
8. ——, "The Mutative Impact of Serious Mental and Physical Illness in a Parent on Family Life," in Anthony, E. J., and Koupernik, C. (Eds.), *The Child in His Family. The International Yearbook for Child Psychiatry and Allied Disciplines*, vol. 1, pp. 131–163, John Wiley, New York, 1970.
9. ——, and BENEDEK, R. (Eds.), *Parenthood: Its Psychology and Psychopathology*, Little, Brown, Boston, 1970.
10. ANTHONY, E. J., and KOUPERNIK, C. (Eds.), *The Child in His Family. The International Yearbook for Child Psychiatry and Allied Disciplines*, vol. 1, John Wiley, New York, 1970.
11. BATESON, G., "The Biosocial Integration of Behavior in the Schizophrenic Family," in Ackerman, N. W., Beatman, F. L., and Sanford, S. (Eds.), *Exploring the Base for Family Therapy*, Family Service Association of America, New York, 1961.
12. ——, et al. "A Note on the Double Bind," *Family Process*, 2:154–161, 1963.
13. ——, et al., "Toward a Theory of Schizophrenia," *Behavioral Science*, 1:251–264, 1956.
14. BELL, J. E., *Family Therapy*, Jason Aronson, New York, 1975.
15. ——, "The Future of Family Therapy," *Family Process*, 9:127–141, 1970.
16. ——, *Family Group Therapy*, Public Health Monograph No. 64, Public Health Service Publication No. 826, U.S. Government Printing Office, Washington, D.C., 1961.
17. BELL, N. W., and VOGEL, E., "The Emotionally Disturbed Child as the Family Scapegoat," in Bell, N. W., and Vogel, E. (Eds.), *A Modern Introduction to the Family*, Free Press, Glencoe, Ill., 1960.
18. ——, (Eds.), *A Modern Introduction to the Family*, Free Press, Glencoe, Ill., 1960.
19. BENEDEK, T., "Parenthood as a Developmental Phase," *American Journal of Psychiatry*, 1:389–417, 1959.
20. BOSZORMENJI-NAGY, I., "The Concept of Schizophrenia from the Perspective of Family Treatment," *Family Process*, 1:103–113, 1962.
21. BOWEN, M., "A Family Concept of Schizophrenia," in Jackson, D. D. (Ed.), *The Etiology of Schizophrenia*, Basic Books, New York, 1960.
22. ——, "Family Relationships in Schizophrenia," in Auerback, A. (Ed.), *Schizophrenia: An Integrated Approach*, pp. 147–178, Roland Press, New York, 1959.
23. BOWLBY, J., "The Study and Reduction of Group Tensions in the Family," *Human Relations*, 2:123–128, 1949; Reprinted in Erickson, G. D., and Hogan, T. P. (Eds.), *Family Therapy: An Introduction to Theory and Technique*, Jason Aronson, New York, 1976.
24. BRUCH, H., "Family Background in Eating Disorders," in Anthony, E. J., and Koupernik, C. (Eds.), *The Child in His Family. The International Yearbook for Child Psychiatry and Allied Disciplines*, vol. 1, pp. 285–309, John Wiley, New York, 1970.
25. ——, and TOURAINE, G., "Obesity in Childhood V. The Family Frame of Obese Children," *Psychosomatic Medicine*, 2:141–206, 1940.
26. BURGESS, E. W., "The Family as a Unity of Interacting Personalities," *The Family*, 7:3–9, 1926; reprinted in Erickson, G. D., and Hogan, T. P. (Eds.), *Family Therapy: An Introduction to Theory and Technique*, Jason Aronson, New York, 1976.
27. CARROLL, E. J., "Treatment of the Family as a Unit," *Pennsylvania Medical Journal*, 63:57–62, 1960.
28. CHRISTENSEN, H. T., *Handbook of Marriage and the Family*, Rand McNally, Chicago, 1964.
29. DUVALL, E. R., *Family Development*, Lippincott, New York, 1957.
30. ELLIS, G., "The Mute Sad-Eyed Child: Collateral Analysis in a Disturbed Family," *International Journal of Psycho-analysis*, 43:40–49, 1962.
31. ERICKSON, G. D., and HOGAN, T. P. (Eds.), *Family Therapy: An Introduction to Theory and Technique*, Jason Aronson, New York, 1976.
32. ERIKSON, E. H., "Identity and the Life Cycle," *Psychological Issues*, 1:1–171, 1959.
33. ——, *Childhood and Society*, W. W. Norton, New York, 1950.
34. ESTERSON, A., *The Leaves of Spring: Schizophrenia, Family, and Sacrifice*, Tavistock Publications, London, 1970.
35. FISHER, S., and MENDELL, D., "The Communication of Neurotic Patterns over Two or Three Generations," *Psychiatry*, 19:41–46, 1956; also in Bell, N. W., and Vogel, E. (Eds.), *A Modern Introduction to the Family*, pp. 616–622, Free Press, Glencoe, Ill., 1960.
36. FLECK, S., "An Approach to Family Pathology," *Comprehensive Psychiatry*, 7:307–320, 1966; also in Erickson, G. D., and Hogan, T. P. (Eds.), *Family Therapy: An Introduction to Theory and Technique*, pp. 103–119, Jason Aronson, New York, 1976.
37. ——, "Family Dynamics and Origin of Schizophrenia," *Psychosomatic Medicine*, 22:333–344, 1960.
38. FLUGEL, J. C., *The Psychoanalytic Study of the Family*, Hogarth Press, London, 1921.
39. FONTANA, V. J., *The Maltreated Child: The Maltreatment Syndrome in Children*, Charles C Thomas, Springfield, Ill., 1971.
40. FREUD, A., *Normality and Pathology in Childhood: Assessments of Development*, International Universities Press, New York, 1965.
41. ——, *The Ego and Mechanisms of Defense*, International Universities Press, New York, 1946.
42. FREUD, S., "Project for a Scientific Psychology," in *The Standard Edition of the Complete Psychological Works of Sigmund Freud* (hereafter, *The Standard Edition*), vol. 1, pp. 283–399, Hogarth Press, London, 1966.
43. ——, "Family Romances," in *The Standard Edition*, vol. 9, pp. 235–245, Hogarth Press, London, 1950; also in *Collected Papers of Sigmund Freud*, vol. 5, pp. 74–78, Basic Books, New York, 1959.
44. ——, "On the Sexual Theories of Children," in *The Standard Edition*, vol. 9, pp. 205–226, Hogarth Press, London, 1959; also in *Collected Papers*, vol. 2, pp. 59–75, Basic Books, New York, 1959.

45. ——, "Analysis of a Phobia in a Five-Year-Old Boy," in *The Standard Edition*, vol. 10, pp. 3–153, Hogarth Press, London, 1958; also in *Collected Papers*, vol. 3, pp. 149–289, Basic Books, New York, 1959.

46. ——, "Infantile Mental Life: Two Lies Told by Children," in *The Standard Edition*, vol. 12, pp. 303–311, Hogarth Press, London, 1958; also in *Collected Papers*, vol. 2, pp. 144–149, Basic Books, New York, 1959.

47. ——, "Fragment of an Analysis of a Case of Hysteria," in *The Standard Edition*, vol. 7, pp. 7–122, Hogarth Press, London, 1953; also in *Collected Papers*, vol. 3, pp. 13–146, Basic Books, New York, 1959.

48. ——, "Three Essays on the Theory of Sexuality," in *The Standard Edition*, vol. 7, pp. 125–234, Hogarth Press, London, 1953; also in *Three Essays on the Theory of Sexuality*, Basic Books, New York, 1963.

49. FRIED, M., *The World of the Urban Working Class*, Harvard University Press, Cambridge, Mass., 1973.

50. FRIEDMAN, A. S., *Psychotherapy for the Whole Family*, Springer, New York, 1965.

51. GALDSTON, R., "Observations on Children Who Have Been Physically Abused and Their Parents," *American Journal of Psychiatry, 122:*440–443, 1965.

52. Group for the Advancement of Psychiatry (GAP): Committee on the Family, *The Case History Method in the Study of Family Process*, vol. 6, Report No. 76, 1970.

53. GIFFIN, M. E., JOHNSON, A., and LITIN, E., "Specific Factors Determining Anti-Social Acting Out," *American Journal of Ortho-Psychiatry, 24:*668–684, 1954; also in "The Transmission of Super Ego Defects in the Family," in Bell, J. E., and Vogel, E. (Eds.), *A Modern Introduction to the Family*, pp. 623–635, Free Press, Glencoe, Ill., 1960.

54. HALEY, J., "The Family of the Schizophrenic: A Model System," *Journal of Nervous and Mental Disease, 129:*357–374, 1959.

55. HARTMANN, H., *Ego Psychology and the Problem of Adaptation*, International Universities Press, New York, 1958.

56. ——, "Psychoanalysis and Developmental Psychology," in Eissler, R. S., et al. (Eds.), *The Psychoanalytic Study of the Child*, vol. 5, pp. 7–17, International Universities Press, New York, 1950.

57. HELFER, R. E., and KEMPE, C. H. (Eds.), *The Battered Child*, 2nd ed., University of Chicago Press, Chicago, 1974.

58. HENRY, J., *Pathways to Madness*, Random House, New York, 1965.

59. HILL, R., "Methodological Issues in Family Developmental Research," *Family Process, 3:*186–206, 1964.

60. HOWELLS, J. G., *Family Psychiatry*, Oliver & Boyd, London, 1963.

61. JACKSON, D. D., "Family Rules: The Marital Quid Pro Quo," *Archives of General Psychiatry, 12:*589–594, 1965.

62. ——, "The Study of the Family: Family Rules," *Family Process, 12:*589–594, 1965.

63. —— (Ed.), *The Etiology of Schizophrenia*, Basic Books, New York, 1960.

64. ——, "Family Interaction, Family Homeostasis, and Some Implications for Conjoint Family Psychotherapy," in Masserman, J. (Ed.) in *Individual and Familial Dynamics*, Grune & Stratton, New York, 1959.

65. ——, "The Question of Family Homeostasis," *Psychiatric Quarterly Supplement, 31:*79–90, 1957.

66. ——, and SATIR, V. M., "Family Diagnosis and Family Therapy," in Ackerman, N., Beatman, F. L., and Sherman, S. M. (Eds.), *Exploring the Base for Family Therapy*, Family Service Assn., New York, 1961.

67. JACKSON, D. D., and WEAKLAND, F. G., "Schizophrenic Symptoms and Family Interaction," *Archives of General Psychiatry, 1:*618–621, 1961.

68. JOHNSON, A. M., and SZUREK, S. A., "The Genesis of Antisocial Acting Out in Children and Adults," *Psychoanalytic Quarterly, 21:*323–343, 1952.

69. JOSSELYN, I. M., "The Family as a Psychological Unit," *Social Casework, 34:*336–343, 1953.

70. KAUFMAN, I., PECK, A., and TAGIURI, C., "The Family Constellation and Overt Incestuous Relations between Father and Daughter," *American Journal of Orthopsychiatry, 24:*266–277, April, 1954; also in Bell, N. W., and Vogel, E. (Eds.), *A Modern Introduction to the Family*, Free Press, Glencoe, Ill., 1960.

71. KEMPE, C., and HEFNER, R. E. (Eds.), *Helping the Battered Child and His Family*, Lippincott, Philadelphia, 1972.

72. KEMPE, C., et al., "The Battered Child Syndrome," *Journal of the American Medical Association, 181:*1, 1962.

73. LAING, R. D., and ESTERSON, A., *Sanity, Madness and the Family*, Tavistock Publications, London, 1964.

74. LEBOVICI, S., "The Psychoanalytic Theory of the Family," in Anthony, E. J., and Koupernik, C. (Eds.), *The Child in His Family. The International Yearbook for Child Psychiatry and Allied Disciplines*, vol. 1, pp. 1–19, John Wiley, New York, 1970.

75. LIDZ, T., "The Family as the Developmental Setting," in Anthony, E. J., and Koupernik, C. (Eds.), *The Child in His Family. The International Yearbook for Child Psychiatry and Allied Disciplines*, vol. 1, pp. 19–41, John Wiley, New York, 1970.

76. ——, *The Family and Human Adaptation*, International Universities Press, New York, 1963.

77. ——, "Schizophrenia and the Family," *Psychiatry, 21:*21–27, 1958.

78. ——, et al., "The Intrafamilial Environment of the Schizophrenic Patient: VI. Transmission of Irrationality," *Archives of Neurology and Psychiatry, 79:*305–316, 1958.

79. ——, et al., "The Intrafamilial Environment of the Schizophrenic Patient: IV. Parental Personalities and Family Interaction," *American Journal of Orthopsychiatry, 8:*764–776, 1958.

80. ——, et al., "The Intrafamilial Environment of Schizophrenic Patients: II. Marital Schism and Marital Skew," *American Journal of Psychiatry, 114:*241–248, Sept. 1957; also "Schism and Skew in the Families of Schizophrenics," in Bell, J. E., and Vogel, E. (Eds.), *A Modern Introduction to the Family*, pp. 595–606, Free Press, Glencoe, Ill., 1960.

81. ——, et al., "The Intrafamilial Environment of the Schizophrenic Patient: I. The Father," *Psychiatry, 20:*329–342, 1957.

82. MIDELFORT, C., *The Family in Psychotherapy*, McGraw-Hill, New York, 1957.

83. MINUCHIN, S., *Families and Family Therapy*, Harvard University Press, Cambridge, Mass., 1974.

84. ——, "Conflict-resolution Family Therapy," *American Journal of Orthopsychiatry, 28:*278–286, 1965.

85. ——, et al., *Families of the Slums: An Exploration of Their Structure and Treatment*, Basic Books, New York, 1967.

86. ——, et al., "The Study and Treatment of Families Who Produce Multiple Acting-Out Boys," *American Journal of Orthopsychiatry, 34:*125–132, 1964.

87. MISHLER, E., and WAXLER, N., *Interaction in Families: An Experimental Study of Family Processes and Schizophrenia*, John Wiley, New York, 1968.

88. ——, "Family Interaction Processes and Schizophrenia: A Review of Current Theories," *Merrill-Palmer Quarterly, 11(4):*269–315, 1965.

89. NEWBERGER, E. H., "The Myth of the Battered Child Syndrome," *Current Medical Dialogue, 30:*327, 1973; reprinted in Chess, S., and Thomas, A. (Eds.), *Annual Progress in Child Psychiatry and Child Development*, pp. 569–573, Brunner-Mazel, New York, 1975.

90. ——, and McANULTY, E. H., "Family Intervention in the Pediatric Clinic: A Necessary Approach to the Vulnerable Child," *Clinical Pediatrics, 15(12):*1155–1160, 1976.

91. PARSONS, T., and BALES, R. F., *Family: Socialization and Interaction Process*, Free Press, Glencoe, Ill., 1955.

92. PAVENSTADT, E. (Ed.), *The Drifters*, Little, Brown, Boston, 1967.

93. PHILIP, A. F., and TIMMS, N., *The Problem of "The Problem Family,"* Family Service Units, London, 1957.

94. RAKOFF, V., SIGAL, J. J., and EPSTEIN, N. B., "Working-Through in Conjoint Family Therapy," *American Journal of Psychotherapy*, 21:782–790, 1967; reprinted in Erickson, G. D., and Hogan, T. P. *Family Therapy: An Introduction to Theory and Technique*, pp. 306–315, Jason Aronson, New York, 1976.

95. RAPAPORT, R., "The Transition from Engagement to Marriage," *Acta Sociologica*, 8:36–55, 1964.

96. RAUSCH, H. L., GOODRICH, D. W., and CAMPBELL, J. D., "Adaptation to the First Years of Marriage," *Psychiatry*, 26:368–380, 1963.

97. RUTTER, M., *Children of Sick Parents*, Oxford University Press, London, 1966.

98. ———, "Sex Differences in Children's Responses to Family Stress," in Anthony, E. J., and Koupernik, C. (Eds.), *The Child in His Family. The International Yearbook for Child Psychiatry and Allied Disciplines*, vol. 1, pp. 285–309, John Wiley, New York, 1970.

99. RYCKOFF, I. M., DAY, J., and WYNNE, L. C., "Maintenance of Stereotyped Roles in Families of Schizophrenics," *Archives of General Psychiatry*, 1:93–98, 1959.

100. SATIR, V. W., *Conjoint Family Therapy: A Guide to Theory and Technique*, Science & Behavior Books, Palo Alto, 1964.

101. SCOTT, R. D., and ASHWORK, P. L., "The Shadow of the Ancestor: A Historical Factor in the Transmission of Schizophrenia," *British Journal of Medical Psychology*, 42(1):13–32, 1969.

102. SPECK, R. V., and ATTNEAVE, C. L., *Family Networks*, Random House, New York, 1973.

103. SPIEGEL, J., "The Resolution of Role Conflict Within the Family," in Bell, N. W., and Vogel, E. F., *The Family*, pp. 361–381, The Free Press, Glencoe, Ill., 1960.

104. ———, and BELL, N. W., "The Family of the Psychiatric Patient," in Arieti, S. (Ed.), *American Handbook of Psychiatry*, Basic Books, New York, 1959.

105. SPITZ, R., "The Psychogenic Diseases in Infancy: An Attempt at Their Etiologic Classification," in Eissler, R. S., et al. (Eds.), *The Psychoanalytic Study of the Child*, vol. 6, pp. 255–274, International Universities Press, New York, 1951.

106. ———, "Hospitalism: A Follow-up Report on Investigation Described in Volume I, 1945," in Eissler, R. S., et al. (Eds.), *The Psychoanalytic Study of the Child*, vol. 2, pp. 113–117, International Universities Press, New York, 1946.

107. ———, "Hospitalism: An Inquiry into the Genesis of Psychiatric Conditions in Early Childhood," in Eissler, R. S., et al. (Eds.), *The Psychoanalytic Study of the Child*, vol. 1, pp. 33–72, International Universities Press, New York, 1945.

108. VOGEL, E., and BELL, N., "The Emotionally Disturbed Child as the Family Scapegoat," *A Modern Introduction to the Family*, pp. 382–397, Free Press, Glencoe, Ill., 1960.

109. WATZLAWICK, P., "A Review of the Double Bind Theory," *Family Process*, 2:132–153, 1963.

110. WEAKLAND, J., "The 'Double Bind' Hypothesis of Schizophrenia and Three-party Interaction," in Jackson, D. D. (Ed.), *The Etiology of Schizophrenia*, Basic Books, New York, 1960.

111. WEINBERG, S. K., *Incest Behavior*, Citadel Press, New York, 1955.

112. WOLFF, S., and ACTON, W. P., "Characteristics of Parents of Disturbed Children," *British Journal of Psychiatry*, 114:593, 1968.

113. WYNNE, L. C., et al., "Pseudomutuality in the Family Relations of Schizophrenics," *Psychiatry*, 21:205–220, 1958; also in Bell, N. and Vogel, E. (Eds.), *A Modern Introduction to the Family*, pp. 573–595, Free Press, Glencoe, Ill., 1960.

114. WYNNE, L. C., and SINGER, M. T., "Thought Disorder and Family Relations of Schizophrenics: II. A Classification of Forms of Thinking," *Archives of General Psychiatry*, 9:199–206, 1963.

115. ZILBACH, J. J., "The Family in Family Therapy," *Journal of the American Academy of Child Psychiatry*, 13, 3:459–468, 1974.

116. ———, "Crisis in Chronic Problem Families," *International Psychiatry Clinics*, 8(2):87–99, 1971.

117. ———, "Family Development," in Marmor, J. (Ed.), *Modern Psychoanalysis*, pp. 355–368, Basic Books, New York, 1968.

118. ZINNER, J., and SHAPIRO, R., "The Family Group as a Single Psychic Entity: Implications for Acting Out in Adolescence," *International Review of Psychoanalysis*, 1:179–187, 1974.

119. ZUK, G., and BOSZORMENYI-NAGY, I., *Family Therapy and Disturbed Families*, Science and Behavior Books, Palo Alto, 1967.

4 / Sociocultural Factors in Etiology

David Looff

Children do not grow up in a vacuum. They cannot be understood apart from the historical, geographic, and socioeconomic characteristics of the area in which they develop. As evaluators, we are reminded, ever and again, that the children we see are members not only of families but also of wider groups whose training patterns affect them a good deal. To do our work well, we need to be aware of these cultural patterns; only then will we be able to understand the child's own functioning and that of his family in an adequate way.

Regional Child Development

The growing-up process of children in any region can be defined operationally as the acquisition of a particular set of facts and skills. One aspect of its success is measured by the rapidity with which the child achieves the goals set for him by his environment. Thus, the structure of adult society and the function of the family unit within this larger framework provide a context within which the growing child interprets his experience. This context also provides a kind of mental set with which both the child and the adult approach new experiences. Viewed in this manner, regional training patterns, which vary from one region or one culture to another, are economical. The consistency with which they are set and maintained is important, of course. It allows us to be comfortable in our own environment. It facilitates the acquisition of the generally efficient behaviors we describe as acculturation or socialization.

The point can be made that these regional training demands are extremely complex and their details vary from one culture to the next. But their outline is universal: the child is expected to master the basic abilities that his environment requires for biologic and social life. In our culture, and most others, these abilities, outlined here as a list of individual personality characteristics of the child, or ego functions, include:[9, 10, 14]

1. Intellectual capacity.
2. Capacity for purposive and coordinated movement.
3. Degree of attainment of the orderly habits of eating and excretion, of regular cycles of sleep and wakefulness, and of a variety of self-help tasks.
4. Degree of attainment of understandable communication and social language.
5. Capacity for object relations with parents, other adults, siblings, and peers.
6. Degree of attainment of well-modulated expression of emotional reactions to the environment.
7. Nature of self-concept, self-awareness, and self-esteem.
8. Reality testing—this includes the child's perceptual capacities, and other cognitive functions.
9. Nature of superego operations (conscience and ego-ideal)—the degree of the child's acceptance of prohibitions and sanctions, prevailing customs, and ideas of decency.

10. Degree of attainment of an orderly pursuit of knowledge and education.
11. Adaptive or integrative capacity—including capacity for meeting and mastering tasks; capacity for understanding and synthesizing the thoughts and feelings connected with events; the capacity for self-observation; the capacity to store tension, which includes the level of frustration tolerance, the level of inner controls on impulses, and the ability to delay gratification; the capacity to sublimate feelings; and the capacity to remember and to recall events.
12. Current level of psychosocial and psychosexual development—with reference to the various stages of development, including an assessment of fixations, regressions, or developmental deviations.
13. Basic personality structure (basic life-style).
14. Areas of psychological conflict—and whether the conflicts in the child are largely external, or internal, or both.
15. Predominant defensive and adaptive capacities (coping, or ego defense mechanisms).
16. Degree of impairment in capacity for physical development, play, learning, or socialization.
17. An assessment of the degree to which all of these abilities, or ego-functions, have been integrated into behavior in the child that is well balanced between the family's and the community's expectations for him and his own self-interest.

In measuring the personality characteristics of an individual child along these, or any other parameters, the clinician draws his impressions both from the character of child development in a particular region and from the results of that development—the mental health or mental disorder of the child himself. In doing this, the clinician presents his perceptions of the ways in which present-day families raise their children in a given region and his clinical conclusions concerning the kinds of adjustments to life that these children are making.

EXAMPLE

The Southern Appalachian region will be used here as a paradigm for the way an evaluator considers the various sociocultural factors in diagnosis. The way of life in this area offers us an example of highly individual cultural patterns. The families provide here training patterns, or models for their children's behavior which are relatively undiluted by social institutions outside the family. The close-knit, interdependent, extended family system is the only major social unit. It therefore holds a unique place as a child training climate. More often than not, the few social institutions available outside the families there have, to date, served merely to reinforce the established training patterns. These patterns appear to have been remarkably consistent within the region through several generations.[15]

At this point, the reader may raise the objection that the use of the Southern Appalachian region (or any other region) as an example of cultural child-rearing practices is too parochial, too limited a model. But the important point that is intended here, through the use of this particular region as a paradigm, is that each clinician must develop an intimate knowledge of the highly individual cultural patterns of the particular region in which he is working, if he is to evaluate adequately the children he sees whose lives are affected by such patterns. Only through an in-depth understanding of how children grow in his region can the clinician gain a valid, balanced perspective of how some cultural practices convert to children's symptoms and psychopathology, but other practices lead the children, at the same time, to function in more adaptive ways.

The point was made earlier that to know the children, wherever we study them, requires some knowledge of the lives of parents, teachers, and the many others upon whom they depend. Thus, perhaps the first step toward understanding the child rearing patterns of a given region is to examine the life style of the adults among whom the child grows.

Regional Adult Life Styles—An Example: At the end of the last century, and more recently in our own time, sociologists and anthropologists have written a great deal about the life style of the Southern Appalachian highlander. In summary, this has consisted largely of a careful cataloguing of the highlander's methods of adapting to his circumstances. According to these writers, the mountaineer's attitudes developed primarily during the last century, but continue to be maintained largely unchanged to the present day. Much of this writing has focused on the life style of the very poor or of the region's working class. However, most of the writers assert that a substantial legacy of values, standards, attitudes, and adaptive methods has come down to Appalachian people of all three socioeconomic classes from their common mountaineer background.* Like legacies anywhere, it is a heritage of both strengths and weaknesses, of attitudes adequate to direct the daily lives of people who habitually use them, and practices that are inadequate for the tasks at hand.

These writers focused initially on the fierce independence that characterized the early settlers in the southern mountains. It was an absolutely essential trait for survival. The hill families lived in geographic isolation. This reinforced the pattern of each individual's depending upon his own talent, strength, and resourcefulness. Thus, cooperative social activities were rare in mountain life; families made their own way. In time isolation, interacting with independence worked a change in the old self-reliance of the highlander. His independence became individualism, a more self-centered trait. Whatever he does, he is himself the focus. Group activities are engaged in only to the extent that his private ends are served.

A second significant trait of the mountaineer is traditionalism. He is bound to the past, its traditions, ideas, and values. Through the years his outlook has been regressive, to the old ways. These traditions maintained the mountaineer in an existence-oriented society, whose goals amounted to meeting only the very basic survival needs. Unlike the contemporary middle-class American, the tradition-oriented highlander is not improvement oriented, nor does he anticipate the future with any measure of confidence.

Within the mountain subculture a third trait, fatalism, was gradually developed. It served to help cope with the chronic sense of failure the highlanders experienced as their land limited and defeated them. Fatalism enabled the mountaineer to feel his life was fundamentally right even when it was discouraging. The trait found no clearer expression than in mountain religion. All Protestant denominations and sects in the region accept hard lives and times as "God's will—He wants it this way. Who am I to complain?"

A fourth characteristic of the mountaineer was his action orientation. Like the natural rhythms of hill life about him, he was episodic and impulsive. These traits, again, were opposed to the routine-seeking orientation of the American middle class. The mountaineer avoided routine-oriented events and institutions as boring, not satisfying. He disliked steady, time-oriented jobs, regular churchgoing, and other activities calling for a methodical application of time and personal effort.

Another characteristic trait was the mountaineer's stoicism. In adapting to the daily apprehensions of his rigorous life with its many stresses, he turned inward, covering his intense anxieties with silence and denial. There are observers who surmise that this underlying fearfulness finds open expression in one characteristic child-rearing practice: children are often made to obey through

* See references 3, 7, 8, 11, 12, 18, 23.

fear. "If you don't mind, something will happen to you—you'll get hit on the road by the truck, or someone will take you away from here." This particular child-rearing practice expresses the mountaineer's long-standing, realistic concern that the outside environment is, indeed, often harsh, cruel, and fear provoking.

A final characteristic of the mountaineer was his person orientation. He personalized his thoughts, words, actions, and relationships. He was oriented not toward objects—outside goals, principles, things, jobs—but toward people. His concern was to be a person within his group, but accepted as an individualist. His constant desire to be noticed and liked by other members of his group in this way was in itself a major life goal. It accounted for the mountaineer's deep sensitivity to real or implied criticism of himself by others. On the other hand, the trait underscored the deep abiding person-to-person relationships that, in time, are often made with others. And it underscored as well the exquisite orientation to and sensitivity about the feelings of others the mountaineer possesses.

Thus, during the transitional period of history between the frontier and today, the Southern Appalachian highlander was required, perhaps inevitably, to develop the personality traits of individualism, traditionalism, religious fatalism, an action orientation, stoicism in manner and speech, and an intense person orientation. These traits enabled him to adapt to the stresses of a time that followed the passing of the frontier. The same traits in essentially unchanged form continue to be shared in today by many present-day Appalachian people. As a result, it is exceedingly difficult for the person possessing these traits to adapt to the relatively impersonal, goal-oriented, routine-seeking ways of most contemporary Americans.

REGIONAL CHILD TRAINING THEMES

Thus, clinicians do well to start their work with children by reviewing the studies of other social scientists such as sociologists and anthropologists, so that they are firmly in context with regard to understanding the life styles of the child-rearing adults in the particular region. Or, as part of their preparation they may include background work of their own with regard to examining the relevant developmental themes for children in a given area. Either way, it is imperative that they explore these critical-for-children's growth themes prominent in any region, each in its turn, and all

in their interaction as they overlap and influence one another. This step is essential before they begin dealing with the clinical problems presented by troubled children. Such a study seeks to define the normal developmental base line in a particular region or subculture. Only from this can the events which represent pathological personality deviations or which represent normality in the children under study be determined. Such factors are critical in so heterogeneous a culture as America.

Example: These same personality traits outlined earlier, taken in aggregate, give characteristic color to all interpersonal relationships in present-day Appalachia. In particular, they permeate the interactions of parents and their children. Those who have worked in the Southern Appalachian region have long familiarity with the strong familistic orientation of the area's lower and middle classes (and to some extent, of the upper class as well). The major dynamic characteristic of these families is their close interdependent functioning. They are markedly inner-directed, with an overriding sense of obligation to extended-family members. Within such a family system, children are taught from birth in both verbal and nonverbal ways to maintain this family closeness. They are taught to do so even at the expense of an individual family member's personal-social maturation. In such a context, the individual's own growth and development are clearly subordinate to the prime task of maintaining the family as a tight knit unit.

The author has elsewhere speculated[15] that this intense familism is trained into the children; it begins with an observable pattern of parental overemphasis on the infancy period itself. This early pattern is strongly reinforced by later events. The families persist in employing infantile modes in the course of relating with their children through subsequent stages of child development. Moreover, as development proceeds, there is a consistent parental pattern of underemphasis on children's autonomy, initiative, curiosity, exploration, and adequate sex-role differentiation.

A second prominent training theme in the Southern Appalachian region emerges from the lower-class families' inability to supervise their wandered-off toddlers, preschoolers, and even older children appropriately. When the children are close by, parents generally display the overprotective, indulgent, permissive behavior characteristic of the children's infancy. The children's response to such treatment is typical: they run free, following any impulse when they are away from adults. And they react with varying degrees of infantility—clinging, whining, demanding, basking in the pleasure of being babied—when they return. As they begin to use the autonomy that the development of motor-muscular skills makes possible, sooner or later these children will actually get out of sight of the parents. At this point, they are often treated by these same parents as though they no longer exist. As a result they frequently get into situations of real or potential danger.

It may be that Southern Appalachian lower-class parents see the child's emerging autonomy as a threat to their complete domination and possession of him; they deal with the threat by denying it. When the child does come to them, this is taken as a sign that he wants them in their familiar caretaking role.

Inevitably, however, these lower-class children continue to grow, and then, for the most part, the adults simply stop playing with them. They supervise them inappropriately, and furnish no positive models or training in setting limits on impulse. They establish no disciplinary controls, and they give no preparation for age-appropriate relating to or talking with other adults. These patterns are most evident in families of the very poor and the working class, but, in a somewhat attenuated way, they hold true for the middle and upper classes as well.

A third prominent training theme in the region emerges from conflicts around sexual development, maturation, and functioning. Although present in all socioeconomic classes, again the conflict seems most acute in lower-class and working-class families. For them, the open overcrowding necessitated by poverty serves in itself to create numerous tensions, sexual as well as nonsexual. It is also true, as several writers have emphasized, that the prevalent strict Protestant ethos is a powerful force in maintaining a conflicted view of sexuality in the region.[13, 21]

The life styles of their parents, the closeness and inner-directedness of the extended-family units, and the operation of the three training themes mentioned above act collectively as a powerful shaping force on the development of very many Southern Appalachian children. As a consequence, they proceed through middle childhood, adolescence, and adulthood in fairly characteristic ways. They are warm, open, personable, friendly, sensitive, feeling-oriented persons who are, nonetheless, frequently overly dependent and overly inhibited with regard to sexual maturation and functioning. In addition, the lower or working-class family children are frequently wild and impulsive and have difficulties in using language as a tool.

This composite picture of a representative child's functioning is based on the training forces at work in families from a given region. As clinicians it gives us essential insights as we prepare to meet with troubled children from the area. Obviously, such representative pictures of children can never set aside our detailed evaluation of the individual child and his family in a clinical setting. Nevertheless, such pictures, and the regional training themes on which they are based, alert the clinician to what he may well find as he assesses the psychopathological problems and ego strengths of the individuals he evaluates.

Regional Psychopathology

The family and the community define "disorder" in a child. They view it as that state in which the child complies poorly or not at all with family training demands. "Pathology" is the manner in which this noncompliance becomes manifest. Usually the younger the child, the less will family and community expect of him, and the less likely will unusual behavior be considered as evidence of disorder. However, as he gets older more is required of him, and, accordingly, the wider the variety of disorders to which he can be subject. What the family and the community do expect reflects their experience with other children of the same age in the community. As he grows up, every child is constantly measured against his peers. His relative successes or failures in defining, meeting, and mastering various tasks are constantly compared with the progress made by other children. But, these peer norms, so publicly derived, cannot be applied, by either the family or the clinician, too rigidly. For not only does the overall rate of development vary widely among children, but the rate of growth for different skills in a given child may be quite uneven.

Since each child's maturation depends on the orderly acquisition of skills, and since each new skill becomes part of the foundation for the next, even a mild slowing or unevenness in development can sometimes give the appearance of gross abnormality. The identification of abnormal behavior in a child is further complicated because behavior that is considered pathologic at one age may be common or even universal at another. For example, headbanging, thumbsucking, and rocking are very common in infants and toddlers. Crying spells, temper tantrums, bedwetting, nightmares, hyperactivity, dialogues with imaginary playmates, and refusing to eat, to go to bed, to greet visitors, or to separate from parents to go to Sunday School are among the many kinds of behavior that are regarded as normal in the child up to the age of four or five. In an older child they would be indicative of a disorder. On the other hand, the overt expression of sexual interest is regarded as normal after puberty but abnormal before that age.

REGIONAL PEER NORMS

Nonetheless, peer norms for the various ego functions are still the best yardsticks against which clinicians can measure children from a given region. Such norms are also the guides used by others. The children referred for mental health evaluation have been designated as having emotional or learning problems by other persons in their cultural setting—parents, teachers, local physicians, public health nurses, courts, and other agencies. The initial designation of these referred children as in some way maladjusted is arrived at by those in the community who know them. It is essentially a culture-determined definition based on peer norms for various behaviors.

REGIONAL CULTURE AND PSYCHOPATHOLOGY

The frequency and severity of various psychopathological symptoms in any given population are probably affected very strongly by social relations and cultural values. Joseph W. Eaton and Robert J. Weil, for example, feel the data they gained from a mental health study of a Hutterite population fits this theory well.[5] Adult patients in the Hutterite group had chiefly those neurotic symptoms which were socially acceptable in their culture. They took their tensions out on themselves by internalizing them as depression or psychophysiologic responses. Phobic and obsessive-compulsive reactions, which would violate strong cultural taboos, were rare. Within their highly structured social system, Hutterite individuals also were sufficiently sheltered and guided to make generalized anxiety reactions rare. A similar study of a Norwegian community has been reported by Johann Brenner.[2] Those who have a strong social learning theory orientation to child development tend to view much of psychopathology as primarily involving learned behaviors, which are reinforced by environmental influences. Those

whose orientation to child development is a psychoanalytic-psychodynamic one, tend to view psychopathology (excluding, of course, acute and chronic brain syndromes) as involving aberrant ways in which the individual internalized the communications, feelings, and behavior characteristics of the significant other persons in his upbringing. Both groups, obviously, are underscoring the rising generation of their children.

Clinicians need to understand how families in a given region raise normal children, what they do that enables children to cope relatively successfully with various development tasks. Such an understanding provides a yardstick; it can be used to make clinical estimates of the successes and failures in life adjustment of the children referred for evaluation.

As time passes, however, work with the children and the families in a given region will progress and more and more clinical data will accumulate. Some linkages will begin to appear between regional developmental themes and both the psychopathology and the ego strengths of the children. Ultimately, what is done in the clinics will rest upon the proposition that to understand the children in a given region, their problems and their prospects, it is necessary to look at the entire field of regional developmental forces. Which ones are involved in change? Which tend to cause stagnation? This kind of knowledge cannot be arrived at simply by speculation. It is necessary for the clinician to look intensively into at least some of the more critical components of regional child development. Only when he does this is he in an optimum position to perceive any of the correlations between development and its outcome—the derivatives of that specific pattern of development for those children.

REGIONAL PSYCHOPATHOLOGY—AN EXAMPLE

A well-known and oft repeated observation of those who have worked in the Southern Appalachian region is the strong familistic orientation of the area's lower and middle classes. To some extent this holds true for the area's upper class as well. Close, interdependent functioning is the major dynamic characteristic of these families. They are markedly inner-directed, and, within such a family system, children are trained in obligatory closeness—from birth on they are taught in both verbal and nonverbal ways to maintain the integrity of this close family system, even at the expense of an individual family member's personal-social maturation.

Clearly related to this, is the frequency with which separation anxiety is a major source of emotional conflict for these children and their parents. Any hint of actual, threatened, or even symbolic disruption in parent-child or in other family relationships begets great concern. During his twelve years of clinic association with the child psychiatry field clinics in the region, the author and his colleagues found separation anxiety the most prominent causal conflict in children who came to clinic with the following psychopathological disorders:

1. *Acute and Chronic School-Phobic Reactions:* Through the years, 20 percent of the field clinic's caseloads represent children of all ages and both sexes who have this disorder—a prevalence figure approximately ten times greater than comparable data from urban clinics in Baltimore, Cincinnati, and Lexington, Kentucky.

2. *Deviations in Social Development:* The infantilized, overprotected preschool child represents another 15 percent of the field clinics' caseloads—a prevalence figure approximately ten times greater than that available from the cited urban clinics.

3. *Overly-Dependent Personality Disorders:* These children from the late middle childhood and adolescent groups make up another 15 percent of the field clinics' caseloads.

4. *Various Psychophysiologic Reactions:* Prominent among these are cyclic vomiting in younger elementary-school-age children, and bleeding duodenal ulcers in adolescent girls.

5. *Interactional (symbiotic) Psychosis:* As a form of psychosis in young children, this condition is only rarely seen in urban clinic populations. In one decade eight Southern Appalachian children with this disorder were found; and this was only from among those who attended field clinics held in just four rural counties—having a total population of approximately 74,000 persons (of all ages)—in Eastern Kentucky.

A study was conducted of the current interactional patterns and earlier training patterns of families of each such child. In each case, marked evidence of training in obligatory closeness was found, coupled with rigorous training in avoiding any separation that would disrupt the close family system. The conclusion was drawn that this training trend in the clinic families could best be understood in terms of the regional pattern of child rearing. It represented an exaggerated degree of, or pathogenic overuse of, that focus on infancy and training in closeness that had been noted in previous surveys of Southern Appala-

chian child development, both by the author and by others.[6, 15]

An equally striking finding was the absence of certain conditions: the primary behavior disorders, or impulse-ridden personalities. These conditions tend to arise wholly or, in large part, from emotional deprivation in infancy. Such disorders simply did not appear in these Southern Appalachian clinic children.

These data seem to suggest the following hypothesis: the normal regional familism (training in close, interdependent family functioning) can be overused by families in the course of child rearing. It then acts as a strong, specific force that shapes those later psychopathological disorders in the children which are based on dependency themes and related separation anxiety. Furthermore, this same familism prevents the formation of those specific types of children's psychopathology that arise from extreme emotional deprivation in infancy.

It has been noted that a second prominent training theme in the Southern Appalachian region emerges from conflicts in the area of sexual development, maturation, and functioning. In a survey of normal child development in this area, this was present in the great majority of the families studied. Although noted in all socioeconomic classes, the conflict seemed most acute in lower-class and working-class families. In these homes, the open overcrowding necessitated by poverty created many tensions, sexual as well as others. The youngsters who emerged from this background had greater problems in inner-impulse controls. It is also true that the strict Protestant ethos is a powerful force in maintaining a conflicted view of sexuality in the region.

There is a relatively frequent occurrence of emotional disorders in Southern Appalachian children and adults based primarily on sexual conflict. The clinical findings suggest that in some families this is clearly related to a pathological exaggeration of the regional sexual attitudes. In particular, sexual conflicts were prominent in those children presenting with the following psychopathological disorders: hysterical or conversion reactions; dissociative reactions; hysterical personality disorders (in adolescent girls); and various other types of personality disorders (as in adolescent boys with underlying psychosexual identity problems).

Clinicians and researchers who have studied hysteria in different population groups have sometimes found sources of conflict other than sexuality to be prominent in persons having these disorders. One writer, for example, felt that in a series of adult men studied in an eastern-seaboard Veterans Administration hospital, conflicts over hostile, aggressive impulses were crucial to the development of various conversion reactions.[22] This would suggest that sexual conflict is probably not a universal etiologic factor in hysteria. There are many clinicians[1, 16, 20] who view hysteria as primarily a disorder of communication, resulting from the inability of the afflicted person to verbalize his conflicted feelings. The conflicts themselves vary from one individual to another. Moreover, in an overwhelming majority of those who develop hysteria in the Southern Appalachian region, the field data support the thesis that sexual conflict, regionally determined, is present. In another region, sexuality may not be so conflictual, or other themes may be more conflict-laden.

Earlier it was mentioned how frequently verbal communication is a problem among Southern Appalachian families. This regional taciturnity constitutes a third prominent training theme. Many Southern Appalachian children and adults, particularly from among the lower class, have enormous difficulty in using words as tools. Both school data and clinical experience illustrate the problem. The sparseness of the language training provided by many families in the region seems clear enough. Evident, too, are the resulting deficiencies in language performance. One can wonder how regional language disorders of this magnitude come about.

The first consideration regarding language usage grows out of the characteristic functioning of the lower-class Appalachian family. This family system is held together by norms of obligation and not necessarily by bonds of affection. Close, interdependent family ties involve training of the children in obligatory closeness; closeness frequently becomes a training end in itself. Situations that are viewed as potentially disruptive of close family ties are warded off. The existence of this trained-in feeling of obligation toward other family members, coupled with an absence of or at least an attenuation of ties based on affection, places a severe emotional strain upon each individual. This includes a sense of guilt; the person does not feel as he thinks he should toward other family members. This state of strain may help to explain some of the intensive internal conflicts as well as some of the striking lack of verbal communication inside families.

Presumably, then, the most severely stressed families would show the greatest lack of verbal communication. Many feel that this explains why the families having the greatest strains from many sources, have the greatest problems in using words as tools. As one impoverished mother put it: "I can't speak, when all my burdens sit so heavy on my chest." This would also explain, the author feels, why the most socially isolated families have children whose emotional problems, such as elective mutism, involve nonverbal themes. These children had fewer experiences of talking matters over with anyone other than their siblings. Their social contacts had been largely limited to their own strained, silent families.

There are frequent occurrences of emotional disorders in Southern Appalachian children and adults based wholly or in large part on the afflicted individual's inability to express conflicted feelings in words. In some of the families this seems to be related to a pathological exaggeration of the regional verbal conflict. Nonverbality was found to be prominent in the very large group of field clinic children having psychophysiologic, dissociative, and conversion reactions. In these conditions the communication problem is as essential for the development of the disorder as are the underlying dependency or psychosexual conflict themes. Nonverbality was also of prime etiologic importance in those children presenting with elective mutism. Overall, these were conditions that could be regarded primarily as disorders of communication. In addition to the available clinical data, school experience demonstrates that many children from the lower class in the area are very poor readers and talkers. This would tend to confirm the adverse effects of regional nonverbality on the course of intellectual-cognitive development in these cases.

A fourth prominent training theme was also mentioned earlier. It has to do with the failure of Southern Appalachian lower-class families to train their young children in acquiring a capacity to store tension. These children very frequently grow up to be wild, impulsive (albeit warm, personable, outgoing, and friendly) older children, adolescents, and adults. They are not trained to acquire inner controls on their impulses. As a result, they present problems that arise from their impulsiveness, problems for themselves and, primarily, for others. For example, they abruptly might wander into and out of marriages, jobs, and other major life tasks. They often strike out at others aggressively or steal what they want, acting on the sudden whim of the moment. Should they marry and have their own children, their impulsiveness often presents a problem for their families. Their employers, the courts, and other social agencies typically find themselves coping with similar difficulties.

These four child-developmental patterns—training in dependency, training in psychosexual conflict, training in nonverbality, and training resulting in poor impulse controls—are prominent in the Southern Appalachian region. They may also be found throughout the rural South as well as in some other countries and cultures. Taken together, the four themes have a joint importance. They form the basis for much of the psychopathology observed in the Appalachian field clinics over the past twelve years. This is underscored by the following figure: roughly 90 percent of all the children seen in the field clinics during this period came with disorders arising from one or more of these four themes.

Regional Personality Strengths

To emphasize that certain regional training forces can lead to psychopathology is to present only half the developmental picture. As specific regional training themes are examined closely, they are found to be two-edged swords. One edge clearly has to do with the cultural shaping of mental disorders. But the other edge is also of critical importance. It involves the cultural shaping of healthy aspects of personality functioning. These are basic to ego strengths with which individuals solve their problems and overcome their difficulties.

SOUTHERN APPALACHIAN FAMILY AND INDIVIDUAL STRENGTHS—AN EXAMPLE

In every phase of work in the Southern Appalachian region, again and again, one finds it almost impossible to overemphasize the significance of regional familism. As it operates through the close, extended-family or kinship system, its influence frequently takes the form of providing strength for the area's families. The traditional tendency of the Southern Appalachian is to cope with stress of all kinds by turning inward upon his close family system. Hence, in times of need or crisis, people in this region will share themselves and their often-meager resources with one another. Such a turning-to-each-other provides a very real basis for continued emotional and economic support for many individuals. More than that, it also engages the extended family in delightful reunions and other get-togethers. These are of enormous importance in assuring the individual's place in a person-oriented society.

Thus, regional familism stabilizes many aspects of Southern Appalachian family life. It makes for coherent family structure and provides a model for its functioning. This positive side of familism makes for a certain steady state. This holds true even for very poor families whose manifold problems are the most vexing, both for themselves and for others. In this respect the Appalachian poor are unlike the socially disorganized poor in the urban slums. The mountain dwellers possess a strength that can be tapped to assist their lives in many areas. Indeed, regional familism accounts for two further strengths in the Appalachian individual's personal functioning.

The first is a marked capacity for essentially trusting relatedness. In and out of the clinics, when one meets Southern Appalachian adults and children, initially they tend to be shy, reserved, and somewhat suspicious toward outsiders. They soon drop this initial guardedness, however, and relate in ways that are quite personal and often very intense. In time, the adults and children made good use of the relationship aspects of treatment; they were able to involve themselves in interviews with remarkable warmth and candor. Many of these families were geographically and culturally outside the mainstream of county life. Nonetheless, they related with the clinic staff generally with no sense of personal isolation. In fact, their relatedness often combined such warmth, openness, and earthiness that it suggested the traditional spontaneity of young children. There were none of the layers of sophistication that so often mark and impede initial treatment interviews with other families. Such qualities of relatedness enabled the interviewers to focus very quickly on family functioning.

Many of the families referred to the mental health clinics were action oriented, primarily in search of symptomatic relief for crisis situations. As a result, the mutual capacity for relationship of interviewer and parents had to be utilized quickly as the basis for helping a given family redirect its efforts with the children. Parents tried out redirective suggestions more readily because they had quickly established a bond with this outside person.

It is of considerable clinical interest to note that the basic capacity for relatedness seemed to cross socioeconomic class lines. For example, the often grubby, ragged children of the lower class who came to clinic were frequently wild, impulse ridden, and manipulative. But along with these traits was a warm way of reaching out to others that had the quality of an essential relatedness.

A review of the developmental backgrounds of many of these children led to the conclusion that they are well trained in basic relatedness from infancy on. However, they are not trained nearly as well in acquiring controls over their aggressive impulses. As babies and older children these lower-class children are well liked; but in many areas they are allowed to do just as they please. Beyond infancy, appropriate developmental supports involving a balance between gratification of need and capacity to delay along with the achievement of limits and controls are not readily maintained by the lower-class families in the area. This seemed to account for the difficulties that beset many of the older lower-class children; they had trouble with perceptual skills needed for orienting to a new environment, with communication skills, and with capacities to delay gratification and to establish internal impulse controls. But during infancy, the lower-class as well as the middle- and upper-class families gave freely of themselves to their children. As an outgrowth of this, the children retained a considerable measure of the ability to relate with others in spite of difficulties with other capacities.

There is a second strength that is also a positive derivative of regional familism. For both the Southern Appalachian adult and child, an unusual feeling-orientation emerges from this background, a capacity to experience deeply and to differentiate exquisitely the feeling-content of one's experiences. The early training in family closeness and relatedness seems central here. An outgrowth of this early training is the skill in observing and correctly interpreting the often subtle nonverbal behavior of people who are often relatively silent. Early in such training, the child learns to pick up feeling-oriented cues from the behavior of adults, rather than from their words. Often enough, with some support from a competent interviewer, people from the region who have been trained to have this exquisite feeling-orientation can be helped to verbalize what they so accurately perceive.

These capacities for relatedness and feeling-orientation have implications for the mental health field that should not be underestimated. All forms of mental health intervention involve giving and receiving help in an interpersonal context. In this connection, the relationship capacities and feeling-oriented skills of Southern Appalachian families are very real indeed, nor are these capacities dimmed by the families' migration to other settings. Presumably, then, those who work in any helping capacity with such families, either in their region or elsewhere, will find this feeling-oriented mutual relationship a powerful factor in the undertaking.

Regional Shifts in Psychopathology

Not infrequently, certain disorders in children occur largely as a result of cultural shifts. The consistently presented regional training patterns make for learned, efficient behaviors as long as the people remain within their cultural setting. By the same token, however, these training processes can also make it stressful for the individual when change is called for.

EXAMPLE

Thus, an infantilized Southern Appalachian child may adapt quite comfortably to an overprotective home environment during his preschool years. Once he starts school, however, he may become anxious when the previously learned dependent behaviors run counter to the school's request that he function more assertively and more autonomously.

Those who have worked with Southern Appalachian migrants in urban settings are aware of this same phenomenon. After the family changes cultural location it may occur in one or more family members. Clinical work with one particular patient, a former coal miner from the Southern Appalachian region, provided an unusual insight into the kind of struggle many migrants experience.

At the time, this forty-two-year-old construction laborer was seen weekly at a mental health clinic in Cincinnati, Ohio. One year previously, he had moved his family from a coal-mining town in southeastern Kentucky to a working-class suburb of Cincinnati. The family was referred for mental health care when the oldest son manifested an adolescent identity crisis and at the same time the man's wife became psychotically depressed. The boy felt strange and different among his new high school classmates. He developed acute anxiety attacks and dissociative reactions. His mother, a silent, apathetic person, had been accepted by her Southern Appalachian neighbors as overly-inhibited and mildly depressed. After the family's move to Ohio, her new working-class neighbors pressed her for interpersonal participation in a bowling league and their kaffeeklatches. She could not easily adapt to the new role that the community expected her to play. Anxiety mounted, leading to despair and eventually to her depressive illness.

Her husband had been raised in a coal-mining family. His father was a silent person who expressed himself by direct aggressive action. Thus, when this man acted rebelliously during his early adolescence, his father would knock him off the cabin porch with his fist or a two-by-four. The man identified strongly with this action-oriented model. In his own marriage he cuffed his wife about and beat his children. Through talks with his neighbors and fellow workers in Ohio he gradually became aware that such role behavior was not altogether acceptable. This demand for change in his behavior versus the inflexible training pattern of his youth created considerable conflict for him. He developed anxiety attacks in his therapist's office as they talked about it.

Thus, a family of this sort may adjust for years in a marginally satisfactory way within the culture of origin. Overt psychopathological symptoms might never appear until after a move to a cultural setting which demands new behaviors. This particular family was significant in that all three key members experienced difficulties adjusting to their new setting.

Effects of Regional Social Class on Mental Health

The more we know of the external forces involved in mental illness, the more we understand the complex connection between individual and social pathology. Generally, it may be said that the effects of social class on mental health, including children's psychopathology, are uneven and complex. The author, among others, is suspicious of viewpoints espousing one-to-one relationships between class position and mental illness. Three writers[19] summarized similar viewpoints about the effects of poverty on psychopathology. They felt that analysis of the poor is best directed at a thorough appraisal of various subgroupings rather than at the disadvantaged as a whole, or at any common denominator thereof.

EXAMPLE

This point is certainly confirmed by the personality and attitudes of the Appalachian lower class. Their hard lives give rise to personal attitudes of fierce individualism, traditionalism, and fatalism. On the other hand, unlike many of the very poor elsewhere in the United States, the very poor in the Southern Appalachian region retain their basic relatedness and their capacity for basic trust. In this respect, the quality of their interpersonal relationships is like the object-relationship capacities displayed by the stable working-class families studied in several urban settings. Another way of stating this is to indicate that the very poor in the Southern Appalachian region are not essentially socially disorganized; thus, they are unlike the lower-lower-class, or very poor, families studied in Boston by one writer.

Pavenstedt and her co-workers found that the parents in the stable working-class group actively participated with their children in the evolution of basic relationships to each other as differentiated, trusted, cherished individuals. These parents and their children were capable of evoking satisfying action from each other in times of need and displaying mutually responsive communication and affective exchange. The children developed autonomously with the appropriate mastery of skills in the toddler period and basically sound foundations of sex-role differentiation in the later preschool period. Closely related to this emotional-personality development were age-appropriate language and intellectual-cognitive skills, with the exception of some cultural-stimulation lags about the time of entering first grade.

By contrast, the children of the socially disorganized group, she and the others studied, did not develop basically trustful object relationships in infancy. Their chaotic, impulse-ridden parents frequently rejected them or related in intensely ambivalent, inconsistent ways. The children grew to be hypersensitively alert to rejection and to real and anticipated dangers in the environment. These children became "immature little drifters." Paralleling this personality disorganization were lags in language and intellectual-cognitive development.[17]

Coles and his co-workers longitudinally followed Negro and Caucasian children of various ages in several southern cities in the early 1960s. That both groups of children were eventually able to overcome acculturated prejudicial veneers under stressful conditions of school desegregation was attributable, Coles felt, to each group's basically sound object relationships learned at home. Both groups of children eventually allowed themselves to respect and trust one another.[4]

The very poor in Appalachia share the hard lot of the very poor elsewhere in the nation. However, they have to face another characteristic as well: the interacting, reinforcing factors of physical, mental, and cultural isolation operate to hold them in disadvantaged areas, frequently resisting changes that would bring them into more effective contact with the outside world.

Conclusion

In this section, the point has been made that clinicians need to examine how very early in the life cycles of children various cultural processes act to influence child rearing. This is particularly important in regard to differences that exist between regions. Some problems so derived begin long before children reach school age. Other culturally determined factors may exert specific influence at later stages of the child's development.

In making such a detailed study of regional training factors, clinicians must determine whether cultural patterns offer minimal, partial, or fully supportive assists to growth. What solutions do they provide for mastery with regard to the child's succeeding developmental tasks? The goal of such study is to determine if there are constructive and creative directions available in the region, sites for the investment of the child's emerging strengths and skills in all areas of his functioning.

Or, there may be negative cultural processes at work that are significant determinants of the child's developmental experiences. In such instances personality patterns may well result which will persist from generation to generation and which will act to lock in the child's inner forces as well as perpetuate self-defeating attitudes. If these forces are combined with regional problems of economics and geography, they may provide the basis for enormous resistance to change. This, in fact, has blocked numerous attempts at intervention which have sought to modify the attitudes and life styles of persons raised under these conditions. In the final analysis, many children are born with rich potentials which are all too often never realized.

By contrast, as specific cultural processes are examined, there are also training forces available which do aid children to develop into individuals who can meet and master a variety of tasks, who can make choices, and who are able to accept change.

Summary

The clinician who evaluates a child brings a variety of skills to the diagnostic process. He possesses knowledge of human behavior, gained from the rich admixture of his own life experiences and his professional training. He sees individual human development as a continuum, from infancy through the multiple levels of childhood, adolescence, and adulthood. He knows that his study of the individual child has its foundation in the current basic information about the unfolding of personality.

In addition, he comes to the evaluation with some knowledge of the psychodynamics operating in the lives of children and their families, and with some awareness of the psychopathology of childhood. He focuses on the families' patterns of thinking, feeling, and behaving, and he considers the impact of these patterns on the lives of their children. And he is weighing as well the myriad varieties of problems to which these children must adapt.

Furthermore, he is aware of the importance of cultural patterns in child development, and thus is alert to the ways in which specific patterns have contributed to the life of the child before him. From this standpoint he is in a position to examine whether or not these cultural patterns offer minimal, partial, or full support to the child's need for mastery. He studies this in relation to the youngster's physical and intellectual equipment, inborn impulses, specific developmental anxieties, and, on a more complex level, in terms of the child's problems, difficulties, fears, interests, hopes, plans, and pursuits.

The clinician seeks to understand the child and his family, to clarify situations, and to assist the parents in redirecting certain aspects of their child's growth. He is sensitive to the parents' feelings, and he is likely to be alive to the emotional experiences of their children as well as liking them. All of this is his preparation.

Added to this background, is the clinician's understanding that the diagnostic study itself is a dynamic process. It offers new relationships and potentially valuable experiences to both child and parents as they are helped to face their problems together. It is based on a sound knowledge of both normal and pathological development, a grasp on ongoing personality function, and an awareness of the continuous interaction of all the psychobiological and psychosocial forces. This understanding demands a multifacted approach. No unilateral study can effectively reveal the crosscurrents and significant forces in a total family situation. Sufficient historical data about physical, psychological, and social factors are needed. At the same time, there must be an adequate evalua-

tion of the child's current levels of physical and psychological functioning, and valid appraisals of his native physical equipment and his intellectual endowment.

Thus, overall, the evaluator of the child assumes the responsibility of synthesizing the various diagnostic data from all these areas—biological-constitutional factors, family factors, and sociocultural factors—into a comprehensive diagnosis of the child in his environment. And, surely, this is one of his finest challenges.

REFERENCES

1. ABSE, W., "Hysteria," in Arieti, S. (Ed.), *American Handbook of Psychiatry*, pp. 272–292, Basic Books, New York, 1959.

2. BRENNER, J., "A Social Psychiatric Investigation of a Small Community in Northern Norway," *Acta Psychiatrica et Neurologica, 62:*50–51, 1957.

3. CAMPBELL, J., "The Southern Highlands and His Homeland," Russell Sage Foundation, New York, 1921.

4. COLES, R., "Southern Children Under Desegregation," *American Journal of Psychiatry, 120:*332–344, 1963.

5. EATON, J., and WEIL, R., *Culture and Mental Disorders, a Comparative Study of the Hutterites and Other Populations*, p. 135, Free Press, Glencoe, Ill., 1955.

6. FORD, T., "Discussion of Loof, D., Psychiatric Perspective on Poverty," in Weaver, T., and Magid, A. (Eds.), *Poverty: New Interdisciplinary Perspectives*, Chandler Press, San Francisco, 1969.

7. ———, *Health and Demography in Kentucky*, The Univerisity Press of Kentucky, Lexington, 1964.

8. ———, *The Southern Appalachian Region: A Survey*, The University Press of Kentucky, Lexington, 1962.

9. GLASER, G., PINCUS, J., and PROVENCE, S., "Psychiatric Illness in Children," in Detre, T. P., and Jarecki, H. G. (Eds.), *Modern Psychiatric Treatment*, Lippincott, Philadelphia, 1971.

10. Group for the Advancement of Psychiatry (GAP), *Psychopathologic Disorders of Childhood: Theoretic Considerations and a Proposed Classification*, Report No. 62, Group for the Advancement of Psychiatry, New York, 1966.

11. JOHNSON, C., et al., *Mountain Families in Poverty, Department of Sociology Bulletin, 29*, The University Press of Kentucky, Lexington, 1967.

12. KEPHART, H., *Our Southern Highlands*, Outing Publishing Co., New York, 1913.

13. LA BARRE, W., *They Shall Take Up Serpents: The Southern Snake Cult*, Duke University Press, Durham, N.C., 1956.

14. LOOF, D., "The Diagnostic Process: An Overview," in Loof, D., *Getting to Know the Troubled Child*, University of Tennessee Press, Knoxville, 1976.

15. ———, *Appalachia's Children*, University Press of Kentucky, Lexington, 1971.

16. ———, "Psychophysiologic and Conversion Reactions in Children: Selective Incidence in Verbal and Nonverbal Families," *Journal of the American Academy of Child Psychiatry, 9(2):*318–331, 1970.

17. PAVENSTEDT, E., "A Comparison of a Child Rearing Environment of Upper-Lower and Very Lower Lower Class Families," *American Journal of Orthopsychiatry, 35:*89–98, 1965.

18. PEARSALL, M., *Little Smokey Ridge*, The University of Alabama Press, Tuscaloosa, 1959.

19. RIESMAN, F., et al. (Eds.), *Mental Health of the Poor*, Free Press, New York, 1964.

20. SZASZ, T., *The Myth of Mental Illness*, Hoeber-Harper Press, New York, 1961.

21. WEINSTEIN, E., "Cultural Factors in Conversion Hysteria," in Finney, J. (Ed.), *Culture Change, Mental Health, and Poverty*, The University Press of Kentucky, Lexington, 1969.

22. ———, Personal Communication, 1967.

23. WELLER, J., *Yesterday's People: Life in Contemporary Applachia*, The University Press of Kentucky, Lexington, 1965.

5 / Behavioral/Learning Theory Formulations

John S. Werry

Definition

Unfortunately, terminology tends to have a will of its own and for better or for worse, the term "behavioral" is now accepted parlance in child psychiatry *for a way of conceptualizing etiology and of practicing treatment derived from learning theory.* This is how it will be used here, even though behaviorally oriented clinicians seldom are concerned only with "behavior" in the narrow sense of externally observable receptor or effector events.

Learning theory also requires some defining since strictly speaking, Freud was a learning theorist, as are ethologists such as Bowlby. As commonly used, however, learning theory has come to mean the particular theories derived from experimental psychology and currently involving only two sub-theories: *Pavlovian, classical, or respondent learning* and *instrumental or operant learning.*

To define *learning* or its synonym, *conditioning,* is not easy, and there are many definitions. But embodied in most, are notions of some change from a previous state of responding, with linking of an antecedent external or internal environment event (stimulus) with some organismic effector process so that stimulus and response occur sequentially to a degree significantly greater than chance, or in short, predictably.

Though the notions of stimulus and response (the simplified form of which is seen in the reflex) are fundamental to learning theory, it does the behavioral approach a disservice to think that it never rises higher than the simple reflex arc.

Historical Roots

Only the twentieth century will be considered here (though the roots of learning theory and behavioral approaches are much older). The behavioral approach, as we know it now, is derived from the mainstream of Russian and American psychology in the twentieth century. While Pavlov came to psychology accidentally through gastric physiology, American learning theorists such as Thorndike and Watson developed their psychology in the search for a mental science independent of philosophy and of the traditional introspective method of deriving knowledge. It is not surprising then that both Russian and American psychology have shown what almost amounts to an obsession with empiricism and objectivization.

Since, unlike psychoanalytic theory, learning theory was born in the laboratory and, with few exceptions, remained there until the 1950s, it has other distinguishing characteristics besides objectivization. The principal one is the use of the experimental method, the essence of which is the attempt to discover systematic relationships between variables to enable predictions to be made. To achieve this degree of precision, limitation of the scope of the theory, of its testing in the child, or of the factors to be manipulated experimentally, is necessary (often clinicians might argue to the point of triviality). On the other hand, while the scope of the clinically-derived theories, such as the psychoanalytic ones, are more ambitious and, because of this, are often more acceptable clinically, they have generally not led to studies of an acceptable experimental and objective standard. Also, their use has beeen one of understanding rather than of prediction and their wisdom much more that of hindsight.[21]

While, apart from Watson, learning theorists generally stayed in their laboratories, the forties and fifties showed a slow emergence into the clinical world. Psychologists, such as Mowrer, Sears, Dollar and Miller, attempted to translate psychoanalytic concepts into learning theory or vice versa.[7, 11, 16] Since the sixties, however, behavioral approaches (e.g., Eysenck, and Ulmann and Krasner)[8, 20] have rejected this attempted marriage, and, just as their forebears rebelled against philosophy, so have they against psychoanalytic and medical approaches in a search for a separate identity.

Learning theory has never been a single theory nor has it been static. Few learning theorists, for example, accept Skinner's radical behaviorism (empty organism) except perhaps as an expedient in certain simple situations such as severe autism or mental retardation or in the understanding and treatment of simple problems or symptoms. Most consider learning theory an insult to the complexity of the human organism and an example of gross reductionism.

While psychologists have long been interested in children, the last two decades or so have seen the growth of a relatively new offshoot of psychology—experimental child psychology. This differs from the older child psychology or child development which was mostly descriptive in its use of the experimental approach. A perusal of a current text[12] shows it is much concerned with learning as a basic component of development, particularly the impact of early learning. It is interesting to note that Hebb[10] and his associates, arguing from psychological theory, began their studies of early experience independently, about the same time that Bowlby was developing his own theories about maternal deprivation from clinical observation.

While the impact of experimental child psychology upon child psychiatry is not yet very great, its importance is likely to grow, particularly since it is concerned with important areas such as perception, language, cognition, memory, socialisation, emotion, and so on.

Russian or Pavlovian psychology is not as well understood in the West, yet it, too, has tried to grapple with levels of human behavior well above the reflex level and with psychopathological phenomena. However, its impact in the west, above the simple conditioned reflex, appears to have been slight.

In summary, then, learning theory applications in child psychiatry are recent and show their parentage in experimental child psychology, namely, micro rather than grand in scope, precise, experimental-manipulative, and prediction oriented. Whether or not they are better or worse than clinically derived approaches depends on the questions asked (e.g., heuristic, or clinical value). Freud and Skinner, however, had one thing in common. They were both scientists who believed in the scientific method of observation, induction of an hypothesis and deduction or predictions from the hypothesis. Their differing backgrounds, epochs, and employment situations have led to vastly different theories, but they have far more in common with each other than those who claim that each individual is unique and that human behavior is some kind of elemental mystery that defies understanding. The enemy of the advance of knowledge is not the behaviorist or the psychoanalyst but the anti-intellectual and the anti-scientific.

Basic Assumptions

Behavioral notions of etiology make certain basic assumptions explicitly, or more commonly, implicitly, most of which are qualitatively if not quantitatively, similar to those of psychoanalytic or other clinical theories.

1. *A Normality/Abnormality Dichotomy is Useful:* While there has been much criticism of the notion of abnormality, particularly the way it is used by medically trained clinicians,[20] nevertheless notions of this type are well-embedded in the behavioral approach. Whatever each may call it, behaviorist and psychoanalyst alike assume that children should behave in an age, sex, and culturally appropriate way *and* be happy most of the time while doing so. If the child is not doing this, he is judged to be deviant or to engage in maladaptive behavior and to be worthy of programs to try to correct this.[13, 20] Any difference between deviant and abnormal is more semantic than real.

2. *There Is a Physical Limitation on Potential:* Less often stated is the second assumption that there is a species or biologically determined potential or repertoire of behaviors.

Not much effort has been expanded to explain why children have not learned to fly and why fish cannot speak or read. There is, however, much more controversy about the universality and invariance of the human potential as epitomized by Watson in his statement "Give me a child. . . ." This is not, however, a peculiarity of behaviorally oriented clinicians. Along with many clinicians who work with children, behaviorally oriented persons generally adopt a well justifiable position that it is better to assume potential than dismiss it without trial. Any difference perhaps lies in the forcefulness with which the latter express it, though most now recognize individual variation, having worked not only with normal children but with the severely autistic and retarded.

3. *Development is Predictable:* The third assumption is that children develop in an orderly and basically predictable fashion and that some of their development is due to physical maturation. Psychoanalysts, child developmentalists like Gesell, or in the cognitive area like Piaget, have

used the convenient model of stages of development as a kind of metaphor, but, while behaviorally oriented clinicians at first avoided the stage model, there has been some emergence of it lately. For example, Bijou and Baer[5] talk of the "universal stage" (0-2 years) (infancy) and the basic stage (2-5 years) while Thompson's[18] three stages of learning are also indicative. Generally speaking, however, while stages do not figure importantly in behavioral approaches, increasingly, *development* does, though still to a limited degree.

4. *Early Learning Is Critical:* The fourth assumption is that early learning affects later learning, sometimes, that it is qualitatively different from later. Also, that the mother or other primary caretaker is critical for early learning. Differences from psychoanalytic theory would, however, be in the reversibility of early learning, its lesser importance and the extent to which others, notably peers, can influence it.[9]

5. *Abnormal Behavioral Obeys the Laws of Learning:* By this is meant that behavior is never qualitatively abnormal but is learned or unlearned like any other behavior. What gives behavior its abnormality or otherwise is its *social significance.*

This is probably the most important underlying assumption for the behaviorally oriented clinician, though if we examine it closely, it will be seen that it is actually elemental to psychoanalytic theory too, and differs significantly only from medical (perhaps better described as biogenic) views of psychopathology though even these allow some learning (pathoplastic) factors. Again, it would seem to be the forcefulness of its expression rather than the concept itself which is distinctive.

6. *Immediate Etiology Is More Important than Remote Etiology:* Put another way, the behavioral approach asks "what is keeping this behavior going or preventing its occurrence if a deficit?" rather than "how did this come about?" (Of course, the interest of the psychoanalytic approach in remote etiology is only insofar as it sees this as the key to present etiology).

7. *"The Symptom Is (or the Symptoms Are) the Neurosis":*[8] This denies the notion of an underlying cause and leads to a symptomatic, better called *problem oriented*, approach to diagnosis, etiology, and treatment.

8. *Consciousness, Awareness or Other Mentalistic Concepts Such as Motives Are Unnecessary:* This is not so much a rejection of the notions —behaviorally oriented clinicians make obvious use of a child's consciousness—as their superflousness to the strictly empirical demonstration of cause and effect relationships between one externally observable event, the stimulus and another the response (S-R). While the behavioral approach recognizes so-called mediating processes (i.e., an S—O—R sequence), they are not presently easily encompassable within the theory.

Theoretical Aspects

RESPONDENT LEARNING

This is one of the two basic learning mechanisms. Respondent, classical, or Pavlovian conditioning or learning occurs when a previously neutral stimulus, the conditional stimulus (CS), acquires the capacity to elicit a naturally occurring response or unconditioned response (UCR), usually a reflex of varying complexity, by being repeatedly presented shortly *before* the naturally occurring stimulus or the unconditional stimulus (UCS) for that reflex. When the CS can elicit the UCR, the latter is then called the conditioned response (CR). The CR ordinarily is similar but not precisely the same and somewhat weaker than the UCR. Presentations of the UCS shortly after the CS must be given from time to time. If this is not done and the response is repeatedly evoked, it ultimately fades or is *extinguished.* The CS usually has a range of values or variations called the *stimulus generalization gradient* over which it can evoke the CR, the power to do so being a function of the similarity of these stimuli to the original CR. This concept of stimulus gradient is fundamental to Wolpe's behavior therapy technique of systematic densensitization, which begins with stimuli evoking the CR (e.g., the phobia) only weakly and working ever closer to the strongest.

Pavlovian conditioning typically involves, primarily, responses mediated through the autonomic nervous system and, as such, are often accompanied by nonspecific changes in the level of arousal and changes in emotional states important to survival of an individual or species. It is, therefore, the type of learning more often involved in the etiology of psychiatric conditions where emotional symptoms predominate, as in phobias and depression. According to Thompson[18] it is developmentally predominant in the second developmental stage, the affective meaning zone (see below). It is a more primitive, more global type of learning often lacking the fineness and complexity of operant type learning. It is also essentially reactive or passive rather than active or problem solving.

OPERANT LEARNING

Operant learning is the second basic learning process. Operant, instrumental, or Skinnerian type conditioning (or learning) actually long antedates Skinner, being fundamental to Freud's pleasure principle and Thorndike's Law of Effect. In contrast to respondent learning, in operant conditioning, the animal is active and chooses from among two or more responses the one most desirable (to it) in terms of the consequences. For operant learning to occur, there must be: (1) a discriminant stimulus (SD) preceding the response (R) which indicates what is to happen after the response is made; (2) an organism which is actually or potentially capable of making the response required; and (3) a consequence to the behavior which has some meaning to the organism. In practical terms this usually means: (1) the occurrence of something which is rewarding or pleasurable to the child (*positive reinforcement*); (2) the cessation of something unpleasant (*negative reinforcement*); and/or (3) the occurrence of something unpleasant (*punishment*).

Other basic concepts are shaping, successive approximation, fading, extinction, counterconditioning, and scheduling. *Shaping* (the response) means guiding the behavior gradually towards the final form desired by reinforcing *successive approximations* to it, as for example, in teaching a child to read beginning initially with shapes, then letters, then simple, then complex words. *Fading* is a technique used in shaping behavior in which a stimulus which causes the desired response but is inappropriate or undesirable in the long term (such as presence of mother in introduction to kindergarten) is gradually faded out along the stimulus generalization gradient (e.g., duration of mother's stay) until the response is independent of it. As in respondent learning, *extinction* means the permanent abolition of the stimulus-response sequence. In the operant situation this is achieved by removing reinforcement and, sometimes, by adding punishment as well. *Counterconditioning*, a term again common to both types of learning, means attaching a new response to the stimulus of a type which is incompatible with the original response and which thus prevents its occurrence. For example, in the behavior therapy technique of systematic desensitization of anxiety responses, muscular relaxation is counterconditioned to the phobic stimulus, thus, hopefully, preventing anxiety.

Schedules (of contingenies) are the pattern in which reinforcement or punishment is made to follow the response: (1) continuous, if after every response; (2) fixed, if following in some regular way, say every second time; (3) variable, if irregular or erratic; (4) ratio, if determined by the number of responses; and (5) interval, if by some interval of time, say every five-minutes interval. A schedule may thus be continuous, fixed ratio, fixed interval, variable ratio, variable interval, or various other combinations. Naturally occurring types of schedules in a child's world are ordinarily either variable ratio or, more commonly, variable interval. This is not the same as inconsistent, a term commonly applied to parents, which implies sometimes reinforcing, sometimes punishing the same behavior. Each schedule has its own characteristics as far as acquisition, rates of responding, and resistance to extinction are concerned, most of which are fairly commonsense. For example, a fixed interval schedule such as end of semester exams, tends to result in a low level of responding (studying) at first, increasing rapidly as the contingency (success or failure) draws nigh. Variable schedules, by their unpredictability, take longer to induce learning but are, by the same token, more resistent to extinction.

Demonstrating etiological relationships: As pointed out earlier, the behavior approach shows its parentage in experimental psychology by a concern with demonstrating cause and effect relationships. While respondent learning has often used the common experimental method of averaging results across a group of individuals, operant learning has preferred the single subject design or case studies.[13] This, of course, is particularly suitable for clinical work but makes demonstrating cause and effect relationships more difficult but not impossible. This is done typically either by the baseline-intervention-baseline (A-B-A) or by the reversal (A-B-C) methods. In the A-B-A method, the behavior is first measured in the natural or *baseline* state (A) and then the naturally occurring reinforcement (or punishment) is withheld (B) during which the behavior changes are predicted, then to complete proof, a return to baseline is effected and the behavior returns. The reversal method is an extension of the A-B-A method. In this, a third phase (C) which is the *opposite* of what was done during the first intervention (B) is added (e.g., A-B-C-A). As with the case study, the single subject design has the problem of demonstrating universality of etiology. For example, while it could be used to demonstrate that the etiology of a child's tantrums lay in their highly effective manner of melting parental resolve, it would not prove that tantrums in all or most children were so caused. In some children they might well represent simple emotional type behavior devoid of any purpose. The techniques are, however, very useful in the treatment situation where one is primarily concerned with individual patient progress.

What has been described so far has shown how the behavior in question is controlled or caused by the systematic manipulation of independent (etiological) and dependent (effect) variables. Implicit in this, is the assumption that both can be measured reasonably accurately. While there are other ways of doing this, the behavioral approach has made predominant use of the *time sampling* technique in which behaviors are accurately defined and their frequency counted at stipulated intervals (see Ross).[14, 15]

While establishing the etiology of *positive* psychopathological symptoms can be done in the aforementioned way, behavioral *deficits* present a very different problem, since teaching the condition does not prove its absence was caused similarly. Thus, for example, the very successful method of treating enuresis, (that is, a deficit of nocturnal continence) by the bedbuzzer does not mean that enuresis is caused by the absence of bedbuzzers in most homes. Rather, a search for factors inimical to learning would have to be instituted, and, then, these varied systematically to see if they are etiological. It is hard to see how this could be done except through more traditional methods, particularly comparisons between *groups* of children. This is implicit in the suggestions by Baer (1973) for establishing variables critical for normal development: first, subject developmental behaviors to behavior modification; second, if such behavior can be modified, inspect the usual environment in which they develop to see if similar contingencies operate there; and third, manipulate these contingencies to see if they are functionally related to the acquisition of these behaviors. We might add a fourth step, then, inspect environments in which learning has not occurred and see if these contingencies are absent or interfered with.

Developmental Aspects

OVERVIEW

Since behavioral approaches in child psychiatry are relatively recent, so are behavioral theories of psychopathology. This is particularly so in what

might be called abnormal developmental and abnormal child psychology, which is mostly what child psychiatry is about. What is needed is a theory which not only explains how particular symptoms come about but fits them into some overall development framework. Whatever its weakness, psychoanalytic theory is above all this.

The pioneering work of Dollard and Miller,[7] Mowrer,[11] Sears, Maccoby and Levin[16] was largely isolated and is now considered obsolete because of its reliance on unpopular drive reduction learning theory and its attempt to utilize psychoanalytic concepts. The theory of Thompson[18] described in detail later, though not widely known in child psychiatry or derived with abnormal behavior in mind, seems promising for a behavioral theory. Not only does it incorporate learning theory concepts within a developmental framework, but it provides a way of utilizing existing clinical observations and is readily applicable to the learning of emotional behavior. It is, however, only a skeleton and needs much elaborating. The more detailed discussion by Bijou and Baer[5, 6] does some of this but only for infancy and with overemphasis on operant learning.

Also noteworthy is Harlow's theory[9] of the development of the five affectional, perhaps better called interactional, systems (mother-child, child-mother, peer-peer, heterosexual, and paternal). Though this is much better worked out than Thompson's theory, incorporating much of child psychology and child development, it is basically atheoretical, telling little of the fundamental learning processes involved. It deals only with the situations which result in normal or aberrant learning. Also, it is restricted to affectional learning. Bandura and Walters[3] and Ullmann and Krasner[20] offer learning theory views of personality and of psychopathology, which, while richer in detail, are not developmentally but rather process oriented. What is needed is an attempt to meld development, process, typology, and the now numerous behavioral case studies into a single body of knowledge.

A DEVELOPMETAL THEORY

Thompson's theory[18] attempts to incorporate what is known about physical postnatal development, modern learning theories and observations, experimental and otherwise, of the psychological development of children, though its major concern is with early learning. (See figure 5-1)

The first developmental stage, called the *temperament-adaptation* zone, occurs in the neonate

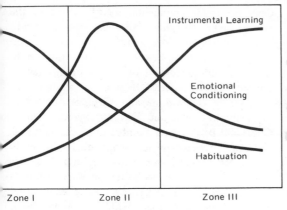

FIGURE 5–1
Critical zones during development defined in terms of three types of storage mechanisms: Zone I, temperament-adaptation; Zone II, affective-meaning; Zone III, instrumental meaning.

Reprinted with permission of the Springer Publishing Company, Inc. from "Early Experimental and Genetic Influences on Flexibility," by W. R. Thompson, in *Experience, Structure and Adaptability*, ed., O. J. Harvey, Fig. 5, p. 83 Copyright 1966 by the Springer Publishing Company, Inc., New York.

when the level of physical maturation is so primitive that the infant is not capable of sensory discrimination or of differentiation in response. This is a stage of simple reactivity or arousability, exemplified in later life by the orienting response to novel, interesting or noxious stimuli. Thompson postulates that this stage establishes temperamental reactivity, the foundation upon which all later behavior is built. While evidence suggests that reactivity is partly genetic or constitutional, work with animals has shown that this reactivity can be increased or decreased by various experiences such as gentling. It follows from this demonstration of ability to influence reactivity in animals, that, if it is also valid for humans (which seems likely), infants can be made more or less reactive by experience such as quality of mothering, physical illness and discomfort, etc. A fortunate early infancy (and a good heredity) should lead to adaptation or *habituation* to the environment as a predictable, secure place while the opposite leads to *sensitization* as a hostile or frightening place. The analogy to Erickson's basic trust versus mistrust is fairly apparent. What makes Thompson's theory an improvement on Erickson's is its linkage to well documented observations and experiments in young animals and, to a lesser extent, in human infants.[18, 19]

The second stage Thompson calls *affect-meaning* zone and occurs when the rapidly developing special senses, especially vision, allows complex discriminations about the environment to be made.

Yet, because of motor immaturity and the abscence of language, effector responses are relatively undifferentiated compared to sensory processes. It is postulated that the basic process here is that of classical or respondent learning in which the child is passive and the responses, learned or conditioned, involve the autonomic system (including the emotions) and involve basic life-maintaining processes.

The omnipresence of the mother, by mid-infancy a visually and auditorily discriminable stimulus, and her intimate association with pleasure and reduction of discomfort obviously give her a primary role in the modification of both fundamental reactivity and of the assigning of affect and meaning to particular elements of the environment, beginning with herself. Like habituation, however, the process of affect-meaning does not stop when the effector apparatus matures but continues throughout life, both actively and as a second foundation stage upon which later years must build.

With the maturation of the motor and other effector apparatus (e.g., language systems), the third stage, the *instrumental-meaning* zone and the basic process operant (sometimes also called instrumental) learning or conditioning become predominant. In contrast to the respondent learning process, the organism is able to choose what solution to bring to bear upon a situation, a simple example being whether to touch or not touch depending on the consequences of the action. In this way the child learns what aspects of the environment can be acted on or manipulated and what are the consequences of such action. Elemental to this voyage of discovery and route to autonomy are the development of cognition, language, and complex motor skills. And it is here that the areas of greatest intellectual effort currently in experimental child psychology could be ultimately incorporated, possibly with the addition of further stages and further learning processes based on say, cognition.

None of these three processes ever terminates, only their relative importance changes. Thompson gives the example of throwing a child into water—reactivity might be increased by the sudden fright making the child generally more fearful, affect-meaning might be changed by the development of a specific fear of water, and instrumental meaning might result in his learning to swim! None of these concepts is new, being part of psychoanalytic theory. What is novel is their relationship to a body of empirical observation, experimentation, and systematic theory. Also they provide an heuristic framework for behaviorally oriented clinicians to study human psychopathology within a developmental context.

Behavioral Psychopathology

While, as discussed earlier, there are several assumptions in the behavioral approach to etiology, the most important and central one is:* There are only two kinds of abnormal behavior, those that represent the failure to learn (behavioral deficits) and those that are the result of learning the wrong thing (maladaptive or deviant behavior).

A derivative of this assumption is that in looking for etiological factors, attention must be directed, in the case of behavioral deficits, to factors (past or present) preventing learning and, in the case of maladaptive behavior, to factors shaping and maintaining the behavior in question. In this analysis, often called behavior analysis, the laws and technology of learning theory are applied. This working hypothesis is deceptively simple, because though anyone can learn principles and technology in a few days, their application requires the usual mysterious ingredients, common to any approach, clinical sensitivity, and ingenuity. A poor clinician is a poor clinician, independent of theoretical orientation and the behavioral approach is no exception.

A BEHAVIORAL CLASSIFICATION

Most nosological systems in child psychiatry are syndromal. The classification offered here is etiological, behavior (or problem), and treatment oriented. This does not mean that it is superior to other classification systems or that painfully acquired knowledge about prognosis or other treatments such as chemotherapy should be jettisoned—rather this system is intended to complement syndromal nosologies. It is derived directly from the assumption, central to the behavioral approach, that psychopathological symptoms represent either failure of, or wrongful learning. It incorporates and assumes some knowledge of learning theory principles discussed previously.

1. DISORDERS OF TEMPERAMENT/ADAPTATION

While most behaviorally oriented clinicians conveniently ignore temperament, it is quite clear from learning theory that it must be considered.

* See references 2, 8, 14, 20.

Thompson's developmental theory is one of the few to make it explicit, but every operant conditioner knows that the first thing a rat does on entering a Skinner box for the first time is to defecate and the extent of this is often used to measure "emotionality." Numerous studies (see reviews by Thompson and Grusec[19] including those by Bergman and Escalona,[4] and Thomas, Chess and Birth[17] have pointed to fundamental individual differences in temperament. Pavlov early recognized basic temperamental differences in his dogs which made them better or worse subjects for his studies, and every dog fancier knows that breeds differ in temperament. Unpopular as it may be, nowadays there is good evidence, too, that there are minor gender differences in emotionality. While one must not underestimate the influence on any differences of later learning, the evidence of fundamental differences in reactivity in neonates and infants is now pretty convincing.[18, 19] Apart from a few studies such as those by Thomas and his colleagues,[17] there has been little interest or study of this type of disorder until recently, so that much of the comment here is speculative. It seems probable that disorders of temperament could take two forms, lack of reactivity, e.g., (in autism) and over-reactivity (such as "colic" in the infant and catastrophic reactions in autistic or brain damaged children).

It follows from Thompson's delineation of stages (based on the organisms's ability to differentiate sensorily and motorically) that pure disorders of temperament are likely to be most important in the first weeks of life; or, in short, in the psychopathology of the neonate and infant. However, from a practical point of view, as the longitudinal studies of Thomas and his colleagues[17] suggest, their role is likely to be most important in influencing later learning rather than in producing pure disorders which would be predicted to emerge only in highly novel situations of a stressful nature (e.g., catastrophic reactions, homesickness). Even then, catastrophic reactions rapidly lead to escape or removal from the situation or if not, as with homesickness, some degree of adaptation soon results. So these pure disorders would be shortlived.

2. DISORDERS OF RESPONDENT (CLASSICAL) CONDITIONING

Deficit Disorders: These are failures to learn, or instances of premature extinction or unlearning. It is important to point out that deficit disorders are diagnosed solely on whether or not function is absent or diminished. Thus enuresis is

TABLE 5–1

A Behavioral Etiological Classification

	Age of Maximum Prevalence	Example
1. Disorders of Temperament/Adaptation		
1.1. Deficit Disorders	0–2 years?	Passivity? Autism?
1.2. Surplus Disorders	0–2 years	Colic First tantrums Catastrophic reactions Homesickness Shyness
2. Disorders of Respondent Learning		
2.1. Deficit Disorders	½–6 years	Affectionatelessness Fearlessness Enuresis Autism
2.2. Surplus or Maladaptive Disorders	½–6 years	Fears Phobias Nightmares? Tics?
3. Disorders of Operant Learning		
3.1 Deficit Disorders	2+ years	Distractibility Hyperactivity Cultural Deprivation Autism
3.2. Maladaptive/Deviant Disorders	2+ years	Depression? Elective mutism Aggression Compulsions Later tantrums Negativism Delusion

not a positive symptoms but a failure to learn nocturnal continence. Their etiology can be sought in an analysis of the respondent learning process.

For learning to occur, a stimulus which the infant or child can perceive as distinctive must be presented closely and regularly (within a second or two) preceding some naturally occurring stimulus capable of eliciting a definite autonomic (including emotional) response. The organism must be capable of responding, and occasional refresher applications of the unconditioned stimulus must be given to prevent extinction. For all practical purposes, disorders of respondent conditioning of interest to child psychiatrists are emotional . in type, so that pathogenic processes with examples in parentheses can now be delineated: (a) Stimulus factors—absence (maternal deprivation), ambiguity (double bind), subthreshold, overcomplex; (b) organismic factors—states inimical to learning (anxiety, satiation), lack of ability to perceive

the stimulus (sensory, intellectual deficits), or to make the response (unlikely for simple emotional responses); (c) learning procedures—timing of conditioned stimulus, too few learning trials or attempts, failure to prevent extinction through topping up presentations of the unconditioned stimulus.

Examples of this kind of disorder are offered in Table 5-1 and readers are invited to apply these principles to an example such as affectionlessness which is generally accepted to be due, in Western society, to some failure in the mother-child relationships in the first year or so of life. Possible distortions of this process are brilliantly summarised by Harlow[9] in extensions of his monkey isolation studies.

Surplus or Maladaptive Disorders: Here, in contrast to deficit disorders, the child has learned an emotional response which is considered pathological by virtue of its intensity, its inappropriateness, or its generality. For example, while a four-year-old would be forgiven fear of a fierce German shepherd dog, a paralyzing fear of all dogs or of a small placid lap dog would not be socially acceptable.

Pathogenesis from the behavioral view would be analyzed under the same categories as for deficit: (1) Stimulus factors would be restricted to inappropriateness of type (e.g., lap dog) to be paired with a naturally occurring reflex such as fear; (2) organismic factors would be emotionality, high anxiety level from other causes, or in the case of sexual deviations, erotic arousal from some other cause; (3) learning factors could be overlearning through too many trials or avoidance tactics so that natural extinction did not occur, as in phobias.

The time scale of examples of respondent disorders set out in Table 5-1 is purely hypothetical based upon Thompson's theory of developmental learning stages. The limits are elastic, and while respondent learning declines in importance largely because the world becomes increasingly comprehensible and masterable, it remains as an ever-present process which is likely to assume importance whenever high states of emotion occur. A complicating factor, however, is that, because of increasing mastery of the environment, surplus or maladaptive respondent disorders are likely to be obscured by action to escape (e.g., tantrums), avoid (e.g., school refusal), or to attain (e.g., sexual assault), the emotional state, or in short, *lead to second order but more obvious and disturbing operant type behavior* for which the conditioned emotional state acts as the often inconspicuous reinforcer (positive or negative). Further, this development of a second order operant response prevents the natural extinction of the conditioned response by counter-conditioning. For example, overcoming fear of dogs by playing with them, (not running away). It is thus not surprising that most of the interest in the behavioral approach with children centers on operant type disorders.

3. OPERANT LEARNING DISORDERS

Deficit Disorders: Again, it must be emphasized that diagnosis of a deficit disorder requires a behavioral deficit such as dyslexia not a positive learned disorder like elective mutism.

Stimulus factors here are basically similar to those outlined for respondent learning deficits. In the operant situation, however, they do not actually *evoke* the response, they merely provide cues.

These cues suggest, but do not compel, a line of action and indicate the consequences which will follow. There is much more room for complexity in cuing than than evoking, so that language and cognition become critical for correct cuing. Similarly, operant responses (for instance, language and highly skilled motor behaviors) are potentially much more complex than a simple respondent and, the more complex the learning process, the more vulnerable it is to interference.

Learning may be impeded by absent, ambiguous or unclear cuing. Organsmic factors include limitation of the sensory, motor, or cognitive ability of the individual (as in mental retardation or autism) or by disruptive states such as anxiety. Though it is only one part of the operant learning process, great emphasis is placed on the critical role of reinforcement or other contingencies in learning and there has been demonstration[13, 14, 15] that deficit disorders, such as inattentiveness, are often due simply to the failure to reinforce good behavior effectively or often enough (conforming is expected of children, often only naughtiness merits attention). Much of the success in behavior modification rests simply on rewarding unnoticed good behavior and thus making it more frequent.

Other sources of failure to learn, premature extinction or often, simply low rates of emission, lie in faulty teaching; failure to shape the behavior (expecting too much too quickly), to use prompts, models or other devices for guiding the child in his attempts to make the right response, and in proper scheduling of learning trials (infrequent or fatiguing or boring) and the reinforcement type (uninteresting) or pattern (initially as frequent or consistent as possible then thinning and irregularising).

Maladaptive or Deviant Disorders: Here the child does have a behavior or skill but its appearance is inappropriate to the situation, excessive (e.g. screeching) or otherwise unsuitable to the child, parent, or social setting.

While theoretically this can be due to stimulus, organism, or reinforcement factors, in practice most of the interest in analysis of a deviant behavior or establishment of its immediate etiology has centered on the search for reinforcement which is assumed as a matter of course to be present. Experience has shown that this is most likely to be attention from significant others (parents, peers, teachers) though a wide range of reinforcers such as food, money, the opportunity to do something of greater interest, satisfaction of curiosity, or problem solving, may be involved. Generally speaking, there is less interest etiologically in how the deviant behavior came about than in *what is maintaining it now* and how it can be changed (see section on behavioral approaches to treatment).

Examples of operant disorders of both types are given in Table 5-1. Again, the list is illustrative only and is neither comprehensive nor are behaviors listed certainly, invariably or exclusively of this etiology. Further examples can be found in reviews by Risley and Baer,[13] Ross,[14, 15] Werry and Wollersheim[22] and other sections in this book (q.v.) Suffice it to say at this point that operant techniques have been applied to the correction of a wide range of deficit disorders of imitation, motor skills, language, reading, social behavior, self-care skills, and to a panoply of deviant behaviors such as aggression, psychotic behaviors, soiling, crying, tantrums, echolalia, elective mutism, anorexia nervosa, obesity, self-mutilating behaviors, self stimulation, and so on.* All have demonstrated the validity and utility of the behavioral-learning view of pathogenesis.

Summary and Conclusions

The behavioral approach is a relative newcomer to child psychiatry, derived from experimental psychology and from learning theory in particular. It shows its origins in an emphasis on objectivity, a rejection of the medical notion of underlying etiology, and an assumption that the process by which psychopathological symptoms are acquired, or if deficit, not acquired, is through the laws of learning. Abnormality is seen to be based solely in

* See references 1, 13, 14, 15, 22.

value judgments about the behavior or deficits made by parents, teachers, or other social evaluators. Learning theory embraces notions of temperament/adaptation and two basic learning processes: emotional learning or respondent conditioning and instrumental learning or operant conditioning.

Its differences from psychoanalytic theory are less than commonly claimed but real enough. In general, the behavioral approach to etiology is more precise and, therefore, more prediction and treatment oriented, but it is narrower in scope. The psychoanalytic approach on the other hand is less precise but more explanatory (especially post hoc) and more satisfying clinically (but not more useful) because of greater scope. The behavioral approach has been applied to a wide variety of psychopathological conditions, processes, and symptoms, with clear demonstration of the universal validity of the laws of learning in their development, maintenance, and modification. It has added significantly to our understanding of childhood disorders, their measurement and their treatment.

The shortcomings of the behavioral approach lie in the relative neglect of the developmental approach, the minimizing of coexistent physical etiological factors and limitations of potential and its preoccupation with simple behaviors, simple organisms (autism, severe mental retardation, very young children) and simple processes. The distinguishing features of the human organism lie in language, cognition, and intelligence, areas of great activity in experimental child psychology (see Reese and Lipsitt[12]) which the behavioral approach must incorporate if it is to advance beyond a simple, symptom-oriented technology.

REFERENCES

1. ASHEM, B. A., and POSER, E. G., *Adaptive Learning—Behavior Modification With Children*, Pergamon, New York, 1973.
2. BAER, D. M., "The Control of Developmental Process: Why Wait?" in Nesselroade, J. R., and Reese, H. W. (Eds.), *Life-span Developmental Psychology*, pp. 185–193, Academic Press, New York, 1973.
3. BANDURA, A., and WALTERS, R. H., *Social Learning and Personality Development*, Holt, Rinehart and Winston, New York, 1963.
4. BERGMANN, P., and ESCALONA, S. K., "Unusual Sensitivities in Very Young Children," in Eissler, R. S., et al. (Eds.), *The Psychoanalytic Study of the Child*, vols. 3/4, pp. 333–343, International Universities Press, New York, 1949.
5. BIJOU, S. W., and BAER, D. M., "Universal Stage of Infancy," *Child Development*, vol. 1, Appleton-Century-Crofts, New York, 1965.

6. ———, "A Systematic and Empirical Theory," *Child Development*, vol. 1, Appleton-Century-Crofts, New York, 1961.
7. DOLLARD, J., and MILLER, N. E., *Personality and Psychotherapy*, McGraw-Hill, New York, 1950.
8. EYSENCK, H. J., "Learning Theory and Behavior Therapy," *Journal of Mental Science, 105*:61–75, 1959.
9. HARLOW, H. F., *Learning to Love*, Albion, San Francisco, 1971.
10. HEBB, D. O., *The Organization of Behavior*, John Wiley, New York, 1949.
11. MOWRER, O. H., *Learning Theory and Personality Dynamics*, Ronald, New York, 1970.
12. REESE, H. W., and LIPSITT, L. P., *Experimental Child Psychology*, Academic Press, New York, 1970.
13. RISLEY, T. R., and BAER, D. M., "Operant Behavior Modification: The Deliberate Development of Behavior," in Caldwell, B. M., and Ricciuti, H. N. (Eds.), *Review*

of Child Development Research, vol. 3, pp. 283–329, University of Chicago Press, Chicago, 1973.

14. Ross, A. O., *Psychological Disorders of Children— A Behavior Approach to Theory Research and Therapy*, McGraw-Hill, New York, 1974.

15. ———, "Behavior Therapy," in Quay, H. C., and Werry, J. S. (Eds.), *Psychopathological Disorders of Childhood*, pp. 273–315, John Wiley, New York, 1972.

16. Sears, R. R., Maccoby, E. E., and Levin, H., *Patterns of Child Rearing*, Row Peterson, Evanston, Ill., 1957.

17. Thomas, A., Chess, S., and Birch, H. G., *Temperament and Behavior Disorders in Children*, New York University Press, New York, 1968.

18. Thompson, W. R., "Storage Mechanisms in Early Experience," in Hill, J. P. (Ed.), *Minnesota Symposia on Child Psychology*, vol. 3, pp. 97–127, University of Minnesota Press, Minneapolis, 1968.

19. ———, and Grusec, J. E., "Studies of Early Experience," in Mussen, P. (Ed.), *Carmichael's Manual of Child Psychology*, 3rd ed., vol. 1, pp. 565–654, John Wiley, New York, 1970.

20. Ullmann, L. P., and Krasner, L., *A Psychological Approach to Abnormal Behavior*, Prentice-Hall, Englewood Cliffs, N.J., 1969.

21. Wenar, C., *Personality Development from Infancy to Adulthood*, Houghton-Mifflin, Boston, 1971.

22. Werry, J. S., and Wollersheim, J., "Behavior Therapy With Children—A Broad Overview," *Journal of the American Academy of Child Psychiatry*, 6:346–370, 1967.

PART B
Nosology

6 / Nosology and Diagnosis

J. Gary May

noso-, a learned borrowing from Greek meaning "disease" . . .

nosology (no sol'o je), *n.* 1. the systematic classification of diseases. 2. the knowledge of a disease . . .

. . . there are no diseases, only sick people

Armand Trousseau

A rose by any other name would smell as sweet.

William Shakespeare,
Romeo and Juliet

The scientific purist, who will wait for medical statistics until they are nosologically exact, is no wiser than Horace's rustic waiting for the river to flow away.

Major Greenwood

The wit of man has rarely been more exercised than in the attempt to classify the morbid mental phenomena covered by the term insanity. The result has been disappointing.

Daniel Hack Tuke

Introduction

CURRENT ISSUES IN DIAGNOSIS

"There are two kinds of people. There are those who divide people into two groups and those who don't." This remark attributed to Robert Benchley accurately describes the current state of child psychiatry. The controversy which rages around diagnosis in children involves an ongoing debate between those who classify and those who do not. It is a fact that classification, regardless of whether it is done on the basis of historical study, descriptive evaluation, statistical clusters, functional determination, computer techniques, or other means of assessment, always tends to have a certain arbitrary and pejorative quality. A diagnosis requires that some simplification take place, that a high value be placed upon certain indicators and a low one upon others. Hence, it cannot totally and adequately describe any individual patient.

For many a clinician, the controversy over classificatory schemata may seem to be distant and to impinge little upon his practice. Nonetheless, diagnosis has a continuing utilitarian value in clinical practice. In the final assessment, although the basis and even the ethics of the classificatory process may be stoutly debated, this pragmatic value is responsible for the continued use of such schemata.

THE DIAGNOSTIC AND STATISTICAL MANUALS OF THE AMERICAN PSYCHIATRIC ASSOCIATION

The official classification system, the Diagnostic and Statistical Manual of the American Psychiatric Association, has extensive use and influence in the United States. Although The Diagnostic and Statistical Manual, second edition (DSM-II), is being extensively revised, the first two editions are of considerable historical importance. The DSM-III is projected for official use following January of 1979.

DSM-I: The first diagnostic and statistical manual (DSM-I) was edited by Dr. Raines and published in 1952. In the introduction to the first edition, Raines reviewed the history of diagnostic classification in the United States, pointing out that the development of a uniform nomenclature was a comparatively recent event. Psychiatry had been represented on the committee to develop the first edition of the Standard Classified Nomenclature of Disease published in 1933. Between 1933 and the second World War, many teaching centers had developed modified systems of nomenclature for their own use; however, with the casualities of World War II, American psychiatry was faced with an increased psychiatric load. The system developed prior to World War II was primarily for the use of public mental hospitals but the military psychiatrist found that only approximately 10 percent of the total cases he saw fell into the categories listed in his nomenclature. Many minor conditions became classified as "psychopathic personality," and it was clear that the official system was untenable. Beginning in 1944, the Navy, then the Army, and finally the Veterans Administration revised the nomenclature. There followed, in 1948, a revised international nomenclature using terminology similar to that of the armed forces.

The first committee on nomenclature and statistics of the American Psychiatric Association, which Dr. Raines chaired, met between 1946 and 1951 and included many well-known names in American psychiatry. They developed the DSM-I. The committee distributed mimeographed copies of the proposed nomenclature to approximately 10 percent of the membership of the American Psychiatric Association and solicited their comments. The final revision was published in 1952.

The DSM-I is remarkable for several reasons. The concepts and approach which it includes represented a major step forward. It reflected an awareness of the need for qualifying phrases, including the designation of severity. It addressed itself to the question of related diagnoses and authorized the use of multiple psychiatric diagnoses when they were logical; it also recognized that certain diagnoses were incompatible with other diagnoses, such as the simultaneous use of psychoneurotic and psychotic reaction. It recognized the importance of premorbid personality and predisposition; and recognized, as well, the value of some indication of stress and its relationship to the onset of the condition.

DSM-I demonstrated a total lack of any special consideration of children in its listings. Mental deficiency was considered. The committee acknowledged the problem it had with a classificatory system for mental retardation; a problem that is not entirely resolved even to this day. Nevertheless, by developing a new system of classification more related to the style in which the psychiatrist was currently working, the DSM-I made an important contribution. Moreover, it recognized dynamic and psychoanalytic principles which made it far more usable than any previous system. The psychiatric manifestations themselves were now the most important aspect of the classification system rather than the severity or degree of organic brain syndrome. The system thereby recognized that the degree of psychiatric impairment may not be related on a one-to-one basis with the extent of the organic lesion.

The DSM-I recognized that mental deficiency produced by paranatal factors or in the formative years of infancy and childhood belong under the chronic brain syndromes. Where the primary clinical problem appeared to be a disorder of intelligence, the diagnosis could be mental deficiency. The committee noted their difficulty in finding another word for this condition and they regarded the term, *mental deficiency*, as a legal term, similar to "insanity," with little psychiatric meaning.

DSM-II: The second diagnostic and statistical manual was copyrighted in 1968. Some substantial changes were made whose merit is still being debated. DSM-II used a style which would be compatible with the International Classification of Diseases (ICD). Some use was made of the allowance by the World Health Organization for some modification of the ICD by individual countries.

The DSM-II had a profound impact on the diagnostic nomenclature *officially* available for cases of children and adolescents. It is interesting to note that there is virtually no discussion of that change in the forward to the DSM-II by Gruenberg (chairman of the committee) or by Kramer in his Introduction to the DSM-II. There was merely mention that, "Dr. Leon Eisenberg, the child psychiatrist, was also added to the subcommittee (on classification of mental disorders)."[2]

There has been an enormous outpouring of discussion and criticism of the DSM-II, much of it related to the general psychiatric sections. However, there has been a relatively universal sense of negative response to the listing of behavior disorders of children and adolescents. There is considerable recognition of a need for a separate section regarding childhood and adolescence.

Spitzer and Wilson[103] review the history of

DSM-II. Like the DSM-I, the DSM-II was developed by a committee of the American Psychiatric Association on Nomenclature and Statistics, and the manual was circulated to 120 psychiatrists. There were a number of changes in the DSM-II, including alteration and organization of sequence. Jenkins, a member of the committee which developed the DSM-II, points out that the DSM-II, by including adolescence in the 308 section, allows for a separation of behavior disorders of childhood and the behavior disorders of adolescence. He states that the subdivision has its origin in the groupings which have been seen repeatedly in statistical clusterings of children brought to child guidance services and clinics. The major works cited in support of that contention are those primarily of Jenkins[50, 51, 53] and his associate Hewitt,[54] along with Kobagashi,[61] Shamsie,[96] and Shinohara.[98]

Jenkins states that the groupings of the categories have been developed purely by descriptive clustering. Albeit inadvertently, this contention may fuel the fire of those who condemn classification systems as related to social class, economic classification, or worse, ethnic labeling. He states that the groupings were derived by a purely descriptive clustering, but he examined the family backgrounds, economic status, family structure, and neighborhoods of children with disorders of behavior and found patterns which fit various diagnostic categories.[50] For example, Jenkins felt that the unwanted illegitimate children and only children were common in the runaway reaction category.

At the same time the DSM-II recognized the specific disorders of childhood and adolescence. By using this particular classificatory system, the DSM-II has given credence to those who would state that the classification is potentially unfair and actually damaging to the child.[46] To further complicate the problem, the classification is derived almost entirely on the basis of behavior with little emphasis on the internal forces which are at work within the child. Although family membership and economic status may fall into statistically significant clusters, it is dangerous to make the child's diagnosis dependent upon his family. To compound the problem, such a formulation may lead to an immediate reaction or "treatment" which can disrupt the family. In several of the categories, Jenkins states that placement may be necessary or mandated. That may be true in individual cases, but to link placement with a diagnostic category can be unfortunate. Since the publication of the DSM-II, the criticism of diagnosis by symptom clusters and factor analysis is widespread. It appears that a wide circle of child mental health professionals found this approach to diagnosis unacceptable, and the negative reactions to the DSM-II's approach to children and adolescents followed quickly. Numerous authors* have commented upon the serious problems for children and adolescents which the DSM-II has fostered. One of the most effective criticisms was that by Silver[99] who takes thoughtful and well-reasoned issue with the DSM-II. He points out that the DSM-II did attempt to rectify the problem of the DSM-I by including a separate section on child and adolescent psychopathology. He points out the logical inconsistencies of the diagnostic schema (such as the DSM-II), which recommends the use of an adult category if the underlying psychopathology or etiology of the condition is understood. It means that the categories which remain for childhood have little value and represent only the most superficial examples of descriptive diagnosis. Silver points out examples of the problem. For instance, the patent placed in the category of "overanxious reaction of childhood," if fully diagnosed, would have to go into another category. Silver offers the analogy of a physician's diagnosing a patient with increased blood and urine glucose as "carbohydrate reaction of childhood." Although it would be descriptively correct, the diagnosis would be of very little value. He points out the difficulties associated with the hyperkinetic reaction of childhood and notes that if one completely understood what was going on and attempted to make a thorough study of the patient, he will utilize either, "the organic (brain syndrome) or functional (neurosis) diagnosis." He discusses the problems associated with runaway reactions of childhood and brings forward the issue of diagnostic adequacy in a developing, ever-changing individual such as the child or adolescent. He notes that the DSM-II did not choose to utilize the 1966 GAP categories and thereby turned away from a more functional diagnostic schema. Silver concludes that the DSM-II, "neither facilitates communication nor reduces confusion and ambiguity . . . thus many psychiatrists have difficulty accepting or using it."

Silver's prophecy has come to pass. Many child and adolescent psychiatrists have difficulty accepting and using the DSM-II. Other criticism abounds. Jackson[49] is very critical of the DSM-II. He is particularly critical of the classification, the psychotic disorders of childhood. He feels

---

* See references 8, 27, 28, 41, 80, and 99.

TABLE 6–1

DSM-II

I. MENTAL RETARDATION
310. Borderline
311. Mild
312. Moderate
313. Severe
314. Profound
315. Unspecified

With each: Following or associated with
.0 Infection or intoxication
.1 Trauma or physical agent
.2 Disorders of metabolism, growth or nutrition
.3 Gross brain disease (post natal)
.4 Unknown prenatal influence
.5 Chromosomal abnormality
.6 Prematurity
.7 Major psychiatric disorder
.8 Psycho-social (environmental) deprivation
.9 Other condition

II. ORGANIC BRAIN SYNDROMES (OBS)
  A PSYCHOSES

Senile and pre-senile dementia
290.0 Senile dementia
290.1 Pre-senile dementia

Alcoholic psychosis
291.0 Delirium tremens
291.1 Korsakov's psychosis
291.2 Other alcoholic hallucinosis
291.3 Alcohol paranoid state
291.4* Acute alcohol intoxication*
291.5* Alcoholic deterioration*
291.6* Pathological intoxication*
291.9 Other alcoholic psychosis

Psychosis associated with intracranial infection
292.0 General paralysis
292.1 Syphilis of central nervous system
292.2 Epidemic encephalitis
292.3 Other and unspecified encephalitis
292.9 Other intracranial infection

Psychosis associated with other cerebral condition
293.0 Cerebral arteriosclerosis
293.1 Other cerebrovascular disturbance
293.2 Epilepsy
293.3 Intracranial neoplasm
293.4 Degenerative disease of the CNS
293.5 Brain trauma
293.9 Other cerebral condition

Psychosis associated with other physical condition
294.0 Endocrine disorder
294.1 Metabolic and nutritional disorder
294.2 Systemic infection
294.3 Drug or poison intoxication (other than alcohol)
294.4 Childbirth
294.5 Other and unspecified physical condition

  B NON-PSYCHOTIC OBS
309.0 Intracranial infection
301.13* Alcohol* (simple drunkenness)
309.14* Other drug, poison or systemic intoxication*
309.2 Brain trauma
309.3 Circulatory disturbance

309.4 Epilepsy
309.5 Disturbance of metabolism, growth, or nutrition
309.6 Senile or pre-senile brain disease
309.7 Intracranial neoplasm
309.8 Degenerative disease of the CNS
309.9 Other physical condition

III. PSYCHOSES NOT ATTRIBUTED TO PHYSICAL CONDITIONS LISTED PREVIOUSLY

Schizophrenia
295.0 Simple
295.1 Hebephrenic
295.2 Catatonic
295.23* Catatonic type, excited*
295.24* Catatonic type, withdrawn*
295.3 Paranoid
295.4 Acute schizophrenic episode
295.5 Latent
295.6 Residual
295.7 Schizo-affective
295.73* Schizo-affective, excited*
295.74* Schizo-affective, depressed*
295.8* Childhood*
295.90* Chronic undifferentiated*
295.99* Other schizophrenia*

Major affective disorders
296.0 Involutional melancholia
296.1 Manic-depressive illness, manic
296.2 Manic-depressive illness, depressed
296.3 Manic-depressive illness, circular
296.33* Manic-depressive, circular, manic*
296.34* Manic-depressive, circular, depressed*
296.8 Other major affective disorder

Paranoid states
297.0 Paranoia
297.1 Involutional paranoid state
297.9 Other paranoid state

Other psychoses
298.0 Psychotic depressive reaction

IV. NEUROSES
300.0 Anxiety
300.1 Hysterical
300.13* Hysterical, conversion type*
300.14* Hysterical, dissociative type*
300.2 Phobic
300.3 Obsessive compulsive
300.4 Depressive
300.5 Neurasthenic
300.6 Depersonalization
300.7 Hypochondriacal
300.8 Other neurosis

V. PERSONALITY DISORDERS AND CERTAIN OTHER NON-PSYCHOTIC MENTAL DISORDERS

Personality disorders
301.0 Paranoid
301.1 Cyclothymic
301.2 Schizoid
301.3 Explosive
301.4 Obsessive compulsive
301.5 Hysterical
301.6 Asthenic

TABLE 6–1 *(continued)*

301.7	Antisocial		306.1	Specific learning disturbance
301.81*	Passive-aggressive*		306.2	Tic
301.82*	Inadequate		306.3	Other psychomotor disorder
301.89*	Other specified types*		306.4	Disorders of sleep

Sexual deviation

302.0	Homosexuality		306.5	Feeding disturbance
302.1	Fetishism		306.6	Enuresis
302.2	Pedophilia		306.7	Encopresis
302.3	Transvestitism		306.8	Cephalalgia
302.4	Exhibitionism		306.9	Other special symptom
302.5*	Voyeurism*			

VIII. TRANSIENT SITUATIONAL DISTURBANCES

302.6*	Sadism*		307.0*	Adjustment reaction of infancy*
302.7*	Masochism*		307.1*	Adjustment reaction of childhood*
302.8	Other sexual deviation		307.2*	Adjustment reaction of adolescence*

Alcoholism

303.0	Episodic excessive drinking		307.3*	Adjustment reaction of adult life*
303.1	Habitual excessive drinking		307.4*	Adjustment reaction of late life*
303.2	Alcohol addiction			
303.9	Other alcoholism			

IX. BEHAVIOR DISORDERS OF CHILDHOOD AND ADOLESCENCE

Drug dependence

304.0	Opium, opium alkaloids and their derivatives		308.0*	Hyperkinetic reaction*
			308.1*	Withdrawing reaction*
304.1	Synthetic analgesics with morphine-like effects		308.2*	Overanxious reaction*
			308.3*	Runaway reaction*
304.2	Barbiturates		308.4*	Unsocialized aggressive reaction*
304.3	Other hypnotics and sedatives or "tranquilizers"		308.5*	Group delinquent reaction*
			308.9*	Other reaction*
304.4	Cocaine			
304.5	Cannabis sativa (hashish, marihuana)			

X. CONDITIONS WITHOUT MANIFEST PSYCHIATRIC DISORDER AND NON-SPECIFIC CONDITIONS

304.6	Other psycho-stimulants			
304.7	Hallucinogens			
304.8	Other drug dependence			

Social maladjustment without manifest psychiatric disorder

VI. PSYCHOPHYSIOLOGIC DISORDERS

305.0	Skin		316.0*	Marital maladjustment*
305.1	Musculoskeletal		316.1*	Social maladjustment*
305.2	Respiratory		316.2*	Occupational maladjustment*
305.3	Cardiovascular		316.3*	Dyssocial behavior*
305.4	Hemic and lymphatic		316.9*	Other social maladjustment
305.5	Gastro-intestinal			

Non-specific conditions

305.6	Genito-urinary		317*	Non-specific conditions*
305.7	Endocrine			

No mental disorder

305.8	Organ of special sense		318*	No mental disorder
305.9	Other type			

XI. NON-DIAGNOSTIC TERMS FOR ADMINISTRATIVE USE

VII. SPECIAL SYMPTOMS

306.0	Speech disturbance		319.0*	Diagnosis deferred*
			319.1*	Boarder*
			319.2*	Experiment only*
			319.3*	Other*

* Categories added to ICD-8 for use in U.S. only.
NOTE: Reprinted by permission of the publishers from American Psychiatric Association, committee on Nomenclature and Statistics, *Diagnostic and Statistical Manual of Mental Disorders*, 2nd ed., (DSM-II), American Psychiatric Association, Washington, D.C., 1968. © 1968 by The American Psychiatric Association.

that the term "childhood psychosis" is more desirable than "schizophrenia," feeling that the child with childhood psychosis does not necessarily become the adult schizophrenic, nor does the condition necessarily phenomenologically represent adult schizophrenia. He recommends that there be two distinct classification systems, one for child and one for adult psychiatry, which would be "organized along analogous yet autonomous classificatory lines."

One attempt was made to develop a correlation table between presenting symptoms and eventual diagnosis. This hypothesis asserted that if the DSM-II categories of behavior disorders were hard and fast, the children should cluster together in equivalent groupings. They did not.[8]

DSM-III: Beginning in September of 1973, under the leadership of Robert Spitzer, M.D., a new task force began to shape the DSM-III. The target date for publication has been set for January

TABLE 6–2

Draft of Axes I and II of DSM-III Classification* as of March 30, 1977

ORGANIC MENTAL DISORDERS

1. This section includes those organic mental disorders in which the etiology or pathogenesis is listed below (taken from the mental disorders section of ICD-9-CM).

Senile and pre-senile dementias
Code organic mental disorder in fifth digit as 1 = (uncomplicated), 2 = with delirium, 3 = with delusional features, 4 = with depressive features, 9 = unspecified.

290.0x	Senile dementia
290.1x	Pre-senile dementia
290.4x	Repeated infarct dementia

Drug induced
  Alcohol
291.60	intoxication
291.40	idiosyncratic intoxication (Pathological intoxication)
291.80	withdrawal
291.00	withdrawal delirium (Delirium tremens)
291.30	withdrawal hallucinosis
291.10	amnestic syndrome (Wernicke-Korsakoff syndrome)

  Barbiturate or related acting sedative or hypnotic
292.01	intoxication
292.81	withdrawal syndromes
292.31	amnestic syndrome

  Opioid
292.02	intoxication
292.82	withdrawal

  Cocaine
292.03	intoxication

  Amphetamine or related acting sympathomimetic
292.04	intoxication
292.14	delirium
292.44	organic delusional syndrome
292.84	withdrawal

  Hallucinogen
292.05	intoxication
292.45	organic delusional syndrome
292.65	organic affective syndrome

  Cannabis
292.06	intoxication
292.46	organic delusional syndrome
292.76	organic personality syndrome

  Tobacco
292.87	withdrawal

  Caffeine
292.08	intoxication (caffeinism)

  Other, mixed, or unspecified drug
292.09	intoxication
292.19	delirium
292.29	dementia
292.39	amnestic syndrome
292.49	organic delusional syndrome
292.59	hallucinosis
292.69	organic affective syndrome
292.79	organic personality syndrome
292.89	withdrawal
292.99	unspecified organic brain syndrome

2. This section includes those organic mental disorders in which the etiology or pathogenesis is either noted as an additional diagnosis from outside of the mental disorders section of ICD-9-CM (Axis III) or is unknown.

293.00	Delirium
294.10	Dementia
294.00	Amnestic syndrome
293.20	Organic delusional syndrome
293.30	Hallucinosis
293.40	Organic affective syndrome
310.10	Organic personality syndrome
294.80	Other or mixed organic brain syndrome
294.90	Unspecified organic brain syndrome

DRUG USE DISORDERS (including alcohol)

Code course of illness in fourth (Alcoholism) or fifth digit as 1 = continuous, 2 = episodic, 3 = in remission, 9 = unspecified.

303.x0	Alcohol dependence (Alcoholism)
305.0x	Alcohol abuse
304.1x	Barbiturate or related acting sedative or hypnotic dependence
305.4x	Barbiturate or related acting sedative or hypnotic abuse
304.0x	Opioid dependence
305.5x	Opioid abuse
304.2x	Cocaine dependence
305.6x	Cocaine abuse
304.4x	Amphetamine or related acting sympathomimetic dependence
305.7x	Amphetamine or related acting sympathomimetic abuse
305.3x	Hallucinogen abuse
304.3x	Cannabis dependence
305.2x	Cannabis abuse
305.1x	Tobacco use disorder
304.7x	Combination of opioid type drug with any other dependence
304.8x	Combinations of drug dependence excluding opioid type drug
304.6x	Other specified drug dependence
304.9x	Unspecified drug dependence
305.9x	Other, mixed, or unspecified

SCHIZOPHRENIC DISORDERS

Course of illness may be coded in fifth digit as 1 = acute, 2 = subacute, 3 = subchronic, 4 = chronic, 5 = in remission, 9 = unspecified.

295.1x	Disorganized (Hebephrenic)
295.2x	Catatonic
295.3x	Paranoid
295.7x	Schizo-affective, depressed
295.8x	Schizo-affective, manic
295.9x	Undifferentiated
295.6x	Residual

PARANOID DISORDERS

297.10	Paranoia
297.30	Shared paranoid disorder (Folie à deux)
297.00	Paranoid state
297.90	Unspecified paranoid disorder

TABLE 6–2 (*continued*)

AFFECTIVE DISORDERS

Episodic affective disorders

Code severity of episode in fifth digit as 1 = mild, 2 = moderate, 3 = severe but not psychotic, 4 = severe and psychotic, 5 = in partial remission, 6 = in full remission, 9 = unspecified.

Manic disorder
- 296.0x single episode
- 296.1x recurrent

Depressive disorder
- 296.2x single episode
- 296.3x recurrent

Bipolar affective disorder
- 296.4x manic
- 296.5x depressed
- 296.6x mixed

Intermittent affective disorders

- 301.11 Intermittent depressive disorder (Depressive character)
- 301.12 Intermittent hypomanic disorder (Hypomanic personality)
- 301.13 Intermittent bipolar disorder (Cyclothymic personality)

Atypical affective disorders

- 296.80 Atypical depressive disorder
- 296.90 Atypical manic disorder
- 296.70 Atypical bipolar disorder

PSYCHOSES NOT ELSEWHERE CLASSIFIED

- 298.80 Brief reactive psychosis
- 298.90 Atypical psychosis

ANXIETY DISORDERS

Phobic Disorders
- 300.21 Agoraphobia with panic attacks
- 300.22 Agoraphobia without panic attacks
- 300.23 Social phobia
- 300.24 Simple phobia
- 300.29 Unspecified phobia
- 300.01 Panic disorder
- 300.30 Obsessive compulsive disorder
- 300.02 Generalized anxiety disorder
- 300.09 Atypical anxiety disorder

FACTITIOUS DISORDERS

- 300.15 Factitious illness with psychological symptoms
- 300.16 Chronic factitious illness with physical symptoms (Munchausen syndrome)
- 300.17 Other factitious illness with physical symptoms
- 300.18 Unspecified factitious illness

SOMATOFORM DISORDERS

- 300.81 Somatization disorder (Briquet's disorder)
- 300.11 Conversion disorder
- 307.80 Psychalgia
- 300.70 Atypical somatoform disorder

DISSOCIATIVE DISORDERS

- 300.12 Amnesia
- 300.13 Fugue
- 300.14 Multiple personality
- 300.60 Depersonalization
- 300.19 Other or unspecified

PERSONALITY DISORDERS

Note: These are coded on Axis II.
- 301.00 Paranoid
- 301.20 Asocial (Schizoid)
- 295.50 Schizotypal (Latent, Borderline schizophrenia)
- 301.50 Histrionic
- 301.81 Narcissistic
- 301.70 Antisocial
- 301.83 Unstable (Borderline personality organization)
- 301.82 Avoidant
- 301.60 Dependent
- 301.40 Compulsive
- 301.88 Other, mixed, or unspecified

PSYCHOSEXUAL DISORDERS

Gender identity or role disorders

Indicate sexual history in the fifth digit of Transsexualism code as 1 = asexual, 2 = homosexual, 3 = heterosexual, 4 = mixed, 9 = unspecified.

- 302.5x Transsexualism
- 302.30 Transvestism
- 302.61 Gender identity or role disorder of childhood
- 302.62 Other gender identity or role disorders of adult life

Paraphilias
- 302.81 Fetishism
- 302.10 Zoophilia
- 302.20 Pedophilia
- 302.00 Dyshomophilia
- 302.40 Exhibitionism
- 302.82 Voyeurism
- 302.83 Sexual masochism
- 302.84 Sexual sadism
- 302.85 Other

Psychosexual dysfunctions
- 302.71 with inhibited sexual desire
- 302.72 with inhibited sexual excitement (frigidity, impotence)
- 302.73 with inhibted female orgasm
- 302.74 with inhibited male orgasm
- 302.75 with premature ejaculation
- 302.76 with functional dyspareunia
- 302.77 with functional vaginismus
- 302.78 other
- 302.79 unspecified

Other psychosexual disorders
- 302.90 Psychosexual disorder not elsewhere classified

DISORDERS USUALLY ARISING IN CHILDHOOD OR ADOLESCENCE

This section lists conditions that usually manifest themselves in childhood or adolescence. However, any appropriate adult diagnosis can be used for diagnosing a child.

Mental retardation

Code a 1 in the fifth digit to indicate association with a known biological factor which must be coded on Axis III. Otherwise code 0.
- 317.0x Mild mental retardation

TABLE 6–2 (*Continued*)

318.0x   Moderate mental retardation
318.1x   Severe mental retardation
318.2x   Profound mental retardation
319.0x   Unspecified mental retardation

Pervasive developmental disorders
299.00   Infantile autism
299.80   Early childhood psychosis
299.20   Pervasive developmental disorder of childhood, residual state
299.90   Unspecified

Attention deficit disorders
314.00   with hyperactivity
314.10   without hyperactivity

Specific developmental disorders
Note: These are coded on Axis II.
315.00   Specific reading disorder
315.10   Specific arithmetical disorder
315.30   Developmental language disorder
315.40   Developmental articulation disorder
315.50   Coordination disorder
Indicate course in the fifth digit as 1 = primary, 2 = secondary, 9 = unspecified.
307.6x   Enuresis
307.7x   Encopresis
315.60   Mixed
315.80   Other
315.90   Unspecified

Stereotyped movement disorders
307.21   Motor tic disorder
307.22   Motor-verbal tic disorder (Gilles de la Tourette)
307.29   Unspecified tic disorder
307.30   Other

Speech disorders not elsewhere classified
307.00   Stuttering
307.91   Elective mutism

Conduct disorders
Code severity in fifth digit as 1 = mild, 2 = moderate, 3 = severe, 9 = unspecified.
312.0x   Undersocialized conduct disorder, aggressive type
312.1x   Undersocialized conduct disorder, unaggressive type
312.2x   Socialized conduct disorder

Eating disorders
307.10   Anorexia nervosa
307.51   Bulimia
307.52   Pica
307.53   Rumination
307.58   Other or unspecified

Anxiety disorders of childhood or adolescence
309.21   Separation anxiety disorder
313.20   Shyness disorder
313.00   Overanxious disorder

Disorders characteristic of late adolescence
309.22   Emancipation disorder of adolescence or early adult life

313.60   Identity disorder
309.23   Specific academic or work inhibition

Other disorders of childhood or adolescence
313.50   Oppositional disorder
313.70   Academic underachievement disorder

REACTIVE DISORDERS NOT ELSEWHERE CLASSIFIED
309.81   Post traumatic disorder

Adjustment disorders
300.40   with depressed mood
309.28   with anxious mood
309.24   with mixed emotional features
309.82   with physical symptoms
309.30   with disturbance of conduct
309.40   with mixed disturbance of emotions and conduct
309.83   with withdrawal
309.90   other or unspecified

DISORDERS OF IMPULSE CONTROL NOT ELSEWHERE CLASSIFIED
312.31   Pathological gambling
312.32   Kleptomania
312.33   Pyromania
312.34   Intermittent explosive disorder
312.35   Isolated explosive disorder
312.38   Other or unspecified impulse control disorder

SLEEP DISORDERS
Non-organic
307.41   Temporary insomnia
307.42   Persistent insomnia
307.43   Temporary hypersomnia
307.44   Persistent hypersomnia
307.45   Non-organic sleep-wake cycle disturbance
307.46   Somnambulism
307.47   Night terrors
307.48   Other non-organic dyssomnias
307.49   Unspecified non-organic sleep disorder

Organic
780.51   Insomnia associated with diseases elsewhere classified
780.52   Insomnia with central sleep-apnea
780.53   Other organic insomnia
780.54   Hypersomnia associated with diseases elsewhere classified
780.55   Hypersomnia associated with obstructive or mixed sleep-apnea
780.56   Other organic hypersomnia
780.57   Organic sleep-wake cycle disturbance
780.58   Organic dyssomnias
780.59   Unspecified organic sleep disorder

OTHER DISORDERS AND CONDITIONS
Unspecified mental disorder (non-psychotic)
307.99   Unspecified mental disorder (non-psychotic)
Psychic factors in physical condition
Specify physical condition on Axis III and degree of psychological component in the fourth digit as 1 =

TABLE 6–2 (*Continued*)

probable, 2 = prominent, 9 = unknown or unspecified degree.	V61.20 Parent-child problem
	V62.81 Other interpersonal problem
316.xo Psychic factors in physical condition	V62.20 Occupational problem
	V62.82 Simple bereavement
No mental disorder	V15.81 Noncompliance with medical treatment
V71.00 No mental disorder	V62.88 Other life circumstance problem
Conditions not attributable to known mental disorder	*Administrative categories*
V6520. Malingering	799.90 Diagnosis deferred
V71.01 Adult antisocial behavior	V70.70 Research subject
V71.02 Childhood or adolescent antisocial behavior	V63.20 Boarder
V61.10 Marital problem	V68.30 Referral without need for evaluation

° The traditional neurotic subtypes are included in the Affective, Anxiety, Somatoform, and Dissociative Disorders.
NOTE: For multiaxial diagnosis, each patient is coded on each of the five axes.
NOTE: Reprinted by permission of the publisher from American Psychiatric Association, Committee on Nomenclature and Statistics, Diagnostic and Statistical Manual of Mental Disorders, 3rd ed., (DSM-II), draft version as of March 30, 1977.

1979 but may be extended. (All the material in this chapter regarding the DSM-III comes from the draft of April 15, 1977, Robert Spitzer, M.D., Chairman, American Psychiatric Association Task Force on Nomenclature.) There will be major changes throughout the document. Changes from their first announcement have created much controversy. In the general section changes include a minimal use of the word "psychosis," the abandonment of the use of the term "neurosis," and the movement of psychophysiological disorders entirely to the realm of physical diagnosis. However, there has been added an expanded group of *Disorders arising in childhood or adolescence.*

The changes generated by the DSM-III Task Force go much deeper than just the names of disorders. The changes include the introduction of a multi-axial system of diagnosis, a format which attempts to mandate a much more specific set of criteria to be used for each diagnosis, and a description of each disorder which includes: Sensual features; Associated features; Sex ratio, prevalence in age at onset; Course, impairment and complications; Familial pattern; Predisposing factors; Differential diagnosis; and, Operational criteria.

For all of the controversy surrounding the DSM-III the task force deserves credit for the involvement of many professionals in this development and the use of extensive field trials for its completion. Of particular interest is the child and adolescent section. This section emphasizes disorders usually *arising* in childhood and adolescence. The stress is upon the origin of the disorders, so that these diagnoses may be used with adults. In the same sense, the general disorders may also be used, when appropriate, with children and adolescents.

The inclusion of a multiaxial system is of special importance for children and adolescents. The five axes suggested by the DSM-III are:

Axis I	—	Clinical psychiatric syndrome(s) and other conditions
Axis II	—	Personality disorders (adults) and specific developmental disorders (children and adolescence)
Axis III	—	Nonmental medical disorders
Axis IV	—	Severity of psychosocial stressors
Axis V	—	Highest level of adaptive functioning past year

It is gratifying to see the inclusion of a multiaxial system in the DSM-III. The multiaxial system is an extension of the work of the participants in ten yearly seminars conducted under the auspices of the World Health Organization (WHO). Rutter[90] described the triaxial system which then was extended in scope by the DSM-III.

The childhood and adolescent section has many important changes. Mental retardation will no longer include the borderline retardation category. There will be some new areas and regroupings including stereotyped movement disorders (tic, Gilles de la Tourette), speech disorders (stuttering, elective mutism), and eating disorders (anorexia nervosa, bulimia, pica and rumination). Where these classifications may not create great controversy there will be serious differences of opinion over some of the other disorders described.

The attention defects disorder category will probably receive much attention. The two subcategories are: With hyperactivity and Without hyperactivity. The committee made a deliberate attempt to not presume an etiology or support one or another view of "hyperactivity" or "minimal brain dysfunction." Much research is being done in this area. The division into *with* and *without* hyperactivity is important. These include a concept of a disorder without hyperactivity but with problems in concentration, mental organization, and impulsiveness.

The specific developmental disorders are very specific, including disorders related to reading, arithmetic, language, articulation, and coordination. These also include enuresis and encopresis.

Conduct disorders are divided into two groups: *unsocialized* and *socialized*. Unsocialized include *aggressive* and *nonaggressive* types. These are controversial categories. Psychiatry has had much difficulty classifying antisocial behavior. The unsocialized aggressive type of disorder is fairly self-explanatory. Antisocial, in the DSM-III, implies a lack of concern for the feelings of others and poor relationships with all but a few peers. The unsocialized conduct disorder, nonaggressive type, implies the same antisocial relationships (or lack of relationships) without open aggressive behavior, although there may be stealing, lying, disobedience, etc. The socialized conduct disorder is of special interest. It requires antisocial behavior in the company of others. It including gang and group antisocial activity. It also implies some "meaningful" relationships with a few selected people, usually peers.

The inclusion of a category for adolescent disorders is a major step forward. The DSM-III refers to these as "disorders characteristic of late adolescence." These categories include: Emancipation disorder of adolescence or early adult life; Identity disorder; and Specific academic or work inhibition.

Although the names of the disorders are fairly descriptive, some interesting points are made in the DSM-III description regarding the specifics of these conditions. In the emancipation disorder there is a requirement that the patients have made a recent change in situation in which they have become more independent of the parents. The disorder is characterized by the development of symptomatology which may include: Problems making decisions; Increased dependence upon parental advice; New concerns about parental permissiveness, expression of value in opposition to the parents, or homesickness, "which the individual finds inconsistent with the conscious wish to stay away from home;" and New marked dependence upon peers.

Identity disorder requires a sense of subjective distress related to identity and future issues in the absence of other diagnosable mental disorder.

This specific academic or work inhibition occurs in the face of apparent ability to do the work.

It also requires that there be a conscious desire and intention to perform adequately.

The DSM-III makes a substantial contribution to the classification of the disorders of childhood and adolescence. Even with a greatly expanded separate section for children and adolescents, with a multiaxial system, and a more definite descriptive style, the DSM-III must be seen as a changing and incomplete system—a system which will require future modification. It is a system for general use and, more specific in detailed nosology, will continue to be developed for the special needs of children and adolescents. Some systems which address these issues address children and adolescents more specifically are now discussed.

THE GAP SYSTEM

The introduction to the GAP (Group for Advancement of Psychiatry) Report, *Psychopathological Disorders in Childhood: Theoretical Considerations in a Proposed Classification*, states:

As yet, no all-encompassing, unequivocally accepted conceptual framework exists within which the intricate interrelationships among somatic, intellectual, emotional and social processes and phenomena in the developing child can be comprehended and organized in a thoroughly logical, all-inclusive fashion. (p. 173)[38]

Perhaps the nomenclature which comes closest to that ideal is the GAP classification system.

The classification was developed by a distinguished committee chaired by Dane G. Prugh, M.D. and included Anna R. Benjamin, Leon Eisenberg, George E. Gardner, Othilda Krug, Reginald S. Lourie, Eleanor Pavenstedt, Eveoleen Rexford and J. Franklin Robinson. Dr. Stella Chess was a consultant to the committee. The report was published in 1966 and has since received considerable attention. In view of this, it seems appropriate to examine the report in terms of its basic framework and to study the differential diagnostic considerations it presents in some detail. A number of these issues will also be discussed in the individual chapters which follow in this section. Suffice to say that this widely used classification system represents the most substantial and perhaps most useful approach yet developed.

The committee attempted to devise a comprehensive framework which included concepts and factors acceptable to professionals from different schools of thought. These basic concepts embraced three dimensions: (1) The psychosomatic dimension—involving the unity of mind and body;

(2) The developmental dimension; and (3) The psychosocial dimension.

The committee sought to establish operational definitions of the clinical categories and to reduce the implications of the category in the areas of etiology, prognosis, and treatment to a minimum. It was recognized that some professionals would be interested in developing diagnostic classifications along axes of special interest such as dynamic-genetic, parent-child, family-demographic, socio-cultural, or etiological. In the GAP Report, there is a suggested approach to a dynamic-genetic formulation. The GAP committee viewed its diagnostic system as an evolving structure in which future change is expected as a result of future knowledge.

A special feature of the GAP classification is the inclusion of a symptom list specific to children. The committee noted that the symptom list of the Standard Nomenclature is more appropriate for adults than for children. In presenting the symptom list, diagnosis is nicely differentiated from mere description. A specific symptom may thus be listed under several diagnostic-nosological headings. As an example there is a discussion of enuresis. They state,

Thus enuresis may be shown as an age-appropriate phenomena in a young preschool child under the heading *healthy response*; as a symptom of a regressive nature in a *reactive disorder*; as a continuing feature of a *developmental deviation*; as part of a neurotic picture involving *conversion mechanisms*; or as one symptom in a *chronic personality disorder* or *psychosis.* (p. 211)[88]

The GAP classification system is summarized in Table 6–4.

Each of the disorders will be discussed in detail throughout this volume. It is important to highlight some of the major diagnostic concepts associated with the GAP system. An initial overview demonstrates several obvious features. The order of presentation is reversed from that of most previous systems; that is, it lists the most healthy, adaptive, and least pathological disorders first. This stands in contrast to other systems (DSM-II, "Australian," etc.) which emphasize the most serious and chronic disorders by placing them first.

There has been considerable discussion of this system since its introduction. In 1970, one clinic reported its experience with twelve months use of GAP.[8] The new categories of healthy response and developmental deviations were found to be particularly useful. It was found, however, that the GAP did not clarify the diagnosis of the hyperactive or minimally brain damaged child. In addition, the adolescent with a severe identity crisis may be too severely disturbed to fit into the category of healthy reaction: developmental crisis. Nonetheless, GAP was found to be superior to the DSM-II in the diagnosis of children.

The system has been utilized in many settings. Shaw and Lucas[97] have employed it in their text. It was later reevaluated by the chairman of the committee and his colleagues[82] in a chapter in Hobbs' massive work. Prugh urges a combination of GAP with the WHO schema.[90] He emphasizes the need to extend diagnosis to include both a psychosocial and a functional classification. Prugh's concept is explained in detail later in this chapter.

"THE AUSTRALIAN SYSTEM" OF
J. V. ASHBURNER

A particularly interesting and well-thought out approach to the diagnosis of children was presented by Ashburner.[5] The paper deals in a constructively critical way with some major issues of classification as reflected in the GAP system.

Ashburner felt the GAP was "useful as a basis of formulation, but is not in its present form a good classification system." He separates the questions of classification and diagnosis and feels that one may go in either of two directions, as shown in Figure 6-1.

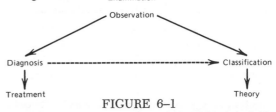

FIGURE 6–1

NOTE: Reprinted by permission of the publisher from J. V. Ashburner, "Some Problems of Classification, with Particular Reference to Child Psychiatry," *Australia and New Zealand Journal of Psychiatry*, 2:244–250, 1968. © 1968 by *The Australia and New Zealand Journal of Psychiatry*.

There may be interconnections between the two systems but they may also be completely isolated from each other. For example, "diagnosis and treatment may go on without classification, and many clinicians would prefer this in the present state of knowledge." Also, there can be classifications without diagnosis. The example Ashburner offers is the defining of offenders by their offenses; it may tell something about crime but nothing about the pathology of criminals.

He states that the usual approach to classification in child psychiatry is to assign an individual to a class according to some dominance rules: See Figure 6-2.

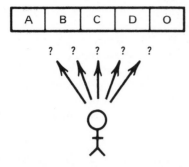

FIGURE 6-2

NOTE: Reprinted by permission of the publisher from J. V. Ashburner, "Some Problems of Classification, with Particular Reference to Child Psychiatry," *Australia and New Zealand Journal of Psychiatry*, 2:244–250, 1968. © 1968 by *The Australia and New Zealand Journal of Psychiatry.*

Another approach is one which is binary in nature and allows multiple diagnoses. This, he feels, is more related to traditional methods of taxonomists and is illustrated in Figure 6-3.

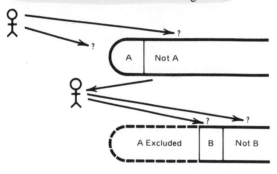

FIGURE 6-3

NOTE: Reprinted by permission of the publisher from J. V. Ashburner, "Some Problems of Classification, with Particular Reference to Child Psychiatry," *Australia and New Zealand Journal of Psychiatry*, 2:244–250, 1968. © 1968 by *The Australia and New Zealand Journal of Psychiatry.*

Ashburner also allows for the possibility of a "classificatory grid" with two or more axes of classification.

The system presented by Ashburner is offered as a means of classification, not diagnostic. He recommends using the major class and subclass headings of the GAP but changes the order (as follows). If two or more class headings apply, the case is classified in the first applicable class.

0. Retardation—moderate to profound
1. Brain Syndrome
2. Personality Disorder
3. Psychotic Disorder
4. Psychoneurotic Disorder
5. Psychophysiologic Disorder
6. Developmental Deviation
7. Reactive Disorder
8. Other Mental Disorder
9. Retardation, Other
10. Healthy Response

Developmental deviations would include the DSM-II category of "special symptoms." Reactive Disorders and Healthy Response would subsume DSM-II "transient situational disturbances."

The criteria for a sensible classification system and the important differentiation of classification versus diagnosis is part of Ashburner's contribution. The utilization of a binary concept with primacy of classificatory category is also valuable. However, the mere rearrangement of the category list of GAP does not satisfy the demand for a more accurate and clinically useful approach to diagnosis.

THE PSYCHOSOCIAL SCHEMA (PRUGH)

As noted, Dr. Dane Prugh was chairman of the GAP Committee on Classification (which produced the GAP system). He participated in the development of some of the most recent advances in diagnostic approaches to children. He was, thus, particularly aware of the absence of emphasis on function and development in classification systems. Prugh developed an approach to psychosocial disorders[80] which has considerable relevance to the current trends in systems of nosology for children.

In his presentation of the psychosocial schema, he briefly reviews the many theoretical forces at work in behavioral disorders. He also looks at advances in the "medical model" which had been extended to a "psycho-physio-social" model.

Prugh emphasized the complexity of "illness" in children in the context of an adaptive equilibrium (or "dynamic steady state"). This intricate process is summarized as follows:

— Stressful stimuli of physical, psychological or social nature may impinge upon the individual . . . stressful stimuli are relative—not absolute . . . the nature and degree . . . are determined by heredity, constitutional, developmental, and experimental factors.

— [The adaptive capacity of the child is] influenced by his own innate characteristics as well as his past experience, the reaction of key persons . . . and the degree of noxious influence of the current stimulus . . . [along with family considerations].

— [Etiology:] Multiple etiologic or "shaping" forces, of predisposing, precipitating, contributory, and perpetuating nature.

— Degree of vulnerability where the child's particular developmental phase ("critical periods") or situation. (p. 340)[80]

Prugh states that the definition of psychosocial dysfunction is somewhat arbitrary and dependent upon the factors listed above, along with some

TABLE 6-3

*Dimensions of Personality Development: Physical, Psychological, Social, Schematic Representation** *

PERIOD	AGE	PSYCHOSOCIAL TASKS (CRISES)	PSYCHOSEXUAL STAGES	RADIUS OF SIGNIFICANT RELATIONS	CENTRAL VALUE ORIENTATION	STAGES OF INTELLECTUAL DEVELOPMENT
	Birth					Sensory-Motor
INFANCY	3 mo.	Trust vs. mistrust (I am what I am given)	Oral-Respiratory Sensory-Kinesthetic (Incorporative role)	Maternal Person	Hope	The infant moves from a neonatal reflex level of complete self-world undifferentiation to a relatively coherent organization of sensory-motor actions. He learns that certain actions have specific effects upon the environment. Minimal symbolic activity is involved. Recognition of the constancy of external objects and primitive internal representation of the world begins.
	6 mo.					
	9 mo.					
	1 yr.	....			....	
PRESCHOOL	18 mo.	Autonomy vs. Shame, Doubt (I am what I "will")	Arel-Urethral Muscular (Retentive-Elminative Modes)	Parental Persons	Will	
	2 yr.					....
	3 yr.	....			....	Preoperational Thought (Prelogical)
SCHOOL AGE	4 yr.	Initiative vs. Guilt (I am what I imagine I can be)	Genital Locomotor (Oedipal) (Intrusive, Inclusive Modes)	Basic Family	Purpose	The child makes his first relatively unorganized and fumbling attempts to come to grips with the new and strange world of symbols. Thinking tends to be egocentric and intuitive. Conclusions are based on what he feels or what he would like to believe.
	5 yr.					
	6 yr.	....		Neighborhood, School	....	
ADOLESCENCE	7 yr.	Industry vs. Inferiority (I am what I learn)				.... Concrete Operational Thought
	8 yr.		"Latency"		Skill	Conceptual organization takes on stability and coherence. The child begins to appear rational and well organized in his adaptations. The fairly stable and orderly conceptual framework is systematically brought to bear on the world of objects around him. Physical quantities, such as weight and volume, are now viewed as constant despite changes in shape and size.
	9 yr.					
	10 yr.					
	11 yr.	....	Puberty	Peer In-Groups and Out-Groups	....	....
EARLY ADULTHOOD	12 yr.					
	13 yr.	Identity vs. Identity Diffusion (I know who I am)	Early Adolescence	Adult Models of Leadership		Formal Operational Thought
	14 yr.					
	15 yr.		Middle Adolescence		Fidelity	The individual can now deal effectively not only with the reality before him but also with the world of the abstract, propositional statements, and the world of possibility ("as if"). Cognition is of the adult type. The adolescent uses deductive reasoning and has the ability to evaluate the logic and quality of his own thinking. His increased abstract powers provide him with the capacity to deal with laws and principles. Although egocentrism is still evident at times, important idealistic attitudes are developing in the late adolescent and young adult.
	16 yr.					
	17 yr.		Late Adolescence			
MIDDLE ADULTHOOD	18 yr.	....			....	
		Intimacy vs. Isolation		Partners in Friendship, Sex Competition, Cooperation		
			Adulthood (Genitality)		Love	
		....			....	
LATE ADULTHOOD		Generativity vs. Self-Absorption or Stagnation		Divided Labor and Shared Household		
			Maturity		Care	
		....			....	
		Integrity vs. Despair, Disgust	Menopause Male Climacteric	"Mankind"	Wisdom....	

TABLE 6–3 (continued)

Dimensions of Personality Development: Physical, Psychological, Social, Schematic Representation*

PERIOD	AGE	PHYSICAL GROWTH	DEVELOPMENTAL STEPS (LINES)	DEVELOPMENTAL PROBLEMS
INFANCY	Birth	RAPID (SKELETAL)	"Normal autism" (0–3 mo.) Anticipation of feeding	Birth defects Feeding disorders: colic, regurgitation, vomiting, rumination, failure to thrive, marasmus, pylorospasm, feeding refusal, atopic exema
	3 mo.	Muscle constitutes 25% total body weight	Symbiosis (4–18 mo.)	
	6 mo.	Aeration maxillery and ethmoid sinuses	Stranger anxiety (6–10 mo.)	Extreme stranger anxiety Early infantile autism
	9 mo.	Eruption of deciduous central incisors (5–10 mo.)	Separation anxiety (8–24 mo.)	Physiologic anorexia
	1 yr.	Anterior fontanel closes (10–14 mo.)	Separation individuation (12–28 mo.) Self-feeding	Sleep disturbances: resistance or response to over-stimulation Extreme separation anxiety
		Eruption of deciduous first molars (11–18 mo.)	Oppositional behavior Messiness Exploratory behavior	Interactional psychotic disorder Bronchial asthma Pica Teeth grinding Pseudo-retardation
		Increase in lymphoid tissue		Temper tantrums, negativism
PRESCHOOL	2 yr.		Parallel play Pleasure in looking at or being looked at Beginning self-concept	Toilet training disturbances: constipation, diarrhea Excessive feeding Bedtime and toilet rituals
	3 yr.	SLOWER (SKELETAL) Deciduous teeth calcified	Orderliness Disgust Curiosity Masturbation Cooperative play Fantasy play Imaginary companions	Speech disorders: delayed, elective mutism, stuttering Petit mal seizures Nightmares, night terrors Extreme separation anxiety Excessive thumb sucking Phobias and marked fears Developmental deviations: lags and accelerations in motor, sensory, and affective development
	4 yr.	RAPID (SKELETAL)		Food rituals and fads
	5 yr.		Task completion Rivalry with parents of same sex	Sleepwalking School phobias Developmental deviations: lags and accelerations in cognitive functions, psychosexual, and integrative development
	6 yr.	Eruption of permanent first molars (5½–7 yrs.)	Games and rules	
		Eruption of permanent central incisors (6–8 yrs.)	Problem-solving Achievement Voluntary hygiene	Tics Psychoneuroses Enuresis, soiling and excessive masturbation
SCHOOL AGE	7 yr.	SLOWEST (SKELETAL) Frontal sinuses develop	Competes with partners Hobbies Ritualistic play	Schizophreniform psychotic disorder Nail-biting Learning problems
	8 yr.	Cranial sutures ossified Uterus begins to grow	Rational attitudes about foods	Psychophysiologic disorders Personality disorders: compulsive, hysterical, anxious, overly dependent, oppositional, overly inhibited, overly independent, isolated and mistrustful personality, tension discharge disorders, sociosyntonic personality disorders, and sexual deviations
	9 yr.		Companionship Invests in: community leaders, teachers, impersonal ideals	
	10 yr.			Pre-delinquent patterns
	11 yr.	Budding of nipples in girls Increased vascularity of penis and scrotum		
	12 yr.	Pubic hair appears in girls SPURT (SKELETAL)		Legal delinquency Anorexia nervosa
	13 yr.	(Girls 1½ yrs. ahead) Pubic hair appears in boys	"Revolt"	Dysmenorrhea Sexual promiscuity
ADOLESCENCE	14 yr.	Rapid growth of testes and penis	Loosens tie to family Cliques	Excessive masturbation Pseudopsychotic regressions
	15 yr.	Axillary hair starts Down on upper lip appears	Responsible independence Work habits solidifying	Suicidal attempts Acute confusional state
	16 yr.	Voice changes Mature spermatozoa (11–17)		
	17 yr.	Acne in girls may appear	Heterosexual interests	
EARLY ADULTHOOD	18 yr.	Acne in boys may appear	Recreational activities Preparation for occupational choices	Schizophrenic disorders (adult type)
		Cessation of skeletal growth	Occupational commitment	
		Involution of lymphoid tissue		
MIDDLE ADULTHOOD		Muscle constitutes 43% total body weight Permanent teeth calcified Eruption of permanent third molars (17–30 yrs.)	Elaboration of recreational outlets Marriage readiness	Affective disorders: manic-depressive psychoses
			Parenthood readiness	
LATE ADULTHOOD				Involutional reactions: depression, suicide
				Senile disorders, chronic brain syndrome, etc.

TABLE 6–3 (*Continued*)

Dimensions of Personality Development: Physical, Psychological, Social, Schematic Representation°

PERIOD	AGE	ADAPTIVE MECHANISMS	EEG DEVELOPMENT	CNS MATURATION	DEVELOPMENTAL LANDMARKS
INFANCY	Birth		Neonate: Low amplitude and polyrhythmic 4–6 and 6–8 cycles per second appear	Brain weight: 350 grams Level of neural function: sub-cortical	Social smile (2 mo.) 180° visual pursuit (2 mo.)
	3 mo.			Transitory reflexes present (i.e., moro, sucking, grasp, TNR)	Reaches for objects (4 mo.) Rolls over (5 mo.)
	6 mo.	Incorporation Imitation Denial Avoidance	Spontaneous K complexes appear (evidence of cortical response to stimulation)	Brain weight: 600 grams Brain stem in advanced or complete state of myelination	Raking grasp (7 mo.) Crude purposeful release (9 mo.)
	9 mo. 1 yr.			Transitory reflexes disappear Brain weight: 900 grams Cranial nerve myelination complete Progressive integration of sub-cortical and cortical areas	Inferior pincer grasp (10 mo.) Walks unassisted (10–14 mo.) Words: 3–4 (13 mo.)
		Regression			Builds tower of 2 cubes (15 mo.) Scribbles with crayon (18 mo.)
PRESCHOOL	18 mo.	Withdrawal Inhibition Displacement	Subalpha 5–8 cycles per second become more evident Anterior fast activity disappears	Babinski reflex extinguished Bowel and bladder nerves myelinated Brain weight: 1000 grams	Words: 10 (18 mo.)
	2 yr.	Projection			Uses 3 word sentences (30 mo.)
		Undoing	Alpha development more dominant Irregularities in rhythms and distortions in waves give EEG "abnormal look." Sleep spindles may appear "spike-like." Drowsy record may show slowing paroxysms. Distorted sleep patterns can appear.	Spinal cord and cerebellum myelination complete	Names 6 body parts (30 mo.) Uses appropriate personal pronouns, i.e., I, you, me (30 mo.)
	3 yr.	Suppression			Rides tricycle (36 mo.) Copies circle (36 mo.) Matches 4 colors (36 mo.)
		Acting out in play and fantasy			Talks of self and others (42 mo.) Takes turns (42 mo.) Tandem walks (42 mo.)
	4 yr.	Repression		Beginning single finger localization	Copies cross (48 mo.) Throws ball overhand (48 mo.)
	5 yr.	Identification		Beginning right-left orientation Cerebrum myelination complete	Copies square (54 mo.) Copies triangle (60 mo.)
SCHOOL AGE	6 yr.	Isolation Pseudo-compulsions in thought, play Turning of emotions into the opposite	14–6 per second positive spikes start to appear. Transient disorganization of awake and sleep tracings is common.	Level of neural function: cortical Body image solidifying	Ties knots in string Prints name Ties shoelaces Simple functional similarities Rides two-wheel bike
	7 yr.	Reaction formation Sublimation			Copies diamond Simple opposite analogies Names days of week
	8 yr.			Cerebral dominance evident (laterality)	Repeats 5 digits forward Can define brave and nonsense
	9 yr.				Knows seasons of the year Able to rhyme
	10 yr.	Rationalization	Increase in alpha voltage and regularity	Brain weight: 1300–1400 grams (adult size)	Repeats 4 digits in reverse Understands: pity, grief, surprise Difficult functional similarities
	11 yr.				Knows where sun sets Can define nitrogen, microscope, shilling
ADOLESCENCE	12 yr.	Intellectualization		(Growth in thickness of myelin sheaths continues for life)	Knows why oil floats on water Can divide 72 by 4 without pencil and paper
	13 yr.	Regressions			Abstract similarities Comprehends belfrey and espionage
	14 yr.	Asceticism	14–6 per second positive spikes begin to disappear		Knows meaning of C.O.D.
	15 yr.				Can repeat 6 digits forward and 5 digits in reverse
	16 yr.		Gradual evolution of stable adult patterns at all levels of consciousness		
	17 yr. 18 yr.				

°NOTE: Reprinted by permission of the publisher from D. G. Prugh, "Psychosocial Disorders in Childhood and Adolescence: Theoretical Considerations and an Attempt at Classification," in Joint Commission on Mental Health of Children, *The Mental Health of Children; Services, Research and Manpower*, Report of Task Forces IV and V, Harper & Row, New York, 1973. © 1973 by Harper & Row.

sociocultural factors including the cultural group's tolerance (or lack thereof) of "sick" or deviant behavior. Prugh states that psychosocial dysfunction includes:

. . . Marked behavioral *regression* to a more safely established level of adaptation in the face of stressful stimuli; *fixation* at a particular level and different dimensions of development; a significant developmental *lag*, and serious *retardation*, or a blunting or *distortion* in one or another aspect of personality development; *limitation and function* that physical, psychological or social levels, or *adaptive breakdown*, as an overwhelming physical illness, severe emotional disturbance, or mental disorder.[80]

Human development in its physical, psychological, and social dimensions are summarized by Prugh in Table 6-3 which follows (Prugh's chart).[80] The Table is especially useful in helping place diagnosis in developmental perspective; it includes the major developmental classification systems side-by-side (except of course, the DSM-III which was developed later).

Prugh also developed a straightforward and useful system of function-dysfunction. Many complex systems have been suggested, but the system Prugh offers is not dependent upon the discipline of the examiner nor upon the use of special rating scales. In his original presentation, the material is divided according to age and each group is discussed as to the type of disorder which is likely to be seen by the clinician, the type of treatment and agencies which may be involved, and the prognosis as related to diagnosis and level of functioning. Prugh's function-dysfunction levels are: (1) Optimal functioning; (2) Functioning but vulnerable; (3) Incipient dysfunction; (4) Moderate dysfunction; and (5) Severe dysfunction.

This approach is clear enough to serve most clinical functions and yet not so complex as to make the use of the scale tedious. It may not be as tightly compartmentalized nor as minutely scaled as necessary for some research efforts. Nonetheless, it appears to be a particularly useful approach to function and will be utlized through the remainder of this chapter.

Diagnosis in Perspective

Having now observed the complexity of the diagnostic question, there remains the necessity for synthesizing the many approaches to diagnosis into a useful and pragmatic scheme. This should have relevance to the clinician and to others involved in the care of children and adolescents, yet should lack undue prejudice or any tendency to determine the fate of the child improperly.

Since 1966 much discussion has centered around the GAP system. Attempts have been made to extend it in such a way as to encompass additional factors which could advance its objectivity and further serve the needs of the child.

It would be most presumptuous for any one person to suggest a system that should receive universally recognized use. As Anthony said, "taxonomy is not one man's business."[4] It will only be through the continual and extensive negotiations between the official bodies of professionals that an effective official diagnostic schema for children will evolve. Even when there is a revision of an international system such as the ICD, it will be necessary to examine it and subject it to critique. It is inconceivable that there will ever be a final diagnostic system for children.

For the purposes of this chapter, however, and based upon current knowledge and conception, the following diagnostic schema is offered for discussion. There remain areas which require considerable extension, such as the inclusion of infant psychiatry and of a more elaborated adolescent diagnostic schema. In order to be complete, the diagnosis must include a reference to the child's developmental state and functional level. Although the schema offered in this chapter is somewhat more elaborate than the GAP system, it is not particularly more complex. Its utilization will require only the noting of information about development and function. For the most part, such data will have already been gathered in the process of making the more traditional diagnosis. The schema requires simply that a notation about the child be made in each of the four areas on the diagnostic wheel. (See Figure 6-4—Diagnostic Wheel). It is also possible to conceive of a diagnostic box similar to a box of sugar cubes in which the child may be represented by one particular cube out of the three-dimensional box. This "cube" would then be the primary diagnosis. Additional diagnoses may also be included by adding the appropriate cube. To construct the diagnostic box, one combines the etiological and descriptive categories into one dimension. (See Figure 6-5—Diagnostic Box.)

THE DEVELOPMENTAL DIMENSION

Numerous authors[73, 82] have emphasized the importance of developmental assessment as a part of diagnosis. Nonetheless, the developmental as-

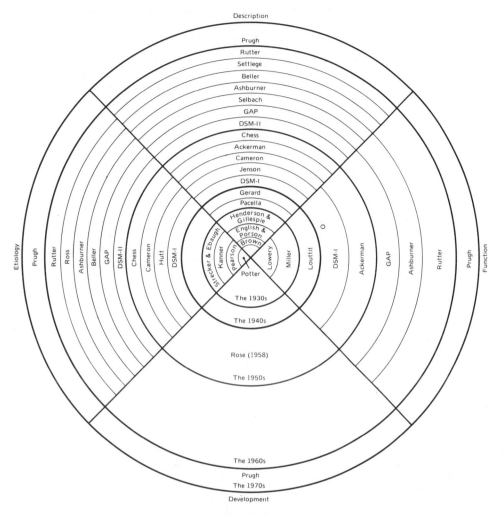

FIGURE 6–4
Diagnostic Wheel

pect of any official diagnostic schema still remains to be included. Earlier, note was taken of the many potential developmental schemata and factors outlined by Prugh on his chart. It is clear that chronological age is not in and of itself a reliable measure of development. More is required. The developmental schema based upon the work of Piaget has great merit, particularly in the cognitive sphere. Currently, this is of special value with minority children.[18] IQ measures have been advanced by Rutter and others in association with the Tri-axial system.[90] Unfortunately, such figures tend to leave out as much about development as they indicate. IQ is especially unreliable in minority and poverty children,[69] and thus lends itself to abuse. To include it in a diagnostic schema is questionable. Anna Freud's Developmental Profile[32] and the concept of lines of development are

valuable, but too complex for most diagnostic schemata. The developmental profile is particularly useful where more complete formulations can be undertaken with individual cases. However, it does not lend itself to a practical diagnostic system which will find early international use.

The straightforward approaches of Erikson[24, 25] with a neo-analytic exposition of basic psychoanalytic developmental concepts is quite useful and is particularly valuable clinically. In terms of the diagnostic schemata that have been described in this chapter, the Erikson psychoanalytic-psychosocial model of development has particular appeal. Adolescence has been divided into three parts to facilitate its discussion as a rapidly changing developmental phase. This should serve as well to encourage the recognition of the importance of the psychodynamics which are at play at each of

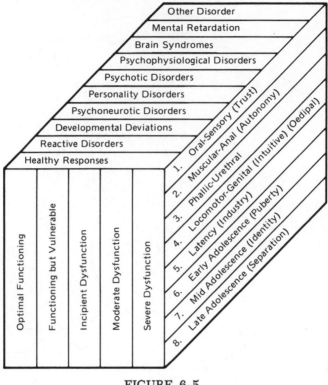

FIGURE 6–5
The Diagnostic Box

these developmental substages. It is also important to note that similar developmental subdivisions will eventually be necessary in infancy. The subspecialty of infant psychiatry is in the process of taking form. As it does, a more thorough appreciation of substage development will eventually be included in diagnostic approaches.

The utilization of a stage-related schema is to profile the developmental aspect of a child being under consideration in relationship to other aspects of the diagnosis. The developmental and chronological ages may not coincide. Thus, a psychotic child of eight may be operating on an oral-trust level of development, whereas an eleven-year-old neurotic girl may be functioning primarily in an area of early adolescent psychodynamic issues and conflicts. When it is not in phase with the child's chronological age, development may be delineated more accurately by utilizing the GAP developmental outline:

1. Maturation (overall sweeping developmental deviation)
2. Motor development
3. Sensory development
4. Speech development
5. Cognitive development
6. Social development

7. Psychosexual development
8. Affective development
9. Integrative development
10. Other developmental deviations

For example, for the psychotic eight-year-old noted above, one may state: "Development—functioning at an oral level with severe lag in overall maturation and particularly behind in speech." For the neurotic eleven-year-old described above, a statement may be made such as: "Development—precocious psychosexual and social development, conflicts occurring in early adolescent level with superior development in cognitive and motor areas."

The diagnosis should reflect the *primary* current operational status of the child; i.e., it may specify delayed development, but it may also give an account of current regressive developmental features. For example, a six-year-old with a reactive disorder following hospitalization becomes obstinate, seclusive, and loses sphincter control. He may thereupon be regarded as operating at an autonomous (anal) level of development and be so diagnosed. As he improves, there may be a rapid return to a previous higher level of development, one which will require a different developmental diagnosis.

One may argue that this kind of diagnosis should be made at the highest level of development achieved, regardless of whether regression has occurred. However, one could assert with equal logic that the diagnosis should reflect the current condition, and that in the nature of things, the developmental diagnosis should be expected to change rapidly. The same is true in clinical pediatrics. If a young child has a simple fracture of the forearm, that fracture may heal rapidly, and in a short time there may be little evidence that the fracture occurred. Obviously the diagnosis of fracture does not continue, although it was valid when it was made. The same may be true of a number of the healthy and reactive disorders of childhood. The clinician should be prepared to change the developmental diagnosis fairly frequently.

There may be better approaches to the developmental dimension, but they will not find popularity unless they are straightforward, describe the child in a clinically useful manner, are fairly easily learned, are based upon relatively universally agreed upon (or at least generally taught) definitions, fit within nosological subclassifications which have widespread acceptance, and are simple to use.

There appears to be no question that child mental health professionals will be increasingly insistent upon the addition of developmental dimensions to official diagnostic schema over the next several decades. This area seems to be particularly difficult to understand for the professional working just with adults. To those not working with children, the responsibility for making a developmental diagnosis may appear to be a complex and burdensome business. In part this is because development is inherently intricate; a more static, less changing organism is far easier to comprehend that a rapidly changing and growing young person. Nonetheless, the necessity for this diagnostic dimension will remain, and many will continue to insist upon its being considered.

THE FUNCTIONAL DIMENSION

In many respects, it is surprising that child psychiatrists have gone so long without insisting on a classification of function-dysfunction. The functional classification is necessitated by the ability of some children to function in the face of serious problems, as compared to other children who will become severely incapacitated in the face of fairly minor environmental stresses

and in spite of their having a more "benign" diagnosis.

It is not easy to describe function. The classification of disorders of function could be quickly expanded to require specific detailed delineation of every aspect of the child's life. Each area of function can be subdivided; for example, school function may be divided academically in terms of reading, math, spelling, music, etc. Such complexity will defeat the diagnostic purpose of functional designation; it is best reserved for a detailed formulation of the child's individual problem.

Many functional classifications have been developed for special clinical or research purposes. These employ rating scales and other measures which offer a substantial nosological classificatory contribution.

This model is an extension of that of Prugh.[80] The categories are fairly clear and self-explanatory. Particularly useful is the category of "functioning but vulnerable": which implies the need for a more preventive approach to the child. It can be applied to many disorders, particularly the reactive, developmental, personality, and psychophysiological disorders.

The category of incipient dysfunction is synonymous with mild disorder and implies some functional impairment. The category of moderate dysfunction is the more generic and probably the least precise of the categories. Many children will fall into this category, and in the future, there may be a need to subdivide this large group.

The combination of a developmental and functional diagnostic dimension can be tied to the GAP classification system. With some modifications, this appears to be a useful clinical and teaching approach to diagnosis. This is found in "Axis V, Highest Level of Adaptive Functioning." This axis indicates the highest level of functioning in the past year. It ranges from "1" (superior) to "7" (grossly impaired). The DSM-III has not included a solid developmental scale for children and adolescence. There is "Axis II, Personality Disorders (adults) and Specific Developmental Disorders (children and adolescents)." There is still no solid official nomenclature which includes a major developmental dimension. The DSM-III looks at "Disorders" but not at developmental positioning. This may require separate categorization of the psychiatric disorders of children, but even if that is necessary, one would question where resistance to inclusion of such categorization might come from. Surely as we grow, medicine comes to understand the classifications of heart disease or the subcategories of endocrine disease, and one would anticipate that these would enter the diagnostic schemata fairly quickly. The same should be true of psychiatric disorders of childhood and adolescence.

Special Problems of Diagnosis

THE HEALTHY CHILD

The problem of how and when to diagnose health in a system based primarily on pathology is worth careful consideration. Indeed, one might argue that ultimately there may be more to be gained from the study of health than from the study of the disease.

Those who have seen themselves as being the "Third Force" (the first two being psychoanalysis and behavioral psychology) in psychology have placed considerable and proper emphasis on healthy functioning. Maslow[67] has studied excellence and creativity as have others.[34] There is a point to be made about the need for contrast as a prerequisite to vision. The dichotomy between health and disease allows each to be studied against the contrasting background of the other. A diagnosis of health, i.e., an absence of notable pathology, is not a diagnosis to be made lightly. It can be too reassuring, it can imply too favorable a prognosis, and future events may demonstrate the limitation of the professional's prophetic power.

The GAP describes healthy reactions which are not necessarily the same as health. The baby whose anxiety is related to eight-month stranger anxiety[101] is nonetheless anxious. This diagnosis is much like the question of an infant who is "cutting" teeth and in much pain. Is that painful condition "health"? The answer is yes and no; it is "normal" developmentally, but painful in the present. With teeth coming through, aspirin may be helpful; with eight-month anxiety, it may also be helpful to consider how many new people the baby can tolerate before bringing him into a large house party. In short, "health" may be relative.

The Triaxial schema[90] included "normal-variation" as related to "transient problems." The category of healthy responses may include children and adolescents at all developmental levels. It will seldom include conditions more severe than moderately dysfunctional. If the condition is rated as "severe," it must be very brief in duration.

The DSM-III may include "no mental disorder." The GAP system includes a category of healthy responses not generally present in other major diagnostic schemata. However, Chess[14] did include a category for "healthy child" in her system as did Ross[88] (whose work predated the GAP Report). The committee stated,

This category is presented as the first on the list in order to emphasize a need for assessment of positive strengths in the child whenever possible and to avoid so far as possible a diagnosis of healthy states by the exclusion of pathology. (pp. 219–220)[38]

The importance of this statement is its realistic perception that all human stress, psychic pain, developmental struggles, reaction to change, and defense against anxiety are not synonymous with disease or pathology. This is of special importance with children and adolescents.

The committee recognized that the criteria for health do not require the absence of conflict. They stated,

The application of such positive personality criteria (i.e., intellectual functioning, social functioning, emotional functioning, and personal and adaptive functioning) would appear in the present state of our knowledge to be more appropriate than reliance upon the presence of such mental states as contentment, happiness, and freedom from fear or inhibition, or reliance upon the existence of certain personality patterns or traits. (p. 220)[38]

Where Freud emphasized as criteria for mental health the ability to work and to love, the child would be assessed on a more developmentally based measure. GAP uses a criterion of "stage-appropriateness" where "stage" is synonymous with the level of psychosocial development appropriate for the child's chronological age. Here the importance of the clinician's knowledge of development is crucial. Development is considered by Eisenberg as the "basic science" of the pediatric-psychiatric disciplines. In studies of childhood, a thorough knowledge of just what is "stage-appropriate" is the foundation for a diagnosis of healthy reaction, reactive disorder, and developmental disorder. This stands in contrast to other more statically descriptive diagnoses such as neurosis, personality disorder, or psychosis. A knowledge of the details of development is required to establish the differential diagnoses of childhood effectively. This includes cognitive development as outlined by Piaget and summarized well by Flavell,[31] stages of psychosocial development,[24, 25] stage-related vulnerability,[82] early stage-related development,[101] and general summaries of development such as those regarding childhood by Mussen, Conger and Cagan[72] and adolescence.[17]

The commonly used pediatric adage, "He'll grow out of it" has meaning and accuracy only when the clinician can fully assess the developmental status of the child or adolescent and be assured that his diagnosis of the condition is accurate. Perhaps most children and adolescents will "grow out of" the healthy reactions. However, one must assess whether or not the individual may "grow out of it" more easily and with less conflict with a bit of professional help.

When making a diagnosis the GAP committee also emphasized the importance of assessing the child's or adolescent's *psychosocial functioning* ("a degree of trust, autonomy, initiative, industry, identity, intimacy, etc."). This denotes the place of the child within the framework of his family and environment.

The subcategories of healthy reaction are of some interest:

Developmental crises are common, but often perplexing. The committee notes that these are of "a brief and presumably transient nature;" yet who has ever really gotten over his adolescence, or some of the other "developmental crises." Examples of developmental crises include eighth-month anxiety, the beginning of school, preschool phobias, compulsivity in school age, and the identity crisis in adolescence.

The *Situational crises* include grief and mourning, reactions to separation and hospitalization, and other acute situational happenings. These reflect external environmental change and crisis.

Thus the "healthy responses" may be said to comprise the common, garden variety of problems seen by the pediatrician, family physician, school psychologist or social worker, or others working with large numbers of children and adolescents. Nonetheless, the diagnosis "healthy response" rests upon a thorough assessment which meets very complex criteria, integration with a solid theoretical knowledge of development, and a detailed understanding of the individual child and his situation. It is not an "easy" diagnosis; nor is it a "snap" decision. As noted earlier, a symptom and diagnosis are not synonymous. Healthy reaction is a diagnosis made on the basis of positive findings and not just upon the absence of pathology. Although it may be influenced by expected outcome, (being a transient disorder with the expectation that the symptom(s) will disappear with time) it must be made in the present, based upon current data. If the decision is made not to treat the child on the basis of a diagnosis of healthy response, that is an active step which can have profound effect upon the child and his future. Under the circumstances, the decision must reflect a substantial, carefully thought out diagnosis.

REACTIVE DISORDER

The diagnosis of "reactive disorder" is one of special nosological interest. It places an emphasis upon an environmentally derived etiological event. In certain respects it resembles a "situational disorder," but is a somewhat more specific category. The GAP committee stipulated that these are disorders "in which the behavior and/or symptoms shown by the child are judged to be predominantly a reaction to an event, a set of events, or a situation" (p. 222).[38]

This disorder involves a conflict which is primarily conscious. However, a reactive disorder may be superimposed upon other, more crystallized conditions such as psychoneurosis, psychosis, developmental disorders, personality disorders and the like.

The DSM-III will probably use the phrase "Adjustment Disorders" with the following subcategories:

With depressed mood
With anxious mood
With mixed emotional features
With physical symptoms
With disturbance of conduct
With mixed disturbance of emotions and conduct
With withdrawal
Other or unspecified

There is also the suggested classification "Post Traumatic Disorder."

As with healthy reactions, GAP emphasizes that this diagnosis be based upon positive criteria rather than upon exclusion. Examples of reactive disorders would be the symptoms occurring following illness, separation, accidents, death of important objects, school pressures and "premature, excessive, or inadequate stimulation." This category may encompass a number of designations found in the older literature including behavior disorders, conduct disturbances, habit disturbances, neurotic traits, etc.

This can be a very useful diagnosis, but requires careful deployment. Whether it will serve as it stands or require further subcategorization will depend upon the experience of professionals over the next several decades. It encompasses diagnostic problems which have been of concern for many years. Some of these have been made especially complex by the introduction of multi-factored clusters of interactional variables inherent in the nature of this reactive disorder category. There is a complex interplay of internal psychodynamic considerations with external, situational and family happenings to be viewed within the framework of the developmental assessment of the individual child. For example, the GAP committee felt that although reactive disorders may occur at any age, they "are more likely to be seen in infants and preschool children because they are less likely to have the capacity to repress affect, internalize conflict and ability to develop a structured psychopathology" (p. 224).[38] They felt that the major determinant of the "picture" seen in the reactive disorder will be the developmental capacity of the involved child.

To make the diagnosis of reactive disorder, the etiology must be clear, i.e., there must be an identifiable event, and the condition must have a positive prognosis (it usually leads to recovery without the formation of an ongoing structuralized disorder). However, the symptoms may vary considerably; there will be a function of the individual child, his development, his internal psychodynamic structure, and his experiences. The severity may vary considerably, extending from a functioning but vulnerable condition to one which is severe and incapacitating.

At times the reactive disorder is deceptively simple; by definition the conflict must be conscious. It can lead the therapist into a false sense of intellectual sureness for he may feel he understands the condition while failing to understand the child.

This group of disorders deserves continued elaboration, attention, and research. This diagnosis should not be accepted without question but the GAP committee has done the field a considerable service. It has brought together the many diffuse labels previously utilized, put them under one rubric, and provided a set of rational diagnostic guidelines. The emphasis upon positive criteria for diagnosis will enhance the usefulness of the category. The challenge for the future will be to further dissect these disorders in terms of the interaction of the environment with the psychic and developmental aspects of the child and the adolescent.

DEVELOPMENTAL DEVIATIONS

These disorders are the special province of child and adolescent medicine and psychiatry. Development reflects the subtle complexity of working with young people. Unlike the adult classification system which emphasizes a rather static, descriptive, discontinuous view of emotional disorder, the developmental problems require diagnosis by comparison to a model and quantification. These are disorders of too much or too little, too early or too late; they are the diagnoses which challenge both the training and experience of the therapist. With these disorders, one's diagnostic acumen grows with time and thoughtful experience. The more children one has seen, the more thoroughly one has observed them, the more perceptive and accurate will be one's ability to diagnose the developmental deviations precisely.

The specific developmental disorders of the DSM-III are very specific. They include the following very specific disorders, as noted before in the earlier discussion on the DSM-III. These disorders are also recorded in the DSM-III on Axis II. The more general developmental conditions are not included, such as disorder of maturation, psychosexual function, sexual development, etc.

The GAP committee, also recognized the importance in these cases of the specific delineation of just which function, or part function, is seen as being deviant.

The GAP subcategory "deviations of maturational patterns" applies to disorders which have serious, broad, almost total development lags. The inclusion of deviation of social, psychosexual, affective, and integrative development presents certain difficult diagnostic problems. In spite of this, these certainly have a place in the developmental deviation category.

In the past, child psychiatrists have probably been overly inclined to place many of the developmental disorders in other categories, such as a neurotic personality, or behavioral disorder. These are more structuralized with implied fixed pathology. This practice has recently received its proper and overdue criticism. Historically, the long use of adult classificatory systems took much of the developmental dimension out of diagnosis in child psychiatry; this tended to perpetuate a view of the child's problems as more fixed and unchanging than they might have been. The child may be defined as a person in transition. Development is therefore the heart of this discipline.

For many, the diagnostic approach to childhood has been characterized by stereotyped, culturally rooted values which have led to the ignoring of certain problems. The culture simply regarded them as "non-problems." For example, in the area of social development, the inhibited, shy, dependent child may have been seen as deviant or even "neurotic," but the special problems of the socially precocious child have been ignored.

The problem of "excessive" sexual interest on the part of children and adolescents has been extensively diagnosed and discussed, but little attention has been given to the psychosexually inhibited, the sexually retarded and ineffectual child or adolescent. Perhaps the culture has defined such a child as "a good child," and has hence failed to recognize the impact that such developmental deviation may have upon the child's future sexual and marital adequacy as an adult.

Many children, whose affective behavior has been predominantly depressive or withdrawn, have been inappropriately labeled as having a *neurotic* or *personality disorder*. Children who have become euphoric or hypomanic at times may have been seen as "hyperactive" and having "minimal brain dysfunction." The hyperactive diagnosis gives an implication of a more static, organic, unchanging condition than may be true; this detracts from the importance of development. The label then leads to the expectation of a crystallized disorder in which the child is seen as a "sick" individual who is treated as such by his family and school.

The proper use of this diagnostic category may protect the child from having to bear the more pejorative label of a permanent condition.

PSYCHONEUROTIC DISORDERS

Although this diagnosis will be discussed at length within this volume, there are several considerations associated with differential diagnosis. The psychoneuroses have been the traditional province of psychiatry; moreover, the psychoanalytic understanding of the nature of neurosis has placed special importance upon childhood factors at the beginning of the neurotic condition. The GAP committee properly points out that the diagnosis requires "unconscious conflicts over the handling of sexual and aggressive impulses which though removed from awareness by the mechanisms of repression, remain reactive and unresolved" (p. 229).[38] The regression and repetitive quality of the neurotic condition is noted. These are disorders which seldom occur before school age. The symbolic symptoms may be accompanied by behavioral symptoms which complicate the differential diagnosis. The traditional term "neurosis" has been abandoned by the DSM–III and replaced with anxiety, affective, somatiform, and dissociative disorders.

The descriptive and diagnostic aspects of psychoneurosis are discussed in detail in a later chapter in this volume.

PERSONALITY DISORDERS

As related to children and adolescents, personality disorder presents special problems of differential diagnosis. The question remains as to when personality becomes so formed and crystallized as to provide the possibility of a "personality disorder." This is discussed by the GAP committee. It is also discussed at length in chapter 13 of this volume. The GAP criteria delineate specific considerations which deserve attention. They define the personality disorder as "characterized by chronic or fixed pathological trends, representing traits which have become ingrained in the personality structure" (p. 237).[38] Some emphasis is laid upon the fact that in the personality disorders, the usual symptom formations seen in the psychoneurotic patient are not present. Moreover, the disorder becomes more ego-syntonic. That is to say, the symptoms do not cause considerable conscious stress or a sense of anxiety within the individual child or adolescent. This differs from the psychoneuroses where the ego-alien quality of the anxiety is clearly perceived. Indeed, it is very much a part of many childhood neurotic situations.

These concepts are not entirely mutually exclusive; ego-syntonic versus ego-alien does not alone determine the diagnosis of neurosis versus personality disorder. Nonetheless, it is an important consideration. The GAP committee felt that it would be unusual for a personality disorder to be seen prior to the late school age period of life. They do emphasize, however, that beginning in infancy and early childhood, certain "premonitory patterns" are often seen which contribute to the nature of the subsequent personality disorder. The severity of the condition is of importance; it may range from a relatively well-organized personality that blends well with most of the child's environment, to severe forms which markedly interfere with the child's functioning.

The GAP committee makes the important point that the total personality picture of the individual must be considered, and that the occurrence of a single symptom or behavior is not enough for the diagnosis. (See Table 6–4.)

The use of alcohol, drugs, or toxic substances is considered to be a symptomatic manifestation. It may fit with a diagnosis of overdependent personality or impulse-ridden personality, but may also fall into a number of other categories. GAP points out that stress-related disorders seen in childhood and adolescence often properly belong under healthy responses or reactive disorders.

133

TABLE 6–4

GAP Classification

1. Healthy Responses
   a. Developmental crisis
   b. Situational crisis
   c. Other responses
2. Reactive Disorders
3. Developmental Deviations
   a. Deviations in maturational patterns
   b. Deviations in specific dimensions of development
      1) Motor
      2) Sensory
      3) Speech
      4) Cognitive functions
      5) Social development
      6) Psychosexual
      7) Affective
      8) Integrative
   c. Other developmental deviation
4. Psychoneurotic Disorders
   a. Anxiety type
   b. Phobic type
   c. Conversion type
   d. Dissociative type
   e. Obsessive-compulsive type
   f. Depressive type
   g. Other psychoneurotic disorder
5. Personality Disorders
   a. Compulsive personality
   b. Hysterical
   c. Anxious
   d. Overly dependent
   e. Oppositional
   f. Overly inhibited
   g. Overly independent
   h. Isolated
   i. Mistrustful

   j. Tension-discharge disorders
      1) Impulse-ridden personality
      2) Neurotic personality disorder
   k. Sociosyntonic personality disorder
   l. Sexual deviation
   m. Other personality disorder
6. Psychotic Disorders
   a. Psychoses of infancy and early childhood
      1) Early infantile autism
      2) Interactional psychotic disorder
      3) Other psychosis of infancy and early childhood
   b. Psychoses of later childhood
      1) Schizophreniform psychotic disorder
      2) Other psychosis of later childhood
   c. Psychoses of adolescence
      1) Acute confusional state
      2) Schizophrenic disorder, adult type
      3) Other psychosis of adolescence
7. Psychophysiologic Disorders
   a. Skin
   b. Musculoskeletal
   c. Respiratory
   d. Cardiovascular
   e. Hemic and lymphatic
   f. Gastrointestinal
   g. Genitourinary
   h. Endocrine
   i. Of nervous system
   j. Of organs of special sense
   k. Other psychophysiologic disorders
8. Brain Syndromes
   a. Acute
   b. Chronic
9. Mental Retardation
10. Other Disorders

NOTE: Reprinted by permission of the publisher from Group for the Advancement of Psychiatry, Committee on Child Psychiatry, *Psychopathological Disorders of Childhood: Theoretical Considerations and a Proposed Classification*, vol. 6, Report No. 62, Group for the Advancement of Psychiatry, New York, 1966. © 1966 by The Group for the Advancement of Psychiatry.

The DSM–III has included personality disorders in its general section. The personality disorder categories may be used beginning in adolescence or earlier.

The GAP subgroupings which are utilized in personality disorders are of particular interest. Some are fairly clear-cut and descriptive in and of themselves, such as the compulsive personality, hysterical personality, and anxious personality. It should be noted that under the category of hysterical personality, conversion symptoms may occur but are not required for the diagnosis. Some of the descriptive terms utilized in this classification are specific and direct in their definition although they are fairly new as classificatory adjectives. These include *overly dependent personality, op-*positional personality, overly inhibited personality,* and *overly independent personality*. The categories which require more elaboration represent a more creative and new conception of personality disorder which can have considerable clinical usefulness. The isolated personality is of particular interest in childhood because these are distant, detached, cold children. The GAP committee points out that many such children are quite capable of achieving successfully in certain areas, particularly in intellectual pursuits. They also make the point that only a small portion of these children appear to be "pre-schizophrenic" and there does not appear to be any latent schizophrenia. Therefore, they suggest the term schizoid personality is apropriate. -

A mistrustful personality is seen as an individual, usually an adolescent, who shows some isolation but whose personality is primarily characterized by "patterns of suspiciousness beyond the adolescent norm" with intense mistrust of others and marked rigidity in thinking" (p. 245).[38] This is a condition which is seldom seen in childhood, usually occurring in late pre-adolescence or early adolescence. As a rule this does not appear to progress to an adult paranoid state, and the use of the term, paranoid personality, therefore, appears to be unwarranted in child and adolescent psychiatry.

There is a specific section which the GAP committee has added which has created some controversy but has great clinical relevance and value. This is the category of tension-discharge disorders. These are children who act out their aggressive, antisocial, destructive, and sexual feelings rather than repressing or inhibiting them. This category has encompassed many previously used terms including

antisocial personality, psychopathic personality, impulsive character, sociopathic personality, dyssocial personality, affectionless character, acting out personality, neurotic character disorder, primary behavior disorder, neurotic behavior disorder, and conduct disorder. (p. 245)[38]

All of these terms have been used by various authors to classify this type of child. In changing the terminology, the committee felt that the words previously used implied too fixed a pattern for children, carried moral judgments that were not clinically appropriate, and did not integrate the behavior with the dynamic condition upon which the behavior was predicated.

The committee also pointed out that

aggressive, destructive or antisocial behavior may of course be seen in many children exhibiting reactive disorders, developmental deviations, or developmental crises in adolescence. Such behavior may occur as a part of a picture involving brain damage, mental retardation, or psychosis. Furthermore, some children in economically deprived, urban areas may show behavior which is in conformity with the group code or mores of the neighborhood or gang, but which may be regarded as antisocial by society at large. (p. 246)[38]

The committee developed two subcategories in this classification, *impulse-ridden personality* and *neurotic personality disorder*. The importance of differentiation can be seen in the way in which these children respond. The *impulse-ridden personality disorder* will be associated with children who have considerble difficulty controlling their impulses, who tend to discharge their impulses

immediately and impulsively without delay or inhibition, often without regard for consequences, and who show little anxiety, internalized conflict or guilt.

The children with a neurotic personality disorder, however, may display symptomatology that is similar to that of the impulse-ridden personality. In their case, however, the behavior appears to be under the strong influence of earlier "repressed neurotic conflicts." Under these circumstances, the behavior takes on a more repetitive character with a more symbolic quality. At the same time there appears to be some underlying anxiety or guilt in which the child "at times unconsciously (seems) to invite limits or punishment." These children are capable of warm and meaningful relationships although these relationships are often highly ambivalent.

The GAP included a new and valuable personality disorder entitled *sociosyntonic personality disorder*. There may be some overlap with the *tension-discharge disorders*. These are children whose behavior and personality may be culturally deviant but subculturally congruent. They defy the larger social set, but fit in with their family, neighborhood, gang, or subculture. This may apply to children coming from urban areas in which gangs and ethnic subcultures abound, they may be children from isolated rural setting who have hallucinatory experiences, or children who belong to cults in which specific religious beliefs apply such as voodoo possession or special religious practices.

The DSM–III includes a category of conduct disorders, discussed in detail earlier in this chapter, which also subdivides the patients who may be seen in the GAP system or as tension-discharge disorders.

Also under the area of personality disorder, the GAP committee has included *sexual deviation*. (In the DSM–III these are the psychosocial disorders.) It is important that this diagnosis be applied with care, and only when the deviation is "regarded as the major personality disturbance with such a degree of chronicity and pervasiveness in personality function as to dominate the individual's orientation to a social life" (p. 250).[38] Some sexual behavior, such as certain homosexual experiences, or the abundance or relative absence of sexual interest and activity may not present a primary diagnosis in and of itself; indeed, during the course of development one may expect that it will change. The committee felt that this category should rarely be used in childhood, and handled with considerable care in adolescence.

PSYCHOTIC DISORDERS

The subclassification system which the committee used for psychosis is simple and straightforward. Here the diagnostic usage changes with the age of the child. It includes psychosis of infancy or early childhood, psychosis of late childhood, and psychosis of adolescence. There are a number of alternative systems for the characterization of psychosis in childhood. The system used by GAP does have certain clinical usefulness and value; descriptively, psychosis varies a great deal with age.

Under the psychosis of infancy and early childhood, early infantile autism is given as a specific subdiagnosis, and other diagnoses, including "symbiotic" psychoses, are included as interactional psychotic disorder. The interactional psychotic disorder is a diagnosis generally made after the first year of life; it is related principally to the symbiotic child-parent relationship so typically present in this disorder.

The psychoses of later childhood include only schizophreniform[56] psychotic disorder. This condition is normally seen between the ages of six and twelve or thirteen years. It often has a gradual onset associated with the use of primitive defenses, considerable looseness in thought process, hypochondriacal tendencies, loss of emotional control associated with temper outbursts, etc. These children seldom have hallucinations and often present with bizarre and stereotyped behavior. There is considerable deviancy in the development in most of these children, and the committee chose to use the word schizophreniform rather than schizophrenia in order to emphasize the developmental differences between children and adults with psychotic disorders. They also sought to point out that children with this "disorder do not necessarily develop a later form."

There are children with milder intermittent thought disorders who might otherwise resemble the "borderline" or so called "pseudoneurotic" disorders of adults. It was recommended that they might be best classified under personality disorders, with a qualifying statement regarding congitive symptoms drawn from the symptom list.

In discussing the psychoses of adolescence, they list two major psychoses. One is acute confusional state.[13] This is a category which needs to be included in the nomenclature. It is a developmentally related, isolated disorder which occurs in adolescence. It begins abruptly with severe anxiety, depression, confused thinking, and depersonalization. There is usually an absence of a true thought disorder or marked breakdown of reality testing. Meaningful emotional relationships may continue. It generally has a good prognosis for immediate recovery, although other disorders may be found to underlie the acute picture. It should be differentiated from schizophrenia and dissociated reactions as well as from the anxiety, depression, or depersonalization which may be seen in normal adolescents.

The schizophrenic disorder, adult type, is typical of that condition. In discussing it, consideration should be given to the developmental level of the patient.

In 1964, Gold and Vaughan[37] expressed the need to develop a satisfactory classification for childhood psychosis, stating that "very few formal attempts have been made to classify these disorders." Their words barely predated something of an explosion in classificatory schemata for these disorders. Gold and Vaughan themselves offered a solid classification system based on the use of the major diagnostic headings and subtypes. Soon after, many classification efforts of considerable merit followed.

TABLE 6-5

I. Psychoses associated with impairment of brain tissue function
  A. Associated with intoxication (atropine, bromides, stramonium, cortisone, etc.)
  B. Associated with metabolic disorders (pellagra, amaurotic idiocy, etc.)
  C. Associated with degenerative disorders (Schilder's disease, dementia infantilis, etc.)
  D. Associated with infections (juvenile paresis, encephalitides, etc.)
  E. Associated with convulsive disorders (temporal lobe epilepsy, dysautonomia, etc.)
  F. Associated with trauma
  G. Associated with neoplasm
II. Psychoses without known brain tissue impairment
  A. Autistic psychoses
    1. Early infantile autism (Kanner)
    2. Symbiotic psychosis (Mahler)
  B. The schizophrenias
    1. Simple
    2. Acute undifferentiated
    3. Paranoid
  C. Psychoses associated with maturation failure
    1. Atypical child (Rank)
    2. Childhood psychosis (Szurek)
    3. Childhood schizophrenia (Bender)
    4. *Pfropfhebephrenia* (Weygandt and Kraepelin)
  D. *Folie à deux*
  E. Manic-depressive psychosis

NOTE: Reprinted with permission by the publisher from L. Eisenberg, "The Role of Classification in Child Psychiatry," *International Journal of Psychiatry*, 3:179–181, 1967. © 1967 by *International Journal of Psychiatry*.

An interesting, useful, and complete system for classifying the psychotic disorders of children was offered by Eisenberg[21] and is reproduced in Table 6–5. The separation of disorders with known brain impairment from those without known brain impairment is similar to that of Howells;[47] this author divides adolescent (and childhood) disorders into two groups. Howells' groups are "psychonosis" ("a morbid process of mind") and "encephalonosis" ("a morbid process of brain").

Eisenberg properly underscores the importance of identifying central nervous system disease, if present. Such identification and proper treatment may be life saving; even when treatment is not possible, the correct diagnosis may spare the family futile and clostly attempts at treatment. The other diagnostic entities Eisenberg lists will be discussed elsewhere in his volume. However, the diagnosis of atypical child, pfropfhebephrenia, and folie à deux deserve a bit of attention.

Rank[83] described the "atypical child" as one who was very disturbed by descriptive and functional criteria, regardless of the etiology of the condition. The children included in this group may therefore be schizophrenic, suffer from a chronic brain syndrome, display some aspect of mental retardation, be severely neurotic, or exhibit some combination of these conditions. The diagnosis is useful as long as it is recognized as a phenomenological classification which does not reflect a specific etiology. This may be a valid way to speak of psychosis and the adult category of schizophrenia where there is frequent argument over the etiology. The category of atypical child obviates that argument.

The term, *pfropfhebephrenia*, is not new, only forgotten. It was (per Eisenberg) coined by Kraepelin "to characterize the psychotic states observed in a colony of mental defectives." The category's usefulness is obvious to child psychiatrists who have worked with the severely retarded. The child with severe behavioral problems which are "more" than accounted for by the retardation may fit into this category.

As a childhood diagnosis, folie à deux is of special interest. It is important to consider this diagnosis when one sees psychotic pairs such as parent-child or sibling-sibling. The criteria for diagnosis require that the healthy partner's symptoms resolve when he is separated from the psychotic partner. Separation may, therefore, be the treatment of choice early on.

In another article, Eisenberg[19] defends the value of making the organic diagnosis when present and also speaks for the desirability of noso-

logical subtypes in childhood psychosis; i.e., the virtue of "splitting" rather than "lumping."

Fish and her colleagues[30] have developed a classification system for two- to five-year-old psychotic children in which the degree of language disturbance is the major indicator of the diagnostic subcategory. The psychotic children are listed in five groups, A through E. There are two groups developed for nonpsychotic children, groups C prime and D prime, which are important as part of the differential diagnosis. See Figure 6–6.

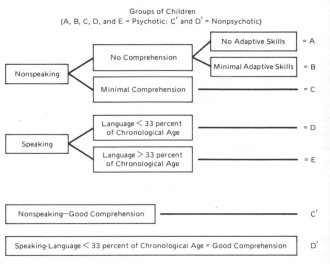

Groups of Children
(A, B, C, D, and E = Psychotic: C′ and D′ = Nonpsychotic)

FIGURE 6–6

NOTE: Reprinted by permission of the publisher from B. Fish, et al., "Classification of Schizophrenic Children Under Five Years," *American Journal of Psychiatry*, 124:1415–1423, 1968. © 1968 by *The American Journal of Psychiatry.*

The two categories under the nonpsychotic group include Group C prime who have no speech but have good comprehension and whose behavior is organized and adaptive. Group D prime can speak, but with sparse communicative language and with a vocabulary of less than thirty-three DQ (developmental quotient); these are children who nonetheless have good comprehension. This system of diagnosis appears to have more relevance to prognosis and treatment than do the equivalent APA diagnostic categories. In the DSM-II, the latter includes mental deficiency, severe, with psychotic reactions; childhood schizophrenia; passive-aggressive personality with retarded speech development; and depressive reaction with retarded speech development. There is an implied relationship between this nosological schema and developmental stages, particularly in respect to patterns of arrest and deviation of sequencing. It allows the nosology to be tested and its validity questioned scientifically.

Fish's classification applies only to those children falling within a three year chronological age range; the important differences between psychotic children in this group and other psychoses in later years, however, cannot be underestimated. With its lack of attention to development, the DSM–II does a great disservice to children such as those described by Fish. This schema may be a prototype for the more rigorous effort that will be needed over the next several decades to develop a solid, complete and effective nosology.

Many additional classification systems have been put forth over the last decade for psychotic children. "Atypical" children were subdivided on the basis of follow-up studies at the Putnam Center.[84] Clusters of signs and symptoms of early infantile autism led to a subclassification approach[75] with very specific delineation of indications for diagnosis.

The problems of subclassification of the psychoses of adolescence has yet to be fully explored. The importance of quite severe, yet transient, psychotic states in adolescence has been noted. The GAP includes these as "acute confusional states." Others have referred to similar states as "episodic behavioral disorders"[71] or "remitting schizoprenias"[116]

The use of the term, *psychosis*, has been avoided by the DSM–III. Instead the phrase, *pervasive developmental disorders*, has been used. The terminology appears to have some merit and may be a useful descriptive alternative to the traditional use of the term, psychosis. Psychosis may be better used as a descriptive term to describe the present condition or function of an individual. The DSM-III classification may be suitable for a general schema; however it is likely that additional research may point to additional categories or subcategories which may later be added, or for more intensive use, a more detailed system such as that of Fish[30] may better serve the need of the specialist.

It appears that the clear direction of the future in the categorization of psychosis is to dissect out and then describe more precisely circumscribed categories. With the clustering techniques available, the opportunity is at hand to handle data in a way that will validate these subcategories scientifically (for example, see the cluster analysis techniques of Tryon and Bailey.[114] There is a definite trend in the direction characterized by Eisenberg as "splitting rather than lumping."

PSYCHOPHYSIOLOGICAL DISORDERS

Although there is considerable discussion of these disorders elsewhere in this volume and they have been thoroughly summarized by Prugh,[81] there are several points which may be made concerning their differential diagnosis. The disorders usually involve organ systems associated with autonomic or involuntary innervation by the central nervous system. In contrast to the conversion disorders which are usually associated with voluntary innervated structures and carry a strong symbolic quality, the symptoms in these conditions are physiological rather than symbolic. It is important to note that structural change can occur in the organs affected by psychophysiological disorders; indeed, this can be of such degree that the pathology may be irreversible and life threatening. Biological predisposing factors may be related to the specificity of the condition, and the disorders may involve more than one organ system.

These disorders can be secondary to other conditions, and should then be added to that diagnosis. They are also to be differentiated from a reactive disorder arising in response to an acute or chronic illness. In the GAP classification, the disorders are named according to which physiologic system is involved. There are a number of disorders which occur in children, and many of the rest occur with both adults and children. The DSM-III places these disorders under their primary physical disease categories.

Brain Syndromes: The brain syndromes are divided in classical fashion between acute and chronic brain syndrome; the overlap between the two is noted. The GAP system recommends that if mental retardation is present, it should be specified in the diagnosis.

Mental Retardation: In the section on mental retardation, the GAP committee dealt only briefly with the related major diagnostic questions. They recommended consultation with two previous publications by GAP.[39, 40]

There are three large groups into which it was felt that the etiological factors associated with mental retardation might fall. These include biological, environmental, and intermediate. Emphasis was placed on the importance of not relying entirely upon psychological testing, and they recommend that a diagnosis of retardation should not be made on the basis of one test. They were particularly concerned about the utilization of a numerical IQ score in order to determine the level of retardation and they underlined how important it was to recognize the relationship of developmental deviation and retardation. There are children with mild mental retardation where a significant hereditary or somatic factor is involved.

A major step by the DSM-III Task Force is to remove the category of borderline retardation from the official nomenclature. This is a courageous step designed to protect the interests and rights of the child from a label of questionable validity.

THE ETHICS OF CLASSIFICATION

There is emphasis in the current literature (see for example, Hobbs[46]) on the ethics of classification of children. The potential harm and dangerous social implications of diagnosis are of concern to all thoughtful child mental health professionals. Of course, the problem applies to adults as well. But children are dependent and vulnerable; they have a long life ahead of them and their development may change their clinical picture.

Of special ethical concern is the potential of nosology to be seen as "labeling"—often pejorative labeling. There is the danger that the label will force the child to live up to the label, to become what the label expects. It is this danger that often prevents the clinician from using the more accurate diagnosis, favoring the less specific and more benign diagnosis to protect the child from the potential harm of being called perhaps "psychotic," "retarded," "sociopathic," "hysterical," or "sexual deviant." These are names with great power; power that can be used against the child.

Sometimes the label will determine the fate of the child. A "neurotic" adolescent may go to a treatment facility while a "sociopathic" companion may go to reform school. Some individuals in schools, social agencies, and society feel that retardation automatically means institutionalization. Some physicians feel that "hyperactivity" always indicates a need for medication.

A potential danger associated with diagnosis is a misunderstanding of the purpose of diagnosis. There is a danger that the clinician may confuse diagnosis with a full dynamic understanding of a child. Diagnosis is a step on a road to understanding. Diagnosis alone is not enough to make a clinical decision regarding treatment, nor is it the same as a full dynamic formulation of the mental mechanisms operative within that child.

There is the danger of making diagnoses for socioeconomic purposes and confusing that with clinical reasons. The diagnosis usually requested and expected by hospital administrators, insurance companies, and similar agencies are diagnoses from the official nomenclature. They seldom require elaborate formulations or full case reports. To present a more complete or elaborated diagnosis under such circumstances presents serious ethical problems. It is important to have clearly in mind the function of the diagnosis, to whom the diagnostic communication is directed, and what use will be made on the diagnosis. The ultimate question is whether the diagnostic process is in the patient's interest.

It is important to maintain a respect for the individuality of the child, particularly as reflected in his cultural background. The clinician must be aware of the child's background and culture when making a diagnosis and take that into consideration within the diagnostic process.

We must be constantly alert to the abuses of categories and labels as applied to children and the fact that inadequate, uncoordinated and, at times, even harmful services directed toward children may arise from the use of diagnostic labels.

We must be constantly aware that categories and labels can predetermine the fate of children. This is particularly true in state institutions, schools, courts, etc. Consider what systems often do with "autistic children," "retarded children," "sociopathic children," "hyperactive children," etc. The diagnosis should serve to enhance the helping process, not label, prejudge, or encapsulate the child.

In the midst of these warnings and concerns it may be suggested that we abandon the classification process altogether; yet as an option it is probably too simplistic and too naive. It is essential that we maintain a classification system in order to develop services, to test validity and effectiveness of treatment processes and programs, and to communicate clinical data effectively. Even Hobbs[46] did not feel that the abuses of classification and labeling could be eliminated by not classifying. He emphasized that instead we must be certain that classification is in the interest of children.

There will be a continuing debate as to whether or not there should be a separate classification system for children aside from that utilized in general psychiatry (in which children and adolescents are but a part). Undoubtedly professionals working with children and adolescents will continue to refine and develop specific diagnostic categories and extend the official nomenclature in a way that is more appropriate and more effective for the population which they treat. It is likely that alternate and more extensive, thorough and specific classification systems for children and adolescents will continue to develop. This should be encouraged. There is room for more than one system. The official system has many uses, particularly in the realm of socioeconomic uses of diagnosis. The inclusion in the DSM-III of a more extensive child and adolescent section, the use of a multiaxial approach and the attempt to develop more specific diagnostic criteria for each category, all will be helpful but child and adolescent diagnosis will not end with the publication of the DSM-III. Those working with children will continue to be aware of and advocate the special needs of children and adolescents, and undoubtedly the diagnosis in the future will reflect that process.

The question of the ethical use of classification is not answered by a reluctance to classify or by utilizing the most benign category but by the continued process of developing an accurate, logical, and effective nosology for children and adolescents. It is this process of continued development, scrutiny, and review that makes classification an ethical endeavor. As long as the individual clinician is continually aware and sensitive to the questions of the use of the classification systems that he applies, the ethical question will be resolved. Diagnosis becomes a matter of questionable ethic only when there is laxity in that vigilance and sensitivity.

Conclusion

The history of medical diagnosis begins in the seventeenth century with an abortive attempt to classify the cause of death of children under six. This thread has been followed to the beginnings of the twentieth century, when efforts to classify the psychiatric disorders of children began, and then traced to the current system of nosology. In retrospect, one is struck with the continuing inadequacy of the general (adult) nosology to serve children adequately. This remains an area of tension between adult and child psychiatrists. The child-oriented professional is aware that children's disorders require a more comprehensive classification which includes consideration of age, devel-

TABLE 6–7

Major Landmarks in Diagnostic Systems for Children

1920 —	Pearson	1955 —	Cameron
1931 —	Strecker and Ebaugh	1957 —	Hutt
1931 —	Lowrey	1958 —	Rose
1932 —	Henderson and Gillespie	1959 —	Jensen
1933* —	Brown, et al.	1959 —	Chess
1934 —	Potter	1960 —	Selbach
1935 —	Kanner	1962 —	Beller
1936 —	Miller	1964 —	Settlage
1937 —	English and Pearson	1964 —	Ross
1937 —	Brown, et al.	1964* —	Thorne
1945 —	VanOphuijsen	1966* —	GAP
1947 —	Louttit	1968* —	Ashburner
1947 —	Gerard	1968 —	DSM-II
1948 —	Pacella	1969* —	Rutter, et al.
1952* —	DSM-I	1973* —	Prugh
1953 —	Ackerman		

(* denotes reference not included in GAP (1966) review of previous classifications.)

opment, and function. There are specific categories for childhood disorders which will be added to the general systems currently in use (the ICD-8 and the DSM-II).

Regardless of the outcome of the legalistic problems, diagnosis of children and adolescents will continue to require care and consideration. The purpose of diagnosis must be kept continually in mind. The dangers of the pejorative use of diagnosis lurk behind each case.

The concept of a diagnostic box has been advanced in which the three dimensions of diagnosis—developmental, functional, and etiological-descriptive—are tied together in each formulation. Within the framework of this conceptualization, the diagnosis must include all three dimensions in order to be complete.

The complexity and tedious quality that attend the construction of diagnostic schemata for children are not unlike the developmental process in the growing child. The process is analogous to the developmental progression described by Piaget, a sequence of assimilation and accomodation. As a given schema begins to find acceptance, the process of its change has already begun.

The murky quality of diagnosis will remain. But it will continue as an important part of clinical practice because it is most useful and functional. Stromgren[106] summarizes the state of darkness, as in current diagnostic conceptualizations, with the feeling that it is better to accept a certain obscurity or even a wrong definition because they will eventually clash with reality and that clash will take the field forward.

The clinician needs diagnosis in order to care for his patient. The nosology used is perhaps less important than the quality of the observations made, the logic and rigor imposed by the clinician on those observations, and the knowledge of and involvement with the patient implied in developing an adequate and accurate diagnosis. The diagnosis remains a bridge at the beginning of the journey in the care of the patient. When it is carefully and properly determined, it can aid appreciably in bringing that patient the most specific help possible at the least expense.

REFERENCES

1. ACKERMAN, N. W., "Psychiatric Disorders in Children—Diagnosis and Etiology in Our Time," in Hoch, P. M., and Zubin, J. (Eds.), *Current Problems in Psychiatric Diagnosis*, Grune & Stratton, New York, 1953.

2. AMERICAN PSYCHIATRIC ASSOCIATION, Committee on Nomenclature and Statistics, *Diagnostic and Statistical Manual of Mental Disorders*, 2nd ed., American Psychiatric Association, Washington, D.C., 1968.

3. ———, Committee on Nomenclature and Statistics, *Diagnostic and Statistical Manual of Mental Disorders*, American Psychiatric Association, Washington, D.C., 1952.

4. ANTHONY, E. J., "Taxonomy is Not One Man's Business," *International Journal of Psychiatry*, 3:173–178, 1967.

5. ASHBURNER, J. V., "Some Problems of Classification, with Particular Reference to Child Psychiatry," *Australia and New Zealand Journal of Psychiatry*, 2:244–250, 1968.

6. BALDWIN, J. A., "Statistical Classification in Psychiatry and New International Diagnostic Code," *International Journal of Psychiatry*, 7:378–384, 1969.

7. BELLER, E. K., *Clinical Process: A New Approach to the Organization and Assessment of Clinical Data*, Free Press, Glencoe, Ill., 1962.

8. BEMPORAD, J. R., PFEIFER, C. M., and BLOOM, W., "Twelve Months' Experience with the GAP Classification of Childhood Disorders," *American Journal of Psychiatry*, 127:658–664, 1970.

9. BRILL, H., "Nosology," in Freedman, A. N., and Kaplan, H. I. (Eds.), *Comprehensive Textbook of Psychiatry*, pp. 581–589, Williams & Wilkins, Baltimore, 1967.

10. BROWN, S., POLLACK, H. M., and POTTER, H. W., *An Outline for the Psychiatric Classification of Problem Children*, New York Department of Mental Hygiene, State Hospital Press, Utica, N.Y., 1933.

11. BROWN, S., et al., *Outline for Psychiatric Classification of Problem Children*, rev. ed., State Hospital Press, Utica, N.Y., 1937.

12. CAMERON, K., "Diagnostic Categories in Child Psychiatry," *British Journal of Medicine and Psychology*, 28(1):67–71, 1955.

13. CARLSON, H. B., "Characteristics of an Acute Confusional State in College Students," *American Journal of Psychiatry*, 114:900–909, 1958.

14. CHESS, S., *An Introduction to Child Psychiatry*, 2nd ed., Grune & Stratton, New York, 1969.

15. ———, *An Introduction to Child Psychiatry*, Grune & Stratton, New York, 1959.

16. COLE, J. O., "Classification and Research on the Prediction of Response to Specific Treatments in Psychiatry," in Katz, M. M., Cole, J. O., and Barton, W. E. (Eds.), *The Role and Methodology of Classification in Psychiatry and Psychopathology*, pp. 143–147, National Institute of Mental Health, Chevy Chase, Md. 1965.

17. CONGER, J. J., *Adolescents and Youth*, Harper & Row, New York, 1973.

18. DEAVILA, E. A., HAVASSY, B. E., and PIAGET, A. N., "Alternative to I.Q.: Mexican-American Study," in Hobbs, N. (Ed.), *Issues in the Classification of Children*, vol. 2, pp. 246–266, Jossey-Bass, San Francisco, 1975.

19. EISENBERG, L., "The Classification of Childhood Psychosis Reconsidered," *Journal of Autism and Childhood Schizophrenia*, 2:338–342, 1972.

20. ———, "Psychotic Disorders. I: Clinical Features," in Freedman, A. M., and Kaplan, H. I. (Eds.), *Comprehensive Textbook of Psychiatry*, pp. 1433–1438, Williams & Wilkins, Baltimore, 1967.

21. ———, "The Role of Classification in Child Psychiatry," *International Journal of Psychiatry*, 3:179–181, 1967.

22. ENGEL, M., "Dilemmas of Classification and Diagnosis," *Journal of Special Education*, 3:231–239, 1969.

23. ENGLISH, O. S., and PEARSON, G. H. J., *Common Neuroses of Children and Adults*, W. W. Norton, New York, 1937.

24. ERIKSON, E. H., *Childhood and Society*, W. W. Norton, New York, 1950.

25. ——, "Identity in the Life Cycle," *Psychological Issues, 1:*1–171, 1959.

26. FEIGHNER, J. P., et al., "Diagnostic Criteria for Use in Psychiatric Research," *Archives of General Psychiatry, 26:*57–63, 1972.

27. FINCH, S. M., "Nomenclature for Children's Mental Disorders Need Improvement," *International Journal of Psychiatry, 7:*414, 1969.

28. FISH, B., "Limitations of the New Nomenclature for Children's Disorders," *International Journal of Psychiatry, 7:*393–398, 1969.

29. ——, "Problems of Diagnosis and the Definition of Comparable Groups: A Neglected Issue in Drug Research of Children," *American Journal of Psychiatry, 125:*900–908, 1969.

30. ——, et al., "Classification of Schizophrenic Children Under Five Years," *American Journal of Psychiatry, 124:*1415–1423, 1968.

31. FLAVELL, J. H., *The Developmental Psychology of Jean Piaget*, Van Nostrand, New Jersey, 1963.

32. FREUD, A., "Assessment of Pathology in Childhood" in *Research at the Hampstead Child-Therapy Clinic and Other Papers, the Writings of Anna Freud*, vol. 5, pp. 26–59, International Universities Press, New York, 1962.

33. GALLEMORE, J. L., and WILSON, W. P., "Adolescent Maladjustment or Affective Disorder?," *American Journal of Psychiatry, 129:*608–612, 1972.

34. GARDNER, J. W., *Excellence*, Harper & Row, New York, 1961.

35. GARMEZY, N., "Process and Reactive Schizophrenia: Some Conceptions and Issues," in Katz, M. M., Cole, J. O., and Barton, W. E. (Eds.), *The Role and Methodology of Classification in Psychiatry and Psychopathology*, pp. 419–466, National Institute of Mental Health, Chevy Chase, Md., 1965.

36. GERARD, M., "Psychological Disorders in Childhood," in Harms, E. (Ed.), *Handbook of Child Guidance*, Child Care Publications, New York, 1947.

37. GOLD, S., and VAUGHAN, G. F., "Classification of Childhood Psychosis," *Lancet*, pp. 1058–1059, November 14, 1964.

38. Group for the Advancement of Psychiatry, Committee on Child Psychiatry, *Psychopathological Disorders in Childhood: Theoretical Considerations and a Proposed Classification*, vol. 6, Report No. 62, Group for the Advancement of Psychiatry, New York, 1966.

39. ——, Committee on Mental Retardation, *Mental Retardation: A Family Crisis—The Therapeutic Role of the Physician*, Report No. 56, Group for the Advancement of Psychiatry, New York, 1963.

40. ——, Committee on Mental Retardation, *Basic Considerations in Mental Retardation: A Preliminary Report*, Report No. 43, Group for the Advancement of Psychiatry, New York, 1959.

41. GRUENBERG, E. M., "How Can the New Diagnostic Manual Help?" *International Journal of Psychiatry, 7:* 368–374, 1969.

42. ——, "Epidemiology and Medical Care Statistics," in Katz, M. M., Cole, J. O., and Barton, W. E. (Eds.), *The Role and Methodology of Classification in Psychiatry and Psychopathology*, pp. 76–97, National Institute of Mental Health, Chevy Chase, Md., 1965.

43. HEBER, R., *A Manual on Terminology and Classification of Mental Retardation*, Monograph Supplement, American Journal of Mental Deficiency, vol. 64, No. 2, 1959.

44. HENDERSON, A. S., KRUPINSKI, J., and STOLLER, A., "Epidemiological Aspects of Adolescent Psychiatry," in Howells, J. G. (Ed.), *Modern Perspectives in Adolescent Psychiatry*, pp. 183–208, Brunner-Mazel, New York, 1971.

45. HENDERSON, D. K., and GILLESPIE, R. D., *A Textbook of Psychiatry*, 3rd ed., Oxford University Press, London, 1932.

46. HOBBS, N., *The Futures of Children*, Jossey-Bass, San Francisco, 1975.

47. HOWELLS, J. G., "Classification of Psychiatric Disorders: Consideration of Adolescents and All Age Groups," in Howells, J. G. (Ed.), *Modern Perspectives in Adolescent Psychiatry*, pp. 209–236, Brunner-Mazel, New York, 1971.

48. HUTT, M. L., and GIBBY, R. G., *Patterns of Abnormal Behavior*, Allyn & Bacon, Boston, 1957.

49. JACKSON, B., "Reflections on DSM-II," *International Journal of Psychiatry, 1:*385–392, 1969.

50. JENKINS, R. L., "Classification of Behavioral Problems of Children," *American Journal of Psychiatry, 125:*1032–1039, 1969.

51. ——, *Breaking Patterns of Defeat*, Lippincott, Philadelphia, 1954.

52. ——, and COLE, J. O. (Eds.), *Diagnostic Classification in Child Psychiatry*, American Psychiatric Association, Washington, D.C., 1964.

53. JENKINS, R. L., and GLICKMAN, S., "Patterns of Personality Organization Among Delinquents," *Nervous Child, 6:*329–339, 1947.

54. JENKINS, R. L., and HEWITT, L., "Types of Personality Structure Encountered in Child Guidance Clinics," *American Journal of Orthopsychiatry, 14:*84–94, 1944.

55. JENSEN, R. A., "Child Psychiatry," in McQuarrie, I., and Kelly, V. C. (Eds.), *Brenneman's Practice of Pediatrics*, W. F. Prior, Hagerstown, Md., 1959.

56. JORDAN, K., and PRUGH, D. G., "Schizophreniform Psychosis in Childhood," *American Journal of Psychiatry, 128:*323–331, 1971.

57. KANNER, L., *Child Psychiatry*, 4th Ed., Charles C Thomas, Springfield, Ill., 1972.

58. KANT, O., "A Comparative Study of Recovered and Deteriorated Schizophrenic Patients," *Journal of Nervous and Mental Disease, 93:*616–624, 1941.

59. KATZ, M. M., "A Phenomenological Typology of Schizophrenia," in Katz, M. M., Cole, J. O., and Barton, W. E. (Eds.), *The Role and Methodology of Classification in Psychiatry and Psychopathology*, pp. 300–320, National Institute of Mental Health, Chevy Chase, Md., 1965.

60. KESSLER, J. W., "Nosology in Child Psychopathology," in Rie, H. E. (Ed.), *Perspectives in Child Psychopathology*, Aldine Atherton, Chicago, 1971.

61. KOBAGASHI, S., MIZUSHIMA, K., and SHINOHARA, M., "Clinical Groupings of Problem Children Based on Symptoms and Behavior," *International Journal of Social Psychiatry, 13:*206–215, 1967.

62. KRAMER, M., "Classification of Mental Disorders for Epidemiological and Medical Care Purposes: Current Status, Problems, and Needs," in Katz, M. M., Cole, J. O., and Barton, W. E. (Eds.), *The Role and Methodology of Classification in Psychiatry and Psychopathology*, pp. 99–115, National Institute of Mental Health, Chevy Chase, Md., 1965.

63. LEHMANN, H. E., "Empathy and Perspective or Consensus and Automation? Implications of a New Deal in Psychiatric Diagnosis," *Comprehensive Psychiatry, 8:* 265–276, 1967.

64. LORR, M., "A Typology for Functional Psychotics," in Katz, M. M., Cole, J. O., and Barton, W. E. (Eds.), *The Role and Methodology of Classification in Psychiatry and Psychopathology*, pp. 261–277, National Institute of Mental Health, Chevy Chase, Md., 1965.

65. LOUTTIT, C. M., *Clinical Psychology of Children's Behavior Problems*, rev. ed., Harper & Brothers, New York, 1947.

66. LOWREY, L. G., "Some Principles in the Treatment of Behavior Problems in Children," *Journal of Nervous and Mental Disease, 73:*62–65, 1931.

67. MASLOW, A. H., *Farther Reaches of Human Nature*, Viking Press, New York, 1971.

68. MATTSSON, N. B., and GERARD, R. W., "Typology of Schizophrenia Based on Multidisciplinary Observational

Vectors," in Katz, M. M., Cole, J. O., and Barton, W. E. (Eds.), *The Role and Methodology of Classification in Psychiatry and Psychopathology*, pp. 507–532, National Institute of Mental Health, Chevy Chase, Md., 1965.

69. MERCER, J. R., "Psychological Assessment and the Rights of Children," in Hobbs, N. (Ed.), *Issues in the Classification of Children*, vol. 1, pp. 130–158, Jossey-Bass, San Francisco, 1975.

70. MILLER, E., "Classification of the Disorders of Childhood," in Rolleston, Sir Humphrey, (Ed.), *British Encyclopedia of Medical Practice*, Butterworth, London, 1936.

71. MONROE, R. R., "Diagnosis of Mental Disorders," *American Journal of Psychiatry, 126:*162–163, 1969.

72. MUSSEN, P. H., CONGER, J. J., and CAGAN, J., *Child Development and Personality*, 4th ed., Harper & Row, New York, 1974.

73. NEUBAUER, P. B., "Psychoanalytic Contributions to the Nosology of Childhood Psychic Disorders," *Journal of the American Psychoanalytic Association, 11:*565–604, 1963.

74. NUSSBAUM, K., SCHNEIDMUHL, A. M., and SHAFFER, J. W., "The Psychiatric Assessment of the Social Security Program and Disability Insurance," *American Journal of Psychiatry, 126:*897–899, 1969.

75. ORNITZ, E. M., and RITVO, E. R., "Perceptual Inconsistency in Early Infantile Autism," *Archives of General Psychiatry, 18:*76–98, 1968.

76. OVERALL, J. E., and HOLLISTER, L. E., "Studies of Quantitative Approaches to Psychiatric Classifications," in Katz, M. M., Cole, J. O., and Barton, W. E. (Eds.), *The Role and Methodology of Classification in Psychiatry and Psychopathology*, pp. 277–297, National Institute of Mental Health, Chevy Chase, Md., 1965.

77. PACELLA, B. L., *Behavior Problems in Children: The Medical Clinics of North America*, W. B. Saunders, Philadelphia, 1948.

78. PEARSON, G. H. J., "Classification of Psychological Problems of Children," in Christian, H. A. (Ed.), *The Oxford Medicine, Psychiatry for Practitioners*, vol. 7, Oxford University Press, New York, 1920.

79. POTTER, H. W., Mimeographed outline given to medical students, College of Physicians and Surgeons, Columbia University, New York, 1934.

80. PRUGH, D. G., "Psychosocial Disorders in Childhood and Adolescence: Theoretical Considerations and an Attempt at Classification," in Joint Commission on Mental Health of Children, *The Mental Health of Children; Services, Research and Manpower*, Report of Task Forces IV and V, Harper & Row, New York, 1973.

81. ———, "Towards an Understanding of Psychosomatic Concepts in Relationship to Illness in Children," in Solnit, A. J., and Provence, S. A. (Eds.), *Modern Perspectives in Child Development*, pp. 246–367, International Universities Press, New York, 1963.

82. ———, ENGEL, M., and MORSE, W. W., "Emotional Disturbance in Children," in Hobbs, N. (Ed.), *Issues in the Classification of Children*, vol. 1 pp. 261–299, Jossey-Bass, San Francisco, 1975.

83. RANK, B., "Intensive Study and Treatment of Pre-School Children Who Show Marked Personality Deviations or 'Atypical Development' and Their Parents," in Caplan, G. (Ed.), *Emotional Problems of Early Childhood*, p. 491, Basic Books, New York, 1955.

84. REISER, D. E., and BROWN, J. L., "Patterns of Later Development in Children with Infantile Psychosis," *Journal of the American Academy of Child Psychiatry, 3:*650–667, 1964.

85. RITVO, E. R., et al., "Correlation of Psychiatric Diagnoses and EEG Findings: Double Blind Study of 184 Hospitalized Children," *American Journal of Psychiatry, 126:*988–996, 1970.

86. ROBINS, E., and GUZE, S. B., "Establishment of Diagnostic Validity in Psychiatric Illness: Its Application

to Schizophrenia," *American Journal of Psychiatry, 126:* 983–987, 1970.

87. ROSE, J. A., "The Emotional Problems of Children," in *Psychiatry for the General Practitioner*, abstract from the Seminar Series, The Carrier Clinic, Philadelphia Mental Health Educational Unit of Smith, Kline and French Laboratories, 1958.

88. ROSS, D. C., *A Classification in Child Psychiatry*, privately printed at 4951 McKean Avenue, Philadelphia, 1964.

89. RUTTER, M., "Classification and Categorization in Child Psychiatry," *Journal of Child Psychology and Psychiatry, 6:*71–83, 1965; also in *International Journal of Psychiatry, 3:*161–172, 1965.

90. ———, et al., "A Tri-Axial Classification of Mental Disorders in Childhood," *Journal of Child Psychology and Psychiatry, 10:*41–61, 1969.

91. SAFIRSTEIN, S. L., "Discussion Regarding Passive-Aggressive Personality Disorder: A Search for a Syndrome," *American Journal of Psychiatry, 126:*981–983, 1970.

92. SANTOSTEFANO, S., "Beyond Nosology Diagnosis from the Viewpoint of Development," in Rie, H. E. (Ed.), *Perspectives in Child Psychopathology*, Aldine Atherton, Chicago, 1971.

93. SELBACH, H., Cited by E. Stengel in "Classification of Mental Disorders," *Bulletin of the World Health Organization, 21:*601–663, 1960.

94. SETTLAGE, C. F., "Psychologic Disorders," in Nelson, W. E. (Ed.), *Textbook of Pediatrics*, 8th ed., W. B. Saunders, Philadelphia, 1964.

95. SHAKOW, D., "The Role of Classification in the Development of the Science of Psychopathology with Particular Reference to Research," in Katz, M. M., Cole, J. O., and Barton, W. E. (Eds.), *The Role and Methodology of Classification in Psychiatry and Psychopathology*, pp. 116–143, National Institute of Mental Health, Chevy Chase, Md., 1965.

96. SHAMSIE, S. J. (Ed.), *Adolescent Psychiatry*, Schering Corporation, Pointe-claire, Quebec, 1968.

97. SHAW, C. R., and LUCAS, A. R., *The Psychiatric Disorders of Children*, 2nd ed., Appleton-Century-Crofts, New York, 1970.

98. SHINOHARA, M., and JENKINS, R. L., "MMPI Study of Three Types of Delinquents," *Journal of Clinical Psychology, 23:*156–163, 1967.

99. SILVER, L. B., "DSM-II and the Child and Adolescent Psychopathology," *American Journal of Psychiatry, 125:*161–163, 1969.

100. SMALL, I. F., et al., "Passive-Aggressive Personality Disorder: A Search for a Syndrome," *American Journal of Psychiatry, 126:*973–981, 1970.

101. SPITZ, R. A., *The First Year of Life*, International Universities Press, New York, 1965.

102. SPITZER, R. L., and WILSON, P. T., "DSM-II Revisited: A Reply," *International Journal of Psychiatry, 7:*421–423, 1969.

103. ———, "A Guide to the American Psychiatric Association's New Diagnostic Nomenclature," *International Journal of Psychiatry, 7:*356–367, 1969.

104. STRECKER, E. A., and EBAUGH, F. G., "Practical Clinical Psychiatry for Students and Practitioners," 3rd ed., Blakiston, Philadelphia, 1931.

105. STROEBEL, C. F., and GLUECK, B. C., "Computer Derived Global Judgements in Psychiatry," *American Journal of Psychiatry, 126:*1057–1066, 1970.

106. STROMGREN, E., "Uses and Abuses of Concepts in Psychiatry," *American Journal of Psychiatry, 126:*777–788, 1969.

107. TARJAN, G., and EISENBERG, L., "Some Thoughts on the Classification of Mental Retardation in the United States of America," *American Journal of Psychiatry, 128 (Supplement):*14–18, May, 1972.

108. TARJAN, G., et al. "Classification and Mental Retardation: Issues Arising Out of the Fifth WHO

Seminar on Psychiatric Diagnosis, Classifications and Statistics," *American Journal of Psychiatry, 128(Supplement)*:34–45, May, 1972.

109. TEINKIN, O., "The History of Classification in the Medical Sciences," in Katz, M., Cole, J. O., and Barton, W. E. (Eds.), *The Role and Methodology of Classification in Psychiatry and Psychopathology*, U.S. Department of HEW, PHS Publication 1584, National Institute of Mental Health, Chevy Chase, Md., 1965.

110. THOMPSON, E. T. (Ed.), and HAYDEN, A. C. (Assoc. Ed.), *Standard Nomenclature of Diseases and Operations*, 5th ed., McGraw-Hill, New York, 1961.

111. THORNE, F. C., *Diagnostic Classification and Nomenclature for Psychological Status*, Clinical Psychological Monograph, vol. 20, supplement 17, 1964.

112. TIZARD, J., "A Note on International Statistical Classification of Mental Retardation," *American Journal of Psychiatry, 128(Supplement)*:25–29, 1972.

113. TRAMER, M., *Lehrbuch Der Allgemeinen Kinderpsychiatrie*, 3rd ed., pp. 342–343, 401–404, Basel, Schwabe, 1949.

114. TRYON, R. C., and BAILEY, D. E., *Cluster Analysis*, McGraw-Hill, New York, 1970.

115. U.S. Department of Health, Education and Welfare, *International Classification of Diseases*, 8th ed., adapted for use in the United States, 1967–68.

116. VAILLANT, G. E., "The Natural History of the Remitting Schizophrenias," *American Journal of Psychiatry, 120*:367–376, 1963.

117. ———, "The Prediction of Recovery in Schizophrenia," *Journal of Nervous and Mental Disease, 135*: 534–543, 1962.

118. VAN KREVELEN, D. A., "Prognosis of Childhood Neurosis and Psychosis," *Acta Paedopsychiatrica, 34*:104–111, 1967.

119. VAN OPHUIJSEN, J. H. W., "Primary Conduct Disorders: Their Diagnosis and Treatment," in Lewis, N. D. C., and Pacella, B. L. (Eds.), *Modern Trends in Child Psychiatry*, International Universities Press, New York, 1945.

120. World Health Organization, "Fifth Seminar on Psychiatric Diagnosis Classification and Statistics," *American Journal of Psychiatry, 123*:3–14, 1972.

121. WORTIS, J., "Comments on the ICD Classification of Mental Retardation," *American Journal of Psychiatry, 128(Supplement)*:21–24, May, 1972.

122. YUSIN, A., SAINA, R., and NIHIRA, K., "Adolescent in Crisis: Evaluation of a Questionnaire," *American Journal of Psychiatry, 129*:574–577, 1972.

123. ZIGLER, E., and PHILLIPS, L., "Social Competence and Outcome in Psychiatric Disorder," *Journal of Abnormal and Social Psychology, 63*:264–271, 1961.

124. ZILBOORG, G. A., *A History of Medical Psychology*, W. W. Norton, New York, 1941.

7 / Differential Diagnosis

Melvin Lewis

Introduction

Differential diagnosis aims at distinguishing between the various conditions which may have similar symptoms. The purpose of this differentiation is to arrive at an accurate diagnosis as a basis for specific treatment and preventive measures, communication, and research.

Difficulties arise in child psychiatry because symptoms, the conditions from which they derive, and the causes of these conditions, are often poorly defined.[37] In practice, the term symptom in child psychiatry has come to mean almost any behavioral manifestation that comes to the attention of the observer. When certain traits, signs or behaviors are particularly prominent and occur together frequently, conventional labels are commonly applied defining a condition or syndrome; e.g., the cluster of short attention span, hyperactivity, labile emotions, and clumsiness is conventionally represented by the label "minimal brain dysfunction." These labels, in turn, may imply an etiology, a specific treatment, or a prognosis. However, in many cases the etiology is multivariate; the treatment, untested; and the prognosis, unknown. In the example given, genetic, congenital, traumatic, infective, neoplastic, metabolic, psychodynamic, and environmental factors may give rise to the identical behavioral manifestations. The treatment is generally nonspecific and the prognosis, wide-ranging. Further, in many instances each factor which enters into such a symptom cluster is often in itself complex and interacts with the other cluster members in a complex manner. In any case, the validity of any such grouping will depend on the accuracy with which each symptom is defined initially.

A second class of difficulties arises because there is no satisfactory or universally accepted classification of diagnostic entities.[1] Many attempts have been made to improve the definition and classification of diagnoses.[10, 12, 29] However, the problem remains unsolved.

Yet a third order of difficulties arises because methods of eliciting data are either inadequate or not standardized. This leads to loss of reliability and, consequently, in validity.[28] Reliability, measured by the degree of agreement between independent, trained observers, refers to the consistency with which children are classified, however unsatisfactory the classification system. Attempts have been made to improve reliability through meticulous and standardized interview structures and rating scales.[15, 33, 35] The skill of the observer and the context, or setting, within which the observations are made must also be taken into account. Observer bias is particularly troublesome. A common bias is one that operates against children who are functioning at a dull, normal or retarded level of intelligence. Physical deformity and marked aggression also tend to arouse strong defenses in the observer, leading to biased judgments. Again, there is at present no universally agreed upon method of data collection, and further studies are needed.

Perhaps a fourth order of difficulties arises from the fact that the same maladaptive behavior may have been arrived at by different routes.[27] That is to say, the maladaptive behavior may have been caused by primary factors such as deprivation, rejection, hostility, inconsistencies, and bizarre parental behavior acting upon a child at specific stages in development; or, it may have been caused by an intrinsic defect or immaturity in the child, rendering him vulnerable to normal demands in the family, school, and society, and leading secondarily to the same maladaptive behavior. Frequently, both kinds of factors are at work, along the lines of Freud's concept of the complemental series.[11]

The immediate task in differential diagnosis is to define as carefully as possible the behavior in question and assess its significance. This raises the question of normality. Normality is behavior that conforms to the expectations of the majority in a given society at a given time. It is not an absolute; it is rather a function of prevailing historical, cultural, and social factors. By the same token, disordered behavior in a child is that which the majority of adults considers inappropriate either in form, frequency, or intensity under the particular conditions in which the behavior occurs. In effect, the child psychiatrist is sanctioned by society to make a judgment about normality, much as a judge (and jury) is sanctioned to make a judgment about guilt or innocence.

Unfortunately, the criteria for all such judgments are often nebulous. The reliability of the witnesses,

the tolerance of the child, family, school, and community, and the context of the psychiatrist's observations, as well as his own biases and thresholds, must all be taken into account by the child psychiatrist in reaching a judgment. Further, as Ross[26] has pointed out, "behavior that is observed at any point in time represents the end point of the interaction of four variables: genetic constitutional endowment, past learning, the individual's current physiological state, and his current environmental conditions." The practical question then becomes: under what conditions does the so-called abnormal behavior appear? For example, even when a definite organic condition, such as psychomotor epilepsy, is present, the precipitation of a seizure may tend to occur only under certain conditions. These may be as various as stress, anxiety, fatigue, rage, and excitement.

Assessments of the nature, sources, and conditions under which a problem arises need to be carried out systematically. The work-up should include the pediatric and psychiatric history, the mental status of the child, an evaluation of the parents and the family relationships, an assessment of the school and community environments, and confirmatory studies such as neurological examination, EEG, psychological tests, and educational tests. Data from such an exploration should enable one to make a diagnosis.

However, there remain a considerable number of cases in which the data do not fit neatly into the diagnostic categories suggested by the available classifications. Indeed, most of the descriptions of syndromes depict a more or less typical, or prototypical, clinical picture. In practice, however, most cases either lack all the diagnostic features of a given syndrome, or present additional features that are not ordinarily considered part of that syndrome. Further, there appears to be a gradient of exactitude in syndromes, extending from certain clear-cut conditions, such as the Gilles de la Tourette syndrome, to increasingly amorphous categories, such as the "atypical child" or the "borderline child." The more amorphous the given category, of course, the less satisfactory is its use. Nonetheless, it may retain some limited communication value for clinicians, particularly in a specific setting. For example, the label "borderline" might be a useful rubric for clinicians in a residental treatment center. They are working with children whose ego is unstable, and whose behavior is characterized by unpredictability and marked fluctuations. Such children, for example, have immature object relations and poor social relationships. They have temper tantrums during

Department of
Health, Education, and Welfare

CHILD BEHAVIOR CHECKLIST - - For ages 4 — 16

CHILD'S AGE	CHILD'S SEX	RACE	PARENT'S TYPE OF WORK *(Please be specific—for example: auto mechanic, high school teacher, homemaker, laborer, lathe operator, shoe salesman, army sergeant.)*
	☐ Boy ☐ Girl		

FORM FILLED OUT BY: DATE

☐ Mother

☐ Father

☐ Other *(Specify):*

FATHER'S
TYPE OF WORK: _____

MOTHER'S
TYPE OF WORK: _____

I. Please list the sports your child most likes to take part in. For example: swimming, baseball, skating, skate boarding, bike riding, fishing, etc.

☐ None

a. _____

b. _____

c. _____

Compared to other children of the same age, about how much time does he/she spend in each?

Don't Know	Less Than Average	Average	More Than Average
☐	☐	☐	☐
☐	☐	☐	☐
☐	☐	☐	☐

Compared to other children of the same age, how well does he/she do each one?

Don't Know	Below Average	Average	Above Average
☐	☐	☐	☐
☐	☐	☐	☐
☐	☐	☐	☐

II. Please list your child's favorite hobbies, activities, and games, other than sports. For example: stamps, dolls, books, piano, crafts, singing, etc. (Do not include T.V.)

☐ None

a. _____

b. _____

c. _____

Compared to other children of the same age, about how much time does he/she spend in each?

Don't Know	Less Than Average	Average	More Than Average
☐	☐	☐	☐
☐	☐	☐	☐
☐	☐	☐	☐

Compared to other children of the same age, how well does he/she do each one?

Don't Know	Below Average	Average	Above Average
☐	☐	☐	☐
☐	☐	☐	☐
☐	☐	☐	☐

III. Please list any organizations, clubs, teams, or groups your child belongs to.

☐ None

a. _____

b. _____

c. _____

Compared to other children of the same age, how active is he/she in each?

Don't Know	Less Active	Average	More Active
☐	☐	☐	☐
☐	☐	☐	☐
☐	☐	☐	☐

IV. Please list any jobs or chores your child has. For example: Paper route, babysitting, making bed, etc.

☐ None

a. _____

b. _____

c. _____

Compared to other children of the same age, how well does he/she carry them out?

Don't Know	Below Average	Average	Above Average
☐	☐	☐	☐
☐	☐	☐	☐
☐	☐	☐	☐

512
Rev. 12-77

PAGE 1

T.M. Achenbach, Ph.D., NIMH, Bethesda, Md. 20014

FIGURE 7–1

NOTE: Reprinted with permission of the Department of Health, Education, and Welfare, from *Child Behavior Checklist*, by T. M. Achenbach, National Institute of Mental Health, Bethesda, Md.

V. **1. About how many close friends does your child have?** ☐ None ☐ 1 ☐ 2 or 3 ☐ 4 or more

    2. About how many times a week does your child do things with them? ☐ less than 1 ☐ 1 or 2 ☐ 3 or more

---

VI. **Compared to other children of his/her age, how well does your child:**

	Worse	About the same	Better
a. Get along with his/her brothers & sisters?	☐	☐	☐
b. Get along with other children?	☐	☐	☐
c. Behave with his/her parents?	☐	☐	☐
d. Play and work by himself/herself?	☐	☐	☐

/II. **1. Current school performance—for children aged 6 and older:**

☐ Does not go to school

	Failing	Below average	Average	Above average
a. Reading or English	☐	☐	☐	☐
b. Writing	☐	☐	☐	☐
c. Arithmetic or Math	☐	☐	☐	☐
d. Spelling	☐	☐	☐	☐
Other academic subjects: e. _____	☐	☐	☐	☐
(for example: history, science, foreign language, f. _____	☐	☐	☐	☐
geography). g. _____	☐	☐	☐	☐

2. Is your child in a special class?

☐ No ☐ Yes—what kind?

---

3. Has your child ever repeated a grade?

☐ No ☐ Yes—grade and reason

---

4. Please describe any academic or other problems your child has had in school.

☐ None

VIII. Below is a list of items that describe children. For each item that describes your child *now* or *within the past 12 months*, please circle the *2* if the item is *very true* or *often true* of your child. Circle the *1* if the item is *somewhat* or *sometimes true* of your child. If the item is *not true* of your child, circle the *0*.

0	1	2	1.	Acts too young for his/her age	0	1	2	31. Fears he/she might think or do something bad
	1	2	2.	Allergy (describe): _____				
					0	1	2	32. Feels he/she has to be perfect
				_____	0	1	2	33. Feels or complains that no one loves him/he
0	1	2	3.	Argues a lot	0	1	2	34. Feels others are out to get him/her
0	1	2	4.	Asthma	0	1	2	35. Feels worthless or inferior
0	1	2	5.	Behaves like opposite sex	0	1	2	36. Gets hurt a lot, accident-prone
0	1	2	6.	Bowel movements outside toilet	0	1	2	37. Gets in many fights
0	1	2	7.	Bragging, boasting	0	1	2	38. Gets teased a lot
0	1	2	8.	Can't concentrate, can't pay attention for long	0	1	2	39. Hangs around with children who get in trouble
0	1	2	9.	Can't get his/her mind off certain thoughts; obsessions (describe): _____	0	1	2	40. Hears things that aren't there (describe):
0	1	2	10.	Can't sit still, restless, or hyperactive	0	1	2	41. Impulsive or acts without thinking
0	1	2	11.	Clings to adults or too dependent	0	1	2	42. Likes to be alone
0	1	2	12.	Complains of loneliness	0	1	2	43. Lying or cheating
0	1	2	13.	Confused or seems to be in a fog	0	1	2	44. Bites fingernails
0	1	2	14.	Cries a lot	0	1	2	45. Nervous, highstrung, or tense
0	1	2	15.	Cruel to animals	0	1	2	46. Nervous movements or twitching (describe)
	1	2	16.	Cruelty, bullying, or meanness to others				
0	1	2	17.	Day-dreams or gets lost in his/her thoughts				
0	1	2	18.	Deliberately harms self or attempts suicide	0	1	2	47. Nightmares
0	1	2	19.	Demands a lot of attention	0	1	2	48. Not liked by other children
0	1	2	20.	Destroys his/her own things	0	1	2	49. Constipated, doesn't move bowels
0	1	2	21.	Destroys things belonging to his/her family or other children	0	1	2	50. Too fearful or anxious
0	1	2	22.	Disobedient at home	0	1	2	51. Feels dizzy
0	1	2	23.	Disobedient at school	0	1	2	52. Feels too guilty
0	1	2	24.	Doesn't eat well	0	1	2	53. Overeating
0	1	2	25.	Doesn't get along with other children	0	1	2	54. Overtired
0	1	2	26.	Doesn't seem to feel guilty after misbehaving	0	1	2	55. Overweight
0	1	2	27.	Easily jealous				56. Physical problems without known medical cause:
0	1	2	28.	Eats or drinks things that are not food (describe): _____	0	1	2	a. Aches or pains
					0	1	2	b. Headaches
					0	1	2	c. Nausea, feels sick
				_____	0	1	2	d. Problems with eyes (describe):
0	1	2	29.	Fears certain animals, situations, or places, other than school (describe): _____	0	1	2	e. Rashes or other skin problems
					0	1	2	f. Stomachaches or cramps
					0	1	2	g. Vomiting, throwing up
0	1	2	30.	Fears going to school	0	1	2	h. Other (describe): _____

0 1 2	57.	Physically attacks people	0 1 2	84. Strange behavior (describe): _____
0 1 2	58.	Picks nose, skin, or other parts of body (describe): _____		_____
		_____	0 1 2	85. Strange ideas (describe):
0 1 2	59.	Plays with own sex parts in public		_____
0 1 2	60.	Plays with own sex parts too much	0 1 2	86. Stubborn, sullen, irritable
0 1 2	61.	Poor school work	0 1 2	87. Sudden changes in mood or feelings
0 1 2	62.	Poorly coordinated or clumsy	0 1 2	88. Sulks a lot
0 1 2	63.	Prefers playing with older children	0 1 2	89. Suspicious
0 1 2	64.	Prefers playing with younger children	0 1 2	90. Swearing or obscene language
0 1 2	65.	Refuses to talk	0 1 2	91. Talks about killing self
0 1 2	66.	Repeats certain acts over and over; compulsions (describe): _____	0 1 2	92. Talks or walks in sleep (describe):
				_____
			0 1 2	93. Talks too much
0 1 2	67.	Runs away from home	0 1 2	94. Teases a lot
0 1 2	68.	Screams a lot	0 1 2	95. Temper tantrums or hot temper
0 1 2	69.	Secretive, keeps things to self	0 1 2	96. Thinks about sex too much
0 1 2	70.	Sees things that aren't there (describe):	0 1 2	97. Threatens people
			0 1 2	98. Thumb-sucking
		_____	0 1 2	99. Too concerned with neatness or cleanliness
			0 1 2	100. Trouble sleeping (describe):
0 1 2	71.	Self-conscious or easily embarrassed		
0 1 2	72.	Sets fires		_____
0 1 2	73.	Sexual problems (describe):	0 1 2	101. Truancy, skips school
			0 1 2	102. Underactive, slow moving, or lacks energy
			0 1 2	103. Unhappy, sad, or depressed
		_____	0 1 2	104. Unusually loud
0 1 2	74.	Showing off or clowning	0 1 2	105. Uses alcohol or drugs (describe):
0 1 2	75.	Shy or timid		_____
0 1 2	76.	Sleeps less than most children	0 1 2	106. Vandalism
0 1 2	77.	Sleeps more than most children during day and/or night (describe): _____	0 1 2	107. Wets self during the day
			0 1 2	108. Wets the bed
0 1 2	78.	Smears or plays with bowel movements	0 1 2	109. Whining
0 1 2	79.	Speech problem (describe): _____	0 1 2	110. Wishes to be of opposite sex
			0 1 2	111. Withdrawn, doesn't get involved with others
		_____	0 1 2	112. Worrying
0 1 2	80.	Stares blankly		113. Please write in any problems your child has that were not listed above:
0 1 2	81.	Steals at home		
0 1 2	82.	Steals outside the home	0 1 2	_____
0 1 2	83.	Stores up things he/she doesn't need (describe):	0 1 2	_____
		_____	0 1 2	_____

which they are out of contact with reality and act as if they are warding off an attacker; at moments they may even become quite paranoid and regressed. Their behavior is like that of a younger child: when they feel unloved, they will either withdraw or become hostile or aggressive. They need the presence of the love object to maintain their hold on reality, i.e., they have a limited "reality span." They are often obsessional and have difficulty in thinking abstractly. The particular usefulness of this clustering under the heading of "borderline" is that it can lead to specific interventions within the residential setting.

Thus, diagnosis is a means and not an end, and differential diagnosis begins with a differentiation of symptoms. In childhood the range of behavior, while wide, is not infinite. Most behavior items are covered in the list shown in Figure 7–1.

When clusters of these items occur with some regularity, they give rise to the so-called syndromes. Beyond the small, subtype clusters that constitute the syndromes, larger correlations of symptoms may also occur. For example, in a factor-analytic study by Achenbach,[2] phobias, stomach aches, fearfulness, and pains had a high correlation with one another, constituting a group of so-called "internalizing" symptoms. Other symptoms found in this group include shyness, worrying, seclusiveness, withdrawal and apathy, headaches, nausea and vomiting, obsession and compulsions, crying and preoccupation with fantasy. The number of girls in this internalizing group was twice that of boys.

At the other pole, symptoms such as disobedience, stealing, lying, fighting, cruelty, destructiveness, vandalism, firesetting, inadequate guilt feelings, swearing, temper tantrums, showing off, hyperactivity, truancy and running away constituted a group of "externalizing" symptoms. "Externalizers" tended to have poorer school performance and a more frequent history of psychiatric, school, and police problems. Aggression, in fact, was more poorly controlled in this group. In this "externalized" group, the number of boys was twice that of girls. Interestingly, the parents of this "externalized" group of children more often tended to have psychiatric and criminal records. The family histories spoke of alcoholism, divorce, neglect, desertion, and illegitimacy.

This categorization, of course, is too global for clinical purposes. Many of the symptoms subsumed under either category may have multiple etiologies. Symptoms such as "daydreams, gets lost in his thoughts," "impulsive, acts without thinking," "nervous movement, twitching," "often feels dizzy," "stares blankly," "sudden changes in mood or feelings," "talks or walks in his sleep," may have a variety of underlying causes.

From a systematic point of view it should be possible to construct an index of differential diagnosis of symptoms in child psychiatry. As illustrations, some symptoms, or symptom clusters, that commonly require a differential diagnosis follow.

Reading Difficulty

Children who have difficulty in learning to read may be suffering from visual or auditory perceptual handicaps, mental retardation, psychological disturbances, maturational lag, inadequate teaching, adverse family environment, linguistic problems, or a specific reading disability. The etiology of a specific reading disability may include those factors associated with minimal brain dysfunction. It is obvious that each of these causes must be considered and investigated. The work-up must, therefore, include tests for hearing and vision, a careful neurological examination, the Wechsler Intelligence Scale for Children, Rorschach and TAT, the Bender Visual Motor Test, evaluation of child, family and school, and specific reading tests such as the Wide Range Achievement Test. Psychiatric interviews alone are rarely insufficient.

Pure, although by no means simple, developmental dyslexia usually presents after the first grade. Many of the children with this problem have to repeat this grade. Clinically, reading is an effort for the child, with many omissions and guesses. Comprehension is poor. The child's handwriting is poor, with many rotations, confusions, and transpositions. All-around frustration, anxiety, and anger are almost inevitable. There are usually no convincing neurological findings.

The rare syndrome of hyperlexia is occasionally encountered, predominantly in boys.[32] These children are often "clumsy," and have a marked apraxia (inability to copy simple figures). They also have some difficulty in comprehension, with an impaired ability to relate speech sounds to meaning, poor relationships, and such language disorders as echolalia, idioglossia, and pronoun reversal. These symptoms are also found in childhood autism; in fact, a common neuropathology, possibly in the parietal lobe, has been postulated for both.[16]

Language and Speech Dysfunction

The general signs of a language dysfunction include reduced vocabulary, especially for abstract concepts such as feelings; delay in the acquisition of two-word sentences (usually acquired by twenty-four months of age); overuse of concrete nouns and verbs; and underuse or omission of abstract word classes such as adjectives, adverbs, prepositions, articles, and conjunctions, giving rise to "telegraphic" or unintelligible speech. Subsequently, some children may also avoid speaking and tend to have "interpreters" who speak for them.

Language dysfunction may arise as a result of hearing loss, understimulation, mental retardation, psychosis, central nervous system impairment, and anatomical defect in any of the apparatuses serving speech. These are the major conditions the practicing child psychiatrist must consider. Screening for these conditions has as a minimal requirement a detailed history, physical examination, hematological assessment, psychiatric evaluation, and psychological tests. Depending on which condition seems most probable, more specific studies will then be required.

Certain associated speech patterns may reflect the level of integration at which the central nervous system is affected. For example, aphonia may occur when the neuromuscular level is involved, including such apparatuses as the lips, tongue, larnyx, and medulla oblongata; dysarthria at the cortico-bulbar level; scanning, explosive, and monotonous speech when the cerebellum is affected, and agnosia (failure in understanding symbols) as well as aphasia (failure to understand the spoken word and/or use of speech) at the level of the cerebrum. Dysrhythmias such as cluttering, stuttering, and/or stammering, and rapid speech may be exaggerations of normal errors of speech. Idioglossia occurs typically among twins.

Specific language dysfunctions, such as echolalia, idioglossia, and pronoun reversal may occur in childhood autism and hyperlexia.

Short Attention Span
(and Hyperactivity)

These terms are usually descriptive rather than truly quantitative. Short attention span is frequently a result of fatiguability, which in turn is a function of the amount of effort the child has to expend in overcoming any difficulty he has in distinguishing background from foreground or in trying to hold on to more units of data than he is capable of managing. Similarly, so-called "hyperactivity" is usually a form of disorganized motor activity that becomes worse in a 1:30 classroom situation, rather than an excess (whatever that may be) of normal, organized behavior. Anxiety may account for this behavior. However, in addition the child may have signs of clumsiness, extraneous movements, confusions of "right and left," "front and back," "before and after," together with so-called soft signs, particularly asymmetries of reflexes or fine finger-hand movements. In such instances, organicity may be present.

Psychiatric interviews, classroom observations, the Bender-Gestalt test, neurological examination, and, if necessary, an EEG, will help in deciding between these possibilities.

Temper Tantrums

The differentiation of the symptom of "temper tantrum" requires attention to the following clinical points. Temper tantrums that represent motor discharge occur typically in young children and are accompanied by screaming and hand flailing. This motor behavior usually occurs before speech becomes available to the child. It is also found in children for whom other, more ego-syntonic, channels are not available, such as certain atypical or autistic children. However, the atypical or autistic child will almost certainly be markedly deviant in other ways, whereas the normal infant will not.

Anger and frustration are the basic causes of temper tantrums. When the tantrums give rise to violent and aggressive behavior with destructive components, they become clinical issues. The frustrations may be the normal frustrations encountered in growing up, but they may also be chronic frustrations arising out of a feeling of being unloved, deprived, or excessively stimulated. A search for these sources of frustration is the first step toward a solution of the problem.

Panic or anxiety may present as temper tantrums. In a sense, they produce "terror tantrums." Usually other signs associated with the cause are present, e.g., decompensating phobic or obsessional symptoms, signs of minimal brain dysfunction, or signs of a borderline disturbance.

In some cases, the tolerance level of the parent may be too low, leading them to describe an item of behavior as maladaptive when, in fact, the behavior is normal, or at any rate, characteristic of a particular child.

Further, even when the behavior is of a magnitude that suggests the possibility of a problem, the behavior may still be adaptive; for example, a child may be appropriately enraged at a frustrating social situation, while not yet mature enough to bring about a change in a more effective way.

Sleep Disturbances

Sleep disturbances may be primary or secondary. The major primary sleep disorders include somnambulism, nightmares, and night terrors, Delta wave disturbance with enuresis, narcolepsy, and hypersomia.[19]

Secondary disturbances, of which insomnia is the most common, may be associated with physical discomfort, anxiety, excitement, depression, neurosis (particularly depressive-compulsive neurosis), and psychosis (including borderline disturbances and schizophrenia).

Sleepwalking, found more often in boys than girls, usually occurs in stage three or stage four sleep, and lasts for a few minutes. There is often some awareness during the episode, but usually no memory of the event once the child is awakened.

Children who are sleepwalkers also commonly have night terrors, which consist of intense anxiety, outbursts of screaming and thrashing around, rapid heart rate and deep, rapid breathing, all lasting for a few minutes, but again, with little or no memory after awakening. Night terrors, like sleepwalking, occur early in stage four sleep. Both conditions have been considered to be "arousal disorders," consisting of delayed or impaired arousal out of stage three or four sleep, perhaps as a result of delay in maturation.[6]

Spontaneous remission usually occurs as the child grows older. It is comparatively unusual to find any pathognonomic psychopathology in these children. However, of those who remain sleepwalkers during young adulthood, approximately one-third are schizophrenic.[34]

In contrast to sleepwalking and night terrors, psychological problems are relatively frequent in children who have nightmares. Essentially, these problems consist of readily remembered frightening dreams, occurring during REM sleep from which the child is easily aroused.

Bedwetting may be a symptom of a sleep disturbance. In general, bedwetting may be familial, organic, or psychological. Diurnal, as well as nocturnal, enuresis, associated with dysuria, may indicate the presence of an organic disorder, such as posterior urethral valve obstruction, double ureter, cystitis, etc. Psychological causes are likely when there has been a history of having been successfully toilet trained. After a dry interval, enuresis begins, following psychological stress associated with, say, the birth of a sibling, the loss of a parent, or illness.

Maturational delay may occur when there has been inadequate expectation for dryness.

At the same time, and perhaps most commonly, familial, maturational lag in sleep patterning may give rise to bedwetting. Characteristically, the child is in stage four NREM sleep when a burst of delta waves occurs and the sleep pattern changes to stage two or one, during which the micturition occurs.[13] Dreaming during REM sleep may occur subsequently, in which case the wetting may be incorporated into the dream. In these cases of maturational lag, there is often a strong family history of bedwetting, with a specific age at which the symptom ceased in the family members.

Delinquent Behavior

Poor socioeconomic conditions,* as well as psychodynamic factors† must be evaluated as possible causes of delinquent behavior. However, Lewis[20] has pointed out that important psychiatric and neurological factors may give rise to delinquent behavior. The severity of the offense is an unreliable guide. The absence of any memory for violent acts should raise the possibility of some form of seizure disorder, including psychomotor epilepsy. A history of birth difficulty, cerebral infection, or head injury may be important forerunners of an organic condition resulting in poor impulse control or a seizure disorder. Similarly, a history of early interpersonal difficulties and behavior problems at school may be important harbingers of later psychotic symptomatology, including hallucinations and paranoid thinking associated with delinquency.[22] A history of psy-

* See references 7, 8, 23, 24, 31.
† See references 3, 14, 17, 18, 30.

chiatric disturbance in the family is important. The influence of living with a psychiatrically impaired relative may be a contributing factor. Further, antisocial behavior is sometimes the child's way of calling attention to the parent's disturbance. The label "sociopathic" should be avoided.[21] Rather, a specific psychiatric and/or neurological diagnosis is required. Depression may be an important component of the child's antisocial behavior.

Stealing

The symptom of stealing may arise from many causes. Sometimes the symptom is due to a failure in distinguishing between "what's mine" and "what's not mine." The failure in turn may be due to immaturity. If there is in addition an organic component, the compulsive defenses that are usually prominent in such children will lead to an exaggeration of the "hoarding" tendency of young children. This may prepare the ground for the child, who subsequently feels unloved and ungratified, and who then steals to obtain love. If the child is also frustrated and enraged at the ungiving love object, he will steal specifically from that love object, representing in part the mixed dependency and hostility felt toward what is usually an ambivalently regarded caretaker. When there has been a considerable distortion of ego development, and more particularly superego development, the child may steal because there have been no parental sanctions against stealing. In such cases the child rarely experiences guilt.

Indiscriminate, repeated stealing is often a sign of inadequate impulse control. This is particularly true in those children who have poor parental models, who are deprived, or who live in a subculture where stealing has other meanings. Sometimes this is an attempt to find a place in, and identify oneself with, a peer group of equally deprived children who roam and steal.

When stealing is accompanied by guilt, it is usually a search for punishment, the expression of a harsh superego. The form of the stealing in these cases is such that there is a strong likelihood of being caught and punished.

Stealing may first appear, or become aggravated, when the child is under stress; in this sense, it is a regressive phenomenon, much as enuresis may at times be a regressive phenomenon.

Thought Disorder

The process of thinking has three major clinical dimensions; actual thought content, speed of thinking, and ease of flow. A variation in any of these dimensions may be of such a degree and duration as to constitute a thought disorder.

Disordered content may take the form of neologisms and idiosyncratic logic, including transductive reasoning (things that are related in time or space are believed to be causal), difficulty in discerning differences and similarities, problems in distinguishing the relevant from the irrelevant, and excessive concreteness.

Disordered speed of thinking may take the form of retardation or a push of thinking and speaking.

Disorders of flow may take the form of blocking, muteness, and excessive repetitions of words and sentences.

A child may experience any of these manifestations subjectively as being alien, out of his control, and, sometimes, as frightening.

There may be an associated disorder of mood (depression, elation, inappropriateness, paranoid rage), of behavior (disorganized, regressed, aggressive, withdrawn, bizarre), or of perception (delusions, hallucinations).

Thought disorder is thus another example of a cluster of symptoms, which is not, in itself, a diagnosis. The possible causes of this cluster may be classified clinically as follows:

1. Psychological; e.g., the psychoses of childhood.
2. Genetic; e.g., inborn errors of metabolism, such as Hartnup's disease and Kuf's disease.
3. Traumatic; e.g., postconcussion syndrome.
4. Infective; e.g., viral encephalitis, brain abscesses.
5. Neoplastic; e.g., brain tumor.
6. Toxic; e.g., amphetamines, steroids, bromism.
7. Deficiencies; e.g., pellagra.
8. Endocrine; e.g., thyrotoxicosis.

The examples given are illustrative rather than comprehensive. The important point here is to think of the classes of possible causes. For example, under the category of psychological, the psychoses of childhood represent a large group of disorders which in turn may be classified as shown in Table 7–1.

The symptom, or rather the cluster of symptoms constituting a thought disorder, should lead to a systemic review of these possible causes. Obviously, some causes will be readily eliminated, while others will immediately suggest themselves as more likely possibilities. Once the field has been narrowed in this way, a more detailed study can

TABLE 7–1

Classification of Childhood Psychoses

A. Early Childhood
   1. Early infantile autism (Kanner)   0–2 years
   2. Anaclitic depression (Spitz)   6 months
      Grief and mourning (Bowlby)
   3. Symbiotic psychosis (Mahler)   2–5 years
   4. Atypical child (Rank)
   5. Children with unusual sensitivities
      (Bergman and Escalona)   2–7 years
B. Later Childhood
   1. Psychosis associated with, though not
      necessarily caused by,
      a. organic brain disease and/or
      b. mental retardation
   2. Schizophrenic-like psychosis, acute and
      chronic states of severe maldevelopment
      or disorganization, comparable to some
      adult forms
   3. Bipolar depression
C. Psychosis of Adolescence
   1. Relatively benign, acute adolescent turmoil
   2. Organic syndromes
   3. Syndromes comparable to most, if not all,
      adult forms of schizophrenia
   4. Bipolar depression

lead to a further narrowing. For example, the associated presence of hallucinations (see below) may give a cross-differential diagnosis of specific syndromes, e.g., childhood autism, symbiotic psychosis, schizophrenia.

Hallucinations

Hallucinations in childhood are almost always pathological. A clinical differentiation can provide clues to their etiology, as follows.

DRUG TOXICITY

Numerous drugs are potentially hallucinogenic, including marijuana, mescaline, psilocybin, LSD, STP, amphetamines, barbiturates, bromides, MAO inhibitors, antihistamines, and atropine-like drugs. At the same time, children and adolescents who take drugs may have an antecedent psychiatric disturbance.[25] Sometimes the timing and form of the hallucinations suggest the possibility of drugs. Other symptoms of drug ingestion may be present including drowsiness, paranoid behavior, confusion, restlessness, excitement, violence, dilated pupils, ataxia, dysmetria, tremor, dysarthria, dyskinesia, akathisia, and hypotensive signs. One must ask about possible drug ingestion.

Urine and blood samples must be tested when drug ingestion is suspected.

SEIZURE DISORDERS

Hallucinations, particularly in the form of hypnagogic hallucinations, may occur in narcolepsy and other seizure disorders. Usually this history will suggest a seizure disorder. Acute febrile illnesses, especially in young children, may give rise to hallucinations. Previous encephalitic illnesses may present much later with hallucinations as the first symptom of degeneration. Neurological examination and EEG are required.

METABOLIC DISORDERS

Metabolic disorders which may give rise to hallucinations include adrenal cortical hypofunction, thyroid and parathyroid disease, hepatolenticular degeneration, porphyria, beri-beri, hypomagnesiumemia (secondary to prolonged parenteral fluid replacement, diuretic therapy, excess vitamin D intake, diabetic acidosis). Signs of the primary metabolic disorder are usually present.

INFECTION

Encephalitis, meningitis, and acute febrile illnesses may, of course, give rise to hallucinations.

IMMATURITY AND STRESS

Precocious motor development, combined with immature ego development, may be part of the symbiotic psychosis syndrome, with secondary hallucinations.

Disturbed superego function, perhaps as a result of the death of a parent at the time of superego formation, may give rise to hallucinations. Usually these hallucinations are auditory and consist of admonitions and prohibitions attributed to the dead parent.

Hallucinations following severe anxiety may occur when the anxiety level overwhelms the child. Young children who are under severe stress and resort to the defense mechanisms of repression, projection, and displacement may also experience hallucinations. The hallucinations appear to be part of a regressive phenomenon, in which the distinction between fantasy and reality is temporarily lost. Often the stress is sexual, and the child may have been exposed to excessive stimulation. The content of the hallucination may suggest the underlying psychological conflict.

In older children, external conflicts rarely, if ever, give rise to hallucinations. However, if the stress is of massive proportions and overwhelms the child, it can lead to profound regression. Circumstances in which this occurs include severe and sudden illness. For example, a previously healthy fifteen-year-old girl suddenly developed hemolytic uremic syndrome, with acute renal shutdown necessitating immediate hemodialysis. While on the machine, she began to hallucinate. Occasionally, active children are suddenly confronted with forced immobilization as a result of treatment for a fractured limb; such youngsters may hallucinate during moments of acute anxiety.

In some instances, severe cultural deprivation *together* with a disturbed parent-child relationship, may determine the prevalence and form of hallucinations. The hallucinations in this group are said to be localized, orderly, and related to reality, consisting of forbidding voices and overt wish fulfillments.[36] Often the hallucinations here are consistent with the superstitions of the parents. The child may appear to be well organized in other ways. However, there is usually evidence of a personality disturbance in the child, and psychosis in the parent, suggesting at least the possibility of a genetic or organic component as well as powerful socio-cultural influences.[9]

Cultural: In fundamentalist sects a high valuation is placed on being possessed by the spirit. Hysterically inclined children and youths may lend themselves to this experience and "hear voices."

Psychosis: When hallucinations are more fragmented, incoherent, and bizarre in content, there is a greater likelihood of a primary psychosis being present.[5] Bodily complaints and paranoid delusions may be associated with the psychosis. Children are often frightened and secretive about these hallucinations. There are usually other signs of psychosis present, including disordered illogical thought processes and inappropriate affect. A history of psychiatric disturbance in the family and maternal deprivation during infancy are often present. Sometimes the child presents with delinquent behavior.[20] Psychological testing, particularly projective tests, are indicated. Precipitants for the psychotic behavior must next be explored.

Seizure Behavior

A frequent and important differential diagnosis is between a paroxysmal epileptic disorder and conversion reaction.

In a conversion reaction there is rarely any aura, and consciousness, while impaired, is not lost. Sequential movements are uncommon. Loss of bladder or bowel control, or tongue biting, does not usually occur. The attack may end suddenly, and there is no post-ictal confusion. The EEG is normal.

Young children under the age of six may hold their breath during a crying spell, become cyanotic, and then lose consciousness. In epilepsy the cyanosis follows the seizure. In hysterical adolescents, hyperventilation may give rise to fainting, presenting as a transient loss of consciousness. Actual loss of consciousness, especially if prolonged, suggests the presence of epilepsy. Syncope, of course, may precipitate a seizure in an epileptic child. Some adolescents are prone to sudden, irresistible, brief attacks of shallow sleep (narcolepsy), often accompanied by sudden, fleeting attacks of loss of muscle tone (cataplexy). This is especially likely to occur during strong emotional states, such as anger. The child is easily aroused from this sleep and has no post-ictal confusion. Consciousness is not lost in cataplexy. Children who have a history of sleepwalking, nightmares, and bedwetting may later develop psychomotor seizures.[4]

Conclusion

It can be seen that even a differential diagnosis of symptoms or symptom clusters does not lead directly to a diagnosis. Such an approach merely opens up possibilities to be considered. In the final analysis, the actual diagnosis depends upon a careful and meticulous assessment of all the available data. These must be judged within the context of the child's equipment, vulnerabilities and developmental level, the family and other environmental factors, and the circumstances of the evaluation process itself.

REFERENCES

1. Achenbach, T., *Developmental Psychopathology*, Ronald Press, New York, 1974.
2. ———, *The Classification of Children's Psychiatric Symptoms: A Factor-Analytic Study*, Psychological Monographs, vol. 80, no. 615, 1966.
3. Aichorn, A., *Wayward Youth*, Viking Press, New York, 1935.
4. Aird, R. B., Venturini, A. M., and Spielman, P. M., "Antecedents of Temporal Lobe Epilepsy," *Archives of Neurology, 16:*67–73, 1967.
5. Bender, L., "Imaginary Companion: Hallucinations in Children," *A Dynamic Psychopathology of Childhood*, Charles C Thomas, Springfield, Ill., 1954.
6. Broughton, R. J., "Sleep Disorders: Disorders of Arousal," *Science, 159:*1070–1078, 1968.
7. Cloward, R. A., and Ohln, L. E., *Delinquency and Opportunity: A Theory of Delinquent Gangs*, Free Press, New York, 1960.
8. Cohen, A. K., "The Sociology of the Deviant Act: Anomie Theory and Beyond," *American Sociological Review, 30:*5–14, 1965.
9. Esman, A. H., "Visual Hallucinosis in Young Children," in Eissler, R. S., et al. (Eds.), *The Psychoanalytic Study of the Child*, vol. 17, pp. 334–343, International Universities Press, New York, 1962.
10. Feighner, J. P., et al., "Diagnostic Criteria for Use in Psychiatric Research," *Archives of General Psychiatry, 26:*57–63, 1972.
11. Freud, S., "Three Essays on Sexuality," in *The Standard Edition of the Complete Psychological Works of Sigmund Freud*, vol. 7, pp. 135–243, Hogarth Press, London, 1953.
12. Group for the Advancement of Psychiatry (GAP), *Psychopathological Disorders in Childhood: Theoretical Considerations and a Proposed Classification*, Report No. 62, Group for the Advancement of Psychiatry, New York, 1966.
13. Gastaut, H., and Broughton, R. "A Clinical and Polygraphic Study of Episodic Phenomena During Sleep," in Wortis, J. (Ed.), *Recent Advances in Biological Psychiatry*, vol. 7, pp. 197–221, Plenum Press, New York, 1964.
14. Glueck, S., and Glueck, E., *Toward a Typology of Juvenile Offenders: Implications for Therapy and Prevention*, Grune & Stratton, New York, 1970.
15. Goodman, J. D., and Sours, J. A., *The Child Mental Status Examination*, Basic Books, New York, 1967.
16. Huttenlocher, P. R., and Huttenlocher, J., "A Study of Children with Hyperlexia," *Neurology, 23(10):*1107–1116, 1973.
17. Jenkins, R. L., and Hewitt, L., "Types of Personality Structure Encountered in Child Guidance Clinics," *American Journal of Orthopsychiatry, 14:*84–94, 1944.
18. Johnson, A. A., "Sanctions for Superego Lacunae of Adolescents," in Eissler, K. R. (Ed.), *Searchlights on Delinquency*, International Universities Press, New York, 1949.
19. Kales, A., and Kales, J., "Sleep Disorders," *New England Journal of Medicine, 290(9):*487–499, 1974.
20. Lewis, D. O., "Diagnostic Evaluation of the Juvenile Offender: Toward the Clarification of Often Overlooked Psychopathology," submitted for publication, 1975.
21. ———, and Balla, D., " 'Sociopathy' and Its Synonyms: Inappropriate Diagnoses in Child Psychiatry," *American Journal of Psychiatry, 132(7):*720–722, 1975.
22. ———, et al., "Psychotic Symptomatology in a Juvenile Court Clinic Population," *Journal of the American Academy of Child Psychiatry, 124:*660–675, 1973.
23. Merton, R. K., "Social Structure and Anomie," *American Sociological Review, 3:*672–682, 1938.
24. Matza, D., *Delinquency and Drift*, John Wiley, New York, 1964.
25. Paulsen, J., "Psychiatric Problems," in Blum, R. H., and Associates (Eds.), *Students and Drugs*, pp. 291–304, Jossey-Bass, San Francisco, 1969.
26. Ross, A. O., *Psychological Disorders of Children*, McGraw-Hill, New York, 1974.
27. Rubin, E. Z., et al., *Cognitive Perceptual Motor Dysfunction*, Wayne State University Press, Detroit, 1972.
28. Rutter, M. L., and Graham, P. J., "The Reliability and Validity of the Psychiatric Assessment of the Child. I. Interview with the Child," *British Journal of Psychiatry, 114:*563–579, 1968.
29. Rutter, M. L., Shaffer, D., and Shepherd, M., *A Multi-Axial Classification of Child Psychiatric Disorders*, World Health Organization, Geneva, 1975.
30. Schmideberg, M., "The Psychoanalysis of Delinquents," *American Journal of Orthopsychiatry, 23:*13–19, 1953.
31. Shaw, C. R., and McKay, H. D., *Juvenile Delinquency and Urban Areas*, University of Chicago Press, Chicago, 1969.
32. Silberberg, N. E., and Silberberg, M. C., "Hyperlexia: Specific Word Recognition Skills in Young Children," *Exceptional Children, 34:*41–42, 1967.
33. Simmons, J. E., *Psychiatric Examination of Children*, Lea and Febiger, Philadelphia, 1974.
34. Sours, J. A., Frumken, P., and Inderwell, R. R., "Somnambulism," *Archives of General Psychiatry, 9:*400–413, 1963.
35. Spitzer, R. C., Fleiss, J. C., and Cohen, J., "Psychiatric Status Schedule: A Technique for Evaluating Psychopathology and Impairment in Role Functioning," *Archives of General Psychiatry, 23:*41–55, 1970.
36. Wilking, V. N., and Paoli, C., "The Hallucinatory Experience," *Journal of the American Academy of Child Psychiatry, 5(3):*431–440, 1966.
37. Zigler, E., and Phillips, L., "Psychiatric Diagnosis: A Critique," *Journal of Abnormal and Social Psychology, 63:*607–618, 1961.

8 / A Developmental Approach to the Classification of Psychopathology in Infancy and Early Childhood

*Stanley I. Greenspan, Reginald S. Lourie
and Robert A. Nover*

As of today, the classification of infant psychopathology has not yet jelled. It involves taking into account a large number of complex issues, e.g., biological, social, genetic, constitutional, and environmental variables. It is not surprising, therefore, that such a nosology still awaits formulation.

Such a formulation must consider multiple lines of development, including cognitive development, the development of human relationships, and the flexibility of organizing and differentiating internal and external experience. This involves coping styles and the integrity of the emerging basic personality functions. Such functions include organizing basic rhythms and cycles; habituating to stimuli; constructing the basic schemata for self-object differentiation, causality, and the organization and regulation of affect; and the organization and regulation of communication.

In addition, the caregiver(s) role must also be considered. This involves multiple functions, such as the ability to provide physical care, the ability to recognize basic states of pleasure and displeasure, the capacity for forming a basic attachment, the capacity to perceive different age-appropriate communications coming from the infant, the capacity for empathetic reception of these communications, and the capacity for differential age-appropriate, flexible responses. The inanimate environment, the family environment, and the larger cultural and social milieu are also vital to the infant's development. Thus, there are many complex clusters of variables affecting the infant's development, all interacting in developmental phase-specific contexts.

Various theories, models, and research approaches have focused on one or another set of variables. For example, psychoanalysis has focused on the development of the drives, object relationships, and the formation of internalized psychological structures (e.g., the development of the ego and superego). Piaget's cognitive psychology has focused on the development of cognition (intelligence) mostly in relation to the inanimate world. Empirical researchers (e.g., Ainsworth,[1, 2]

Sander,[12] Stern[15]) have studied certain discrete *measurable* behavioral patterns. The approach presented in this chapter is a step toward a framework compatible with the understanding of development generated from each of these areas of study, and which, at the same time, complements the standard diagnostic classification schemata.

In psychiatry, the general strategies of nosology have been either to describe a symptom-complex or to list conditions according to etiology. Traditionally, psychopathological syndromes of infancy and early childhood have given rise to a number of terms: autism; symbiotic psychoses; anaclitic depression; metabolic depression (marasmus, failure to thrive); hyperactivity; colic; the hypersensitivities; cyclic vomiting; auto-erotic rumination; overprotection (vulnerable child syndrome); maladaptive role assignments; anorexia and feeding problems (hunger, Kwashiorkor, negativism); sleeping problems (separation anxiety); stranger anxiety; separation anxiety (eating problems, aggression); negativism (superego distortions, passive-aggressive personality, anorexia); early forms of aggression (biting, crying, oral sadism, "bad" image, destructive impulse control); gender distortion; superego distortions; beginning negativism; projection of unacceptable impulses; two selves; passivity; psychopathic personality nucleus; constipation-diarrhea; narcissistic personality; masochism; pica syndrome; poor self-image; and habit patterns (thumbsucking, tongue or cheek sucking, body rocking, head banging, hair pulling (trichotilomania)).

A less fully developed, but potentially more useful, approach to diagnosis is the application of a structural developmental model. Here it is assumed that each infant has unique individual methods of dealing with internal and external experience (or stimuli). These modes of coping are considered according to their developmental structural characteristics. The most desirable structure facilitates progressive development. It does this through fostering the full range of age- and phase-appropriate human experience without significant compromises in functioning. For example, the ability of the infant to regulate himself must be viewed in the context of the infant's capacity to begin engaging and relating to the world around him.

This approach does not exclude etiological or symptom-complex diagnosis. Indeed, what is needed is a three-column statement. In the middle is the developmental structural diagnosis. This describes the developmental stage-specific method of organizing and processing experience. To the degree that there are distortions or defects in this structure, one can list, in column one, symptom configuration (e.g., autistic psychosis), and in column three, (where possible) specific etiologic agents (e.g., infection, a traumatic environmental event). The developmental structural approach, in a sense, seeks a final common pathway. It defines the product of the interaction between etiological or causal agents and constitutional patterns. It sets forth the dynamic and structural characteristics of the personality. As such (according to the principle of multiple determination), one should not expect one-to-one correspondences between the developmental level of organization and specific symptoms. (This is true even though certain symptom complexes may be more characteristic of one type of developmental disorder than another.) For each disorder of structural organization, the various causal factors, from genetic and constitutional to dynamic and familial, must each be considered in its own right in relationship to the combined effect of all on this "final pathway." This is the way in which the evolving personality deals with developmental phase-specific experience. While the categories will be presented as discrete entities, it should be emphasized that development is not discontinuous. Early experience may lead to an impairment in a "latter category." This comes about when the organism's inability to deal with phase-appropriate experience shows up in the area of functioning described by that category. The following is a brief and preliminary outline of nosology for the earliest years of life.

Disorders of Homeostasis

Perhaps the first task in which one may observe difficulties in the newborn infant is in its attempt to achieve homeostasis. This task involves the ability to regulate state and form basic cycles and rhythms (sleep, wake, alertness), to organize internal and external experience, (e.g., implement certain stimulus thresholds, habituate to stimuli, organize initial response patterns, develop motor integrity, gaze, etc.), and to integrate a number of modalities into more complex patterns such as consoling oneself and coping with noxious stimuli. An optimal homeostatic experience in the early weeks and months of life involves all of these, together with the work of integrating them and bringing them into balance.

There are often precursors to an infant's failure to achieve homeostasis. These may be apparent while the infant is still in utero. At birth, the infant's first task is to adjust to the extrauterine environment, both animate and inanimate. This includes adapting to changes in his own physiologic functioning. Gross physical or neurological defects, immaturity of the central nervous system, difficulties in early patterns of integration,[3, 12] certain environmental conditions, organ sensitivities (gastrointestinal problems), and allergies are a few of the factors that may contribute to a homeostatic disorder. For example, there is the excitable infant who cannot habituate to stimulation, the infant with specific sensitivities (auditory, tactile), and the infant with immature motor responses who cannot orient, or accept soothing from the caregiver. Then there is the hyperstimulating caregiver who keeps the infant too aroused, or the one who misses all the baby's cues. While gross deficits in perceptual apparatuses (e.g., blindness or deafness) will make an infant more prone to a disorder of homeostasis, other integrative capacities may compensate and comparatively successful homeostatic experience may still become possible.[6]

It should be emphasized that the capacity for homeostasis is not simply the capacity for a state of calm or rest. Rather, the optimal capacity for homeostasis involves the integration of developmentally facilitating life experiences in the fullest sense. This occurs within the context of taking in stimulation through the available sensory modalities, organizing these several inputs in a rich, developmentally appropriate manner (e.g., cycles and rhythms and states of alertness and relaxation), and reaching a state of organized experience. This will foster the initiation of human relationships and interest in the world. Even in the absence of manifest symptoms (excessive irritability, withdrawal, etc.) and/or in the face of stress, one can observe the degree to which an infant fully organizes a homeostatic experience. For example, the infant who is alert, oriented, and engaged in the animate and inanimate world in an organized manner in the context of established patterns of sleeping-wakefulness and eating, may be contrasted with the infant who can be calm only at the expense of an optimal state of alertness and engagement. To the former, a mild stress (illness) may result in a temporary change in sleep patterns, while to the latter, a similar stress may result in intense apathy and lack of engagement in the animate world.

Disorders of Human Attachment

The capacity for achieving a homeostatic experience characterizes the first few months of life. By age two to four months, a higher level of organization emerges[5, 13] and is visible as an evolving capacity for human attachment (e.g., the social smile).

The capacity for attachment is shown in the nature of the homeostatic equilibrium achieved between the infant and primary caretaker(s), and in the quality of feeling and reciprocal interactions they exchange. The reciprocal use of multiple sensory modalities (holding, tactile, sucking, proprioceptive, visual, auditory), the degree of contingency in the interactions (e.g., how much caretaker and infant respond to one another),[15] the organization and complexity of the early communication patterns (e.g., rich, varied, increasingly complex interactions), and the depth and phase appropriateness of feelings experienced and expressed by the dyad (e.g., warm, joyful satisfaction or mechanical, intermittent excitation) are all parameters which may be used to gauge the quality of attachment. The degree to which stress (e.g., infant's hunger, mother's being upset) compromises this quality provides a measure of the integrity of the early attachment patterns.

The most severe attachment disorder is autism. Because of genetic or constitutional difficulties or severe early environmental trauma, the autistic youngster never fully achieves homeostasis. It therefore does not move on to the second task, that of human attachment. Disorders of human attachment also arise when depressed mothers cannot reach out to their infants, when their quality of relationship seems shallow and insecure. Another variety comes about when the infant's individual constitutional differences make physical touch or other kinds of human stimulation painful; such a child may be all too vulnerable to a disorder of attachment. Anaclitic depression, psycho-

physiologic difficulties (vomiting, rumination), failure to thrive (metabolic depression, marasmus), and feeding and sleeping disturbances may all be related to this type of disorder. In general, disorders of human attachment should be characterized along the dimensions described earlier and, where possible, with reference to specific causal factors.

Disorders of Somato-Psychological Differentiation

Once a secure human attachment is achieved through the mutual cuing and reciprocal responses of infant and primary caregiver(s), there occurs a process of emotional differentiation. This is similar to the process of differentiation in sensory-motor development. Through this process, basic schemes of causality are established which underlie the most fundamental aspects of reality testing. While the infant is having internal "emotional" sensations and experiences, however, these do not exist at an organized psychological or mental representational level.

The child's capacity to differentiate between his own actions and the consequences of his actions may be observed in the somatic-psychological sphere. It occurs when the infant begins to distinguish one person from another (this will reach a noticeable level at eight months, at what has been called stranger anxiety),[13] to sort out different somatic-psychological states (e.g., hunger from other need states such as affection or dependency), and to discriminate among moods or communications (anger) from its primary caregiver(s). The infant, now less dependent on internal states (e.g., not just a victim of its own hunger, weariness, or tiredness) is more of a social, interactive being.[5, 14]

Differentiation is facilitated through social interaction, as well as by interaction with the inanimate world. For example, contingent responses help the infant appreciate his role as a causal agent and thereby to distinguish means from ends in interpersonal relationships. Not only obvious patterns of interaction, but subtle emotional and empathetic interactive patterns undergo their own differentiation. However, all these advances need not occur simultaneously. It is possible to have an infant undergo differentiation in the areas of gross motor responses and general interpersonal causality and yet remain undifferentiated at a subtle, empathetic, emotional level. For example, if there is no empathetic, emotional interaction between caregiver and infant (because mother responds in a mechanical and remote manner or projects her own feelings onto her baby)—the infant may not learn to appreciate basic causal relationships between people at a level of feelings as compared to acts (feeling angry can cause another to feel bad).

During this stage one can observe the shift from magical causality (e.g., an infant pulls a string to ring a bell which is no longer there) to consolidation of simple causal links, to the beginning of more complicated means-ends differentiation, e.g., use of substitutes, detours, and intermediary devices. With this, the foundation for flexibility of coping style has been initiated.

Somatic-psychological differentiation should be studied in the context of the many phase-appropriate dimensions of differentiation. Some of these are cognition, human relationships, affects, and the flexibility to deal with stress (without compromising developmentally facilitating behavior). An example of an extreme defect in differentiation is the infant who does not respond to different environmental events with different responses of its own and has not developed age-appropriate contingent behavioral and emotional responses (a basic sense of causality as the foundation of reality testing). This may be due either to his own constitutional make-up, events in his earlier development, or because of a withdrawn or overly intrusive (projecting) primary caretaker. A less severe problem exists when only one aspect of emotional differentiation (because of the character of contingent responses) is compromised, e.g., anger is ignored or leads to withdrawal.

Many symptoms may be related to disorders of somato-psychological differentiation. These include sensory-motor developmental delays, apathy or intense chronic fear (stranger anxiety), clinging, lack of explorativeness and curiosity, flat or nonresponsive emotional reactions to significant caregivers, as well as specific maladaptive patterns of relatedness such as biting, chronic crying, and irritability.

Disorders of Internalization
(Behavioral Organization and Initiative)

Eventually the stage of somato-psychological differentiation reaches an organizational level at which the infant is able to differentiate clearly and subtly the significant others in his interpersonal sphere. As this takes place, there is an increase in the process of "taking in" or internalizing, evidenced by increased imitative behavior. Along with this, certain emotional systems become organized, e.g., affiliation, separation, fear and wariness, curiosity and explorativeness.[1] The study of attachment[2, 10] as a complex "high order" behavioral system illustrates the development of constructs that match the infant's greater organization of behavior at this time.

Initiative and exploration are enhanced by the capacity for combining schemata into new behavioral organizations that are goal directed (e.g., further use of detours, substitutes, delays and intermediary devices). The infant's capacity to take the initiative and to organize behavior and feeling states is enriched by, and in part further facilitates, his capacity to internalize. For example, progressively more imitative behavior appears which, in turn, facilitates organized exploratory behavior from the secure base of the primary caregiver(s). The gradual individuation which occurs is perhaps best described in Mahler's account of the practicing subphase of the separation-individuation process.[9]

The capacity for creating new forms of behavior emerges from the many factors that may now be combined. These include existing schemata, complex behavioral patterns (tertiary circular reactions), trial-and-error explorations, the traces retained by the enhanced memory, and the internal presences that arise from the gradual shifting from imitation to identification. Taken together, these bring about a much greater sense of the toddler as an organized human being who initiates activities (e.g., pulling parent somewhere). There is also evidence for the beginning of a psychological sense of self.[8]

Disorders in behavioral organization and internalization may compromise the beginning of internal "psychological" life. Behavior remains fragmented, related to somatic or external cues. Intentionality and sense of self are "nipped in the bud," so to speak.

A severe disorder at this phase will therefore affect the basic capacity for forming mental representations. One can see the results of such a structural defect when adult patients enter into states of fragmentation (where their internal representations are disorganized).

Specific disorders of this phase are evidenced by a wide range of problems. These can vary from a complete lack of imitation, intentionality, and organized emotional and behavior systems to circumscribed limitations in certain emotional or behavioral systems, e.g., the child cannot assert himself or has difficulties with affiliative behavior. Symptoms may include chronic temper tantrums, inability to initiate even some self-control, lack of motor or emotional co-ordination, extreme chronic negativism, delayed language development, and relationships characterized by chronic aggressive behavior.

Disorders of Organizing Internal Representations

Subsequent to this initial period of internalization and behavioral organization, about eighteen to twenty-four months, the youngster should be able to organize mental representations (object permanance).[4, 9, 11] However, because the youngster can now see himself more accurately in a psychological sense[9] as separate and small, there may be some emotional regression.

Disorders of the organization of internal mental representations have a profound influence on functioning in all basic areas of the ego; this is often seen in the psychopathology of adult psychotic and borderline cases.

The establishment of an internal sense of self and object occurs along with the initial ability to conserve internal representations of animate and inanimate objects. As this proceeds, it produces changes which are visible in the increased behavioral, emotional, cognitive, and interpersonal repertoire of the two-year-old (e.g., the ability to say "No," the development of personal pronouns, ability to recall, ability for organizing mental images and searching for inanimate and animate objects, memory for emotional experience, locating experiences that pertain to the self and nonself, and the beginning of cognitive insight combining internalized schemata, being able to identify the various parts of self, relating in a diminishing need-feeling manner, and the beginnings of cooperation and concern for others).

Disorders of this phase are evidenced by the lack of psychological life (internal representations), and may be observed in symptoms involving severe regressive behavior (disorganized emotional and motor responses), chronic unrelenting clinging with complete disruption of explorative behavior, chronic primitive aggressive behavior (biting, scratching, throwing things), chronic fearfulness, and either interpersonal promiscuity or withdrawal.

Disorders of Psychological Differentiation

Following the capacity to organize internal mental representations (of the object, and the self), there occurs further differentiation, now at the level of mental representation or psychological life. Whereas earlier there was a somato-psychological differentiation (e.g., sensorimotor), there is now a differentiation at the level of mental representation. This involves symbol formation and the corresponding capacity for language development.

Between eighteen and twenty-four months, the ability develops for organizing representations. In the young child these images exist in the context of "magical thinking" or "primary process thinking." At this point there are organized perceptions of feelings, behaviors, and aspects of self and nonself. However, these can be combined or distorted according to need or drive state, thereby distorting reality. Over time there is a differentiation of the self from nonself. Concomitant with this, at a representational or psychological level, there is a differentiation of various feeling states and behavior. The culmination of this process is the establishment of libidinal object constancy.[9] With this, there emerge delineated self and object representations which form the foundation for many basic ego functions. These include reality testing, organization and regulation of impulses, organization and regulation of thought, and integration of thought and affect. Ultimately, there is an ongoing delineation of the sense of self, and it becomes ever more coherent. Eventually it reaches a stage where it is not undermined by brief separations or intense feeling states such as anger.

Disorders of psychological differentiation are seen at two levels. At the more severe level are those syndromes consistent with the borderline to psychotic states of personality organization. There is a capacity for some organized internal psychological life, but it is extremely vulnerable to stress (separation, strong feeling states). Along with this, primary process or magical thinking predominates. There is a fixation at the stage of psychological differentiation.

At a less severe level, basic differentiation does occur, but at a price. This includes major distortions in personality or character formation, i.e., an overall inability of the personality to engage fully in life's major endeavors. Here are the beginnings of the severe personality disorders, such as the very negativistic, withdrawn, schizoid, paranoid, or very depressed or apathetic youngsters.

This becomes visible in a number of ways. Thus, it characterizes the child who is moving toward self-object differentiation and the establishment of basic ego functions, but when the shift from fantasy to reality is not taking place; or when under emotional stress, severe distortions in reality-oriented thinking occur; or when there is a continued lack of organization and regulation of emotions and impulses; or when chronic patterns of disorganized aggressive or regressive behavior are present. Distortions in character formation can be discerned when the negativism only gets worse; the withdrawal from human relationships increases; the ability to care for bodily functions does not become established; the tendency to blame others becomes more intense; and the fears of loss of self, security, love, and bodily injury are so severe, that progressive development is experienced as dangerous (e.g., intimacy, assertion, curiosity, and self-control are relinquished).

Disorders in the Consolidation Level of Integration and Flexibility of Basic Personality Functions

Disorders in the consolidation and further differentiation of basic ego functions are seen in vulnerability to regression, states of anxiety and depression, and moderate to mild characterologic constrictions, e.g., moderate obsessive-compulsive patterns, hysterical patterns, patterns of impulsive behavior, or patterns of externalization.

If development has progressed optimally through the phase of object constancy and the differentiation of the self from nonself, the youngster then moves on to more complex human relationships, triangular patterns, and the oedipal phase of psychosocial development. Difficulties in this and later phases can result in regressions along limited lines, e.g., in the libidinal or aggressive realms, and may take form as certain encapsulated disorders commonly thought to fall within

the neurotic range (although more major regressions can occur).

Later experience during latency, adolescence, and adulthood builds on the existing structure and ultimately determines the overall level of organization of the personality.

The capacity to shift from simply organizing differentiated internal self- and object representations to forming new and original derivative representational systems at various developmental levels serves as the foundation for the developmental level of defenses and the ultimate flexibility of the personality.[7]

Clinical Illustrations and Conclusion

The framework presented here describes a series of developmental stages and implied tasks that can organize understanding of what may at times appear to be groups of unrelated symptoms. The developmental disorder is the final common pathway for a variety of etiological factors and their related symptoms. For example, consider the following illustrative, abbreviated clinical excerpts from cases the authors have worked with:

Case 1: Jane was constitutionally mildly apathetic. In her own exceedingly calm, slow manner however, she was able to engage the world and regulate herself. When her mother would become tense, Jane would withdraw and sleep for long periods of time. Mother became increasingly phobic and "felt unloved" because "Jane never gets joyful with me." An attachment formed that was shallow and mechanical. There were no contingent responses, visual or vocal interactions; only some minimal tactile contact. Jane's weight gain, growth, and development came to a halt. Medical work-up was negative. "Failure to thrive" was diagnosed from a symptom-complex perspective, and a "disorder of attachment" was diagnosed from a developmental perspective.

Treatment which focused on mother's underlying depression and feeling of "being rejected," together with helping her understand her baby's special constitutional characteristics, led to a relatively rich reciprocal attachment. Weight gain, growth, and development resumed.

Case 2: David was constitutionally sound, mildly hyperalert, and developing well. There was a rich, deep attachment between him and his loving but somewhat engulfing mother. About eleven months of age he began to show signs of sensorimotor retardation (e.g., no crawling, sitting, or pulling himself up). A neurological work-up was negative. A psychiatric work-up, however, revealed an over-protective, "symbiotic" mother who projected her own feelings and fears onto her son. Although "attached," she did not respond differentially or contingently to any of David's communications and emerging development. Out of fear of injury, she even kept him from playing with toys and other inanimate objects. David was therefore not being responded to (and was not receiving differentiated or contingent feedback) from the animate or inanimate aspects of his environment. David's communications were gradually becoming less varied as he would vacillate between states of global frustration (crying, etc.) and mild apathy. While the symptom-complex diagnosis was "delayed or retarded maturation," the developmental diagnosis was disorder of somato-psychologic differentiation. Behavioral, emotional, and basic motoric differentiation was not occurring.

A treatment program which helped mother to understand and deal more adaptively with her aggressive and dependent strivings (e.g., not to project them onto the baby and his development) and to "read" and respond to David's different communications reversed the symptoms and promoted differentiation. Six months later David was above age level according to psychological testing (Bayley) and clinical observation.

Case 3: Allen was a premature baby with attentive and loving parents. Initially, however, he would not sleep unless rocked for hours and would not establish regular sleeping patterns. He was mildly hyperalert, hyperexcitable, and a fussy eater. While Allen evidenced a mild disorder of "homeostasis," his parents' ability to "adjust" to

him (they changed their schedule to meet his) helped Allen to a healthy adjustment, so that by six months he was in a regular sleep pattern and was developing normally.

Case 4: Kate began spitting up most of her food shortly after her twelfth month. Organic causes were ruled out and it was observed that she used her mouth as a primary mode of exploring the world (e.g., put most new objects in her mouth). Mother had at this time begun working full time and because of her separation from Kate had become somewhat depressed without acknowledging it. She was emotionally unavailable to Kate, even in the evenings after work.

Kate's lack of imitative behavior, organized emotional and communicative patterns, and an overinvestment in the inanimate world led to a diagnosis of "disorder of internalization, behavioral organization and initiative." A relatively simple recommendation for mother to work part time alleviated some of mother's depression and permitted her to spend additional time with Kate. By fourteen months, Kate was eating normally and evidencing stage-appropriate behavioral and emotional patterns.

According to the three-columned approach described in the introduction, the four cases may be viewed schematically in Table 8–1.

While the cases presented and schematized are somewhat oversimplified versions of complex clinical situations, they are intended to illustrate the usefulness and overall goals of a developmental approach to diagnosis in infancy and early childhood. The framework presented in this chapter attempts to facilitate the understanding of diverse symptomatology and forms the basis for developmentally specific, dynamically-oriented treatment plans.

TABLE 8–1

ETIOLOGICAL FACTORS	DEVELOPMENTAL DIAGNOSIS	SYMPTOM DIAGNOSIS
Case 1 Maternal depression and withdrawal	Disorder of attachment	Failure to thrive
Case 2 Maternal overprotection, exaggerated symbiosis	Disorder of somato-psychological differentiation	Sensorimotor delay or retardation
Case 3 Immaturity of CNS integrative capacities	Disorder of homeostasis (mild)	Sleep disturbance
Case 4 Maternal separation and unavailability	Disorder of internalization, behavioral organization, and initiative	Eating disturbance Rumination

REFERENCES

1. AINSWORTH, M., "The Development of Infant-Mother Attachment," in Caldwell, B., and Ricciuti, H. (Eds.), *Review of Child Development Research*, vol. 3, University of Chicago Press, Chicago, 1973.

2. AINSWORTH, M., BELL, S. M., and STAYTON, D., "Infant-Mother Attachment and Social Development: Socialization as a Product of Reciprocal Responsiveness to Signals," in Richards, M. (Ed.), *The Integration of the Child into a Social World*, Cambridge University Press, Cambridge, 1974.

3. BRAZELTON, T. B., *Neonatal Behavior Assessment Scale*, Lippincott, Philadelphia, 1973.

4. DECARIE, T. C., *Intelligence and Affectivity in Early Childhood: An Experimental Study of Jean Piaget's Object Concept and Object Relations*, International Universities Press, New York, 1965.

5. EMDE, R., GAENSBAUER, T., and HARMON, R., *Emotional Expression in Infancy: A Biobehavioral Study*, Psychological Issues Monograph Series, 1976.

6. FRAIBERG, S., *Insights from the Blind; Comparative Studies of Blind and Sighted Infants*, Basic Books, New York, 1977.

7. GREENSPAN, S. I., "Intelligence and Adaptation: An Integration of Psychoanalytic and Piagetian Developmental Psychology," *Psychological Issues*, International Universities Press, New York, December, 1978 (in press).

8. LEWIS, M., and ROSENBLUM, L. (Eds.), *The Effect of the Infant on Its Caregiver*, John Wiley, New York, 1974.

9. MAHLER, M. S., PINE, F., and BERGMAN, A., *The Psychological Birth of the Human Infant, Symbiosis and Individuation*, Basic Books, New York, 1975.

10. MAIN, M., *Exploration, Play, and Cognitive Functioning as Related to Child-Mother Attachment*, Unpublished doctoral dissertation, Johns Hopkins University, Baltimore, Md., 1973.

11. PIAGET, J., *The Origins of Intelligence in Children*, International Universities Press, New York, 1952.

12. SANDER, L., "Issues in Early Mother-Child Interaction," *Journal of the American Academy of Child Psychiatry, 1*:141–166, 1962.

13. SPITZ, R., *The First Year of Life. A Psychoanalytic Study of Normal and Deviant Development of Object Relations*, International Universities Press, New York, 1965.

14. SROUFE, L. A., and WATERS, E., "The Ontogenesis of Smiling and Laughter: A Perspective on the Organization of Development in Infancy," *Psychological Review, 83*:173–189 (a), 1976.

15. STERN, D., "Mother and Infant at Play: The Dyadic Interaction Involving Facial Vocal and Gaze Behaviors," in Lewis, M., and Rosenblum, L. (Eds.), *The Effects of the Infant on Its Caregiver*, John Wiley, New York, 1974.

PART C

Syndromes

9 / Normality as a Syndrome

Humberto Nagera and Ronald M. Benson

Normalcy in children may be the least often used diagnosis of clinicians. The Diagnostic and Statistical Manual of Mental Disorders of the American Psychiatric Association[1] has no special code for normalcy. In the Group for Advancement of Psychiatry's proposed classification of childhood psychiatric diagnoses,[4] the first category is "Healthy Responses," with subcategories of developmental crises and situational crises, depending upon the predominant source of stress from within or from the environment.

Their description of this syndrome in their monograph concedes that the assessment of healthy responses are subjective and impressionistic, but that a positive, as opposed to exclusionary diagnosis, can be made in terms of partial functions in the relationship to total functioning allowing for developmental levels.

GAP's criteria include intellectual, social, emotional and personal, and adaptive functioning. Also included are stage appropriateness and allowance for developmental and situational stress.

As Offer and Sabshin[9] have demonstrated, the evaluator's philosophic point of view may play an important role in his diagnosis of normality. These authors have synthesized four concepts or assumptions about normality prevalent among mental health workers. Implicitly a given professional may subscribe to one or another of these philosophical assumptions at the expense of the others, and his critical judgment of what is normal, as opposed to deviant or pathological, could be as much determined by his unrecognized decision as by the observational data.

The first of Offer and Sabshin's four concepts is "normality as health." This view holds that if there are no gross "symptoms" in the clinical picture, the patient is normal. This view conceives of most people as normal and is the viewpoint associated with traditional descriptive psychiatry.

"Normality as utopia" is a second category described by the aforementioned authors. Subscribers to this concept think of normality as an ideal, or at least relatively ideal state of mental functioning, and variations from this state are considered disturbances. This viewpoint is often associated with the writings of psychoanalysts.

The third approach is "normality as average." This mode of thought is based on the statistical distribution within a population. Extremes in either direction from the center of the normal curve are considered deviant.

The final concept is "normality as process." Here normality is considered a typical, describable, and predictable progression over time. This viewpoint is, in fact, at a different level of abstraction than the first three and could be subsumed under any of them.

In a sense these four viewpoints are, like the metapsychologic viewpoints in psychoanalytic theory (i.e., dynamic, economic, structural, genetic, and adaptive), all necessary to make a complete statement about the normalcy of any given child or segment of behavior of any child at a stated moment in time.

Indeed, all clinical and pragmatic judgments about whether or not what is observed is or is not normal involves a complex gridwork of overlapping considerations. Every level of organization, from a molecular and biologic to psychologic, familial, social and political, and even evolutional (i.e., the grand scheme of things) contains within it certain thoughts and assumptions about normality.

The recent attention to homosexuality and its classification as normal variant, pathologic symptom, syndrome, or free choice, which led to a referendum within the American Psychiatric Association, highlights the complications involved in judgments of normalcy. Gay activists view the problem in one light, traditional descriptive psychiatrists and some psychoanalysts in another, sociologists in another, historians in another, and perhaps cultural anthropologists in yet another still. To attempt a comprehensive, cohesive, and synthetic approach to this question of the normalcy or nonnormalcy of homosexuality provides an intriguing and challenging exercise which will reward those who attempt it by revealing the complexity of conflicting considerations.

It is, in fact, at this stage in the development of child psychiatry as a discipline, not possible to describe a "syndrome of normalcy." Not only are there competing and conflicting concepts of normality, but there is, as yet, an insufficient literature of studies about normal children and adolescents from developmental, biologic, social, cultural and familial, psychologic, and outcome perspectives. For example, developmental studies about some variables are quite complete, such as the development of EEG patterns from birth through adolescence. Brain development studies from a biochemical viewpoint, however, are, for obvious technical reasons, much less complete. Studies of object relations are quite good in early childhood and adolescence but sparse in latency. Family studies of some social groups are relatively plentiful while other groups remain absent from the literature. Integrative studies over time are rare and limited in scope, although some efforts have been made (e.g.,[4, 9, 6] Gesell, Offer, Kagan). Overall, however, no comprehensive longitudinal or cross-sectional studies of normality in children are available to provide the clinician with a fixed point upon which to hang his diagnosis.

Since there does not exist a simple and encompassing definition of normalcy in children, all that can be undertaken is an examination of the variables which influence normality and the methods the child clinician can use to approach such a diagnosis.

The situation with children is much more complex than with adults, but even with adults no clear-cut concept of the "normal person" has yet been described. Freud[3] considers the line between normality and pathology to be very indistinct; he asserted that any given individual might well traverse it back and forth several times during a lifetime, or even in the course of one day. This view is consistent with current epidemiologic concepts.

A commonly accepted and clinically useful criteria for normality in adults is the ability to work well, a good sexual adjustment including good interpersonal relationships, and the capacity to enjoy leisure. These pragmatic and useful criteria, which may be justifiably valuable to general psychiatrists and adult analysts, are essentially not useful to the clinician asked to evaluate the emotional and psychological health of a group ranging in age from birth to the onset of adulthood.

Descriptive statements are particularly misleading and useless when considering normalcy in a child. With an adult, the clinician deals with a more or less finished product. The adult at a given point in time, at least viewed as a "black box," can either deal with an average range of environmental, interpersonal, and intrapsychic demands by adequate adaptation or he cannot. It is, then, the precise definition of "adequate adaptation" which provides the principal obstacle to a simple definition of normalcy.

A clinician can, for example, reasonably assume that both the structure of the brain and mind are relatively constant and that the adult's functioning, while limited by the state of the organism at a given moment and while pervasively limited by pathology, is still a relatively fixed quantity. That is to say, an observation today and next week of the same person might be different, but the difference would not reflect fundamental changes in the organism, assuming no progressive pathological process or active therapeutic intervention. The differences, then, represent either a change in the environmental circumstances acting upon and within the adult or a change in state within the person because of biological or psychological factors of a relatively evanescent nature, such as fatigue, anxiety, or toxicity.

With children, the situation is totally different. They are in a constant process of very active development. This implies rapid changes taking place

166

simultaneously in all areas of personality along numerous lines of development. The different areas of the personality need to interact with one another constantly in the process of living and growing up. There are balances and imbalances in all these lines of development. At each different age and stage of development this creates a constantly changing disequilibrium in terms of the nature, quantity and quality of the conflicts, stresses, etc. As a result, the emerging phenomena are extremely complex. What is descriptively normal during the first year of life may be considered quite inappropriate during the second. Thus, the clinical picture for any given age is much more variable and dynamic than is the case with adults. Evidently the developmental point of view is an essential consideration when trying to assess the child.

These considerations apply generally throughout the child's development. In addition, there is the complicating presence of a child's capacity to imagine, to fantasize, and to use defenses that distort the reality of any given situation. These are coupled with the child's ego immaturity, limited capacity for abstract thinking (in the earlier years), and limited fund of information. Together these factors set the stage for the multiple individual variations of what is descriptively normal at any given age as well as for possible psychopathological developments. Furthermore, they highlight the innumerable weaknesses and dangers involved in the developmental processes and the more than ample opportunities for both "normal" and "abnormal" variations.

Biologic Factors

An organic maturation of the brain reaches completion somewhere before two years of age. Up to that point, there exists a special relationship between the *genetic potential* of any given brain and the amount of stimulation that it receives. Early in life such stimulation comes largely from mother's ministrations. This input is essential if the brain is to unfold ideally and reach its optimal genetic potential.

Formerly it was believed that only internal genetically determined embryological maturational forces defined the degree of quality and maturation the brain would attain. Increasing evidence from animal experimentation and "fate experiments" in human infants tend to show in quite a

compelling manner that such an assumption is incorrect. These maturational forces alone cannot bring a brain to achieve whatever its ideal potential might be. To reach that "ideal" potential, external stimulation of the immature brain is required. These patterns of stimulation—usually provided by the mother—seem to influence brain development and its quality by at least three different mechanisms.[7] Thus:

1. Appropriate forms of external stimulation at the right time seem to increase the degree of vascularization in various areas in the brain. Generally speaking, for any organ, better vascularization means better functional abilities.
2. Appropriate forms of external stimulation at the right time seem to increase the amount of dendritization that takes place. This means more potentially available functional pathways and, as such, possibly a "better," more capable brain.
3. Appropriate forms of external stimulation at the right time seem to increase the rate at which myelinization takes place. The relationship between myelinization and function seems reasonably well established, though, here too, there are many unanswered questions.

Conceivably the effect of all the above processes is cumulative and may contribute to what determines the "quality" of the brain for any given human being. These basic organic structures sustain psychological function. They are the biological determinants of later human behavior. It follows that the assessment of the developmental normalcy of a young infant must include considerations of this type.

The assessment of the developmental normalcy of a very young infant is not an easy matter. For example, by six or eight months, a child may descriptively show unmistakable signs of developmental retardation. We cannot simply conclude that the child's brain is abnormal per se, especially in the common situation when there is an absence of clear neurological signs. We have to discriminate between functional retardation due to a lack of stimulation and a host of other possibilities. The latter will range from malnutrition (either during the pregnancy or early life), to diseases in the mother during the pregnancy that might affect brain development, birth traumas or damage, genetic defects or abnormalities, etc. The diagnostic and prognostic significance of such differential diagnoses is self-evident. In those cases that fall within the so-called critical perods, the brain may be potentially normal. The situation may then still be reversible by the provision of nutrients either in the physical or psychological sense. Where the damage to the organic structure is already established or the damage to the functional capabilities of the brain has become irreversible, a totally different assessment of current and future normalcy will ensue.

Micro-social Factors

Although neither adults nor children are islands unto themselves, this is particularly true of children. Every child, especially every infant, is an integral part of a complex system. At the outset, the system consists essentially of baby and mother. Mother, in turn, is dependent on other support systems such as her husband, her family, her own mother, etc. As development progresses, such systems modify and enlarge themselves. A more influential role is extended on the child's normal (or abnormal) developmental progression by such people as the father, siblings, grandparents, etc. In short, the child develops within a special social system, the family unit. As growth continues, such systems and the elements that constitute them continue to change and presently, in latency, they include teachers and the community of peers. The latter acquire enormous importance by the time the child reaches adolescence.

Inevitably all the elements in such systems serve in some measure to determine the shape of the child's developmental progression (or the lack of it and its multiple variations). Once "behavior" or "pathology" is determined to be outside the normal range for a child of a given age, it is essential to ascertain what is at fault with the youngster's particular system.

Let us consider a case of developmental retardation in a nine- or ten-month-old baby. He was late smiling and holding his head up. His hand-eye coordination was poor, he could not sit appropriately, etc. Such a clinical picture could be explained in various ways including the possibility of some organicity. On the other hand, it might be determined that this is an unwanted child, left very much to himself; his interaction with mother reduced to the most basic functions to sustain life; and in short, neglected, understimulated and sensory deprived. This would also explain the nature of his developmental retardation.

This situation bears on other aspects of the nature of normality. In terms of several viewpoints of normality this child is "abnormal," not in a "healthy state" (i.e., not progressing in a timely way, not statistically normal, far from ideal), since he is developmentally retarded. At the same time there is nothing intrinsic to the child that determined such developmental retardation. The child was "potentially" capable of developing normally; might still be able to do so. He was normal and in a way is normal now; developmental retardation is a "normal," i.e., expectable and predictable, though not healthy response to the conditions of understimulation and sensory deprivation to which he was subjected. If this child were provided with the necessary stimulation, the situation would reverse itself and the child "catch up" developmentally (as Spitz and others demonstrated long ago and Selma Fraiberg most recently). (I am ignoring, for the moment, the possibility that there may be critical periods beyond which some permanent damage to certain aspects of the personality may accrue, even if the child seems to catch up milestone-wise.)

Manifest Variability

Conceptually and empirically, "normality" implies a very wide frame of reference statistically within which much variation can take place. All these variations are perfectly compatible with "normality." Thus, some children will start walking as early as eight or nine months of age while others may not do so until they are close to the second year of life. The same is of course true of speech. Some children are capable of sentence formation and fluency in the first half of the second year of life; others do not achieve that degree of proficiency until they are three or older. In addition, there seem to be significant but "normal" statistical differences between girls and boys in this area. Nor is it uncommon for children to move into the phallic-oedipal stage as early as two and a half years of age. Such youngsters show clear concerns, interests, and anxieties in terms of triangular relationships although other similarly normal children who are less precocious may not do so until three and a half or four years of age.

Dynamic Factors

To complicate matters further, it is typical for normal children to go through what has been described elsewhere[7] as developmental conflicts.

These conflicts are both numerous as well as characteristic for every age and stage of development.

Like any other conflicts of children and adolescents, developmental conflicts create stresses, anxiety, and guilt. Typically, they lead to symptom formation and behaviors of various kinds that in and of themselves, or when observed in any other context, would be considered "abnormal." Hence, a paradoxical situation emerges where it is "normal" for "normal children" to produce symptoms and behaviors to go through developmental conflicts that the inexperienced clinician or the lay person could consider as clear indications of pathology. It is somewhat surprising that every child psychiatrist and pediatrician will occasionally label such symptoms or behaviors as abnormal or psychopathological in essentially normal children.

The best example of this, but not the only one by any means, is what psychoanalysts have referred to as the infantile neuroses. Somewhere between two and a half and five, children of both sexes start to show abnormal manifestations of different degrees of intensity. These behaviors and symptoms are the expression of the typical (and quite normal) developmental conflict for that age group. Thus, these children may start displaying various forms of sleep disturbance. These characteristically take the form of nightmares or night terrors. They wake up in a panic and attempt to sleep in the parental bed, or have one or another of the parents come to their room or sleep in their beds, etc. Fears of a large variety are common, most typically fears of the dark, monsters, "ghosts," and burglars. This is frequently accompanied by anxious requests that they be allowed to sleep with their lights on, or to sleep in the parental bedroom, or to have their bedroom doors open, etc. Related requests are posed for yet another story to be read at bedtime, or another glass of water, or another kiss, or still another trip to the bathroom. A different variation is the fear of somebody hiding in the room with evil intentions of coming through the window to attack the child and harm or kidnap him, etc. Many other phobic symptoms afflict the minds of these children, such as fears of animals, especially those that can bite such as dogs, cats, lions, tigers, etc. Much (castration) anxiety is observed, usually expressed as concerns about hurts, injuries, accidents and possible damage to their bodies. Often there are marked reactions on seeing a crippled person, a blind person, etc. Associated behaviors include an increase in masturbatory activities, brief or more extended recurrences of bedwetting, etc. Many bedtime ceremonials and rituals, as well as other forms of obsessive-compulsive behavior, are not infrequent.

Depending on the intensity of all this the child is handicapped to some degree while the developmental conflict endures. Similarly, parental concern and reactions to the child will vary with the severity, pervasiveness, and intensity of the symptoms. Often enough there is a disturbing effect on the marital couple's activities.

Thus, for children of such an age and at such a stage of development, a very visible disturbance is considered the "normal condition" provided that it is kept within reasonable limits. Again, the paradoxical situation of a child showing plenty of "symptoms" and "abnormal behaviors" that by their very existence actually stamp him or her as a perfectly normal little boy or little girl!

One most significant difference between the manifestations of a developmental conflict such as this and those related to other forms of pathological conflict is that the one is transitory and the other permanent. In other words, in the case of the developmental conflicts the developmental imbalances that led to the stresses, tensions and conflicts responsible for the symptoms are corrected spontaneously as development progresses. However, this is not a likely outcome in any other conflictual situation with the exception of the type of phenomenon to be described next.

Children's development is constantly being interfered with in a variety of ways. Developmental interference[7] has been defined as that action arising in the child's environment which disturbs the typical unfolding of development. Usually this refers to a gross external or environmental interference with the needs and/or rights of the child. It applies as well to situations in which excessive or unjustified demands are made of the child. The reverse occurs as well when the necessary demands (according to age and stage of development) are not made of the child. This is especially true with those parents or, more especially, with those mothers who tend to prolong the babyhood of their children. The parents who make, or fail to make, the type of demands we are discussing here tend generally not to take into account the fact that the child may well lack the necessary ego development at that point to comply with such demands or to cope.

Such inappropriate interventions can create stress situations that the child cannot handle. This may result in symptom formation and/or behavior on the surface that is only similar to what occurs in the case of neurotic conflicts. Yet there are significant differences between them.

In any case, the type of disturbance created by a developmental interference can sometimes affect development in a positive manner. For example, it might speed it up. Of course, in any given case, that type of outcome may or may not be desirable. In general, however, such developmental interferences usually affect development in undesirable ways.

The degree of impact on the child is dependent on various factors. Among these are age, the stage of development, the nature of the interference, and the amount of time it has been in operation. Naturally, the interferences can occur at any point in the child's development. Let us consider a few examples. A severe prolonged postpartum maternal depression may interfere with the mother's ability to care for and stimulate her child appropriately. Such a situation will have a number of repercussions. Another example is recurrent exposure to hunger, either through primary neglect or because of the rigid feeding time tables that were so popular with pediatricians not long ago. Other examples include painful illnesses, prolonged hospitalizations that can act as an interference because of the separation itself or because of the trauma of painful medical manipulations. In particular, surgical interventions such as a simple tonsillectomy or appendectomy (performed between the ages of two and a half to five) may trigger traumatic floods of castration anxiety and act as the nucleus for the pathological growth of an infantile neurosis. Interferences can take the form of rigid toilet training with much conflict between parents and child, or training that is either started too early or unnecessarily postponed. Death of parents, siblings, or other important members of the family can affect the child's development in a variety of ways. A sexually provocative or seductive mother can have such an impact during the phallic-oedipal phase or even during adolescence. In fact, there is an inexhaustible list of possible developmental interferences, all of which will influence how the child appears in terms of "normality" or "abnormality." There are some interferences that are accidents of fate, and others that are actively introduced in the life of the young by the world about them.

To further complicate the assessment of what is "normal," the same type of interference may well produce a wide variety of results and reactions in different children. Clearly, there are some distinct general tendencies related to the nature of the interference and the stage of development. Yet, each case needs an individual evaluation since different genetic endowments, different backgrounds, different previous experiences, different internal circumstances (i.e., a better capacity to handle anxiety, more sublimatory potential and capacity, etc.) will either tend to determine where the damage, if any, will be done, or to reinforce or soften the effects of any particular interference.

The effects of such interferences are various and multiple. Children do react to the stresses created by developmental interferences with "abnormal" manifestations. These frequently resemble the symptoms observed in the cases of neurotic conflicts or neurosis proper (as was also true for the developmental conflicts). Thus, for example, much anxiety can be present on the surface, or multiple forms of regression can be observed affecting either the child's instinctual development (i.e., regression to bedwetting) or his ego. In the latter case the result may be the giving up of certain ego achievements such as speech, regression to baby talk, etc. Further, many other "abnormal" behavioral manifestations or symptoms may be present.

But in spite of this superficial identity there are important differences as well. Many of the "symptoms" resulting from interferences, especially early on in life, are not the compromise formations with symbolic unconscious meanings and contents that are found in the neuroses. They are instead reactions to the stress and anxiety produced by the interference. As such, they lack the advantages that a conflict solution achieves even if it takes the form of symptom formation. In other words, many such symptoms are not responsive to interpretations of content and are not helped by "treatment" in the form of the various psychotherapies. On the other hand, interventions aimed at the removal of the interference like advising a parent to stop pressing for premature toilet training will restore the dynamic equilibrium within the child and improve the mother-child relationship. As soon as that happens, the symptoms tend to disappear. This is a most important distinction from the symptoms of neurotic disorders where no amount of manipulation of the environment, or easing the pressures on the child will remove the symptom.

Thus a child may present clinically as highly "symptomatic and abnormal" but a closer look will demonstrate an essentially normal child, or whom unmanageable stresses have been forced from the outside. The child cannot regulate this excessive tension and reacts by producing symptoms. Such symptoms are not the expression of inherent "abnormality" *but of the abnormal expec-*

tations and demands that the child's environment is placing on him.

Many factors contribute to increase the difficulties of this type of assessment. If the interference has been present long enough or has been severe enough, it may further affect personality development well beyond the production of transient symptoms and abnormal behavior. This may mean that removal of the interference may resolve those symptoms or behaviors that are due to that stress. Nonetheless, these may be a more permanent impact on certain aspects of development. Indeed, the final form of the child's personality structure may well be decisively shaped by the long acting interference. Certain forms of interference may affect specific ego functions. If these events occur early in life, those affected functions and the ego itself may take after their form. Such changes may or may not be compatible with eventual "normality." In any case, such interferences may in fact be among the significant factors which shape development. They could account for many individual variations in functioning and for the even wider range of variations of normality. They may also contribute to the outcome of subsequent developmental conflicts, neurotic conflicts, the infantile neuroses, etc. They may play a role as well in the establishment of fixation points at different levels. These in turn create weaknesses in the personality that become visible only at later stages. They appear when the child is confronted by some of the later typical developmental conflicts that impose a heavy burden on personality resources.

Macro-social Factors

In considering the criteria of normalcy, an added complication emerges. This concerns some special situations that are bound to influence how the child develops. They are in a way a caricature or a paradigm of something that to some degree is true of all cases. Consider, for example, the special conditions surrounding a child raised in the ghetto.

It is inevitable that for any society, "normal" behavioral and ethical standards are substantially determined by the values of the dominant social or cultural group. Since there are many subgroups and subcultures with more or less organizations that persist within the larger dominant group, it follows that conflicts between subcultural and dominant cultural values are quite common, particularly for certain groups of children.

This is a pattern of so-called asocial, unethical, amoral, promiscuous, and delinquent behavior present in some ghetto children. This definition is applied by those who assess behavior with the standards of middle-class America. Yet, within the ghetto subculture that same behavior may have to be considered "normal" since it has adaptive and survival value, both in the psychological and physical senses of the word. Thus, the question of normal or abnormal has to be followed frequently by the question for which cultures, groups, subcultures and according to whose criteria.

Children raised in the ghetto may well have internalized the ethical values and standards or behavior offered to them by parents, relatives, other peers in the community or, in short, by the subculture. According to the middle-class standards, behavior that is perfectly "normal" in the subculture is totally unacceptable and is considered "abnormal" by this larger group.

Cases of this type point to some of the added difficulties in considering normalcy. The problem here is that normality can be defined simultaneously from various points of view and with different conceptual tools. Thus, a given child may be regarded as psychologically "normal," but from the sociological point of view is considered "abnormal." In other words, what is normal psychologically may be considered abnormal in the sociological sense. It is unfortunate that psychiatrists are frequently expected to treat or to correct ills at the root of which we find negative sociological, economic, and/or political factors. Naturally, such influences affect the final form of the human beings subjected to their impact. This bears directly on any given child's final "psychological make-up." Under the circumstances, this personality structure is not only expectable but "normal." Yet, from the sociological point of view the behavior may be highly undesirable or downright inappropriate.

The Handicapped or Gifted Child:

A Special Case

The same thinking applies to the variety of possible physical handicaps that children can suffer. The development of a child born blind can differ significantly from that of a normally sighted infant. The difference will be even more marked if no special efforts are made to provide stimulation to compensate for the lack of sight or to deal with the ensuing distortions in the parent-child relationship, such as parental guilt and the associated reactions.

Thus, when sight is lacking, development will deviate in ways that are typical and "normal" for children blind from birth, but are "not normal" for the sighted ones. For example, there are the so-called blindisms in children lacking sight from birth. Similar behaviors would have rather ominous diagnostic connotations if observed in the sighted child.

As we can see, the determination of what is "normal or abnormal" for any given age is an extraordinary complex exercise for which there are no reliable short cuts. The very experienced child psychiatric clinician may find it somewhat easier to make such determinations since he will have automatized the identification of gestalts that are basic to differential diagnosis. Such gestalts are not established magically. They are always the distillate of a laborious, and at the beginning, very slow process of systematic examination of the child itself and the child as a function of the previously described multiple variables.

On occasion a very gifted and experienced clinician may conclude that a child is or is not normal after a very "limited" examination. In such instances he is employing many unconscious engrams and gestalts that allow him to come to a rapid definition of the problem in a very impressive and accurate way. Asked to explain how he formed his opinion, he would find himself hard put to do so. But if he were to spell it out, he would presently be traversing the many difficult paths of differential diagnosis in the several areas outlined here.

Finally, it is appropriate to underline the value of Anna Freud's contributions in this regard.[2] She rightly questions the reliability of symptoms and behaviors as adequate indicators of normalcy and/or pathology in the case of children and adolescents. She approaches this issue from the developmental point of view and concludes that an assessment of "normalcy" in children should be closely correlated with the child's capacity to continue his development progression unimpeded. If his developmental path is clear of "unusual" obstacles that may distort it, hinder it, interfere with it, or halt it, the child's potential normalcy is there. Development itself frequently takes care of much "pathology." Thus, in a sensitive manner, she balances the excessive weight given by some to the actual presence of symptoms and abnormal behaviors at any given time during the child's development.

REFERENCES

1. American Psychiatric Association, Committee on Nomenclature and Statistics, *Diagnostic and Statistical Manual*, 2nd ed., American Psychiatric Association, Washington, D.C., 1968.

2. FREUD, A., "Indications for Child Analysis," in Eissler, R. S., et al. (Eds.), *The Psychoanalytic Study of the Child*, vol. 1, pp. 127–149, International Universities Press, New York, 1945.

3. FREUD, S., "Analysis of a Phobia in a Five-Year-Old Boy," in *The Standard Edition of the Complete Psychological Works of Sigmund Freud*, vol. 10, pp. 3–149, Hogarth Press, London, 1955.

4. Group for the Advancement of Psychiatry (GAP), Committee on Child Psychiatry, *Psychopathological Disorders in Childhood: Theoretical Considerations and a Proposed Classification*, vol. 4, Report No. 12, Jason Aronson, New York, 1974.

5. KAGAN, J., and MOSS, M. A., *Birth to Maturity: A Study in Psychological Development*, John Wiley, New York, 1962.

6. KNOBLOCH, H., and PASAMANICK, B., *Gesell and Amatruda's Developmental Diagnosis*, 3rd ed., Harper & Row, New York, 1974.

7. NAGERA, H., *Early Childhood Disturbances, the Infantile Neuroses, and the Adult Disturbances*, The Psychoanalytic Study of the Child, Monograph Series, vol. 2, pp. 28–47, International Universities Press, New York, 1966.

8. OFFER, D., *The Psychological World of the Teenager*, Basic Books, New York, 1973.

9. ———, and SABSHIN, M., *Normality*, Basic Books, New York, 1966.

10 / **Reactive Disorders**

Edwin S. Kessler

Name of the Syndrome and History of Its Identification

As behavioral manifestations came to be understood in a developmental framework, the attempt to define the boundaries between normal and pathological responses was increasingly reflected in schemes of classification. The American Psychiatric Association's Diagnostic and Statistical Manual of Mental Disorders (DSM-II) describes transient situational disturbances as one of the ten major categories. Specifically 307.0–307.2 are called adjustment reaction of infancy, childhood, and adolescence. Possibly influenced by the earlier GAP report,[10] Psychopathological Disorders in Childhood, DSM-II states that these conditions "occur in individuals without any apparent underlying mental disorder and represent an acute reaction to overwhelming environmental stress."

A prognostic quality is implied in the assumption that "if the patient has good adaptive capacity his symptoms will recede as the stress diminishes. If, however, the symptoms persist after the stress is removed, the diagnosis of another mental disorder is indicated."

The GAP report was the first to give official name to reactive disorders, to place them between healthy responses and developmental deviations, and to define the category accordingly. The term reactive disorders was chosen to avoid the problems posed by having to assess fixity and transience of symptoms. Langford[12] stated that "the committee considered the whole grouping of transient situational reactions, . . . abandoned this and returned to reactive disorders. There seems to be no doubt that in many children these may go on from conflicts with the external environment, which have not as yet been internalized, to develop into internal conflicts, or personality disorders, or they may clear up very rapidly." Wisely, no prognostic assumption of recovery was made and progress to a more stable and complex disorder did not necessitate a revision of the diagnosis. If the outcome were unfavorable this could be related to the underlying vulnerability of the child and to the history of interaction of the child with the environment. Thus a number of reactive disorders might have been classified in the earlier literature under the headings of behavior disorders, conduct disturbances, neurotic traits, habit disturbances, and even anaclitic depression.

By avoiding any emphasis on classification by symptom description, the GAP report reserves this category for those disorders in which the behavior or symptoms shown by the child are judged to be primarily a reaction to an event or a situation in the external environment. To distinguish these disturbances from situational crises occurring in the course of healthy development, the disturbances must be considered to be of pathological degree. The child's reaction is predominantly a conscious attempt to cope with the stress and not a result of internalized conflict.

Description of the Syndrome

The GAP report is outstanding in clarity and succinctness. The following delineation of the syndrome is a liberal mix of summary and direct quotations from its contents. A great variety of events or situations may precipitate or perpetuate a reactive disorder. Some of the more common factors are excessive or inadequate stimulation; illness, accident or hospitalizaton; prolonged absence or loss of a parent; hostile or misguided attitudes of caretakers, especially parents; school pressures, etc. The acuteness or chronicity of the situation will influence the nature of its impact on the child. A situation arising suddenly may be highly traumatic, while a more gradual evolution may allow sufficient time to adapt to the stress and master it. A difficult situation may be tolerated for a short period of time, but if it is prolonged, eventually it can lead to disorder.

In making the diagnosis of reactive disorder, the dynamic state of the child and the nature of his reaction should be emphasied rather than the kind and degree of stress. A relatively mild stimulus such as a scolding by a teacher may produce a reactive disorder in a particular child depending upon its meaning to the child and his parents, his original endowment, his level of development, the nature of his past experiences, and the adaptive resources he has available at the time. A situation such as a three-week absence of the mother, which will have a profound effect upon a two-year-old, may have relatively little impact upon a latency-age child. On the other hand, an event which interferes with the older child's struggle to achieve the task appropriate to his level of development will have more impact than it might have had earlier.

The GAP report describes the wide variety of responses to sudden loss of adequate mothering. "The infant . . . may react with apathy, eating and sleeping disturbances and failure to thrive. The older child may react with disturbances in conduct and may try to punish or coerce his environment by active aggressive behavior or by passive resistance. He may withdraw into himself for solace, developing habit patterns such as thumb-sucking or manipulating parts of his body. He may continue infantile patterns or regress to them, as with wetting or soiling. He may show overt panic or other psychological reactions such as excessive day-dreaming and pre-occupation with fantasy."

Use of the term "Reactive Disorders" as applied to children and adolescents really starts with the GAP report, and as we have seen is somewhat different from the term "Adjustment Reaction" as used by DSM-II. However, a group of occurrences quite similar to reactive disorders are described by Nagera[14] as "Developmental Interference." More precisely, he is speaking about the impact of certain events upon the course of the child's development rather than the manifest reaction of the child to these events. But there is little doubt he has the same issues in mind. He states that "the terms may be reserved to describe those situations that involve gross external (environmental) interferences with certain needs and rights of the child." He points out that the child may not have the ego capacity to comply or cope with such environmental demands. The examples he offers are sometimes accidental, such as long separations of mother and child due to prolonged illness or hospitalization of the mother, or may be culturally determined, such as early and rigidly imposed toilet training or feeding on a fixed, inflexible timetable at certain points on the clock. As in the criteria for GAP's "Reactive Disorders," Nagera notes that "children react to the upheavals created by the developmental interfer-

ences with abnormal manifestations which in many instances greatly resemble those observed in the case of neurotic conflict or neurosis proper." This is the crucial issue. Although the "symptoms" appear identical on the surface, "closer examination shows that there are important metapsychological differences between these symptoms. The "symptoms" occurring early in life are frequently not compromise formations with symbolic unconscious meaning and content (the symptom itself implying a certain amount of unconscious gratification), rather, they are specific reactions and are devoid of any of the advantages that a conflict solution by means of compromise formation in the form of symptoms achieves."

All developmental interferences are not presumed automatically to be damaging to the structure of the personality or to lead necessarily to ultimate developmental deviations. However, they may indeed lead to developmental conflicts, from which they must then be distinguished. In this classification, a developmental conflict occurs when certain specific demands of the environment are made when the child is at the appropriate developmental phase, and he must cope with them. These parallel the "situational crises" of the GAP report which are found in "Healthy Responses." Toilet training in the anal phase of development is an example. It may be carried out at the correct time, but it can be done in improper or traumatic ways. When that happens, it can be transformed into a serious developmental interference which leaves its trace on personality and may provide a nidus for what may ultimately become organized as a neurotic conflict.

Neubauer[15] raised pertinent questions suggesting that reversibility might be a key concept in differentiating reactive disorders from neurosis and character disorders. When points of interference with development are found, can they be undone? Will development then return to its original direction without further sign of interference? However, he used the term reversibility in the sense of the developmental process rather than simply of the symptom. By this measure, a reactive disorder would be one that permits ongoing normal development once the stress (developmental interference) is removed.

Settlage[18] also suggests two categories of disorder in children that appear when the conflict is not fully internalized. He uses the terms "Developmental Disorders" and "Situational Disorders." Both are due to conflict between the child and his environment. Developmental disorders, like Nagera's developmental conflicts, "occur quite normally in relation to the inevitable and characteristic conflicts associated with the successive stages of ego and psychosexual development. Situational disorders occur in reaction to environmental pathology or a pathological situation in excess of that associated with normal development." The latter clearly parallels the GAP reactive disorders and the developmental interferences of Nagera. It is interesting that these constructs were all presented between 1964 and 1966. The work of Anna Freud[6, 7] and her developmental assessment of childhood pathology were seminal to these concepts.

Special consideration of the concept of vulnerability is pertinent at this point. Anthony[1] describes four theoretical factors which determine the degree of vulnerability in a child. There are at birth rudimentary apparatuses of perception, memory, motility, and other primary autonomous functions of the ego which prepare the child for dealing with reality even before it has the experience of reality.[11] Secondly, the so-called "protective barrier" against stimuli is a theoretical construct used by Freud as a probable antecedent of later defense mechanisms. Bergman and Escalona[3] employed this concept in their description of children with a "thin" protective behavior who accordingly have unusual sensitivities to certain environmental stimuli. The result is a precocious ego development with attendant high vulnerability.

The third theoretical factor in the genesis of vulnerability is the capacity to postpone and control discharge in relation to stimulation. Anna Freud[8] regarded this as an essential, innate feature of the human ego. A fourth factor[4] is the presence of a "primary positive response" of the infant to the world; this occurs alongside the primary negative ones. Anthony states that there is some evidence to link these positive attitudes to the positive object relationships developing later.

There is also evidence to attest that there are wide variations among infants with respect to these postulated structures and functions as a constitutional "given." In addition, the impact of deprivation or trauma in this earliest period may significantly interfere with their future evolution and thereby lead to an increase of vulnerability. (p. 4)[1]

This would logically extend to a vulnerability of the defense system.

The diagnosis of reactive disorder may pose a nosological dilemma when ordinary stress is brought to bear on the vulnerable child. The relatively invulnerable child[2] can bring about adaptive reactions as described under Healthy Personality (GAP report).[10] But suppose the child is more vulnerable; that is, even though no manifest psychopathology exists, his adaptive ego functions are less competent! Ordinary stress may then cause a more severe or less easily reversible disturbance. In fact, one may still diagnose this as a reactive disorder, albeit fleeting and rapidly evolving into another category. The development of a neurotic structure which remains after the reduction of stress would then be indicative of a greater degree of vulnerability. However, there is probably no clear dividing line between the outbreak of a reactive disorder in a vulnerable personality on the one hand, and the onset of a neurosis following a precipitating event on the other.

Another category of disorder, the traumatic neurosis, also occurs in reaction to an event in the environment, and differs from the classical neurosis in a similar fashion in that the symptoms are not the result of an internalized structural conflict. Rather, its manifestations are due to the ego's attempt to avoid disorganizating helplessness in the face of overwhelming stress or subsequent threat of such stress.

Because of this, post-traumatic disorders are better classified with the reactive disorders than with the neuroses. They differ from the usual reactive disorder in that the stress is of such intensity and suddenness that the ego is overwhelmed with excitation, is unable to use its more highly adapted coping mechanisms, and responds with primitive reactions such as regression, or flight.

The concept of the protective barrier is basic to the theory of the traumatic neurosis. Freud[9] suggested the analogy to the surface of an organic vesicle, suspended in the atmosphere, receiving haphazard bombardment of stimuli from all around. There would be gradual toughening and thickening of the surface through cornification. The outer layers would be changed and the vesicle would become increasingly resistant to stimuli. The inner processes, like the mental apparatus, would no longer be so subject to forces from the environment impinging upon it. In the same manner, the psyche of the human infant is protected by a relatively "thin" barrier but is additionally shielded by the solicitude and protection of nurturing adults. It has already been noted that some infants may be relatively less well equipped with a protective barrier and depend more heavily on the caretakers to avoid disruptive penetration of the shield.

In a traumatic neurosis, the suddenness and intensity of the assault breaches even a normal protective barrier, and the capacity of the mental systems to maintain organization and integration of functions is momentarily overcome. Or, the ego may continue to operate for a time in orderly fashion with hypercathexis of some emergency functions and temporary suspension of full awareness of the dangers. In either case there follows a massive flooding of the ego apparatus with painful stimuli which are experienced as an overwhelming threat to integrity. All sorts of symptoms may then appear. Eventually the stress abates and/or the ego adapts and begins once more to seek an even keel. In the phase of reorganization there may be a full integration of the experience into the personality with subsequent recovery of adequate function, or even added resilience and confidence in the ability to cope with stress. However, the emergency defensive reactions may affect the processes of reorganization. Regression in particular may characterize various ego functions and the sense of vulnerability may come to dominate the mental life of the individual. Such pathological reorganization is often manifested by diffuse anxiety, phobic avoidance, and increased dependency feelings accompanied by shame.

An eleven-year-old boy was referred for treatment following a serious accident near his home. He had just left the school bus when a car struck him; he suffered a fracture of the leg, arm, and shoulder, and a broken rib which lacerated the liver. He was soon near death from shock, and emergency surgery was required. In the hospital he was uncomplaining, but moody. He recalled all the details of the accident and talked about them with ease. However he was desperately unhappy about being in a hospital room with another boy patient. His explanation was simple; he was afraid there might be a storm and the other boy would see his fear. The orthopedic surgeon at this point convinced the parents to seek psychiatric help for a storm phobia of ten months duration.

The previous August, the family had chartered a boat for a fishing trip in the Chesapeake Bay. A sudden squall with high winds, driving rain, lightening and thunder threatened to capsize the boat. The relatively inexperienced captain became panicky and was calmed by the mother. The father secured the three boys with life jackets and tried to comfort Michael who was weeping and trembling. The two older boys were "cool." The storm blew over before any serious accident occurred, and the family returned home shaken, but exuberant. As compared to the others, however, Michael, then ten years of age, was rather solemn.

A few days later he was left to stay with a friend. A storm arose and the parents were called during the night to come for Michael who was weeping uncontrollably. Following this, he would not be away from home at any threat of a storm. He checked weather reports daily. If it began to rain while he was at school he complained of a stomachache and went to the nurse's office. His mother had to be always available by phone to pick him up.

Past history was unremarkable. There were close family feelings, and Michael had always been fairly outgoing and sociable. He was somewhat more sensitive than his next older brother, Dennis, who frequently provoked and ridiculed him. Michael enjoyed athletics but was not as competent as Dennis.

Mother felt some resentment about Michael's anxiety, but aligned herself to a degree with Michael's attempts to conceal it and supported his sporadic attempts to overcome it. Father had frequent trips away which placed further emotional burdens on Mother.

Michael was seen once in the hospital, two times at home, and then, after a month, for twice weekly therapy. As a result of psychiatric evaluation it was felt that this was essentially a traumatic neurosis rather than a traumatically precipitated psychoneurosis. Although he was very reluctant to talk about the boat episode or his reactions to threatening weather, his symptoms caused such discomfort that he did not resist therapy. A combination of desensitization therapy and play therapy was employed. He had to "work" at least half the appointment before he would be released to free play. Altogether these were nine more appointments, and during the last two, he "worked" the entire time. During the last appointment he achieved deep relaxation and a warm skin response measured with a dermal thermistor while listening to the recording of a crashing autumn storm. He and the therapist agreed to see one another in three months, or after the next storm, whichever came sooner. Mother was seen three times and further communication was managed by phone. In fact, they did not have a subsequent appointment. Six months later, Michael was visting with friends and showed only slight traces of uneasiness (which Mother could detect) during an actual storm.

The rapid dissolution of the phobic reactions by gradual confrontation with and mastery of the anxiety is supportive evidence for the diagnosis of traumatic neurosis. There was no apparent intrapsychic conflict that supported the symptom. In fact the conflict between his ego and ego-ideal as a result of the symptom supported his earnest efforts to work in therapy. It is no mean feat for an active eleven-year-old boy to lie on the floor and develop progressive skeletal muscle relaxation to the point of somnolence! His case demonstrated several cardinal features of the post-traumatic neurosis: sudden, overwhelming danger from the environment; loss of a sense of invulnerability even in the presence of reassuring, familiar protectors; disorganization of ego controls; and subsequent reorganization at a regressed level characterized by phobic avoidance and increased dependency. In the reorganization, some aspects remained at a more mature level; the ego-ideal strivings appropriate to his age resisted the regressive pull of his ego. Shame added some severity to his symptoms and produced the appearance of a more severe neurosis.

In summary, the use of the term Reactive Disorder is recommended for those disorders which are judged to be primarily a reaction to an event or a situation in the external environment. The assessment of significant stress at a particular time must take into account the dynamic state of the child in his ongoing environmental situation. The resulting disturbance would be judged to be of pathological degree, but would occur as a result of the child's attempt to cope with the stress and not a result of unconscious internalized conflict.

Frequency and Distribution

The incidence of reactive disorders is universal; it is difficult to conceive of a human being progressing from infancy through adolescence without trauma sufficient to interfere, at least temporarily, with psychosocial development. One might even speculate that the absolute absence of such stress would find our "fortunate" young adult vulnerable and poorly equipped to cope with the realities of his life. Such is the impossible borderline between normality and pathology. The frequency and severity of reactive disorders will vary in individuals. There is a complex interaction between the impact of the deprivation or assault on the organism and the environmental supports and biological strengths with which it struggles to deal with stress. So intricate is this interlocking process that all predictions become inherently uncertain.

A study of a nonclinical group of children from twenty-one months to fourteen years old was carried out by MacFarlane, Allen, and Honzik.[13] They demonstrated the presence of a high frequency of behavioral problems in this group. Their approach to classification was essentially empirical; they classified the frequency of behavioral problems according to age and sex and data on each type of problem. By noting the decreasing incidence with age, increasing incidence with age, and the peak age period, they were able to demonstrate the relationship of age to conflict. They made no attempt to classify the underlying factors or causes; in their data, however, they were able to provide findings that support the concept of varying reactions to stress at different levels of development.

It would be simplistic to assume that a setting of social injustice always results in more psychological trauma. Children who have been toughened by adversity and who have experienced deprivation of significant social and material needs may still be fortunate enough to get the kind of good support that sees them through. They might possibly be better equipped to survive and grow in an unpredictable and chaotic future life than more fortunate youngsters who escaped multiple early traumata. On the other hand, when life unfolds in a stable culture, without surprises, the child of adversity will surely be handicapped in comparison with his advantaged counterpart.

Although reactive disorders occur at all ages, the infant and preschool child are more vulnerable to a wider range of environmental assaults or lack of support. They have fewer coping devices and less structured psychological apparatus with which to manage the stress or to bind the resulting conflict. Loss of mother at nine months can have a devastating, sometimes a fatal impact. Yet the very plasticity of the relatively undifferentiated organism allows for more recovery and reversibility than would a similar loss at age four. For example, the nine-month infant may die; or he may recover from his anaclitic depression with an appropriate substitute. The four-year-old who has suddenly lost his mother will not develop marasmus, but the already structured ego will have been so injured that scars of this experience will be embedded in his personality thenceforth. By late adolescence the possibility of true mourning provides an additional means for coping with the disorder in the course of time. (Wolfenstein[22] raises the question whether true mourning is possible even in adolescence if the adolescent has not previously experienced this phase-specific depression of final separation-individuation from parents.)

Clinical Course

Reactive disorders are readily recognized when a disturbing event jars the equilibrium of a normally developing child and is followed by behavior that is atypical for this younger or for any youngster at his level of development. We also know that the source of major character disorders, neuroses, and most likely borderline states can be traced in careful anamnesis to early traumatic events, or to repeated affronts on the child's ability to handle stress at his then level of development. This would imply a diagnosis of reactive disorder in the past that progressed to serious illness. As mentioned earlier, this need not change our concept of reactive disorder. Rather, we must be alert to the possible serious consequences of sudden overwhelming insult or of stress that is less intense but longer sustained. This is especially true in the younger individual whose repertoire of coping mechanisms is limited and within whom the spread of excitation and anxiety is rapid because of the immature psychic structure available to handle it.[19] The reaction will be more severe, but the reversibility will be greater.

Older children suffering from a reactive disorder where the stress is not soon relieved are more likely to bind the anxiety by the development of some form of fixed psychopathology. The relief of the stress may not lead to reversibility as readily as in the case of the younger child.

The subsequent course of the disorder will also depend upon the suddenness and duration of the stress. A small child separated from his mother for a frightening hour in a crowded department store may react with nightmares, bedwetting, and clinging for a few days afterward, but with no sequelae.

However, the provocation to the child may be more subtle and gradual in development. The resultant disturbance should still be classified as a reactive disorder, although it would probably go unrecognized and is all too likely to progress to internalized conflict. For example, a mother, who has enjoyed her son's infancy and his early moves towards individuation and relative autonomy, may nonetheless react to manifestations of his sexual interests and phallic pride with increasing hostility. If this should chance to be intensified by current resentments toward her husband whom the boy admires, her attitudes may squelch his developing assertiveness and healthy motility. The change in his behavior might be noted but its cause go altogether unrecognized. If his disturbance were sufficiently marked to create concern, appropriate intervention might be initiated to ameliorate the situation. At that point the recognition of reactive disorder will be established. Unfortunately, it is far more likely that such a reactive disorder will escape notice. The external situation will remain unchanged, and lasting alterations in the developing child's personality will occur.

There is still another possibility. A resourceful child whose development to this point has been adequate will go through a period of anger, rebellion and behavior that is challenging and provocative to mother. And mother may take stock of the situation, recognize her reactions as incongruent with her overall feelings towards her son, and learn to avoid head-on collisions and unrealistic demands for his passivity.

It should be noted that while reactive disorders are usually, and most easily, diagnosed in normal individuals, they can also occur in youngsters suffering from previous psychopathology. A comparison of two case examples will illustrate this point. In the first, there was an unusual opportunity to examine a normally developing youngster in the course of a developmental crisis (Healthy Reaction). Eight months later he then developed a true reactive disorder which was amenable to treatment. The second case is of a girl in late adolescence already showing evidence of passive-aggressive personality disorder with depressive trends. However, the depressive reaction for which she was brought in was recognized as a reactive disorder. Instead of prescribing long-term psychotherapy, which would have disrupted her life situation, brief psychotherapy was undertaken which enabled her to recover from the depressive reaction and proceed with her developmentally appropriate plans to go away to school.

THE CASE OF TIM

Tim was not quite four years of age when his parents called hesitantly for advice. Both were concerned that he was now refusing to give up the bottle even though he had previously been without one from age sixteen months to around thirty-four months. Mother realized that she was uneasy about handling some aspects of his education, but she was particularly uncomfortable about his return to the bottle.

For the first six weeks of his life, Tim had had severe colic every evening from seven to eleven o'clock; even a pacifier gave no relief. It ended suddenly, and he developed a cheerful, easy-going disposition. At sixteen months he had severe diarrhea, and the chubby youngster, recently weaned and with no eating problems, became finicky and lost weight. He returned to the bottle for about a week and gave it up again. Between two and three, toilet training was accomplished without stress, except for periods of diarrhea of unknown origin. His brother Eric was born when he was thirty months of age. The parents had been embarrassed by Tim's frequent use of the pacifier, so a few months later they removed it. They then found that the heretofore occasional request for the bottle now became increasingly insistent until he was regularly taking three a day. Although still sunny in disposition and affectionate towards Eric, there were occasional unpredictable temper tantrums often around the issue of clothing. The call for therapeutic help had actually been stimulated by an hysterical one and a half hour of screaming refusal to dress himself. He cried, "Mommy, I need you; I want you; I want Daddy." Father had had to leave in the midst of it. The parents were puzzled since the clothing had been selected and put out the night before as usual, and although he attended nursery school three mornings a week, this was not such a morning.

During the initial interview a few issues stood out. Father was earnest and concerned, but in recent months had been very much away from home because of the opening in his private law practice. Mother was intelligent, empathic, very loving to her children, and aware of their individual differences. She was most uncomfortable about their experiencing anxiety or deprivation. Both parents spoke disapprovingly and disparagingly to Tim about his use of the bottle, but they never told him clearly that they wished him to give it up. They did not recognize that his protective concern for Eric's welfare was a reaction formation against his envy and rivalry. They were more delighted with Tim's sweetness than with his assertiveness.

Tim was interviewed one week later. He was a wide-eyed, trusting, very appealing, very verbal four-year old with slight speech immaturity. He played an imaginative game with the telephone and then announced with pride, "I'm four and of course I drink from a cup now." His play was inventive and lively. He enjoyed drawing pictures and used color freely. He particularly liked a board game called *Trouble*. He read game directions from the box; his reading was easily at a third-grade level.

The parents confirmed that they had explained their wish for him to give up the bottle and that he no longer needed it. He displayed little resistance. They commented that since that time he has also been more outgoing with his friends, although he still preferred to have them visit his house rather than for him to leave home in order to visit them. The parents were reassured that Tim was not too fragile to move on from his temporary regressive position; but it was also explained that he needed more approval for assertiveness and, when possible, more time with Father. It was suggested that after about six months it might be wise to see how he was progressing and for them to call.

Mother did call about eight months later. Tim had been having nightmares and bedtime fears for about a month. Eric, although just over two, had become tough, aggressive, was relatively impervious to pain, and appeared stronger than Tim. Tim gave way to him a good bit and had been having tantrums when frustrated. Just recently he had complained of a "bad boy" at school who hurts him and on one occasion, while playing with a friend, he suddenly asked his mother to send the friend home. However, the call had in fact been precipitated by Tim's comment to her the previous evening, "Do you remember that doctor I went to see who played *Trouble* with me? Could I see him again?"

Tim greeted the doctor warmly and immediately told that he had trouble at school and it was from wrestling. "I get backaches from Gary. He wrestles when I don't want it." He sometimes wrestled with his friends but not when he didn't want to. He also talked about his fears. At night he thought that a dinosaur "might come in and eat me up. I cover up my head." He was asked if that helped and replied: "No." He talked more about the bad kids and about how Eric was sometimes bad. It was decided to continue interviews with Tim and he was seen weekly for the next two months. Contact with parents was maintained by somewhat less frequent visits and phone calls.

The parents readily understood the relationship between Eric's aggressiveness, Tim's overcontrol supported by the parental "you're older than he is" attitude, his restraint of aggression with other youngsters, and the projection of his own hostile impulses at night.

Tim described his problems very directly and also expressed a good many of his aggressive feelings in therapy. This time the parents supported his growing assertiveness and reported gradual disappearance of the night terrors. By the end of school, in their last interview, the parents reported that Tim was openly more hostile to Eric and holding his own. He was more engaged with neighborhood friends, although he would on occasion wander off and leave them. They then went on to describe their concern about Eric who was very advanced, competitive, and motorically active. There was more concern about him now than about Tim.

Tim's reactions could be traced to a moderate degree of sadness and regression following Eric's birth. Having always received supportive responses for his sweet nature and cheerful disposition, he mobilized his energy for the reward of parental love through passivity and the control of aggressivity. It is also true that both he and his parents enjoyed his creativity and intellectual ability.

When first seen, he was employing mild regression as a way of coping and occasional temper tantrums from pent-up resentment. The parents were concerned about his "immature way" and, being somewhat knowledgeable about child psychology, decided to seek consultation. This provided an opportunity to see a normally developing youngster confronted by a rather common problem (sibling rivalry) that he was handling in a manner quite appropriate for his level of development, temperament, and home environment. No treatment was suggested and minimal advice and interpretation resolved the problem of that moment.

However, it had not been sufficient to protect him from the more severe reaction accompanying the demand upon him to remain passive and to continue to suppress aggression despite increasing provocation from his brother. Without intervention it is possible that the resultant reactive disorder would have developed into a personality trait disorder, or, depending upon unforeseeable complex interactions, a childhood neurosis.

THE CASE OF SARAH

By contrast, Sarah, age seventeen, was not without problems. She was living at home with her mother, a clinical psychologist, and a ten-year-old younger half-brother. Mother had divorced her second husband. Despite bouts of physical ill health, mother was energetic, driving, somewhat impatient, and domineering. She was aware of her own characteristics, the needs of her children, and the difficulties confronting them.

Sarah's father had formerly kept in regular communication with her; each summer she would join him and his second wife for vacations. Following the vacation four years earlier, he had

inexplicably stopped writing or calling. Finally, one year ago, she received a postcard casually mentioning that they had had a baby daughter.

Sarah tended to be slow and passive-aggressive, and she defeated her mother in many little ways. She was a successful student but rather careless and unimaginative about her appearance and only moderately involved with friends. She got along fairly well with her brother but was more clearly ambivalent towards her mother whom she correctly perceived as hard-working, intense, considerate but impatient and demanding. Although not particularly indulgent, mother did support Sarah's consuming interest in breeding and showing her valuable pet dog.

Mother called me at the end of Sarah's senior year of high school. She was concerned that Sarah had become increasingly sloppy, lethargic, and weepy. Father's present wife was expecting a second child, but she didn't know if Sarah was aware of it. Sarah had given up an advanced placement English class and had done so poorly in chemistry that she had to be given an "Incomplete" and was repeating it in summer school. She has been unable to mobilize herself for college applications. Without the help of a friend who worked with her on the necessary essays and forms, she would not have completed any of them. As it was she completed only one, to an excellent school in the Midwest where she had been accepted on early decision. Sarah agreed to be seen, but sat glum-looking and silent in the chair facing the doctor. She appeared rather unkempt and unattractive. Her responses to questions were appropriate if somewhat flat. Discussion seemed to go nowhere, and the psychiatrist had to be very active to keep the interview alive.

Sarah acknowledged that she needed help. Her mother had confronted her with her destructive lethargy, and she agreed that something was wrong. She couldn't understand what had happened in school. The AP English class was really not very good; she didn't mind the transfer out of it into the regular class, and she had done well enough. However, in chemistry she simply let things go. This she could not understand. Although she liked the course and thought the teacher was excellent, she gave up trying and completed very little work. In response to questions about her family, she told about the last vacation she had had with her father and his wife in New England which had as usual gone quite well. And then there was nothing until the card one year ago! She wept profusely and added that she heard that they were expecting a second child. During most of the first interview the doctor found himself withholding an urge to push for answers. Long silences left him wondering whether she had heard the comment or had any intention of answering, but despite her slowness she eventually did answer and in appropriate fashion. However, in no subsequent interview did we have to cope with her passive-aggressive style to that degree. In fact she became increasingly enthusiastic, chatty, and bright-eyed. She paid more attention to her dress and grooming and revealed an attractive smile.

This brief summer psychotherapy consisted of six appointments over a two-month period. On several occasions it was pointed out how much she was avoiding emotionally meaningful issues by filling in with stories of dog shows etc. She acknowledged this, and would get back to looking at her style of interaction with people, her sorrows, her wishes, her values, etc. Two additional factors influenced the course of the work. Very early, by fortuitous circumstances, the doctor was able to recognize the existence of a true reactive disorder superimposed on her passive-aggressive, depressive personality organization. The description of the chemistry teacher in the second interview struck him with a shock of recognition. He asked, "Do you attend X school and is your teacher Mrs. G?" It was. As it happened, three years earlier he had known two students who had suffered with the same syndrome; a sense of utter defeat, helplessness, and self-blame, coupled with insistence that, "She's a very good teacher, and I was learning a lot, but I just didn't put in the work." Characteristically Mrs. G. would give long assignments and then pop tests on unassigned, suggested outside reading. Tests were graded arbitrarily so that on some occasions there might be one A, one B and all the rest lower, while on other occasions over half the class might receive an A. Pop quizzes and major tests were rated equally. Shame and frustration were often experienced by students; yet classroom teaching was stimulating, exciting, and rewarding to bright students. One of the previous patients, also a student in Mrs. G's class, had deteriorated in all his classes and come close to dropping out of school following a sense of utter humiliation. Because of complaints from a fair number of students and their parents, Mrs. G. was no longer teaching advanced placement classes; nevertheless, she was known throughout the school as difficult, a tough grader, but the best chemistry teacher in the city.

Sarah began to describe the impossibility of feeling any success, any self-worth. She recognized in retrospect how thoroughly her previously valued self-concept as a student had been damaged. She was currently doing exceptional work in her summer chemistry class, generally achieving near perfect scores on her examinations. She finished the course with an A+ but also realistically acknowledged that this teacher wanted the students to do well and that her competition was less keen.

Quite early Sarah seemed to lift out of the low point of her depression and gain confidence and enthusiasm. The therapy was continued because it was felt that she needed understanding, admiration and respect from a father-like person. She talked about possible future problems of loneliness, of her tendency to be stand-offish with acquaintances, and of her inclination to withdraw and sulk.

It was reassuring that six weeks after the start of her school, the doctor received a letter from her that reflected cheerfulness, a pleasure with academic success, and the miraculous discovery that she could meet so many people who were friendly and attractive. "In the past few weeks I think I've come to know as many special people as I've known in 17 years. Maybe it's me, maybe it's the select population, probably both." About her mother she said, "It's been good to get away from home. My mother is a very difficult, to put it mildly, person to live with; I realize her specialness and love her more now. I think I am also more like her now, organized, studious, shoulder-to-cry-on than before. It has taken a separation for me to gain a perspective and see that I can be me without being the opposite of her."

Sarah appeared to have profited from the clarification of the school trauma which had intensified her problem of underlying depression, feelings of worthlessness, and suppressed rage. This was the reactive disorder. The response to the doctor's paternal, affectionate, yet reality-appraising interest filled a need, albeit temporarily, which helped her to risk moving forward in her development as a young woman.

In summary the supportive therapy helped restore her self-esteem by differentiating reality trauma from inner sense of failure and by facilitating the developmental thrust of this period. It is likely, however, that more definitive treatment is indicated for the underlying personality disorder.

Organic Etiological Factors

It is evident by definition that no specific organic etiology is involved. However, stress may be physical, psychological, or social; in Engel's[5] unitary concept, health is more than the abscence of disease. In children, health represents a phase of successful adaptation and ongoing growth and development. Disease represents a failure of adaptation or a breakdown in the attempt of the human organism to maintain an adaptive equilibrium. During this phase, disturbances or failure may occur in the growth, development, or adjustment of the organism as a whole or in any of its systems. Thus organic disease will also have its impact on the psychological and social levels of adaptation in response to factors other than the severity of the illness.

For example, forced immobilization in a body cast will have a great impact on a two-year old. This is when his rapidly developing ego is exploring the environment and exulting in the motility which helps him channel aggression and promote individuation from mother. Coping with this trauma would be more manageable for a youngster of quiet temperament than for one who has been highly active and impatient. Thomas and his colleagues[20] have demonstrated the importance of individual temperament on the child's development and subsequent interaction with the environment in both health and illness.

Illness, hospitalization, and surgery frequently provoke reactive disorders in children and adolescents. These have accordingly been studied with special care in order to anticipate those reactions which might be almost universal and to develop means for handling them more effectively. Prugh[16] emphasizes that the stress on the child is relative rather than absolute, and depends upon his basic endowment, constitutional characteristics, developmental capacities, and the nature of his past experiences, including his experience with disease.

Acute illness or injury cause effects that are both direct and reactive. The former include listlessness, frustration, disturbances in sleep and appetite, and irritability. More specific to children are restlessness, hyperactivity, feeding problems, night terrors, and sleeping problems. The more striking reactive effects are various forms of regression which may vary from the temporary giving up of newly acquired skills to a marked return to immature, dependent, or aggressive behavior. Depression and mood swings may occur.

A common phenomenon is misinterpretation of the meaning of the illness with consequent emotionally charged reactions. Prugh also comments on the frequent occurrence of physiological concomitants of anxiety, conversion reactions, dissociative reactions, and perceptual motor lags that may persist for several weeks or months after the illness without apparent damage to the central nervous system.

Chronic illness is more likely to have deep seated and long-range effects on personality. This is especially true because of the unrelenting pressure from a complex of factors involving treatment procedures, parental reactions, effect on body image, and isolation from the normal stream of social development.

Children with various diseases or handicaps display personality effects that range from overdependent, overanxious and passive, or withdrawn patterns utilizing secondary gain, to overindependent, aggressive patterns with strong tendencies to deny illness. These forms of adaptation may reach unhealthy extremes. A middle group shows realistic dependence, acceptance of limitations, with adequate social patterns and compensatory outlets.

Although to some extent the specific illness and/or injury are likely to determine the form of the disorder, the basic concept that underlies this approach is that of a whole individual responding to psychological stress of whatever origin, organic or interpersonal.

Psychodynamic Factors and Therapeutic Methods

It is peculiarly true of the reactive disorders that the therapeutic approach and psychodynamic understanding must be discussed together. The basic concept of reactive disorders is that they are disturbing manifestations of the organism's effort to cope with greater stress than usual. The conflict is not waged between intrapsychic forces. It is, rather a struggle between the ego at its particular level of development and one or more of a myriad of interfering external forces. Therefore there can be no general formulation applied to the condition that fit the classical psychodynamic model.

Instead we must look for an understanding of the responses of a particular individual confronted with a stress that markedly upsets his former relatively stable equilibrium. To do this we have to focus on several questions: (1) what is the child's level of development, and more especially what internal psychological resources and vulnerabilities does he bring to his current state of adequate equilibrium; (2) what are his current biological strengths and vulnerabilities; (3) what familial and extrafamilial social structures contribute to his equilibrium; and (4) lastly, regardless of its conventionally accepted significance or lack of significance, how much disruptive power does the newly intruding stress actually exert upon this dynamic equilibrium?

If we postulate an individual within the normal range of temperamental organization, the interaction will be between X temperament in Y setting under Z current state of good enough equilibrium confronted by A injury or B traumatic event, acute or chronic. This multifactorial situation makes room for a wide variety of responses (symptoms); nevertheless these tend to fall in clusters at certain levels of development. Only by elucidating and studying the interactions of these variables can we identify a reactive disorder and differentiate it from developmental deviations or true psychopathology.

Although these same issues are considered in the evaluation of every patient, we are here emphasizing that the appearance of pathology is due to the disruptive impact of the stress rather than to the pathological psychic structure. It seems likely that we are also describing what may become the initial phase of psychological illness not related to primary developmental deviations.

Treatment must be preceded by identifying the nature and the source of the stress. One cannot simply dismiss concerns about treatment by the obvious recommendation that the cause of the disorder be removed. One cannot "remove" a crippling injury or repair a family broken by death or divorce. Even when a stress can be removed, the use of an inappropriate coping mode might persist in the child, and this would still have to be managed.

Various modalities of treatment are available. A therapist should have his own special skills along with an understanding of other possible methods. Particularly with children, a combination of approaches may be desirable, even though the emphasis is likely to be on those with which the therapist has most familiarity.

In the case of Tim, previously described, the pressure of an aggressive, competitive younger brother disrupted a personality style with an emphasis on gentleness, consideration, and intellectual achievement. This style was in comfortable equilibrium with Tim's own activity pattern as well as with parental values. However, at some point, the parents unwittingly continued to reward the inhibition of aggression and the child's immature ego internalized the implied prohibition. Here it is difficult to say whether we have a reactive disorder or an incipient neurosis. What does matter is that effective intervention should permit a resumption of healthy development.

With Tim, brief individual psychotherapy combined with assistance to parents in modifying their pressures revealed the ready reversibility of the condition. However, had the parental style been more firmly fixed because it was rooted in Mother's abhorrence of male aggressivity or in some interaction between Mother and Father wherein both had a neurotic stake in keeping Tim passive and the younger more aggressive, then the brief therapy would not have sufficed.

Various approaches might have been tried, and various methods or combinations might have been successful. Some possibilities can be suggested:

1. Individual therapy with Mother by same therapist or collaborator.
2. Collaborative therapy, with both parents being seen.
3. Family therapy, in any of its numerous forms: (a) entire family seen together; (b) parents only seen, with emphasis on systems approach; and (c) seeing one parent only based on the presumed ability of that individual to be most effective in altering the pathological family system.
4. Group therapy for Mother, or parents together.
5. Behavioral Modification training program with parents. In addition, there are still additional therapeutic modalities that could be involved: (a) medication for Tim, such as 25 mg imipramine at bedtime, and (b) school consultation, home visits and other direct environmental manipulations.

Here is where a broader vista is important. School consultation, medication, and reassurance to parents would be insufficient. However, the relative success or failure of individual, group or family psychotherapy would depend upon the accurate understanding of the dynamics, the skill of the therapist grounded in his own modality, and the judicious use of compatible other approaches.

REFERENCES

1. ANTHONY, E. J., "The Syndrome of the Psychologically Vulnerable Child," in Anthony, E. J., and Koupernik, C. (Eds.), *The Child in His Family: Children at Psychiatric Risk*, vol. 3, John Wiley, New York, 1974.

2. ———, "The Syndrome of the Psychologically Invulnerable Child," in Anthony, E. J., and Koupernik, C. (Eds.), *The Child in His Family: Children at Psychiatric Risk*, vol. 3, John Wiley, New York, 1974.

3. BERGMAN, P., and ESCALONA, S. K., "Unusual Sensitivities in Very Young Children," in Eissler, R. S., et al. (Eds.), *The Psychoanalytic Study of the Child*, vol. 3/4, pp. 333–352, International Universities Press, New York, 1949.

4. BUHLER, C., "The Reality Principle," *American Journal of Psychotherapy*, 8:626–647, 1954.

5. ENGEL, G. L., "A Unified Concept of Health and Disease," *Perspectives in Biology and Medicine*, 3:459–485, 1960.

6. FREUD, A., "Normality and Pathology in Childhood," *Assessment of Development*, International Universities Press, New York, 1965.

7. ———, "Assessment of Childhood Disturbances," in Eissler, R. S., et al. (Eds.), *The Psychoanalytic Study of the Child*, vol. 17, pp. 149–158, International Universities Press, New York, 1962.

8. ———, *The Ego and the Mechanisms of Defense*, International Universities Press, New York, 1936.

9. FREUD, S., "Beyond the Pleasure Principle," *The Standard Edition of the Complete Psychological Works of Sigmund Freud*, vol. 18, Hogarth Press, London, 1953.

10. Group for the Advancement of Psychiatry (GAP), *Psychopathological Disorders in Childhood: Theoretical Considerations and a Proposed Classification*, vol. VI, Report No. 62, Group for the Advancement of Psychiatry, New York, 1966.

11. HARTMANN, H., *Essays on Ego Psychology*, International Universities Press, New York, 1964.

12. LANGFORD, W. S., "Reflections on Classification in Child Psychiatry," *Diagnostic Classification in Child Psychiatry*, pp. 1–21, American Psychiatric Association Research Report, 1964.

13. MACFARLANE, J. W., ALLEN, L., and HONZIK, M. P., *A Developmental Study of the Behavior Problems of Normal Children Between 21 Months and 14 Years*, University of California Press, Berkeley, 1962.

14. NAGERA, H. C., *Early Childhood Disturbances, The Infantile Neurosis, and the Adulthood Disturbances*, International Universities Press, New York, 1966.

15. NEUBAUER, P., "Normal Development in Children," in Wolman, B. (Ed.), *Manual of Child Psychopathology*, McGraw-Hill, New York, 1972.

16. PRUGH, D., "Towards an Understanding of Psychosomatic Concepts in Relation to Illness in Children," in Solnit, A., and Provence, S. (Eds.), *Modern Perspectives in Child Development*, p. 246, International Universities Press, New York, 1963.

17. ———, and ECKHARDT, C., "Children's Reactions to Illness, Hospitalization, and Surgery," in Freedman, G. C., Kaplan, H., and Saddock, V. S. (Eds.), *Comprehensive Textbook of Psychiatry*, vol. 2, Williams and Wilkins, Baltimore, Md., 1975.

18. SETTLAGE, C., "Psychoanalytic Theory in Relation to the Nosology of Childhood Disorders," *Journal of the American Psychoanalytic Association*, 12(4):776–801, 1964.

19. SHIRLEY, H., *Pediatric Psychiatry*, Harvard University Press, Cambridge, Mass., 1963.

20. THOMAS, A., CHESS, S., and BIRCH, H. G., *Temperament and Behavior Disorders in Children*, New York University Press, New York, 1963.

21. TITCHENER, J. L., and ROSS, W. D., "Acute or Chronic Stress as Determinants of Behavior, Character, and Neurosis," in Arieti, S., and Brody, E. (Eds.), *American Handbook of Psychiatry*, 2nd ed., vol. 3, pp. 39–60, Basic Books, New York, 1974.

22. WOLFENSTEIN, U., "How is Mourning Possible? in Eissler, R. S., et al. (Eds.), *The Psychoanalytic Study of the Child*, vol. 21, pp. 93–123, International Universities Press, New York, 1966.

11 / Developmental Deviations

Milton Engel

Introduction

In a discussion of Rutter's[39] comments on the GAP classification, E. J. Anthony comments on the struggle with classification and diagnosis over the past half century.

He compares the world of psychiatrists to that of ancient Gaul, a nation divided into three parts. We have the organic division, the psychodynamic division, and a group in between; moreover, there is little communication across the boundaries.

Developmental deviation is a classification where all three divisions may come together.

With increasing awareness of constitutional factors, it may in time be recognized more often both as a primary diagnosis and as a secondary one.

The Name of the Syndrome

Developmental deviation is a category of disturbance listed in the GAP Report No. 62 of June, 1966.[1] It does not appear as such in the DSM-II; in that context these disturbances are covered under VII. Special Symptoms (306):

306.0   speech disturbances
306.1   unspecific learning disturbances
306.2   tic
306.3   other psychomotor disorders
306.4   disorders of sleep
306.5   feeding disturbance
306.6   enuresis
306.7   encopresis
306.8   cephalalgia
306.9   other special symptoms

and possibly under IX. Behavior Disorders of Childhood and Adolescence (308)

308.0   hyperkinetic
308.1   withdrawing

In the literature various authors have used different terms to describe these same problems:

Cameron[11]—developmental variance
Settlage[45]—developmental disorders
A. Freud[22]—developmental disturbances
Chess[13]—developmental disturbances
Prugh[38]—developmental variations
Rutter[42]—developmental disorders and specific developmental disorders
Shaw and Lucas[46]—specific learning disabilities
Silverman and Ross[47]—developmental disturbances
Harrison and McDermott[28]—developmental disorders
Neubauer[35]—ego deviations
Rexford and Van Amerongen[40]—developmental disturbances and developmental irregularities and failures
Sobel[48]—developmental disorders
Cohen[15]—developmental disabilities

Description

PRIMARY

The syndrome refers either to deviation in the overall maturational rate or sequence, or to specific aspects of personality development. The GAP Report suggests the syndrome be broken down as follows:

3. Developmental Deviations
    A. deviation in maturational pattern
    B. deviation in specific dimension of development
        1. motor
        2. sensory
        3. speech
        4. cognitive function
        5. social development
        6. psychosexual development
        7. affective
        8. integrative
    C. other developmental deviations

Since the committee had already inserted "Healthy Response" as one of the ten basic diagnostic categories, it was here stating that these developmental deviations must be reserved for those youngsters whose problems by definition fall outside the healthy range.

At the same time, it is important to note that this group of deviations is not necessarily fixed in nature; any one of them may pass spontaneously with no assistance. However, they may also require some assistance. In any case a specific developmental deviation will have some effect on development and may, thus, later give rise to a more structured disorder.

As outlined under the GAP Report, this term refers to conditions where biological factors, heredity and constitution, are very prominent.

Some deviations involve almost the total maturational timetable. Others involve a number of part functions; while still others apply only to selected aspects of development. The broad categories will now be discussed.

A. DEVIATIONS IN MATURATIONAL PATTERNS

This refers to broad overall unevenness of development which takes the form of precocity or lags in maturation. An example would be the case of a three-year-old boy who was referred for delayed onset of speech. Upon examination it was noted that many of his milestones had been consistently delayed. Crawling and walking began late. He was very infantile in his relationship with his mother and did not reach out to other children nor explore. His cognitive functions were immature—all of this was present, in addition to the delayed onset of speech. Such children can also exhibit delay in their capacity to attain control of their vegetative patterns, such as sleep, eating, bowel and bladder functions. In contrast to this group are the youngsters who seem to do everything early; they smile, sit up, walk, talk, and manage all sorts of adaptations far earlier than is usual.

B. DEVIATIONS IN SPECIFIC DIMENSIONS OF DEVELOPMENT

1. *Motor Development:* This refers to children who show a continual lag in their psychomotor development, or who are hyperactive. There may be difficulty in coordination or delay in development of handedness. Gross brain damage is not a factor. If there is a place in the overall diagnostic categories for the syndrome of minimal

brain dysfunction, some of these children might have to be diagnosed under this category. Those children whose increased activity is mainly caused by anxiety, however, would not be included here.

2. *Sensory Development:* This category refers to children who have difficulty monitoring sensory stimuli including any of the five senses.

3. *Speech Development:* This category includes the children who have significant delays in the onset of speech. It would not include children where deafness, oppositionalism, elective mutism, gross brain damage, or early childhood psychosis cause the delay in the onset of speech. In addition to delayed onset, the category also is used for those children with a disorder of articulation, rhythm, phonation, or comprehension of speech. With these, an infantile pattern of speech persists in the absence of somatic abnormalities. This category can also be used for children with a marked precocity of speech development. Stuttering and the normal echolalia which occurs with the onset of speech would not be included.

4. *Cognitive Functions:* This refers to lags and deviations in the capacity for symbolic or abstract thinking. Some children will show persistent prelogical thought processes or a delay in the ability to repress primitive fantasies. These interfere with the neutralized processes of cognitive development. It is suggested that other deviations of cerebral integration without gross brain damage be included here, along with those conditions where the children appear to be pseudoretarded. It should also be used for children who show precocious or accelerated intellectual development. These children function as if there were a hypertrophy of one aspect of development with the result that there is an overall unevenness in the way they grow. The idiot savant, some borderline children who show compensatory hypertrophy of certain cognitive capacities, and the street wise, pseudo-hypermature ghetto child are examples of individual variations in these deviations.

5. *Social Development:* This category includes those patterns of social capacity that develop unevenly, be they delayed or precocious. It embraces children whose true personality disorders have not yet crystallized. Some characteristic traits that might be present are marked shyness, excessive dependency, inhibition, difficulties in separation from the parent, and the kind of immature aggressive behavior that is so often reflective of the delayed achievement of autonomy.

6. *Psychosexual Development:* This category applies to children who show precocious or delayed heterosexual interest. This would include significant deviations in the timing of appearance of sexual curiosity with a persistence of infantile autoerotic patterns. It is also intended for children in whom there is some internalized conflict without the presence of a crystallized neurosis or more chronic personality disorder. An example is the young boy who exhibits marked passive dependent behavior. Later he may develop learning inhibitions which reflect an imbalance between more aggressive strivings for independence and earlier dependency patterns.

7. *Affective Development:* These are children who appear moderately anxious and show emotional lability of a type less mature than expected at their level of development. There can be overcontrol of affect, apathetic tendencies, or mild depression. However, neither a structural psychoneurotic reaction nor a personality disorder is present. The cyclical patterns of euphoria and hypomania alternating with depressed moods and diminished activities also belong here.

8. *Integrative Development:* This refers to those children in whom there is a moderate deviation in development of impulse control or frustration tolerance. They display an uneven or overactive use of certain defense mechanisms such as projection or denial without the presence of personality disorder or psychosis.

This deviation as well as those mentioned previously will have to be distinguished from similar tendencies found under the personality disorders.

C. OTHER

This includes developmental disturbances not specified in the previous two categories.

SECONDARY

Developmental deviations are usually recognized as primary conditions; under certain circumstances they can appear as secondary conditions. This would be true especially for neurosis or personality disorders where early deviations in development were among the factors which crystallized into a neurosis or led to the more chronic personality disorders. Examples of this would be children in whom a delay either in motor or integrative patterns evoked defenses to cope with the discomfort that resulted from the delay. These conceptualizations might be helpful with latency children who have been made to feel that their rate of development was both not acceptable and out of line with that of their peers. All too often they become depressed and show low self-esteem and poor self-concept.

The History of Its Identification

Developmental deviation represents the category or syndrome which attempts most actively to bring together the concepts of psyche and soma. The crystallization of the syndrome by the GAP Committee is intertwined with the development of ego psychology over the last fifty years. In the nineteenth century the notion of emotional problems and personality development was dualistic and static. The concept of a deviation in development has only come about with the evolution away from this view to one of a continuum between abnormal and normal behavior and normal personality functioning with variations and exaggerations.

As reviewed in the GAP Report,[25] the system of classification advanced these attempts to address past classifications of children's disorders and to come to terms with the varied approaches used by different workers in the field. It is within this framework that the syndrome of developmental deviation was defined. The syndrome reflects the committee's wish for a theoretical structure which embraces three concepts—psychosomatic, developmental, and psychosocial. This syndrome is the one most bound up with the committee's concern for maturation and development. While paying attention to the general curve of development, which already included variations in each developmental stage, the committee felt that the concept of developmental deviation would address those variations that were beyond the normal range, and which reflected the presence of a disordered biological template (a term suggested by Edwin Kessler).

English and Pearson[17] list speech disorders under which one finds an inability to speak clearly due to damage either in the auditory receptive mechanism or in the associative sensorimotor speech mechanism. They also list inhibition of social behavior. Brown[10] refers to educational disabilities.

Margaret Fries[23] describes her attempts to understand differences in endowment as manifested by congenital activity patterns. She uses the term "core" for the interaction of the genetic endowment, the intrauterine experience, and the birth process. The "congenital activity type" is the core's sensorimotor response. "We found that children of different congenital activity types need to be handled differently in order to develop their ego strength, facilitating rather than frustrating their ability to cope with the world."

She cites "Harold" as a case example. From birth this boy was busy and active. Psychological testing at five and one half revealed an intelligent child with a "pseudo-adult quality, suggesting that a maturity to which he is not equal has been forced upon him." When Harold was seen almost twenty-five years later by Dr. Robert Prall, there was a struggle between independence and dependency strivings and active versus passive yearnings which could have been predicted at age five and one half. He was still a man of action and impulsive decisions. Prall guessed that the level of motor activity had been high in this young man's childhood and that his parents had probably enjoyed and fostered it early in life. This is an example of how a deviation in motor development, a precocity, facilitated the turning to the motor system for conflict resolution and resulted in a less than optimal development of other ego functions.

Bergman and Escalona's[8] classic paper on unusual sensitivities in children, and Beres[7] work on aggression in children were often used as the basis for further understanding ego deficits in childhood psychosis. Their work, however, may also be seen as building blocks toward an appreciation of developmental deviations.

Lourie[30] reported on rhythmic functions in several groups of children. He did not speculate on a possible relationship between the varying clinical pictures of these rhythmic activities and deviations either in drive capacity or in the ego's ability to contain the drives. He did, however, refer to investigations which linked these activities to discrete sensory functions.

Chess[13] and coworkers have studied nine characteristics of temperament and their relationship to behavior disorders over the past twenty years. Even though she referred to "biological irregularity' as being a component in understanding the temperamental characteristic (usually an exaggerated one), she was clear that she did not view this as reflecting a developmental deviation. This term she reserves for gross brain damage or mental retardation.

Cameron[11] described several trends in constructing a classification of diagnostic categories. His first category turned out to be developmental and included problems related to "physiological maturity or development" and "intellectual handicaps."

Provence and Ritvo[37] discuss a specific kind of developmental deviation found in institutionalized infants. They show that in spite of the presence of maturationally intact ego apparatuses, deprivation has a very damaging affect upon the development of various ego functions.

Anna Freud[22] wrote of developmental disturbances that were *not* disturbances reflecting a developmental deviation; these are ". . . mental disturbances . . . caused by the child's dependence and . . . the strains and stresses of development itself" (p. 154). In addition, however, she does refer to the "nonorganic disturbances of vital body needs . . . and excessive delays in acquiring vital capacities such as control of mobility, speech, cleanliness, learning." (p. 153) The term "nonorganic" would seem to refer to the absence of gross brain damage; this, then, suggests a form of disturbance similar to a developmental deviation.

Nagera[34] makes only a brief reference to developmental deviation. ". . . as many other forms of disturbances were . . . studied . . . some . . . differed from the normal not merely in quantitative terms. . . In some of these disturbances there were essential differences of a genetic and developmental nature. . . . These manifestations are rather dependent on a set of etiological factors that lead to deviations in development in one or many areas of the personality and finally to "atypical development. . . ." (p. 23) Thus his concepts of developmental interference, conflict, and disturbance are not related to developmental deviation.

Settlage[44] refers to the developmental disorders as "due to the inevitable and characteristic conflict associated with the successive stages of psychological development." His position appears to be similar to that of Nagera and A. Freud.

Rutter,[43] in a detailed study in 1969, reviewed the WHO Seminar on psychiatric disorders of 1967 along with a comparison of the GAP Report and stated "developmental disorders were especially important in relation to early childhood." He noted that there was good agreement, for instance, in how to apply the term to an eight-year-old youngster with greatly delayed development of speech and language. At the same time there was a great deal of discussion about the nature of the disorder, and much theoretical disagreement. He reserved the term developmental disorder for those abnormalities related to biological maturation; these were generally much more common in boys, and were not secondary to any other psychiatric syndrome. Thus, the category would include certain delays or distortions in development of speech or language. In addition, he would include examples of specific learning disorders, abnormal clumsiness, cases of enuresis or encopresis where the abnormality existed in isola-

tion and was not part of any other psychiatric syndrome. Rutter proposed a triaxial classification reserving developmental disorder for specific delays in development or for those abnormalities of development which were related to biological maturation and were not secondary to any other psychiatric syndrome. He suggested eight subcategories: (1) hyperkinetic; (2) delays or distortions in the development of speech and language where these were not part of a structured neurological disorder nor part of other psychiatric syndromes. Some examples might be: in the comprehension of sound as in developmental receptive aphasia or a developmental defect in the production of spoken language (developmental executive aphasia), or a developmental word-sound difficulty (disorder of articulation of speech); (3) other specific learning disorders; (4) abnormal clumsiness; (5) enuresis; (6) encopresis; (7) tics; (8) stuttering.

Ashburner[4, 5] suggested that developmental deviations be viewed as overlapping categories 306 and 308 from DSM-II. He saw reactive disorders and developmental deviations as two "polar clusters within one big class." Disagreeing with the GAP definition, however, he suggests that some deviations such as those of social skills, psychosexual development, affective development and the integrating function might be within the variation of normal.

Bemporad[6] studied the use of the GAP Report as a diagnostic classification for one year in his clinic, and found it useful. Developmental Deviations were diagnosed in 15 percent of cases.

Cohen[15] cites the need for recognizing developmental disabilities as reflecting the interaction of biological disorders, experiential, and environmental factors. In his view, these conditions are the expression of a complex combination of a biological endowment, maturation, and the nature of interpersonal experience.

Freeman[20] reported a study on the reliability of psychiatric diagnoses in childhood and adolescence. He analyzed the data obtained by a GAP subcommittee in 1968 using forty-four case histories, and reviewed the degree of agreement. The category of developmental deviation was used rarely and with a high rate of disagreement. Prugh and his colleagues[39] cited the aforementioned studies and considered the GAP classification, with its developmental framework useful. He stated that developmental deviations described those lags or precocities in motor, sensory, cognitive, social and other dimensions of development that were conceived to be based on inborn or innate individual characteristics, largely biological in origin, transcending the boundaries of the child and his environment.

Frequency, Incidence, Prevalence, Distribution and Cross-cultural Information

There are very few studies which yield concrete data. The general impression is that early in life far more boys than girls are observed to have developmental deviations. It also appears that there are more developmental deviations in the lower socioeconomic groups, but there are no hard figures.

The incidence of emotional disorders in early childhood is largely unknown. Studies of high-risk target groups, however, such as children in day care centers, reveal that at least one-third are viewed by teachers and clinicians as having mild problems which interfere with development. Another one-third show transient difficulties (Population Study of a Day Care Center, Child Development Center, Pre-School Liaison Project, New York City, January 1967. Another group revealed 23 percent before age six identified by mothers and psychiatric evaluation as having problems more significant than the normal range of transient difficulties.

Age of Onset: Developmental deviations occur more often in young children, specifically in the areas of speech, language, and motor development. Thus, the likelihood of a diagnosis being made is greater in the toddler and the pre-school child than with the older child. One might add that with a growing awareness of the need for thinking about developmental deviations and certainly with the possibility of employing it as a secondary diagnosis, it may appear more frequently.

Distribution Within Sibling Patterns: No data are available.

Special Studies: In the Bemporad[6] study of 310 children seen at the clinic during one year, the diagnosis of developmental deviation was made in 46 children (14.9 percent). In the Freeman study[20] such rough agreement as was obtained centered mainly around two of their forty-four cases. This fraction, less than 5 percent, were the only children viewed as suffering primarily from developmental deviation.

Clinical Course of the Condition

Much of the following material is based on Settlage's[44] work.

Characteristic features at each level of development will now be presented.

During the first year of life, the main features of the condition will be generalized signs of distress such as excessive crying, refusal to suck or excessive sucking, excessive regurgitation or vomiting, disturbance in bowel pattern, and disturbance of sleep. During the second and third years of life, as the child begins to crawl and walk, deviations in the motor sphere become apparent, such as poor coordination, jerky movements, and exaggerated temper tantrums. With the emergence of speech, there may be stuttering, unusual sounds with poor modulation, and other language difficulties such as lisps. Sleep disturbances may occur including nightmares and refusal to go to sleep without the presence of a parent. Delayed toilet training may represent a neurological lag as well as a delayed capacity to integrate body sensations, impulses, and the wish to please the parent. During the oedipal period, fear of the loss of the parent's love persists and tends to be expressed in fantasies of injury to the genitalia. These may heighten previously noted sleep disturbances or cause them to begin anew. Phobias are common as children advance through each phase of development; along with the advances, the possibility of regression to earlier phases increases. There may be lapses in bladder or bowel control; some children become excessively clinging and dependent. For the school-age child, the most common way for developmental deviation to appear is through some kind of school problem, either in learning or in behavior. Thus a child might not be able to sit still, or cannot integrate himself into the school group. In addition, there can be symptoms such as destructiveness, bullying, or stealing. Symptoms of earlier stages such as phobias, sleep disturbances, or problems with bladder or bowel control may persist.

One needs to distinguish between a developmental deviation and other disorders. In the first year of life, one must rule out the normal variation of healthy responses, as well as the possibility of disturbances related to an organic insult such as birth trauma, infection, or gross brain damage. With increasing age, a reactive disorder must be ruled out and more attention paid to environmental influences. As the child reaches the oedipal phase, neurotic problems need to be differentiated, and later still, the emergence of character disorder. Developmental deviations may become manifest over a period of months, but on the other hand, may not be apparent for a long time especially if only a single parameter of development such as motor or sensory growth is involved. A more global maturational deviation involving a general lag, unevenness, or precocity would be evident earlier. The deviations which include the capacity for control and integration in bodily functions such as eating, sleeping, speech, bowel and bladder function are usually easily noted. Those which involve only the motor system include the hyperactive, hypoactive, and poorly coordinated child. Time is often needed to evaluate fully the nature of the problem. Deviations involving the sensory system are often missed until a very careful history is taken which reveals that the youngster is either over-reactive to or apathetic in the face of various stimuli.

The most common developmental deviation is seen in the area of speech. Here deafness, oppositional behavior, elective mutism, brain damage or early childhood psychosis must be ruled out. During the third and fourth year of life disorders of articulation, rhythm or phonation, and a persisting infantile type of speech with poor comprehension become more evident. Disturbances involving only the cognitive functions usually are not apparent until the youngster enters school; at that point the differential diagnosis between mental retardation and developmental deviation often requires careful observation. Irregularities in social development with delayed capacities to handle brief separations from parents early in life often persist as the child grows, and take form as patterns of marked shyness, dependence, and inhibition, or immaturely aggressive behavior.

A deviation of psychosexual development may manifest itself as a persistent infantile autoerotic pattern or as markedly precocious or delayed heterosexual interests.

A deviation in affective development often can underlie moderate anxiety and excessive emotional lability, especially in the younger child. As the child grows older, one would need to differentiate between a growing obsessive-compulsive neurosis and a marked overcontrol of emotions stemming from a lag in affective development.

A deviation in integrative development often may underlie a profound lack of impulse control or poor frustration tolerance. The accompanying uneven use or overuse of various defense mechanisms may be helpful in discerning the presence of such a condition. It is important to keep in mind the possible applicability of this concept to certain aspects of the minimal brain dysfunction syndrome.

Regression itself, especially in the very young child, may reflect a developmental deviation in the capacity for integration. Some children seem to regress in the face of the slightest conflict or frustration, while other children respond with an attempt to develop more age-appropriate coping skills.

In addition, a predisposition to severe regression such as occurs in childhood schizophrenia may reflect an underlying developmental deviation, as reported in a case by Jordan and Prugh.[28]

Three case examples follow.

CASE #1. DEVELOPMENTAL DEVIATION—
DEVIATION IN MATURATIONAL PATTERN,
ESPECIALLY IN THE MOTOR SPHERE,
INTEGRATION, AND SPEECH

John was an almost four-year-old Caucasian boy referred to a therapeutic nursery school because of hyperactivity and immature speech. He was an only child. His parents, middle-eastern nationals, worked for an embassy as domestics. They occupied a one-room basement apartment where John was often kept in a crib for long hours.

Pregnancy and birth history were described as normal. John was not toilet trained.

At the referring center, he was described as frantic, refusing to follow directions, crying all the time, having tantrums, and into everything.

At the clinical center he was impulsive and clumsy, often knocking down toys and other children inadvertently. He didn't seem to realize the consequences of his actions as he went about pathetically trying to make friends. He always seemed surprised, as though everything was so new—toys, activities, people.

The initial formulation mentioned developmental deviation but it also included reactive disorder. The staff pondered over the history of inadequate stimulation bordering on sensory deprivation and wondered what effect it might have had upon his development.

Treatment was begun and, within several months, he was greatly improved. There were fewer tantrums, more responsive behavior, no crying, eagerness to attend school, and increased relatedness to peers and adults. Speech was better but still immature, and his hyperactivity, although reduced, still made him clumsy and impulsive.

It was felt that the reactive component of his

behavior had been neutralized by the therapeutic setting; what remained was the clinical picture of a developmental deviation in maturational patterns.

CASE #2. MENTAL RETARDATION, PSYCHOSIS, AND CHRONIC BRAIN SYNDROME

Bobbie was seen at age eleven for consultation. The specific request was for help with medication and appropriate placement.

He was the younger of two children. His older brother had been born with a cleft palate. Mother was pregnant during the 1964 rubella epidemic; otherwise birth history was normal. Bobbie was considered "fine" until he was one-year old, when he became acutely agitated, clawing at his skin. During the next two years his developmental milestones were delayed. He was taken for evaluation at age three because he was "unable to communicate." He was described as frenzied, putting everything into his mouth, and not relating appropriately to peers or adults. An EEG was normal.

From age four through eight he was enrolled at a therapeutic nursery-day center where various diagnoses including developmental deviation were considered. He was described as hyperactive, distractible, agitated, disorganized, with short attention span, poor speech, and deficits in fine and gross motor movements. He was tried on various medications, including stimulants and phenothiazides, all with only temporary relief.

Although various examiners felt there was improvement, over the years his course was essentially one of emotional arrest at around age three.

By age eleven, he was best described as retarded socially and intellectually, and psychotic. He needed haloperidol (Haldol) and almost constant one-to-one attention to make him manageable. Placement in a residential training school was recommended.

CASE #3. DEVELOPMENTAL DEVIATION IN MOTOR AND INTEGRATIVE DEVELOPMENT— ALSO, PSYCHONEUROTIC DISORDER, DEPRESSIVE TYPE, MILD

Richard, age five, was referred from his nursery school with poor impulse control. He had been considered a discipline problem at age two and was ejected from another nursery school at age four for poor behavior.

He was the youngest of four children and was considered "mother's baby." Pregnancy and birth history were normal. As an infant, he had been described as mildly restless. Around age two he became the "wild man." He had tantrums, wouldn't leave mother's side, was always on the move, and would listen only to father.

In nursery school, he punched other children, ran away, and could not ask for or accept help.

Psychological tests revealed a bright boy who was angry, depressed, hyperactive, and lacking in controls. In addition to being afraid of being hurt, there was a growing sense of falling apart. The psychologist was impressed with the constitutional aspect of his poor controls, and felt that this was reflected by the pronounced scatter on subtests in his psychological evaluation.

He was treated with methylphenidate hydrochloride (Ritalin) and once-weekly psychotherapy. His mother was seen regularly although less often and there was close contact with his teachers who were both sensitive and very cooperative. After one and one-half years, he was able to go to a normal private school. The medication and psychotherapy were stopped.

At age eight, he is doing well, is at the top of his math class, and seems very happy.

Organic Etiologic Factors— Endogenous Factors

Developmental deviations are due largely to endogenous factors which are currently poorly understood. It is in this area that work in the coming decades will help to elaborate more specifically the etiology of these deviations. It is to be hoped that forms of treatment or specific medications will be found to help with the course of development by compensating for the deviation, be it lag or precocity. Kessler[29] has introduced the concept of the "growth template" to highlight the biological factor which underlies these deviations.

Ritvo and his colleagues[41] report on a patient, Jerry, similar to Harold, described by Fries.[23] He was a thin, wiry child, almost constantly in motion. They comment on the interaction of the child's constitutional predisposition with that of his environment: ". . . both parents were observed using the child to a marked and unusual degree as an object to arouse and stimulate their own impulses and upon whom they could discharge both their sexual and aggressive impulses to an abnormal and unusual extent." (p. 117) They quote Escalona and Leitch: "Marked discrepancies between maturity of behavior in different areas of development reflect developmental deviations and are associated with disturbances of the child's adaptation to the social, biological, and physical environment. Irregular levels of maturity displayed within a single test may also reflect a disequilibrium in the child's adaptation to the demands of every day existence." They felt their patient used his motor equipment as an avenue of discharge for both loving and hostile feelings which often increased his state of disorganization. One of the results of this was that language became a game rather than a necessary skill in the service of communication. They comment that the degree of disorganization under stress was another indication of the child's ego disturbance. Since the patient's development appeared excellent the first nine months of life, they inferred that his "equipment" was adequate. They also wrote, ". . . there can be genetically or constitutionally determined disturbances in development which appear only after months or years." (p. 126)

This patient's difficulty resulted from developmental deviations both in the motor sphere where precocity was evident, and in the area of control, where development was decidedly below age level. Together these resulted in a decreased capacity for sublimation of his instinctual strivings.

Blodgett[9] reported the case of a five-year-old boy whose presenting symptoms included: delayed motor development, poor muscle tone, lack of coordination, general retardation, delayed bladder and bowel function, and delayed speech. Blodgett cited studies demonstrating a relationship between the patient's psychological state and the activity of his adrenal cortex. The author postulates that his patient's retardation of growth was related to hyperactivity of his adrenal cortex. This in turn he felt was induced by the emotional disturbance that stemmed from the child's relationship with his mother.

Psychodynamic Factors

INDIVIDUAL

Meers[32, 33] has made detailed studies through the psychoanalysis of several black ghetto children. He concludes, ". . . that the psychological microscopy of this work has outlined severe ego impediments which includes both subtle and gross distortions of perception and memory, and extends to chronic self-devaluation that affects motivation." In addition, he states, "the technique of psychoanalysis extends such psychiatric and social research in facilitating discriminations between developmental defects, developmental arrests, and neurotic inhibitions of ego functions." The presence or absence of a biological component would appear to be the key to the differentiation. His work, however, points to the possibility that with severe stress and distortion, a clinical picture simulating a developmental deviation can occur.

FAMILIAL

Codling[14] discusses developmental deviation in a group of children studied at Yale. These were youngsters in whom developmental problems, noted in the earliest months of life, had resulted in a disturbance of the mother-infant interaction. She stresses that our increasing understanding of the reciprocal interaction between child and parent makes us assume that these early problems adversely affect the development of normal satisfying relationships and mutual adaptation between child and parent. She cites a group of children in whom the constitutional factors cause the normal process of development to become either delayed or uneven. Some of these constitutional difficulties are due to early severe or chronic illnesses including prematurity, reactions to a difficult birth, or congenital defects of metabolism. She emphasizes the reactions of parents to youngsters with developmental deviation, noting "in some instances the parents react to a deviation of the child's normal development with a distortion of their perception of him that is far out of proportion to the reality situation." She gives the example of five-year-old Andy, who had been extremely uncomfortable in the first months of life with persistent colic, constant crying, and irritability. The parents were unable to comfort him and Andy reflected their attitude in this sad self-appraisal—"they don't like me much."

Another example is a four-year-old boy whose impulsive provocative behavior was uncontrollable in home and neighborhood. Treatment, including placement in a nursery school, was successful. The patient's attention span in play increased, and there was a modification in his impulsive behavior. As his behavior improved, his mother's depression increased and the mother began to question her own attitude in response to the patient. It was noted that the mother-child relationship was a receptacle for the mother's own conflicts about her marriage and her own parents. The patient's particular constitution and activity problems were reinforced by the mother's reaction to him; the circular spiral interacted and continued until they came for treatment.

REFERENCES

1. ACHENBACH, T., *Developmental Psychopathology*, Ronald Press, New York, New York, 1974.

2. ANTHONY, E. J., "Behavior Disorders in Childhood," in Mussen, P. (Ed.), *Carmichael's Manual of Child Psychology*, 3rd ed., vol. 2, pp. 667–764, John Wiley, New York, 1970.

3. ———, "Taxonomy Is Not One Man's Business," *International Journal of Psychiatry*, *3(3)*:173–178, 1967.

4. ASHBURNER, J., "Classification in Child Psychiatry," *Australian and New Zealand Journal of Psychiatry, 4*: 7–14, 1970.

5. ———, "Some Problems of Classification With Reference to Child Psychiatry," *Australian and New Zealand Journal of Psychiatry*, 2:244–249, 1968.

6. BEMPORAD, J. R., et al., "Twelve Months' Experience with the GAP Classification of Childhood Disorders," *American Journal of Psychiatry, 127*:118–124, 1970.

7. BERES, D., "Clinical Notes on Aggression in Children," in Eissler, R. S., et al. (Eds.), *The Psychoanalytic Study of the Child*, vol. 7, pp. 241–263, International Universities Press, New York, 1952.

8. BERGMAN, P., and ESCALONA, S. K., "Unusual Sensitivities in Very Young Children," in Eissler, R. S., et al. (Eds.), *The Psychoanalytic Study of the Child*, vols. 3/4, pp. 333–352, International Universities Press, New York, 1949.

9. BLODGETT, F., "Growth Retardation Related to Maternal Deprivation," in Solnit, A., and Provence, S., (Eds.), *Modern Perspectives in Child Development*, International Universities Press, New York, 1963.

10. BROWN, S., et al., *Outline for Psychiatric Classification of Problem Children*, rev. ed., New York State Hospital Press, Utica, 1937.

11. CAMERON, K., "Diagnostic Categories in Child Psychiatry," *British Journal of Medical Psychology, 28*: 67–71, 1955.

12. CHESS, S., *An Introduction to Child Psychiatry*, Grune & Stratton, New York, 1969.

13. ———, "Healthy Responses," in Freedman, A., and Kaplan, H. (Eds.), *Textbook of Psychiatry*, 1st ed., chap. 40, Williams and Wilkins, Baltimore, 1967.

14. CODLING, L. V., "Psychiatric Clinics for Children," in Solnit, A., and Provence, S. (Eds.), *Modern Perspectives in Child Development*, International Universities Press, New York, 1963.

15. COHEN, D. J., et al., "Mental Health Services for Children in Issues in the Classification of Children," in Hobbs N., (Ed.), *The Future of Children, I.*, Jossey-Bass, San Francisco, 1975.

16. ENGEL, M., "Dilemmas of Classification and Diagnosis," *Journal of Special Education, 3*:231–239, 1969.

17. ENGLISH, O., and PEARSON, G., *Common Neuroses of Children and Adults*, W. W. Norton, New York, 1937.

18. FINCH, S., *Fundamentals of Child Psychiatry*, W. W. Norton, New York, 1960.

19. FISH, B., "Limitations of New Nomenclature for Children's Disorders," *International Journal of Psychiatry, 7*:393–398, 1969.

20. FREEMAN, J., "A Reliability Study of Psychiatric Diagnosis in Childhood and Adolescence," *Journal of Child Psychology and Psychiatry, 12*:43–54, 1971.

21. FREUD, A., "The Symptomatology of Childhood," in Eissler, R. S., et al. (Eds.), *The Psychoanalytic Study of the Child*, vol. 25, pp. 19–41, International Universities Press, New York, 1970.

22. ———, *Normality and Pathology in Childhood*, International Universities Press, New York, 1965.

23. FRIES, M., "Congenital Activity Types," in Eissler, R. S., et al. (Eds.), *The Psychoanalytic Study of the Child*, vol. 8, pp. 48–63, International Universities Press, 1953.

24. ———, and WOOLF, P., "The Influence of Constitutional Complex on Developmental Phases," in McDermott, J., and Settlage, C. (Eds.), *Separation-Individuation*, International Universities Press, New York, 1971.

25. Group for the Advancement of Psychiatry (GAP), Committee on Adolescence, "Psychopathological Disorders in Childhood," Report No. 62, vol. 6, Group for the Advancement of Psychiatry, New York, 1966.

26. HARRISON, S. I., and McDERMOTT, J. F., *Childhood Psychopathology*, International Universities Press, New York, 1972.

27. Joint Commission on the Mental Health of Children, "Mental Health from Infancy Through Adolescence," *Report of Joint Commission on Mental Health of Children*, Harper & Row, New York, 1973.

28. JORDAN, K., and PRUGH, D., "Schizophreniform Psychosis of Childhood," *American Journal of Psychiatry, 128*:323–330, 1971.

29. KESSLER, J., "Nosology in Childhood Psychopathology," in Rie, H. E. (Ed.), *Perspectives in Child Psychopathology*, Aldine-Atherton, Chicago, 1971.

30. LOURIE, R. S., "The Role of Rhythmic Patterns in Childhood," *American Journal of Psychiatry, 105*:653–660, 1949.

31. MEEKS, J., "Behavior Disorders in Childhood," in Freedman, A., and Kaplan, H. (Eds.), *Comprehensive Text of Psychiatry*, 2nd ed., vol. 2, Williams and Wilkins, Baltimore, 1975.

32. MEERS, D., "Psychoanalytic Research and Intellectual Functioning of Ghetto Reared Black Children," in Eissler, R. S., et al. (Eds.), *The Psychoanalytic Study of the Child*, vol. 28, pp. 395–417, International Universities Press, 1973.

33. ———, "Contributions of a Ghetto Culture to Symptom Formation," in Eissler, R. S., et al. (Eds.), *The Psychoanalytic Study of the Child*, vol. 25, pp. 209–230, International Universities Press, 1970.

34. NAGERA, H., *Early Childhood Disturbances*, International Universities Press, New York, 1966.

35. NEUBAUER, P., "Disorders of Early Childhood," in Arieti, S. (Ed.), *American Handbook of Psychiatry*, 2nd ed., vol. 2, pp. 51–67, Basic Books, New York, 1974.

36. ———, "Panel Report on Diagnosis of Childhood Disorders," *Journal of the American Psychoanalytic Association, 11*:595–604, 1963.

37. PROVENCE, S., and RITVO, S., "Effects of Deprivation on Institutionalized Infants, in Eissler, R. S., et al. (Eds.), *The Psychoanalytic Study of the Child*, vol. 16, pp. 189–205, International Universities Press, New York, 1961.

38. PRUGH, D., "Psychosocial Disorders in Childhood and Adolescence," in *Mental Health of Children*, Harper & Row, New York, 1973.

39. ———, et al., "Chapter X in Issues in the Classification of Children," in Hobbs, N. (Ed.), *The Futures of Children I*, Jossey-Bass, San Francisco, 1975.

40. REXFORD, E., and VAN AMERONGEN, S., "Psychological Disorders in Grade School Years," in Arieti, S. (Ed.), *American Handbook of Psychiatry*, 2nd ed., vol. 2, pp. 68–84, Basic Books, New York, 1974.

41. RITVO, S., et al.,"Some Relations of Constitution, Environment and Personality," in Solnit, A., and Provence, S. (Eds.), *Modern Perspectives in Child Development*, International Universities Press, New York, 1963.

42. RUTTER, J., "Classification and Categorization in Child Psychiatry," *Journal of Child Psychology and Psychiatry, 6:*71–83, 1965.

43. ———, et al., "A Tri-Axial Classification of Mental Disorders in Children," *Journal of Child Psychology and Psychiatry, 10:*41–61, 1969.

44. SETTLAGE, C., "Psychologic Disorders," in *Nelson's Textbook of Pediatrics*, 10th ed., W. B. Saunders, Philadelphia, 1975.

45. ———, "Psychoanalytic Theory in Relation to the Nosology of Childhood Psychic Disorders," *Journal of the American Psychoanalytic Association, 12:*776–801, 1964.

46. SHAW, C., and LUCAS, A., *Psychiatric Disorders of Childhood*, 2nd ed., Appleton-Century-Crofts, New York, 1970.

47. SILVERMAN, J., and ROSS, N., "Mental Disorders in Childhood," in Wolman, B. (Ed.), *Handbook of Child Psychoanalysis*, Van Nostrand, New York, 1972.

48. SOBEL, R., "Adjustment Reactions of Infancy and Childhood," in Freedman, A., and Kaplan, H. (Eds.), *Textbook of Psychiatry*, 2nd ed., vol. 2, Williams and Wilkins, Baltimore, 1975.

49. THOMAS, A., and CHESS, S., *Temperament and Behavioral Disorders in Children*, New York University Press, New York, 1968.

50. THOMAS, A., et al., "A Longitudinal Study of Primary Reaction Patterns in Children," *Comprehensive Psychiatry, 1:*103–112, 1960.

12 / Psychoneuroses

Paul L. Adams

Definition and Introduction

The psychoneuroses of childhood are a special class of disordered behavior. Since categories are designed to meet the needs of behavioral scientists, the conventional classification, albeit generally useful, does not always match the picture the patient presents. Popular everyday usage is little better. It tends to label "neurotic" every behavior regarded as nonoptimal. In fact, however, "neurosis" is not synonymous with "deviance." A child's neurosis is more definite and more structured than a vague malaise, or a ripple of disobedience or fear. Technically, the term "psychoneurosis" refers to a distinctive—although, as childhood suffering goes, moderate or mild—type of patterned behavioral deviation of childhood. In common medical parlance, it is said that children with psychoneuroses show definite symptoms. For a neurosis to form, such symptoms have to occur; the deviation then becomes crystallized around them. Sometimes the term assigned is exactly "symptom neuroses" to separate these conditions from "character" deviations.

The symptoms in the neurosis are usually conceived of as originating in the child's efforts to cope with fear and anxiety and as continuing to express underlying inner conflict. This formulation is too simple, but it is a good starting definition. Some neuroses, in some children, are highly structured; others are not, and all these will be discussed presently. Neuroses may be primary, secondary, and partial or latent.

PRIMARY PSYCHONEUROSES

If childhood neuroses are sensibly conceived of as syndromes of behavior centered on anxiety, how is anxiety manifested behaviorally? Assuredly some forms of registering anxiety are not easily apparent to others. Nor is the child always aware of such feelings; he may find a way to hide the outward manifestations of felt fear. As a result tracking the subtle effects of anxiety can sometimes be very difficult. The involved anxiety is in fact, organismic: it is evidenced by changes in the locomotor (fight, flight), vegetative (pallor, galvanic skin response), endocrine (elevated blood pressure), mimetic (grimace), and phonatory (nervous talk) systems of the child's body. In many cases, but not in all, it is also experienced subjectively as tension, fear, strain, panic, or various disturbing visceral sensations. At the very least, there are vegetative and endocrine changes associated with every instance of anxiety in a child. Generally speaking, however, anxiety is guarded against and concealed; only in the psychophysiological laboratory or in an intimate clinical setting it is overtly observable. Nevertheless, it is present covertly, and inferences of its existence can be made by studying the varied strategies of defensive coping. These tactics are usually called *defense mechanisms*. Under proper circumstances they are readily apparent and can be evaluated and made use of in formulating a diagnosis about the kind of primary neurosis present.

As the child's introspection, insight, and candor develop, the child can report that he senses that something is amiss or "dumb" about his way of living, or that something creates a nagging sense of inconsistency or perplexity within him. This feeling of unpleasure can be considered as both cognitive strain and emotional ambivalence. Cognitively, it may be only a dim perception of a repetitive but fruitless method of problem solving and coping. From the emotional standpoint, the child experiences being anxiety-driven and dysphoric. The neurotic child's thinking seldom becomes grossly disorganized and rarely entails a major misperception of reality. Still, he may experience the distress of all that subjective discomfort, unrest, and unpleasure which attend neurotic behavior.

Of course, not all anxiety is neurotic. It is a feeling which develops in a complicated symbolic milieu. Distinctively human (although something quite akin to anxiety may be seen in other mammals) anxiety is experienced early in the life of each human child. "The source of anxiety is existence itself."[22] Nonetheless, even in infancy, anxiety can coalesce into definite behavioral symptoms; and the primary neuroses of childhood have been found to form at any time from infancy through adolescence.

SECONDARY PSYCHONEUROSES

The fear (anxiety) itself, as well as the derivative defensive activities connected with the fear, may occur in multiple, diverse behavioral contexts. Brain injured and psychotic children, as well as children with developmental deviations, must grapple with fears and anxieties, and may secondarily develop psychoneurotic symptoms—particularly anxiety attacks, depression, morbid fears, tics, obsessions and compulsions. Again, as Lauretta Bender[19] long ago described, the pseudoneurotic schizophrenic adolescent may present himself as if he were a sufferer from severe, mixed neuroses. It is appropriate to regard such a youth as primarily schizophrenic and only secondarily neurotic.

There are frequent instances of mixed neurosis. Thus, severe obsessives may have a few depressive and phobic symptoms. In all such instances, again by convention, the major set of the more serious symptoms is used to formulate the principal or primary diagnosis. For example, a diagnosis may be recorded (for statistical purposes) as "depressive neurosis with hypochondriacal features," or "anxiety neurosis with hysterical features."

PARTIALLY PSYCHONEUROTIC CONDITIONS

The sociopathic or delinquent child may present hints and *Anlagen* of neurotic symptoms that give the disorder a more hopeful prognosis. Especially when working with delinquents, the clinician looks carefully for signs of latent depression or obsession, for he knows that delinquents who have neurotic conflicts are more readily helped.

Without remediation, there are some five conditions which may develop into behavioral states that phenomenologically resemble the psychoneuroses, at least in part. These "latent forms" of childhood psychoneuroses are: the *personality disorders* (e.g., the compulsive personality may become symptomatic and engage in rituals); the *reactive disorders* (after reinforcers have come to impinge repeatedly on the child's behavior); the *psychophysiologic disorders*; the *developmental deviations*; and even the persistent, unattended, and unresolved, *crisis-coping* responses which may develop a neuroticlike fixity and rigidity.[68]

In Western societies, the inner conflicts borne by a neurotic child pertain to the internal elaboration of such emotions as fear, anger, dependency longings, sexual desire, and sadness. Different psychiatric schools single out and emphasize different emotions. Any emotion may function to trigger anxiety for the child.

Compared to many other patients, the psychoneurotic child is not a profoundly damaged person. Although he is unhappy, his suffering is usually contained within the societal norms of children's behavior. Such a child ordinarily does not need to enter a hospital or other segregated institution with special programs for behavioral control and therapy. To be sure, some childhood neuroses are totally incapacitating; they then fall into the category of chronic diseases that seriously diminish the full possibilities of human childhood. These are, however, the extreme cases. For the most part psychoneurotic conflict hampers and hurts, but does not totally cripple, the child. Neurotic conditions are often regarded as personal and individual (intrapsychic), entailing only mild to moderate social deviance. Even when they are moderately severe, they do not provoke general concern since their interpersonal roots and ramifications seldom spread beyond the child's immediate household. Still, other face-to-face contacts experienced by the child within primary groupings—with peers, playmates, teachers and neighbors—may be brought into the orbit of the child's psychoneurosis, and these significant others may both become aware of and be emotionally touched by the child's suffering. Eventually, they are often enough the people who take the child to an agent of healing to seek relief from his troubles. Thus the suffering can communicate and, in its own quiet way, affect the social realities that surround the child.

Classification in Child Psychiatry

For practical clinical purposes, a useful approach to nosology would be one that merely distinguished the group of neuroses—because they are presumed to be rather benign and are known to be learned—from the graver psychotic disorders that are organic or, at any rate, have more malign prognoses. In the first edition of his textbook, Leo Kanner[88] adopted a practical and common-sense Meyerian approach to the neuroses. The vocabulary he employed was not very familiar; he called these conditions the "minor psychoses," and tried to differentiate them from "the not essentially organic and not specifically oligergastic, parergastic, or thymergastic reaction patterns," that is, not organic, retarded, schizophrenic, or manic-depressive.

A TRI-AXIAL CLASSIFICATION

A Tri-Axial Classification has been proposed as a way to enhance not only the child psychiatrist's understanding of children but also his communication with his colleagues in other child-centered disciplines. Simply put, the three axes proposed by the World Health Organization 1967 Seminar on Psychiatric Disorders, Classification and Statistics[130] were: (1) the clinical psychiatric syndrome (one of which is "Neurotic disorder"); (2) the level of intellectual functioning; and (3) associated or etiologic factors, both psysical and environmental.

That such an approach would have great utility seems certain. If the International Classification of Diseases (ICD) does adopt these three axes of description of childhood disorders, then it seems likely that the forthcoming American Psychiatric Assocation revision of the DSM will try to bring American praxis into line with ICD. Such international agreement on diagnostic usage would undoubtedly be a step forward. Accomplishing this agreement, however, is not simple and easy. There are political ideologies that might become aroused and ruffled if a controversial diagnosis were given. For example, in some parts of the world, poverty, it is claimed, has been abolished as an etiological circumstance. Or, in America, there is the example of the removal of homosexuality from the list of psychiatric deviances. That is a matter on which ancient pieties clash with contemporary liberation movements. Diagnosis, therefore, is not devoid of political significance, especially when the prospect of societal etiology is invoked for serious consideration.

Since those who have written most about childhood neuroses have been governed less by rough-and-ready canons of clinical utility than by a concern for hairsplitting distinctions, there has grown up a profusion of fine nosologic terms that do little to enhance the clinician's work with distubed children. Hence, the novel approach taken by those preparing DSM–III[145] when they dropped the term "neuroses" entirely from children's disorders! Equally striking was Eysenck's "Ockham's Razor" approach, contending that the symptom itself is the disorder[47] and that one need not go further than the symptom.

Fish and Shapiro[50] studied forty-five children and derived inductively four major empirical types of childhood disorder:

Type I: Autistic-Disjunctive
Type II: Immature-Labile
Type III: Anxious-Neurotic
Type IV: Sociopathic-Paranoid

Their Types III and IV showed greater ego integration, better prognosis overall, higher IQ, and better response to placebo and environmental reinforcements than did their Types I and II. Thus a natural pooling of Types I and II, and again of Types III and IV, seemed to emerge, drawing distinctions that made a difference, clinically, as well as for research purposes. Presently, Types III and IV, the anxious-neurotic and sociopathic-paranoid, will be considered here.

The great humanistic philosopher, Wilhelm Windelband, a Heidelberg professor, described in his Strassburg lectures of 1900 (p. 27ff)[155] the distinction between *nomothetic* and *idiographic* knowledge, a distinction that has merit for study of childhood neuroses today. The former mode of understanding contemplates the general principles that emerge from a large number of observed cases, while the idiographic mode is concerned with what can be learned by detailed study of the unique individual. The work of Sigmund Freud exemplified the nomothetic, or generalizing, approach. Although he dealt with individual cases in great detail, he always viewed them as providing data for a more sweeping "project in scientific psychology." In his view, individuals acted out drives common to the species. Gordon Allport espoused the merit of a different viewpoint wherein the concrete individual is the sole focus of scientific work:

The most rigid tests of scientific procedure, fully admitted by nomothetists, are *understanding, prediction* and *control* above the levels achieved by unaided common sense . . . [T] hese rigid tests are met as readily by knowledge of the single case (secured often by means of personal documents) as by knowledge of nomothetic laws. (p. 59)[10]

In psychiatry and psychoanalysis, solitary cases have been very influential in making broad generalizations and in developing the contemporary theory of neuroses. If a case is striking, and behavior is dramatically and successfully changed, that single case becomes accepted as the prototype and an attempt is made to fit all others into its pattern (p. 259).[121] Freud's report on little Hans is an example of such a single case of childhood neurosis that became determinative of much of the child analysis to follow its 1909 appearance. Freud wrote of the Hans case[58] as if issuing a forewarning, that he was "tempted to claim for this neurosis of childhood the significance of being a type and model."

APPROACHES TO CLASSIFYING THE CHILDHOOD NEUROSES

According to psychiatric convention (under psychoanalytic influence) the five major subclasses of neuroses affecting children have come to be:

1. Actual neuroses: anxiety neurosis, neurasthenia, hypochondria, and depersonalization neurosis (Federn)
2. Psychoneuroses (also called symptom neuroses, or defense neuroses): (a) transference neuroses —Phobic, obsessive-compulsive and hysterical neuroses, and (b) narcissistic neuroses—melancholic depression (Helene Deutsch)
3. Character Neuroses
4. Traumatic Neuroses
5. Experimental Neuroses

These five subclasses will be described briefly.

The actual neuroses were those for which Freud "could find neither psychic causations nor psychic mechanisms."[117] He ascribed them to a misdirecting or misdeploying of more strictly somatic and sexual energies, rather than to the intrapsychic elaborations and structuring of those energies. This Freudian view was more widely accepted and applied more fully to children by Wilhelm Reich than by the less extreme Freudians. Reich seemed to insist that *all* neuroses are actual neuroses. Children could suffer from actual neuroses, indeed, if they masturbated or experienced forms of sexual tension for which they had no possible orgasmic discharge. They might then become panicky, ridden with fears, or steeped in hypochrondriasis. Children reared in sexual repression become neurotic, Reich insisted.[123] Even the more orthodox Freudians conceded that, when they were chronic, actual neuroses could be transformed into psychoneuroses, to wit, anxiety neurosis blends into phobic neurosis and neurasthenia into conversion hysteria. Hypochondria often turns into a schizophrenic psychosis.[117]

The *psychoneuroses* of childhood, originally considered by a socially critical Freud[123] to indicate a conflict between id and outside world, are often considered nowadays to be purely inner (thereby leaving out all reference to the anti-humanist aspects of society). They are thought to have oedipal conflicts at their core; they are felt to be amenable to cure by analysis of transference (unless the child is too narcissistic), and they include the classical (and common) symptom pictures such as phobic, obsessional, and hysterical patterns. These *psychoneuroses* will be the focus of this chapter.

Some children suffer from narcissistic wounds but lack the overt symptoms of psychoneurosis. They might nonetheless manifest partial internalization of external demands and develop *character neuroses*. In adults, these have been described by many writers from Abraham, Reich and Glover to Franz Alexander and Fromm; in children the character neuroses have been listed by the Group for the Advancement of Psychiatry[68] under the rubric of "personality disorders."

Traumatic neuroses in children were described best in Freud's early views that children often were seduced and molested by adults, and in Otto Rank's views about the traumatic quality inherent in every separation experienced by a growing child. When the upset is persistent and pervasive, (or merely overwhelming for the child —as in war and violent revolution, or in being subjected to physical abuse by one's parent, or suffering shipwreck, earthquake, tornado) the child shows a strong tendency to reexperience the trauma, often in the form of frightening dreams. His behavior becomes disordered, but according to Freudian theory, *without containing a masked infantile wish*. It is this combination of precipitating trauma plus lack of the id wish or longing that produced the earmarks of the traumatic neurosis.

Experimental neuroses have seldom been intentionally inflicted on children, although J. B. Watson's conditioning of Albert to fear furry objects was an exception.[153] Because of the ethical restraints, experimentally induced neuroses usually have involved cats, rats, dogs, and monkeys, but usually not children. As a part of the procedure of behavior therapies, however, something analogous to experimental neuroses does occur. Under certain circumstances, when neurotic symptom removal from children is accomplished, it is followed by a *reinstating* of the neurotic symptom (as the acid test showing the symptom's tie to reinforcers). In such instances there is a formal analogy to experimentally induced neuroses in childhood.[90]

CONCEPTS OF CHILDHOOD NEUROSES CHANGE

The Diagnostic and Statistical Manual of Mental Disorders, Second Edition (DSM–II) was published in 1968 by the American Psychiatric Association,[69] replacing the first DSM which appeared in 1952. In DSM–II, the neuroses of childhood were in no way separated from the neuroses of adults; and, as shown by parenthetical enclosure in the following list, this was echoed by the child psychiatrists in the Group for the Advancement of Psychiatry:[68]

300	Neuroses (GAP: Psychoneurotic Disorders)
300.0	Anxiety neurosis (GAP: Anxiety type)
300.1	Hysterical neurosis
300.13	Hysterical neurosis, conversion type (GAP: same)
300.14	Hysterical neurosis, dissociative type (GAP: same)
300.2	Phobic neurosis (GAP: Phobic type)
300.3	Obsessive-compulsive neurosis (GAP: Obsessive-compulsive type)
300.4	Depressive neurosis (GAP: Depressive type)
300.5	Neurasthenic neurosis (Neurasthenia)
300.6	Depersonalization neurosis (Depersonalization syndrome)
300.7	Hypochondriacal neurosis
300.8	Other neurosis

The GAP Committee on Child Psychiatry proposed even fewer categories of neuroses than had the APA-sponsored DSM–II. When psychiatrists find themselves becoming attached to a particular diagnostic system, they often proclaim: "After all, diagnosis is a vital analytic process, not a static entity; *diagnosis* from its Greek derivation means *thorough understanding*." DSM–II made sufficient modifications on DSM–I to give evidence that dynamisms are involved in diagnosis; and recently DSM–III entered the stream of diagnostic classification[145] and promised to make further alterations. Some of the proposed changes signified an evolving theory and practice, while other changes attempted actively to alter (not merely to reflect) the course of theory and practice.

In the late seventies, the field stands at an interesting juncture in notions about classifying and labeling children. Two potent and countervailing forces are at work in Western psychiatry. On the one hand, there is a growing movement to set forth the sociological view that labeling is a form of social control whereby societal definitions of behavior as *insane* or *mad* are imposed upon relatively powerless individuals, thereby impelling them to take up roles which perpetuate the stigmatizing behavior. According to extreme proponents of labeling theory, such as Howard Becker, Thomas Szasz, and Ronald Laing, labeling as such is sociogenic of madness. All this was critically reviewed in 1976 by Jane M. Murphy.[115] On the other side of the attack on labeling is a tendency embodied in the current framers of DSM–III, whose efforts are to discard all labels which have not been supported and validated by research. They seem to say, let us keep only those labels that make a real difference. That is a clean sweep approach that could in the long run have salutary effects on child psychiatry generally and the classification of the childhood neuroses in particular. Some practitioners will be distressed that the preciosity of a long list of neuroses, often more metatheoretically based than research-proven, will drop out of usage. Certain practitioners will hesitate to depart from the past, regardless of whether the tradition is actually "tried and true." That is not to overlook a rather sturdy tradition among psychoanalysts to reduce their diagnostic work to a very scanty operation, since they feel it sets up a self-fulfilling prophecy for the therapist.

Common Neurotic Types

Traditionally, the common neuroses of children include:

Two Actual:	anxiety neurosis (anxiety reaction)
	hypochondriasis
Four Defense:	phobic neurosis
	conversion hysteria ("Briquet's syndrome")
	dissociative hysteria
	obsessional neurosis
One Narcissistic:	depressive neurosis

There are also depersonalization and neurasthenic neuroses in childhood, but they are rarer than the seven types listed. These seven patterns will be described as they emerge in various ages and life conditions. Taking off from that base in more or less sound psychiatric tradition, the discussion will move later into some of the newer concepts concerning the neuroses of childhood.

ANXIETY NEUROSIS

The child is said to be suffering from this condition when unvarnished fear bursts forth in his life, in the form of repeated attacks of panicky feelings (anxiety) that somehow are not defended against with the "ego defense mechanisms," i.e., the usual devices of repression or denial. Anxiety neurosois is probably the most frequent form of neurotic "nervousness" in both children and adults. Sometimes young infants early become adept at showing fear and anxiety, both because they pick it up from their caretakers and because of temperamental differences that manifest themselves early in the life cycle. Initially, the child with anxiety neurosis seems always skittish and on the verge of panic; ultimately he resolves into a child with more workable but neurotic defenses that "bind anxiety" into conversion hysteria, phobic neuroses or others.

The classic description, made four and one-half decades ago by Katherine M. Banham Bridges, told how the neonate shows the emotion of *excitement*, the three-month-old child *distress*, and the six-month-old infant *fear*.[24] That is, she showed how anxiety or *fear* appeared in the growing child only at six months of age, how at that age it differentiated out of *distress* which, in turn, had emerged from a prior generic *excitement* that held sway (from an emotional standpoint) from birth to almost three months of age. Hence, a more general excitement, not a recognizable anxiety,

seemed to be observable in neonates, all poetry about birth canal anxieties notwithstanding. Chess and her associates[32] delineated the components of the *anxious* infant, perhaps, in their description of the *difficult* infant—irregular rhythms, withdrawal from new stimuli, frequent negative mood, intense reactions, and slow adaptability to change. Such an infant is discernable by two to three months of age and brings its own temperamental dynamics into its developmental encounters with the world around.

The difficult children not only have the jitters but make others jittery. Their agitation and hyperkinesis are out of the ordinary, and are detected as such by nursery school and kindergarten teachers as well as by the parents. As the children grow older, an episodic and formal pattern comes to show itself in their times of panic, often consisting of feelings of "tingling" or as one hyperkinetic child once described it, "a crawly electric feeling." The newer structuring and constellating deserves the name of *anxiety neurosis*. If the hyperkinesis is blatant, sexual unrest or fear of neglect and abandonment are usually the driving forces. (See also Chapter 20.)

The fullblown textbook picture of the emotional state and behavioral problems in anxiety neurosis is one of: impending doom; inadequacy feelings; indecisiveness; insomnia; irritability; restlessness; school problems; and unease. As always happens in emotional expression, there is autonomic alerting demonstrated by the following signs and symptoms: diarrhea; dilation of pupils; dizziness; dryness of mouth; fear of imminent death; nausea; palpitations; sweating; and trembling.

To illustrate this condition, Lucy was an anxiety-ridden little girl. She was the third child of a plumber and a mother who worked in a textile mill. Her two older sibs were males and a sister was one year younger. Lucy was nine when she was brought to the psychiatry clinic by her alcoholic father, who, when sober, proved to be her closest ally in the household. Father remarked, "Lucy is catered my way and gets upset when her mother fusses at me. My wife is a very high strung person. Since I got back from overseas I have noticed that all three of the girls are nervous and high strung. (This was no slip of the tongue for he considered his wife on a par with his two daughters.) My wife and I spat and that tears Lucy to pieces. She (the wife) goes all to pieces if my plumbing business does not bring in a steady income. She fusses a lot at me for trying to have a shop of my own, but by now I've had it for six months, and it is beginning to go better. My wife thinks she's a better Christian than I am, and that makes Lucy worry if I'll go to heaven. Lucy wants to stick with me all the time and that makes my wife mad—she wants Lucy to go on outside. . . . Lucy did very well in school right up to this year. This year she barely gets by, and seems to have a horror of school." Father, seen initially, as well as Lucy, gave a story of these additional problems: a feeling that nobody liked her at school, worry about the family's inability to provide candy and clothes and material possessions, fear of going to sleep at night (particularly if father was out of the house, because then he was usually drinking), frenzied hunting for father's Antabuse pills (he hid them when he wanted to set out on a binge of drinking, and the family tried to find them in order to force him to take them regularly).

Lucy was fretful and lived in fear that her father might murder her mother when he became drunk. "I'm afraid he'll get drunk and run in on Mommy and hurt her. They used to beat up one another, but he is way stronger than Mommy is. I don't want either one to get hurt. I don't like one of them more than the other one. My mother gets me more things when she gets paid, but my Daddy gives me my way except when he's drinking. I stay scared that somebody will get killed when he drinks. I had a dream that Daddy got killed in a fight with a man with a funny name I had never heard. It sounded like a foreigner's name. I forgot what it was. But I said to myself when I saw Daddy dead, in the dream, 'From now on, he'll be home every night.' I rushed and buried him, before my Mommy got home, between the pine tree and the light pole . . . I hope my Daddy don't get hurt. I hope that bad dream never comes true. I don't like my mother no more than my Daddy. He furnishes groceries and she furnishes me clothes, and it's important to be dressed and to have something to eat, both. I can't take sides, because if I did then they'd give my sister and brothers something without giving it to me. So I have to look like I ain't on neither one's side."

It seemed a fortunate circumstance that Lucy and her parents received some help just as her anxiety-neurotic picture was settling into a more fixed structure, with prominent hysterical and phobic features. As it was, her naked anxiety was available to be dealt with, and she obtained relief from "ego-oriented" parental guidance and individual psychotherapy—a total of some forty contacts spread over fourteen months.

HYPOCHONDRIACAL NEUROSIS

This form of narcissistic/actual neurosis is seen in the sometimes frail but often robust child who complains of both emotional and physical complaints as if they were belovedly embraced parts of the self. These children have a lowered capacity to achieve insight as to the contexts in which their troubles arise. They have adopted a very simple form of reasoning that goes something as follows, "I am sick. Do not try to make me out to be anything but sick. I am not pretending, my sickness is real. I hurt. I do not know conflict; I am not tense or fearful—I simply hurt." They do,

however, have troubles which, like other neuroses, arise from and are aggravated by stressful interpersonal relations. Although they cling tenaciously to the somatic symptoms, these really carry little intrinsic import. However, they do give out messages to the child's parents and other intimates of needs that are otherwise suppressed and unspoken.

Since many psychotherapists do not like hypochondriacs very much, they find it difficult to decipher the child's transmitted message. In many cases, a brief and confronting therapeutic approach to the parents, individually or together, helps to soften up the hard core of somatic preoccupation within the family; it thereby makes subsequent treatment of the child easier. In eclectic and flexible clinical experience, these children are served better if the psychiatrist does periodic physical examinations and uses the physical contact to bridge over the relatedness gap between the obsessively concerned child and the often rather indifferent and irritated doctor. The doctor tenaciously resists the child-parent effort to badger him into sending the child to a round of unnecessary consultants, and is piqued by the unflattering suggestion that the doctor may be "overlooking something important." The case vignette that follows illustrates how hypochondriasis may arise without physical illness, reflect family conflicts, accrue both primary and secondary gain, and be treated by skillful phasing of the work with parents and child.

W. R. was an eight-year-old firstborn son of a career soldier (sergeant rank) and a mother who was a sickly, nagging, complaining housewife. The parental pair had been married for ten years. By the time they brought eight-year-old Willie to a child psychiatry clinic, they had borne two daughters who were three years old and six months old, respectively. The family was pervaded by discord between mother and father. The promiscuous father was actively accusatory and jealous of his frigid wife in ways that bordered on paranoid delusions. The mother was, in reality, "faithful" to her despised spouse. With a family history that included four generations of "nervous breakdowns," the mother's enjoyment of bad health included belief that she had a displaced coccyx, ulcerative colitis, a bladder infection, a chronic vaginal discharge, and bouts of "sick headache." Both mother and father were of working-class backgrounds. Both came from families with health concerns but who had been unable to pay for the best health care. The father rebuked mother for being a spendthrift, a coddler and sissifier of little Willie, and he decried her as a wife who could not be warmed up by any of his "Kama Sutra" strategies and his techniques of foreplay and coitus that worked supremely well with his casual, extramarital lovers. Father moved about quickly, for, in addition to his military position, he worked as an electronics repairman at nights, and still managed some extramarital sexual activity.

Little Willie learned well, for his age, how to enact depression, complaining, passive aggression, and projection. He complained incessantly of stomachaches, headaches and nervousness. Since his dad beat him cruelly when he was crossed, Willie gave his father a wide berth. Father accused mother of alienating Willie's affection.

Mother responded indulgently to every one of the boy's physical symptoms and attributed them to nervousness induced by the father's maltreatment of both the son and her. She petted, massaged, and medicated the boy as if she were nourishing an ailing prince who she hoped would get strong enough one day to avenge her with a parricidal gesture. Willie expertly played the role of a slowed, depressed, fragile little flower *most of the time* . . . until he became a firesetter, undeterred by his father's brutal fisticuffs. Firesetting was the symptom which prompted father and mother to bring their son to the clinic. Willie's hypochondriasis, marked by depression-withdrawal alternating with acting out (firesetting, abuse of the three-year-old sister), was unrelieved until marriage therapy for the parents led them into an improved conjugal relation. Soon thereafter, their parenting improved and brief individual therapy brought dramatic improvement to Willie's hypochondriasis.

PHOBIC NEUROSIS

Formerly called *anxiety hysteria*, the phobic neurosis of childhood is ordinarily regarded as one of the "transference neuroses" and is placed somewhere between (conversion and dissociative) hysteria and obsessive neurosis. The phobic child, said to be caught in an oedipal situation, strives to mute the anxiety he feels, first by detaching it from the actual situation, or person or idea or thing, which is feared. The second step is to displace the anxiety onto a symbolic situation, person, idea, or thing. He is then free to be comfortable with the source of the anxiety, and to be afraid of the symbol. In short, a neurotic fear symptom has developed. It is important to recognize that the anxiety symptom is economical, thus: the little boy fears horses to symbolize the father—after all, it is far easier for him to avoid horses than to avoid father; the little girl fears spiders to symbolize the punitive, devouring mother, and again the advantages of such an arrangement are obvious. Similarly, the adolescent male fears appearing in public to symbolize his wish to exhibit his enlarging genital; the adolescent female fears high places because they symbolize her longings to be sexually promiscuous; for each, it is far better to face the one fear than even allow themselves to think about the other. As long as the phobic situation is avoided, which can be exhausting and nerve-wracking enough (to both child and family members), there is no panic. But as soon as the phobic "thing" is too proximate, dread breaks out; the restricted, over-controlled world of the phobic collapses, and a state bordering on panic or agitation ensues.

Freud's reflection on and study of childhood phobias caused him to alter his views about anxiety. These, briefly put, changed greatly from his early view that the life energy, *libibo*, became fixated at various pregenital phases and because libido was "dammed up" and not expressed genitally, a transformation of libido occurred to produce anxiety. Later, Freud in 1926 decided that this did not ring true clinically, and modified the earlier formulation as follows: Not blocked libido but an overwhelming inflow of stimuli (especially aggression) accounts for anxiety. Freud gave the experience of birth, and its significance for the neonate, as the prototype of triggering this traumatic anxiety that overwhelmed the infant. Thus far, his view did not remove him too far from his earlier views about traumatic anxiety. However, a distinctly novel modification lay in his introducing *signal anxiety*, namely, the anticipatory anxiety of the "burned child who avoids the fire." The child, once traumatized and bathed in traumatic anxiety, learns to anticipate in fantasy a traumatic happening and to become fearful before the trauma strikes. This latter anxiety was learned (not reflexive and automatic), took place as an ego operation (even if it attempted to ward off id forces), and originated in death energy (Thanatos or *mortido*)—aggression discharged against the self.

Freud differentiated between (1) objective anxiety (*Realangst*) in the face of an external agent inducing terror and (2) neurotic anxiety which sprung from internal representations of impulses which threatened imperiously to overwhelm the person. Both of these forms were distinguished from (3) moral anxiety which entailed superego-initiated punishment. Neurotic anxiety, as meticulously explained by Freud, could either be *free-floating*, that is, relatively unattached, or *phobic* and specifically, and intensely, attached to a substitute object, *or panic* in which one fears a demolition of the ego apparatuses by naked impulse.

Phobic anxiety often held, Freud contended, a fear of castration or genital injury at its innermost core. At the heart of many neuroses is the castration complex, derived in the case of the male from a boyish egocentrism, expecting all human beings to have penises, and from a belief that parents disapprove of the boy's genitality.

Similarly, the castration complex of girls emerges directly, Freud suggested, from the girl's discovery that she lacks a penis, from the subsequent penis envy felt by her, and from her tendency to accept the clitoris as a small penis, partly making up for her lack of the larger organ, and in some analyzed cases of frigidity, from her inclination to become fixated on clitoridal sensations, blocking her from maturing to the level of "vaginal orgasm." A vignette of a seven-year-old boy will illustrate some of the characteristics of a phobic child.

Isaac S. was the older of two sons. Mother had divorced their father six years earlier when Isaac was one year old and the little brother was still unborn. Since that time she had slept in one bed with both sons in a household run by the maternal grandmother, a great aunt and a great uncle. The boys' father showed not a flicker of interest in their upbringing and support. They lived in a small southern town where Isaac's mother worked in a cotton mill. The younger brother was outgoing and an easy child for the mother, but Isaac was a "scaredy cat." He was afraid to go to school when a schoolmate threatened to bring a knife the next day. He lived in constant dread of being struck on the nose and dying of nosebleed. He developed elaborate precautions against being hit—he would walk up to complete strangers and say, "I like you. You won't hit me, will you?" His mother said that he begged her "not to switch him when he makes noise. He's got this fear of his nose bleeding him to death. The other night I didn't whip him but just made him sit in the corner. He acted plumb crazy. He had this crying fit, saying he knew he was about to die. He don't act like a normal child at them times."

In the playroom Isaac seemed to be testing his own bravery, for he loved aggressive shooting and dart-throwing. At times, however, his counterphobic devices fell down and he would say odd things, such as, "Let me slow down and take off my jacket so I don't get too tired. I may get sick or get a nosebleed." In the first interview he gave these three wishes: (1) "I wish I had a car, a big grownup's car to drive. Little boys are too little to drive, but I'd wish for a car so I could go fishing and go to see Myrtle" (a relative who lived in another city); (2) "I'd wish for a farm with a horse on it, but more than a horse I'd like a big bunch of cows to milk;" (3) "I wish that I had power like Jesus who made us all, so I could make it warm when I wanted, or cold, or make it rain."

It was soon a matter of clear consensus between mother and her therapist that Isaac had too many bosses, especially too many grandparental figures. But what could the mother do? She could not afford to move out of the household. She could not manage to pay baby sitters when she worked. She was stuck, she said. She slept in a double bed with both boys, and in the same room where the maternal grandmother and great aunt slept together in a second double bed, with the maternal great uncle in a single bed. That was the only room they could afford to heat in wintertime. The boy slept next to mother, and in consequence of his close attachment to her,

he had seen her menstrual flow on her gown as well as on the menstrual pads. He did not speak of this to her but he thought "it meant she had been injured." Shortly afterward, he developed his phobia of uncontrollable epistaxis.

CONVERSION HYSTERIA

Hysterical children show five features with considerable regularity:

1. An enchanted world view. They are given to more primitive, or magical, or infantile, perspectives than their normal agemates. In social traditions, the child with conversion hysteria today is usually not urbanized, but peasant.

2. Extreme expressions of emotion. These children are overly dramatic, like ham actors, and display a pervasive egocentrism. Their emotional repertoire is not as substantial as it is flamboyant. Emotions of self-regard are frequently defenses against feelings of unimportance, lack of substance, and a compulsion to keep up a "good act" so as to ward off *nonexistence*.

3. Increased suggestibility and identification. They are conformist "copy cats" who more quickly identify with, than empathize with, another person. This accounts for their frequently adopting the symptoms of relatives and schoolmates, and becoming slavishly attached to a mentor.

4. Disturbed sensorimotor functions. Their symptoms run from deafness or blindness to choreas and paralyses. Paradoxically, toward their conversion symptoms, they display a lack of worry or flamboyance as if they are now playing an acceptable sick role. This is the well-known primary gain. Their conceptions of anatomy are crude to nonexistent, thus, their anesthesias follow no sensory distribution known to a freshman medical student. Psychoanalysts emphasize how the conversion symptoms lessen the pangs of anxiety while they symbolize, at the same time, the now unconscious (repressed) wish. The paralyzed hand is the one that would, if gratification were possible, masturbate, or carry out a physical assault, or thumb a nose.

5. Altered consciousness. They are, for example, indifferent to and unaware of what is going on around them—even to the point of detaching from their sense of reality—as in a hysterical anesthesia. Their attentional priorities are often given over to fantasies about taboo matters; these, however, too readily put them in touch with drives that are real, so they quickly divert their attention as well as they can to self-obliterating repression.

Hysterical children conspicuously display cognitive strain and communication deficits. They live in households where there is a big discrepancy between what people long for (or practice) and what they preach. According to Angyal,[13] the families adopt a method of vicarious living in which everyone's real self is subdued in order to put forth a substitute self—this is ordinarily described as "repression." An example of discordance between practice and preachment is Freud's case of the Wolf Man. There, the parents punished and proscribed lust and sexuality for the children right alongside their own enjoyment of frequent, fun-filled and "fancy-frilled" sexual behavior. Another example, well described by James Proctor,[122] is the dissonance produced by a dull life of stolid conformity and privation lived out simultaneously with ideologies about hell-fire-and-damnation contrasted with heavenly bliss on streets paved with gold. The apocalyptic visions that, over and over, have inspired the weary poor and oppressed may provide other examples of the discrepancy between practice and preachment, or the real and the substitute self, which furnishes the basic life situation for inducing his neurosis into a hysterical child.

Preschool children furnish vivid instances of the rapid-fire spread of hysteroid symptoms from one child to an entire nursery group. All of them want to urinate at the same time; one gets hurt and they all limp and whimper as if a single noxious stimulus had been brought to bear on one undifferentiated mass child. And boys freely copy girls and girls copy boys at the age of three to six years.

By *elementary school age,* there is more structuring of sex role, with a preponderance of hysterical adaptations among females that endures throughout the remainder of the life cycle.

Early adolescence is a time "made for" hysterical formations, in a sense, since the common plight is one of leaving behind some old roles and identities before the new formations have crystallized. Asking "Who am I?" the adolescent is anxious, imitative, and hysteria-prone. This is true, many clinicians aver, for both male and female. The author has worked with two young adult male hysterics who, when the respective wives became pregnant, became blind, in one case, and paralyzed, in the other. Hysteria knows no particular gender or season in the life cycle.

The following vignette illustrates some of the typical phenomena of hysteria first appearing in childhood.

B. A., a rather seductively self-conscious, young black woman of seventeen years complained: "I am nervous. I have some kind of nervous spells. Last night my father carried me to _____ Hospital with one of these nervous spells and they referred me here. I had a spell like that when I was up in New Jersey last month . . . I just begin to get cold when the spell comes on. I feel all shook up and want to run. I don't want to be where it is dark or closed up. I don't want to be inside the building. But before I can run I fall out, black out." Her spells consisted of deep breathing, stiffening, foaming at the mouth, and tongue-chewing. Her symptoms dramatized her powerlessness. The EEG was normal.

This adolescent had her first episode of "falling out" at six years of age. She was helping her mother wash and dry dishes when her mother harshly reprimanded her, "Get outa my way!" At age ten her second "spell" occurred, and the third at age fourteen (before her mother's death in that same year). She then stayed free of the spells until her father's remarriage when she was sixteen. She completed high school at age seventeen, and during the summer following high school graduation she "went north" to work as a waitress, hoping to earn enough money to support herself in college. Her vocational plan was abandoned when she had a passing-out spell. Her favorite brother, Johnny, was in the army overseas. He had promised to help her pay for college, but she had not wanted to depend too heavily on his generosity.

Ms. B. A. had attempted sexual intercourse one time in the autumn of her senior year, enjoying it "not a bit" but "a little glad to get it over with," since she saw it as a badge of mature womanhood. In the past, she had undertaken to perform tasks precociously because, she said, she wanted to grow up fast. She was a diligent student, and the youngest person in her class. At fourteen, when her mother died, she carried on, as if grown up, to perform housework and schoolwork and to serve her father and sibs faithfully. The stepmother was a woman who "goes to church a lot and she thinks we ought to. Sometimes she is nice but then she'll be . . . well, I don't know how to say it. Before I got sick she thought I was bad and that I ought not to go to teenage dances on Friday nights. She has two girls of her own, not by my Daddy, and she don't worry about them doing bad as much as she does about us." The stepmother urged B. A. to go to faith healing sessions at church, but her father opted for a psychiatric approach in addition to the religious one. Fortunately, a free psychiatric clinic was available to her.

The psychiatrist deemed it necessary to demystify an experience that seemed, to the adolescent patient, to have no origins and to make no sense at all. He therefore took a highly directive, confronting approach. She was encouraged to try to remember when and where her spells came on, what feelings she was having, and toward whom. She was further instructed to try at once to change the symptom-course by going outside, even by running, if that seemed to forestall the fainting spell. In addition, she was given the promise (never taken up) of some pills (a minor tranquilizer) if she could not get rid of her "falling out," thus offering a bridge to support her self-esteem as she tried to move from a symptomatic to nonsymptomatic state. In order to de-repress and better integrate her conflicting interpersonal roles, demands, and messages, effort was made to continue exploring for the meaning of her "unpleasure." She became more honest and candid about her real feelings, acknowledged more of the ambivalence in her relations with father, favorite brother, stepmother and therapist. Pretense and vicarious gratification thereupon lessened. Especially with stepmother, she learned ways other than symptoms to "get that witch off my back." She worked with dreams and claimed them as another part of her more direct, fuller life. She became symptom-free, relative to her falling-out episodes, but stopped treatment before she had become fully orgastic or had been financially able to enroll in college.

DISSOCIATIVE HYSTERIA

According to the American Psychiatric Association's second edition of the *Diagnostic and Statistical Manual of Mental Disorders* (DSM–II) the hysterical neuroses are subdivided into conversion hysteria and dissociative hysteria. The same children who suffer from conversion reactions may also develop dissociative reactions, since both disorders grow out of a hysterical personality and a hysterical family milieu in which vicarious living is prized. Although the full range of dissociative reactions is rarely seen nowadays, they do constitute about 5 percent of all childhood neuroses. There are four principal forms of dissociative reactions that are still seen occasionally (chiefly among "nonstandard" culture groups). These include amnesia, fugues, multiple personality, and somnambulism. In all forms, however, there are certain threads that run a common course. The main ingredients of childhood's dissociative neuroses are:

1. Disturbances in consciousness. Since the earliest descriptions by Pierre Janet and William James, the splitting of experience into a part that is aware and a part that is outside awareness or consciousness has been given a great deal of emphasis. The dissociation in consciousness is what makes this form of hysteria so highly dramatic, whether the disturbance occurs as twilight states, narcolepsy, trances, stupor, or pseudodelirium.

2. Personality disorganization. The breakup in the self may be temporary, but it is comprehensive. The child exhibits intense disavowal, or denial (unlike repression), disclaimer and even amnesia for things that he has done. The personality structure is usually said to be weakened or split, in response to a drastic sense of threat or stress upon the self-concept. The patterns of cracking up range from depersonalization to multiple personality.

3. Odd motor expressions. The overt behavior of the child may cover a gamut from aimless running and pacing, to catalepsy, narcolepsy, cataplexy, and to fugue states. Neurotic "somnambulism" has been greatly publicized but should be carefully distinguished from children's sleepwalking which is not hysterical. Nonhysterical sleepwalking takes place in non-REM stages of sleep and is overcome by "outgrowing it."

W. J., a ten-year-old white girl from the Appalachian mountains, had an ecstatic religious experience at a midsummer Holiness revival meeting. Theretofore shy, she "turned on" at the revival meeting, envisioned herself alternately reposing in the arms of Jesus and preparing to be a warrior for Christ in readiness for Armageddon. She spoke in a loud, firm voice that surprised her mill-working mother but also gave the mother great pleasure. She writhed, appeared to have an orgasm, spoke in strange tongues and shouted out that she had been *saved*. The next day she seemed aloof and serene, but had total amnesia for the preceding evening.

A month later she was missing from the bedroom she shared with a younger sister and two brothers and could not be found for more than a week. She was absent on the opening days of school. This was surprising since she had apparently always liked school, although she had been only a fair student during the first four grades. When found in a knob town some twenty miles from her home she insisted that she had a different name, and when she was taken back home, she did not seem to recognize her mother and father or her sibs. Her first look of recognition came as she asked her father to promise not to beat her any more. By the following morning she had "snapped out of it" and disclaimed any memory for anything that had happened to her during the whole week of her departure from home and subsequent return.

OBSESSIVE-COMPULSIVE NEUROSIS

The child with obsessional neurosis shows these essential features in the clinical picture:

1. Intrusive ideas, images, and impulses
2. A subjective feeling that these "mental events" are forced (compulsion, anancasm)
3. A feeling at the same time that the compulsion must be resisted.

To this elaborate formulation, psychoanalysts have added traits of obstinancy, frugality, and orderliness, which give even more complexity to the intricate picture shown by the suffering obsessional child or adolescent. Others have described the clinical picture as one in which dynamisms of alternating defiant rage and guilty, fearful yielding are called upon to explain what the child is doing in his anguished state. Some have regarded the basic defect of the obsessive child to be a lack in spontaneity and naturalness.

A search for moral superiority in a family context where a specific variety of pretense, fakery or "hypocrisy" reigns seems to dominate the symptomatic picture of most obsessive children. The goal of most therapeutic interventions, whether psychodynamic or behavioral is to replace the elaborate defensiveness of the illness by a training in naturalness.[3]

A case vignette will indicate the manner in which the phenomena of obsessive disorder express themselves in children.

S. C. was eleven years old when he was brought by his professional parents for psychiatric evaluation. He had suffered for more than a year at that time from phobias, obsessions, and compulsions. He called the latter "my promptings," to refer both to their imperious and exogenous flavor. He fought to the point of exhaustion against the very promptings that drove him to step on imaginary dots on the floor. Having stepped on them once, he felt obliged to step again, and usually did not feel "un-driven" until he had gone through a three-time ritual. "I go back and add two to make it come out five or ten. Sometimes I'll intentionally trip, just so's to have a minor to ward off a major." He thought the dots on the floor might be fecal in nature, although he conceded they were not really there, and he was preoccupied with the idea that some toxin would enter his body through his anus. Early in his psychiatric care there was a rapid augmentation of his worries about germs, dirt, feces, decay, death, bodily harm; his sexual unrest, insomnia, and ritual making led him very nearly to a psychotic state.

S. C. was the eldest child and the only male in a sibling group of four. His younger sisters were disinclined to give way to his obsessive behavior, but the mother allowed herself to be caught up in it deeply. The boy's feelings about his mother were starkly dual and ambivalent, displaying a cyclicity between angry defiance and anxious yielding, begging forgiveness. His dreams dealt with wars in which the two opposing sides were led by queens; he spoke with the cadence and intonation of a victorian southern belle with "the vapors" so that even when he was fairly expressive, it was at first merely a pose of effeminacy. His dream characters were queens, monsters, petrified cavemen, deformed torturers, biting snakes, tigers, giant frogs with monkey faces, the sun exploding, and snails struggling to shed their shells.

DEPRESSIVE NEUROSIS

It has been postulated that depression in childhood is one of the two basic conditions affecting children. Thus, neurotic children are considered to be understood either as showing the fundamental adaptive (in reality, maladaptive) paths of anxiety and hyperalertness or else as showing depression-withdrawal. Complicating matters considerably is the empirical observation that depressed children who suffer losses, who fear abandonment, and who crave unrequitedly to be nurtured and protected in their feelings of infantile helplessness, are not always "nice kids;" on the contrary they may be aggressive, hateful children. Many delinquents function from a position of emotional depression, many agitated and restless children are more sad and lonely than jazzed up or cunning. This substantiates the ancient clinical maxim that what meets the eye is not the basic dynamism but only the most effective behavior available to the child under the circumstances. Reaction formation operates in the narcissistic neurosis of depression just as it operates in the transference or defense neurosis of obsession. Depressed children, however, are usually less narcissistic than depressed adults. Mild depressions are generally taken to be neurotic, whereas severe depressions are considered to be psychotic. A child whose self-concept is impaired or threatened will be fertile ground for a depressive neurosis.

If a lowered self-esteem exists, the child who suffers any loss (real or fantasied) mobilizes his anxiety less than his hatred. And hatred mobilized in the face of a loss is promptly transmuted into self-hatred and self-laceration. Despite the fact that many adults would respond with psychomotor retardation, the fact remains that a child becomes energized during depression. In childhood, he strikes out against the environment just as readily as he becomes punitive toward himself.

The child who acts out is giving a message to the people around him just as certainly as he would send a message if he sat mutely brooding about his lack of worthiness and his guilt. The people around a depressed child often have superlative empathy for the child's sadness which lurks under his tough and antisocial exterior. That does not always bring relief to the neurotically depressed child, however, for the child may long in his heart of hearts to be punished—not understood. Frustrated dependency may rapidly become destructiveness.

Depression of an anaclitic variety occurs in infancy; it is termed *marasmus* by pediatricians. The marasmic child is almost always the child who is maternally deprived, with the ages of five to sixteen months seeming to constitute a replica, of sorts, of an ethologist's "critical phase" for the imprinting of animal behavior patterns. Deprivation of care and attention during these months of the infant's life deprive him of the ability to feel that he can depend on and trust others, that he can be loved without deserving love, that he can be accepted merely because he is himself—human, alive, in the world, and experiencing the "*condi-*

tion humaine." The marasmic child, with anaclitic depression, is the product of a failure of dependency, a child who has not learned that the human species can give physical care with love and protection to its young. Such a child may die if nobody cares enough to form the attachments that promote the life of a human infant.

During "latency" the child who is depressed shows the feelings of inferiority that stamp the underachiever, the slow learner, the child with learning disabilities. The child feels inferior and obtains no validation of his worth from either family or peers. That is a feeling of a little girl (or boy) lost. That such a child may be as steeped in hatred as in sadness is shown in the following case of a depressed eleven-year-old Caucasian girl.

Sally Y. was born in Europe to an American Catholic father and a German Lutheran mother who had escaped from a Russian prison camp in East Germany. The mother had not wanted a baby, but the father forbade her to have an abortion and although she acquiesced, she subsequently rued her compliance for more than eleven years. Sally's mother, Mrs. Y., was a self-absorbed person; she openly declared that she resented the good fortune that Sally enjoyed, namely, receiving food, shelter, clothing, and even toys and games, without doing anything to earn them. She had a low opinion of herself, or to be more accurate, of the larger part of self, and identified that bad part with Sally. The daughter too was always splitting herself into good and bad, and this appeared to her young psychiatrist to be a hopeful sign initially—she might be able to make a therapeutic alliance and make progress in therapy, the doctor surmised. The doctor had not made adequate allowance for the deeply narcissistic setting in which both mother and daughter dwelled; ultimately this made therapy very difficult.

Sally's communications went like this: "I keep being bad. I try not to be bad, and say 'I am going to be good.' I want to be good, but I keep getting into trouble. I keep on being bad. I love my mother *so much*. I'd like to be good . . . She is at work when I get home from school. My Daddy works too. So I stay with my [maternal] grandmother and grandfather till they get through work. They moved here from Europe and live across the street . . . Mother teases me a lot. She keeps me guessing about what kind of presents I am gonna get. She always asks me what I think I'll get. I kept a lizard in my room, but it died. What I *really* want is a little monkey. I asked her for a fish, but she says they die too easy. I don't want a fish, anyway. I would rather talk to a monkey or a dog, or scratch him. Laddie belongs to the whole family; but I would rather have a dog for myself, just for myself. I told her if I could have a dog or a monkey, I'd take good care of it, and I could even put it in a cage in my room so it wouldn't mess up the house. She said, "We'll put *you* in a cage and pen you up.' " Sally's crimes consisted of lying (usually when backed into the trap her mother had laid for her), of stealing (usually of candies from a neighborhood store), of begging (in order to buy small trinkets and sweets for herself), and of troubles with other children. Sally only played occasionally with younger children, whom she dominated, and with older boys (twelve to fifteen years) with whom she had intercourse or on whom she practice fellatio. She lived essentially friendless and isolated and spent her late childhood "feeling lonely and helpless in a hostile world"—Horney's term for the basic neurotic core.

During six months of contact with this family and this young girl, it became very clear that the mother wanted to be rid of the daughter. "My mother is mad at me, and today said she didn't want to waste every Saturday running me in to see you at the clinic. She said if you couldn't do anything to make me good, she would send me to an orphanage and get rid of me . . . She asked me the other day how I would like it if we all went to Germany and left me here with some stepmother and stepfather. I told her I wouldn't like that because even if I act bad I think sometimes I'd like to be with my family. She said the other ladies in her office bragged on their little girls, but she couldn't find one good thing to say about me. . . . She said today she was through with psychiatry, that from now on she would beat me for every thing I do wrong—I forgot to take my underwear over to get it ironed at my grandmother's—and she was not gonna waste her time coming here, and she'd kick me outa the house when I was thirteen or fourteen. She keeps asking me how I'd feel if I was sent away. I don't want to be sent away, but sometimes I think I may be better off away from my mother."

The family tried foster home placement and placement in a parochial correctional school; finally they decided to stop taking her to the psychiatry clinic. The mother herself was offered psychiatric help and declined. Most observers of human behavior would not be astonished to learn that at age twelve years, Sally attempted suicide in boarding school.

Differential Diagnosis

Children's psychoneuroses have to be differentiated from several other behavioral disturbances, a number of which are much more serious. The important categories for differential diagnosis include the following eight. The major differential features of each are noted:

1. The *psychoses*, whose severely and pervasively deviant behavior (in respect to the child's age) is accompanied by impaired reality testing.

2. Those behavioral disorders associated with *organic brain syndromes*—whose symptoms indicate acute or chronic central nervous system dysmaturation, injury, or dysfunction.

3. Those disorders called acting out, socio-

pathic, or *antisocial*—that is, the child is "delinquent," in trouble with law and court officers. He consistently violates laws regarding property, obedience toward parents, school attendance, and other norms.

4. Those *personality disorders* that are not manifested in delinquent deviance nor in symptoms reflecting internalized conflict but, by contrast, show up as highly idiosyncratic "character armoring"—compulsive, hysterical, overanxious, overly dependent, overly independent, overinhibited, oppositional, isolated, and mistrustful personality disorders.

5. Those *reactive disorders* whose forms of behavioral deviance are bound to specific events or situations—for example, a child who is mute only at school, an infant with anaclitic depression, and so forth.

6. Those behavioral disorders which are called "developmental interferences"[57] or developmental deviations[68] because the disordered behavior is untimely, either precocious or retarded, and inappropriate for the given child's actual age and gender. This assortment includes such a disparate group as precocious genitality, delayed speech, long sustained hyperactive motor patterns and similar aberrations.

7. *Psychophysiologic disorders* in which emotional upset and its vegetative effects are accompanied by morphologic lesions. This occurs in many cases of migraine, asthma, anorexia nervosa, neurodermatitis, colitis, and peptic ulcer.

8. Those *crisis-coping responses* of essentially healthy children—who mourn when a parent dies, who develop transient phobias at age four years, who strive to "find themselves" as adolescents. The deviance may be gross but, either because of its transience or its "having a point," it lacks ominousness and indeed connotes health.

History of Childhood Neuroses

Until the psychoanalysts began to emphasize early childhood, psychiatrists were generally little inclined to give attention to disturbed children, much less to neurotic ones. When they did consider children, psychiatrists usually minimized the possibilities of children's becoming "insane." They took only severe madness seriously, sought for biogenic origins whenever disorders were present, and transferred, although somewhat reluctantly, the labels used for adults directly to children, if

the latter behaved slightly similarly.[42] Both today and in the past, in classifying children's behavior, the values of the categorizer are always at work. In the past, the welfare of children, and the possibility that they might possess a complex inner life, were not taken very seriously by psychiatrists and other adults. If children showed deviance, it was not considered to be a function of their dynamic make-up or their interpersonal relations; instead it was a playing out within them of species-wide imperatives or drives, including original sin, witchcraft, and the influences of the bad seed.

As early as 1690, John Locke, and by 1762, Jean-Jacques Rousseau had begun to plead that children should be educated according to their individual drives and capabilities, and that children should be observed and understood by the adults who wished to mold them. Nevertheless, Immanuel Kant, a foremost figure of the Enlightenment, in his 1798 treatise on *Classification of Mental Disorders* said nothing of children's psychopathology.[159] Early efforts at including children in the Freedom movement were sporadic and scattered.

In his 1867 text[101] Henry Maudsley devoted a chapter to children's disorders, and included their neuroses. He called these conditions "instinctive insanity" and "moral insanity," but symptoms of hysteria and dissociation abound in all his categories of "mania" and "epileptic insanity," "melancholia," "monomania," and others. Maudsley was attacked so effectively that by the 1880 edition of his book, he had backtracked, according to Kanner,[85] deleting most references to children. By the third edition, children were left out completely. Charles Darwin joined many other gifted writers who were keeping diaries of the events and activities of infants throughout the latter part of the nineteenth century.[37] None of these contained any efforts to describe neurotic behavior as it would be depicted today.

In the 1880s, G. Stanley Hall conducted questionnaire research wherein thousands of parents were queried about their children's behavior, including neurotic symptoms. Hall was a psychologist, the president of Clark University, and the host of Sigmund Freud (in 1909) and Adolf Meyer (1909 and earlier). Hall knew that parents underestimate their children's problems, as later demonstrated by Lapouse and Monk,[93] but his great contribution lay in the construction of a data base of norms for the behavior of young children at specific ages. Also, in the United States, Spitzka, by 1883, described childhood disorders in some detail, alleging, in keeping with his *Zeitgeist*, that they were due to heredity, fright, sudden changes of temperature, and masturbation.[86] Late in the nineteenth century psychiatrists such as Emminghaus, Moreau de Tours, Ireland, and Manheimer similarly discussed childhood neuroses; yet Emil Kraepelin, in his 1894 textbook, (and again in 1904)[36] continued the neglect of children in the manner shown by Kant one hundred years earlier.

Lloyd de Mause[40] classified attitudes toward children during history. He speaks of *infanticide*, from antiquity to the fourth century A.D.; *abandonment*, from the fourth to the thirteenth century: *ambivalent coexistence*, from the fourteenth to the seventeenth centuries; *intrusiveness* in the eighteenth century; gentler but fuller *socialization*, nineteenth to mid-twentieth century; and *helping, in empathy*, beginning at the middle of the current century. Currently, there exists an assortment of attitudes, some more modern, some vestigial. In general, current cultural values are essentially demeaning of childhood; the child is used largely as a screen onto which adult projections are freely thrown. It is no wonder, therefore, that psychiatry has paid small heed to children. On the other hand, even if this is not the "Century of the Child," as predicted by Ellen Key, it is at least the first era in which significant voices in the culture ask that children be treated as valued beings, to be served, understood, and respected. Enriched by contributors from many disciplines, childhood neuroses are considerably better understood today than in earlier eras. Finally, this is *the century of child psychiatry*, a specialty whose involvement with childhood neuroses has been of a crucial character.

THE CLASSIC CASES OF FREUD

In the year 1900 (sometimes he cited the year as 1899), Freud began psychoanalytic treatment of Dora. He had seen this young woman earlier in 1898 (when she was sixteen years old) for hoarseness and cough. Dora's dynamics, psychogenetics, and symptoms came to be regarded as typical examples of the hysterias. Freud contended that her neurosis had its onset when she was eight years old. The variable physical complaints from which she suffered in subsequent years were viewed as conversion symptoms of her unresolved infantile neurosis (case published 1905).

In 1906 Freud commenced his largely indirect contact with five-year-old "Hans" (the nominal disguise given to Herbert Graf, who later became an eminent operatic stage director) for Hans's phobia of horses. The Hans case report was published in 1909. Little Hans had been threatened with penile amputation when his mother found him masturbating, and his parents, although "progressive" for the turn of the century, encouraged Hans to overcome—indeed to "break himself" of—his masturbatory habit. There is disagreement with Freud's conclusions, both by post-Freudians such as Fromm[54] and by behavior therapists,[157] but Freud asserted that Hans showed an Oedipus complex behind his neurosis, that the phobia was a compromise between internal and external demands, that Hans had been seductively dealt with by his mother, and that the true essence of his problems lay buried under a mass of repression. When Freud met the young Graf at nineteen years of age, about 1920, he repeated his view that all his earlier opinions had been vindicated.[105]

In 1907 Freud began treatment with the "Rat Man," a famous case published in 1909. This young man suffered from an obsessional neurosis. He felt that a young woman friend and his father (although deceased) would have rats gnaw into their ano-rectal areas. Freud interpreted his symptoms as indicative of the patient's death wishes toward his father in early childhood—the familiar Oedipus complex—from which regression to anality and homosexuality had occurred.

By 1910, when he began psychoanalytic treatment with the "Wolf Man," and, more conspicuously, by the time the case was published in 1918, Freud sought to show up the errors of Adler and Jung by his interpretations of the meaning of the case. The "Wolf Man" case involved a prolonged analysis of a mixed neurotic picture. The gist of the case was that at age one and one-half years, the "Wolf Man" had seen his parents having intercourse in "an especially favorable posture" to trouble an infant's fantasy, namely, the maternal vagina received the penis from the rear. At age three and one-fourth years, the child had been seduced by his older sister; soon thereafter he had masturbated in the presence of his nurse who threatened to castrate him; at age four he dreamed of six or seven white wolves sitting calmly in a walnut tree outside his bedroom; influenced by his sister he developed a wolf phobia from four to four and one-half; from four and one-half to ten years he developed Christian scrupulosity and a fullblown obsessional neurosis. His anality had the unconscious meaning of his being "castrated" like his mother and penetrated anally by the paternal penis. The "Wolf Man," then, corroborated for Freud the existence of the form of infantile sexuality and childhood notions about sexuality that Freud had propounded, along with the central place of the Oedipus complex and the soundness of his crystallizing views about childhood neurosis.

LATER FREUDIANS

The concept of neurosis as a constellation of symptoms deriving from the oedipal or post-oedipal phases of development is a viewpoint long propounded by psychoanalysts. It reached its clearest critique and expictation in the formulations of Humberto Nagera and the Anna Freud group. Nagera[116] tried to broaden the original view that an infantile neurosis underpins virtually every form of deviant behavior in childhood and adulthood. Under the influence of ego-analytic thinking, Nágera agreed with Hartmann[73] that if "every naughtiness . . . is considered as 'neurotic' then the term has lost all real value in psychologic discourse." Nágera insisted that the "neuroses proper" of childhood are not the same as *neurotic conflicts* (which are transitory), or as *developmental conflicts*, or as *developmental interferences*, during childhood. The net effect of Nagera's approach is to sharpen the diagnostic thinking about neurosis and to regard fewer children as truly neurotic. Likewise, Nagera pointed out the importance of "latency neurosis, prepuberty neurosis, adolescent neurosis [and] adulthood neurosis" as well as "infantile neurosis." Since 1966, most psychoanalysts seem to have accepted the broadened and clarified view of the Anna Freud/Nagera group.

Melanie Klein and her followers appear to hold similar views, but tend to move the emerging components of the oedipal phase back into earlier infancy. As clinical experience with very young children has advanced, for many analysts the Kleinian viewpoint has taken on ever more credibility. Whereas Hartmann, Erikson, and Anna Freud placed emphasis on the ego and the outer world, Melanie Klein[89] and her disciple, Hanna Segal,[36] emphasized the id and superego more than they did the ego. This resulted in a greater surface orthodoxy on the part of the Klein group, but it concealed a more radical development away from the Freudian mainstream—in the greater Kleinian attention to the mother, to the earliest feelings and images of the infant, and paradoxically to ego-and-other "object relations."[70]

Certain of the post-Freudians, however, notably Chodoff and Fromm-Reichmann, have totally cast aside the classifical Freudian stress on the father and on oedipal conflicts as originating and structuring neurosis. Fromm-Reichmann[33] raised the possibility that certain class-bound and ethnicity-bound Viennese family configurations and styles may breed Oedipus complexes, but they do not breed all forms of neurosis, nor all forms of human suffering.

DEVELOPMENTS BESIDES PSYCHOANALYSIS

As early as 1903, Adolf Meyer had developed his own version of analyzing the neurotic constitution. He contended that neuroses were personality imbalances resulting from faulty or disorganized habits. In order to study them, he developed his life chart, a form of psychobiography, in keeping with his theory. By the 1920s, Meyer was calling neuroses "merergasias," partial dysfunctions, and "kakergasias" meaning bad-abnormal-poor-faulty reactions.

In 1909, a few years before the "Wolf Man" case was published, and in the very same year that Freud had published his case studies of both Hans and the "Rat Man," a clinic had been set up in Chicago by William Healy and associates. It was associated with the Juvenile Court and designed for the direct study of deviant children. The concept of psychiatrists' and their associates' observing and working directly with children caught on rapidly, and, *pari passu*, so did the sociogenic or interpersonal perspective on childhood neuroses.[87] William Healy examined all these developments in his 1915 book on the "neurotic" delinquent, a text more familiar today to social science students than to medical students.[74] Healy proved to be a giant in the history of child psychiatry in general and childhood neurosis in particular. He was a student of Meyer, William James, and G. Stanley Hall, and a proponent of Freud. Healy's thinking generously admitted new and divergent ideas. Under his influence child guidance became a pluralistic, multidisciplinary project directed toward neurotic delinquents.

Following Healy's pioneering work, a continuing flood of productive work concerning neurotic children emerged from Chicago, particularly under the auspices of the Institute for Juvenile Research. Child guidance clinics soon appeared in many regions: for example, one began in Louisville in 1913, the Thom Clinic opened in Boston in 1921, and from 1922 to 1927 the Commonwealth Fund sponsored pilot clinics (in only eight cities in 1922) all across the United States. By 1930, there were over 500 child guidance clinics in existence. To train personnel to staff them, an Institute for Child Guidance in New York City opened in 1927 and closed in 1933. Most of the clinics were in the Meyerian "mental hygiene" tradition. They adapted readily to Freudian, Jungian, Rankian, and Adlerian concepts. They were community-centered, and they incorporated the orthopsychiatric team in their study of and services to children. Eventually, in many settings, these clinics came to deal almost exclusively with neurotic children. Only in a few cities did their work continue to focus on delinquents. Whatever the limitations of theory, training, and practice concerning childhood neuroses, from 1920 to 1960, and beyond, nearly everything accomplished was done in association with these American community child psychiatry facilities.

On the continent of Europe, *Kinderpsychiatrie* (or *psychiatrie infantile*, or *psiquiatría infantil*) developed close to hospitals. These child psychiatry enterprises tended to follow either an organicist-empiricist bent or, in quite a divergent way, to operate exclusively under the aegis of the psychoanalytic institutes (especially the Vienna, and later on, the London Institute). Anna Freud and Melanie Klein were outstanding leaders in the field of child analysis, the former enlarging the mainstream of Freudian orthodoxy and the latter ostensibly narrowing and perfecting the same orthodoxy. During the same first half-century, in the USSR, Krasnogorski[91] and others continued the orthodox Pavlovian tradition with little progress in the realm of childhood neuroses.

In the United States, however, some interesting developments of learning-conditioning theory (relevant to child neuroses) were appearing in the work of John B. Watson and others.[83] Watson's 1920-reported case of eleven-months-old Albert was the account of a child conditioned (by respondent learning in Pavlovian style) to fear furry objects. This was accomplished by the simultaneous presentation of furry things and harsh noises.[153] It is one of the great classics of learning theorists. American behavioristic psychologists such as Hull, Spence, Guthrie, Hilgard, and Marquis remained within the Pavlovian camp but did not stress the nervous system as much as had the Russian master. There were many efforts (by Kubie, Alexander, and French, for example) among psychoanalysts to "integrate" psychoanalysis with Hullian and other neo-Pavlovian learning theories; the best-known work of this kind was accomplished by John Dollard and Neal Miller of Yale, in 1950.[43]

Since the thirties, Burrhus F. Skinner, working mainly with pigeons, but always ready to extend his behavioral experimentation to human animals, took up another avenue for the study of the learning process, namely, operant conditioning. Laboratory based and logicoempirical in methodology, operant conditioning was confined largely to the work of Skinnerian experimental psychologists until the 1960s. During this period neurotic children (as well as retarded and other severely damaged children) came into the limelight for an unusual degree of public recognition during the presidency of John F. Kennedy. In that era, greater numbers of experimental psychologists "turned clinical" than had done so during all earlier times. Those who were interested in operant conditioning (also known as behavior modification or behavior therapy) joined forces with practitioners of desensitization and deconditioning to help change the face of clinical practice with neurotic children. As mentioned before, the phobic children were those most often studied and treated in behavior therapy. However, it was not among the neurotics so much as among retarded, delinquent and psychotic children that behavior therapy was employed most frequently and with the greatest efficacy.[11]

These were new developments in the approaches to nosology as well as new interventions. A rather indirect approach to the psychopathology of childhood, and to childhood neuroses, is the factor-analytic approach. This involves the survey of large numbers of children, in order to find out inductively what general factors stand out as valid clusters of behavior. In several such attempts, the results have been inconsistent, depending on the traits inherent and specific to the population studied. There has been little progress in advancing the survey approach of G. Stanley Hall, of Ralph Dreger,[44] and T. M. Achenbach.[1] Achenbach found that when he surveyed for the presence of ninety-one pathognomonic symptoms of disordered behavior, two principal factors appeared in the age groups four through nine years and ten through fifteen years. The first factor he called "Externalizing-Internalizing." It was bipolar, and consisted of one pole of "acting out," and the other of "acting in." The second factor dealt less with neurotic type behaviors and he called it "Severe and Diffuse Psychopathology." Achenbach's work has been replicated by Shechtman[138] who found that the boys in her subject group displayed more externalizing-internalizing behavior than did the girls. She further found that with increasing age there was a progressive tendency for both sexes to be more externalizing, although a notable number of older boys became more internalizing. Shechtman wisely cautioned that only gross categories can be derived from such studies of a large age span. Moreover, she observed that taxonomy based thereon did not handle the problem of the longitudinal study of the developmental progression of symptoms throughout childhood and into adulthood.

Frequency of Childhood Neuroses

Far too little is firmly known about childhood psychopathology in general and, specifically, about the frequency of neurotic symptoms among children. In particular, there is a serious lack of data about what happens to those symptoms and those children as development proceeds. It is known that parents underestimate them.[93] Rutter and his colleagues[129] found that some of the commonest childhood "symptoms" such as nail-biting or thumb-sucking have no predictive value whatsoever. In general, the "acting-in," neurotic symptoms are more frequent. But they are so much more benign than the "acting-out" symptoms, that many behavioral scientists have tended to regard *only antisocial and aggressive symptoms* as truly high-risk childhood behavior.[124, 125, 182] Nevertheless, during these early years, the misery and anguish experienced by the child then and there are universally held to warrant treatment of neurosis in childhood. (See the later volume on "Treatment.")

Most studies of the prevalence of childhood neuroses, as well as other disorders, have been studies on small populations. Cantwell's[30] survey of a group of military dependents is one example. It showed a surprisingly high prevalence of disorders (viz., 35 percent). Ten percent of the children were neurotic with more girls than boys falling into this category. If this is typical, a staggering number of children may need psychiatric aid.

In a study of 158,000 psychiatric outpatient clinic terminations of children in the United States, Rosen and associates[127] found that 6.1 percent of the male patients under eighteen years old and 8.4 percent of the females suffered from psychoneuroses—7 percent of all terminated outpatient children were neurotics. By contrast, 20.7 percent of all the children hospitalized (N=17,815) in psychiatric units of general hospitals were diagnosed as psychoneurotic, while only 2.6 percent of all children in private psychiatric and 3.7 percent of all children in public psychiatric hospitals were so designated.

Clinical Course

NEUROTIC FEATURES IN GENERAL

As neurotic children mature, they exhibit a wide range of morbidity. In this sense, they comprise a heterogenous, and even "unstable" coterie. Many recover spontaneously, and others worsen severely. The majority probably carry some pathologic features throughout their life. Some other aspects of their problems are resolved. Ultimately, however, they carry a fixed core of neurotic difficulty on into maturity. In brief, childhood neuroses are often the expression of serious inner problems with a tendency toward repetitiveness, chronicity, or fixity.

Some neuroses can arise during infancy and in the preschool eras. Nonetheless, the peak time of onset is during elementary school. Perhaps another peak period is in late adolescence or early adulthood, a time when the YAVIS is highly valued in this society. (YAVIS refers to the Schofield rubrics of adult patients who are *young, attractive, verbal, intelligent,* and *successful,*[134] as opposed to the non-YAVIS patients who are middle-aged or older, physically run-of-the-mill or ugly, verbally inhibited, intellectually mediocre or lower, and economically from the working class or below.)

The Freudian conceptual formulation of childhood neuroses has been widely held and very influential. To recapitulate briefly, this conception is as follows. Psychoneuroses are disturbances derived from unconscious conflicts. The conflicts involve sexual and aggressive drives (or erotic and death instincts). Although these drives and conflicts are out of awareness, they are regnant and insistent. The conceptual structures, id, ego, superego, and external objects are all invoked, and all are depicted in terms of specific strivings and functions. The superego, for example, is said to reject certain id forces, thus resulting in ego prohibitions and conflict. If the id forces are potent and the defenses of the ego and superego relatively weak, the wishes threaten to emerge into awareness; the threat provokes anxiety. This in turn signals the ego to bind the psychic energy of the id more and more firmly. If this binding function is unsuccessful in part or in whole, neurotic symptoms emerge. The defenses are multifaceted, however. They oppose the instincts and the wishes of the id in the service of pleasing important others—such as the child's parents—but they also let some of the id wishes sneak forth under disguise and compromise in order to please the important self. The compromise that forms in this way is the symptom. Hence, every neurotic formation does double duty: it is both a prohibition of id wishes and a discharge of id wishes. Furthermore, the neurotic symptom shows some effort to heal and solve conflict as well as to fix and enthrone conflict. It is obvious that many metaphors are employed in this formulation. At the same time, it has the necessary degree of complexity to begin to account for clinical experience.

With the onset of a neurosis, a partial breakup of the child's behavior is seen, since some regression does take place; reality testing however, is not grossly impaired. In Freud's formulation, the neuroses are held to be the results of a fixation at, or regression to, one of the phases of infantile sexuality—oral, anal, or phallic oedipal. The severity of the symptom picture depends on the rigidity and primitiveness of that fixation or the depth of the regression. This conflictful situation does not necessarily give rise to symptoms outright; at times only "neurotic character traits" will occur.

DEVELOPMENTAL ASPECTS OF NEUROSIS

In the first year of life, it is usually felt that the child's personality has not developed sufficiently to structure a neurosis. Sometimes, phobic neuroses do appear, however, and fulfill the basic metapsychologic criteria of this condition. That is, inner mental representations of conflict appear to have formed, the dread object seems to have acquired symbolic significance, anxiety appears, and defenses are mobilized. Only some of these can be observed directly while others constitute hypotheses which cannot be verified empirically. For the rest, during these early months the child displays what John Rose[126] called "primary tension disturbances" (such as colic, sleep difficulties, gastrointestinal difficulties, eczema, and other allergies) and "primary deprivation syndromes" (developmental failure, failure to thrive, apathy and detachment, repetitive movements, etc.). All of these developmental problems are more diffuse and global than the neuroses, but they hold within them the seeds of neurotic formations. They are often termed "latent neurotic pictures." (See early subsection on "Partially Psychoneurotic Conditions.")

From age twelve months to thirty months the child may show behavior that is more closely allied to neurotic symptoms, but most of the diffuseness of the first year persists. Again, it is the phobic responses that predominate, but other more or less clear-cut neuroses are seen, such as obsessive-compulsive and anxiety neurosis.

From thirty months to six years of age the same trend continues. Neuroses may appear and some may be full blown, but in general, the more diffuse and global disturbances prevail. During this era, more Kleinians than followers of Anna Freud have identified and treated neurotic children.

After five or six years of age, there seems no doubt that neurotic symptom pictures can be identified as well as neurotic trait disturbances and neurotic characters. In each stage of childhood there may be recrudescences and exacerbations of old conflicts and new neurotic constellations may be set in motion. Indeed these may occur as important events in the process of treatment. It lends a hopeful note to observe that resolutions and progressions occur at each phase.

CLINICAL VARIETIES IN A SIMPLIFIED VIEW

The clinical varieties of childhood neuroses have been described in several different ways. Freud's views were fashioned on the model of the Apollonian and the Dionysian. In the one, overcontrol is the obvious feature as seen in obsessive-compulsive neurosis, and in the other, overreaction is the outstanding trait, as in hysterical neurosis. E. James Anthony[16] followed the lead of George Engel in recognizing that the supercharged, stirred up, neurotic child is not the same as the child manifesting depression and withdrawal. Depression is more narcissistic, hysteria more subject to transference. Anthony's description of the major variants of neurosis subdivided these conditions into those marked by anxiety and those marked by depression. A somewhat broader and more empirical parceling was that developed by Barbara Fish and Theodore Shapiro,[50] who found likenesses and yet differences between the anxious-neurotic and sociopathic-paranoid type of child. Their dichotomy is reminiscent of the early psychoanalytic distinction between those who act-in and those who act-out, groups called by Achenbach and others[1, 138] *externalizers* and *internalizers*.

What seems to be called for is a usable division of neurotic children, and, ideally, a division which is both logical and empirical. To begin with, there seems to be a group of children who do incorporate the constraints and values of family members and others with whom they have face-to-face intimate relations. These are the youngsters who do not bother others as much as they bother themselves, and who have many unhappy feelings. They suffer not from anxiety (or cognitive strain) alone but also from loneliness, sadness, despair, apathy, demoralization, tension, unfulfilled dependency longings, guilt-ridden sexual desire, and anger. All of these feelings are held in and bottled up, producing stressed and disturbed functioning. This kind of child, perhaps, best deserves being called the *internalizer*; and his unpleasure is manifest mainly as fear and sadness. The other kind of neurotic child then may be called an *externalizer*. He attributes a good part of his trouble to agents and forces outside of himself and usually imputes blame to those people who dwell in his intimate interpersonal network. When he obtains insight he does not say, "I see what I am doing to myself." Instead he says, "I see what they are trying to do to me." His insight is that type which psychiatrists have been prone to label sick or paranoid. It is often a valid type of illumination that comes to certain neurotic children who are indeed victimized and oppressed. It is militant, and may be more abrasive than the reactions of the more docile neurotic type. It does not have the ethical warmth of the Judeo-Christian virtue assigned traditionally to self-blame, to working toward atonement and self-purification; but it may have an untapped utility in healing some of the hurts of neglected, abused, impoverished, and regimented children in an era of urbanized, secularized modernity. The quasi-paranoid and quasi-antisocial bent seem partially to promote health in some urban ghetto dwellers, thus fulfilling the time-honored canon that every neurotic development shows an effort toward health. For many children, externalizing seems more relevant and serviceable than does an anxious-depressive form of insight. Advantages multiply for the externalizing child who is in pain, if he is lucky enough to know an August Aichhorn, or Paul Federn, or William Glasser, or Adelaide Johnson. The externalizer is full of utopian possibilities, just as the internalizer is full of ethical potential.[2] Further, as the Jungian paradox indicates, these two modes serve each as the shadow of the other, and a healthy life style would combine some features of both without overexaggeration of either.

The internalizing neurotic children are those who suffer from (1) the more conflict-laden syndromes—hysteria, obsessive-compulsive, phobic, depersonalization and anxiety neuroses; and (2) the more narcissistic and withdrawing syndromes —hypochondriacal and depressive neuroses. Externalizing neurotic children may include those who are usually labeled as neurotic delinquents,

neurotic characters, and paranoid personalities. In addition, some obsessive and phobic children are not far from these externalizing children. Perhaps the older school phobic is more likely to be an internalizer. In the material that follows, each group will be described briefly. Finally, the school phobic child will be dealt with as exemplary of the unsteady state of contemporary anthropology, nosology, symptomatology, dynamic theory, etiology, therapy, and prognostication with neurotic children.

Internalizers "ponder things in their hearts" and have active fantasy lives. Those with anxiety neuroses can be quickly characterized as children who show episodes of fear or panic but know not why. Sometimes an anxiety neurotic in a state of high cognitive discord and strain is hard put to articulate his fear-dread-apprehension. Many therapists play down the cognitive repair needed by such neurotic children, since they feel that it is not wise to launch a frontal attack on this area of difficulty. They claim that a "depth" approach to fantasies and affects will in any case yield the desired cognitive gains as a by-product. Children with phobias do select a specific object to be the focus of their fears, an object that is often ludicrous even to the child. But willy nilly the object is dreaded and avoided. The internalizer is certainly not outgoing. In contrast to this phobic stance, hysterical neurotics with conversion symptoms appear virtually fearless. They seem to opt for a rather naive, direct escape from anxiety by adopting the sick role, replete with denial and repression. After all, the infirmity accounts for every shortcoming—one's inadequacy, dependency, immaturity, lack of fun—and besides, the child is often winsome and dramatic, evoking attentive sympathy if not empathy from many adults. Indeed, as analysts have long noted, hysterical-conversion types of children become more jittery when their symptoms are being removed than they were formerly when the paralysis or tic or fainting tendency held sway. All the internalizing children will produce many fears and fantasies if an adult is willing to encounter them.

Children with hysterical dissociative reactions are not as bland as those with conversion symptoms. Their hurts are more evident, their whole repertoire of behavior may look as if it had become unglued. They show amnesia, fugue and twilight states, automatisms, depersonalization, and multiple personality and even excitements and posturings that border on catatonia (see "Common Clinical Pictures" earlier in this chapter). Obsessive compulsive neurotic children also look tense and fearful, very "uptight." This is most marked when they are interrupted in the overcontrolled rituals they have developed in their search for ways to feel less driven, if not happy. Functionally, this behavior serves to disguise from themselves, as well as from others, the "unacceptable" feelings that originally sent them into their spiraling funk. Obsessive children are mired in an endless vacillation between enraged defiance and queasy guilt. In brief, for the internalizing neurotic child, in some measure, thought, word, and deed, as well as feelings, are all awry. These youngsters respond to placebo and suggestion, and learn rather readily. They have problems that cry out for relationships with understanding and helpful adults, and even if they do not form intense bonds with a therapist, they can more readily enter into healing relationships than can the narcissistic-withdrawing neurotic children.

Depressed neurotic children are a different matter; they are not usually the overtly sad and slow people that neurotically depressed adults are likely to be. They are more inclined to show irritability and jitteriness (as will some agitated adults). Depressed neurotic children may be hyperactive, and at times their disturbance may evidence its presence in the form of stealing, parental disobedience, fitful school truancy, and sleeping difficulties. The child may compose a note suggesting suicide, but the whole aura of it is, "you will be sorry when I am dead." Such a child shows in the clearest possible manner that he not only feels cut off from important people whom he earlier loved, but also that he experiences a hatred, one that he finds fearsome, toward these same persons. The internalized conflict or ambivalence seen in such a child is not a matter of guesswork; it is really there. Warmth is lacking in the depressed child; his love is withheld. He alternates between denunciation of others and self-blame. Apathetic silence, that can amount to an active avoidance of communication and relatedness, may be the only outward clue to his mood state of depression. This child is an internalizer who readily externalizes.

The depressed child is said to be narcissistic because he has pulled back from relationships and turned in toward himself. Physical complaints may also signify social withdrawal, for the child who has headaches, backaches and bellyaches is a child who has turned inward, away from others, as surely as has the depressed child. In fact, in some instances, hypochondriacal neurotic and depressed neurotic children may be one and the same, for the hypochondriacal symptoms may function as depressive equivalents. To the degree that both types of neurosis are narcissistic (in terms of libido theory, the cathexis is withdrawn from objects and invested in the ego) the children may show touchiness or hypersensitivity, and such a high level of suspicion that they come close to resembling those with externalizing neurotic problems. From the perch of narcissism, a child can lash out against others as readily as he can lacerate himself. The point is, the overlap in actual childhood neurotic constellations knows no limitations that neat theory or nosology may wish to impose.

Externalizing neurotic children are reminiscent of children in the "paranoid position" described by Melanie Klein. With or without libido theory, it is evident that a child's conflicts with others (with "objects," with "external reality") may just as easily lead to a paranoid as to a depressive stance, to externalizing as readily as to internalizing. The conventional view is that the externalizer is a child whose conflicts are outer-directed, centered between ego and outside world and who is therefore best seen as having a "primary behavior disorder." In contrast to this, the theory regards children with "psychoneuroses" as those who tend to contain and internalize conflicts by forming symptoms. To take cognizance of those children who are symptomatic, but who are also angry at significant adults and hence antisocial, the theory has to be bent so as to conceptualize either: (1) a combined neurosis and behavior disorder; (2) a neurotic character disorder, or (3) a behavior disorder with fragmentary neurotic traits. As Leo Kanner pointed out, however, nowadays neuroses are considered to be predominantly sociogenic disorders, emerging and receding within interpersonal contexts.[87] As more has been learned about neurotic children and, in particular, about their relations to parents, childhood neuroses have come to be regarded as not strictly intrapsychic. Instead, as Sullivan[148] stated, they are viewed as "interpersonal" as well—something observable, not merely guessed at, or wished for, as in "the illusion of personal individuality." The acting-out neurotic child is just as conflicted as the acting-in neurotic child. He is just as unawares, as alienated, and as demoralized. Adelaide Johnson[80] showed that he is just as much locked into an interactive system with his parents and family; he may even have as many "inner" conflicts concerning anger, lust, envy, loneliness, security longings and sadness; he may have as elaborate a fantasy life if an adult will go to the trouble of showing interest in it. Indeed, he may be caught up in ego-dystonic suffering, to the same extent as and sometimes even more so, than the internalizer.

Coming at the issue from another angle, it seems that the depressed neurotic, obsessional neurotic, phobic neurotic, and any one of many others, may show up predominantly either as an externalizer or as an internalizer. After all, in Achenbach's factor analytic work[1] the behavioral items fell into a bimodal cluster, full of overlapping elements and sharing many common ingredients. It is suggested that no useful contribution is made by clinging to the notion that only internalizers are neurotic, while the externalizers are something quite different.

AN EXEMPLARY CHILDHOOD NEUROSIS

School phobia can be taken as a prototypic childhood neurotic cluster. A rapid review of this syndrome will illustrate the imprecision of current diagnostic procedures, the Babel of etiologic declarations,[137] the prescientific state of clinical research, the primitiveness of some efforts at tracing natural history, and finally the controversy that currently rages over the direct removal of symptoms.

Dating back to 1941, the syndrome of frantic, fearful avoidance of school has been regarded as a distinctive pattern of childhood disturbance.[81] Little attention has been given by psychiatrists to the compulsory quality of schooling. They share the widespread inclination to accept compulsory education as a positive value, one to which the child and parents must be required to comply. It seems safe to say that mental health professionals today value compulsory education as highly as did the social reformers of one hundred years ago who were fighting child labor in the mines, mills, and fields. Even writers with a pronounced *laissez-faire* orientation toward child therapy have emphasized the value of a prompt, coercive return of the child to regular school attendance. From within that social orientation, school phobia is generally regarded as a neurotic disorder. Still, in some cases, allowance is made for the operation of character deviations and for a strong interactive component between parent and child. Mother, especially, is viewed as communicating separation fears to child. Aside from highlighting separation, many authors have stressed bisexual, depressive, and sado-masochistic features. Melitta Sperling devoted a great deal of thought to school phobia.[144] Operating within the Freudian framework, she declared school phobia to be a pregenital neurosis, a form of anal-sadistic constellation. She said school phobias—and all phobias—are intermediate between hysteria and compulsive neurosis, but closer to compulsive neurosis. As she viewed it, the core conflict has to do with fears of separation from the sado-masochistic bondage of child to mother. She ridiculed the idea that prompt return to school is good for the neurotic problem and urged that the total neurosis be treated analytically. She divided school phobias into an *acute* variety where, in an almost existentialist vein, she saw the danger as a loss of control, and, ultimately, as a fear of death. For her, a symbolic precipitant is always present in this type. The acute syndrome, she stated, is a "traumatic neurosis with school phobia as the presenting symptom."

In contrast to the acute type was the *induced* school phobia, for which an obvious precipitant was lacking. For this, Sperling proposed indirect treatment for the child by giving active treatment to the parent. This method was best from preschool to late latency or prepubertal age, whereupon, especially for chronic cases of induced school phobia, she proposed direct treatment of the child concomitantly with the parent. For adolescents, she recommended seeing only the adolescent, with the parent being sent to another therapist.

Edward Hampe and associates[71] have also divided school phobics into two types similar to those enunciated by Sperling. They feel that the age variable is probably critical but note that some older children—over eleven—will be in their acute Type I, and some younger children may be in their more chronic Type II.

Waldron and associates[152] undertook a worthwhile logicoempirical approach when they formulated four types of school phobia:

Type 1. Family interaction: separation anxiety and sadomasochistic clinging
Type 2. Classical phobia: displacement, projection and externalization marked
Type 3. Acute anxiety: dread of impending harm or destruction at home
Type 4. Situational-characterological: dread of school itself as a threat to self esteem.

Selecting thirty-five children with school phobia who were no more seriously disturbed than neurotic, they obtained a matching group of thirty-five children no sicker than neurotic who did *not* have the school avoidance symptom. In that way, they were set up to see in what way school phobics had distinctive symptoms, and statistically significant ones.

The features on which school phobics were unlike other neurotics consisted of the former's (1) significantly higher level of separation anxiety, (2) significantly excessive dependency, (3) significantly greater depression, (4) unrealistically high self-expectations, (5) greater blaming (projecting, externalizing) aggression onto people outside the family, (6) greater inhibition of fantasy, and (7) greater school maladjustment.

These writers found no statistically significant difference between school phobic and other neurotic children on "need to control others." (This feature is often imputed to school phobics but is, in fact, found as frequently in other neurotic children.) About the parents and family, there were some surprises: Mothers of other neurotics were as ambivalent and hostile as the mothers of school phobics; the two groups of mothers were similarly distant and unavailable; actually *fewer* parents of school phobics than of other neurotics cohabited with their own parents. Yet school phobics' parents *differed significantly* from the parents of other neurotics in: (1) difficulty in separating from the child, (2) difficulty in recognizing the child's need for separateness, (3) resenting the child's demands, (4) scapegoating the child, and (5) (mothers') regarding the child as more important than the spouse.

The several types these authors described were not mutually exclusive. Thus, Type I school phobia, with its prominent themes of family participation in separation anxiety and sado-masochistic bonding, included two-thirds of the cases. Type 4 school phobia, their "situational-characterological" category, with school bound up in issues of self-esteem, involved over one-half of the cases. Type 2 cases, typically phobic in nature, usually clustered with Types 1 or 4, but also covered 9 percent of the cases that did not fall into Types 1 and 4 groups. All of the hypothesized Type 3 cases (fear of harm at home) fell into either the Type 1 or Type 4 aggregates. As a result, Type 3 did not truly differentiate among the school phobics. Also, to inject a note of additional complexity (seldom lacking when psychopathology is empirically studied), Waldron and his collaborators noted that 18 percent of the entire assemblage of school phobics did not show the familial dynamisms of Type 1 children, yet only another 18 percent *did* show Type 1 characteristics in pure form, *without overlapping the other types*. Therefore, the story is a familiar one, in that as soon

as one undertakes to control bias and to examine a larger number of cases, one begins to learn. The lesson is that complexities generally outweigh simplicities, that pious dynamic formulations can oversimplify without illuminating, and that some metapsychologic postulates have skimpy reference to the real world of suffering children.

The situation with epidemiology, natural history and follow-up work on school phobic children is also instructive. Albeit one of the dramatic, and rather frequent, emergencies seen by child psychiatrists, school phobia is undoubtedly a rare occurrence (less than 1 percent) among large populations of school age children. Even when their treatment was free, and transportation and timing were freely accommodated, Miller and associates[109] were unable to obtain a sample adequately representative of blacks, Catholics, lower class, and "middle socioeconomic status children." Hence, clinical experience is not thorough and not representative; if it were, one would not have concluded so naively that school phobics are brighter children by IQ tests.[4] Actually, it is now known that school phobia is not correlated with high IQ but is normally distributed along with IQ.[71]

A tentative conclusion can be made that natural remissions occur in school phobia, and that the prognosis is best in children under ten or eleven years old. It also appears rather likely that for both younger and older school phobics, earlier intervention is more effective strategy for changing the course of school phobia. The type of treatment provided seems to be a matter of relative indifference, for *rapid* intervention *early* in the course of the school phobia—whether by behavior therapy or by brief or longer term psychotherapy—appears to be the critical criterion.

Some children with school phobia may be showing the prodrome of mood disorders which generally crystallize in adult life. Imipramine, an anti-depressant drug, brings relief of school phobic symptoms significantly more often than does placebo over a six-week period of treatment. Further, some follow-up studies of school phobics have suggested that they suffer from depressive illness as they become adults.

All in all, a study of school phobia is a study of the state of science, art, and craft in the whole realm of childhood neurosis. It is possible that some of the requisite research will soon be done to enrich and confirm whatever there is in current theory that is plausible, logical, and empirically testable.

Etiology of Childhood Psychoneuroses

When etiology is studied, attention is given to the assessment of childhood neuroses on three levels: (1) predisposing or readying conditions, (2) precipitating events or mobilizing factors, and (3) necessary and sufficient causes or conditions. *Predisposing background conditions for childhood neuroses* include such biologic factors as the child's temperament, physique, intelligence, and gender; environmental factors such as the parents' patterns of child rearing, communication, and psychopathology. There are many detailed aspects of each dimension that can be scrutinized, e.g., the gene pool which has been tapped in the given individual child, the accumulated experience or learning of the child, and others. *The precipitating events* may be physical ailments, psychic traumata, or broad socio-cultural disruptions in the life of the child. *The necessary conditions* for developing a neurosis may include a certain basic maturational level, a specific pattern of intrafamilial interactions and values, and so on. *The sufficient causes* may reside in the piling up of strains and inner fantasies to such a degree that one reaches that "straw that breaks the camel's back," or a specific trigger for anxiety is reached, or an emotion that is unacceptable to child and parents has been evoked. It is generally assumed that in human activities, the biologic foundations furnish the necessary conditions but not the sufficient ones: the latter arise from within culture and society.

The etiology of childhood neuroses is imperfectly understood, and only some vague approximations of sensible causal analysis are at hand. The systems theory approach will be considered briefly here with a limited discussion of organic etiologic factors and of psychosocial dynamisms.

SYSTEMS APPROACH

Instead of thinking of causes arranged in a linear pattern, the one leading to the other and thus finally to effects all in a similar straight line, both modern physics and psychiatry have inclined toward adopting a different view of causation. This approach recognizes a complex system of interactive and mutually interdependent variables. General systems theory has tried to formulate a unified theory of human behavior that takes cognizance of the neurotic child, for example, as knowable at the cellular, organ, organism, group, societal, and supranational level. At each level,

the system is a set of interrelated units. Up to the level of the organism the child's component parts are at issue, but above the organismic level the larger environmental conditions within which the individual interacts come to play on the child.

Most commentators regard Freud's formulations as expressions of a closed system. Living systems are more aptly seen as relatively open, with rather free exchange of matter/energy and communication back and forth across their borders or boundaries.[107] Gordon Allport[9] objected that the relatively open system, even as defined by James G. Miller and Norbert Wiener, is usually not conceived of as open enough, and that systems theory (also communication theory and equilibrium theory) cramps and diminishes the human being. Nevertheless, James Miller has traced numerous applications of general systems theory to psychiatry, as have Karl Menninger and his associates.[106] Their logic regards anxiety as information and considers pathology to arise from overloads and inadequate inputs and outputs of information.

ORGANIC ETIOLOGIC FACTORS

The major organic factors known and presumed to bear on childhood neuroses are two endogenous types, namely, Genetic-Constitutional and Neural-Congenital, and one fairly common exogenous type, i.e., Post-Traumatic. Paul Schilder and his wife, Lauretta Bender, are among the foremost theorists of organic contributions to behavioral deviations.[19, 133] Bender and Schilder held that central nervous system dysmaturation, maturational imbalances (embryonal lags), infections, traumata and many other organic insults may aggravate or induce a neurotic reaction. Leo Kanner similarly stressed symptomatic neurotic behavior that was set in motion following an organic illness of the child (often reported to be a participant of school phobias, incidentally). Anna Freud[57] has made the same declaration about regressed, hospitalized children.

At times, writers have discussed the genetic-constitutional conditions of children's neuroses in loose terms, much as pediatricians discuss the genetic familial background of juvenile diabetes mellitus. Sundby and Kreyberg,[149] for example, indicated that 14 percent of the neurotic group of children they studied showed "hereditary taint" by virtue of the presence of psychotic or psychopathic disorders in their close relatives: 71 percent of the mothers of this group of neurotic children were mentally ill, and 32 percent of fathers were mentally ill (mostly "nervous" and "neurotic"). Cammer provided a more explicit statement when he found that manic-depressive parents had more obsessive children than was to be found in the general population.[27] There is conflicting evidence about the increased familial incidence and therefore, presumably, the likelihood of genetic influence on childhood neurosis.

It is of interest that Slater and Cowie[140] found no significant difference between 342 controls and 330 offspring of psychotic parents on "neuroticism" or "extraversion" or on the adjustment scores of the children as adjudged by their parents. It may be that it is asking the wrong question to explore the genetics of neuroses. This was suggested by Shields[139] who found, from studies of 62 same-sex twin pairs (36 were monozygous, 26 dizygous) between ages 12 and 15 years, that the evidence is stronger for genetical determination of *personality traits* than of frank neurotic symptoms. Neurotic symptoms would presumably be more sociogenic.

Or, in asking the genetic questions, one should perhaps direct them to very specific types of neuroses. I.I. Gottesman[64] examined thirty-four monozygous and thirty-four dizygous pairs of twins among normal school children via the MMPI. He concluded that (1) hysterical and hypochondriacal neuroses have little or no genetic component, but (2) those neuroses with features of anxiety, depression and obsession have a "substantial genetic component" under the environmental terms governing his study sample. Eliot Slater[141] contended in 1971 that neuroses results from more than one genetic factor, with dissimilar effects dependent on the particular neurosis type, or with overlapping effects producing more than one type of neurosis. In sum, at present there is little room for any dogmatic assertion in this matter.

Head trauma will serve as an example of the role played by exogenous organic etiologic factors in neurosis. Slater and Cowie[141] found a significant incidence of irritability, depression, hydrochondriacal, and hysterical symptoms following head trauma.

Psychosocial Dynamisms in Childhood Neurosis

With the admittedly poor and conflicting evidence available at present, psychoneuroses are plausibly taken to be sociogenic in the main. The Freudian view of individual dynamics has been summarized already. (See the foregoing sections on "Approaches to Classifying the Childhood Neuroses," "The Classic Cases of Freud," "Later Freudians," and "Neurotic Features in General.") Greater attention will be devoted now to three early non-Freudians and to psychodynamics and sociodynamics in interpersonal, familial, and sociocultural spheres. Some additional material on sociogenic factors in neuroses will appear in the subsequent section on "Specific Therapies for Childhood Psychoneuroses."

Adler, Jung, and Rank were early figures associated with Freud who later departed the Freudian ranks. Nonetheless, their psychodynamic views were often rather close to those of Freud. After 1924, the views of Adler and Rank deviated more than did the Jungian views. This seems to be true at least in the case of those Jungians who work with children. Probably the classic Jungian child therapy and theory text remains that of Frances Wickes, *The Inner World of Childhood*.[154] For Jung and the Jungians, libido was regarded as a generic "life energy" and not exclusively the motive power supplied by Eros. In much the same way as was true for adults, children showed broad temperamental differences that the Jungians assessed in a global way, or, at times, tested for. The temperamental phenotype was considered to be either introverted or extroverted. If the libido took an extroversive direction, the child showed an outgoing drive toward others, and toward things. If the libido was expressed in an introversive mode, the child was more introspective, self-aimed, and subjective.

Like other analysts, Jungians seemed to hit it off better with introverted patients than with those who were extroverted. However, since each temperamental phenotype carried its obverse, the *shadow* of introversion was extroversion. Within this system, the child's behavior was subsumed under two pairs of functions: (1) sensation and intuition; and (2) feeling and thinking. One may appear as Sensation dominant/Feeling or thinking auxiliary, or as Intuition dominant/Feeling or thinking auxiliary. Jungians have been very sensitive to all overdone or compulsive behavior, advocating in its stead a life of more naturalness and balance. The child whose full potential was not lived out and actualized was, for Jungians, a tragic figure. They therefore sought to help neurotics more than all other types of children. Just as Freudians stressed insight, conflict resolution, and ego mastery, the Jungian search was always for balance and consistency.

The collective unconscious was a Jungian formulation to account for common themes in myths and legends and human practices everywhere. It served as a way of showing the need, even of young children, to have a sense of family and tribe, and to commune with "the 2-million-year-old man within" every person's psyche. This gave support for the individuating work that Jung, presaging Rank, set up as the quality that pervaded the developmental course of the human child from birth to maturity: the child emerged progressively from collective to individual. Archetypal images and complexes (including Mother, the shadow), the soul images of *anima* and *animus*, and the *mandala* were Jungian efforts—sometimes extreme efforts—at formulating the kind of phylogenetic mental preprogramming that Freudians attributed to children mainly through id and the sequential development of the "instincts." Both in England and the United States, Jungians adapted readily to child guidance strategies of teamwork, where attention was given abundantly to the familial, and the tribal or social, aspects of neurotic disorders.

In the final analysis, both Jung and Freud advocated greater activation and actualization of consciousness and regarded true insight as the healer of neurosis.[82] Jung more than Freud, however, saw wholesome possibilities for the unconscious as well. Neither spared children from the heavy yoke of fate's unpredictable but immutable dealings.

Adler had left Freud in 1911, but he had been unfaithful still earlier. Adler questioned libido theory and repudiated the idea of a sexual basis for behavior. In 1908 he wrote a paper on "Aggressionstrieb"[7] in a Freudian tone, but quickly recanted. The Freudians, on the other hand, clung to the notion of a basic aggressive drive, which they regarded as more palatable than the Freud-enunciated death instinct, Thanatos.

Adler loved and trusted people, and liked café fare and talk. In keeping with this, he had begun his career as a socialist general medical practitioner in working class areas of Vienna. He placed a sensible and modern emphasis on social, societal, and class conditions in the life of the neurotic child and his family. Sometimes this entailed a playing down of fantasies in the child's troubles. At the last, Adler came to emphasize sociability, or social feeling (*Gemeinschaftsgefuehl*), instead of inferiority and superiority. Self-esteem and social feeling were the dominant themes in the Adlerian system of psychodynamics. These primary motifs could be endangered by three classes of etiologic circumstances: (1) organic inferiorities and diseases that make the child feel ashamed and incompetent; (2) neglect which breeds neglect, aloofness, and an inflated goal of security and superiority; and (3) pampering.

Adler took a commonsense interest in the social situation, both as it existed objectively, and as it was perceived through the eyes of the child. Though the Freudians called Adlerism *superficial* in its approach to child guidance and to parental life-style analysis, the Adlerians retorted that they were watching the head and body of the psychodynamic peacock, while the Freudians overvalued the florid tail of metatheory. In Austria, child psychiatry has inclined to be more Alderian than Freudian.

Adler did not value the anamnesis and historiography of a neurotic child when it was done within a theoretical framework of intricate metapsychology. In his own terse dogmatic way, he saw the basic issues as, not *whence*, but *whither*? He introduced the use of the child's earliest recollection as psychiatric datum, regarding it as a clue as to the child's *current* goals and style, including his self-concept. Holistic before Karen Horney wrote down her holistic theses, Adler was perhaps a proper member of Maslow's Third Force, concerned with pilot movement, expansion, and growth. Thus, the purpose of Adlerian psychiatric work with a neurotic child was to move the patient from a "relatively minus" to a "relatively plus" position.[15]

Otto Rank did not personally work with children but wrote in considerable quantity about childhood neuroses and child "education." His first wife, Beata Rank, worked with very seriously impaired atypical children, and his friend and biographer, Jessie Taft, did a great deal of therapy with children who were neurotic and wrote at length about her findings. From Taft and Frederick H. Allen, with some contributions from John A. Rose and Clark Moustakas, the Rankian tradition of work with neurotic children has continued.

Rank apparently wished to mediate among the Jung, Adler, and Freud groups while making some fitful attempts to set up a Rank group both in Paris and the United States. The Rankians do not deprecate the neurotic child for his pathology, but laud him for his achievement of a creative step beyond the ordinary. *Neurosis, they said, is better than mediocrity and automaton conformity.* Taft, Rank, and Allen, all stressed the need for symptom improvement as essential to the feeling of relief that makes therapy truly therapy. The healing relationship with the therapist makes the child feel better, less neurotic. For Rankians, the important motive of the human being was not to achieve security (by belonging, love, respite from striving and anxiety) but to *accomplish selfhood* (by self-assertion, the achievement of prestige or self-esteem, and the acceptance of one's being different from others). Rank counterposed the striving for union against the striving to emerge as a unique individual (first articulated as birth trauma, the aboriginal separation fear rooted in biology). Though the child's affiliative longings are recognized as great, Rankians have tended to value individualistic strivings even more. Rank and followers also stressed the child's mother-relatedness. Half a century ago this was a very heterodox doctrine for Freudians, who at the time universally believed that the father and the oedipal complex developed around him were the *sine qua non* of neurosis.

SULLIVANIAN CONCEPTIONS OF CHILDHOOD NEUROSIS

It is interesting to turn now from Rank, who carried individualism to an almost absurd extreme, to Harry Stack Sullivan, who might be said to have denied individuality to an almost absurd extreme. This demonstrates something of the polarities that prevail in the whole perspective of the psychodynamics of childhood neurosis as a sociogenic disturbance. It seems odd that Sullivan is reported to have made the formal move to oust Rank from the International Psychoanalytic Association. Sullivan's views on child development were very advanced for his day. He rephrased some of the Freudian viewpoints on the psychosexual stages, but with his emphasis on relationships, he also added a new dimension. This view was derived from the social psychology of the 1920s and 1930s; *interpersonal relations* has more warmth, just on the face of it, than *object relations* or *libidinal phases*. Sullivan attempted to reinterpret some of Freud's views and to put them into a language that was understandable to social psychologists and acceptable to his own followers. In child development, his greatest contributions appear to have been his incorporation of the work done by Jean Piaget, his emphasis on communication within the original family, and his detailed attention to the preadolescent phase of childhood. He regarded anxiety and pain as great curses of mankind, but he stated that, in this epoch in history, alienation and loneliness with their primordia emerging in preadolescence were equal blights on personality development. Sullivan's per-

ception was that people who do not form chumships, with loving bonds to culturally similar peers during the "late latency" or preadolescent era, are the ones who develop paranoid orientations in later life.

Sullivan's ecological views were highly congenial to a large segment of the field of orthopsychiatry and social psychiatry. Family therapy owes much to Sullivan, and his formulations of the childhood of the obsessive-compulsive remain fruitful today. Sullivan described the pattern that Jackson, Bateson, and others were later to label the double bind, and he inspired the entire transactional analysis school of Eric Berne, Claude Steiner, and others. Two rather popularly oriented books that show Sullivanian inspiration are *Games Children Play* by A. H. Chapman[31] and *Understanding Children* by Richard Gardner.[59] *Learning Psychotherapy* by the child analyst Hilde Bruch[25] is also a Sullivanian opus. Raymond Sobel and Barbara Fish have carried Sullivanian influences into their research on children; and Stanislas Szurek has acknowledged his indebtedness to Sullivan's interpersonal approach in the realm of work devoted to schizophrenic children and adolescents.

Sullivan added little (except his more social viewpoint and his careful attention to obsessives) to what Freud had accomplished in the exploration of childhood neuroses. For that reason, it makes sense to call Sullivan a neo-Freudian, while Karen Horney and Erich Fromm are more aptly labeled post-Freudian, neo-Adlerian. Sullivan did not use libido theory; instead he looked at human motives and dynamics in a much more social way. For Sullivan the basic drives were (1) the pursuit of bodily satisfactions and (2) the pursuit of security. Anxiety was the master foe of security; however, Sullivan ascribed anxiety not to intrapsychic events but to an interpersonal field. He emphasized the ways in which neurotic children strive, albeit unsuccessfully, to allay both the tensions associated with their pursuit of bodily satisfactions and the anxiety connected with seeking security. The tensions of anxiety are usually experienced distortedly ("in the parataxic mode"), and the tensions of bodily needs are usually experienced in both syntaxic (i.e., undistorted) and parataxic modes. It was a post-Freudian viewpoint, to say that an anxious child shows more parataxic distortions than does a child feeling bodily needs. The talking animal, man, was not given consideration when biology and physiology reigned, according to Sullivan's system. Sullivan traced out in detail, moreover, the ways in which even the satisfaction of bodily needs are warped and molded by anxiety.

Sullivan took a pre-Skinnerian stance against speculations about the inner mind's "black box." He referred to this as "the immutably private"—intrapsychic, unobservable, and therefore, not to be studied. The self-system or self-dynamism was, for Sullivan, something that developed in the course of the life cycle. The earliest fundamentals laid down in infancy were borrowed from the mother and "significant others" to such a degree that Sullivan disputed the uniqueness of the individual. Sullivan saw the self as but a "reflective appraisal by others."

Erich Fromm is another member of the Washington School of Psychiatry in which Sullivan was an early leading figure. Fromm has been called both neo-Freudian and neo-Adlerian, and has had wide influence on the sociogenic theory of childhood neurosis. Fromm too (like Freud, Sullivan, Jung, and Rank) worked not with children but only with adults; in them, however, he discerned the childhood problems that lead to their adult neuroses.

Fromm's training as a sociologist gave him a societal grasp and breadth that was lacking in many analysts—though Abram Kardiner, Géza Róheim, Wilhelm Reich, George Wilbur, Warner Muensterberger, Erik H. Erikson, and George Devereux would all be important exceptions. Fromm rejected the universality and biological preprogramming of the Oedipus complex. He rejected libido theory as well and emphasized ontogenetic learning and culture as more important than any phylogenetic programming. Fromm did sound pioneering work on "social character" or "basic personality" (Kardiner's term). The focus here was on child rearing, the values of the family of origin, the class perspective of the family, and the ways in which individuals were enculturated in a class system. Very early, Fromm asserted that the central issue in childhood neurosis is the child's grappling with irrational authority, the latter defined as an authority imposed without any warrant except that the adult is stronger and will demand obeisance from the inferior child. Fromm stated that it was this encounter of a child with irrational authority, rather than the specificity of an Oedipus complex, which accounted for the building of a childhood neurosis.

For Erich Fromm, the central problem for all psychology is the problem of human relatedness, relation to the world, to others and to oneself. The problem of alienation, seen not from an orthodox Marxian slant but from that of a humanistic socialist, guided Fromm's thinking through *Escape from Freedom* to many other works. In all, Fromm examined the growth of individuality in Western societies (a Rankian notion) and the ways individuals attempted to escape from acceptance of their individuality, namely, sadomasochism or authoritarianism (a Reichian derivative), destructiveness toward one's opponents, and automaton conformity (Jungian and Rankian). In Fromm's views of the pathology of normalcy are concepts reminiscent of Carl Jung and Otto Rank, although in 1943, Erich Fromm, later a guru and apostle of love, denounced Rank as a "crypto-fascist." Fromm is mainly concerned with adults, not children; he argues vigorously for a socialist reconstruction of society[55] linked with pervasive respect for the integrity of the individual. Fromm contends that when that occurs, the Oedipus complex will disappear into the patriarchal and unjust past.

Karen Horney put anxiety at the center of her dynamics, for she felt that anxiety set in motion all the forces of defense and coping for both the neurotic and the normal. Horney sounded the clarion call for new approaches in psychoanalysis, without libido theory. As precipitators of anxiety, Horney stressed the role of hostile impulses and feelings. Cultural taboos against hostility only made it all the more anxiety-producing. Horney had evolved by 1950[77] the three main styles of living which for many have become the hallmark of Horneyan thought. These were moving *toward* people, moving *away from* people and moving *against* people. The neurotic's major strivings were: exaggerated helplessness (toward), or isolation (away from), or hostility and aggression (against). Horney was often said to have founded the "cultural school" since she showed how certain character problems and neurotic traits were culturally sanctioned and promoted in bourgeois United States society.[76] But Horney did not evolve many very convincing developments beyond Freudian views, so that today the Horneyan analysts are not very different from those orthodox Freudians who might have peeked into Adler's writings. Horney herself did not work with children, and her unitary or holistic viewpoint has not found a vocal advocacy among child psychiatrists. Nonetheless, Frederick H. Allen, Leo Kanner, and many other child psychiatrists have recognized the seminal influence of this woman analyst from Germany who, whether in Chicago or New York, wrote so clearly that her books were on the recommended list of the Society for General Semantics.

HUMANISTIC VIEWS

Still another trend among post-Freudians is that exemplified by the existentialists and humanists. Each existentialist is different from every other and their world-weariness and *Angst* have not been as systematically translated, or transposed, into a psychodynamic theory as have some other systems. They have thus far had little impact on research or treatment with children. Hanna Colm[35] is a notable exception, for her existentialist writings about children have been numerous. Ludwig Binswanger[22] too has elucidated some ways that children can be understood with the aid of an existentialist perspective. A brief example of the ontologic approach adopted by Binswanger is contained in his report on a five-year-old child with a *heel phobia*. A shock came to this little girl when she suddenly experienced a moment of discontinuity and separateness. It happened when she pulled off a skate and her shoe heel stuck in the skate. Theretofore, her outlook had been one of safeguarding herself against anxiety by pretending that the world was one of only smooth transitions. The phobia served to buttress her illusion that her restricted, impoverished world was one ruled purely by connectedness. By development of phobic symptoms she stayed on guard against suddenness, against the discontinuous, the separate; she maintained a falsely reinforcing "motionless world-clock" in her cognitive perspective. The neurotic symptoms, said Binswanger, kept her fixated on a restricted vista and prohibited her from developing an expanded world-view. Her phobia was merely part of her insistence that her life-realm was emptier, smaller, simpler, and more stable than her sudden loss of the shoe heel had shown it actually to be.

Existentialists often state that neurosis is an escape from a fuller, more vital experiencing of life. Hence, the neurosis causes a growth failure in personal potential. As Maslaw stated this point,[103] "We fear our best as well as our worst."

Arthur Burton[26] has given one of the most understandable versions of the humanistic-existential viewpoint since Rollo May's *Existence*.[104] Existentialist and humanistic psychodynamic views have influenced many of the followers of Freud, Jung, Adler, Rank, Horney, Fromm, Sullivan, Carl Rogers, and Abraham Maslow. Since Maslow's views are ordinarily neglected, a short introduction to them might well be in order.

Kurt Goldstein had observed that the only way to know a brain damaged person was to know his whole personality and life style, his "way of being in the world." This had influenced Abraham Maslow deeply. Goldstein[63] reported experiments with brain damaged people which proved that the whole person indelibly influenced even so simple an example of behavior as the knee jerk. Moreover, Goldstein went further than a holistic view —he contended that *self-actualization* is the key to all human behavior. Self-actualizing is a basic motive, then, representing the person's effort to grow into full potential and to realize the full range of his capabilities. By that criterion, neurosis is indeed a growth failure.

Maslow seized on the concept of self-actualization and advanced the idea that actualizing is not a slow process; sometimes it comes suddenly in the form of a *peak experience*. Maslow's psychodynamic theory[103] puts needs (or drives, or values) into a hierarchical ordering. At the base of the Maslovian pyramid is the *physiologic* level, hunger or the need for food, for example. Next above are what could be called the *safety* needs of the child, the needs to be free from fear and pain and to experience considerable security in his world as caring, meaningful, and orderly. Next above these are the needs *for love*. Maslow insisted that unless the basic needs at levels 1 and 2 (levels focused on by Marxists) are met, the needs (for love) of level 3 will never be satisfactory. Hence the pyramidal structural model. Maslow regarded the level 3 need for love as the Freudian focus. The still higher level 4 needs were the Adlerian focus, the needs for *esteem*. Finally, at the apex of the pyramid stood the Maslovian/Goldsteinian level 5 needs, for self-actualizing, and for self-transcending.

As Maslow envisioned these pyramiding levels, the preceding level must be gratified before any available driving force can operate at the next higher level. Also, according to Maslow, as soon as one level is satisfied, the next higher level is activated at once and becomes the motive life of the person. Humanistic psychologists have become increasingly numerous in the child care field, a field where it is frequently said that child advocacy is as appropriate as child therapy. The influence of Maslovian dynamic theory has been to restore the growing and expanding person to a central place in psychodynamics. Perhaps that is a needed corrective in a day when a more "social" psychiatry is in vogue among the intellectuals but with scarce support from the nation's centers of real power.

FAMILY DYNAMICS IN CURRENT
PSYCHIATRIC THEORY

Most psychiatrists have seen neurosis as a family affair, and numerous writers have described neurotigenic family types. Salzman and Fromm-Reichmann early depicted the neurosis-inducing family as a special phenomenon of bourgeois Western civilization. They became neo-Freudian or post-Freudian partly, it is said, in order to employ more freely the Freudian genius, to be able to seek an ampler understanding of dynamic pictures that differed from the Freudian model. Nathan Ackermann was a child psychiatrist who early freed himself in order to apply the gist of analytic thought to the family. He viewed it as a small group with a specific set of dynamisms that varied for each individual family. Erich Fromm, too, placed the problem of the child's submission to irrational authority at the heart of neurosis, and neurosis became thereby the outcome of an intrafamilial process. Family theorists grew more influential within the ranks of both general and child psychiatrists during the quarter century between 1950 and 1975. At the beginning, there was only a strong determination to regard the unit of treatment as the family, not the individual. Oftentimes, however, their practice outran their simple Rankian theory, and well before they had developed a clear system or rationale for doing so, they had begun seeing members of families in groups instead of individually.

The family is often regarded to be a relatively closed system, in equilibrium or homeostasis on three counts—role taking, verbal communication, and deep emotional longings. Hence, families came to be described by some theorists as a sort of blob, a membrane, that existed for hatching individuals but which often failed in its hatching function. Murray Bowen called this the *undifferentiated ego mass*[23] of a family. Lyman Wynne and co-workers referred to the overall constellations of rigid role-taking in families under the terms *pseudo-mutuality* and *pseudo-hostility* (terms used to denote, respectively, those families that pretend all is sweetness and togetherness, and those who repudiate love and mutuality). Both polar types, it is said, induce neurosis (or worse) through blocking differentiation and separation. Families showed a spectrum that ranged between full differentiation and failure of differentiation when they arrived at their homeostatic style. R. D. Laing added, from Marx, the idea that *mystification*, imposing an ideology and a mystique, is one of the sick purposes of some families. Laing contended that families try to impose on children what the children feel, think, want, need, and believe.[92] Concomitantly with these brain washing efforts, the family negated or *invalidated* the child's own views and *inducted* the child into fuller collusion in the parental mystique. Stierlin gave a fast-moving review[147] of family theory in 1974.

Stierlin's own views are important, since they deal with the transactional modes of binding, expelling, and delegating. Any of these modes may become pathogenic. Binding refers to the creation of dependency at the id level, to mystification at the ego or cognitive level, and to a pervasive feeling of loyalty and guilt at the superego level. The combined effect is that any inclination to break away mobilizes deep guilt and a sense of disloyalty. *Expelling* refers to the activities of neglectful parents who push their children into premature separations. And *delegating* depicts the multitudinous compromises arrived at in families whereby some centrifugal force is permitted but the child is given "only so much rope" so that only a restricted orbiting can occur. In effect, it is a blending of expelling and binding.

Family therapists, it may be noted, showed a penchant for working with families where one child was schizophrenic. Hence, in many of its formulations, family therapy theory is more oriented to schizophrenia, much as behavior therapy is oriented mainly toward phobias. There are trends in the field of family theory, however, in which family approaches are applied to psychosomatic disorders (such as anorexia nervosa), to character problems and to neuroses—indeed to any and all problems that had formerly been regarded as the proper realm of individual psychopathology. Jan Ehrenwald[46] was one early theorist who showed that at least three generations make up the family and person psychopathology, and if any real reconciliation is to occur, a three-generation purview must be taken. Clinical child psychiatrists have found the three-generation compass a congenial one, for it gives emphasis to grandparents as well as parents and provides a wider range for helping.

Family theory sometimes shares the very shortcomings it attributes to the intrapsychic theories it is supposed to supplant—according to a frequent allegation—it is culturally blind. It vaunts the position of the father and sees the restoration, or inclusion, of the father as a sign of healthy family change. Some family theorists have been accused of holding male chauvinist views, of being bourgeois, of being outmodely patriarchal in ideology, and of adding to the child's weakness and insignificance by overvaluing the power of the parents in relation to the child. Salvador Minuchin and associates,[110] however, have shown the adaptability of family theory and therapy to slum families with mother and grandmother but without fathers, as well as to more traditional families with pervasive problems arising from poverty.

DYNAMISMS OF NEUROSIS ACCORDING TO LEARNING THEORY

Compared to family theory, learning theory seems to have still less in the way of speculative and assumptive underpinnings and concomitants. The biologic theory is certainly simply, hardly more than an assertion that an organism acts and responds within a system of environmental stimuli. Activity ("behavior") is functional because it is responsive. It is motivated. Responses are given to stimuli. The reflex arc is the model. According to learning theory, in order to understand how learning occurs, we need to scrutinize either the *organismic* responses (conditioned or unconditioned) or the *environmental* stimuli or reinforcers (and contingencies for others' responses) or both organismic and environmental conditions. The responses of organism "A" may serve as reinforcers of the responses of organism "B". Learning theory gives a prominent place to "interpersonal" relations and influences. Likewise, it is child oriented, applied more to a diversity of children's problems than to adults' problems. In practical terms, in the United States it is applied mainly by nonprofessional women.

The symptom, the behavior itself, is of central importance for learning theory. Hence, the symptom's baseline frequency, the setting in which it occurs, its changes in frequency, indeed, everything about it, are all basic data to be recorded and studied by the behavior therapist. Outcome figures are readily comparable with onset figures, and the base in quantitative behavioral data (counting) serves well as an index of efficacious outcome. There is a longstanding and often repeated assertion that removal of a symptom only results in symptom substitution, but most clinicians who believe this have not tested their belief. Occasionally, when behavioral items that are said to be neurotic symptoms, such as bedwetting, are removed by Mowrer's alarm system, the weight of the evidence is overwhelming that symptom substitution does *not* occur. For that matter, most follow-up studies do not show any predictive merit in a symptom such as bedwetting. In other words, by whatever approach the bedwetting is stopped, the child seems to proceed with his development no better, and no worse, than if he had not been enuretic. Before behavior modification had been formulated, Otto Rank emphasized the essence of therapy as a release from the oppressive burdens of neurosis. Rank thought a hastening of symptomatic relief was a worthwhile objective, and so did many of the child-therapist Rankians such as Jessie Taft and Frederick Allen.

For learning theory, the crux of the neuroses is that they are patterns of behavior containing some elements that are not adaptive or desired. The symptom picture does not have to be ironed out so that it fits a theoretical framework; it only has to be counted and ranked so that the worst symptoms can be given a place of special priority as targets for extinction. For most behavior theorists, the focus of their work is not a complex neurotic syndrome but specific behavioral items in uncomplicated clusters—fear of the dark, bedwetting, tantrums, tics, and so on. Behavioral theory does not value intricate metatheory. Instead it seeks the formulation that is the most frugal, simple, and clear.

From this standpoint, a functional analysis of the problem behavior, of the factors that control it, and of the ways to change it are all that are needed in the pursuit of "causes" and dynamisms. As charged, behavior theory strives to be as poor as possible in "theory" (meaning axioms, assumptions, postulates, inferences, guesses, speculations, and wild flight of fancy). Again, as charged, behavior theory does not reject any information but tends to give priority to current events instead of remote recollections. The live child, acting in the present, is enough to go on. Behavior theory is highly interactive with behavioral research and therapy. And, as a last point, as is often charged, behavior theory carries several metaphysical assumptions that it merely omits to mention. Behavior therapists, armed with different approaches and explanations—underlining respondent or operant or continuity learning—get results from their efforts. In that, they remind one of many other therapists (with contradictory notions) who seem to help children with a diversity of problems.[11]

Specific Therapies for Childhood Psychoneuroses

The treatment of the neuroses of childhood is the end purpose of diagnosis. In another context than treatment of neurotic children, Abraham Maslow divided contemporary schools of psychology into:

1. Traditional Freudian psychoanalysts
2. Behaviorists or learning theorists
3. A Third Force of Alfred Adler, Carl Jung, Otto Rank, Carl Rogers, Gardner Murphy, J. L. Moreno, Frederick Perls, Charlotte Bühler, Erich Fromm, Kurt Goldstein, Karan Horney, Clark Moustakas, Henry Murray, and Abraham Maslow.

The third force described by Maslow had the common trait of a less mechanistic view of man, and many in the third force see both Freudians and learning theorists as conceiving the human person as a robot, whereas the third force sees the person as a pilot. The pilot is more alive than a robot; he is constantly involved, making choices and living in interaction.

It must be noted that Maslow's values have not received as much support as the work of many others. Julius Segal and associates[158] examined the therapy research support given by the National Institute of Mental Health for the year 1972-73. NIMH did not identify that part of the psychotherapy research devoted to child therapy, but the apportionment itself is of interest: $6.85 millions were spent totally. Of these funds 55 percent were spent for behavior therapy research, specialized therapies 19 percent, individual psychotherapy 13 percent, group therapy 7 percent, and psychoanalysis 6 percent.

PSYCHOANALYTIC THERAPY FOR CHILDHOOD NEUROSES

The conventional wisdom that governs child psychiatry today states that the treatment of choice for neurotic children is psychoanalysis or psychoanalytically oriented psychotherapy. Some of the psychoanalytically-oriented therapies are more like the Third Force than the First, Freudian psychoanalysis, and will be discussed later, even though their adherents call themselves analysts.

A few analysts differentiate sharply between diagnosis and therapy, but for the most part the diagnostic assessment made by an analyst is not totally different in style from the way the analytic treatment proceeds. If it were not rather similar, the child would probably feel confused by the abrupt change in style. The diagnostic work done by the analyst usually includes early history that has been obtained during separate interviews with the parents (often the mother and for some at least a token session, or several, with the father). Also, the early meetings give a chance to set in operation some pattern of interchange between adult and child (some familiarity and beginning relationship), as well as a preliminary consensus with the child and/or the parents about the working diagnostic formulation, the need for the analysis, and some of the practical arrangements for the analysis.

One practical arrangement of more than passing import is the frequency and regularity of the sessions. Many contend that if they do not occur four or more times weekly, it is not in fact psychoanalysis. The diagnostic formulation guiding the analyst is usually based upon a dynamic assessment of core conflicts, major coping and defending maneuvers, ego functions, id strengths and fixations, levels of drive development achieved (both libidinal and aggressive), structure of interpersonal relations, phenomenology of symptoms, and perhaps even a "surface" diagnosis within the classification scheme currently in use. If the cost of child analysis is to be paid for by third parties, the analyst's future use of conventional diagnostic labels may become more common. Still, for analytic therapy, it is the diagnostic-genetic profile that has the greater utility, and not the label.

Where necessary, play is used as a vehicle for the interaction within the sessions. There is a lot of evidence accumulating that progress (the learning, perhaps) is greatest when the therapeutic sessions have not relied primarily on fantasy play but have made connections with cognitive force as well as serving a cathartic function.[53] Hence, most analyses tend toward verbal dialogue between child and analyst, an activity from which the child may take refuge by playing. Children's dreams, drawings, and other imaginative materials are brought into the analytic work. Expressions of transference are obviously present, and because they are so easily analyzed—after all, the real parent(s) are immediate and dominant realities in the child's life—some writers have insisted that nothing resembling adult-style transference transpires during a child analysis. A meaningful relationship can grow, however, and, in general, there is a progressive diminution of the neurotic symptoms consonant with the increase of insight resulting from the analyst's work. This will include clarification, identification, reassurance, advising, confronting, imparting information, and, finally, the analytic chief stock in trade, interpretation. Analytic interpretation is a special form of insight that comes when the child's symptoms or otherwise relevant behavior are illuminated by an exposition of the associated ego defenses, by an understanding of the hidden id wish, by a reconstruction of the etiologic early infantile experience, and by connecting all these with the related contemporary transference fantasies.

A therapeutic alliance is initiated when the child sees that his immediate troubles are not the whole story, and that, with the analyst's help, he can grow well. Resistances and reluctances, regression and backsliding, will tend to recur repeatedly because change toward health is not an easy path for a child to walk. Usually however, the neurotic child opts ultimately for enduring symptom removal. In the analyst's view, he gives up his libidinal and his ego regressions. To get well, resistance must be surmounted, even by the child analysand who did not (chances are) want the treatment in the first place. Ultimately, the resistances are in fact character defenses; to the extent that the more infantile forms of defense are interpreted and given up, the child becomes ever more free to grow.

Psychoanalysis of children with neuroses is rather well charted, although the foregoing description is surely too brief and perhaps too biased. The neuroses remain the childhood behavioral disturbances that lend themselves most readily to analytic understanding and to analytic helping or cure.

BEHAVIOR THERAPY FOR CHILDHOOD NEUROSES

There are several behavior therapies that must be considered for the childhood neuroses, bearing in mind that, save for phobias, behavior therapy has not been employed mainly for neuroses. The types to be considered herein are:

1. Classical or respondent conditioning
2. Systematic desensitization, flooding; negative practice
3. Operant conditioning

Classical, respondent, Pavlovian conditioning was exemplified in the work of Watson and Raynor.[153] In 1920, they conditioned an infant's phobic responses to furry objects by simultaneously presenting him with the furry objects and a harsh sound. They showed that phobic responses could be learned. Then Mary C. Jones[83] demonstrated that these responses could be deconditioned or unlearned by simultaneously presenting the feared object and a pleasant stimulus. The thinking here was rather close to the mechanistic materialism of Pavlov, employing cognitive models based on the neural tissue responses involved in reflex arcs. Later on, the learning itself came to be focused on, with less stress given to the body-brain issues. A quip holds that behaviorists lost both minds and brains.

Systematic desensitization has been developed mainly by Joseph Wolpe.[156] It has been used more with adults than with children, but its target symptom is anxiety. The basic notion is to pair the anxiety provoking stimuli with a response antagonistic to the anxiety. The pairing weakens the linkage between the evocative stimuli and the experience of anxiety, and, in many instances, the symptom reduction is facilitated beyond what can be achieved only by repeated exposure to the stimuli. This is an extension of Mary C. Jones's work in the 1920s. She had removed fear by pairing anxiety-provoking stimuli with pleasurable stimuli of even greater intensity.

In practice, systematic desensitization takes a highly systematic, rational, and clinical approach to the fear-producing stimuli. The anxiety-provoking stimuli are parceled out, graded for severity and ranked. Then the symptom-producing stimuli are presented in a sequence of gradually increasing severity. At the same time, they are simultaneously accompanied by stimulation which counters anxiety. For example, a school phobic child may be taught to relax, to mobilize "counterphobic" fantasies and affects, and then gradually to be drawn nearer and nearer the school he fears. This becomes a better example if the school phobia is a typical phobia and not based on separation anxiety or characterologic disturbance, as cited in the foregoing material on "An Exemplary Childhood Neurosis." Children who are more articulately verbal and introspective may not require actual physical approximation to school; they may simply be taught to relax progressively and to "imagine" in fantasy a progressing series of steps toward the feared situation, namely, being at school and away from home. Lazarus and Abramovitz[95] have used "emotive imagery" to treat neurotic symptoms in children. The progressive relaxation training of Jacobson[78] is a favorite technique for helping achieve systematic desensitization. The relaxed habitus allows graded doses of anxiety to be mastered, until finally the symptom has been removed in the consulting room. A high degree of transfer from the clinic to the outside world has been demonstrated repeatedly. But, if possible, all other things being equal, an *in vivo* intervention is preferable to one given *in vitro*.[102] Systematic desensitization and analytically oriented psychotherapy have been used together (by the same therapist) with neurotics, and, instead of relaxation, short-acting barbiturates have been used to good advantage.

Flooding and *paradoxical intention* are related procedures that deserve momentary mention as behavior therapy devices. In flooding, the goal of preventing an avoidance or fear response is reached through exposure to the very cues that elicit the unwanted, neurotic behavior. The exposure is done through imagery or through actual, real life exposure. The latter appears to be more effective. When properly conducted, this approach has been found not to be harmful, for in periods of time (lasting usually no more than twenty minutes) the patient's anxiety is reduced to bearable levels. It is important to have the therapist maintain the "holding attitude" of reassurance until anxiety has been truly diminished, because premature ending of a session can lead to a strengthening of the anxiety, instead of its removal. Less systematic but similar to flooding is paradoxical intention, the technique popularized by Victor Frankl. According to numerous anecdotes, however, it has also been employed by good teachers for generations—August Aichhorn, Sylvia Ashton-Warner, Fritz Redl. Tics, compulsions, and other neurotic symptoms have been treated by paradoxical intention or *negative practice*. The procedure in brief is to identify the symptom, count its frequency and then have the child "overdo" the symptomatic behavior. By this deliberate repetition, repeated in, say, thirty-minute sessions ten times per week, the child masters and then extinguishes the "faulty" behavior. In studies of negative practice, its efficacy has been reported only as moderate.

Operant conditioning or instrumental conditioning emphasizes another aspect of learning and of behavior. Instead of a focus on responses, the therapist's interest here is directed to the environmental reinforcers of responses—those things that follow or succeed an emitted behavioral response. Because they follow it, the probability increases that they will take control of the response. So it is not the *behavior* directly that is to be manipulated or changed, it is the contingencies, *the consequences of behavior*, that must be manipulated. Hence, "operant" or naturally occurring behavior (including compulsions, obsessions, fears, depressive speech, aggression, conversion symptoms), and not artifically elicited or induced behavior, is what engages the concern of the operant conditioner. Thereafter, the shift is quickly made to the reinforcers and the contingencies under which the reinforcers come into play. When that is done, and the behavior itself has been counted, the next process is to alter the contingencies and to change the reinforcers with the expectation that the behavior itself is now modified. More technically and accurately, a four-step sequence occurs: (1) a *discriminative stimulus* exists, functioning as a signal that the reinforcer will follow the response; then (2) the *operant response* is emitted, so (3) the *reinforcer* goes into action and (4) a *consummatory response* comes about.

Lazarus and associates[96] reported a case of school phobia in which respondent techniques (systematic desensitization) were employed first and then followed by operant techniques. Behavior therapists are clinicians, and like other clinicians, when they are not doing primarily investigative work, they are flexible and use a variety of approaches. Since pragmatism reigns, almost anything that affords quick relief is used in preference to something that delays the behavioral change, the relief of suffering.

It has often been argued, but seldom demonstrated, that relief of symptoms, "without getting to the intrapsychic root causes of the neurosis," will be of little benefit to the child. One reason adduced is that the child will merely replace the symptom that has been extinguished with an equally symbolic, equally pathologic equivalent symptom. The shortest answer to this objection is that such replacement is usually not found. Indeed, when a problem behavior is extinguished and healthy behavior is reinforced, there is no vacuum left in the child's behavioral repertoire. In reality, other symptoms are more likely to fall off than to increase. Behavior therapy sometimes aims to enrich a fearful child's expansiveness and freedom of expression. This is usually called "assertiveness training" and is one way to augment the range of healthy behavior. Some children are so timid and inhibited that they may need a prelude of desensitization before assertive training can be commenced. Assertive training has been used with both internalizing and externalizing children. Lazarus in *Behavior Therapy and Beyond*[94] described the ways in which people who inhibit positive feelings can be "trained in emotional freedom." The aspect of behavior therapy that involves accentuating the positive has been especially well depicted by the psychiatrist George Saslow.[132]

THIRD FORCE AND ASSORTED PSYCHOTHERAPIES

As stated earlier, these psychotherapies are a wide assortment of post-Freudian, neo-Freudian, neo-Adlerian, existentialist, and humanistic therapies, individual and group. A selected sample will be considered, not for representativeness but for sketchy exemplification.

Adlerian Psychotherapy: By 1934, Alfred Adler and a small devoted group had been able to set up thirty child guidance clinics in Vienna, manned by paraprofessionals and working closely with school teachers. These were closed with the arrival of the Nazis. Adler, himself, always valued work with children, and his followers have kept that tradition alive.[45] Adler considered the obsessive child to be the prototypic neurotic, in contrast to Freud who gave that laurel to the hysterical youngster. Adler's formulation of the compulsive's problems ran thus: the compulsive fights fake battles, on the "useless side of life," where his private victories do almost nothing to forward his sense of affiliation with others. He feels inadequate in practical and realistic matters and inflates his achievements in useless matters. He strives superhumanly because he is insecure in his humanness. He is forever accomplishing and then undoing in order to be unaware of his imperfections, to try to maintain his prestige, and to kill time. For Adler, all neuroses were a wallowing in uselessness.

Ansbacher[14] has been the most persistent popularizer of Adlerian methods of therapy. His summary listed four phases of Adlerian therapy: (1) *Achieving and sustaining a positive relationship with the patient.* Adler stressed the behavior therapy principle of encouragement, reinforcing the child's positive assets. Rapport and social feeling are both the goal and the means of psychotherapy for Adler. (2) *Gathering data* on early childhood is a part of therapy because it illuminates the percepts of the child now. For Adlerians, the fact finding is a important phase of therapy. It is important to inquire and study because the study shows us the private valuations, the personal meanings of the reported events, thereby enabling a dynamic assessment of the overarching life style. (3) *Interpretation* for Adler was different from analytic interpretation. It was a more educative device, sharing with the patient the therapist's understanding of the child's goals, cravings, and longings as they progress and change. The therapist listens for the exact opposite of what the child says; as when he talks of his obstacles and defeats, one listens for his grandiosity and his attempts to preserve his "fictive superiority." (4) *Active reorientation and reconstruction.* The child's new insights are operationalized, and at the same time that he is undergoing alteration of self-concept and life style, the family members will ordinarily be undergoing a simultaneous readying for support of the healthier behavior the child enacts. Adlerian injunctions regarding psychotherapy are deceptively commonplace and directive.

Jungian Psychotherapy: Eve Lewis,[98] Michael Fordham,[52] and Frances Wickes[154] are three prominent Jungian writers on child therapy, whose works provide a detailed account of Jungian techniques for treating neurotic children. Jungians seem more and more drawn, as do the Horneyans, back toward the psychoanalytic fold. For Jungians, this has been expedited by the advent of ego psychology among the Freudians. Jungians reiterate that synthesis, not analysis, is often needed in therapy with neurotic children. For the Jungian, synthetic work is done in line with the internal processes of the growing child himself, the child who is viewed by Jungians as wanting to grow big, as liking to acquire more and more skills of all kinds, and finally as undergoing "unconscious maturation processes," thanks to his humanity and the collective unconscious.

Jungians are perhaps more open, more educative than Freudian psychoanalysts; they seem to discuss more, give more advice, suggestions, and explanations than do Freudians, (with the Kleinians exempted). Jungians, according to Fordham (in 1969), move into three areas of special expertise when working with children: (1) making a family diagnosis as well as a child diagnosis in order to start the therapy, (2) use of play techniques, and (3) continual monitoring and management of the parent-child psychopathology. Interestingly, within this framework, parent-child relations proceed on an unconscious level where projections and archaic longings rage; these were attended to as carefully in 1925 as in 1975 by Jungian analysts. At the latter date, more Jungians were explicitly proposing family group sessions, but there was a persistence and viability, one feels, in their view that *The Father* and *the Magna Mater* "are the dominants that rule the preconscious soul of the child." And as Jung wrote, when these generic archetypes are projected onto the child's human parents, the latter take on "monstrous proportions."[154] The collective unconscious stretches farther than cradle joys or bad upbringing, and it was in respect to its ultradepth operations that Jungian child analysis differed from other therapies.

Sullivanian Psychotherapy: Maurice R. Green[65] made one of the few attempts to spell out ways that Sullivanians may conduct psychotherapy with neurotic children. Other essays have been presented by Richard A. Gardner in his *Understanding Children*[59] and particularly in the twelve cassette tapes, *Techniques of Child Psychotherapy*,[60] and by Arthur Harry Chapman in his book, *Games Children Play*,[31] and Hilde Bruch in *Learn-*

ing Psychotherapy.[25] Green laid down two aims of therapy for the Sullivanian: (1) to help the child as he grows to enjoy intimacy, with a differing and ever widening circle; and (2) to help the child achieve competence wherever it has been diminishd by interpersonal problems. From a technical standpoint, the Sullivanian's attention to transference and counter-transference is in many ways more Kleinian than ego-analytic. At any rate, the attention is unfaltering, and the distortions of both child and adult are examined; at the same time they are expected and accepted not as something dreadful, but as ineluctably human. Sullivanian therapists, to dredge up one additional distinction, seem to place greater emphasis on more open use of the self of the therapist than do some other schools. However, openness and naturalness by the therapist must be for the good of the patient, not the therapist. Indeed, as Bruch wrote,[25] the therapist is constantly looking at what transpires between him and the patient so that he can see what the patient needs "in disguises that may not coincide with conventional psychodynamics."

Transactional Psychotherapy: It is easy to follow the stepwise movement from Adolf Meyer and Freud, to Sullivan, and thence to Eric Berne[21] and contemporary Transactional Analysis therapies (TA). Berne went further than Sullivan in inspecting the communications, manifest and latent (and between the lines), of interacting persons. Chapman[31] applied many of Berne's concepts, with Sullivan's, in his examination of the "games" utilized by children, neurotic and normal. Claude Steiner[146] has developed the Bernean notion of script analysis, whereby the usual and customary communications which become stylized for each person are subjected to scrutiny and analysis. Aptly enough, Berne regarded Adler as the original "script analyst," since Adler was keep to analyze life styles and scripts. The linkage between Adlerism and TA is not difficult to detect. Alvyn M. Freed[51] has spelled out self-enhancing techniques for pre-school and early primary-grade children in his *T. A. For Tots*, and for older children in *T. A. for Kids*. Conventional psychodynamics and classification do not interest most of the popularizers of transactional analysis. Their therapy goals are intimacy, awareness, and spontaneity whether the analysis is done individually or in a group.

In Steiner's view, TA is a radical therapy. It assumes that people are capable of living in harmony with self, others and nature; that troubled people are worthy and intelligent beings; and that

cure, as quickly as possible, is the goal of all therapy. This same optimistic spirit about the human stuff of children comes through in TA writings about work with children. The three modes of ego state, Parent, Adult and Child, are easily translated into psychoanalytic and Sullivanian constructs, but indeed something gets lost in the translation, as when a "Pig Parent" in the TA lexicon becomes a "strict and archaic superego" for the Freudian, or induces a "malevolent transformation" in the language of Sullivans. Think too of "stroke starvation" as a metaphor in comparison to the paler "striving for consensual validation" of Sullivan, or the "image of the holding mother" of Winnicott. The neurotic child may be expected to benefit greatly from TA as it is ideally carried out, whether that child is an internalizer or externalizer. Indeed, TA has gone farther than most of the current therapies in giving some credence and merit to the outlook of the paranoid child.

Will Therapy or Relationship Therapy: Otto Rank has had considerable influence on the therapy of neurotic children in North America. Rank's imprint is seen on Jessie Taft and the functional school of social work, on Carl Rodgers and nondirective and "growth movement" approaches, on Frederick H. Allen and John A. Rose, as well as William C. Adamson and Exie Welsch, in child psychiatry and child guidance, and on Margaret Mahler in child analysis—all these show Rank to have been a truly seminal force in empathetic helping of neurotic children. The classic Rogersian work with mildly disturbed children remains the work of Virginia Axline.[17] Jessie Taft's *The Dynamics of Therapy/in a Controlled Relationship*[150] is another classic of time-limited relationship therapy in a pronouncedly Rankian mode. Frederick Allen's *Psychotherapy With Children*[8] and the related book *Psychotherapy with Children: The Living Relationship* by Clark Moustakas[113] share the view that the relationship between child and therapist, rather devoid of intellectual reasoning, is simultaneously means and end. The relationship is the significant growth experience. The child is seen separately from mother and father in order to enact the messages of separation and individuation, of birth and death, of fusion and separateness. The neurotic child is respected, both for his neurosis (*artiste manquée*) and for his potential for autonomy and self-determination. Struggle will occur and it is not an unfavorable sign connoting resistance and breach of contract; instead, it is a favorable sign of the play of indomitable will on the part of the child.

Gestalt Therapy: Drawing in a general way on the Gestalt psychology of Wolgang Kohler, and the field theory of Kurt Lewin as it was worked into application for the National Training Laboratories ("applied behavioral science"), the anarchist poet Paul Goodman joined with Frederick S. Perls and Ralph Hefferline to write *Gestalt Therapy*.[19] Perls quickly changed from a rather pedestrian psychoanalyst (who with help from Ernest Jones founded the first Institute for Psychoanalysis in Johannesburg, South Africa) to a spiritual font and guru of Gestalt therapy. He moved to New York in 1946 and founded the Institute for Gestalt Therapy there in 1952. Perls and his associates held that the main goal for the neurotic was to achieve an "organismic balance" through heightened awareness. Unfinished play or work, interruptions of any sort, are the bane of Gestaltist existence. The abundant splits and dichotomies of everyday life are the targets of their therapy.

Therapy aims to restore awareness and promote encounter and dialogue. Encounter is a term rife with meanings; generally it connotes self-acknowledgment and self-acceptance. The splits and polarities in life are totally accepted by the neurotic child. Janet Lederman's *Anger and the Rocking Chair*[97] along with *Born to Win: Transactional Analysis with Gestalt Experiments*[79] by Muriel James and Dorothy Jongeward contain an abundance of Gestalt therapeutic leads for child therapy. Dreamwork as done in Gestalt therapy has proved readily adaptable in other kinds of individual psychotherapy. Its effectiveness lies in its belief that a dream is not taken as "a letter unopened" but as a message full of drama to be reenacted then and there and fully relived. Each sequence and each character are considered to be a part of the self that the child has been splitting off but needs to reintegrate into a Gestalt.

Psychodrama: As early as 1911, Jacob L. Moreno originated psychodrama in Vienna out of his work in Spontaneity Theater for children. Samuel R. Slavson later began group psychotherapy based (it seems) on his Morenean learnings.[67] Beginning with impromptu play, Moreno found that dramas made up on the spur of the moment by disturbed children had a cathartic effect. In these dramatic scenes, the plots, situations, and roles were all reflections of the children themselves. They created the characters out of their own imagery and projections and obtained release as a result. What Moreno did looked very much like the "release therapy" later developed by David M. Levy, though Moreno's child's play was in many ways less contrived, more spontaneous, and more projective. Psychodrama by its very nature was a group endeavor. It bore fruit not only in psychodrama but also in group psychoanalysis for children, in encounter groups, in role playing for children, in sensory awareness exercises, and many other approaches. As Eric Berne wrote,[20] since "nearly all known 'active' techniques were first tried out by Dr. J. L. Moreno in psychodrama, . . . it is difficult to come up with an original idea in this regard." Richard de Mille[41] proposed a group of "children's imagination games" which have some of the flavor of psychodrama and some of the aura of a children's "emotive imagery" group. In addition, they bear a title that reflects some of the brightness and creativity of the whole imaginative enterprise—*Put Your Mother on the Ceiling*. A spate of devices to help neurotic children to acknowledge their real feelings seems to be part of the current *Zeitgeist*. They have a high degree of surface validity.

Family Group Therapy: This method of dealing with neurotic children is utilized, but to a more limited degree than with psychotic, delinquent, retarded, and brain damaged children. Family group therapy as a general treatment modality is described elsewhere in this handbook, and the reader is referred to those sections.

Analytic Group Therapy with Neurotic Children: In 1934, Samuel R. Slavson[143] began working with school age children in activity group therapy. Holding to the idea that disturbed children suffered from "neurotic conflicts" in some form, Slavson's method at first was group recreational activity, in which the leader assisted, playing the parental-observer role, every ready to make explanations based on psychoanalytic understandings. Ideally, externalizing children obtained corrective emotional experience from the opportunity to enact hostility that was manageable and meaningful when the group therapist had given explanations of the rages. At the same time, ideally, the internalizing child was given an opportunity to be more expressive, less fearful and withdrawn into himself.

Slavson became influential in the American Group Psychotherapy Association, an organization countering to some extent the Moreno-inspired American Society of Group Psychotherapy and Psychodrama. Both groups appeared to shift their major emphases to adults, but a strong current of group psychotherapy with children and adolescents remains in both camps. The work of Haim Ginott during the 1950s and early 1960s carried forward the Slavsonian attitudes and ways of conducting group therapy with disturbed children. Ginott[61] took cognizance of the many facets of group work, including reality testing, educational enrichment, reassurance, relationship, catharsis, sublimation, modeling, and insight. Ginott's group observed rules about attendance, encouraging verbalization against violent behavior, forbidding destruction of the clinic property, and so on. With groups of children and adolescents, sometimes purposefully unscreened and unselected, i.e., "heterogeneous" groups, many community mental health centers have adopted the activity group and play group as a modality for giving sometimes inexpert aid to numbers of neurotic and other children. When peer socialization, pure and simple, is a need, such groups may work effectively for certain neurotic children.

Reality Therapy: The name of William Glasser as the author of *Reality Therapy*[62] became a familiar name during the decade between 1965 and 1975. Glasser's orientation is admittedly toward delinquents, mainly adolescents, and his work is especially welcomed by youth correction workers. Reality Therapy is a group endeavor, oriented to the here and now and to the promotion of a sense of responsibility and moral accountability on the part of the group members. The view that neurosis and other forms of mental disorder are merely learned decrement, or leaned helplessness, and sometimes learned immorality has a premodern intonation that is more reminiscent of Benjamin Rush than Camilla Anderson. The reality therapist is truly involved, even immersed in the group interaction. In some correctional settings, reality therapy has been combined with a scheme of total confrontation (akin to that employed at "Synanon" for drug addicts) called "guided group interaction." This has sometimes been known to have a devastating effect on young people who are not as tough as the stereotyped delinquent may be thought to be.

Camilla Anderson Therapy: In the context of a vigorously directive and stringently moralistic therapy such as Glasser's, one perhaps should include a brief word about the diametrically opposite approach to moral accountability developed by the child psychiatrist, Camilla Anderson.[12] Anderson worked within the psychodynamic traditions that Glasser rejected, even working primarily with individuals. Like Glasser, she set as her goal the reality-orientation of the cured neurotic, but she got to that goal quite differently. Anderson (like Horney) saw the ubiquity of pride and guilt and conceived of both as flips of the selfsame neurotic coin. Her intention, therefore,

was to free the child from the conscience of others, and perhaps to help him find one of his own. Morally judgmental attitudes possessed by the patient when coming to treatment had to be extirpated and replaced by critical conceptual judgments (a form of cognitive repair) and realistic appraisals. As a result, psychotherapy was a liberation from a moral value-orientation and a reorientation toward realistic appraisals that are conducive to warmer, more vibrant social relations. In some ways, both Anderson and Glasser lay claim to a "reality therapy" but with very different styles.

PHARMACOTHERAPY WITH NEUROTIC CHILDREN

Child psychiatrists do not have a complete and objective overview of neurotic children and their treatments. First, the numbers of neurotic children who come to medical attention are preselected according to economic class, and many lower-class neurotics may never enter any doorway of the established medical care system. Depending upon the degrees of inaccessibility of scientific medicine and on the availability of folk cures (*santería, curanderismo,* and so on) these patients will usually find nonscientific help if they find any. Further, of those children who do become identified as fearful, anxious, depressed, phobic, hysterical, obsessive compulsive, and otherwise neurotic, a majority is probably seen exclusively by pediatricians and general family practitioners. That is, referral to child psychiatrists never takes place. Hence, it is reasonable to conclude that some forms of effective drug treatment do occur at the hands of nonpsychiatric, primary-care physicians. It has been estimated by numerous clinicians that hydroxyzine (Atarax, Vistaril), (a minor tranquilizer) is the great subduer of childhood neurosis in North America. Everyday observation indicates that hydroxyzine is a much used form of psychopharmacotherapeutic intervention for children with any kind of neurotic or "neurotic-like" symptom. In some parts of the United States, a pediatric referral to child psychiatry will never be made without the pediatrician's having prescribed hydroxyzine prior to the referral. That circumstance assuredly tells all concerned that hydroxyzine, although often helpful, is not a panacea.

Many of the students of Lauretta Bender and Schilder, on quite empirical grounds, have employed rather large dosages of diphenhydramine (Benadryl) for tense, jumpy, irritable, and anxious children. Diphenhydramine is not the sole avenue taken, usually, but is employed in conjunction with other therapies. Barbara Fish,[49] and Magda Campbell,[28] and Theodore Shapiro[29] have done exemplary work in this area with neurotic and still more severe disorders.

Only one other class of pharmacotherapeutic agents will be alluded to, namely the antidepressants, particularly the tricyclics, which have been used when children show depression outright or in the guise of school phobia, regressive bed wetting, and hyperkinesis of a neurotic type. Some largely uncontrolled and anecdotal work has been done with a combination of amitripty-line and perphenazine to block the worsening spiral of ritualistic behavior such as tooth-brushing in obsessive youths.

In general, pharmacotherapy has been as seldom studied by double blind methodology (the best way to study drug effectiveness) as have the psychotherapies been studied by the best available methodologies for their appraisal.

The clinician does not always do his best scientific work as he hastens to do clinical work with neurotic and other children. As a result, childhood neurosis is not as fully charted and understood as would seem to be called for.

REFERENCES

1. ACHENBACH, T. M., *The Classification of Children's Psychiatric Symptoms: A Factor-Analytic Study*, Psychological Monographs, vol. 80(7), no. 615, 1966.

2. ADAMS, P. L., *A Primer of Child Psychotherapy*, Little, Brown, Boston, 1974.

3. ———, *Obsessive Children: A Sociopsychiatric Study*, Brunner-Mazel, New York, 1973.

4. ———, McDONALD, N. F., and HUEY, W. P., "School Phobia and Bisexual Conflict: A Report of 21 Cases," *American Journal of Psychiatry, 123*:541–547, 1966.

5. ADLER, A., *Superiority and Social Interest*, Northwestern University Press, Evanston, Ill., 1970.

6. ———, *The Science of Living*, Doubleday, New York, 1969.

7. ———, "Der Aggressionstrieb im Leben und in der Neurose," *Fortschritte der Medizin, 26*:577–584, 1908.

8. ALLEN, F. H., *Psychotherapy with Children*, W. W. Norton, New York, 1942.

9. ALLPORT, G. W., *Personality and Social Encounter*, Beacon Press, Boston, 1960.

10. ———, *The Use of Personal Documents in Psychological Science*, Social Science Research Council, New York, 1942.

11. American Psychiatric Association Task Force, *Behavior Therapy in Psychiatry*, Jason Aronson, New York, 1973.

12. ANDERSON, C., *Beyond Freud*, Harper, New York, 1957.

13. ANGYAL, A., in *Neurosis and Treatment: A Holistic Theory*, Hanfmann, E., and Jones, R. M. (Eds.), John Wiley, New York, 1965.

14. ANSBACHER, H. L., "Goal-Oriented Individual Psychology: Alfred Adler's Theory," in Burton, A. (Ed.), *Operational Theories of Personality*, Brunner-Mazel, New York, 1974.

15. ———, and ROWENA, R., " The Increasing Recognition of Adler," in Ansbacher, H. L., and Rowena, R. (Eds.), *Superiority and Social Interest: A Collection of Later Writings of Alfred Adler*, Northwestern University Press, Evanston, Ill., 1970.

16. ANTHONY, E. J., "Neurotic Disorders," in Freedman, A. M., Kaplan, H. I., and Sadock, B. J. (Eds.), *Comprehensive Textbook of Psychiatry*, vol. 2, Williams and Wilkins, Baltimore, 1975.

17. AXLINE, V. M., *Play Therapy*, Ballantine Books, New York, 1972.

18. BENDER, L., "The Concept of Pseudopsychopathic Schizophrenia in Adolescents," *American Journal of Orthopsychiatry, 29*:491–512, 1959.

19. ———, "Schizophrenia in Childhood—Its Recognition, Description and Treatment," *American Journal of Orthopsychiatry, 26*:499–506, 1956.

20. BERNE, E., "Book Review of Gestalt Therapy Verbatim by Frederick S. Perls," *American Journal of Psychiatry, 126*:163–164, 1970.

21. ———, *Transactional Analysis in Psychotherapy: A Systematic Individual and Social Psychiatry*, Ballantine Books, New York, 1961.

22. BINSWANGER, L., "The Existential Analysis School of Thought," in May, R., Angel, E., and Ellenberger, H. F. (Eds.), *Existence: A New Dimension in Psychiatry and Psychology*, Basic Books, New York, 1958.

23. BOWEN, M., "Family Psychotherapy with Schizophrenia in the Hospital and in Private Practice," in Boszormenyi-Nagy, I, and Framo, J. L. (Eds.), *Intensive Family Therapy*, Harper & Row, New York, 1965.

24. BRIDGES, K. M. B., "Emotional Development in Early Infancy," *Child Development, 3*:324–341, 1932.

25. BRUCH, H., *Learning Psychotherapy: Rationale and Ground Rules*, Harvard University Press, Cambridge, 1974.

26. BURTON, A., *Modern Humanistic Psychotherapy*, Jossey-Bass, San Francisco, 1967.

27. CAMMER, L., "Schizophrenic Children of Manic-Depressive Parents," *Diseases of the Nervous System, 31*: 177–180, 1970.

28. CAMPBELL, M., *Psychopharmacologic Treatment in Children*, paper presented to International Symposium on Psychopharmacology, University of Louisville School of Medicine, February 15, 1975.

29. ———, and SHAPIRO, T., "Therapy of Psychiatric Disorders of Childhood," in Shader, R. I. (Ed.), *Manual of Psychiatric Therapeutics: Practical Psychopharmacology and Psychiatry*, pp. 137–162, Little, Brown & Company, Boston, 1975.

30. CANTWELL, D. P., "Prevalence of Psychiatric Disorder in a Pediatric Clinic for Military Dependent Children," *Journal of Pediatrics, 85*:711–714, 1974.

31. CHAPMAN, A. H., *The Games Children Play*, G. P. Putnam's Sons, New York, 1971.

32. CHESS, S., et al., *Your Child Is A Person: A Psychological Approach to Parenthood Without Guilt*, Viking Press, New York, 1965.

33. CHODOFF, P., "A Critique of Freud's Theory of Infantile Sexuality," *American Journal of Psychiatry, 123(5)*:508–517, 1966.

34. COLBY, K. M., *An Introduction to Psychoanalytic Research*, Basic Books, New York, 1960.

35. COLM, H., "The Self-Defeating Search for Love,"

in Moustakas, C. E. (Ed.), *Existential Child Therapy*, Basic Books, New York, 1966.

36. CRAMER, J. B., "Common Neuroses of Childhood," in Silvano, A. (Ed.), *American Handbook of Psychiatry*, vol. 1, pp. 797–815, Basic Books, New York, 1959.

37. CRUTCHER, R., "Child Psychiatry: A History of Its Development," *Psychiatry*, 6:191–201, 1943.

38. CUNNINGHAM, J. M., WESTERMAN, H. H., and FISCHOFF, J., "A Follow-Up Study of Patients Seen in a Psychiatric Clinic for Children," *American Journal of Orthopsychiatry*, 26:602–612, 1956.

39. DAI, B., "Obsessive-Compulsive Disorders in the Chinese Culture," *Social Problems*, 4:313–321, 1957.

40. DE MAUSE, L., "The Evolution of Childhood," in de Mause, L. (Ed.), *The History of Childhood*, Harper Torchbooks, New York, 1974.

41. DE MILLE, R., *Put Your Mother on the Ceiling: Children's Imagination Games*, Viking, New York, 1973.

42. DESPERT, J. L., *The Emotionally Disturbed Child*, Doubleday, New York, 1970.

43. DOLLARD, J., and MILLER, N. E., *Personality and Psychotherapy: An Analysis in Terms of Learning, Thinking and Culture*, McGraw-Hill, New York, 1950.

44. DREGER, R. M., "A Progress Report on a Factor-Analytic Approach to Classification in Child Psychiatry," in Jenkins, R. L., and Cole, J. (Eds.), *Psychiatric Research Reports of the American Psychiatric Association*, 18:22–58, 1964.

45. DREIKURS, R., *Psychodynamics, Psychotherapy, and Counseling*, Alfred Adler Institute, Chicago, 1967.

46. EHRENWALD, J., *Neurosis in the Family and Patterns of Psychosocial Defense: A Study of Psychiatric Epidemiology*, Harper & Row, New York, 1963.

47. EYSENCK, H. J., "Learning Theory and Behavior Therapy," *Journal of Mental Science*, 105:61–75, 1959.

48. FANON, F., *The African Revolution*, Grove Press, New York, 1967.

49. FISH, B., "Drug Use in Psychiatric Disorders of Children," *American Journal of Psychiatry*, 124:31–36, 1968.

50. ———, and SHAPIRO, T., "A Typology of Children's Psychiatric Disorders: I. Its Application to a Controlled Evaluation of Treatment," *Journal of the American Academy of Child Psychiatry*, 4:32–52, 1965.

51. FREED, A. M., *T.A. For Tots*, Jalmar Press, Sacramento, 1954.

52. FORDHAM, M., *Children as Individuals*, Hodder and Stoughton, London, 1969.

53. FRAIBERG, S., "A Comparison of the Analytic Method in Two Stages of a Child Analysis," *Journal of the American Academy of Child Psychiatry*, 4:387–400, 1965.

54. FROMM, E., *Crisis of Psychoanalysis*, Fawcett Publications, Greenwich, Conn., 1970.

55. ———, *The Revolution of Hope: Toward a Humanized Technology*, Bantam Books, New York, 1968; also see, Fromm, E. (Ed.), *Socialist Humanism*, Doubleday, Garden City, N.J., 1965.

56. ———, *Man for Himself*, Fawcett, Greenwich, Conn., 1947.

57. FREUD, A., *Normality and Pathology in Childhood*, International Universities Press, New York, 1965.

58. FREUD, S., "Analysis of a Phobia in a Five-Year-Old Boy," *The Standard Edition of the Complete Psychological Works of Sigmund Freud*, vol. 10, Hogarth Press, London, 1955.

59. GARDNER, R. A., *Understanding Children*, Jason Aronson, New York, 1973.

60. ———, *Techniques of Child Psychotherapy* (12 Cassette Tapes), Behavioral Science Tape Library, Fort Lee, N.J.

61. GINNOTT, H., *Group Psychotherapy with Children*, McGraw-Hill, New York, 1961.

62. GLASSER, W., *Reality Therapy*, Harper & Row, New York, 1965.

63. GOLDSTEIN, K., *The Organism*, American Book Company, New York, 1935.

64. GOTTESMAN, I. I., "Differential Inheritance of the Psychoneuroses," *Eugenics Quarterly*, 9:223–227, 1962.

65. GREEN, M. R., "The Interpersonal Approach to Child Therapy," in Wolman, B. B. (Ed.), *Handbook of Child Psychoanalysis: Research, Theory and Practice*, Van Nostrand Reinhold, New York, 1972.

66. GREEN, A. W., "The Middle-Class Male Child and Neurosis," *American Sociological Review*, 2:31–41, 1946.

67. GREENBERG, I. A. (Ed.), *Psychodrama: Theory and Therapy*, Behavioral Publications, New York, 1974.

68. Group for the Advancement of Psychiatry (GAP), Committee on Child Psychiatry, *Psychopathological Disorders in Childhood: Theoretical Considerations and a Proposed Classification*, Group for the Advancement of Psychiatry, New York, 1966.

69. GRUENBERG, E. M., et al., *Diagnostic and Statistical Manual of Mental Disorders*, 2nd ed. (DSM-II), American Psychiatric Association Committee on Nomenclature and Statistics, Washington, D.C., 1968.

70. GUNTRIP, H. J. S., *Psychoanalytic Theory, Therapy, and the Self*, Basic Books, New York, 1971.

71. HAMPE, E., et al., "Intelligence and School Phobia," *Journal of School Psychology*, 2:66, 1973.

72. HARRIS, I. D., "Differences in Cognitive Style and Birth Order," in Westman, J. C. (Ed.), *Individual Differences in Children*, pp. 199–210, John Wiley, New York, 1973.

73. HARTMANN, H., and KRIS, E., "Problems of Infantile Neurosis: A Discussion," in Eissler, R. S., et al. (Eds.), *The Psychoanalytic Study of the Child*, vol. 9, pp. 31–36, International Universities Press, New York, 1954.

74. HEALY, W., *The Individual Delinquent*, Little, Brown, Boston, 1915.

75. HENDERSON, L. J., "The Study of Man," *Science*, 94:1–10, 1941.

76. HORNEY, K., *The Neurotic Personality of Our Time*, W. W. Norton, New York, 1937.

77. ———, *Neurosis and Human Growth*, W. W. Norton, New York, 1950.

78. JACOBSON, E., *Progressive Relaxation*, University of Chicago Press, Chicago, 1938.

79. JAMES, M., and JONGEWARD, D., *Born to Win: Transactional Analysis with Gestalt Experiments*, Addison-Wesley Publishing Company, Menlo Park, Calif., 1973.

80. JOHNSON, A. M., and SZUREK, S. A., "The Genesis of Antisocial Acting Out in Children and Adults," *Psychoanalytic Quarterly*, 21:323–343, 1952.

81. ———, et al., "School Phobia," *American Journal of Orthopsychiatry*, 12:702–711, 1941.

82. JONES, E., *Free Associations: Memories of a Psycho-Analyst*, Basic Books, New York, 1959.

83. JONES, M. C., "The Elimination of Children's Fears," *Journal of Experimental Psychology*, 7:382–390, 1924.

84. JUDD, L. L., "Obsessive Compulsive Neurosis in Children," *Archives of General Psychiatry*, 12:136–143, 1965.

85. KANNER, L., "Historical Perspective on Developmental Deviations," *Journal of Autism and Childhood Schizophrenia*, 3:187–198, 1973.

86. ———, "Childhood Psychosis: A Historical Overview," *Journal of Autism and Childhood Schizophrenia*, 1:14–19, 1971.

87. ———, *Centripetal Forces in Personality Development: The Seventh Annual Karen Horney Lecture*, read before Association for the Advancement of Psychoanalysis at New York Academy of Medicine on March 25, 1959.

88. ———, *Child Psychiatry*, Charles C Thomas, Springfield, Ill., 1935.

89. KLEIN, M., *Contributions to Psycho-Analysis 1921–1945*, McGraw-Hill Books, New York, 1964.

90. KRASNER, L., and ULLMANN, L. P., *Research in*

Behavioral Modification, Holt, Rinehart and Winston, New York, 1965.

91. Krasnogorski, N. I., "Physiology of Cerebral Activity in Children as a New Subject of Pediatric Investigation," American Journal of Diseases of Children, 46:473–494, 1933.

92. Laing, R. D., The Politics of Experience, Ballantine Books, New York, 1967.

93. Lapouse, R., and Monk, M. A., "Fears and Worries in a Representative Sample of Children," American Journal of Orthopsychiatry, 29:803–818, 1959.

94. Lazarus, A. A., Behavior Therapy and Beyond, McGraw-Hill, New York, 1972.

95. ———, and Abramovitz, A. "The Use of 'Emotive Imagery' in the Treatment of Children's Phobias," Journal of Mental Science, 108:191–195, 1962.

96. Lazarus, A. A., Davison, G. C., and Polefka, D. A., "Classical and Operant Factors in the Treatment of a School Phobia," Journal of Abnormal Psychology, 70:225–230, 1965.

97. Lederman, J., Anger and the Rocking Chair: Gestalt Awareness with Children, Viking Press, New York, 1973.

98. Lewis, E., "Initiation of an Obsessional Adolescent Boy," in Moustakas, C. (Ed.), Existenital Child Therapy, Basic Books, New York, 1966.

99. Lewis, H., Deprived Children: The Mersham Experiment—A Social and Clinical Study, Oxford University Press, London, 1954.

100. Malinowski, B., Sex and Repression in Savage Society, Harcourt, Brace & Co., New York, 1927.

101. Maudsley, H., Physiology and Pathology of the Mind, Macmillan, London, 1867.

102. Marks, I. M., "Problems in Exposure (Flooding) Research," British Journal of Psychiatry, 124:103–108, 1974.

103. Maslow, A. H., Motivation and Personality, Harper & Row, New York, 1954.

104. May, R., Angel, E., and Ellenberger, H. F. (Eds.), Existence: A New Dimension in Psychiatry and Psychology, Basic Books, New York, 1958.

105. "Memoirs of an Invisible Man-I, Herbert Graf Recalls a Half-Century in the Theater: A Dialogue with Francis Rizzo," Opera News, 36(11):24–28, 1972.

106. Menninger, K., Mayman, M., and Pruyser, P., The Vital Balance, Viking Press, New York, 1963.

107. Miller, J. G., "Living Systems: Basic Concepts," Behavioral Science, 10:193–237, 1965.

108. Miller, L. C., "Louisville Behavior Check List for Males, 6–12 Years of Age," Psychological Reports, 21:885–896, 1967.

109. Miller, L., et al., "Comparison of Reciprocal Inhibition, Psychotherapy, and Waiting List Control for Phobic Children," Journal of Abnormal Psychology, 79: 269–279, 1972.

110. Minuchin, S., et al., Families of the Slums: An Exploration of their Structure and Treatment, Basic Books, New York, 1967.

111. Morris, D. P., Soroker, E., and Burrus, G., "Follow-up Studies of Shy, Withdrawn Children—I. Evaluation of Later Adjustment," American Journal of Orthopsychiatry, 24:743–754, 1954.

112. Morris, H. H., Jr., Escoll, P. J., and Wexler, R., "Aggressive Behavior Disorders of Childhood: A Follow Up Study," American Journal of Psychiatry, 112:991–997, 1956.

113. Moustakas, C. E., Psychotherapy with Children: The Living Relationship, Ballantine Books, New York, 1970.

114. Mullahy, P., Oedipus, Myth and Complex: A Review of Psychoanalytic Theory, Grove Press, New York, 1955.

115. Murphy, J. M., "Psychiatric Labeling in Cross-Cultural Perspective," Science, 191(4231):1019–1028, 1976.

116. Nagera, H., Early Childhood Disturbances: The Infantile Neurosis and the Adulthood Disturbances, The Psychoanalytic Study of the Child, Monograph No. 2, International Universities Press, New York, 1966.

117. Nunberg, H., Principles of Psychoanalysis: Their Application to the Neuroses, International Universities Press, New York, 1955.

118. Pasamanick, B., The Epidemiology of Behavior Disorders of Childhood, Neurology and Psychiatry in Childhood, Williams and Wilkins, Baltimore, 1954.

119. Perls, F. S., Hefferline, R. F., and Goodman, P., Gestalt Therapy, Dell, New York, 1965.

120. Piaget, J., The Origins of Intelligence in Children, International Universities Press, New York, 1952.

121. Pillsbury, W. B., The History of Psychology, W. W. Norton, New York, 1929.

122. Proctor, J. T., "Hysteria in Childhood," American Journal of Orthopsychiatry, 28:394–403, 1958.

123. Reich, W., Character-Analysis, Farrar, Strauss and Giroux, New York, 1971.

124. Robins, L. N., "The Adult Development of the Antisocial Child," Seminars in Psychiatry, 2:420–434, 1970.

125. ———, Deviant Children Grown Up, Williams and Wilkins, Baltimore, 1966.

126. Rose, J. A., "The Emotional Problems of Children," in Psychiatry for the General Practitioner, abstract from the Seminar Series, Carrier Clinic, Philadelphia Mental Health Educational Unit of Smith, Kline and French Laboratories, 1958.

127. Rosen, B. M., et al., Utilization of Psychiatric Facilities by Children: Current Status, Trends, Implications, National Institute of Mental Health Statistics Series B, No. 1, U.S. Government Printing Office, Washington, D.C., 1968.

128. Rutter, M. L., "Psycho-Social Disorders in Childhood and Their Outcome in Adult Life," Journal of Royal College of Physicians, London, 4:211–218, 1970.

129. ———, Graham, P., and Yule, W., A Neuropsychiatric Study in Childhood, Heinemann, London, 1970.

130. Rutter, M. L., et al., "A Tri-Axial Classification of Mental Disorders in Childhood: On International Study," Journal of Child Psychology and Psychiatry, 10: 41–61, 1969.

131. Sarbin, T. "Anxiety: Reification of a Metaphor," Archives of General Psychiatry, 10:635–638, 1964.

132. Saslow, G., "Application of Behavior Therapy," in Usdin, G. (Ed.), Overview of the Psychotherapies, Brunner-Mazel, New York, 1975.

133. Schilder, P., Contributions to Developmental Neuropsychiatry, International Universities Press, New York, 1964.

134. Schofield, W., Psychotherapy: The Purchase of Friendship, Prentice-Hall, Englewood Cliffs, N.J., 1964.

135. Sears, R. R., "Survey of Objective Studies in Psychoanalytic Concepts," Social Science Research Bulletin No. 51, Social Science Research Council, New York, 1943.

136. Segal, H., "Melanie Klein's Technique of Child Analysis," in Wolman, B. B. (Ed.), Handbook of Child Psycho-Analysis, Van Nostrand Reinhold, New York, 1972.

137. Shapiro, T., and Jegede, R. O., "School Phobia: A Babel of Tongues," Journal of Autism and Childhood Schizophrenia, 3(2):168–186, 1973.

138. Shechtman, A., "Age Patterns in Children's Psychiatric Symptoms," Child Development, 41:687–691, 1970.

139. Shields, J., "Personality Differences and Neurotic Traits in Normal Twin School-Children," Eugenics Review, 45:213–246, 1954.

140. (Cited in) Slater, E., and Cowie, V., The Genetics of Mental Disorders, Oxford University Press, London, 1971.

141. Slater, E., and Cowie, V., The Genetics of Mental Disorders, Oxford University Press, London, 1971.

142. Slater, E., and Slater, P., "A Heuristic Theory of Neurosis," Journal of Neurology and Psychiatry, 7: 49–55, 1944.

143. SLAVSON, S. R., *Analytic Group Psychotherapy with Children, Adolescents and Adults*, Columbia University Press, New York, 1950.

144. SPERLING, M., *The Major Neuroses and Behavior Disorders in Children*, Jason Aronson, New York, 1974.

145. SPITZER, R. L., et al. (Eds.), *Diagnostic and Statistical Manual of Mental Disorders*, 3rd ed. (DSM-III), Draft Version as of Sept. 3, 1975, American Psychiatric Association Committee on Diagnostic Nomenclature, Washington, D.C.

146. STEINER, C. M., *Scripts People Live: Transactional Analysis of Life Scripts*, Grove Press, New York, 1974.

147. STIERLIN, H., "Family Theory: An Introduction," in Burton, A. (Ed.), *Operational Theories of Personality*, Brunner-Mazel, New York, 1974.

148. SULLIVAN, H. S., *Personal Psychopathology: Early Formulations*, W. W. Norton, New York, 1971.

149. SUNDBY, H. S., and KREYBERG, C., *Prognosis in Child Psychiatry*, Williams and Wilkins, Baltimore, 1968.

150. TAFT, J., *The Dynamics of Therapy in a Controlled Relationship*, Dover, New York, 1962.

151. TEXTOR, R., *A Cross Cultural Summary*, HRAF Press, New Haven, Conn., 1967.

152. WALDRON, S., JR., et al., "School Phobia and Other Childhood Neuroses: A Systematic Study of the Children and Their Families," *American Journal of Psychiatry, 132:*802–808, 1975.

153. WATSON, J. B., and RAYNOR, R. R., "Conditioned Emotional Reactions," *Journal of Experimental Psychology, 3:*1–14, 1920.

154. WICKES, F. G., *The Inner World of Childhood*, New American Library, New York, 1968.

155. WINDELBAND, W., *Geschichte und Naturwissenschaft*, Heitz & Muendel, Strassburg, 1904.

156. WOLPE, J., *Psychotherapy by Reciprocal Inhibition*, Stanford University Press, Palo Alto, Calif., 1958.

157. WOLPE, J., and RACHMAN, S., "Psychoanalytic 'Evidence': A Critique Based on Freud's Case of Little Hans." *Journal of Nervous and Mental Diseases, 131:* 135–148, 1960.

158. YAHRAES, H., and National Institute of Mental Health Task Force and Coordinating Committee, *Research in the Service of Mental Health*, Segal, J. (Ed.), National Institute of Mental Health, Rockville, Md., 1975.

159. ZILBOORG, G., and HENRY, G. W., *A History of Medical Psychology*, W. W. Norton, New York, 1941.

13 / Personality Disorders

Stuart M. Finch and Joseph M. Green

Webster defines personality as "the totality of an individual's characteristics," and as "an integrated group of emotional trends, behavior tendencies, etc." The beginnings are surely laid down at birth. Freud stated, long ago, that each individual ego begins "with its own peculiar disposition and tendencies."

The nosology of psychiatric disorders in children and adolescents has been and still remains something of a problem. The broad category of "personality disorders" is an excellent example of this. If one uses the classification of the GAP report, (Psychopathological Disorders in Childhood: Theoretical Considerations and a Proposed Classification),[4] there are a dozen or so personality disorders. Some of these, such as the oppositional personality and the compulsive personality, are commonly seen and the diagnoses are frequently made. Others, such as the mistrustful personality, are so rarely seen and so poorly understood that a busy clinician with many patients may never find an occasion to use them. DSM-II (*Diagnostic and Statistical Manual of Mental Disorders*, 2nd Edition),[1] includes about the same number of personality disorders, most of which are similar to those in the GAP report.

However, since the statement is made, "there are life-long patterns, often recognizable by the time of adolescence or earlier," there is a suggestion that they are not usually appropriately applied to children. DSM-II then adds a separate category of "Behavior Disorders of Childhood and Adolescence," some of which are similar to some of the personality disorders of the GAP classification. The child psychiatrist using DSM-II is likely to turn to the behavior disorders first because they refer specifically to children. (At the time of this writing, DSM-III is being prepared for publication, but has not been previewed by these authors.) We find the GAP classification more complete and more useful to the practitioner who works with children.

Unfortunately, it has not generally been accepted by those in public positions who gather the statistics. They insist on diagnoses from DSM-II, therefore, there is no way of ascertaining the evidence or distribution in the population of the syndromes we are writing about. Clinical hunches are hardly scientific, but are the best we can do in these cases. As a matter of practical fact, even if statistics were available from a wide variety of places, we must recognize that diagnoses are used so differently at different institutions around the country as to be almost useless. As we would view it, a personality disorder is a diagnosis which should be used for children and adolescents only when three conditions are met: definitive aberrations of behavior should be present, the youngster's character should be clearly formed into an identifiable pattern, and transient situations should not be the primary cause of the aberrations. The second of these is the most difficult to ascertain. Indeed, some may argue that personality disorders are adult phenomena and a priori are not appropriate diagnoses for children whose personalities are still fluid and developing.

Any intuitive mother can recognize the constitutional differences in her children, practically from the day they are born. Nor does it take an especially intuitive mother to note the differences. Any observer standing before the window of a newborn nursery will observe that some babies are moving very restlessly, some are protesting angrily, and some are accepting passively.

How often do we hear the remark by parents, "Johnny was a pistol from the first time they brought him to me in the hospital. He has been that way ever since, into everything and never slowing down. His brother is the opposite, quiet and shy, and slow to accept new people or situations." Both children may be quite normal emotionally, but certainly are quite different in psychological makeup.

But if Johnny and his brother are still the way they have always been, there are many other children whose personality at six years is greatly different than even a pediatrician would have predicted on the basis of their behavior in the nursery. As Thomas, Chess and Birch[7] have pointed out, it is the interaction of temperament and environment that fuel the process of personality development, whether normal or disordered. Their New York Longitudinal Study begun in March, 1956 is probably the most comprehensive approach we have to this complicated interaction as it affects personality. They identified several constellations of temperamental traits present in the newborn and correlated them with the development (or lack of development) of certain behavior disorders. They showed how "environmental influences may profoundly modify the expression of temperament." If the interaction leads to maladaptive behavior, a personality disorder is born.[6]

Kris summarized an earlier study in 1957[5] and organized a longitudinal study of personality development at the Child Study Center of Yale University. He and his coworkers hoped to "supply essential data for the understanding of personality and for the early diagnosis, and hopefully prevention, of personality disturbances." They considered the influence of the environment on the predisposition of the child as crucial to personality development. They formulated a specific hypothesis: "that there is a relationship between the innate equipment characteristics of the child and the mechanisms of adaptation the child prefers to use." Brazelton,[2] after discussing the uniqueness of every newborn, selected three babies, whom he described as "average baby," "quiet baby," and "active baby." He followed them, contrasting and describing the babies and their interactions with parents, through each of the next twelve months. He was concerned with normal development and the range of individual expression, but it becomes clear once again that the difference in this early stage of life between the paths that lead to "normal" personalities or to disordered personalities is not great.

While much has been written and said about the constitutional predisposition of children, we have yet to learn why one child chooses an alloplastic (acting out) route and the next child an autoplastic (internalizing) one. The latter tends to become neurotic and to suffer, while the former "acts out" his problems and makes other suffer.

Even this division is oversimplified. To be specific, what is the difference between a child with a compulsive type personality disorder and one with a compulsive neurosis? Or, what is the difference between a child with an hysterical personality disorder and one with an hysterical neurosis? When diagnosing adults, to be precise is extremely difficult and to be so with children and adolescents is often, at best, guess work.

We must, first of all, assume that children or even teenagers are, in the nature of things, in transition. They have come into the world with a "given" constitution. This constitution intersects with the vicissitudes of experience in their particular environment, be it stable and healthy or unpredictable and rejecting. From this interaction comes character, the laying down of the basic structural framework of the self and the psyche. We are concerned, here, with the quality of that structure, the elements of stability in human adjustments, and the enduring patterns that make for certain ongoing ways of life. Personality is the expression of this character structure as it interacts with environment. It refers to the overall manner in which a youngster or adult behaves.

To emphasize this point, let us look for a moment at the patterns of behavior of close friends, classmates, or even spouses. If we knew them well, we can predict with some accuracy how they will behave under given conditions. For example, we recognize that one woman will overreact to any new situation because we have seen her do it time and time again. The next woman, we know, will react without much emotion, but will express many intellectual ideas. We have also seen her do this many times before. These are adults, however, and children are not miniature adults. Their personality patterns are not so firmly fixed.

The diagnosis of personality disorder can rarely be used prior to school age. The intraphysic drives are still in a state of flux prior to this age and character is not clearly formed into an identifiable pattern. Changes can and do occur. The most aggressive, active, hard to manage, three-year-old may become a quiet, docile, overly well-behaved seven-year-old. In retrospect, one can often see the early roots of a personality disorder, but to make the diagnosis in a preschooler is not only difficult but often erroneous. These authors believe that there is rarely any way to distinguish the child who will later develop a personality disorder from the child who will later develop a similar neurosis. As a practical matter, child psychiatrists are rarely called upon to do so. How many preschool children are brought in by their parents because of a budding personality disorder? The principal diagnoses which bring about the psychiatric examination of preschool children are much more serious and are likely to involve psychotic or affective disorders, brain syndromes, or mental retardation.

The next problem, alluded to earlier, is the difficulty of differentiation of certain types of personality disorders from psychoneurotic disorders; for example, it is difficult to differentiate the compulsive, hysterical or anxious personality disorders from their counterparts in the psychoneurotic categories. These conditions are, in many ways, more closely related to each other than are the compulsive, hysterical, and anxious personality disorders related to the antisocial types of personality disorders. A youngster with a compulsive or hysterical personality disorder may develop a compulsive or hysterical psychoneurosis. When stress is increased, anxiety mounts and heretofore hidden or absent neurotic symptoms may become prominent. On rare occasions one can even see the impulse-ridden child become compulsive. This generally tends to occur when the circumstances of the child's life change dramatically and he becomes emotionally attached to an adult whom he wishes to please and desperately hopes not to displease. He overcontrols his impulses, but overshoots the mark and becomes inhibited and compulsive in the process.

Compulsive Personality

The child with a compulsive personality has often been described as "too good" and this term would seem rather apt. Such youngsters are well behaved, pseudomature, and relatively unemotional; they tend to strive for very high goals. They are anxious to please and are thus often well liked by parents and teachers. They display little of the mischievous behavior common to normal childhood. There usually are, however, a few "leaks" in the otherwise rigid system. The classic example is the youngster who may be meticulous about his outer clothing and his appearance, but will wear the same underwear for a week at a time.

Perhaps the most common reason for which such children are referred is temper tantrums. They overcontrol themselves beyond their capacity, and periodically the controls break and the inner turmoil bursts forth as a tantrum. Usually it passes rapidly and the child reinstates the controls.

Children with a compulsive personality are not likely to be referred for mental health care, especially if their personality is fairly intact. On the whole, they please adults and avoid irritating them. This provides the child with acceptance and apparent security, but the price he pays is to remain isolated, perfectionistic, and unable to be close to others. As a result, he misses out on many of the important maturational events that characterize a normal childhood and adolescence.

The psychopathology of the compulsive personality has as one of its main roots excessive, perpetuated anality. Normal anality, as exemplified by the toddler, is expressed in a number of emotional characteristics. These include negativism, selfishness, ambivalence, tantrums, and sadism. There is an increased interest in excretions, and, of course, a shift from oral to anal as the primary erotic zone. The "terrible twos" gained this name for a reason. To a child of this age, "no" is a word used repeatedly (both to the child and by the child); fecal play or play with materials of fecal consistency is common. Cleanliness is not well liked by the toddler and his motto is "the dirtier, the better." He wants what he wants when he wants it and gives little thought to the rights of others. His play is parallel in type and rarely a joint venture with a peer. His sado-masochism is also evident as he showers affection on the household cat one moment and teases it the next.

It is during these preschool years that parents are attempting to "civilize" the child. He is not without his childish omnipotence and only gradually with consistent training does he begin to accept rules and regulations. If the youngster's needs for assertiveness and autonomy are met and properly blended with consistent requirements for conformity, the child normally moves ahead in his development.

During this anal phase, the youngster is particularly concerned with his bodily eliminations. He likes to withhold feces. He then experiences pleasure when he defecates where and if he wishes. His parents, on the other hand, have begun to ask him to use the potty. If there are older siblings, the child may try to emulate them, but if he is the first, this added incentive is lacking. If the parents are patient, consistent, and not punitive, he will gradually conform because of his desire to please them. If, however, a parent is impatient or inconsistent, the child may "refuse" to become toilet trained and also act out in other ways.

In general, then, we see that the child with a compulsive personality disorder retains a considerable residue of inner anal impulses which, in turn, make for a punitive and primitive superego. To the extent that the ego is fixated, it too is not fully developed and has to struggle hard to "mediate" the inner battle. Characteristically, the defenses of isolation and intellectualization tend to predominate.

One question poses itself at this point—how does one differentiate between a well-behaved, good, but normal child and one with a compulsive personality? For instance, many "normal" children during the latency period show mild, transient compulsive patterns. One common children's game is "Don't step on the crack or you break your mother's back." The child who hits every other fencepost provides another example. These children are using the magical thinking normally characteristic of the preschooler to add structure to their lives. The important point here is that their lives are not built around such obsessional or compulsive behavioral sequences. They may occasionally use them, but good relationships with peers and adults are much more prominent. The truly compulsive child tends to be dominated by his perfectionistic and emotionally isolated attitudes. Unfortunately, such a distinction is not easily drawn by many adults, and the compulsive child becomes a welcome addition to the home or classroom.

Youngsters with a compulsive personality usually come from families in which there is either an overdose of rigidity and strictness or a lack of adequate adult control. In the first case, the child adopts or introjects the superego values of the parents. He sets stern standards for himself and then struggles to meet them. His adaptation is rigid and inflexible; he finds it difficult to move easily between the adult demands for academic excellence and peer demands to minimize academics in favor of games and sports. The play activities chosen by latency-age children demonstrate that some compulsive defenses are normal and typical for the age. Rules of the game are extremely important and woe to the child who breaks the rules; soon no one will play with him. It is as though children of this age have only recently left the protection of the family and ventured out into the larger world of potentially hostile strangers. They seek security and predictability in strict adherence to the rules.

In the second instance, where adult control is inadequate, the child lacks reasonable adult boundaries; he sets them for himself. Reality experience tells him what he needs, but it can't offer him a reasonable model to emulate and he overdoes it. There are many other types of families that can produce a child with a compulsive personality disorder. There are those which involve parental inconsistency, and those in which the standards of the grandparents are quite different from those of the parents and where the approval of the grandparents is much sought after, but difficult to obtain. A similar conflictual situation may arise if the standards of the teacher are quite different from those of the parent. The conflict leads to anxiety, and compulsive defenses are mobilized to relieve the pain.

The treatment of a child with a compulsive personality can be difficult in several ways. In the first place, he is usually referred because of a symptom such as temper tantrums or perhaps a vague parental idea that he is not "one of the regular boys." If the symptom can be eradicated, the family is usually quite happy even though the therapist sees much more total psychopathology. Only too often, the family of the compulsive child basically "needs" such a youngster; without help they would not be able to tolerate a "normal" child. The therapist is then on the horns of a dilemma. If he merely extinguishes the symptom, he leaves the road open for future problems in the child. If, on the other hand, he helps his patient toward normality, the child may be in trouble with the parents. Needless to say, the youngster's primary allegiance is to the parents and if he feels they are in disagreement with his therapist, he will not benefit from treatment.

There are various answers, but one which must always be avoided is the "rescue fantasy" in which the therapist tries to become the "good parent" and take the place of the natural but "bad" parents. A better solution would be first to initiate therapy with the child. During concurrent work with the parents, the therapist can strive to help them understand the conflictual situation in which they have placed their child. If this is successful, they will allow their youngster to be a more "regular boy" and give up some of his compulsive defenses, and they will accept him with the changes. When this, or even more intensive treatment for the parents is unsuccessful, it may be necessary to consider brief residential treatment. The latter is used only as a last resort when every other avenue has been explored.

Jerry, age nine, was referred to the child psychiatrist by an alert, intuitive pediatrician. The doctor had taken care of Jerry since birth and knew his parents well. All had gone well from a physical standpoint, and Jerry seemed outwardly happy and healthy. He was the oldest of three children and treated his younger siblings in an almost paternalistic way. He had always been the most willing to follow parental rules.

He was in the fourth grade and academically he was near the top of his class. He had many friends but questioning revealed that he had no really close friends. He was not athletic but participated in some sports when the PE teacher suggested it.

The pediatrician's reason for referral was his concern about the boy's pseudomaturity and apparent psychological brittleness. For example, he always greeted the doctor in a sort of false adult fashion. He submitted to examination, injections, and other procedures without overt anxiety, but the physician could sense the inner tension.

In talking with the parents, the pediatrician brought to light Jerry's emotional isolation. The boy was not happy with himself or his productivity. If he got a B in a course, he felt he should have worked harder and gotten an A. If he got an A, he felt he really did not deserve it. He rarely got into the normal childhood fights but instead would have a sort of temper tantrum and retreat to his room for several hours. Recently he had begun to show an increase in these outbursts. These had been present prior to his school years, but they had continued and increased in frequency. While the earlier episodes occurred almost anywhere, the current ones were usually restricted to his room where he could be overheard to curse, bang the furniture, and finally settle into a quiet sobbing.

On the surface, his parents seemed to be a happily married, upper middle-class couple. They had made every effort to give their children not only love and attention, but almost every material thing they desired. On closer scrutiny, the differences in personality of the two parents became evident. The mother was an efficient, perfectionistic person with many obsessional qualities. She prided herself on "doing the right thing" whether it was child rearing (by the book), keeping an immaculate house, or being the perfect hostess. Her husband was a dynamic professional person, deeply involved in his work but equally involved in hobbies and sports, which he forced on Jerry far too rapidly. The father and mother both put pressure on the boy to measure up to their standards so that he felt he would lose their respect and love unless he excelled in everything. When he produced something good, he was praised mildly and told he could have done better. No matter what he did, he felt it was not good enough and he outdid his parents in placing demands upon himself.

Initially, the parents were bewildered by the pediatrician's request for a psychiatric consultation. Fortunately, the doctor was able to explain his reasoning in a noncondemnatory way and they accepted this. They even accepted the necessity of their being a part of the evaluation and also of treatment if that should be recommended.

The therapy sessions which followed were relatively few in number. Jerry saw the child psychiatrist and the parents met with a psychiatric social worker. The latter helped the parents "slow down" a bit and demand less of Jerry. The boy loosened up in treatment and began to enjoy things on a more basic emotional level. He remained somewhat compulsive but not to the extent that it interfered with his interpersonal relationships and self-esteem.

Hysterical Personality

The hysterical personality in a youngster is a "junior grade" replica of the adult hysterical personality. The latter term was dropped for a few years, but has made its way back into DSM-II, where it is included as one of the personality disorders. It is also included in the GAP listing on the "Psychopathological Disorders of Childhood."

In the GAP classification, several kinds of neuroses are listed which used to be under the broad heading of hysteria. Specifically, these are the phobic, the conversion, and the dissociative types. Within the category of personality disorders only hysterical personality is named.

This seemingly complicated picture means that a child may have a hysterical personality. In the face of emotional stress, he may develop a classical psychoneurosis which will be superimposed on this underlying personality structure. Because of the nature of the child's basic character, the type of neurotic disorder he develops is likely to be one of the three (or a mixture of the three) mentioned previously. If the neurosis responds to treatment, or if there is a spontaneous remission, the hysterical personality is again likely to come to the fore (it is less amenable to change than is the neurosis). As the child is in many ways a preview of the adult, so the hysterical personality, once established, is likely to remain with the person throughout life.

Typically, children with an hysterical personality disorder show a number of characteristics similar to their adult counterparts. They tend to be emotionally labile, overly dramatic, seductive, and generally naive. They are great seekers of attention, often in positive ways, and they love to be on stage. At the same time, they are seemingly unaware that their actions are drawing attention to themselves. After a flirtatious performance, they seem to ask: "Why is everyone looking at me?" Many of the children involved in long-term child molestation are found to have hysterical personalities. Adolescents with this personality make up are likely to act seductively without being aware that they are doing so. Typically, they lead their companions into anticipating sexual favors which they are not prepared to grant. These children are very suggestible and are often dependent on their environment to provide them with the clues to their sense of identity. They take on roles which are indicated to them and are never sure who they are. They differ from those children who find their identity within themselves. While girls with this syndrome probably outnumber boys, it should be remembered that boys with an hysterical bent are by no means uncommon.

Hysteria was, of course, Freud's first avenue into psychoanalysis. In child analysis, "Little Hans" was a hysteric with many phobias.[2]

According to the psychoanalytic model, the hysteric is one who has reached but never resolved his oedipal complex. The complexities of development are such that the cases do not emerge in pure culture. On the contrary, most children will present a mixture of problems. The hysterical child, for instance, will display behavior connected with oral and anal problems, but will be chiefly concerned with distressing phallic phase difficulties. Basic to this is an unsolved oedipal complex and, as a result, the child cannot successfully enter the latency phase. A sound identification with the parent of the same sex has not been completely accomplished, and much of the child's psychic energy remains bound up in a family triangle. Thus, it is not available to invest in peer relationships and in finding one's place in the

larger world. The child elaborates an older and more sophisticated version of the play typical of the oedipal period—imaginative, creative, unlimited by the bounds of reality—rather than enjoying the more typical play patterns of latency aged children. Chronologically, the child may be in latency, but psychologically he has not arrived there.

There is no single family constellation associated with all cases of hysterical personality disorder, but there are several factors which would tend to predispose in this direction. Perhaps one of the most common is a lack of closeness and warmth between the parents. Erotic wishes which would ordinarily have been directed toward the spouse may be unconsciously attached to one or more of the children. Such a parent then becomes overtly or covertly seductive toward the child. For example, the mother who continues to fondle and bathe the child and to display herself before her eight-year-old son will encourage hysterical personality formation. If she is confronted with the sexual overtones of what she is doing, she becomes indignant and refuses to listen—implying that the problem is in the mind of the confronter. Similarly, the father who caresses and amorously teases his ten-year-old daughter in an almost adult manner will increase her possibility of developing in such an hysterical direction. Identification with an hysterical parent is, of course, another likely facilitator for the development of an hysterical personality. In the examples given, the apparent unawareness of the sexual overtones implies some hysterical features in the parental personality. In such a case, the child is in double jeopardy; on the one hand, he must deny the sexual seductiveness in the parent's behavior in order to continue to respond and sustain the relationship, strengthening the hysterical aspects of his own personality, and on the other hand, he is constantly confronted with the hysterical traits of the parent with whom he will identify.

The treatment of a youngster with an hysterical personality disorder is usually sought only when the dramatic flare and seductiveness have reached proportions that cause problems in school and/or with peers. As long as the condition remains relatively mild, the child is considered "cute" and "flighty," but not really ill or in need of treatment. Actual therapy with such a youngster is quite enjoyable, but if they are seriously disturbed, such therapy can be complicated. With their bent for dramatics, they are often active in school plays, but the borderline between being "on stage" and "off stage" gets blurred and the therapist may have difficulty helping the youngster separate the two. To the child, as to the adult counterpart, everything is sort of an act and none of it is for real.

Jane was eleven years old when first referred to the child psychiatrist at the request of the school counselor. She was an attractive, physically precocious girl, intelligent but not learning well in school. The counselor's main concern, however, was her seductiveness and the not infrequent sex play with peers. She was also seductive to all male teachers and to the other men in the school.

Her parents, particularly the father, seemed unable or unwilling to see the problem. It rapidly became evident that the parental marriage was characterized primarily by distance. They did not argue or fight openly but had little in common, and each went his or her own way. Jane, an only child, was literally the apple of her father's eye and he lavished gifts and affection upon her. Mother tried discipline but was ineffective, especially when Jane could turn to her father and get whatever she wanted.

Jane had few friends because she always wanted things her way. She spent hours alone reenacting movies or TV shows. Her life ambition was to become an actress, but she was left out of the school play because she would not follow instructions. She insisted on participating to suit herself.

Treatment was begun with Jane being seen by a child psychiatrist and her parents by a psychiatric social worker. In the beginning, both therapists seemed to have an easy time. The parents appeared cooperative and the child was friendly, although somewhat seductive in manner and dress. After a short while, the marital problems began to emerge, but the parents seemed content to ignore them. Jane, meantime, was attempting to manipulate her therapist in her most seductive manner. Her skirts became shorter and her blouse tighter. When the therapist did not respond as she wished, she became furious and screamed obscenities at him. She told her father the therapist was crazy and asking her "a lot of dirty questions." Needless to say, it took a meeting with both parents and both therapists to calm things down.

Eventually, the youngster was sent to a boarding school which had rigid standards, but which supported the help being given Jane and her family. Finally, when she found she could not manipulate the school or the therapist and that both her parents were alike in their desire for her to change, she began to improve. At the time of termination, Jane was still hysteric, but her behavior had become more acceptable. It is difficult to predict how she will handle adolescence and young adulthood, and the possibility of further personality problems certainly remains. Both she and her parents left treatment with good feelings, however, and one can assume they would seek further help if the need arose.

Anxious Personality

The child with an anxious personality is uncomfortable, but is not incapacitated by anxiety. Certainly he is less upset than the youngster with an anxiety neurosis. Such a child's general approach to the world is cautious and a new situation will probably cause some initial anxiety, but he is not markedly inhibited and generally will handle situations adequately and develop appropriately. Even so, most of the time he is tense.

To understand this personality pattern, one must first comprehend what anxiety is. Subjectively, practically everyone has experienced it at one time or another and knows that it feels like fear. The rapid heart beat, the knot in the chest, the sweaty palms, "butterflies" in the stomach, a feeling of inner strain, and a sense of dread; together, these are anxiety. It differs from fear in that fear represents a normal reaction to a really dangerous situation, while anxiety does not. Anxiety represents a warning against inner psychological danger. Whenever the individual's mechanisms of defense are threatened by the possibility of the breakthrough to consciousness of forbidden unconscious impulses, anxiety results. With fear, one knows the source of the danger and can fight or escape. With anxiety, one has a vague sense of danger, but doesn't know where it will strike. There is no external enemy, no one to fight.

With children, it is sometimes more difficult to separate the two feelings. For example, the youngster who has fallen into a river or swimming pool and been rescued may be apprehensive about water for some time to come. In such a case, it may be difficult to clearly separate anxiety from fear. If, however, the child becomes panicked by water under almost any or all circumstances, it is reasonable to think of anxiety rather than fear. Like the adult, the child often understands the problem intellectually but has not accepted it emotionally. He realizes that what he feels so anxious about is not a real danger, but the anxiety remains.

The youngster with an anxious personality is mildly to moderately anxious most of the time. It rarely becomes severe. If asked, parents will say he is a "nervous" child, fidgety and can't sit still for over a few minutes. He never seems really relaxed and even his sleep is restless, often disturbed by nightmares. In school, he is a problem for the teacher because of his inability to sit still and his daydreaming. He is not so much a disobedient child as an exasperating one. Contrary to the antisocial child who acts out, adults usually feel sympathy for the anxious child even if he poses them a problem. At times, his symptomatology may appear remarkably similar to that of the youngster with minimal cerebral dysfunction, and the two conditions may be confused. The differences are sometimes subtle, but in general, the hyperactivity of the anxious child exhibits a less "driven" quality, and its intensity is more intermittent. The "soft neurological signs" and the visual motor difficulties frequently present in the MBD child are not found in the child with an anxious personality. Both children may present problems at school, but those of the anxious child are more neurotic in character while the MBD child shows diagnosable learning disabilities. While many MBD children respond to stimulant medications, some anxious children do as well. Thus, the response to Methylphenidate hydrochloride (Ritalin) does not differentiate betwen the two. In both cases, time and attention may bring improvement.

The traditional view associated anxiety syndromes with oedipal fixation. In fact, the anxious child does not usually have a preponderant fixation at any one phase of psychosexual development. As a rule, there are various mixtures of oral, anal, and phallic-oedipal residues. Concerns about separation vie with castration fears as sources of the child's pain. The basic issue here is not so much a matter of instinctual arrest. Instead it is the rather loosely organized character of their ego defenses; the chronic anxiety emerges from that.

The family constellations can vary, but a common ingredient is inconsistency or unpredictability. The concept can be translated into Erikson's stages of optimism versus pessimism and trust versus mistrust, with pessimism and mistrust predominating in the personality configuration of the anxious personality.

To the young child, consistency of support is essential. Inconsistency lays the foundation for anxiety. Traumatic events play their powerful role as well in provoking anxiety, especially if they are repeated. This might occur when a child who must endure numerous surgical procedures is poorly prepared and suffers much pain. As is true of other personality disorders, identification with a fearful, anxious, worrying parent will assist the establishment of those personality traits in a child.

Nora was seven years old when first referred by her pediatrician for what appeared to be an incipient, mild school phobia. She attended school under protest and was frequently absent because of "stomach aches." She often asked to go to the nurse's office. Her teacher said she was capable of good school work but seemed to spend much of her time daydreaming or fidgeting. She had few friends because other children saw her as a "whiner." Reluctance to go to school had been present from kindergarten but had been considerably worse for the last few months. The parents also noted that Nora had difficulty in getting to sleep at night,

had occasional nightmares, ate poorly, cried frequently, and bit her fingernails. In recent months those symptoms had also become more severe.

A few months earlier, her father had suffered a coronary. He had required hospitalization, followed by a period of rest at home. The father was only forty-two years old at the time, an ambitious energetic man competing successfully in the business world. He had been advised to seek a less demanding job and was bitterly disappointed at the suggested change. He vacillated between pushing himself too hard and regressing to bed. His daughter became his "junior nurse" and worried about him constantly.

The psychiatrist had to collaborate with the school and with the father's cardiologist. The teacher was able to provide Nora with more support and encouragement. The father's prognosis was good. The psychiatrist was able to help the parents understand the effect of their attitudes on Nora. Through play therapy, he was able to talk more realistically with her about her father's condition. In this way, he helped Nora express her worries and recognize some of the sources of her anxiety. The incipient school phobia disappeared, and the child began to expand her activities.

Nevertheless, Nora remained a chronically anxious child. Her anxiety did not prevent her from going to school, making more friends, and generally seeming much happier. However, she continued to bite her nails, and, in the face of new situations she was always apprehensive. Even in her therapeutic sessions, a certain amount of anxiety persisted. A fine tremor was present and an overtalkativeness that betrayed her tension. During her span of treatment she did not work her problems through completely, but, in time, she achieved a sufficiently comfortable adjustment to allow for termination. She is likely to remain somewhat anxious henceforth, and how she copes with her anxiety will depend on the stresses she is exposed to as she grows older. It is not improbable that further treatment will be needed at a later date.

The Overly Dependent Personality

As the term would indicate these youngsters are excessively dependent, clinging and often whiney and demanding. They show an interest in activities more appropriate for younger children and are generally nonathletic and noncompetitive. What few friends they have are likely to be younger. They are either ignored or scapegoated by peers and easily dissolve into tears when threatened or thwarted. They cling to protective adults such as parents or teachers.

One of the most common causes of this pattern is parental overprotection. Certainly, all children require parental protection and guidance. This is only one dimension of care, however, and should be mixed with encouragement toward independence and the development of new skills. It has been said that if a parent wishes to raise a child to be independent and to have good judgment and common sense when he is twenty-one, the parent should allow him to be one-third independent when he is seven, and two-thirds by the time he is fourteen. Every wise parent realizes that raising children involves taking risks, and there has to be preparation for the time when the child is "on his own."

The overprotective parent, for his own inner reasons, prevents or discourages the child from taking appropriate steps toward autonomy. Sometimes this situation arises from, or at any rate, is aggravated by the presence of a chronic physical illness. One sees this not infrequently in diabetic or asthmatic children. Inquiry usually reveals that the child could do much more but has been excessively overprotected by a fearful or guilty or ambivalent parent.

Joe was twelve years of age when the pediatrician first referred him to the child phychiatrist. He had a history of idiopathic epilepsy which had been successfully controlled by medication for the past five years. While the pediatrician had specified a few activities that would not be wise for the boy, the mother had added many of her own to the list. She felt that Joe should never become excited nor frustrated lest he have a seizure. This meant that the most normal peer activities were forbidden and discipline was almost totally absent.

The father, a passive man, had tried unsuccessfully to loosen the emotional bond between his wife and son, but he eventually withdrew, feeling it was a lost cause.

Therapy consisted of a team effort between the pediatrician, the child psychiatrist, the neurologist, and the social worker. Gradually, with only partial success, Joe began to emancipate himself. He and his father began to enjoy more masculine activities together and he joined the Boy Scouts. The mother was reassured that all the professionals involved were interested and would not push Joe too far. She slowly loosened her close ties with Joe. He, on the one hand, welcomed the changes, but on the other, resented and feared them. His skills in boyish activities were far below those of his age group, and he joined from pressure more than from desire.

He did improve and his mother was given all possible assistance to support her in helping him. The eventual outcome was reasonably good, although he retained some aspects of his dependency and immaturity.

Oppositional Personality

As noted in the GAP report, these children had previously been classified as passive-aggressive personalities. Actually, either term should be ac-

ceptable; in fact, however, the older term has probably been so ingrained into the average psychiatrist and child psychiatrist that it is difficult to replace.

Certain personality organizations are dominated by the issues around compliance with adult requirements. In a certain sense, there are three choices: one can obey all rules and develop a compulsive personality, one can rebel actively and become an antisocial character disorder, or one can say "yes" to the rules but never quite follow them and so become an oppositional personality. Why one child chooses one alternative and the next another is not always clear. There are probably some very powerful constitutional factors that influence or determine personality type. The constitutional factors come first and are the basis for the choice of how to deal with adult requirements.

The child with an oppositional personality develops a passive-aggressive manner of behaving. Basically this implies some form of chronic rebelling against rules and regulations. He begins his pattern quite early in life by sensing the conscious as well as unconscious needs and concerns of his parents. Whether it be eating, toilet training, good manners, or whatever, it is perceived by the child as being of substantial importance to his parents. Once the child determines the "area" of battle, the oppositional war is on. He maintains himself in a child's position and feels that the demands made by parents are excessive or unfair. If, for instance, it is toilet training, he has become aware that his daily bowel movements are of substantial importance to his mother. If he has a bowel movement when and where she wishes, she is happy; if he does not, she is angry and perhaps punitive. One avenue open to him is to utilize the passive-aggressive route. He begins by readily agreeing to go potty, but sits there and nothing happens. His mother tries everything to bring about the desired results. She has a seemingly compliant, nonrebellious child who willingly goes to the potty but does not defecate. She talks to him, reads to him, promises him gifts, or any other inducement she can think of. He continues to absorb her attention but does not produce. She is frustrated but is hesitant to be punitive because he has not openly rebelled. He has, in essence, rebelled aggressively while behaving in a passive manner.

One of the biggest problems that occurs in such a child is that of the oppositional traits tend to become ingrained and to spread to other areas. By the time the true situation is recognized and evaluated, both the child and his parents are unhappy. He is not punctual for school, late with asignments, and lackadaisical about doing home chores. By the fifth or sixth grade, there is a beginning concern about his tendency to procrastinate. One of the most common complaints of teachers is that while such a youngster is usually intelligent, he doesn't work to capacity. Assignments, if completed, are often too late. If there were a code phrase for the oppositional child, it would be, "I'll do it later." His procrastination can spread until it reaches a remarkable degree. One child, for instance, would not only get up late on school mornings but would proceed to put his shoes on the wrong feet. When his exasperated parents thought he was finally ready, they would discover the shoes. He would miss the school bus and a parent would have to drive him, only to find he had "forgotten" his books. Nowhere had he openly rebelled, but he certainly had done so in a passive manner. He had achieved the goal of getting at his parents and without the risk of punishment. Psychodynamically, his orientation is primarily anal. Oppositional traits pervade every area of his life.

Sam was eight years old when the family physician referred him to the child guidance clinic. The chief complaint was that constant strife prevailed between the child and his parents. He had two younger sisters who seemed to be getting along well. The parents reported that Sam had been a "difficult" child to manage ever since he was a toddler. He rarely rebelled openly or lost his temper, but, in a passive way, he managed to not follow through on parental requests. Toilet training was begun at about one year of age by his somewhat over-zealous mother, and he soon learned that a daily bowel movement was important to her. He would dutifully sit on the potty but produce nothing. His mother wheedled and cajoled and finally became angry. The episodes usually ended in a stalemate, and the child was tending toward chronic constipation.

The obstinancy and procrastination began to spread to other areas. He dawdled at the table, he was late getting up in the morning, etc. When he began school, the problems accompanied him. Sam often said, "I don't know," to questions when, in fact, he did know the answer, and the teacher felt he was working well below his potential.

From the beginning of the evaluation, he seemed pleasant and comfortable and remained so. His problem emerged rapidly when he adopted the "I don't know" stance. His therapy was slow and tedious and filled with passive-aggressiveness. Gradually, however, as he began to see what he was doing, and that the therapist could cope with it and did not become angry, he became more cooperative.

Meanwhile, the therapist had also been working with the parents to help them understand their problems and deal with them more effectively. The primary goal was to help them avoid battles with Sam, except in those few instances where it was unavoidable. He was served meals with the rest of the family with no remarks about what or when he ate. He was told that he would be called once on school mornings. If he missed the school bus, he would have to walk and make his own explanation to the teacher, who had been made aware of the situation.

Sam was beginning to experience the results of his opposition rather than of his passivity. As he becomes more fully aware of this, he will be able to mobilize aggression constructively when the goal is important, while realizing what price he must expect to pay for being oppositional.

The Overly Inhibited Personality

According to the GAP report, "these children show superficial passivity, with extreme or pathological shyness, inhibition of motor action or initiative, and marked constriction of personality functions, including, at times, diminished speech or even elective mutism, among other features." As pointed out in the report, they differ from schizoid youngsters in that they do want friendships but don't know how to make them. Both the schizoid child and the overly inhibited child will be outside the circle of peers. But the former child will ignore the peers unless to communicate the message to leave him alone. The overly inhibited child will hungrily look on, fearful and unable to communicate his wish to be accepted by the groups.

Constitutional differences may be a factor in the adjustment of these children, but family patterns are certainly important. A not uncommon pattern seen in such families might be labeled "social isolation." Although this may take many forms, the very closely knit, almost asocial family is apt to produce this syndrome.

Such a family lives as a relatively isolated unit within the larger society and has few, if any, outside activities. There is a family dictum, spoken or unspoken, that "outsiders" cannot be trusted. At every chance, the child seeks the solace of home to avoid the presumed "dangers" in the world outside.

The development of such disorders is influenced by many factors including constitutional predisposition and parental idiosyncracies. For whatever reasons, the parents do not help the child develop self-confidence nor do they foster within him the ability or desire to compete. School performance is usually lack-lustre and contributes to the cycle of poor achievement, causing low self-esteem which further inhibits the mobilization of aggression toward productivity. Suffice it to say, it is improbable that this pattern will develop in a child of an out-going, trusting and friendly family.

Barbara was nineteen years old when first seen by the psychiatrist. Her history showed all too clearly the process by which an overly inhibited personality developed in childhood. She was an only child. Her mother was a tense, anxious person who constantly sent the child double messages. Mother went to the extreme of locking the girl out of the house to force her to seek playmates; more often still, she infantalized her daughter and kept the child close.

The father was an industrious businessman who came home late from work, ate a hurried dinner and went to bed. On the surface, this was a close knit, fond family, but the real message from the mother to the daughter was: don't trust anyone but us. Being a bright girl, Barbara excelled academically and spent much time alone at home studying. She had few friends and failed to develop skills that would allow her to make friends. She became a recluse. She longed for companionship but was fearful of making any overtures to peers which might lead to a relationship. She remained peripheral to the peer group. During adolescence she dated rarely. When she did, she felt awkward and was reluctant to repeat the experience. By the time she reached nineteen, she began to realize that she no longer wished to remain in an isolated trio with her parents but that she needed help to free herself.

Her treatment brought out two aspects of a central conflict. One part of her wanted to go back and being a little, protected girl, but the healthier part wanted to be a young woman. As is true in most such cases, she also had to convince her parents that they would not "lose" her if she matured, but rather that their relationship would be enriched. She needed their permission to become more independent.

She left home and went away to college. This helped loosen the bond with her parents. Initially she buried herself in books, but with the help of the therapist she slowly began a social life. It was not easy because she lacked the experience of her peers, but she did gain a degree of self-confidence, and the ensuing rewards promoted more improvement.

This case illustrates an important problem which constantly faces the child psychiatrist dealing with a youngster who has functional emotional problems. Something in the parents' psyches, conscious or more often unconscious, has been a causative factor in the child's problem. For example, some parents may "need" a compulsive child, others a psychosomatically ill child, and still others an antisocial "acting-out" child. When such inner needs exist in parents, they must be modified if the youngster is to reach his real potential. The child psychiatrist who tries to help a youngster become "normal" while that youngster continues to live in a family which promotes "abnormality" will either fail with the youngster or put him in the awkward position of divided loyalties.

The younger the child, the more closely he is tied to his parents and the greater their influence on his personality development. To the degree that they fail to respond to his constitutional needs, have emotional blind spots, or communicate other distortions in their demands and expectations, the child will suffer. The child psychiatrist and the parents must be striving for the same goals or treatment will not succeed. With an adolescent, it will be even more difficult for the parents to change toward normalcy. The child himself must help them to accept such change, and the additional help of other mental health professionals to work with the parents may be required.

The Overly Independent Personality

These are youngsters who show a tendency toward positive enthusiasm, perpetual activity, and pseudomaturity. Often this is evident from a very early age. It is as if they always wanted to be older and to undertake activities beyond their age level. They are in a great hurry to grow up.

Most normal children perceive the world in terms of their own age level and act accordingly. They accept the fact that the older you get, the more you can master successfully and the more you can do. They are aware of their own limitations and recognize the authority of adults. They use reasonable caution in approaching new and strange ventures.

The child with an overly independent personality is not bound by such rules and caution. He will joyously leap into the deep end of a swimming pool even though he cannot swim and has been warned about it. He may challenge an older and bigger child, not so much out of anger, as out of a sense of omnipotence. One of the most frequent comments his parents make is that "he isn't afraid of anything." Most of these children are injured and punished more often than their peers, but this does not cure the problem nor even dampen their enthusiasm. They tend to share one characteristic with the sociopathic child; neither of them learn by experience.

As the GAP report points out, chronic illness may be a contributing factor, especially when it results in the child being infantalized over a period of time. In other cases, the parents have consciously or unconsciously contributed to perpetuation of the early childish omnipotence. Because of a child's physical illness or for neurotic needs of their own, parents may let a youngster "walk all over them." He then proceeds to follow the same course outside the home—in school and with friends—and it gets him into trouble. If the parents continue to maintain the same attitudinal relationship to the child at home, the child continues to behave in the same manner elsewhere.

Another way this comes about is when one or the other parent has superego lacunae in his character makeup. Such a parent unconsciously encourages the child to precocious, pseudomature, overly confident behavior. The behavior gives vicarious pleasure or satisfaction to the parent. The child repeats it because he senses that the parent desires it and that he will be rewarded in some indirect fashion. This again is similar to an element in the child-parent relationship that is often seen in sociopathic youngsters. However, an important difference should be noted. The overly independent child is not basically angry or antisocial; his behavior is primarily the result of a perpetuated immature feeling of omnipotence.

George was first referred for evaluation at seven years of age. His mother's complaint was, "He is a lovable child but I can't control him. He alienated all his classmates, won't go along with rules and regulations and is always doing something dangerous or foolish. He is a bright, enthusiastic boy but just always carries things too far."

George's parents were financially well-to-do. Each parent was involved in many outside interests, and they had often used nursemaids for George. When they did spend time with their son, they indulged him with many material gifts but demonstrated little real love and almost no consistent discipline.

On the first visit to the child psychiatrist, George behaved in his characteristic "omnipotent" fashion. He greeted the doctor warmly and proceeded to ignore any words of caution about what was allowed, what was forbidden, what was the purpose of his visit, etc. He promptly seated himself in the doctor's chair and began to play with the telephone. When reminded that the phone was "off limits," he paid little attention.

He spent part of the time complaining about his recent birthday presents. He had received a toy shaver and a toy lawn mower when he had actually wanted the real thing. He made numerous statments bragging about his prowess in athletics, although parents had reported that he was mediocre at best. When he could not win a game, he lost interest and quit. He wanted to play a game of checkers but made up his own rules to assure his victory.

It seemed as though he failed to recognize his own limitations vis-a-vis other youngsters and adults. The parents were relatively unaware of George's problems and had accepted the referral only because of pressure from the school. They refused a treatment program which would in any way involve them and sent the boy to a boarding school where he continued to have many of the same problems.

The Isolated Personality

According to the GAP report, these youngsters "tend to exhibit distant, detached, cold or withdrawn attitudes toward family and friends. Frequently they are isolated and reclusive or "isolating" persons; they experience difficulties in competition and in expression of even healthy aggressive impulses, although they may show occasional unpredictable outbursts of bizarrely aggressive or sadistic behavior."

The report goes on to suggest that these children have no very deeply meaningful relationships. They prefer their isolated existence and satisfaction seems to come to them from fantasy and autistic reveries. Not only are they isolated emotionally, but even physical isolation is frequently sought. They do not seek relationships with others, and they do not respond to emotional outreach from others. It is as if this child were living in a glass cage which neither allows him to move out nor others to move in.

A few of these youngsters exhibit latent schizophrenic qualities, although many do not. Considering how relatively little we know about schizophrenia in adulthood, and that we know even less about latent schizophrenia in childhood, this diagnosis seems to be an instance of splitting hairs. These youngsters may or may not be latent schizophrenics; the boundaries are often vague and ill-defined with much overlap.

Such children may be of low, medium, or high intelligence. One is often hard pressed to be accurate in prognosis. Some of these youngsters, particularly under the stress of puberty and adolescence, become overtly psychotic. Others retain their isolated lives, but do not decompensate and are able to function in society.

Joe was a fourteen-year-old boy when referred by the juvenile court for evaluation. On two occasions he had approached women and made obscene remarks and gestures. No actual physical contact was made.

The history revealed that he was the second of four children. He had always been a "loner," had few friends and always remained at the periphery of peer activities. His school work was marginal, although his intellect was in the average range. There was no history of other antisocial acts.

During the interview, he answered questions rather openly, but said he had no idea why he accosted the women. He had no girl friends and could not bring himself to touch girls even in a jesting way. All of his answers seemed logical except when speaking of the incidents with the women. He knew that his actions had been wrong, but when pressed, seemed unsure whether he would do it again. He agreed he should have more friends and do better in school. Near the end of the interview, he was asked how much feeling had gone into what he had been saying and he replied, "very little." He did not seem schizophrenic nor bizarre; indeed he was really quite logical. The main problem was that the words he said had little conviction behind them and therefore had little real meaning to him. He was not only emotionally distant from the therapist, but also from his peers and even from the members of his own family.

Outpatient psychotherapy and concurrent chemotherapy were recommended and initiated. He was a model patient in that he was always punctual, reasonably verbal and quite willing to discuss his past and present. His answers and comments were always correct and logical, but he continued to show lack of real feeling for anything he said. He recognized the emotional distance between not only himself and the therapist, but himself and everyone.

Gradually, his previously absent emotions began to show slightly. He started dating girls, but this made him feel extremely awkward and uncomfortable. He did join a few group activities with his peers but remained close to the periphery of the group and failed to develop any close friendships.

In general, his adjustment improved, but the isolation was still paramount. He had a certain mistrust of closeness stemming from early childhood. The roots were deep and difficult to eradicate.

The Mistrustful Personality

This disorder is rarely seen in children and is not common to adolescents. It approaches, but is not so severe as, a paranoid personality. It lacks the factor of projection which figures so prominently in the personality of the paranoid adult.

Leaving aside the usefulness of the diagnosis, a word should be said here about Erikson's concept of trust and mistrust. This has its roots in early childhood and is of critical importance to general personality development. Consider the stranger anxiety in the preschooler. It is a type of mistrust that is almost universal. Or consider the widespread distrust of psychiatrists shown by adolescents. Many feel that seeing a psychiatrist is proof of what they have feared, namely, that they are crazy. Another example of "normal" mistrust is the feeling of a lower-class family from a minority subculture when the school refers them to a large psychiatric facility. They are fearful of possible consequences and distrustful of the mental health personnel. Finally, there is that large group of adults who basically distrust others and cannot get close to them emotionally.

The roots of mistrust are laid down during childhood and adolescence and require careful scrutiny by the child psychiatrist. The youngster whose parents provide him a regular, predictable, and warm atmosphere is prone to rely on others and become basically trusting. Conversely, the child whose parents are unpredictable and frequently do not meet the child's emotional needs may well produce a person who cannot get close to or trust anyone. Such a child will probably never receive a diagnosis as a mistrustful personality. The very nature of his problem is likely to prevent his coming to a mental health facility. Such a diagnosis, since it is hardly ever applied to a patient, becomes more important in understanding the various aspects of child development than for its clinical applicability.

Sociosyntonic Personality Disorder

Although the GAP report delineates two subdivisions of this syndrome, it appears that the subdivisions are merely variations of symptomatology stemming from differences among subcultures. In essence, these are youngsters whose behavior is consonant with the values in their subculture but is deviant or troublesome to society as a whole. The child feels no conflict or guilt about his behavior. It is syntonic with the social sub-systems within which he lives and to which he owes his allegiance. Indeed, if he rejected the behaviors that define the symptoms of this personality disorder, he would in turn be rejected by his peers and considered deviant by the standards of the subculture to which he belongs. For example, certain modes of action may be quite acceptable for a family in the neighborhood of a defined subculture, but not outside of it. The city child from a poverty-stricken neighborhood may have to learn certain patterns of behavior such as fighting, lying, and stealing merely to survive. Altercations are expected to be "resolved" by violent methods and to do otherwise would cause ostracism. In Appalachia, hysterical-like phenomena are common and hardly considered by neighbors and friends to be symptoms of mental illness. In a Mexican-American barrio, symptoms of psychosis are believed by many to be the result of a hex, and help is sought from a *curandero* rather than from a psychiatrist.

In many ways, youngsters with such behavior are at once psychologically healthy but culturally deviant. In the past, they have been called dyssocial personalities. They often come from families in which the ingredients for building a "normal" personality are present, but the more the family or subculture mores deviate from the larger group-accepted norm, the more chance the child has of being labeled a sociosyntonic disorder. By definition, then, this diagnosis does not indicate intrapsychic problems, but rather a style of living that works well at home but not in the larger society.

A Mexican-American family moved from a crowded, poverty-ridden barrio into a rather sedate, white, middle-class neighborhood. The parents were hard working and upward-striving people who loved their children. Problems appeared very soon, first in the form of shouting and yelling between parents and children, as well as between siblings. Battles seemed to erupt at least once a day, sometimes settled with shouting and other times with spanking. Although obviously anxious to make friends, the children were loud and rough with neighborhood children. The same thing happened on the playground at the new school, where their overt aggression and name-calling lost them friends and identified them to the teachers as problem children. The school requested a consultation with a child psychiatrist. After reviewing the situation, he asked to meet with the parents and the children himself; a variation from his usual role of consulting with the school personnel.

He found the parents cooperative and mystified by the consultation request. They felt they had a happy marriage and that their children had always adjusted well both at home and in their previous school. The children seemed intelligent, well dressed, and polite.

It was only after the psychiatrist had observed the children in school and the social worker had made a home visit, that the situation became clear. This was a loud, vociferous family with a high level of emotional output. Their behavior was not unusual in the neighborhood from which they had come.

This case raises questions so often posed in our society today. With increased mobility and moves toward integration, old patterns are failing and new avenues of adjustment must be sought.

Summary

As can be seen from the foregoing pages, a diagnosis of some types of personality disorder in a child or an adolescent can be difficult and the possibility of error is large. Children and teenagers are in a state of flux, and what originally seems to be an alloplastic disorder may eventually become an autoplastic one.

While it is true that almost every adult with a personality disorder had problems as a child, it remains that hindsight is better than foresight. The general psychiatrist working with adult patients can usually uncover childhood idiosyncracies that were the origins of the eventual problems. The point to be made is that during childhood and adolescence, the mental health worker should be convinced of the seriousness and permanency of aberrations in behavior of his youthful patients before labeling them with some type of personality disorder.

REFERENCES

1. American Psychiatric Association, *Diagnostic and Statistical Manual of Mental Disorders*, 2nd ed. (DSM-II), p. 41, American Psychiatric Association, Washington, D.C., 1968.
2. BRAZELTON, T., *Infants and Mothers: Differences in Development*, Delacorte Press, New York, 1969.
3. FREUD, S., "Analysis of a Phobia in a Five Year Old," *Collected Papers of Sigmund Freud*, vol. 3, Hogarth Press, London, 1953.
4. Group for the Advancement of Psychiatry (GAP), Committee on Child Psychiatry, *Psychopathological Disorders in Childhood: Theoretical Considerations and a Proposed Classification*, Group for the Advancement of Psychiatry, New York, 1966.

5. KRIS, M., "The Use of Prediction in a Longitudinal Study," in Eissler, R. S., et al. (Eds.), *Psychoanalytic Study of the Child*, vol. 12, pp. 175–189, International Universities Press, New York, 1957.
6. RITVO, S., et al., "Some Relations of Constitution, Environment, and Personality as Observed in a Longitudinal Study of Child Development: Case Report," in Solnit, A., and Provence, S. (Eds.), *Modern Perspectives in Child Development*, pp. 107–143, International Universities Press, New York, 1963.
7. THOMAS, O., CHESS, S., and BIRCH, H., *Temperament and Behavior Disorders in Children*, New York University Press, New York, 1968.

14 / Psychoses of Childhood

Barbara Fish and Edward R. Ritvo

Name of the Syndrome, Alternative or Historical Name, DSM-II Name and Number, and GAP Terminology

Unless it is further qualified or defined, the term childhood psychosis covers a heterogeneous group of severe disorders occurring between infancy and twelve years. It is a generic term, which includes both the psychoses associated with definite organic brain syndromes (OBS) and the group without localizing signs of brain pathology. In the latter group, symptoms suggestive of central nervous system (CNS) dysfunction may or may not be present to a varying degree, but the nature of any underlying brain disorder has not yet been identified.

This chapter will focus primarily on children with psychosis in which there is no definite evidence of a specific OBS. In the DSM-II,[2] this group is called "Schizophrenia, childhood type" (295.8). The GAP classification uses the terms: "Early Infantile Autism," "Interactional Psychotic Disorder," and "Schizophreniform Psychotic Disorder."[105] How the various terms are used here and by other authors will be discussed. For convenience, when the general term childhood psychosis is used without further specification, it will be in this more limited sense, referring only to the broad group of childhood psychoses without specific OBS.

The most commonly used terms for these conditions are childhood schizophrenia and infantile autism.[64, 92, 133] Different authors have used these terms and a variety of synonyms in different ways; some to encompass the entire range of these conditions, and others to refer to segments of the affected population.

In the literature of the 1940s and 1950s, the patients were usually defined in a gross way by brief case descriptions or lists of major clinical symptoms. Since the 1960s, there have been increasing attempts to use specific diagnostic criteria.

However, these criteria are rarely spelled out in operational terms which others could use in a reliable way. Furthermore, almost none of the authors have indicated which criteria they consider to be necessary and sufficient for the diagnosis, i.e., symptoms which are universally present in that disorder, are confined only to that condition, and differentiate it from other disorders. Because of this, if the reader wished to determine the boundaries of the population being described and the degree of overlap with populations in other studies, he would have to analyze the case material in detail. At best, this is a difficult and uncertain task.

In this chapter there is an analysis of the characteristics of the populations used in the major studies of childhood psychosis. This clarifies significant resemblances and differences among groups of children who have been labeled psychotic, autistic, or schizophrenic by various authors. The proposed DSM-III criteria for infantile autism and childhood schizophrenia are spelled out. Infantile psychosis is used as a generic term for psychosis with an onset before two years of age; it may include psychosis with OBS, as used by some authors.

Description of the Syndrome

THE SYNDROME AS PRIMARY

Childhood psychosis (without specific OBS) encompasses a range of severe, pervasive disorders of total personality functioning; these involve characteristic disturbances in the integration of speech and thought, affect and social relatedness. The affected child's perception and comprehension of reality deviate markedly from norms for the child's age and cultural group. There may be poorly integrated development of locomotor, fine motor, and visual-motor skills, resulting in peculiar and erratic patterns of functioning. This is especially likely when the disorder is manifest in the first two years.

Psychotic children may share certain symptoms (e.g., anxiety) with other types of disturbed children. Usually these common symptoms occur in a more severe form in the psychotics (e.g., panic reaction). They also tend to occur juxtaposed to or in rapid alternation with disturbances in the opposite direction (e.g., indifference). This gives the total personality a grossly unintegrated, fragmented, and chaotic quality.

When the fragmentation of personality is extreme, it appears unmistakable and pathognomonic. But the degree of personality disorganization varies at different times, even in the same child. Clinical evaluations of lesser degrees of disorder rest on global judgments and are notoriously subject to disagreement. It is difficult to establish reliable criteria for such global phenomena as "disorganization of personality" or "fragmented ego." The authors will therefore follow the lead of those who are developing specific diagnostic criteria for adults.[215] First the critical symptoms will be defined. These clinical disturbances span a wide range of severity which will be described briefly for each area of personality functioning. Then the necessary and sufficient criteria which are used in the current version (1976) of the DSM-III to diagnose childhood schizophrenia, infantile autism, and "Childhood Psychosis, other type" will be outlined. The variety of clinical pictures within each diagnostic group will be described.

DEVELOPMENTAL AND INTEGRATIVE DISORDERS OF SPEECH, LANGUAGE FUNCTION, AND THOUGHT

Starting with the early descriptions of Potter,[171] Despert,[59, 60] Bender,[18, 19] and Kanner,[123, 124] all authors have considered the profound disorder of speech, language function, and thought to be a critical diagnostic characteristic of childhood psychosis.

Certain characteristics of the speech represent retarded development. Words may never be acquired, or they may appear, and then be lost. In samples of infantile psychosis, 20 to 40 percent of the children are reported as being mute (Table 14–1).

All degrees of retardation occur. Speech may be limited to naming and simple adjectives, or to the present tense, even when past events are referred to. The mean sentence length and the complexity of syntax may lag well behind age norms.[207] However, other psychotic children show precocious language function and are preoccupied with word play.[18]

Absent or retarded speech is found in many other disorders. What is specific to childhood psychosis is the coexistence of jargon and unintelligible speech alongside mature speech.[205] The higher the percent of unintelligible speech, the more retarded is the child compared to age norms and the worse his prognosis.[204]

The *comprehension of speech* is also impaired to a varying degree. The child may be completely oblivious to words, with no evidence that speech is understood. This may be so extreme that younger children are sometimes thought to be deaf, until it is determined that they do respond erratically to sounds other than speech. Or, the child may respond only to the tone and melody of speech, and not to its symbolic content; e.g., he responds in some minimal oblique way to a sharp "no!" or to his name being called, but when nonsense words are spoken in the same tone, he responds identically. Comprehension may be limited to simple verbs and nouns referring to the immediate present context. When retardation is less severe, only the comprehension of subtle or abstract meanings may be impaired.

Nonverbal communication may also be severely impaired. In contrast to other children with speech handicaps, there may be little or no use of gestures or pantomime.[110] The child may only scream, until his mother guesses what he wants. Except for expressions of distress, those socially appropriate facial expressions which ordinarily reinforce meaning are usually absent.

Disorders of the mechanical production of speech may add to the problems of the listener who attempts to understand the communications of the psychotic child. Bender[18] described the "wooden-like" and "ventriloquistic" quality and "mechanical modulation of the voice" in these cases. There are peculiarities of pitch, intonation, phrasing, stress, and volume. Speech may be "chanting" or singsong, with odd prolongation of sounds, syllables, and words. A question-like melody may be used stereotypically, even for propositional statements. Odd respiratory rhythms may produce hollow-sounding speech and "choppy," staccato passages. Frequently, the mouth and tongue show decreased tone and a lack of firm lip closure, resulting in articulation that is mumbled and indistinct. Goldfarb and associates[99] analyzed these peculiarities of phonation and articulation and found that they did, indeed, differentiate the speech of schizophrenic children from that of normal ones. The peculiar-

TABLE 14-1

Distribution of IQ's in Psychotic Children in Percent

AUTHOR (DIAGNOSIS)[a]	PUB. YEAR	n	ONSET (YEARS)	MUTE (0 WORDS)	PERCENT RETARDED					TESTS USED[b]
					TOTAL <50	50–69	TOTAL <70	70–89	≥90	
SCHIZOPHRENIA										
Kolvin (LOP)	1971	30	5–15	0	3	13	16	27	57	WISC/SB
Bender (CS)	1972	50	2–10	0	10	14	24	38	38	WISC
INFANTILE PSYCHOSIS										
Bender (CS)	1972	50	<2	18	36	18	54	30	16	WISC/KB
Goldfarb (CS, NO)	1961	9	<5	—	—	—	22(<75)	11(75–89)	67	WISC
Goldfarb (CS, O)	1961	17	<5	—	—	—	71(<75)	11(75–89)	18	WISC
Fish (CS, speaking)	1968, 1976	27	<2	0	52	44	96	4	0	Gesell, Verbal
Fish (CS, speaking)	1968, 1976	27	<2	0	22	30	52	41	7	Gesell, Perf.
Fish (CS, speaking & mute)	1968, 1976	38	<2	29	66	32	97	3	0	Gesell, Verbal
Fish (CS, speaking & mute)	1968, 1976	38	<2	29	37	26	63	29	8	Gesell, Perf.
Rutter (IP)	1967	63	≤5	40	46	25	71	19	10	MP (Perf.)
Kolvin (IP)	1971	46	<3	28	51	27	78	15	6	MP (Perf.)
Lotter (A, "A")	1967	15	≤4.5	20	67(<55)	20(55–79)	87(<80)	13(≥80)	—	25% PPVT / 75% Perf.
Lotter (A, "B")	1967	17	≤4.5	35	71(<55)	12(55–79)	83(<80)	17(≥80)	—	25% PPVT / 75% Perf.
Knobloch (A)	1975	50	<2	—	60(<35)	25(35–75)	85(<75)	15(≥75)	—	Gesell or other

[a] LOP = Late onset psychosis; CS = Childhood psychosis; CS = Childhood schizophrenia; CS, NO = CS, "nonorganic"; CS, O = CS, "organic"; IP = Infantile psychosis; A = Autistic; A, "A" = A, "nuclear" group; A, "B" = A, lower ratings on autistic symptoms; (S) = Schizophrenic-syndrome or schizophrenic-like.
[b] WISC = Wechsler Intelligence Scale for Children; SB = Stanford Binet; KB = Kuhlmann Binet; MB = Merrill Palmer; PPVT = Peabody Picture Vocabulary Test.
— = No information given.

ities of speech production add to the quality of "oddness" and impair the communication of meaning as well as that of affect.

When speech has developed beyond jargon and single words, the language disorders which are more specific to *childhood schizophrenia* can be identified. There may be rigidly stereotyped, echolalic speech, with an apparent inability to reorganize what is heard and to create new sentences adapted for use in new contexts.[206, 207] Kanner[124] gave detailed descriptions of this "delayed echolalia." "Affirmation is indicated by literal repetition of a question. . . . Personal pronouns are repeated just as heard with no change to suit the altered situation . . . consequently he comes to speak of himself always as 'you' and of the person addressed as 'I.' Not only the words but even the intonation is retained." When this rigidity and delayed echolalia are extreme, it results in distorted syntax and fragmented speech. These disorders of form are as specific to childhood schizophrenia as are the incoherence and formal thought disorder in adult schizophrenia (see "Formal Thought Disorder, 1. Incoherence," p. 253).

Even when the form of speech is less grossly disrupted, there are disturbances in conceptualization and the logic of thought and association which render the speech more or less incomprehensible to others. Words may be used idiosyncratically, or condensed and distorted to create neologisms. Kanner (pp. 245–246)[123] termed these idiosyncratic usages "metaphorical substitution." His examples demonstrated that what was irrelevant to the listener was not irrelevant to the child, but that it was necessary to know the original context to understand the child's association. Bender[18] saw the symbols as reflecting "tendencies for condensation or the . . . mixing of abstract and concrete thinking." For one child, a circle was "a 'rat-cheese-hole,' dealing with his problems of introjection, anality and his anxiety concerning aggression."

Such neologisms represent "metaphor" and "symbol," in the sense that the word stands for something else; at the same time, they manifest a concrete mode of thinking, which is rooted in a specific situation, not an abstract generalization. There is no ability to comprehend common denominators or to conceive of causality.[102] For Kanner's[123] "Paul," a saucepan was still a "peter eater," three years after his mother dropped a saucepan while she recited to him the nursery rhyme about "Peter, Peter, pumpkin eater." The normal child quickly responds to the essential and invariant patterns in his experience, and derives the ordinary meanings and causal relationships from them. To the psychotic child, two items or events which chance to be randomly juxtaposed, become locked in an irrevocable association. The saucepan remains embedded in its initial context and is not differentiated as an ordinary pot. Such fixed associations between random events, with no generalized concept of their essential elements, lead to idiosyncratic meanings and, in a descriptive sense, to irrelevant and noncommunicative speech. Baltaxe and Simmons[6] hypothesized that this occurs because these children can label but "are unable to decode a previously heard utterance in terms of its basic syntactic or semantic relationships. . . . They use the entire utterance as a label for a similar situation" (p. 446).[6]

Hermelin and O'Connor's[110] experiments, comparing autistic children with matched subnormals, demonstrated that the autistic children had better rote recall than subnormals. For the autistics, however, recall depended on an " 'echobox type' memory store," one which relied on "the purely acoustic and phonetic aspects of speech" (p. 86) . . . "Coding and categorizing are deficient, and 'sense' is little better remembered than 'nonsense' " (p. 91). They were "impaired in the appreciation of the grammatically structured aspect of language" and in the "ability to associate words semantically."

The deviant and illogical associations in his speech provide a glimpse into the world of the schizophrenic child. A world composed of an endless succession of randomly juxtaposed events is one basically devoid of meaning or predictability. It is a confusing and incomprehensible experience that cannot be shared by other children or adults.

The noncommunicative characteristic of this speech had been emphasized earlier by Despert.[60] She conceptualized the frequent disparity between the rote recall of large numbers of nursery rhymes and the small vocabulary used for the expression of needs, as a "dissociation between language-sign and language-function." Shapiro and associates,[204, 205, 206, 207] and Baltaxe and Simmons[6] have summarized more recent studies and analyzed the linguistic characteristics of the speech to quantify the deficits of structure, meaning, and communicability.

The British group[52] briefly summarized the diagnostic criteria for speech disorder: "Speech may have been lost or never acquired or may have failed to develop beyond a level appropriate to an earlier stage. There may be confusion of

personal pronouns, echolalia, or other mannerisms of use and diction. Though words or phrases
may be uttered, they may convey no sense of
ordinary communication." This represents an accurate summary, but reliable criteria require more
specific operational definitions. Further, one must
restrict the criteria to characteristics that are not
shared by other immature or retarded children.

The following definitions of diagnostic criteria
for formal thought disorder in schizophrenic children have been adapted from the outline used
for adult schizophrenia in the Research Diagnostic
Criteria of Spitzer and colleagues[215] (hereinafter
abbreviated RDC). These have been changed so
as to conform to the data obtained on schizophrenic children.

Formal Thought Disorder: "Neologisms are not
included because of the general unreliablity of
clinical judgments of these phenomena, and because it is unlikely that these would be the only
manifestations of thought disorder" (p. 3).[215]

1. Incoherence. Understandability of speech is
impaired by distorted grammar, incomplete sentences, lack of logical connections between phrases
or sentences, or sudden irrelevancies" (p. 3).[215]

2. Distorted grammar. In children, distorted
syntax can be identified only in phrases of three
or more words. This should exclude simple developmental errors of inflection or tense, such as
irregular verbs and final s's (p. 42).[205]

3. Simple echoing, i.e., the immediate, exact
repetition of another's remark, should be excluded,
although, to some extent, it represents uncommunicative speech. Only quantitative techniques,[207]
can differentiate the rigidly stereotyped echoing of
young schizophrenic children, which conforms
precisely to the model, from the more flexible
imitation which occurs during the acquisition of
speech in normal young children and in nonpsychotic children with retardation or speech
delays. In contrast to the nonpsychotic children,
the echoing of psychotic children persists after
the stage when vocabulary is rapidly being accumulated. However, there are as yet no qualitative clinical criteria which can differentiate psychotic from normal echoing reliably without using
such quantitative techniques. Immediate echoing,
alone, does not differentiate psychotics from nonpsychotic controls matched for mental age.[197]

4. Habitual pronoun reversal, i.e., confusion of
personal pronouns, and use of the second or third
personal pronoun to refer to the self. This is a
form of echoing, but it involves a more complex
level of speech construction. When nonpsychotic
children reach this level of complexity, they

usually are able to transform the syntactic structure of their imitations.[207] Pronoun reversal
does differentiate psychotic from nonpsychotic
children.[197]

5. Fragmented speech, which may be connected
by inappropriate words. Example:

"No what see to you this now . . . nice loo do I
say those things I say new things a new thing away"
(a four-year, nine-month-old) (p. 527).[59]
"Somebody and no kids can get some everything—
creepy crawlers, I don't know" (a five-year-old) (p.
49).[205]
(Examiner: What's funny about that?) "Because it's
laugh" (an eight-year-old).[71]

6. "Lack of logical connection between phrases
or sentences, or sudden irrelevancies."[215] Since
young children rarely speak in "paragraphs," "irrelevancy" may refer to the absent connection with
the immediately preceding remark of the patient
or of the examiner, or with the contextual framework of the interview. Words and sentences are
triggered by adventitious and idiosyncratic associations and are emitted in inappropriate contexts
as were the previously discussed phrases, "peter
eaters" and "rat-cheese-hole." The greater the
percent of such noncommunicative speech, the
worse the outcome.[204] Delayed echoing usually
falls in this category, also.

7. Loosening of associations. "Repeatedly saying things in juxtaposition, which lack a logical
or inherent relationship, or shifting ideas idiosyncratically from one frame of reference to
another" (p. 3).[215] This may occur in schizophrenic children, but only when they have
achieved more verbal fluency. Examples:

"Gargoyles have milkbags"; "Needle head. Pink
wee-wee. Has a yellow leg. Cutting the dead deer.
Poison deer. Poor Elaine. No tadpoles in the house.
Men broke deer's leg" (while cutting the picture of a
deer from a book) (Elaine, seven-year-old).[124]
"They don't want me to play with them. They
like me a lot. They like me more and more. There
ain't no others. I like them lots and lots and lots. I
am an oddicle person because I belong catching one
before they do" (an eleven-year-old) (p. 50).[18]
(Response to TAT card) "A man with whiskers
and another with whiskers. They went off with their
ears off, both of them. They were walking down the
street with their legs off and they're dead and that's
all. This is dead because his whiskers off and cause
they were out on the street, a car run over them.
They were twins, they lived together. They had to
pay $50" (p. 342).[186]

Disturbances of Thought Content: In psychotic
children with more advanced language, there may
be strange or morbid preoccupations with movement and aggression; with the child's own body

and its functioning; with his disturbances of self-awareness and sense of identity, orientation in time and space, and his relationships to others[18] (e.g., obsessive preoccupation with prehistory, maps, train schedules, etc.). The content reflects the special experiences of childhood and the unique history and problems of the individual child. It is the unusually morbid and bizarre nature of these fantasies, and the child's inability to distinquish them from reality, which differentiate the fantasies of psychotic children from others'.

In the schizophrenic child under ten years, paranoid ideas usually are fragmentary and diffuse and do not meet the criteria of specific schizophrenic delusions established for adults (e.g., thought broadcasting, thought insertion or withdrawal, delusions of control and influence). (pp. 3–4).[215]

Some prepuberty schizophrenic children meet the following criteria for abnormal thought content, adapted from the RDC definition of "bizarre delusions." Judge "the extent to which the belief is patently absurd, fantastic, or implausible" (p. 4).[215]

Bizarre delusions may occur which are patently absurd, fantastic, or implausible, and are evaluated as being deviant, relative to the child's age and cultural background. This would not include more commonly held "implausible ideas such as communicating with God, the Devil, ghosts, or ancestors, or being under the influence of curses, spells, voodoo, or hypnosis" (p. 4).[215] Fantasies regarding supernatural powers, ability to fly, the existence of demons, monsters, etc., which are common content in children's fantasies, should be excluded, even though they have a special fascination for the schizophrenic child. Bizarre delusions in schizophrenic children usually involve ideas of peculiar alterations of body shape and functioning, or ideas regarding fantasied objects, machines, or persons the child experiences as being inside his own body ("introjects").[18]

DISORDERS OF SOCIAL RELATEDNESS

Bradley's[34] review of the literature concluded that autistic withdrawal of interest from the environment and from social contact was the fundamental diagnostic symptom in all reports of schizophrenia in children. It had been noted as an avoidance of eye contact as early as six months of age; later, it led to seclusiveness and bizarre preoccupations.

Kanner[124] emphasized "the children's inability to relate themselves in the ordinary way to people and situations from the beginning of life." He differentiated this from "a 'withdrawal' from formerly existing participation," because "this is not, as in schizophrenic children or adults, a departure from an initially present relationship; . . . There is from the start an extreme autistic aloneness that, whenever possible, disregards, ignores, shuts out anything that comes to the child from the outside." He described the child's response to an intruding hand or foot "which was dealt with per se and not as part of a person. He never addressed a word or a look to the owner of the hand or foot."

Bender[18] was more impressed by the overwhelming anxiety of the young schizophrenic child which "leads him to cling physically and psychologically . . . By contrast with adults one can often make an unusually good contact with schizophrenic children. There is generally a searching, penetrating, even aggressive clinging dependence . . . Failure to get satisfaction from such contact may gradually lead to withdrawal, but not until there has been a long period of illness" (pp. 52–53). She considered withdrawal in children to be a sign of deterioration, leading to the most severe outcome. Withdrawal occurred in two-thirds of her schizophrenic children whose diagnoses had been confirmed independently at follow-up. It significantly differentiated the schizophrenics from matched nonpsychotic controls.[23]

The British group[52] defined the diagnostic criterion of withdrawal as follows: "Gross and sustained impairment of emotional relationships with people. This includes the more usual aloofness and the empty clinging (so called symbiosis); also abnormal behavior towards other people as persons, such as using them impersonally. Difficulty in mixing and playing with other children is often outstanding and long-lasting." This includes the descriptions by both Kanner and Bender, but it requires a more specific operational definition.

Autistic Withdrawal; A Gross and Sustained Impairment of Emotional Relatedness With People: When most severe, there is little human interaction or what there is is bizarre; the child appears preoccupied; attention focus is indefinite, oblique, and vague in direction. The child may appear oblivious of the examiner, if left alone, or may not respond directly through facial expression or behavior to verbal or behavioral approaches, except that eye contact is studiously avoided. The child may passively accept physical contact, even lap sitting or tickling, if this does not require eye contact. Without making eye contact, he may even manipulate an adult's hand to produce some desired action.

With less severe impairment, the child may respond intermittently but does not sustain any interaction; verbal and behavioral responses are very delayed and frequently require forceful social approaches. His responses often appear to be dictated by inner impulses and preoccupations and seem inappropriate to the immediate social context.

There may be diffuse impersonal clinging or mechanically compliant behavior in which adults are treated as interchangeable; the child relates to an unfamiliar person in precisely the same manner as he deals with supposedly familiar figures. In general, the child is markedly aloof and distant. He rarely initiates social contacts and shows an apparent lack of positive interest in people. There is an absence of empathic responses to the feelings of others and a lack of appreciation of humor.

Relationships with peers manifest these disturbances to an even greater degree than relationships with adults. Cooperative interaction and friendships do not develop in early childhood.

DISTURBANCES IN THE RANGE, MODULATION, AND INTEGRATION OF AFFECT

Kanner[124] did not specifically discuss shallow affect except by implication, referring to the indifference with which the child treated others, unless they intruded upon him. However, his case histories frequently mention the children's "blank expression." He described their tantrums as being precipitated by interruption of rituals, and their need for "sameness." Bender[18] was more impressed with the excessive anxiety which these children showed. She considered the loss of anxiety as an ominous prognostic sign; "it is then we speak of deterioration." Diffuse anxiety occurred in two-thirds of her schizophrenic children whose diagnosis was confirmed at follow up, and it significantly differentiated them from the non-psychotic controls.[23]

The British group[52] did not specifically mention shallow affect, except as it might be implied by the "aloof" social relationships. They did include anxiety as one criterion. "Acute, excessive, and seemingly illogical anxiety is a frequent phenomenon. This tends to be precipitated by change, whether in material environment or in routine, as well as by temporary interruption of a symbiotic attachment to persons or things. (Apparently commonplace phenomena or objects seem to become invested with terrifying qualities. On the other hand, an appropriate sense of fear in the face of real danger may be lacking)."

Anxiety is a common symptom in many psychiatric disorders of children. Only the illogicality surrounding its eruption, and its excessively unmodulated quality, distinguish the anxiety of psychotic children from that of less disturbed children.

Fluctuating Affect Which is Shallow and Incongruous: The RDC only defines affect as a criterion for the hebephrenic subtype; "fluctuating affect which is shallow, incongruous, or silly" (p. 8).[215]

1. Affect is shallow and grossly incongruous with concurrent thought content, as expressed in the patients' specific verbalizations.

2. There may be abrupt, unmodulated shifts between extremes of affective expression; flat, underresponsive affect, with little variation in facial or vocal expression, alternates with silly giggling, explosive crying, or undifferentiated states of irritability, excitement, panic or rage. These acute shifts in affect are precipitated by minimal, ordinarily irrelevant changes in the environment, or they arise inexplicably, without any external stimulus discernable to the examiner.[81]

DISORDERS IN THE INTEGRATION OF ATTENTION AND PERCEPTION

There is usually a profound disturbance in the organization of attention and the integration of perceptual experience. Diminished responsiveness to new or obvious stimuli in any sensory modality, as well as excessive responses to minor, irrelevant stimuli, have been observed in the same child at different times.[23, 162] There may be preoccupation with proximal stimuli of touch, taste, and smell, in contrast to more adaptive global exploration using vision and hearing.[97, 202]

The peripheral sensory function appears to be intact in psychotic children. They do not differ from normals in visual, auditory, or tactile acuity, or in color vision.[96] However, they show higher thresholds for free-field speech stimuli than for pure tones.[115] This discrepancy "is evidence that the phenomenon of 'not-hearing,' which is so characteristic of many psychotic children, is not a primary defect of sensory acuity. Rather, it reflects altered attention to or integration of human speech by the children."[92]

The British group[52] included "abnormal perceptual experience (in the absence of discernable organic abnormality)" as one of their diagnostic criteria. They defined this as "implied by excessive, diminished, or unpredictable response to sensory stimuli—for example, visual and auditory avoidance, insensitivity to pain and temperature." They did not include any specific definition of disorders of more complex perceptions as such, but did include "pathological preoccupation with particular objects or certain characteristics of them, without regard to their accepted functions."

These bizarre responses to the environment represent deviations from the usual organization of attention and the ordinary responses to patterned stimulation in the environment. The experiments of Hermelin and O'Connor[110] have elucidated the nature of certain deficits which underlie these behaviors and which differ from the deficits in subnormals. Autistic children fixated on visual displays for much shorter periods than subnormals; they spent more time gazing at the background and made few comparisons between the two figures (pp. 32, 59). Nonspeaking autistics could not learn visual discriminations of shape or direction, which were learned by matched subnormals (p. 34). The autistics relied more on motor strategies in learning position discrimination. They were not able to use visual cues to improve their performance in visual-motor tasks, such as tracking and puzzles; instead, they relied on an efficient use of trial-and-error manipulative cues. Autistics were unable to learn a task which required them to recognize a simple visual pattern, e.g., to place squares in serial order according to size (pp. 75–76). Their preference for proximal receptors apparently is related to their reliance on information from induced and active movements, their limited ability to process and interpret visual data (pp. 124–126), and their inability to integrate visual information with motor and kinesthetic feedback (p. 60).

The following are operational definitions for the bizarre behaviors which comprise one of the DSM-III[1] criteria for the diagnosis of infantile autism.

Bizarre Responses to the Environment: which involve an apparent lack of appreciation of meaningful pattern and structure. This is often combined with the imposition of arbitrary and idiosyncratic patterns on objects and events, which the child adheres to rigidly, appearing distressed if he is prevented from doing so (Kanner's "insistence on sameness"). These peculiar responses may take several forms:

1. An abnormal, stereotyped preoccupation with odd objects or minor details of the environment which significantly precludes more age-appropriate, organized, goal-directed activity. The child rigidly repeats a limited repertoire of behaviors. He is constricted in his attempts at meaningful exploration, and he lacks the ability to adapt flexibly to a wide variety of appropriate activities and organized use of objects. Objects are manipulated without regard for their physical properties or usual functions, or without being combined and exploited for patterned play. For example, there may be an insistence on always carrying about a string, or a particular, peculiar object; there may be perseverative preoccupation with certain features of objects, such as their texture, taste, smell, color, size, or number; or, there may be perseverative preoccupation with minor details, holes, breaks, or irregularities, without regard for the usual use and meaning of these characteristics. There may be perseverative lining up, stacking, inserting or twirling of objects, without regard for gravity or for their size, form, and usual function in play (e.g., dolls or cars are stacked or "stuck" onto walls, pencils are twirled, etc. This does *not* include creative, organized, imaginative play, in which a block may be *used* as a car in a flexible and organized way).

2. Other complex ritualistic behaviors. For example, simple everyday routines, or an apparently haphazard arrangement of toys or other objects, or idiosyncratic ritualistic movements and behavior patterns are reproduced in precisely the same manner over and over, down to the most minute, irrelevant detail of the pattern. Usually this reproduces the initial experience of the child with these objects, or expresses some special preoccupation. Simple repetitive movements (e.g., "hand-flapping," athetoid "finger-twiddling," rocking, whirling) are not included here but would be categorized under motility, unless they are incorporated into a more complex behavior sequence which is then repeated, ad infinitum.

Disturbances of Perception: Psychotic children who are less severely retarded show analogous disturbances in the perception of patterned stimuli which can be elicited by the use of more complex configurations. Bender[18] first described the disorders in spatial orientation, the problems in separating figure from ground, and the fluid and distorted visual-motor patterns which occurred in reproductions of the Bender-Gestalt figures. She found similar disturbances in the schizophrenic child's perception of his own body and its relation to surrounding space. The drawings of the human figure are often distorted with bizarre elaboration of the peripheral details, e.g., hair and extremities, fingers, and so on.[58] Heavy outlining, abnormal detailing, and confusion in spatial orientation characterized the drawings of two-thirds of the schizophrenic children whose diagnoses were confirmed on follow up. These features significantly differentiated them from their matched nonpsychotic controls.[23]

Goldfarb[96] subsequently tested these functions and demonstrated that the performance of schizophrenic children was significantly poorer than normals' in directional discrimination, orientation to time, place, and person, human figure drawings, the integration of body perceptions two-point discrimination, face-hand test,[66] finger localization,[26] right-left discrimination, the integration of visual patterns, figure-ground discrimination, and the response to auditory feedback.

Schizophrenic children manifest other perceptual failures which are qualitatively different from those of children with OBS associated with psychosis. Birch and Walker[29] studied the Block Design performance of childhood schizophrenics and matched controls with OBS and psychosis. The children with OBS recognized their errors; the schizophrenic children could not. Their perceptual recognition was initially correct, but it was disrupted by their subsequent performance errors. This may be related to the increased reliance on motor cues, which Hermelin and O'Connor found in the more severely retarded autistic children.

Children with OBS may show certain impairments on perceptual tasks which also are seen in the productions of psychotic children. What distinguishes the psychotic children is the unusual fluctuation in their level of performance; a juxtaposition of advanced and retarded performance is seen on the same test. Even when the total score for a test is within normal limits, subscores may demonstrate this unusual variability.

For example, in the human figure drawing, the trunk and extremities may be primitive and score at a four- or five-year level; yet, the same figure may show an unusual elaboration of facial detail, with detailed ears, nostrils, mouth, teeth, and especially, eye detail (pupil, iris, lashes, and so on), which may score as high as an eleven-year-old. In addition, there may be bizarre exaggeration and distortion of the orifices and periphery (fingers, toes, hair), as well as transparencies, bodies inside the figure, bizarre distortions of the form, or a mechanical, robot-like appearance.

Similarly, on the Bender-Gestalt, if one scores each figure relative to age norms, one finds excessive circular, almost scribbling forms, typical of a three- to four-year old, in the presence of mature

seven- to ten-year-old diamonds and hexagons. Certain signs resemble those seen in adult schizophrenia. Single patterns are split and fragmented. Figures may be idiosyncratically elaborated and may be incorporated into forms which reflect the patient's special preoccupations. Figure-ground problems may be prominent; the boundaries between figures may be lost, with the figures crossing and interpenetrating each other; all of the figures on the page may merge into a new and often distorted pattern.[18]

Some of these characteristics result in relatively high Koppitz[131] scores for the child's age, reflecting relative immaturity and poor visual-motor perception. "Rotation" is scored as such; the excessively circular forms may yield scores for "distortion of shape;" fragmentation of certain figures (cards A, 3–6) yields scores for poor "integration." Performance may be so poor as to suggest "brain injury" in Koppitz's terms. According to her scoring, confused organization on the page and signs of impulsivity (dashes, increasing size of figures, heavily reinforced lines) may suggest "emotional disorder." But the unevenness of performance and other specific schizophrenic signs are not reflected in the total Koppitz score. Evaluation of the factors requires additional qualitative analysis of the figures.

The Rorschach responses demonstrate analogous problems in integrating visual percepts when schizophrenic children with average IQ's are compared to normals.[7, 98] On this test, the schizophrenics manifested poor perception of form, giving responses which showed little congruence with the stimulus blot (significantly higher W − percent, lower F + percent). They gave fewer popular responses and a greater number of original ones, but the majority of their original responses were unrelated to the reality of the blot forms and indicated that their fantasy material was unusual or even bizarre (higher O − percent). They also made far-fetched generalizations for a single detail to the entire ink blot (higher DW percent) and tended to perseverate the same answers for several blots. A higher percentage of their responses was determined solely or primarily by color, rather than by form (higher C percent and CF percent); this reflected their immature emotional organization and relative absence of rational control.

The Rorschach of a schizophrenic child often shows an unusual variability in the level of form perception; he may unexpectedly drop to a poor form response on cards that are considered easy to interpret.[58] These are generally "queer" answers, resulting from extremely irrelevant associations or peculiar reasoning. There may be contamination of one percept by another and illogical condensations.

The TAT responses of psychotic children showed certain perceptual disturbances which were not seen in a matched group of nonpsychotic disturbed children.[134] Major perceptual distortions and omissions occurred more often in the psychotic group. Unique and absurd distortions, such as seeing people as frogs, or an animal as a skeleton, occurred only in the psychotic group. The psychotic child may make up a fantastic tale which has no relation to the pictures presented, or he may take off from a small incidental element.[58]

DISTURBED PERFORMANCE ON INTELLIGENCE TESTS

Incidence of Mental Retardation in Psychotic Children: Intelligence tests provide a powerful measure of effective cognitive and adaptive functioning. They reflect the disruptive effects of psychosis in a variety of ways. The overall result is a variable degree of impairment in total scores. When matched for socioeconomic status and educational standing of the parents the Intelligence Quotients (IQ's) of psychotic children fall significantly below those of controls.[96]

Low IQ in psychotic children correlates with other measures of severity of the psychotic process. IQ's under 70, and especially those under 50, are associated with: (1) infantile psychosis (onset before two years);[20] (2) more severe early developmental abnormality;[74, 82] (3) more severe non-specific "soft neurologic signs";[96] (4) more severe disintegration of personality and behavior;[81] and, (5) poorer social functioning in adolescence and adulthood.

In any single sample of psychotic children, the distribution of IQ's will therefore reflect the proportion of children with these indicators of severe psychosis. The composition of a sample is affected somewhat by the source of the patients. It is tied directly to the authors' criteria both for selection and for diagnosing children as psychotic.

Table 14–1 summarizes the major studies which reported the incidence of different IQ's in psychotic children. The groups classified here as "infantile psychosis" had onsets before two to five years.

Of these 305 children, 62 to 78 percent had IQ's under 70; 42 percent to 51 percent of these scores were under 50. This underestimates the frequency of retardation in Rutter's,[196, 197] Kolvin,[130] and Lotter's[139] groups; on the Merrill-Palmer, more of the children in these studies had Performance IQ's under 70 than did the children in Fish's[70, 82] group. Almost all of the latter had Verbal IQ's under 70, but there were fewer mute children than in Rutter's, Kolvin's, and Lotter's studies. This was true despite the fact that the members of Fish's group were only two to five years old. This means that in the three older groups, Verbal IQ's would have been lower than in Fish's group. Kanner[124] stated that "all the children did well with the Seguin formboard," but he reported no scores.

The children classified in Table 14–1 as "childhood schizophrenia" had onsets of illness after two to five years. Compared to the infantile psychotics, they had only one-third to one-half as many with IQ's under 70, and one-tenth as many with IQ's under 50. They also had a much higher proportion with IQ's over 90. Kolvin's group included only ten children under thirteen years of age, and is therefore not comparable to Bender's prepuberty schizophrenics.

It is obvious that when IQ's are reported for heterogeneous groups of psychotic children, the proportion of severely retarded children will be higher if more children with infantile psychosis are included. The Verbal IQ is the most objective measure of how severely impaired a psychotic child is and is a critical determinant of outcome. Many of the so-called "contradictions" between different studies of psychotic children are based on spurious comparisons of groups with very different proportions of severely retarded children. Therefore, when the attempt is made here to reconcile the discrepancies in the literature, the reader will be referred to the IQ distributions in Table 14–1.

Stability of IQ: Rutter, who studied a severely impaired group (Table 14–1 and Table 14–2), reported considerable stability of IQ on follow up. The correlation btween initial IQ (Merrill-Palmer) and the scores at follow up (usually the Wechsler), five to fifteen years later, was about 0.80 for the non-speaking children and for the group as a whole.[195] Goldfarb and associates[101] found that the IQ's of children who initially scored below 45 continued to remain low, but in the case of children who scored higher than that, function tended to improve with treatment. Bender[9] reported serial Verbal IQ's obtained over much longer spans of twenty to thirty-five years. Many children with infantile psychosis showed deterioration, especially during chronic institutionalization: some schizophrenic children, however,

TABLE 14-2

Percentage of Pregnancy Complications and Organic Brain Disorders in Psychotic Children

AUTHOR (DIAGNOSIS)[a]	PUB. YEAR	n	ONSET (YEARS)	% IQ's <50[b]	M/F RATIO	PREGNANCY COMPLICATIONS SEVERE[c]	PREGNANCY COMPLICATIONS TOTAL	EPILEPSY FIRST OBS.[d]	EPILEPSY +AT ADOL.[e]	ORGANIC BRAIN DISEASE DEFINITE	ORGANIC BRAIN DISEASE TOTAL (WITH POSSIBLE)
SCHIZOPHRENIA											
Kolvin (LOP)	1971	33	5–15	3	2.6	12	12	12(−16?)	—	27	31
Bender (CS)	1972	50	2–10	10	2.8	8	14	8	4	2	12
INFANTILE PSYCHOSIS											
Bender (CS)	1972	50	<2	36	6.1	28	44	10	6	8	16
Kanner (A)	1953	100	≦2	—	4.1	0[f]	0	0	1	1	1
Goldfarb (CS, NO)	1961	9	<5	—	2.2[g]	0	0	0	—	0	0
Goldfarb (CS, O)	1961	17	<5	—	4.8[g]	35	59	6	—	6	24
Fish (CS, total)	1968, 1976	38	<2	37	2.8	18	32	3	0	3	3
Fish (A)	1968, 1976	9	<2	89	8.0	0	38	0	0	0	0
Creak (S)	1963	100	—	—	3.6[h]	—	—	5	7	14	14
Rutter (IP)	1967, 1970	63	≦5	46	4.2	—	—	3	28	35	63
Kolvin (IP)	1971	46	<3	51	3.3	35	46	19(−22?)	—	39	54
Lotter (A, "A")	1967	15	<4.5	67	2.7	23	—	0	—	7	13
Lotter (A, "B")	1967	17	<4.5	71	2.4	20	56+	24	—	29	47
Knobloch (A)	1975	50	<2	60(<35)	—	56	56+	74	—	100	100
Schain (A)	1960	50	—	(100?)	1.6	6	16	42	—	54	—

a See Table 14–1 footnotes.
b IQ's as on Table 14–1.
c Criteria vary for different studies.
d Incidence when first seen.
e Additional cases of epilepsy beginning at adolescence or after.
f 15% with birth complications; no pregnancy complications reported.
g Goldfarb.[93]
h Ratio from Creak and Ini.[ss]
- = No information given.

rose from Verbal IQ's below 80 to average or superior levels. Finally, although these were the exception, there were a few who rose from untestable levels before five years to scores above 70.

Pattern of Intelligence Test Performance: The British group[52] include as one criterion "a background of serious retardation in which islets of normal, near normal, or exceptional intellectual function or skill may appear." The types of deficits, the degree of variability, and the patterns of relative functioning in different areas must be specified further.

The Wechsler Intelligence Scale for Children provides a standardized measure of the child's effective functioning on critical verbal and performance tasks. It will reflect overall dysfunctions in attention, concentration, and persistence, as well as special problems in logical reasoning and everyday judgments (Comprehension, Picture Arrangement), abstraction (Similarities), problems in auditory and visual sequencing (Digit Span, Picture Arrangement), visual-spatial patterning (Block Design, Object Assembly), and many other problems. The specific profile will vary, depending on the individual child's assets and impairments, so that few patterns distinguish the psychotic group as a whole from normal children.

What is clear is that the subtest scores of schizophrenic children show significantly greater intertest variability than those of controls matched for age and IQ. Wechsler and Jaros[227] studied one hundred schizophrenic children, eight to eleven years of age, whose IQ's ranged between 80 and 120. Their "three by three" test sign proved to be the most discriminating. The "three by three" criterion was reached if three subtests each deviated by three or more scaled score points from the subject's mean. This correctly identified 44 percent to 90 percent of the schizophrenic children in two separate validity studies, at a cost of only 8 percent false positives.

Differences of sixteen points between Verbal IQ and Performance IQ occurred in 16 to 36 percent of the schizophrenic children, ten to twelve years of age, and were significant; but, either Verbal IQ or Performance IQ might be the higher score.[227] Rutter[194] found that at follow up testing in adolescence, psychotic children with retarded speech achieved high scores on Block Design and Object Assembly, relative to the other subtests. This pattern did not occur in the psychotics without retarded speech, and it was not characteristic of schizophrenic children with IQ's over 80.[227] High visual-spatial performance with an extremely low verbal score appears to be a characteristic pattern

only of the very retarded autistic children. When they function at a pre-school level, a similar pattern is seen on the Gesell. There, a high formboard performance is often the only score close to age level.[82, 181]

Intratest variability also is characteristic of schizophrenic children, just as it is of adult schizophrenia. There may be an unexpected failure on an easy item, followed by success on difficult items within the same subtest. These erratic failures often result from some sudden preoccupation with an irrelevant aspect of the task. The main issue is neglected and the response may appear illogical.[58]

Disorders of Motility: Many of these children show poorly integrated patterns of motility. The histories of retarded and irregular gross motor development[18, 21, 77, 80, 83] are discussed below. Awkward, "dyskinetic" motility, with a heavy-footed, wide-based gait, and poorly coordinated associated movements may remain as residues of these early difficulties. The children are significantly poorer than controls on finger-to-finger and finger-to-nose coordination, tests of rail-walking, and on the Lincoln-Oseretsky Battery.[96]

Bender[18] pointed out that many of the bizarre and stereotyped movements seen in schizophrenic children represent primitive reflex patterns which are retained alongside of more mature motor behavior. Choreoathetotic movements of the hands, which are normal patterns for four-month infants, may be incorporated into stereotyped mannerisms of the hands ("hand-flapping" and oscillating) or fingers ("twiddling"), and may be retained until nine years, or even later. These movements occur more frequently in psychotic children who are severely retarded, but they also occur in nonpsychotic retardates.[197] *Whirling* on the longitudinal axis in spontaneous motor play, or after slight passive turning of the head, represent normal behaviors and postural responses until about eight to nine years. These may remain even past puberty as prominent behaviors in psychotic children, especially those with increased motor impulses. Whirling behavior may be elicited simply by having the child watch a spinning top.[162] *Walking on tiptoe* often occurs normally as a transient pattern in the second year, when children begin to walk; decreased suppression of extraneous (including "mirror") movements is a normal characteristic of immature motor organization; motor impulsivity and jumping and darting movements are normal elements in the motor play of pre-school children. In each case, however, these patterns appear more peculiar when they persist as prominent behaviors in the school age psychotic child. *"Motor com-*

pliance"[18] and sinking passively, molding oneself into an unfamiliar adult's lap, might also be considered signs of immaturity, as well as of passivity; normal children, once they have achieved independent sitting and walking, usually assert their physical autonomy. *Head rolling, head banging, rocking, and swaying* are nonspecific repetitive rhythmic behaviors which occur in normal infants and in many nonpsychotic retarded children. They are likely to be especially prominent in the more severely retarded psychotic children.[197]

Kanner[124] mentioned that several of his children "were somewhat clumsy in gait and gross motor performances," but he emphasized the absence of any neurologic or physical stigmata. The British group[52] includes one criterion in this area: "Distortion in motility patterns—for example, (a) excess as in hyperkinesis, (b) immobility as in catatonia, (c) bizarre postures, or ritualistic mannerisms, such as rocking and spinning (themselves or objects)."

The types of motility which are described above as representing immature patterns, tend to occur more often in infantile psychotics, especially those with lower IQ's.* These immature motor signs cannot be considered as diagnostic criteria or "tests" for childhood psychosis. They are not universal, even in severely retarded psychotic children, and they are also found in nonpsychotic children with OBS.

Whirling characterized two-thirds of the schizophrenic children whose diagnosis was confirmed on follow up.[23] This was significantly more than the 10 percent of the matched nonpsychotic controls who whirled. Rachman and Berger[174] confirmed that whirling significantly differentiated schizophrenic children from controls who were matched for IQ as well as for age. Kramer and associates[132] confirmed that the incidence of whirling in normal children decreased with age. At each age, whirling occurred significantly more often in the schizophrenic children and most often in the most severe group of "autistic" childhood schizophrenics. The chronological age norms for assessing such motor "immaturity" were influenced by sociocultural background.[132]

Catatonic posturing, rigidity, immobility, or "waxy flexibility" are rarer and more deviant motor patterns. When they occur, they are much more likely to be found in severely ill childhood schizophrenics than in other disorders. Facial grimacing and oral mannerisms have to be differentiated from specific neurological disorders and Gille de la Tourettes disease.

INTEGRATIVE DISORDER MANIFESTED IN THE ORGANIZATION OF PERSONALITY AND BEHAVIOR

The integrative disorder goes beyond the disorders in separate functions to involve the total organization of personality, or ego function, of the psychotic child. It is reflected in chaotic patterning in all aspects of behavior. Characteristically, there is irregular and poorly integrated functioning of language and cognition, attention and perception, and often of motility, which can be observed during a single psychiatric or psychological examination. The major manifestations in these different areas have been described above. All symptoms may show remarkable variability, fluctuation, and inconsistency. Abrupt and inexplicable shifts in attention, or in the sequences of play, or between opposite extremes of behavior (extreme rage and negativism to bland detachment and automatic compliance), may occur within seconds. An unusual range and combination of symptoms, defense mechanisms, and coping techniques may be seen within a very brief period, or at different stages of the illness.

When the disorder is most extreme, "the children present primarily as fragmented personalities rather than with any predominant adaptive patterning." They "are characterized by grossly unintegrated, erratic, and deviant functioning in all areas. Disturbed functioning is so prominent that the fragmentary attempts at comprehensible goal-directed behavior tend to be obscured by unpatterned behavior not apparently unified by any goal-idea. They frequently appear not to comprehend social or external situations as others do; responses appear to be dictated by inner impulses and experiences and appear 'inappropriate' to external stimuli" (p. 45).[81]

INTEGRATIVE DISORDER MANIFESTED IN THE LONGITUDINAL COURSE OF DEVELOPMENT

Bender[18] first reported histories, and then documentation from parents' "Baby Books"[21] showing that uneven development of somatic growth, physiologic patterns, motility, and cognitive functioning, frequently began in infancy. In these children, there was no period of normal development followed by regression, as in adult schizophrenics, but an onset of "mental illness in the first two years of life, which subsequently proved to be

---

* See references 67, 71, 74, 82, 96, and 197.

schizophrenia."[18] This observation has been confirmed by studies of pre-schizophrenic infants from birth.[71, 73, 76, 77] The nature of the early disturbances in development, as determined by direct observation of infants, is discussed below.

When one must rely on retrospective information, it is easy to miss many early deviations. Except for the exceptional paranoid mother, parents rarely exaggerate early abnormalities. Details are usually forgotten, except for severe degrees of motor retardation or a total absence of play with toys. Records of height and weight, baby books, photographs, and home movies often reveal disturbances that parents and pediatricians have overlooked or forgotten.

Careful histories reveal retarded or irregular development in 55 percent[51, 82] to 80 percent[74] of the children. The irregular course of development is reflected in unusual sequences of retardation, acceleration, and plateaus. Postural-motor landmarks are the most reliable and can be converted readily to developmental quotients (DQ's). Such calculations reveal extreme fluctuations, between DQ's below 70 and over 130, in over one-third of the psychotic children with Verbal IQ's under 70.[74] When such fluctuations can be documented, they indicate an early integrative disorder which differs from that seen in OBS. The most severely retarded young psychotic children usually show fewer high peaks and fluctuations in early development and are more likely to show severe retardation.

ISSUES RELATING TO DIAGNOSTIC CRITERIA FOR THE DIFFERENT CLINICAL SYNDROMES OF PSYCHOSIS IN CHILDREN

The universe of childhood psychosis encompasses clusters of the above disorders, which vary in severity. The psychotic child who has the most severe impairment in all areas would be a mute child with almost no meaningful responses to people or to the environment. Such a child might be differentiated only with difficulty from profoundly retarded children with specific OBS. At the other extreme would be a psychotic child with precocious, although idiosyncratic speech, who is morbidly preoccupied with bizarre fantasies and elaborate obsessional rituals. This child would have to be differentiated from severely neurotic children.

Can these two children be extremes of one continuum? Or must they be separate etiologic entities? One school (Rutter and Kolvin) marshals evidence to support the latter position. Others

(Bender, Goldfarb, Ornitz, and the authors) point out that children show degrees of severity intermediate between these two extremes. Furthermore, the manifestations may change in the same child from an autistic to a schizophrenic form at different stages of development. Whether they are absolute or relative, these subdivisions represent only modal clusters, which help to conceptualize the phenomena. The children come in all shades and varieties of these and do not respect anyone's arbitrary boundaries.

The major current controversy involves the children with infantile psychosis. Some groups of these children have a high incidence of OBS. No relationship to adult schizophrenia is evident in their family histories or in their fate as adolescents. Other groups demonstrate a continuity with adult schizophrenia in both their family histories and their longitudinal course into adulthood. These data are discussed below.

Until there is sufficient data to delineate these etiological subdivisions of infantile psychosis, some common convention must be adopted so that investigators can compare the findings in different studies and have some assurance that they are discussing the same children. This is necessary whether one wants to compare the effectiveness of different treatments, or to understand the meaning of research in the pathophysiology of the disorders. The changing conventions will be discussed further. Periodically, these become crystallized in the official diagnostic classifications (DSM-I and DSM-II).[2, 3]

PROPOSED CLASSIFICATION—DSM-III (1976 VERSION)[1]

For the purpose of this section, categories and criteria will be described which are as nearly like the ones being worked out by the committee on the DSM-III, as possible. The version presented below may only approximate the final official version, since the latter has not yet been formalized or agreed upon. These definitions are stated more rigidly and explicitly than they are in the DSM-II. This should make for greater reliability. It also will result in a larger number of children being classified temporarily as "Psychosis, other type," since many children do not fit these strict criteria. As their symptoms crystallize with age, they may then fit another syndrome in the DSM-III. In any case, the categories and criteria must be seen as arbitrary conventions, limited by current knowledge, and arrived at by many compromises, none of which will satisfy everyone.

This outline of diagnostic criteria is based on four principles:

1. In accordance with the multiaxial scheme of the proposed DSM-III[1], the diagnostic criteria below define only the *clinical* diagnostic categories of psychosis occurring in prepuberty children. For any child, this clinical diagnosis must be accompanied by information on the other axes:

a. A diagnosis of mental retardation, if this exists on the clinical-axis, in addition to the diagnosis of psychosis;

b. The diagnosis of any specific developmental disorders; and,

c. The diagnosis of any non-mental medical disorder.

2. The clinical diagnosis is based on the current episode, as required by the DSM-III. This permits data to be accumulated regarding the change or stability of different clinical syndromes over time.

3. In order to increase agreement among different diagnosticians, the criteria define categories which are mutually exclusive.

4. Criteria which are necessary and sufficient to establish the diagnosis are clearly separated from symptoms which may commonly be associated with the condition, but which are not sufficient for diagnosis.

The necessary and sufficient criteria for infantile autism are drawn from the present version of the DSM-III.[1] These appear to be taken largely from Rutter's study[191, 196, 197] (Table 14-3). Those for schizophrenia have been developed by the authors to conform with the convention adopted by the DSM-III Committee that schizophrenia in childhood must fit the diagnosis as defined for adults. The required criteria for schizophrenia were developed from much research in adult schizophrenia. Unfortunately, they represent a compromise which is ill-adapted to the facts of development in childhood. No doubt, they, too, will be revised when more appropriate and reliable criteria can be agreed upon. The criteria for "Childhood psychosis, other type" define a diagnosis by exclusion of schizophrenia and autism. This latter, and the commonly associated symptoms under all three diagnoses, represent descriptions from the authors' own clinical experience.

SCHIZOPHRENIA (DSM-III: 295.xxx)

1. *Necessary and sufficient symptom:* This diagnosis requires the presence of a *formal thought disorder* typical of schizophrenia (as defined in (1).(a)., above). This should be documented by a verbatim example from the patient's speech.

Schizophrenic children under 9 years rarely have the specific types of Schneiderian hallucinations and delusions listed in the DSM-III as alternative criteria to thought disorder for diagnosing schizophrenia in adults.

2. *Symptoms commonly associated, but not necessary or sufficient for the diagnosis:*

a. Autistic withdrawal (as defined in (2).(a)., above).

b. Affect which is fluctuating, shallow, and incongruous (as defined in (3).(a)., above).

c. Attention and perception show characteristic disorders (as described in (4)., above).

d. Cognitive functioning shows a characteristically erratic and inconsistent pattern (as described in (5)., above).

e. Motility may be disordered (as described in (6)., above), especially in those with an early onset.

f. Development usually shows erratic and variable functioning with irregularity in its longitudinal progression and "scatter" on any one examination (as described in (7). and (8)., above).

In accordance with the DSM-III, patients with a formal thought disorder will be diagnosed as schizophrenic, whether they are children or adults. Schizophrenia in children usually will be diagnosed as "Schizophrenia, unspecified" (295.90x, the sixth digit coding the course as acute, 1, to chronic, 4). A few schizophrenic children fit the adult criteria for the "Disorganized (Hebephrenic)" or "Confusional Turmoil" subtypes. Ordinarily, schizophrenic children under 9 years do not meet the criteria for the "Paranoid" or "Catatonic" subtypes, nor do they have the specific forms of hallucinations or delusions which can also be the basis for diagnosing schizophrenia.

INFANTILE AUTISM (DSM-III: 299.0xx)

1. *Necessary and sufficient symptoms:* a. through d. are required for the diagnosis:

a. *Autistic withdrawal* (as defined in (2).(a)., above).

b. There is a *severe impairment in verbal and nonverbal communication*, but formal thought disorder (as defined in (1).(a)., above) must be absent. The child may be mute, use jargon, or use words, with or without immediate echolalia. The speech of these children usually is at too primitive a level to assess reliably the presence of a formal thought disorder. Communication by gesture and appropriate facial expression is also severely impaired.

c. *Bizarre responses to the environment* (as defined in (4).(a)., above), including either *abnormal stereotyped preoccupations* and/or *complex ritualistic behaviors* (as defined in that section).

d. Symptoms a. through c. have developed prior to 30 months of age.

2. *Symptoms commonly associated, but not necessary or sufficient for the diagnosis:*

a. Affect which is fluctuating, shallow, and incongruous (as defined in (3).(a)., above).

b. Attention and perception are severely impaired (as described in (4)., above).

c. Cognitive function is impaired to some degree (as described in (5).(a)., above).

d. Motility may be disordered (as described in (6)., above).

e. Development may show generally retarded, but possibly erratic and variable functioning, with irregularity in its longitudinal progression and "scatter" on any one examination (as described in (7). and (8)., above).

3. If the current syndrome fulfills the "necessary" criteria in 1. above, but is associated with a *known organic brain disease* (for example, congenital rubella), then the condition is diagnosed in the DSM-III as "*Autistic Syndrome with Organic Brain Syndrome*, associated with congenital rubella," or whatever the disease is.

EARLY CHILDHOOD PSYCHOSIS, OTHER TYPES (DSM-III: 299.8)

1. *Necessary and sufficient symptoms:* a. through c. must be present:

a. *Autistic withdrawal* (as defined in (2).(a)., above) or some *other* form of impaired relatedness to people, producing a disruption of personality organization which is of psychotic proportions.

b. *Formal thought disorder* (as defined in (1).(a)., above) *must be absent*.

c. If the necessary current criteria for *infantile autism* are present (as above), then the onset must be *after 30 months* of age.

2. *Symptoms commonly associated, but not necessary or sufficient for the diagnosis:*

a. Affect may be fluctuating, shallow, and incongruous (as defined in (3).(a)., above).

b. Attention and perception may be severely impaired (as described in (4)., above) so as to disrupt relatedness to the environment and the perception of reality to a psychotic degree.

c. Bizarre responses to the environment may be present (as described in (4).(a)., above), but all the other remaining symptoms which are necessary for the diagnosis of infantile autism are not present.

d. There may be a severe impairment of verbal and nonverbal communication (as defined above for infantile autism), but all the other remaining symptoms which are necessary for the diagnosis of infantile autism are not present.

e. Cognitive function may be impaired to some degree (as described in (5).(a)., above).

f. Motility may be disordered (as described in (6)., above).

g. Development may show erratic and variable functioning with irregularity in its longitudinal progression and "scatter" on any one examination (as described in (7). and (8)., above).

3. If the current syndrome fulfills the above criteria, but is associated with a *known organic brain disease* (for example, congenital rubella), then the condition is diagnosed in the DSM-III as "*Childhood psychosis, other type with Organic Brain Syndrome, associated with congenital rubella*," or whatever the underlying disease is.

This category is for children who manifest sufficient disturbance in one or more of the above areas to be diagnosed as psychotic, but who do not meet the "necessary" criteria for childhood schizophrenia or for infantile autism, and who do not meet the adult criteria for affective disorder, or acute or chronic brain syndromes. If a child meets the criteria for any diagnosis in adults, that term is then used for diagnosing the child, according to the DSM-III.

THE SYNDROME AS SECONDARY OR AS A SYMPTOMATIC EXPRESSION OF AN UNDERLYING CONDITION

There are rare instances in children in which a clinical picture resembling schizophrenia has been found to be a phenocopy produced by an underlying temporal lobe epilepsy. When the episodic changes in behavior are very subtle, the diagnosis may be suspected only by astute clinical observation of the child's subjective change in state, or by encephalography. The diagnosis can be confirmed if the psychotic thought disorder subsides abruptly when appropriate anti-epileptic medication is given. Such children would be diagnosed in the DSM-III as temporal lobe epilepsy with a schizophrenia-like syndrome.

Over the years, much evidence has accumulated regarding the incidence of "soft neurologic signs" in psychotic children. These are non-localizing signs with no evidence of a specific, known organic brain syndrome. As specific tests become available, it is possible that some of these children may then be found to have specific organic brain diseases.

A more difficult problem arises with profoundly retarded children with infantile psychosis. The extreme case is a mute child who gives no evidence of comprehension of speech or gesture. He ignores meaningful patterns in his environment. He attends perseveratively only to irrelevant, minor details of his surroundings, scratching, twirling, or lining up objects, and screams if his routines are interrupted. This child is indistinguishable from other profoundly retarded children who have specific OBS.

Gesell formerly described retarded children, who would now be labeled "infantile autism," under the rubric of "pseudosymptomatic retardation."[90] He noted that they had an alert expression and that their bizarre, stereotyped behavior was often treated psychiatrically under the misconception that it was psychologically induced. He emphasized however that despite these findings their retardation was real. Clemens Benda[8] remarked that "applying psychiatric standards to behavior patterns, the idiot is almost by definition an 'autistic child'." He found children with a picture indistinguishable from this where there was definite evidence of brain damage following encephalitis or neonatal anoxia. Bender[12] stated that "Kanner's syndrome . . . is not a clinical or etiologic entity . . . nor does it indicate a specific type of mental illness . . . it is a defense against disorganization and anxiety in children with many types of pathology," including schizophrenia, congenital rubella, and retrolental fibroplasia.

Only three children in Kanner's[124] first series of eleven autistics were mute; all had Performance IQ's of 75 to 94 on the formboard. Since that time, however, the diagnosis of autism has been applied to large numbers of mute and profoundly retarded children (e.g., functioning with a Performance IQ below 50) (Table 14-1). Many children with OBS fit the DSM-III criteria for infantile autism, and only some authors attempted to exclude organic disorders from their series. The major studies are summarized in Table 14-2 and are arranged in order of increasing mental retardation, as in Table 14-1.

Several characteristics differentiate the children with infantile psychosis. They have much more cognitive impairment (Table 14-1). Most groups have a higher male/female ratio and more pregnancy complications than the schizophrenics (Table 14-2). Schain's group differs from the rest in both these respects. Only Kanner did not note any complications of pregnancy.

However, within the infantile psychotics, there is a major division (Table 14-2). The first five studies* have a relatively low incidence of epilepsy and definite OBS. This is true despite the fact that Creak and Bender included patients whose convulsions began in adolescence. (Two of Creak's[51] patients turned out to have neurolipoidosis at autopsy. None of Bender's[9] four patients, who died before forty, had brain disease at autopsy.) The division is produced by the difference in selection criteria used by the two sets of authors. The first five authors began with the concept of childhood schizophrenia as a disease entity, analogous to or related to adult schizophrenia, or even continuous with it.[20, 71] Therefore, these five authors attempted to separate infantile psychosis from psychosis secondary to organic brain disease, and they excluded children with specific neurologic disorders.

Bender also relied on additional criteria to differentiate childhood schizophrenics with onsets under two years from organically brain damaged children who showed autistic withdrawal. In the absence of speech, she relied on features of the motoric and perceptual disorders which were characteristic of schizophrenia,[18] and which contrasted with the disorders in organic brain damage.[15, 18] She considered the variability and "plasticity" of functioning to be distinguishing features of schizophrenia in children. Fish used similar

criteria and defined specific test profiles of Performance DQ's and the fluctuating longitudinal course, which characterized schizophrenic impairment, as opposed to OBS.* The mute, stereotyped, autistic children who showed only retarded functioning, without these features (Group "A"),[82] were diagnosed as "psychosis with mental retardation" ("autistic" on Tables 14-2–14-6), pending any follow-up evidence that proved them to be schizophrenic.

Rutter took a different approach.† He disregarded etiologic factors and considered autism to be a syndrome, defined only by behavioral criteria. He, therefore, included children whether or not they had organic brain disorders. By selecting only the children unequivocally considered psychotic by every one of several psychiatrists, he apparently culled the most severely psychotic children. This resulted in a group which contained more mute and profoundly retarded children (Table 14-1). A high incidence of manifest neurologic disorders was present in this severely impaired group (Table 14-2). The definite and probably OBS included epilepsy, meningitis, toxoplasmosis, neurolues, lead encephalopathy, etc. The "probable" apparently refers only to the causal relationship between the definite OBS and the psychotic manifestations.[197]

Table 14-3 is adapted from Rutter[191, 197] and lists the incidence of key symptoms which differentiated infantile psychotics from nonpsychotic retardates. Rutter[191] considered these symptoms to be "specific and universal," but they appear to be neither.

Two symptoms are universal (abnormal peer relationships and retarded language development) in the psychotics; however, they also occur in 82 percent and 84 percent of the nonpsychotic retardates. While the differences are statistically significant,[197] these symptoms, obviously, would not help one make a differential diagnosis in an individual child. The symptoms which have a higher specificity (decreased comprehension, pronoun reversal, stereotyped movements) occur in 50 percent of the psychotics, or even less. While they are more specific, occurring infrequently in the nonpsychotics, they are by no means "universal" in the psychotic group.

These data must be kept in mind when using the DSM-III criteria for infantile autism, which apparently were based on Rutter's study.[196, 197] Rutter spelled out Kanner's criteria in more ob-

---

* See references 20, 51, 53, 70, 82, 96, and 121.

* See references 71, 74, 76, 80, and 83.
† See references 193, 194, 195, 196, and 197.

TABLE 14–3

Percentage of Infantile Psychotics and Nonpsychotic Retardates with Symptoms Diagnostic of Autism

"UNIVERSAL AND SPECIFIC SYMPTOMS" (RUTTER, 1974, P. 148)	INFANTILE PSYCHOTICS (RUTTER & LOCKYER, 1967)	NONPSYCHOTIC RETARDATES (RUTTER & LOCKYER, 1967)	INFANTILE PSYCHOTICS (KOLVIN ET AL., 1971)
1. Profound failure to develop social relationships:			
a. Abnormal relations with peers	100*	82	100
b. Autism	90*	13	85[b]
2. Language retardation:	100*	84	88
a. Decreased comprehension; ever thought deaf	35*	11	—
b. Echolalia (% total)	46	30	51
Echolalia (% of speaking)	a	a	71
c. Pronominal reversal (% total)	30*	13	30
Pronominal reversal (% of speaking)	—	—	41
3. Ritualistic or compulsive symptoms:			
a. Any of symptoms listed	90*	54	100
b. Any symptom = marked	62*	13	—
Number of children (no. speaking)	63(—)	63(—)	47(34)

* Significantly differentiated psychotics from nonpsychotic controls (Rutter & Lockyer, 1967, p. 1173).
a Echolalia in "over ¾ of speaking psychotic children, a rate twice that in the control group" (Rutter & Lockyer, 1967, p. 1174). Numbers of speaking children not given.
b Percent gaze avoidance.
— = No information given.

jective, operational terms, permitting greater reliability of diagnosis. But these four criteria (Table 14-3), alone, select an etiologically heterogeneous group. Some children will be similar to Kanner's and Bender's infantile psychotics. Others will share the four "necessary and sufficient" symptoms but will turn out to have specific neurologic disorders. Rutter acknowledged this difference between his population and Kanner's (p. 1180).[197] If he had eliminated the known organics, it would have reduced this heterogeneity, but it is very likely that these four criteria, alone, would not have excluded the children who developed convulsions later in life.

Kolvin patterned his criteria for "infantile psychosis" after Rutter's,[130] considering the key symptoms to be: onset before three years, a self-isolating pattern of social behavior, and either a catastrophic reaction to environmental change (topographical) or gross motor stereotypies. However, in the latter he included head banging and rocking, and these occur in even larger numbers of organically damaged retardates than would whirling and finger flicking. Accordingly, his population of infantile psychotics is at least as severely retarded as Rutter's (Table 14-1), and shows an even higher incidence of convulsive disorders (Table 14-2).

Lotter[139] also used criteria similar to Rutter's

to select a severely impaired group who were still autistic at eight to ten years. His "nuclear group" of autistic children (Group "A") displayed more repetitive, ritualistic behaviors. Most of these were considerably more complex than the stereotyped motor patterns Kolvin used as criteria. Lotter's high scores yielded a fairly "pure" group with no convulsions and very few OBS[138] (Table 14-2). Group "B" had less of the complex ritualistic behaviors, less clearly psychotic speech, and more OBS.

Within Rutter's framework, infantile autism became simply a behavioral syndrome which could include children with known brain disease; no attempt was made to relate this to childhood or adult schizophrenia. As a result, as Benda[8] and Bender[12] had predicted, the severely retarded child with autistic behavior was rediscovered. Schain and Yannet[201] apparently were the first to point out the frequency with which convulsions were associated with autistic behavior in severe retardates. These children had such dissimilar conditions as hydrocephalus, retrolental fibroplasia, and severe brain hemorrhage. The criteria were limited to an unrelatedness to people, which began in the first two years, and an absence of serious motor retardation.

Knobloch and Pasamanick[127] studied retarded

children under two years who failed to regard people as persons, who insisted on sameness, and who failed to use language for communication. This group had the highest incidence of profound retardation at school age (Table 14-2). All had OBS, including cerebral palsy, Schilder's acute disseminated sclerosis, Hurler's disease, trisomy 21, encephalitis, congenital rubella, and others. Knobloch emphasizes that generally children with such marked neurologic disorders are not referred to psychiatrists, but they constitute about 5 percent of retarded populations.

Hauser and associates[107] analyzed cases of possible autism given pneumoencephalograms. These children had failed to develop communicative language, had grossly impaired relationships with people, and had at least two other "points" of the British group. However, the vignettes reveal no psychotic speech; some children showed "excellent reasoning" and "used gestures adeptly" to communicate, and few had any rituals. It is questionable whether most of these children would fit the DSM-III criteria. It is of interest that there were enlarged lateral ventricles, especially widened left temporal horns, in fifteen of seventeen of the children. Since "autism" was defined so loosely, it would be hazardous to apply these findings in general to other groups.

The populations of infantile psychosis discussed above may be divided into those which include many with OBS and those which do not (Table 14-2). Groups with more brain damaged children also have more who are mute and profoundly retarded (Table 14-1). In the DSM-III, it will be necessary to record the IQ and to note the presence of any major or minor neurologic disorders on the biological axis. Studies should be analyzed for these two crucial variables.

The History of the Identification of Childhood Psychosis

Walk[224] presented a scholarly review of the early pediatric and neuropsychiatric literature. He notes that sporadic cases of childhood psychosis, in the absence of apparent organic brain disease, have been reported for at least 200 years beginning with Perfect's report of an eleven-year-old boy he treated in the 1770's. Rubinstein[190] found similar cases in his review of the American literature before 1900. The pre-Kraepelinian literature

suffered from the same problems of diagnosis and classification which plagued adult psychiatry. Until the 1930s, dementia praecox or schizophrenia was diagnosed in children under sixteen, using much the same standards as were being applied to adult patients. This literature has been reviewed elsewhere.[34, 60, 62, 171]

In this country, the modern era of studies of schizophrenia and related disorders in childhood was initiated when the Children's Service was established at New York State Psychiatric Institute in 1929, under Howard Potter; the Children's Psychiatric Clinic was established at Johns Hopkins Hospital in 1930, under Leo Kanner; Lauretta Bender took over the Children's Psychiatric Service of Bellevue Hospital in 1934, and Charles Bradley became director of the Emma Pendleton Children's Home soon after. Reports by Potter,[171] Despert,[59, 60] and Bradley[34] followed within a few years. Table 14-4 summarizes the observations by these authors, compared with later reports of large series by the major contributors to the field. These were selected to represent the different populations and points of view that will be discussed below. The symptoms which are tabulated in Table 14-4 are those which those authors considered significant for the diagnosis, as well as other symptoms which they noted or which were drawn from their case reports. These symptoms, and the authors' varying criteria for them, are discussed more fully above. Two more recent studies[70, 82, 197] noted symptoms which differentiated psychotic children from comparison groups of retarded and developmentally disabled children. The DSM-III criteria for infantile autism and schizophrenia in children, and the associated symptoms, are tabulated for comparison with these major reports.

Potter,[171] Despert,[59, 60] and Bradley[34] reviewed the literature and reported their own cases in order to demonstrate that schizophrenia was not so rare in prepuberty children as had been thought earlier. They agreed that the patients' immaturity modified the usual symptoms of adult schizophrenia. Potter believed that children's limited ability to abstract and to verbalize kept their delusions simple and naive, with only fragmentary evidence of autistic and dereistic thinking. All three found, in agreement with Lutz, that hallucinations occurred only after six years. Potter and Despert observed schizophrenia in children three and one-half years of age but found delusions only in those ten years and older. Potter thought that the term childhood schizophrenia should be confined to those who were largely in the first decade and showed no physical signs of

TABLE 14-4a

Criteria and Symptoms of Childhood Psychosis, 1933–1976[a]

AUTHOR	PUB. YEAR	DIAG-NOSIS[b]	COMPR. POOR	ODD QUAL.	MUTE[c]	RE-TARDED	ECHOL. (NS)[d]	NON-COMMUN.	DELAY ECHOL., PRON. REVERS.	FRAGM. SYNTAX	DIS-CONN.	SEMANTIC CONFUS., IRREL-EVANT	ILLOG., DEREIS-TIC	BIZARRE DELUS.	HALLUC. OR DELUS.
			INFANTILE AUTISM						*LANGUAGE SYMPTOMS — SCHIZOPHRENIC*				*THOUGHT CONTENT*		
Potter	1933	S						*			*	*	+	+	(+)
Despert	1938, 1941	S		+				*		*	*	*	*	+	(+)
Bradley	1941	S						*							(+)
Bender	1947	S		+	+	+	+	+	+	+	+	+	+	*	(+)
Kanner	1943	A			+	+	+	*	*	+	+	+			
Creak	1963	(S)		+	+	+	+	+	+						
Mahler	1949, 1952	IP, Sy (S)								+			*		
Szurek	1956	A, At, S	*		+	+	+	+	+	+					
Brown	1960	At, (S)	*	*	*	+	*	*	*	*					
Goldfarb	1961, 1968	S	*	+	+	+	+	*	+						
Fish	1968, 1976	A	*	O	+	+	O	O	O	O	O	O	O	O	O
Fish	1968, 1976	S	*	+	+	+	+	*	*	*	*	*	+	O	O
Rutter	1967	IP	*		+	+	+	*	*						
Kolvin	1971	IP					(+)	(+)	O				(+)		O
Kolvin	1971	LOP					+	(+)	+			+	*		*
Ornitz and Ritvo	1968	A		+	+	+	+	*	+						
DSM-III	in prep.	A	+	+	*	*	*	*	O	O	O	O	O	O	O
DSM-III	in prep.	S	+	+	O	+	+	+	*	*	*	*	*	*	(*)

[a] Sx = Symptom; + = Sx present; (+) = Sx rare or "not specific"; O = Sx absent; * = Sx considered significant in diagnosis or prognosis (as under "Comments" on Table).
[b] A = Autistic; At = Atypical development; IP = Infantile psychosis; LOP = Late onset psychosis; S = Schizophrenia or childhood schizophrenia; (S) = Schizophrenic-syndrome or schizophrenic-like; Sy = Symbiotic psychosis.
[c] No words developed (not acute pschotic mutism).
[d] Immediate echolalia, or not specified.
[e] Distortion on the Bender-Gestalt, human figure and other drawings, and in perception of Rorschach, TAT, etc., and ordinary stimuli.

puberty. Despite his emphasis on the differences due to their immaturity, Potter's cases were all severe schizophrenics, whom he could categorize as dementia praecox or schizophrenia, predominantly of the catatonic type. Thirty years later, the extreme severity of his cases, as well as the correctness of his diagnosis was confirmed at follow up.[25] Despert[60] noted that the symptoms in children were less differentiated than those in adults, and that even when they resembled adults' symptoms, they were much more "fluid and variable." She called particular attention to the "frequency of the anomaly of speech development," in which the "child had a capacity above normal to retain words and use them in a mechanical way," although "his vocabulary for expression of needs was small" and noncommunicative.[60] Thus, she antedated Kanner by some five years.

1940s: BENDER AND KANNER

A glance at Table 14-4 reveals that beginning with Bender[18] and Kanner,[124] young children who were "mute," e.g., had no formed speech or recognizable words, were identified as schizophrenic or autistic (only acute psychotic mutism had been reported earlier). Moreover, a variety of new symptoms were reported and considered to be pathognomonic. In 1942, Bender reported that childhood schizophrenia, e.g., before eleven years, "reveals pathology in behavior at every level and in every area of integration or patterning within the functioning of the central nervous system, be it vegetative, motor, perceptual, intellectual, emotional or social. This behavior pathology disturbs the pattern of every functioning field in a characteristic way . . . , striking at the substratum of integrative functioning or biologically patterned behavior." In 1947, she detailed the range and variety of clinical manifestations in all of these areas, as seen in the first one hundred children[18] (Table 14-4). The symptoms of the most primitive children in her study overlapped those described by Kanner. Those with the most complex speech were similar to the children described by Potter and Despert (Table 14-4).

Bender's unique contribution was that she studied all these phenomena in a neurodevelopmental context, in the same way she and her husband, Paul Schilder, had previously studied brain damaged children.[15] They viewed perceptual maturation as being inextricably bound up with the neurological development of postural control, vestibular function, and motility. Bender described the schizophrenic child's resulting disturbances in spatial orientation and perceptual patterning, as seen in their visual-motor Gestalt reproductions, human figure drawings, and spontaneous art work. She related these motor and perceptual problems, in turn, to the child's distorted and uncertain perception of his own body and identity. These difficulties were revealed in his behavior and verbal productions and were connected to his inability to identify with and to relate to others.

Having defined all these phenomena in developmental terms, Bender noted the juxtaposition and the shifting back and forth between precocity and primitive, regressed behaviors. She conceived of this fluidity and variability as being, in themselves, the fundamental characteristics of the schizophrenic disorder. This disorganization resulted from an underlying disorder in the integrating capacity of the CNS. The inherited predisposition to the disorder was the same as for adult schizophrenia, the clinical picture being changed by the different ages of onset and the varied defenses to the biological disorganization.

Bender's[16] "pseudodefective" group, where the onset was under two years, was similar to Kanner's early infantile autistics. Those with later onsets had more neurotic, paranoid, and sociopathic symptoms. Some have assumed that she included many nonpsychotic children in her group.[62] However, the case vignettes[11, 13, 18, 87] indicate the psychotic nature of their symptoms. On follow up into adulthood,[20] they proved to be schizophrenic. Bender's work had an enormous historical impact. Her rich clinical descriptions anticipated most later accounts. Her characterization of the disorders of biological and psychological maturation opened the way for subsequent investigations.

In 1943, Kanner reported the first eleven cases of what he subsequently termed early infantile autism. He considered their "aloneness" and "obsessive insistence on sameness" as the two pathognomonic symptoms; later[123] he elaborated on their language disorder and idiosyncratic associations. He related the "aloneness" to autistic withdrawal in schizophrenia, emphasizing that this could occur with no earlier history of normal social relatedness. For the most part, the "sameness" involved elaborate ritualistic behaviors, including complex verbal routines with the mother. Only two of the eleven children were mute, and these had DQ's of 75 and 94 on the formboard. Kanner differentiated these children from the bulk of mental retardates because of their skillful, fine motor manipulation, their usually more adequate performance on the Seguin formboard, their alert "intelligent" facial expression, and the absence of

TABLE 14–4b

Criteria and Symptoms of Childhood Psychosis, 1933–1976[a]

AUTHOR	SOCIAL RELATEDNESS		AFFECT		PERCEPTION		MOTILITY			
	AUTISTIC WITHDRAWAL	IMPERSONAL CLINGING	FLAT, INCONGRUOUS	ANX., PANIC	STEREOTYPIC IRREL. DETAIL	DISTORTED PERCEP.[e]	RHYTMIC; SELF-MUTIL.	DYSKINETIC	STEREOTYPIC; ATHETOID	WHIRLING
Potter	*		*	*	+					
Despert	*			*					+	
Bradley	*		+	(+)	(+)					
Bender	+	*	+	*	+	*		*	*	*
Kanner	*		+	+	*			(+)		
Creak	+	+	+	+	+		+		+	+
Mahler	+	*		*	+					+
Szurek	+		+	+			+		+	
Brown	*		+	*	*		*	+	*	
Goldfarb	*	+		*	+	+	+	+		+
Fish (A)	*	O	+	+	+	O	+	+	+	O
Fish (S)	*	+	+	+	+	*	+	+	+	+
Rutter	*			+	*		*		*	
Kolvin (IP)	*	O			*		*	+	*	
Kolvin (LOP)	+	*			O		(+)	+	+	
Ornitz and Ritvo	*				*		+		+	*
DSM-III (A)	*		+	+	*	(+)	+	+	+	+
DSM-III (S)	+		+	+	+	+		+	+	+

[a] Sx = Symptom; + = Sx present; (+) = Sx rare or "not specific"; O = Sx absent; * = Sx considered significant in diagnosis or prognosis (as under "Comments" on Table).
[b] A = Autistic; At = Atypical development; IP = Infantile psychosis; LOP = Late onset psychosis; S = Schizophrenia or childhood schizophrenia; (S) = Schizophrenic-syndrome or schizophrenic-like; Sy = Symbiotic psychosis.
[c] No words developed (not acute psychotic mutism).
[d] Immediate echolalia, or not specified.
[e] Distortion on the Bender-Gestalt, human figure and other drawings, and in perception of Rorschach, TAT, etc., and in ordinary stimuli.

congenital stigmata and neurological findings. His assumption that these children were not mentally retarded has not been confirmed by psychometrics. When re-examined in adolescence, one-fourth were psychotic and 31 percent were schizoid.[125]

Kanner's group included children with psychotic speech as complex as those called "pseudoneurotic" by Bender.[16] He considered infantile autism to be "the earliest possible manifestation of childhood schizophrenia . . . The basic nature of its manifestations is so intimately related to the basic nature of childhood schizophrenia as to be indistinguishable from it."[122] Its importance consisted in its being a well-defined syndrome and in "the correction of the impression that a compara-

tively normal period of adjustment must precede the development of schizophrenia."[122] He was struck by the children's bland, indifferent expressions as long as they were left alone and viewed the congenital absence of affective-social responsiveness as the primary deficit, one which was constitutional in nature. His emphasis on the "cold, refrigerator," intelligent, highly educated parents[121] led many to assume that he was implying a primarily psychogenic disorder; in fact, he was not.

By 1953, when Kanner had accumulated a series of one hundred autistic children,[121] he noted the absence of mental illness in their families and was more inclined to separate his group

	ORGANIZED BEHAVIOR	OVERALL INTEGRATION			
CATATONIC	STEREOTYPIC RITUAL	BIZARRE, DISCONN.	EXAM UNEVEN	DEVEL. IRREG.	OTHER COMMENTS BY AUTHOR
*		*			Delusions = simple, naive; Fragment evidence of dereistic thought.
+	+	+	*	NC Speech	Hallucinations > 6 years; Delusions > 10 years.
(+)	+	*			Hallucinations > 6 years (Lutz); Anxiety = not specific to S.
*	+	+	*	*	Hallucinations = not specific to S; CNS variability pathognomonic.
	*		+		Autism and stereotypy pathognomonic.
+	+		+	+	
			+		No differentiation of self/world, animate/inanimate.
+	+		+		
+					* Sx predicted poor outcome at follow up.
	+		+		
(+)	+	+	O	O	All mute; * Sx vs. nonpsychotic developmentally disabled.
(+)	+	+	*	+	Mute/speaking; * Sx vs. nonpsychotic developmentally disabled (Verbal IQ's all < 70).
	*		(+)		* Sx vs. nonpsychotic retarded.
	+				* Sx = selection criteria.
	+				* Sx = selection criteria.
				*	
+	*	+	+	+	
+	+	+	+	+	Schneiderian hallucinations, delusions = rare < years.

from the other subgroups of schizophrenia. Subsequently, Kanner expressed dismay that the term autism was being applied too loosely to a vast and heterogeneous group of severely impaired children. Apparently, the problem arose from the fact that he reduced all the phenomenology to his two key symptoms of withdrawal and stereotypy, and did not include the range of behaviors noted in his vignettes (Table 14-4). These limited criteria permitted the inclusion by others of many severely retarded children with organic brain disorders, whom Kanner had excluded. Bender[12] stated that Kanner's key symptoms of withdrawal, stereotyped behavior, and severely retarded or absent speech did not define any disease entity.

To be sure, these symptoms would encompass the earliest onset, most severely retarded schizophrenic children; but they would also include many severely retarded children with organic brain disorders. Rigidity and stereotyped behaviors are characteristic of children with organic brain disease, and withdrawal is simply a primitive defense of a child placed in a situation with which he is totally unable to cope by any more sophisticated mechanisms.

Psychoanalytic Formulations and Treatment: 1950: Following Bender and Kanner, there was an explosion of interest and an exponential increase in the studies of psychotic children. Only some major trends can be sketched here. The reader is referred to more detailed historical reviews* and annotated bibliographies.[38, 100, 220]

From the late 1940s on, a large number of American psychiatrists, who wrote about childhood psychosis, were primarily interested in the psychotherapy of psychotic children. Many prominent psychoanalysts figure in this group. They focused on the psychological meaning of the symptoms for individual children and conceptualized the psychological mechanisms in terms of the abnormal development of instinctual drives and ego functioning. The emphasis on the special meaning of symptoms for a particular child often meant that less attention was paid to diagnosis and to describing the phenomenology shared by psychotic children as a class. However, one can still relate those symptoms were are discussed, and which are described in the case vignettes, to the types of childhood psychosis described above.

Mahler's writings on the symbiotic type of "infantile psychosis" ("schizophrenic-like") have become classics.[145, 146] These children usually had an onset of psychotic symptoms in the third or fourth year, or else "at the height of oedipal conflict" (presumably between four and six). In the first year of life they tended to be irritable rather than severely withdrawn, and their psychosis was manifested by generalized panic reactions, desperate clinging behavior to the mother, dereistic thinking, and often bizarre and obsessional somatic preoccupations[145] (Table 14-4). They appear to be similar to the schizophrenic children with onsets at three and one-half to four, described by Despert[59, 60] and Bender.[18] Some would fit Bender's description of the "pseudoneurotic" type. Later, Mahler[144] wrote that autistic and symbiotic features were often combined, and children should be categorized in terms of the predominant defenses. Mahler[144] continued to develop her ideas on the importance of the "individuation" phase in normal and psychotic ego development and experimented with modified psychoanalytic techniques to treat young symbiotic children. She believed (as did Weil)[228] that constitutional factors underlay the ego deficit in these children.

Szurek[217] was one of the most articulate spokesmen for the position that childhood psychosis "is entirely psychogenic." The large number of schizophrenic, autistic, and "atypical" children he and his colleagues treated at Langley Porter had symptoms which corresponded to those described by Bender and Kanner (Table 14-4); they ranged

from those who were mute to those with more advanced psychotic speech. However, he considered it "unnecessary to draw any sharp dividing lines between . . . psychoneurotic and psychotic" children. Psychotherapeutic work with both the children and the parents convinced him that "the psychotic child manifests in his disorder the incorporation of and identification with the *disorder* of *both* of his parents' personalities."[217] He and Berlin, therefore, emphasized psychotherapeutic work with the parents in their treatment program for the psychotic children.[218]

Rank, Putnam, and their co-workers at the James Jackson Putnam Center characterized the children they studied as suffering from "Atypical Development."[175] These were infantile psychotics[35] which included Bender's childhood schizophrenia, Kanner's autism, and Mahler's symbiotic psychosis. The "atypicality" referred to the fact that some ego functions were arrested, whereas others (music, construction ability, language, physical skill) developed precociously, although isolated from any integrated adaptation. Essentially, this reformulated part of Bender's concept of variable and unintegrated development in the language of ego psychology. It also recalls the "peaks of performance" described by Kanner, Creak, and others. However, in accounting for the fragile ego functioning, Rank[175] emphasized pathological early parent-child relationships, traumatic events, and physical illness as etiological factors rather than constitutional factors. The symptoms and dysfunctions of the children were described in detail by Brown.[37] It is clear (Table 14-4) that the phenomenology overlaps that of Kanner's autistic and Bender's schizophrenic children, except that the schizophrenic disorders of language and thought content which require more complex speech (disconnection, semantic confusion and irrelevance, dereistic thinking, somatic delusions) were not described for these children under six years. Their outcome in adolescence was similar to Kanner's group.

FURTHER DELINEATION OF THE SYNDROMES OF AUTISM AND SCHIZOPHRENIA

During this same period of the 1950s, clinical studies were continuing in an attempt to define the syndromes of childhood psychosis more accurately, in terms of their longitudinal course, associated familial and genetic factors, phenomenology, and subclassification. By 1956, the follow up of Kanner's group into adolescence had been reported,[125] as well as the first follow up

---

* See references 64, 92, 133, 157, and 161.

of Bender's group into their early twenties.[24] Kanner[121] had found an absence of psychosis in the parents of his children, and Bender had found a high incidence of schizophrenia in the parents of hers.[22] Bender also had spelled out operational criteria for "plastic" development in the various areas of behavior and had tested this quantitatively.[23]

Creak[52] collaborated with a group of British psychiatrists in formulating the "nine points" of clinical symptoms which defined the "schizophrenic syndrome." As seen in Table 14-4, these draw from the symptoms described both by Bender and by Kanner. They do not specifically mention the schizophrenic disturbances of speech and thought content, which require the development of more complex language. The results of Creak's studies[51, 53] suggest that her population included more children with infantile psychosis than with later onsets.

Beginning in 1956, the "second generation" of investigators began to publish studies of the phenomenology of childhood schizophrenia and infantile autism. At the Ittleson Center, Goldfarb utilized a large battery of neurologic and perceptual tests to determine which of the symptoms described by Bender differentiated schizophrenics from normal children. He and his co-workers developed tests to study the speech of the children and the functioning of their families. His schizophrenic group was subdivided into "organic" and "nonorganic" subgroups, according to their history and neurologic examination.[96] At least three of the "organics" had a specific neurologic disorder, such as convulsions or expressive aphasia, but most had only nonspecific indications of brain dysfunction. The "organic" children turned out to have greater impairment of IQ, more "soft neurologic signs," and other handicaps, but they had more adequate families. Goldfarb[94, 95, 96] postulated a complementary series of constitutional and environmental factors which could lead to a schizophrenic syndrome.

Fish[67, 71, 76, 77] began her studies of the antecedents of schizophrenia, comparing the development of infants born to schizophrenic and to nonpsychotic mothers. Integrative disorders of development were operationally defined in terms of specific profiles of DQ's on testing and fluctuations in serial DQ's. Bender's predictions from the histories of schizophrenic children were confirmed, but Fish also found milder developmental disorders in other "vulnerable" infants[77] whose later adaptation took the form of severe to moderate personality disorders.[67, 71, 80, 83] Fish postulated that "pandevelopmental retardation" is the expression in infancy of the inherited neurointegrative defect in schizophrenia; for a vulnerable infant, the ultimate outcome depends on the severity of the intrinsic defect and the nature of the child's experience.

In the 1960s, Fish and her co-workers at Bellevue developed subclassifications of schizophrenic children based on the severity of integrative defect and language impairment.[81, 82] The subcategories were found to be significant for the immediate response to milieu and pharmacologic treatments and also predicted five-year outcome.[82] Their mute, psychotic children with only primitive stereotyped manipulation of materials and essentially no "high points," correspond to Kanner's mute autistics (Table 14-4). Children with characteristically irregular functioning were considered to be schizophrenic. At a mean age of three and one-half, one-half had typically psychotic speech (Table 14-4); 80 percent of the remainder developed such speech later (Table 14-1). The descriptive categories were subsequently condensed to define symptoms which were both necessary and sufficient to diagnose schizophrenia and the major behavior disorders.[72]

In 1965, Rutter and his colleagues began to publish their follow-up studies of severely impaired psychotic children seen earlier at the Maudsley, comparing them to nonpsychotic retarded controls.* Unlike his predecessors, Rutter studied infantile psychosis, or autism, as a behavioral syndrome and considered it to be unrelated to schizophrenia.[195] Therefore, he included many children (35 to 63 percent) whose psychosis was associated with definite or probable organic brain disease (Table 14-2). His selection criteria were such, that if any one of the consulting psychiatrists was in doubt about diagnosing psychosis, that child was eliminated. This apparently tended to eliminate the later onset, higher functioning schizophrenic children who are more variable, and about whom there is apt to be more difference of opinion early in their course. What was left was a group with a large number (40 percent) of mute children (Table 14-1). Rutter's infantile psychotics apparently did not display the disconnected speech, semantic confusion, or irrelevancies noted in Kanner's group (Table 14-4). As a result, at follow up, this group resembled Kanner's mute autistics; few (8 percent) were able to function in regular school or jobs, and apparently few were grossly psychotic (Table 14-8). The description of affect, social relatedness,

---

* See references 136, 137, 195, 196, and 197.

and speech of some of the children resembles Kanner's "severe schizoids," but no follow-up diagnoses were reported.[192, 196] The high incidence of psychosis in late adolescence in Kanner's group occurred only in those with speech (Table 14-8).

The symptoms being considered as criteria for infantile autism in the DSM-III are apparently those which differentiated Rutter's infantile psychotics from his nonpsychotic retardates (Table 14-3). These symptoms will select: (1) a group with low IQ's (Table 14-1); (2) definite OBS in anywhere from 10 to 100 percent of the group (depending on the source of patients and additional criteria used) (Table 14-2); (3) a low incidence of familial schizophrenia (depending on the degree of dilution by patients with OBS) (Table 14-6); and (4) a poor outcome in adolescence and adulthood (Table 14-8).

Rutter's selection criteria apparently excluded not only many autistic children with speech, but also most schizophrenic children with onsets after two years,[197] who were among the Maudsley admissions between 1950 and 1958. Anthony[5] describes children whose psychoses began between three and five years and in mid-childhood (Groups "2" and "3"). Since he saw them at the Maudsley between 1952 and 1957, one can only assume that they were eliminated by Rutter's selection criteria. Anthony says of the parents of these psychotic children, "Certainly some in our group could pass as well compensated schizophrenics. One often has the clinical feeling that parent and child suffered from essentially the same psychotic process but that the adult was better equipped to cope with the problem."[5] One gets no hint from Rutter's family data that such parents existed within the families he selected for study.

Therefore, one can legitimately question the basis for Rutter's[192] conclusion that childhood schizophrenia does not exist. He had based this view on the assumption that he studied a representative sample of the universe of young psychotic children. Comparison of his population with the other studies makes it all too clear that his series represents only a profoundly retarded segment of infantile psychosis. Since he restricts the diagnosis of childhood schizophrenia to children with hallucinations or delusions he also excludes a great many children whom U.S. psychiatrists diagnose as schizophrenic. Certainly, if one returned to the pre-1933 pre-Potter criteria, one would diagnose very few childhood schizophrenics. However, even forty-five years ago, hallucinations and delusions were not the only criteria used to diagnose either schizophrenia or dementia praecox. One can eliminate childhood schizophrenia from the DSM-III, as the committee apparently plans to do, but unfortunately it is not so simple to eliminate the psychosis which plagues a large number of children.

In 1967, Lotter published his classic epidemiological study of autistic children in Middlesex County, England. He used specific criteria for retarded or noncommunicative speech, stereotyped and ritualistic behaviors, and severe autistic withdrawal (Table 14-4). He states that his group was necessarily a severely affected one, since it was limited to children who continued to show these symptoms at ten years. This selected the most severely impaired autistics, who had shown little remission or progress by that age. His data are somewhat easier to interpret than Rutter's, since he divided the "nuclear" group ("A") from those with lower scores on the criterion symptoms ("B"). This left a "nuclear" group which had fewer children without speech (Table 14-1) and very few with organic brain disorders (Table 14-2). He added valuable data on the incidence, socioeconomic status, and developmental retardation of this severe group.

Kolvin continued this British tradition in his study of infantile psychosis ("IP") versus late onset psychosis ("LOP").[130] He selected infantile psychotics, using essentially the same criteria as Lotter, and he also required an onset before three years. The infantile psychotics rarely had advanced psychotic language (e.g., semantic confusion, irrelevancy, dereistic thinking) (Table 14-4). They had a higher incidence (78 percent) of Performance IQ's under 70 than did Rutter's group (Table 14-1), and an even higher incidence (39 percent) of definite organic brain disorder (Table 14-2). Like Rutter's group, there was no increased familial incidence of schizophrenia (Table 14-6). The late onset psychotics were those with onsets over five years who showed Schneiderian hallucinations or delusions. Not surprisingly, Kolvin found very few such children with onsets before nine years; only ten of the thirty were under thirteen years. Like Rutter, Kolvin concluded that only these two extremes of childhood psychosis existed—the infantile, severly retarded type, with a high incidence of organic brain disorders; and a type with onsets in late childhood, which closely resembled adolescent and adult schizophrenia. He, too, apparently overlooked the fact that, as a result of his selection criteria, these were the only parts of the universe he had sampled.

In 1965, Ornitz, Ritvo, and their colleagues[162, 163] began to publish their studies of neurophysiological and biochemical deviations in autistic children. They postulated a continuum between autism and childhood schizophrenia,[159, 161] and they used criteria which apparently selected a group which was more etiologically homogeneous than Rutter's. In addition to autistic withdrawal, retarded or noncommunicative speech, and bizarre stereotyped behaviors, they required evidence of unmodulated perceptual responses and irregular development (Table 14-4). This combination of Kanner's and Bender's symptoms appears to have selected a group of severely autistic children who had no complex psychotic language (Table 14-4), but also one with very few (7 percent) specific organic brain disorders.[183] It appears to be closer to Kanner's original conception, and also to Bender's "pseudo-defective" type, than are the groups selected by Rutter's criteria. This may be one reason that these authors found similar neurophysiological abnormalities in autistic and in schizophrenic children.[159]

CHILDHOOD PSYCHOSIS, 1933–1976;
AND THEN WHAT?

In this country and in Britain, there has been a spreading tendency to diagnose "infantile autism," or "autistic children," on the basis of scanty or poorly specified criteria. This has led to the selection of samples of profoundly retarded children, composed almost entirely of those with organic brain disorders. Kanner's contribution in focusing on the earliest onset schizophrenics appears to have taken a paradoxical turn which he neither anticipated nor desired. Using the criteria he proposed, much more heterogeneous groups of children are now being diagnosed as infantile autism. In the DSM-III, the presence of organic brain disease would be noted on the biologic axis; "soft neurologic signs" on the development axis. It is essential to subdivide groups according to these findings, or the DSM-III's infantile autism will become a meaningless assortment of retarded children, unrelated to etiology or outcome.

Conflicting diagnostic definitions and varying standards, therefore, still plague the field of childhood psychosis. Potter, Despert, and Bradley urged the field to recognize that children are not miniature adults and to look for more undifferentiated symptoms in childhood schizophrenics. Bender delineated the symptoms of childhood schizophrenia in terms of the deviations from the normal maturation of motility, perception, and

language. In the 1940s, it was an advance to describe the broad range of symptoms which were important in defining the syndrome. In the next decade, however, the diagnostic pendulum probably swung too far over. Many disturbed children, whom one would consider today to have only borderline or even no psychotic symptoms, were lumped together in an ill-defined category of childhood psychosis. Psychoanalytic writers who were concerned primarily with the inner meanings behind behavior considered diagnosis to be less important.

In the 1960s, child psychiatry had reached a sufficient level of sophistication to begin to move in the direction adult psychiatry was taking[232] and to define diagnostic criteria in more specific terms. It is probable that the position toward which the current DSM-III Committee is moving will turn out to be too restrictive, since schizophrenia in childhood comprises far more than a formal thought disorder. However, for the present it is possible to live with a system which will diagnose a large group of children as "Childhood psychosis, other type." This can serve until reliable criteria are defined with which to diagnose schizophrenic children who have not yet developed a formal thought disorder or other symptoms characteristic of adults. The associated characteristic symptoms in development, motility, and perception should be reported in the developmental axis. A prediction of the future course belongs in the estimate of prognosis. In describing a diagnostic entity, only the first step has been taken when one has specified the clinical syndrome.[232] The next step is to define its unity by its longitudinal course. Childhood schizophrenia has been shown to be such an entity and one which is continuous with adult schizophrenia (Table 14-9). The outcome of infantile autism has not been delineated as clearly, since the independent psychiatric and neurologic diagnoses given to Kanner's, Creak's, Brown's (James Jackson Putnam Center), and Rutter's children in adulthood are not yet known.

The further characterization of a diagnostic entity by familial and genetic factors has been done for childhood schizophrenia, but additional studies are needed which use blind, independent diagnoses of the relatives. Some objective means of categorizing nonpsychotic, as well as schizophrenic relatives, would add to the richness of the genetic data, but such measures have yet to be shown to be valid and reliable. Clinical diagnoses, using strict research criteria,[215, 232] global health-illness scales,[65] MMPI profiles, or other similar measures already used in genetic studies of adult schizophrenics[104, 113, 126] would enable investigators to compare those families with the families of childhood schizophrenics.

The past ten to fifteen years has seen the beginnings of more sophisticated biological and phenomenological research in childhood psychosis. One may hope that in the future autism and childhood schizophrenia will be delineated further by neurophysiological and biochemical characteristics, pharmacologic responses, objective analyses of the characteristics of schizophrenic language and thought in children,* and by additional perceptual and cognitive studies.[110] Such research could specify the diagnostic categories of infantile autism, childhood schizophrenia, and psychoses with organic brain disorders more precisely; in addition, it might well define subgroups within these major disorders which would be significant for treatment.

Frequency, Incidence, Prevalence, and Distribution

Lotter[139] found the prevalence of autistic children, eight to ten years of age, in Middlesex County, England, to be 4.5 in 10,000. Half of these (Group "B") tended to have OBS (Table 14-2). Torrey and associates[221] included some children with more complex psychotic speech and found a prevalence rate of 4.7 in 10,000 in the Collaborative Perinatal Study in this country. An additional 2.0 in 10,000 were psychotic but did not fit all the criteria for infantile autism. Organic brain disorders were excluded in this study.

DISTRIBUTION BY GENDER

All studies of childhood psychosis show a predominance of boys over girls. This appears to reflect the same biological vulnerability of infant males that is seen in their higher rates of mental retardation and other neurologic disorders. The male to female ratio in infantile psychosis ranges from Lotter's 2.5 to 1 to Bender's 6.1 to 1; in schizophrenia beginning after two years, it is 2.6–2.8 to 1 (Table 14-2). Bender found that this changed from 2.2 to 2.0 to 1 for onsets at two to five and six to seven years, to a ratio of 5 to 1 for those onsets at eight to nine years.[20]

* See references 6, 204, 205, 206, and 207.

SOCIOECONOMIC DISTRIBUTION

The socioeconomic distribution of the families of schizophrenic children whose onsets are over two years of age (Table 14-5) is similar to distributions reported for adult schizophrenics.[125] There is a higher incidence of lower-class families than in the general population. This is true for both Bender and Faretra's[20] and Kolvin and associates[130] studies (Table 14-5), although Bender and Faretra's population has two and one-half times as many from the lowest, marginal, and dependent group as Kolvin's.

The findings for infantile psychosis vary somewhat among the several studies (Table 14-5). Goldfarb's[94] is the only study with no increase of upper-class (I) families. The other studies range from Lotter's[139] 12.5 percent to Kanner's[121] 90 percent (of professional parents). Creak and Ini,[53] Goldfarb,[94] Ritvo and associates[183] and Bender and Faretra[20] all have explained the increased incidence of upper-class patients in terms of the different admission policies of the psychiatric institutions represented. Lotter's findings, however, cannot be explained on this basis, since his was an epidemiological study, combing schools and other facilities for children who met his criteria for autism. No satisfactory explanation of this has yet been offered. Ritvo's is the only study which matched autistic with nonautistic inpatients[183] (Table 14-5). The results show no difference in social class. Whatever factors operate to increase the number of upper-class families with infantile psychotic children, these factors are not specific to this condition. Three of the studies[20, 70, 82, 183] show a bimodal distribution. Their increased incidence of the lowest classes resembles the findings for the schizophrenics (Table 14-5).

AGE OF ONSET, USUAL AGE WHEN SEEN, AND AGE OF SPONTANEOUS REMISSION

In psychotic children, disturbed development and behavior are often detectable at birth (Table 14-7). In the beginning, the severe symptoms are similar to those in OBS with severe mental retardation. The milder symptoms are similar to those in children who are vulnerable but who may never show the full clinical picture of childhood psychosis. One can arbitrarily define the age of onset as the period when the child shows all the symptoms necessary for the DSM-III diagnosis.

Infantile Autism: In infantile autism, *autistic withdrawal* may begin at birth. This must be differentiated from a sensory deficit, and from pro-

TABLE 14–5

Social Class Distribution of Families of Psychotic Children in Percent

AUTHOR (DIAGNOSIS)[a]	PUB. YEAR	n	ONSET (YEARS)	SOCIAL CLASS[b]				
				I	II	III	IV	V
SCHIZOPHRENIA								
Kolvin (LOP)	1971	32	5–15	6	9	38	28	19
Bender (CS)	1972	50	2–10	8		40		52
INFANTILE PSYCHOSIS								
Bender (CS)	1972	50	<2	30		32		38
Kanner (A)	1953	100	≤2		90		10	
Goldfarb (CS)	1968	61	<5	7	8	33	34	18
Fish (CS)	1968, 1976	38	<2	16		60		24
Fish (A)	1968, 1976	8	<2	22		56		22
Creak ((S))	1960	102	—	36	23	32	7	2
Creak (census, 1951)	1960	(census, 1951)		3	15	53	16	13
Rutter (IP)	1967	63	<5	24	32	41	3	
Kolvin (IP)	1971	46	<3	17	22	41	17	2
Lotter (A, "A")	1967	14	<4.5	28+	28+	28+	14	
Lotter (A, "B")	1967	16	<4.5	12+	19	56	12	
Lotter (census, 1951)	1967	(census, 1951)		5	19	57		19
Ritvo (A)	1971	74	≤2		36	15		49
Ritvo (controls)	1971	74	—		38	21		41

[a] LOP = Late onset psychosis; CS = Childhood schizophrenia; CS, NO = CS, "nonorganic"; CS, O = CS, "organic"; IP = Infantile psychosis; A = Autistic; A, "A" = A, "nuclear" group; A, "B" = A, lower ratings on autistic symptoms; (S) = Schizophrenic-syndrome or schizophrenic-like.
[b] Criteria vary for different studies.
— = No information given.

found retardation without psychosis, which could produce absent responses. It may be difficult to distinguish these disorders before six months. To meet all the DSM-III criteria for autism, a child must engage in bizarre stereotypic behaviors which are more complex than choreoathetotic hand movements or primitive manipulation. Complex rituals can be more clearly recognized after independent locomotion and exploratory behaviors occur.

Decreased babbling in the second six months and a selective inattention to the human voice should arouse suspicion; but, it is difficult to establish that language is significantly retarded before eighteen months. Therefore, although many symptoms may be present earlier, and by six months one can suspect the diagnosis, a child usually can not meet the necessary criteria until after eighteen months.

In other autistic children, the onset may be less insidious, or else mild early disturbances are overlooked. The "onset" may then be signaled by a relatively acute regression in social, vocal, and affective responses, and often in gross motor and visual-motor development. Children who have earlier appeared to be alert, and even responsive and precocious, suddenly change. Their expres-

sion becomes dull, the focus of their attention becomes oblique, vague, and nonresponsive. They may abruptly go limp and become unable to chew or swallow textured food. These changes may be sufficiently marked so as to be obvious in a succession of baby pictures. This frequently occurs between eight to ten months of age, but it may occur at any time before thirty months.[74, 75] Onset of psychosis after thirty months must be classified arbitrarily as "Childhood psychosis, autistic syndrome, other type" in the DSM-III.

Childhood Schizophrenia: A similarly arbitrary "onset" is established by the DSM-III criteria for schizophrenia. The preschizophrenic infant may show the same disturbances from birth as the autistic infant and may manifest disturbed behavior continuously thereafter. However, the DSM-III diagnosis of schizophrenia could not be made until speech was sufficiently complex to document a formal thought disorder. Some schizophrenic children display typical disturbances of syntax and meaning, with clearly psychotic speech, as soon as they speak in three to four-word sentences. This is rare before two years.

Children who lapse into psychotic speech after a period of relatively normal communication usually have had early developmental symptoms and some previous psychiatric symptoms. Bender has summarized the variety of onsets in the largest series.[20] Onsets of schizophrenia after two years clustered between two to four years, and five to seven years, with another peak at nine to ten years. A minority (30 percent) of the late onset children previously had appeared to be relatively normal, although "overly quiet, model children." Almost all of those with onsets up to seven years had been obviously disturbed before. About 40 percent were withdrawn and autistic; 45 percent presented other forms of disturbed behavior.

Most children have an insidious onset. Concerned parents may seek an early evaluation, but progressively more deviant behavior may not be recognized until later at school. "Onset" becomes an artifact of when the child is interviewed and psychotic material is finally identified.

Some children have a more acute onset. They may abruptly regress in speech and behavior between three and five years of age. Even their motility may become clumsy, requiring differentiation from the organic dementias. Acute onsets in latency often appear to follow illness, injury, or a severe psychological trauma, such as loss of a parent or disruption of the home. Bender and Faretra[20] found the most dramatic onsets in girls between four and seven years.

Rutter[191, 197] and Kolvin and associates[130] found few onsets of childhood psychosis between three and seven years. Most infantile psychosis began before thirty months. Schizophrenia began at seven years and later.[130, 191] The apparent rarity of onsets between two and seven arose because these two authors required Schneiderian hallucinations or delusions for a diagnosis of schizophrenia. Such phenomena rarely occur before nine years. Kolvin found only fourteen out of thirty-three late onset psychoses had onsets before eleven years, and most of these occurred late in childhood. Only 13 percent of these children displayed no "premorbid oddity." One-third of those under eleven had acute onsets. It is difficult to see what is gained by ignoring a large number of children whose schizophrenia begins in early childhood, especially when they fit even the strict DSM-III criteria for schizophrenia.

"Childhood Psychosis, Other Type": Many children under five, with profound autistic withdrawal, do not have sufficiently stereotyped or ritualistic behaviors to be diagnosed as infantile autism. Their speech and nonverbal language is predominantly noncommunicative, but it is too sparse to be characterized as a formal thought disorder with incoherence. According to the DSM-III, they would be diagnosed as "Childhood psychosis, other type." Their onsets are similar to those in infantile autism and early onset childhood schizophrenia.

Usual Age When Seen: Depending on the threshhold of parental concern and the sophistication of the attending physician, infantile autism or schizophrenia may be suspected well before three years of age. If there is little early precocity or agitation, the retardation and unresponsiveness may not be investigated until special schooling is required. The schizophrenic child frequently is not seen professionally until grossly psychotic behavior becomes unmanageable at home, nursery, or grade school. Panic, excitement, or aggression are noticed before aloof, self-isolating behavior and a quiet preoccupation with bizarre delusions.

Age of Spontaneous Remissions: Spontaneous remissions of childhood psychosis may occur at any age. Symptoms may decrease, but only rarely will they disappear completely or permanently. The severity of residual impairment depends on the age of onset and the degree of disruption of normal childhood experiences. Verbal IQ is the single most important determinant of adaptive functioning after remission. It is comparable to the measures of premorbid functioning, which reflect chronicity in adult schizophrenia. The various paths which childhood psychosis may take are discussed below.

DISTRIBUTION OF AUTISM AND SCHIZOPHRENIA AMONG FIRST DEGREE RELATIVES

It has now been established that a genetic predisposition is a necessary condition for the development of schizophrenia in adults.[104, 188, 211] Family and twin studies demonstrate that the closer the genetic relationship to a schizophrenic proband, the greater the risk of a relative developing schizophrenia. Since the concordance rates in monozygotic twins are only in the range of 35 to 58 percent,[104] obviously other factors must contribute to the full emergence of a schizophrenic psychosis. What these factors may be has not yet been determined. The relatively high risk for schizophrenia in the offspring of schizophrenics remains whether or not the children are reared by their own kin at home, or apart from their schizophrenic relatives in adoptive homes.[113] Children of nonschizophrenic parents, who were reared by schizophrenics, do not appear to have an elevated risk for schizophrenia.[229]

Based on her own and Kallman and Roth's[119] data, Bender stated very early[22] that childhood schizophrenia was genetically continuous with adult schizophrenia, but the onset was precipitated earlier, usually by some physiological crisis, and that in some cases, this might be birth itself. Fish[67, 71] later supported this position. At first, Kanner considered infantile autism to be the earliest form of schizophrenia; however, he did not find schizophrenic relatives in the families of his probands.[121] Rutter[192, 196, 197] and Kolvin and associates[130] presented evidence that unlike schizophrenia in late childhood, infantile psychosis was not genetically continuous with adult schizophrenia. Hanson and Gottesman[106] reviewed these conflicting data and concluded that most groups of infantile psychotics seem unrelated to schizophrenia and probably are associated with OBS.

There is good agreement that childhood schizophrenia which begins after five years, and which has clinical features similar to adult schizophrenia, has the same genetic predisposition as adult schizophrenia (Table 14-6). In Kallman and Roth's,[119] Bender and Faretra's,[20] and Kolvin and associates[130] studies, the rates for schizophrenia in the parents of childhood schizophrenics are as high or higher than the rates (4.2 to 4.4 percent) for parents of adult schizophrenics.[188, 211] The incidence of parents hospitalized with schizophrenia was as high for Bender's children with onsets between two and seven years (12.2 percent) as for those with onsets after eight years (11.5 percent).

Kallman and Roth's[119] is the only major study of childhood schizophrenic twins. Children with mental retardation, or onsets before seven, were excluded. If one includes co-twins with a later onset, the 70.6 percent uncorrected concordance rate for childhood schizophrenia in monozygotic

TABLE 14–6

Schizophrenic Relatives of Psychotic Children in Percent

AUTHOR (DIAGNOSIS)[a]	PUB. YEAR	PROBANDS ONSET (YEARS)	% DEFINITE OBS[b]	% SES CLASS V[c]	PARENTS: HOSPITALIZED SCHIZOPHRENIA n	% SCHIZOPHRENIC	SIBLINGS: AUTISM OR SCHIZOPHRENIA n[d]	% AFFECTED
SCHIZOPHRENIA								
Kallman (CS)	1956	7–11	—[e]	—	204	8.8	234	7.7 (S)
Kallman (CS)	1956	7–11					35 Dz	22.9 (S)
Kallman (CS)	1956	7–11					17 Mz	88.2 (S)
Kolvin (LOP)	1971	5–15	27	19	64	9.4	56	1.8 (S)
Bender (CS)	1972	2–10	2	52	100	12.0		
INFANTILE PSYCHOSIS								
Bender (CS)	1972	<	8	38	100	7.0	87	13.8 (S)
Kanner (A)	1953	≦2	1	10(IV & V)	200	0	131	2.3 (A)
Goldfarb (CS)	1962	<5	4	18	84	2.4(−21?[f])	48	8.3 (S)
Fish (CS)	1968, 1976	<2	3	24	70	5.7	44	4.5 (A, S)
Fish (CS)	1968, 1976	<2					2 Mz	100 (A)
Fish (A)	1968, 1976	<2	0	22	16	0	5	0
Creak ((S))	1960	—	14	2	120	1.7(−2.5?[g])	135	0(2.2?[h])
Rutter (IP)	1967, 1970	<5	35	3	126	0	85	0(2.4? A[j])
Kolvin (IP)	1971	<3	39	2	92	1.1	68	0
Lotter (A)	1967	≦4.5	19	13(IV & V)	60	0(1.7–8.3?[k])	62	0(4.8?[m])

a LOP = Late onset psychosis; CS = Childhood schizophrenia; CS, NO = CS, "nonorganic"; CS, O = CS, "organic"; IP = Infantile psychosis; A = Autistic; A, "A" = A, "nuclear" group; A, "B" = A, lower ratings on autistic symptoms; (S) = Schizophrenic-syndrome or schizophrenic-like.
b As in Table 14–2.
c As in Table 14–5.
d Mz = monozygotic twins; Dz = dizygotic twins.
e Psychotic children with MR excluded.
f In addition, 16 (19%?) never hospitalized but diagnosed borderline, ambulatory or pseudoneurotic schizophrenic.
g In addition, 1 (0.8%?) "anorexia nervosa, ?schizophrenic."
h 3 (2.2%?) "psychotic"; 2 with MR.
j 1 (1.2%?) "?autistic;" 1 similar, but "less abnormal;" neither psychotic.
k 1 hospitalized for "delusions and hallucinations, not specific for schizophrenia," diagnosed amphetamine psychosis; 1 reportedly hospitalized as "paranoid psychopath." Not hospitalized, included 2 with "nervous breakdowns," 1 "inadequate psychopath."
m 3 chronically disturbed (4.8%?): 1 "very autistic-like," IQ 65; 1 "anxious and chaotic" at 8, IQ 56, hospitalized at 14, possible "depressive psychosis;" 1 had speech "suggesting a psychotic condition" at 8, perseverative but not grossly psychotic at 12.

(Mz) pairs is raised to 88.2 percent. Similarly, the rates for dizygotic (Dz) pairs (17.1 percent childhood schizophrenia and 22.9 percent total schizophrenics) and siblings are higher when one includes those with adult schizophrenia. In other words, adult schizophrenia tends to cluster in the families of childhood schizophrenics, although most of the illness in siblings and co-twins resembles that in the index cases and occurs before puberty. Rosenthal[188] concluded that "these findings considered collectively make a strong case for the biologic unity of preadolescent and adult schizophrenia and suggested that "preadolescent schizophrenia is a more virulent form which has virtually complete penetrance."

At first glance, the studies of infantile psychosis (Table 14-6) appear contradictory. Bender and Faretra[20] found that 7 percent of the parents were schizophrenic. This is less than the rate for children with later onsets, but it is significantly higher than the prevalence in the general population. Fish found a somewhat lower rate (5.7 percent) in parents of two- to five-year-old schizophrenic children.[70, 82]

On the other hand, six studies have failed to find an increased prevalence of schizophrenia in the parents of infantile psychotics (Table 14-6). The low rate in Kanner's study is not consistent with the relative absence of OBS in his group (Table 14-2) and the 44 percent of his "speaking" group who were psychotic on follow up (Table 14-8). Meyers and Goldfarb[150] reported that 21 percent of parents were schizophrenic, but only 2.4 percent were hospitalized. The remainder included "borderline, pseudoneurotic, and compensated schizophrenics" whom others might consider personalities." Lotter[138] provided some data on relatives who were not officially diagnosed as schizophrenic in hospitals. From his brief vignettes (Table 14-6), 4.8 percent of the siblings appear to be very possibly schizophrenic. While no parent "was known to be schizophrenic," hospital notes were available on only four of the six, and Lotter warns of "the difficulty of obtaining reliable information" on disorders not requiring hospitalization. A careful reading suggests that one to five (e.g., 1.7 percent to 8.3 percent) of these parents might be suspected of having acute psychotic or chronic borderline disorders in the "schizophrenia spectrum."[126] The data are insufficient to make a strong case either for *or* against an increased risk for schizophrenia in these relatives.

These apparent contradictions are not too difficult to understand. It is clear from Table 14-6

that the populations are dissimilar in other ways than their genetic histories. Rutter's[193, 197] and Kolvin and associates'[130] populations have high rates of organic brain disorders. The rates are somewhat lower in Lotter's and Creak's groups but they are still two to six times higher than the OBS in Bender's and Fish's series. One would not expect children with OBS to have families with increased rates of schizophrenia. Hence, it is misleading to calculate parental rates of schizophrenia using populations diluted by a large but indeterminate number of children with OBS. Excluding the children with known and probable OBS would leave much smaller samples on which to calculate rates of familial schizophrenia: a maximum of twenty-three in Rutter's group, twenty-four in Kolvin's, and twenty-two in Lotter's. The actual number of children in each study who are free of OBS is unknown. One should not be surprised to find more familial schizophrenia in populations where organic brain disorders have been excluded more successfully.

These populations also differ with regard to their socioeconomic class composition. The families of Bender's and Fish's infantile psychotics have two to three times more Class V families than the general population, and more than Goldfarb's and Lotter's groups. Kanner's, Creak's, Rutter's, and Kolvin's groups have almost no families in Class V. It has been well established[128] that there is an increased prevalence of schizophrenia in this lowest socioeconomic group. The large number of such families in Bender's and Fish's series[20, 70, 82] is consistent with the family incidence of schizophrenia. The exclusion of Class V families from the other studies, whatever the reasons has apparently eliminated one source of families with high rates of schizophrenia, which was available to the Bellevue studies.

Clinical Course of Childhood Psychosis

CHARACTERISTIC FEATURES AT EACH LEVEL OF DEVELOPMENT

In the vast majority of childhood psychotics deviant development, often from birth, and a variety of disturbed behaviors were present before the onset of the psychosis. These are summarized in Table 14-7. The characteristic features at each level of development, in the life of a psychotic child, depend on the child's maturing abilities and

TABLE 14–7

Developmental Symptoms at Various Ages in Childhood Psychosis

SYMPTOMS	AGE, IN YEARS, MAY APPEAR	INFANTILE AUTISM	CHILDHOOD PSYCHOSIS, OTHER TYPE	CHILDHOOD SCHIZOPHRENIA
Physiological Instability	0–	+	+	+
Growth rate fluctuation	0–	......	+	+
State Behavior and Affect Symptoms				
Excess "quiet," apathy	0–	+	+	+
Irritable, labile	0–	......	+	+
Flat, incongruous	½–	+	......	......
Social Development				
Autistic withdrawal	0–	*+	+	......
Ritualistic behaviors	1–	*+	......	......
Retarded, immature	2–	+	+	+
Gross and Fine Motor Development				
Retarded	0–	+	+	......
Irregular, fluctuates	0–3	......	+	+
Soft neurologic signs	1–	+	+	+
Stereotypic movements	1–	+	......	......
Catatonic posturing	6–	O	O	......
Perceptual Development				
Retarded	0–	+	+	+
Irregular development, variable function	¼–	......	+	+
Bizarre, stereotypic preoccupation with objects	½–	*+	......	......
Distorted percepts (B-G, DAP, TAT, etc.)	4–	......	......	+
Hallucinations specific to schizophrenia	6–	*O	*O	......
Language Development (Verbal and Comprehension)				
Retarded	½–	*+	+	+
Noncommunicative use	1–	*+	+	+
Incoherence 3+-word units)	2–	......	+	+
Incoherence 3+-word units)	2–	*O	*O	*+
Loose, irrelevant associations	2–	*O	*O	*+
Bizarre delusions (somatic)	6–	*O	*O	*+
Paranoid, Schneiderian delusions	9–	*O	*O	......

+ = frequently present; *+ = presence required for diagnosis; O = usually absent; *O = absence required for diagnosis; ...... = may or may not occur.

the severity of the disease. In the first year of life, disorders of motor development and disturbed responsiveness to stimuli are most prominent. Symptoms of more complex functions occur later.

Similar symptoms have been found in all three types of childhood psychosis. A spectrum of deviations in development occurs, with gradations in the severity of the disturbances rather than qualitative differences.* It is stipulated that complex psychotic speech must be present in order to diagnose schizophrenia (as in the DSM-III). This will select out children who have less retarded Verbal IQ's and who are therefore likely to show less severe retardation in other areas. Autistics

* See references 67, 71, 74, 80, 81, 82, and 83.

generally manifest more severe early withdrawal and greater early retardation of development. DQ's under 70 for one or more gross motor landmarks (sitting, standing, walking) were found in one-half of the autistic children studied by Fish[74] and by Lotter,[139] and in one-third of Goldfarb's[96] "organic" subgroup. Fish found milder retardation in one-half of the childhood schizophrenics with higher IQ's.

Lotter[139] and Bender and Faretra[20] reported delayed speech in 50 to 60 percent of infantile psychotics. Kolvin reported that 88 percent of infantile psychotics acquired three-word sentences after three years. Fish and associates[82] found that only infantile psychotics with language DQ's over 30 had used sentences before three. Bender and

Faretra[20] and Kolvin and associates[130] also reported speech delays in about one-half the schizophrenic children with onsets after two years.

Infantile Autism: The very young autistic infant is frequently overly quiet and apathetic. Muscle tone, crying, and activity are decreased, and there is no postural accommodation to being picked up. Other cases are excessively irritable, rigid, and tense, with irregular patterns of feeding and sleeping. Gross motor development is often retarded but may be irregular. For example, the infant may raise his head very early but not sit for months; or he stands as soon as he sits but seems fearful, unstable, and won't walk for months.

There is often an inattentiveness to the face and voice plus a lack of response to other visual stimuli; at the same time there is often an oversensitivity to minor noises. Inattention to toys is succeeded by absent or deviant reaching for and manipulation of objects. These may only be cast or flicked away, or dropped from a limp hand. The infant usually does not develop the differentiated social responses of the second six months; he does not comprehend or imitate gestures, play "peek-a-boo," "pat-a-cake," or wave bye-bye. Babbling and the first words may develop with minimal delay in the second six months, only to be dropped later; or speech may be retarded from the beginning.

These deviations appear more bizarre in the second year. The child remains mute and unresponsive, or speaks only rarely, and then in echolalic fashion. As visual-motor and perceptual development do not progress normally, the child's strange, restricted, and stereotyped manipulation of objects, and his ritualistic behaviors, become more obvious. In severely retarded autistic children, once behavior has reached this level, there may be very little change thereafter. Other cases may progress in a variety of ways including an evolution into a clearly schizophrenic picture.

Schizophrenia in Early Childhood: The preschizophrenic infant may show the same early deviations as the young autistic infant. Here, however, development is more likely to be punctuated by erratic accelerations with more evidence of precocity. The preschizophrenic infant may also be overly responsive, and very demanding of attention; he may seem to be an alert, sociable infant, although usually with increased sensitivity and difficulty in imitative and gestural play.

Disturbed behavior usually becomes prominent in the second year. The child may show an increased withdrawal; he may display severe panic reaction and desperate clinging to the mother; or he may have violent tantrums with minimal or no apparent cause. The severity of these behaviors and the combination of extreme hostility and excessively fearful dependence results in chaotic, frantic behavior, which usually baffles the parents. If emerging speech is obviously noncommunicative and idiosyncratic, the child's psychosis becomes clearly recognizable.

If language is less fragmented, the child may enter school, but his disturbed behavior makes normal peer interaction impossible. Academic performance is impaired or reflects his obsessive preoccupation with certain topics or fantasies. Fantasies generally involve morbid preoccupations with the body's functioning or with introjected persons or objects; or they involve exaggerated preoccupations with oral aggression, with the child's own identity and with his orientation in time and space.[18]

From about five or six on, schizophrenic children may develop severe anxiety states with obsessive and compulsive phenomena, or they can exhibit all manner of persecutory and paranoid symptomatology, becoming withdrawn or violently aggressive and destructive. Any combination of these manifestations may occur. These children must be differentiated diagnostically from children with neuroses and from those with antisocial, aggressive behavior disorders.

Around nine to eleven years, projection begins to replace introjection as a psychic mechanism. The child begins to be aware of hallucinations beyond the body's surface and may organize some of his confusing and disturbing experiences within a persecutory and paranoid framework. However, at this age, hallucinations and delusions still tend to be fragmented and are not as well organized as they are in the adolescent and adult schizophrenic. If school functioning and relationships with peers have seemed adequate up to this point, this adaptation is soon severely disrupted by the overwhelming psychotic preoccupations.

CLINICAL VARIETIES
OF CHILDHOOD PSYCHOSIS

Infantile Autism: The major subdivisions of infantile autism depend first on whether or not a specific organic brain disorder is present. If so, the outcome is generally poorer and depends on the course of the underlying organic pathology. Subdivisions according to Verbal and Performance

IQ's under 30, 50, and 70 are highly predictive of later cognitive and social functioning and reflect the severity of the psychosis. Divisions by IQ make for reliable comparisons of children in different studies.

Childhood Schizophrenia: Primary subdivisions according to IQ's above or below 70 predict outcome and reflect the severity of disruption by the psychosis. Children with IQ's under 70, resemble Bender's[14] "pseudodefective" schizophrenics and those termed "autistic dysjunctive" (Type I) and "immature labile" (Type II) by Fish and Shapiro.[81] They show grossly unintegrated, deviate, and retarded functioning in all areas.

Children with IQ's over 70 can elaborate their psychotic preoccupations. They may resemble Bender's[14] "pseudoneurotic" schizophrenics who present the picture of pan-neurosis with anxiety, phobias, obsessions, compulsions, or hypochondriacal symptoms; in addition they may experience intense concern about body boundaries, body image, identification and orientation in time and space. They display disturbances in thought processes and speech, distortion in all perceptual areas, and exaggerated or unusual introjections and projections. They often display exaggerated insight, precocious verbal and graphic abilities, an unusual capacity for abstract conceptualization, and high intelligence. Children in this group or stage are often recommended for psychotherapy.

Bender's "pseudopsychopathic" type is seen most often in late childhood or adolescence. These children present paranoid ideation, difficulties in identification with peers, and negativistic reactions to authority. They tend to aggressive and antisocial acting out, with persecutory preoccupation.

There is actually much overlapping of symptoms across these three or four major types, with children often showing intermediate forms which share some features of two or more types. The above arbitrary subdivisions establish boundaries along what are actually continua of pathology, maturational, and integrative disorders.[81] The diagnostic subtypes represent modal clusters of symptoms; the children do not come in such neat "packages." Furthermore, as time goes on, many change from a "pseudodefective" to a "pseudoneurotic" type, or from a pseudoneurotic to a pseudopsychopathic or paranoid form.

Continuity, Distribution Along the Life Cycle, Exacerbation and Remission

Follow-up studies should indicate whether childhood psychosis is continuous with adult schizophrenia, or with other adult disorders.

Childhood Psychoses in Adolescence: Five major studies* followed 401 psychotic children until they reached a mean age of fourteen to fifteen years (Table 14-8). Goldfarb's[93] follow up of forty-eight schizophrenic children to a mean age of 16.6 years indicated that 50 percent were institutionalized, and 65 percent were grossly impaired. Outcome (reported according to ratings of ego function) was related to the initial ratings of ego impairment. The "ego" ratings reflected both IQ and severity of psychosis. This method of reporting precluded tabulation on Table 14-8 and any easy comparison with the other studies. No diagnoses were reported.

Of Kanner and Eisenberg's[125] autistics with speech "around four years of age," 44 percent were "clearly psychotic" by the time they reached adolescence. All but one of the others were severely schizoid and eccentric. The "atypical" children followed by Brown[35, 36, 37] and Reiser and Brown[176] had the same symptoms as Kanner's autistics[37] (Table 14-4). Their outcome was similar as well. (Table 14-8). Reiser and Brown[176] report fewer schizophrenics, but the 30 percent who were "severely disturbed" included those considered "comparable to adult hebephrenics" and those who were "between adults with simple schizophrenia and those with severe inadequate personality disorders." "Several" (number not reported) of the schizoids became schizophrenic later.[176] Brown[35] reported five such cases (added to Table 14-8). Havelkova's[108] group had a poorer social and educational outcome (Table 14-8). The follow-up diagnoses of 100 percent psychotic (schizophrenia or autism) were not defined further.

Creak's[51] group appears to have been more like Kanner's nonspeaking autistics (Table 14-8). However, she did not report initial IQ's nor follow-up diagnoses. Rutter and associates[196] group appears to be the most severely impaired of all. Their outcome closely resembles that of Kanner's mute autistics (Table 14-8). Unfortunately, Rutter did not report the psychiatric diagnoses in adolescence. Apparently, at least 10 percent to 16 percent resembled Kanner's severe schizoids, and a large number (not specified) had incoherent speech. No "convincing evidence of hallucinations" or delusions was elicited.

In all of these studies, poor prognosis was related to a low level of intellectual functioning in the pre-school years. No words by "about four years,"[125] no speech when the child was over

---

* See references 35, 36, 37, 51, 108, 125, 136, 137, 176, 196, and 197.

TABLE 14-8

Outcome of Infantile Psychosis in Adolescence

	KANNER & EISENBERG (1955)			BROWN (1960, 1963, 1969); REISER AND BROWN (1964)	HAVELKOVA (1968)	CREAK (1963)	RUTTER & LOCKYER (1967) RUTTER ET AL. (1967)	
	TOTAL	NO SPEECH	SPEAKING				TOTAL	>16 YEARS
Number Followed[a]	42	19	23	129	71	100	63	38
% IQ's < 70 (First Observation)[a]	≧45?[c]	100	—	—	—	—	71	—
% Definite OBS[b]	1	—	—	—	—	14	35	—
Age at Follow-Up in Years—Range (Mean)	8–24(14)	—	—	9–22	8–17	—	(15.7)	>16
% Diagnosis (Adolescence):								
Normal-Neurotic	2	0	4	13	0	—	—	—
Schizoid	31	5	52	23	0	—	—	—
Schizophrenic/Psychotic	24	0	44	11	100	—	—	—
Other Severe Disturbance	0	0	0	30	0	—	—	—
Severe MR (IQ < 35)	43	95	0	23	—	—	≧63?[d]	—
% Adjustment (Adolescence):								
Regular School or Employed	33	5	56	36	24	15	8	8
Special Class or Training Center	0	0	0	11	0	42	33	21
School/Institution For Disturbed	17	11	22	17	30	43	45	53
School/Institution For Retarded	24	37	13	30	46	0	14	18
Home; No School or Job	26	47	9	6	0	—	—	—
IQ's (Adolescence):								
% < 70	—	—	—	63	61	—	—[e]	—
% < 50	≧43?[d]	95[d]	≧0?[d]	41	28	—	63[c]	—

a As in Table 14–1.
b As in Table 14–2.
c No figures reported. We calculated minimum percent from number without speech.
d No figures reported. We calculated minimum percent from description of number who were "markedly feebleminded." Some of "psychotic" may be retarded, also.
e Wechsler Full Scale mean = 76.6 for 17; Vineland mean = 47 for 53 children (Lockyer and Rutter, 1969).

three years old,[37] and Performance IQ's below 60[196] characterized the children who remained profoundly retarded. In Havelkova's[108] study, there was a group who developed useful speech and emerged from an autistic picture to a pseudo-neurotic form of schizophrenia; 69 percent of the children who accomplished this before four and one-half years of age had normal intellect at follow-up.

Childhood Schizophrenia Followed Into Adulthood: Unfortunately, few authors have followed psychotic children into adulthood. Rutter's[193] report of a mail follow up, at a mean age of 21.7 years, provided information on social adjustment and additional cases of epilepsy (Table 14-2), but no other neurologic and no psychiatric diagnoses. Kanner[120] followed only the first eleven cases but gave no diagnoses. Bennett and Klein[25] followed the severe childhood schizophrenics who were originally studied by Potter.[171] On reexamination in their forties, all twelve were indistinguishable from chronic adult schizophrenics (Table 14-9). Only one maintained himself outside a hospital; most were severely deteriorated.

The most detailed information is available on one hundred childhood schizophrenics followed by Bender[9, 20] up to ages twenty-two to forty-five years. Other psychiatrists had diagnosed ninety-four as adult schizophrenics. One had psychosis with psychopathic personality, and five were considered to be organically defective (Table 14–9). Annell's[4] findings were similar, although her follow up extended only to twenty-three years and used stricter European criteria for the diagnosis. Adult diagnoses were the same for children with onsets under two years[20,55] (Table 14–9). While only 50 percent of the infantile psychotics in Dahl's[55] series were diagnosed unquestionably schizophrenic in hospitals as adults, four additional patients (40 percent, for a possible total of 90 percent) appear to be in the "schizophrenia spectrum." Their independent hospital diagnoses were: one diagnosed "schizophreniform psychosis" (at fifteen) and "schizophrenia (pseudoneurosis)" (at eighteen); one diagnosed psychosis secondary to oligophrenia (at fifteen to twenty-two) and schizophrenia (at twenty-eight); one schizoid character disorder; one "psychosis infantilis antea" (whom Dahl personally diagnosed, as he reported in a personal communication in 1976, as borderline schizophrenia).

Bender's[9] detailed report of outcome attests to the severity and chronicity of the disease when schizophrenic symptoms begin early. Compared to schizophrenics first admitted as adolescents or adults, twice as many childhood schizophrenics (63 percent) remain chronically disabled and institutionalized (33 percent). Children with onsets before two years had the highest rate (72 percent) of chronicity, compared to those with later onsets (54 percent chronically institutionalized). To some extent, this increased chronicity resulted from the larger number (83 percent) of early-onset schizophrenics whose IQ's remained below 70, compared to those with later onsets (49 percent).

Bender's[9] tables of the serial IQ's demonstrate the variability of IQ in childhood schizophrenia, which parallels the fluctuating course of illness. Bright children who became mute and catatonic became untestable. Others were untestable early, but matured to levels well above 70. Marked variability was more characteristic of children with IQ's over 50 but occurred in some with lower

TABLE 14–9

*Percentage of Childhood Schizophrenics
Independently Diagnosed Schizophrenic as Adults*

AUTHOR	PUB. YEAR	ONSET (YEARS)	n	PERCENT SCHIZOPHRENIC AS ADULTS (AGE RANGE IN YEARS)
Annell	1963	<2–9	19	85 (15–23)
Bennett & Klein	1966	3.5–10	12	100 (40–45)
Bender	1972	<2–10	100	94 (22–45)
Bender	1972	<2	50	90 (22–45)
Dahl	1976	<2–<14	17	53[a] (20–40)
Dahl	1976	<2	10	50 (20–40)

[a]One-third of these diagnosed chronic "atypical psychosis." "Same characteristics as the schizophrenics," including hallucinations, but less florid symptoms and lower intellectual function.

TABLE 14–10

Adult Adjustment of Childhood Schizophrenics (Onsets < 2 and 2–10 Years) in Relation to the Maximum IQ Before 11 Years

| | MAXIMUM IQ < 11 YEARS | | |
	<70	>70	TOTAL
Number	39	61	100
Percent employed:			
Fully	5	11	9
Partially	0	5	3
Percent dependent or marginally adjusted	8	36	25
Percent chronically institutionalized	87	48	63

SOURCE: Adapted from Bender, L., "The Life Course of Schizophrenic Children," *Biologic Psychiatry,* 2:165–172, 1970.

IQ's. Of those who later adjusted in the community, 52 percent had IQ's which rose 10 to 40 points between two to six years and latency. Only 28 percent of the chronic patients had similar increases.

In Bender's long-term study of these one hundred schizophrenic children,[9, 20] the major factor predicting adult outcome was the maximum IQ achieved before eleven years (Table 14–10).

There were a number of children who attained IQ's over 70 at some time before they were eleven years old. For these individuals full employment as an adult, and marginally to totally dependent adjustments in the community, were eventually much more frequent. However, even among these cases, at some time in the course of their childhood illness (before they were eleven) one of those who became fully employed and one-half of those who made dependent or marginal adjustments had had some IQ scores below 70. Of those whose IQ's never rose above 70 before age eleven, 87 percent remained chronically institutionalized. Given the variability of IQ in childhood schizrophenia, one should not predict chronic institutionalization from a single IQ in childhood. It would be necessary to follow the course of the illness with serial IQ's, to determine whether any significant improvement would occur before eleven.

In this large series of severely ill schizophrenic children, only nine ever became fully employed. Six of these were bright youngsters with onsets after two years, who before eleven had maximum IQ's that ranged from 96 to 154. Three never required hospitalization after their initial treatment. The rest of the children who adjusted at some level in the community included children with onsets before or after two years, and chil-

dren who achieved maximum IQ's of 44 to over 90 before eleven years. Generally, these children were hospitalized for longer periods before they could make any community adjustment. Some have been out since mid-adolescence. The rest were discharged as adults.

Changes in Clinical Symptomatology from Childhood to Adulthood: The variety of clinical courses and the evolution of the clinical picture in those children who have been followed into adulthood can best be illustrated by very condensed vignettes. These are chosen to illustrate the various onsets and eventual outcomes discussed above. Autism remained static or evolved into childhood schizophrenia; the latter changed in form and severity and evolved into adult schizophrenia or a compensated borderline or schizoid state.

1. *Onset under two; autism, no speech: chronically institutionalized.* "Richard"[120, 124] was autistic with no words at thirty-nine months. He responded intermittently to commands. DQ on the formboard was approximately 75. He is reported to have said "good night" at around five. He was institutionalized from nine years. At thirty-three, he was essentially unchanged; nonverbal and withdrawn.

2. *Onset under two; autism; childhood schizophrenia; chronic undifferentiated schizophrenia: chronically institutionalized.* "SB"[9, 11] was autistic; fearful, with tantrums in childhood. At nine, he was characterized as "cataleptic, echolalic, jingling neologisms." IQ's: 47 at seven years; 35 at nine; 49 at eleven. Since adolescence he has been chronically hospitalized. Untestable at nineteen years, at thirty-two years his IQ was 19. At thirty-nine years, he was was disturbed and bizarre.

3. *Onset under two; infantile autism; childhood*

schizophrenia; chronic undifferentiated schizophrenia: dependent in community. "HJ"[9, 11] was autistic; fearful, with tantrums in childhood. Despite an IQ of 86 at six years, he was unable to attend school. At eleven, he became mute, tense, and resistive (IQ 71). After pentylenetetrazol (Metrazol) treatment he went home and attended special classes until eighteen, achieving third grade work. At follow up at thirty-eight years, he had remained at home, continued to be withdrawn, and was dependent on mother.

4. *Onset under two; infantile autism; childhood schizophrenia; schizoid personality disorder: employed.* "Donald"[120, 124] was autistic, withdrawn, with stereotyped behaviors and elaborate verbal rituals. Speech was predominantly psychotic, and characterized by the ejaculation of irrelevant words and phrases. By seven, he was no longer grossly psychotic but was eccentrically obsessive, with occasional metaphorical language. He progressed at a country school, eventually got a B.A. and worked as a bank teller. At thirty-six, mother reported that he was a bachelor living with his parents. He participated in community activities but "takes very little part in social conversations and shows no interest in the opposite sex" (not reexamined).

5. *Onset six years; childhood schizophrenia; borderline schizophrenia: employed.* From two and one-half, "MP"[9, 11, 87] had had prolonged terrors and panic; at four he was phobic. At five, he became mute and at six, was withdrawn, anxious, clinging, and used bizarre language (IQ 76). He improved with psychotherapy and was able to return home (IQ 96 at seven years), but he was unable to get along in school or with peers. At ten he required pentylenetetrazol (Metrazol) treatment, but has been home since then (IQ 79 at fifteen). He graduated high school and then worked as a door-to-door salesman until last follow up at age forty years (IQ 80 at twenty-two). At follow up, he was empty, dreamy, flat; he experienced marked feelings of unreality; was possessed by many obsessive thoughts and somatic preoccupations; and remained in constant conflict with his parents. He apparently had no real relationships with anyone.

6. *Onset six years; childhood schizophrenia; no mental disease; sociopathic personality disorder; chronic paranoid schizophrenia: dependent.* "PA"[9, 11, 13, 87] was always querulous, asocial, and dependent. At six, he developed bizarre grimacing and posturing, complained of bugs and dirt in his food, and was unable to attend school. At nine, he became withdrawn, was preoccupied with auditory hallucinations, and had incoherent speech (IQ 87). He improved at eleven (IQ 99) and appeared normal until fifteen, attending school with many friends and interests. At fifteen, however, he became antisocial and delinquent. One year later, at sixteen, he again became acutely psychotic hallucinating and delusional (IQ 80 to 64). He was in and out of hospitals as a paranoid schizophrenic for the next fifteen years. From thirty-one until the last follow up when he was thirty-eight, he remained at home in a dependent state.

7. *Onset ten years; chronic paranoid schizophrenia: chronically institutionalized.* "JC"[9, 11, 87] was always anxious, seclusive, and asocial. He was hospitalized from ten to fourteen and diagnosed as catatonic schizophrenia. He hallucinated voices in his head telling him to kill (between eleven and thirteen his IQ was 74, 68, 78). From fourteen to twenty, he was in and out of state hospitals, adjusted poorly at school, and was unable to work. He served in the army from twenty to twenty-two. From twenty-three to the last follow up at thirty-eight, he had continued to shuttle in and out of hospitals and was unable to function. He was diagnosed chronic paranoid schizophrenia.

The continuity between childhood schizophrenia and adult schizophrenia has been documented by the follow ups into adult life. Half of Bender's group had their onsets with autism or symbiotic psychosis before two years. The patterns of changing diagnoses as the clinical picture evolves from infancy and early childhood to latency, adolescence, and adulthood are exemplified in the above vignettes and in many other examples in the literature (Bender[11, 87] and references cited in Bender and Faretra[20]). The distinctions between schizophrenic residual state, borderline schizophrenia, schizoid personality disorder, and no mental disease obviously require a careful, independent psychiatric evaluation and cannot be based on reports from relatives. Other follow ups of large series of autistic children* have yet to report the psychiatric and neurologic diagnoses made in adulthood.

ASSOCIATED SOMATIC EXPRESSION

Soft Neurological Signs: Bender[18] was the first to call attention to the pervasiveness of soft neurologic signs in young, schizophrenic children, especially those with onsets before two years. These signs generally represent delayed and re-

* See references 36, 51, 108, 125, 176, 196, and 197.

tarded development or poor integration of CNS functioning; they do not constitute a syndrome which points to any specific localization in the CNS. The soft neurologic signs included delayed motor development, immature and poorly co-ordinated movement, and poor integration of visual, auditory, and proprioceptive perceptions. Their possible etiological significance is discussed below.

Similar soft neurologic signs have been found in adolescent schizophrenics[112] and in adult schizophrenics, especially in those with thought disorders[222] and in those with a premorbid history of asociality.[173]

Congenital Stigmata: Goldfarb[95] reported that compared to normal controls, there was an increased number of congenital stigmata in schizophrenic children. The mean number of stigmata for the schizophrenics was 2.48; that for the normals was 0.65. Thirty-eight percent of the schizophrenics had four or more stigmata each, whereas this was true for only one percent of the normals. Waldrop and Halverson[223] found a similar increase of congenital stigmata in one subgroup of hyperactive boys. This reflects some embryonic and fetal maldevelopment in early onset schizophrenics[95] as well as in a subgroup of hyperactive and developmentally disordered children.

Physical Growth: Bender's[18] clinical impression was that "growth discrepanices are marked. The children are too big or too little, too fat or too thin." Menstruation occurred early in several girls with the onset of schizophrenia and without other gross endocrine anomalies. Precocious or delayed puberty in boys also occurred. She considered that this unevenness in the regulation of somatic growth and the "nonspecific endocrine dyscrasias would seem to explain the dysplastic features of many adult schizophrenics." Compared to matched controls, twice as many schizophrenics had some abnormality in height and weight, but this trend did not reach significance.[23] Goldfarb[96] found no significant differences.

However, Dutton[61] found definite growth failure in a group of boys who had been psychotic from an early age, and who functioned on a mentally retarded level. Compared to standard norms, twenty-five percent had depressed linear growth and seventeen percent had delayed skeletal maturation (below two standard deviations from the mean). Simon and Gillies[209] found bone age to be below the tenth percentile in 34 percent of children; a number also fell below the tenth percentile in height. In sum, a subgroup of psychotic children without OBS showed definite growth failure.

Fish[67, 71, 76] demonstrated that when growth was measured serially in preschizophrenic infants, periods of retarded physical growth accompanied the periods when postural-motor and visual-motor development showed abnormalities. These periods of "pandevelopmental retardation" appeared to reflect active disorganization of CNS maturation. Longitudinal growth curves thus seem to be more sensitive indicators of growth failure than single cross-sectional comparisons between groups.

Other Physiological and Homeostatic Disturbances: Bender described irregular physiological rhythms in the eating, sleeping, and elimination patterns of schizophrenic children, and vasovegetative control which was excessively labile or underresponsive.[18, 23] Children were flushed and perspiring, or had blue, cold extremities. There might be excessive fever with minor infections or normal temperatures with severe illness. If abnormal responses to pain, illness, noise, and vascular responses were combined, one-half of the schizophrenic children showed such abnormalities, and none of the matched controls did. This was significant at the .001 level.[23]

Organic Etiologic Factors

ENDOGENOUS FACTORS

It should be clear from the previous discussions that etiology can be discussed only for specifically defined subgroups of childhood psychosis.

Genetic, Constitutional: Only three subgroups of childhood psychosis have families with an increased number of schizophrenic relatives (Table 14–6):

1. Children whose psychosis began after five years, and who show formal thought disorders, hallucinations, or delusions, which are characteristic for schizophrenia (Table 14–6; Kallman, Kolvin, Bender: "onset over two").

2. Children whose psychosis began before two years, or between two and five years, who show a characteristic schizophrenic formal thought disorder when seen (Table 14–6; Bender, Fish: schizophrenics with speech).

These two groups 1. and 2. would be diagnosed as schizophrenia in the DSM-III.[1]

3. Preschizophrenic children with infantile psychosis. They present no evidence of OBS; they

display absent or primitive and noncommunicative speech when they are seen before five years; and they manifest the disorders of integration, perception, cognition, and irregular development, described as specific for schizophrenia. Using the DSM-III, some fit the criteria for infantile autism. The remainder would be diagnosed as "Childhood psychosis, other type."[1] Such children were included in the groups of infantile psychosis studied by Bender and Fish, who had increased genetic histories for schizophrenia (Table 14–6; Bender, Fish: schizophrenics without speech). At follow up, these children have also proved to be schizophrenic. (Table 14–9.)

Children who would be diagnosed as schizophrenic in the DSM-III (Groups 1. and 2.), therefore share the same genetic predisposition for schizophrenia as do their adult counterparts. Such children have onsets before two years, as well as after. Preschizophrenic children with infantile psychosis share this predisposition (Group 3.), but in the early stages of their illness they would be diagnosed as infantile autism or "Childhood psychosis, other type," according to the DSM-III.[1] Additional studies are needed to accumulate a larger body of genetic data for childhood schizophrenia, as has been done for adult schizophrenia. Data for children in Group 3. should be analyzed separately, until follow up has demonstrated that they meet the DSM-III criteria for schizophrenia in childhood.

Most groups of children diagnosed as infantile autism, according to the DSM-III,[1] will have lower rates of schizophrenic relatives. Indeed, their rate approaches that of the general population (Table 14–6; Kanner, Creak, Rutter, Kolvin, Lotter). The preschizophrenic children described in Group 3. might be included in such groups. However, unless additional criteria are used to select a preschizophrenic sample, these would be diluted by profoundly retarded infantile psychotics who have a high incidence of specific organic brain disorders.

Neurologic, Congenital: A variety of neurologic and congenital abnormalities occur in childhood psychosis. The question is, which of these are specific to childhood psychosis or any of its subgroups? Only then can one consider their possible etiologic significance.

1. Specific Organic Brain Disorders with Infantile Autism

Studies of infantile autistics which did not exclude specific organic brain disorders found such conditions in 30 to 100 percent of the cases (Table 14–2; Rutter, Kolvin, Lotter, Knobloch,

Schain). The frequency was lower if drawn from a population of psychiatric patients, and higher if children were selected from pediatric or neurologic cohorts, or from institutions for the retarded. This difference arises because children with gross neurologic disorders usually are not referred for psychiatric evaluation.

A wide variety of neurologic disorders was found in these studies: many types of epilepsy, as well as cerebral palsy, phenylketonuria, severe brain hemorrhage, toxoplasmosis, neurolues, meningitis, lead encephalopathy, neurolipoidosis, and others. Autism also has been described in children with congenital rubella.[44] Obviously, the vast majority of children with these diseases do not have infantile autism.

The occasional association of aspects of the syndrome with such disorders does raise questions for those interested in the possible brain substrates that underlie autistic symptoms. Schain and Yannet[201] discuss the limbic system as a possible site of dysfunction, which might explain the affective disorder and the seizures. One autopsy showed a dropping out of cells in the hippocampus. Hauser and associates[107] found evidence of temporal lobe disorder in fifteen of seventeen pneumoencephalograms and in one-half of the electroencephalograms. They emphasized the importance of this area in explaining the impaired language function of these children. "Autistics" in these two studies do not appear to meet the DSM-III criteria. Ornitz and Ritvo hypothesized a neurophysiologic mechanism which might produce the syndrome, whether or not it is associated with specific neurologic disorder.

2. Pregnancy Complications and Infantile Psychosis

The studies analyzed above (Table 14–2) indicate that the incidence of pregnancy complications is two to three times higher in infantile psychotics than in those with later onsets. There is also a higher incidence of mental retardation in infantile psychosis (Table 14–1).

Within the infantile group, there is some tendency for higher rates of pregnancy complications to be associated with lower IQ's. Bender and Faretra's[20] "autistic" group had a higher rate (50 percent) than their symbiotic group (33 percent). Fish and associates'[82] schizophrenic children without speech had a slightly higher rate (40 percent) than those with speech (30 percent). The same association between low IQ and pregnancy complications holds true for Goldfarb's[96] "organic" group.

Pregnancy complications appear to add a nonspecific impairment to the clinical picture, which includes a lowering of IQ. This may be similar to the influence of pregnancy complications in many other types of disturbed children.

Two recent studies permit a finer analysis of the pregnancy complications associated with psychotic children and with children genetically vulnerable to schizophrenia. Both utilized the prospective data from the Collaborative Perinatal Study of the National Institute of Neurological Diseases and Stroke. Among the 30,000 children analyzed, Torrey and associates[221] identified twenty children with infantile autism and childhood schizophrenia. Only three had any suspicion of neurological abnormality (abnormal EEG only, or soft neurologic signs). The perinatal data were compared with matched low IQ and normal IQ controls. The only significant difference was an increase in uterine bleeding for the experimental group, especially in the second trimester. It was minimally symptomatic and without any apparent cause.

Rieder and associates[180] compared offspring of schizophrenic parents and matched controls from the same Collaborative Study. Vaginal bleeding or edema of the face and hands during the pregnancies of chronic schizophrenic mothers, or of women married to such schizophrenics, was predictive of a lower seven-year IQ in the child. Low birth weight and poor socioeconomic conditions were not predictive. Schizophrenic fathers as well as mothers were involved, so this was not the adverse affect of a schizophrenic mother on her child in utero. It appeared that these children had a genetic vulnerability which made them more susceptible than their controls to these particular pregnancy complications. This suggests a possible mechanism for the effect of complications on schizophrenic children.

3. Soft Neurologic Signs in Childhood Psychosis

The soft neurologic signs which are found frequently in childhood psychosis have been described above. They involve poor integration and organization of motor and perceptual functions. The manifestations change with age and with the developmental level and cognitive capacity of the child. Therefore, in severely retarded children with infantile autism there are more primitive manifestations present than in bright schizophrenic children.[18] Only some of these signs appear to be specific for childhood psychosis.

The soft neurologic signs which are similar to those seen in OBS and other developmental disorders may have a similar significance when they occur in childhood psychosis. They are more frequent in the severely retarded psychotic children; this suggests that they reflect a general deficit in brain function. The mothers of these children also have the highest incidence of pregnancy complications, a factor which might give rise to soft neurological signs.

However, nonspecific brain damage does not explain the "soft signs" of many bright schizophrenic children. The pattern of their cognitive and perceptual dysfunction differs from that in organic brain damage. It is more variable, and it is characterized by combinations of advanced and retarded functions which are not seen with OBS. In many of these children there is no evidence of any pregnancy or birth complications. Soft neurologic signs in some schizophrenic children appear to be the static "residues" of an earlier neurologic disturbance which is characteristic of preschizophrenic infants, and which differs from the delays seen in organically brain damaged infants.

4. The Neurointegrative Disorder in Preschizophrenic and Vulnerable Infants; Pandevelopmental Retardation

The histories of children with infantile autism and childhood schizophrenia often reveal retarded gross motor and fine motor development. In some schizophrenic children, especially those with IQ's between fifty and ninety, evidence can be found for both accelerated and retarded gross motor development.

Fish studied development prospectively in children of schizophrenic mothers and nonpsychotic mothers*; at the point of the most recent observation, they were sixteen to twenty-three years old. Standard infant tests and measurements were repeated ten times from birth to two years, at key ages. Separate DQ's were obtained for postural-motor, visual-motor, integrative functions, and language development. Behavioral state and caloric vestibular responses were measured. Independent psychologic and psychiatric assessments were made when the children were ten, and again at eighteen years.

There were two children who were later diagnosed as childhood schizophrenics. In both instances, analysis of the developmental curves revealed a major disorganization of neurologic maturation.[71] There was no fixed neurologic defect but rather a disorder of the timing and integration of neurologic maturation from the first months of life. This differed from the usual forms of retardation and precocity. First, there was an

---

* See references 67, 71, 76, 77, 78, 80, and 83.

unusual fluctuation in the rates of postural-motor, visual-motor, and physical development (e.g., the DQ dropped thirty points in two months, and then rose fifty points within three months). Sometimes, there was a temporary loss of a previously acquired ability. Sometimes, they showed a reversed cephalocaudal gradient of postural development, with head control lagging months behind the control of trunk and legs. At times, a "higher" function remained relatively intact while more primitive functions, such as motor ability, were severely retarded. This is the reverse of the pattern in diffuse, chronic brain damage.[168] The erratic functioning on developmental testing is analogous to the disturbance of older schizophrenic patients who fail easy items on an intelligence test and then succeed on more advanced items during the same session.

The most severe generalized retardation involved physical growth, as well as postural-motor and/or visual-motor development. This "pandevelopmental retardation" (PDR) was related to psychiatric morbidity at ten years.[67, 71] It was most severe in the two preschizophrenic infants and most extreme in the one where the onset was earlier, and the cognitive and perceptual impairments more severe. Children whose PDR was milder and shorter, later had severe to moderate schizoid, paranoid, or inadequate personality disorders that fell within the "schizophrenia spectrum." Another group of these children displayed no retardation of physical growth; at ten years, their disorders were even milder. By that same age PDR was significantly correlated with severe to moderate psychiatric disorder. PDR was not related to pregnancy or birth complications. However, there was a significant correlation with a history of schizophrenia in the mother.

In addition to PDR, three abnormal patterns in the first months of life were found in schizophrenics' offspring. The first was an "abnormally quiet" state. These infants did not cry in the first month, even with vigorous postural manipulation. At the same time their responses to visual, auditory, and tactile stimuli were normal or increased. They displayed extreme underactivity, flaccidity, and overextensibility of the joints, with doughy muscle tone but normal, though pendular, deep tendon reflexes. There were several types of severe disturbances of visual-motor functioning: delays in visual fixation on objects held in the hand; severe delays in reaching and manipulation in the first year, with failure of bimanual integration at the midline; apraxia; and retarded form perception in the second year. This was followed at ten years by failures on the WISC Block Design subtest and on other perceptual tests. The "quiet" state and delayed bimanual integration were associated with later psychiatric morbidity.

Decreased to absent vestibular responsiveness was associated with the periods of PDR between birth and two years, with the "abnormally quiet" state in the first month, and with the failures of bimanual integration in the fourth and seventh months. Its transitory nature rules out any organic lesion of the vestibular system. Decreased nystagmus is a sensitive indicator of slight decreases in arousal.[50, 169] This suggests that transitory states of decreased CNS activity (manifested by depression of gross motor, proprioceptive, and vestibular functions, but not of vision or hearing), accompanied periods when CNS integration was disrupted.

Early developmental disorder was correlated with perceptual disorders which, at ten years, constitute soft neurologic signs. PDR between six and nine months was followed by failures on the formboard in the second year. Failure on the formboard was in turn significantly related to failures on the Block Design subtest of the WISC, at ten years, and to other perceptual defects (high Koppitz scores on the Bender-Gestalt, poor fine coordination, and defective finger schema). These perceptual defects and associated specific reading disabilities occurred significantly more often in the schizophrenic offspring, although only one mother had pregnancy complications.

Direct measurement of preschizophrenic infants, therefore, reveals a neurointegrative defect, which results in a dysregulation of maturation at all levels. The profile of successes and failures on any single exam was unlike that seen in chronic brain syndromes. The severity correlated with later psychiatric morbidity. Disorder at critical early ages predicted perceptual defects or soft neurologic signs in latency, which sometimes persisted into adult life.

Biochemical and Hematologic Studies: Over the past several decades, many investigators have attempted to identify neurobiochemical and hematologic abnormalities in adult schizophrenic patients. This work has been extended recently at a few centers to include children with the syndromes of autism and childhood schizophrenia.

In this section, those studies will be reviewed, in chronological order which relate to indoleamines, tryptophan metabolism, catecholamines, and hematologic factors. Unfortunately, three ubiquitous methodological issues limit cross-comparison of research results from these studies.

These issues are: (1) the lack of diagnostic specificity, (2) differences in the biochemical assay techniques employed, and (3) the lack of normative developmental data for many of the measures employed.

1. Indoleamines. In 1961, Schain and Freedman reported on the first study of serotonin levels in the blood of children diagnosed as having "autism" and other forms of mental retardation. They remarked that "consistent, unusual elevations of blood serotonin were found only in children with a diagnosis of autism, although the mean 5-HT level of the other severely retarded children was higher than that of the mildly retarded group."

These findings were confirmed and elaborated upon in a second study by Ritvo and associates.[185] These authors surveyed serotonin levels and platelet counts in twenty-four autistic and thirty-six age-matched comparison children. Results indicated that

both serotonin and platelet were inversely related to age in the normal population; the mean serotonin and platelet counts of age-matched groups of autistics were significantly higher than comparison cases; and, the mean serotonin per platelet values were not significantly different between age-matched groups of autistics and comparison subjects. However, a significantly greater variability of serotonin per platelet was found within the youngest group of age-matched patients, when compared with controls (24 to 47 months).[185]

A third survey of serotonin and platelets in autistic children was reported in 1970 by Boullin, Coleman, and O'Brien.[32] They observed no differences between mean platelet size, "but the number of platelets per milliliter of plasma was significantly increased in the autistic patients. No concomitant increase in serotonin per platelet was noted, rather the concentration was slightly diminished."

In 1971, the authors[234] reported an attempt to observe the circadian rhythmicity of blood serotonin levels and platelet counts in seven autistic and four nonautistic inpatients. The studies were unable to demonstrate any clear circadian variation in platelet counts, blood serotonin concentrations in the autistics, nor differences in variations between patient and control populations.

In 1974, Campbell and associates[43] reported a study on the serotonin concentrations in platelet-rich plasma of eleven autistic patients. They noted that the levels were not significantly different from those in comparison cases. They also made the interesting observation that "low intellectual functioning was the only parameter which seemed to

be clearly associated with higher serotonin levels." This result is consistent with that of Schain and Freedman,[200] who noted that nonautistic, severely retarded comparison groups also had elevated levels of serotonin.

In 1975, Campbell and associates[42] reported another study of serotonin levels, in which twenty-three patients were compared to sixteen age- and sex-matched children. It was found that serotonin levels were higher in the patients than in the controls, although the differences did not reach significance. However, serotonin levels were significantly higher in the subgroup of patients with "florid psychosis, and those with lower IQ's than in patients in remission or partial remission or higher IQ's."

In 1971, the authors[182] attempted to study the effects of lowering blood serotonin. Following a seventeen-day placebo period, four hospitalized autistic boys were given 300–500 mgs of L-dopa per day, for six months. In the three youngest patients, a significant decrease of blood serotonin concentrations was observed along with a significant increase in platelet counts and a similar trend in the others. Urinary excretion of 5-HIAA decreased significantly in one patient, and a similar trend was found in the others. Unfortunately, however, no changes were observed in the clinical course of the patients, nor in their amount of motility disturbances, REM sleep, or endocrine levels (FSH and LH).

In 1976, Campbell and associates[41] reported a second study of L-dopa administration. Their patients were eleven childhood schizophrenics, and the doses given ranged from 900 to 2,500 mgs per day. They also administered levoamphetamine in a crossover paradigm. Their results confirmed the authors'[182] in that L-dopa administration did not alter the course of the disease. However, it did appear to be "stimulating" to the patients, an effect that warrants further study.

In the same year, Campbell and associates also reported a study of MAO activity in platelets of twenty-one schizophrenic and eighteen normal children matched for age and sex. They found no significant differences between the groups. However, in view of the small number of patients, their heterogeneity, and the difficulties in assay techniques, they indicate that the study should be extended before definitive conclusions are reached.

Four groups of investigators have reported on the uptake and efflux of serotonin from the platelets of autistic children. The first study was by Siva-Sankar.[210] He found no differences between patients and controls with respect to: the uptake of norepinephrine by platelets, the uptake of serotonin by red blood cells, nor the uptake of norepinephrine by red blood cells. However, a significantly lower rate of uptake of serotonin by platelets was noted in the autistic group when compared to the "schizophrenic nonautistic" cohort, and to other patient groups. Furthermore, analysis of the data by age revealed a relationship between decreased uptake of serotonin and age (the autistic patients had lower levels, similar to those found in the younger age groups of other patients). This developmentally related finding was consistent with the authors' observation[185] of serotonin and platelets. It also seemed to bear out previous theoretical suggestions of Bender[17] that a maturational lag may exist in children with the syndromes of autism and childhood schizophrenia.

In 1971, Lucas and associates[142] reported a second study of serotonin uptake by platelets. They reported finding no differences between normals and patients.

A third series of studies was begun by Boullin, Coleman, and O'Brien in 1970. In their first report,[30] they noted that "autistic platelets accumulated serotonin to a slightly greater extent than normals, 2.6 times the endogenous content, compared with 2.0 times for normal platelets." They also found that platelet sizes were not different, but that concentrations of platelets were significantly greater in autistics. They found no increase in serotonin levels, but rather that the concentration of serotonin per platelet was slightly diminished. The results of the efflux part of this study revealed that platelets from normal and autistic children lost a similar percentage of the total amount of radioactivity during the resuspension procedure, before reincubation for ninety minutes. However, a two-fold increase in the efflux of radioactive serotonin during the incubation from the autistics represented a "definite abnormality." This apparently did not arise from lack of ATP, since the ATP content of platelets was the same for the autistics and the normals.

In 1971, Boullin and associates[32] reported their second study designed to determine if increased serotonin efflux could be used to predict the diagnosis of autism as determined by the Rimland E-2 parental questionnaire. Both platelet ATP and serotonin uptake by platelets were examined in this study; neither showed any significant difference between the autistic and comparison cases. However, the "efflux ratio" predicted that six children were "autistic" and four were "nonautistic psychotics." The E-2 scores had labeled seven children as autistic and three as nonautistic psychotics.

In 1972, Boullin and O'Brien[31] reported their study, using labeled dopamine rather than serotonin. The results indicated no significant differences of uptake or loss of dopamine between patients and controls, but a greater variation in individual values within the autistic group.

In 1975,[233] an attempt was made to replicate this study of Boullin and associates.[30] Their techniques were employed along with methods designed to minimize platelet damage. Both procedures failed to reveal significant differences either in uptake or efflux rates between the autistics and hospitalized comparison groups or normals. Methodological considerations which could possibly account for this failure to confirm their previous findings were discussed in detail. In particular, it was stressed that differences in subject selection, as well as biochemical assay techniques, may have accounted for the inability to confirm the previous findings of group differences.

Bufotenin (the N-dimethylated derivitive of serotonin) excretion has been studied in autistic children by Himwich and associates[114] and Narasimachari and Himwich.[152] They found that five of six patients who were "suspected of having infantile autism" excreted bufotenin. The excretion of this substance in adult schizophrenics is widely debated in the literature. Although no consensus seems to have been reached, this interesting avenue of research bears further investigation.

2. Tryptophan Metabolism. In 1958, Sutton and Reed[216] reported a study of tryptophan loading in an eighteen-month-old girl with seizures, whom they had diagnosed as "autistic." Their results indicated that during tryptophan loading she excreted decreased amounts of 5-hydroxyindoleacetic acid, indoleacetic acid, and tryptophan. They hypothesized that "the mental aberration" in autism may be the result of "an altered ability to maintain normal brain serotonin levels."

Shaw and associates[208] also studied the effects of tryptophan loading on indole excretion. They tested twenty-one subjects, eleven of whom were "childhood schizophrenics." It was observed that after tryptophan loading, all but three subjects (two schizophrenics and one nonschizophrenic) showed increased excretion of 5-HIAA over their control periods.

In 1965, Heely and Roberts[109] measured the effects of tryptophan loading and amino acid excretion. They reported, "some of the psychotic children had increased excretion of their tryptophan load." Unfortunately, they did not describe their statistical procedures or clinical parameters so that it is impossible to determine the meaning of these results.

In 1970, Jørgensen and associates,[118] in Denmark reported a three-hospital survey of amino acid excretion in the urine of 178 children (ages three to twelve years). Their results indicated "there was no case of specific hyper-aminoaciduria found."

At the present time, it would seem that the final answer to whether abnormal responses to tryptophan loading occur in certain developmentally disturbed children has not been ascertained. Certainly, this area of investigation should be pursued to elaborate the suggestive observations cited.

3. Catecholamines. In 1974, Cohen and associates[47] reported a pioneering study of homovanilic acid (HVA) and 5-hydroxyindoleacetic acid (5-HIAA) in the cerebrospinal fluid of twenty children (nine "autistics," eleven "atypical," and ten with epilepsy). They found significant differences in cerebrospinal fluid HVA and 5-HIAA levels, and they found that these levels were also significantly correlated with each other. No differences were found within the group of "psychotic children" between those labeled "autistic" and those labeled "atypical psychotic but nonautistic."

The urine of some adult schizophrenic patients has been found to contain 3, 4-dimethoxphenylethylamine (DMPEA). It has been labeled "pink spot" since it turns pink when exposed to a modified Ehrlich's reagent. Widelitz and Feldman[231] reported a study of twelve "childhood schizophrenics" and twelve "normals," in whose urine they looked for pink spots. Their results indicated that eight of the twelve schizophrenics excreted pink spots of 5 micrograms or more. Five of six normals also had pink spots, but their total amount per aliquot was less than 2 micrograms. The significance of these results remains uncertain at the present time, and no follow up studies apparently have been conducted.

4. Hematologic Studies. Fowle[85] reported a study of leukocyte patterns in schizophrenic children, normals, and siblings of schizophrenics. She concluded that the schizophrenic children had "an atypical leukocyte pattern which was characterized by higher frequency of several morphologically distinct types of lymphocytes and plasmacytes than are found in the blood of their brothers and sisters and normal control children." This study has not been followed up by others and is in need of replication utilizing the newer techniques that have been developed since its completion.

In 1969, Gittelman and Cleeman[91] reported that they were unable to find differences between mean serum magnesium levels of psychotic and control groups.

In 1969, Saladino and Siva-Sankar[199] reported a study on erythrocyte magnesium and potassium levels. Their results revealed that "schizophrenic-autistic" patients showed "the lowest levels (of magnesium and potassium) and the least variation with chronological growth." They conclude that these results support the hypothesis that there is a "maturational lag" existing in "schizophrenic-autistic patients;" their data, however, were not sufficiently specified to support this statement.

In 1971, Goodwin, Cowen, and Goodwin[102] reported on malabsorption and cerebral dysfunction in children diagnosed as "autistic." They noted that, "there was no significant difference between the groups indicative of any increased stress or altered hormonal stress responses in the autistic subjects."

In 1971, Lucas and associates[142] reported finding a significant difference between childhood schizophrenics and matched nonpsychotic hospitalized comparison patients, with regard to red blood cell cholinesterase activity. So far as is known, this study has not been replicated.

DeMyer and associates[56, 57] have conducted a series of studies of blood macronutrients. Their results revealed greater variablity of free-fatty-acids and plasma glucose levels in psychotic children than in controls; at the same time, the subjects showed normal responses to insulin administration, high carbohydrate diet, and glucose administration. The mean levels of plasma-free-fatty-acids, however, were higher in the psychotic group. They conclude "that a possible reason for free-fatty-acid variability in psychotic children may be a deficiency in the regulatory feedback mechanism at a neurogenic or cellular level."

The final study to be reviewed in this section was reported by Cohen and associates[45] in 1976. They assessed blood lead levels in children with "autism," "atypical development," and their siblings. Their results revealed that the group of "autistics" had significantly higher mean levels of blood lead than the "atypical" children and the normal siblings. They discussed these differences in terms of possible dietary intake habits which might have been responsible.

Even a cursory review, such as this, indicates that many interesting possibilities have been explored and need to be replicated and extended by further studies. Hopefully, such studies will be designed to mitigate difficulties caused by lack of diagnostic specificity. It is also important that they employ the most sophisticated techniques available and focus on the developmental issues implicit in all research with children.

Neurophysiological Studies: Most clinical studies of psychotic, autistic, and schizophrenic children have emphasized their unusual reactions to sensory stimuli. Specific terms have been coined to describe these characteristics ("perceptual inconstancy,"[162] "unusual sensitivities,"[27] "abnormal receptor preferences,"[97] "preference for proximal versus distal receptors,"[203]) and theories have been proposed to explain their occurrences.[219] Unfortunately, extensive application of routine neurological examinations[96] and clinical EEG's[184] have proved of little value. Thus, it has been necessary to await the recent development of sophisticated measures of neurophysiological function that could be systematically applied to groups of patients and controls before such theories could be tested. In this section, the results of several of these studies will be reviewed.

Cross-comparison of neurophysiologic studies is difficult for several reasons. For example, varying criteria have been used for patient selection by different investigators. Also, in some cases, newly developed techniques are incompletely understood; while for others, adequate reliability studies and normal developmental parameters have not yet been developed.

As previously cited,[184] a double blind study of clinical EEG's failed to discriminate eighty-six psychotic patients from ninety-eight matched psychiatrically hospitalized patients. As might have been expected, the clinical EEG was correlated only with the presence or absence of clinical evidence of CNS dysfunction. In other EEG studies, Kolvin and associates[129] and Hutt and associates[117] observed unusually low voltages. They interpreted this as suggestive of chronic hyperarousal. However, in carefully controlled studies, during which stimulus conditions were monitored, Creak and Pampiglione[54] and Hermelin and O'Connor[111] were unable to confirm these findings. In a more recent study, Small[212] compared qualitative EEG measures (voltage integration and auto- and cross-correlations) in seven autistic and seven normal children. Analysis of their data revealed significantly less session-to-session transhemispheric variability in the autistics.

The EEG during sleep has also been studied extensively. Ornitz and associates[164] and Onheiber and associates[154] observed normal sleep cycling and normal amounts of rapid eye movement sleep. However, qualitative assessments of the eye movements revealed that the autistics were more like normal infants than age-matched comparisons, a finding suggestive of a maturational defect.[158, 166, 219]

Studies of the auditory evoked responses during sleep have revealed that inhibition during rapid eye movement bursts was less likely to occur in autistics than in matched normals.[167] Other studies of the recovery cycle of the auditory evoked response during sleep revealed no differences between normals and autistics.[165]

Small and associates[213] demonstrated that the contingent negative variation response (CNV) is intact in autistic children, and when two stimuli were paired together, response occurred. However, unlike the controls, the autistics did not show a differential response to slides of familar versus unfamiliar faces. LeLord and associates[135] reported that in autistic children, they observed large, slow, negative or positive potentials in response to stimulus coupling. These responses were significantly larger than those obtained from normals.

The galvanic skin response (GSR) has been studied with inconsistent results.[28, 151] These investigators first noted that an autistic group gave an inadequate GSR response to both auditory and visual stimuli. When, however, they used changes in heart rate as their experimental measure, they were not able to replicate this finding.

MacCulloch and Williams[143] reported increased variability in heart rate between autistic and normal children. Their findings were confirmed and elaborated upon in a further study by Hutt and associates,[116] in which careful control for activity levels were maintained. Their results revealed greater variability of beat-to-beat heart rate in autistic children during stereotyped behaviors.

Early clinical reports[18, 27] suggested the possibilities of specific disturbances of vestibular mechanisms. This was explored experimentally by Pollack and Krieger[170] in 1958, and by Colbert and associates[48] in 1959. Both of these studies revealed decreased nystagmus. In 1969, the authors designed an extensive study of post-rotatory nystagmus in twenty-eight autistics and twenty-two matched normals. Laboratory conditions utilizing electronystagmography also permitted studying the effects of visual input. The autistics had a significant reduction of post-rotatory nystagmus duration when studied in a lighted room, but not when in the dark.[186] Further studies are underway to clarify the exact nature of the influence of visual input.[165] Results to date indicate that the inhibition of post-rotatory nystagmus most likely depends on interactions between vestibular stimulation and visual input.[155]

NEUROLOGIC AND BIOLOGIC THEORY

Lauretta Bender: The neurologic and biologic theories of childhood schizophrenia developed primarily out of Lauretta Bender's work and concepts. From 1942, she conceived of schizophrenia "as striking at the substratum of all integrative functioning," leading to a characteristic pathology at every level of the CNS. This resulted from the same hereditary predisposition as adult schizophrenia and had to be considered developmentally.[19] After comparing the histories of infant schizophrenics with premature infants,[21] she conceptualized the CNS pathology in terms of "plasticity," referring to the pluripotentiality of the undifferentiated embryo.[10] The neurological hierarchy and control in childhood schizophrenia remain primitive and plastic; it retains the embryonic capacity for regression and acceleration, interpenetration and interchangeability, with a decreased coordination of separate subsystems into the organism's total adaptive function. This gives rise to the physiological instability and the variability of development and of functioning. Even "boundaries between psychological regions tend to shift and be permeated more easily than in the normal child:"[23] symbolic and concrete thinking alternate; percepts and memory traces of objects are distorted by mutual influences; reproductions and drawings become distorted and confused; and associations become idiosyncratic.

The basic, inherited biologic disorganization persisted, whether the child became overtly psychotic (as a result of physiological or other stress), or whether he compensated and showed only residual symptoms. She considered the "all-pervasive pananxiety" to be "the counterpart in awareness of the chaotic and unstable organization of the child's psychobiological system as a whole."[23] The child's problems in achieving a satisfactory patterning of his perceptions of his own body and of the world, led to his problems in identification and socialization, and to the development of neurotic and other defenses. The clinical picture varied with the age of onset and with the unique assets and defenses of the individual child.[14, 18]

At first glance, this is a highly abstract set of constructs. However, the constituent parts can be operationally defined and tested experimentally. This has been done for some of the integrative disorders of motor, perceptual, and cognitive functioning,[23, 96, 110, 227] for development and physical growth,[67, 71] and for neurophysiology.[162] Others have investigated the identical "boundary problems" in the thinking and perceptual disorders of adult schizophrenics. These phenomena are familiar to all clinicians. It is only the super-abstraction of plasticity, encompassing such manifold disorders at all levels of CNS functioning, that is difficult to grasp.

Leo Kanner: Kanner believed that the inability of autistic children "to form the usual biologically provided affective contact with people" was innate, inherited,[121] and related to the "constitutional components of emotional reactivity."[124] However, he never elaborated any theory of this intrinsic constitutional inadequacy.

William Goldfarb: Goldfarb[96] postulated that childhood schizophrenia, like mental retardation, "may represent a range of precipitating causes, genetic, environmental, and neurological." The "behavioral deficiencies . . . can be produced either by a neurological defect in the child or by abnormal conditions in the rearing environment." Accordingly, he subdivided the children into "organic" and "nonorganic." He believed that the degree of neurologic integrity created gradations of ego deficit; but, beyond referring to the impairment as "brain damage,"[96] he never elaborated a theory of the neurologic involvement itself.

Beate Hermelin and Neil O'Connor: Hermelin and O'Connor[110] performed the most sophisticated series of psychological experiments to date on young autistic children. They concluded "that autistic children are deficient in the capacity to appreciate order or pattern where this involves extracting the structure of a sequence of stimuli." They had good rote memory and made efficient use of kinesthetic and motor feedback cues, but their ability to use visual information or the syntactic or the meaningful aspects of language was impaired. They behaved as if all of these structured inputs were random and meaningless. Hermelin and O'Connor regard this inability of autistic children to encode stimuli meaningfully as their basic cognitive deficit, and they hypothesize how this might lead to proximal receptor preference, the ignoring of verbal signals, and to stereotyped and inappropriate responses to complex patterns of sensory input. This body of work provides additional evidence of a fundamental integrative deficit in severely impaired autistic children, and a theory to explain the major symptoms.

Barbara Fish: Fish[75] followed Bender in postulating that a fundamental integrative disorder of

CNS functioning constituted the inherited biological predisposition to schizophrenia. Bender's "plasticity" was operationally defined in quantitative terms. It was demonstrated that preschizophrenic infants showed a fluctuating dysregulation of maturation—or "pandevelopmental retardation" (PDR)—from birth.[67, 71] This involved physical growth; gross motor, visual-motor, and cognitive development; proprioceptive and vestibular responses; muscle tone and arousal.

Fish[67, 71] hypothesized that PDR is the phenotypic expression in infancy of the inherited neurointegrative defect in schizophrenia, and that it serves as an early "marker" for the biologically vulnerable infants. For a vulnerable child, the eventual outcome depends on the severity of his intrinsic developmental disorder, and on whether his experiences exaggerate his inadequacies or help him to compensate and to adapt as a successfully coping "schizotypic"[149] personality.

In the vulnerable infants, certain developmental disorders left residual perceptual defects and soft neurologic signs; these persisted into latency, and even into adulthood. Fish[67, 71] postulated that these were the same neurointegrative defects which were found in large controlled studies of infants[148] and children[147] who were genetically at risk for schizophrenia. Similar neurologic disorders had been found in the controlled studies of children who subsequently developed schizophrenia, especially the more chronic forms.* These soft neurologic signs persisted in many adolescent[112] and adult[173, 222] schizophrenics. Fish concluded that in the affected individuals, the inherited neurointegrative defect showed a continuity from birth to adulthood, although the manifestations changed with maturation. The infant observations suggested that many of the early developmental symptoms might respond to intervention during infancy. Conceivably, this could prevent the cumulative disability and overwhelming feelings of hopelessness and inadequacy, which otherwise ensue.[68]

Psychodynamic Factors

ETIOLOGIC THEORIES

Many theories based on psychoanalytic metapsychology have been proposed over the past several decades to explain the etiology of childhood psychoses. Most postulate that pathological parent-infant relationships occurred during early critical stages of psychosexual development. Others postulate "inherent" ego defects which become clinically manifest as the child develops through the first year or two of life. Within these frameworks, they attempt to explain specific clinical phenomena as resulting from different types and/or timing of postulated psychotoxic events, or disruptions of hypothetically defined normal stages of ego development. These theories have been summarized, extensively reviewed and critiqued many times.[64, 133, 230] Unfortunately, these theories have not lead to objectively definable hypotheses which could be tested by generally accepted scientific methods. Neither have they led to therapeutic techniques which have been demonstrated to affect the course of the disease in patients treated by psychoanalysis or psychodynamically based psychotherapy.

Specific psychotoxic events have, however, been documented to be of etiological significance in certain specific types of disturbed psychosexual development. Such psychologically traumatizing factors include: maternal deprivation, victimization by psychotic or assaultive parents, prolonged isolation, and sense organ pathology. The effects of deprivation of mothering figures on infants raised in institutions have been studied by Provence and Lipton,[172] and on children at home by Coleman and Provence.[49] Rutter[192] and Bowlby[33] also have contributed significantly to the understanding of these syndromes.

In summary, these studies indicate that psychotoxic factors do induce developmental disturbances. They have not been shown to be related to the specific clinical syndromes of autism or childhood schizophrenia. Patients with induced psychotoxic syndromes have shown a positive response to restitution of the expected nurturing environment; this further distinguishes them from patients with autism and childhood schizophrenia.

Strategies and Techniques for Patient Management

The medical management of patients with autism and childhood schizophrenia is a particularly complicated and taxing undertaking, for one is dealing with a total family in which one member has a lifelong disease. Thus, overall management strat-

* See references 153, 178, 179, 187, and 226.

egies must be directed to assessing and managing factors related not only to the patient's illness, but also to parents, siblings, and community factors.

The complexity of this task necessitates three distinct management strategies, each of which requires different tactics. The first strategy deals with assessment of the patient's medical, intellectual, cognitive, psychological, and psychosocial status; the second strategy focuses on choosing, implementing, and coordinating symptomatic therapies; the third strategy deals with periodic reassessments and redirections of treatments.

The first strategy is to obtain data and organize initial diagnostic assessments. Tactics include, among other things, gathering data from interviews with all knowledgeable relatives, teachers, and other significant adults in the patient's life, reviewing home movies and photo albums, home visits, and obtaining all prior medical records. Flexibility and imagination are necessary to complete an historical picture, and one cannot overemphasize the importance of piecing together as complete a picture as possible. Other tactics include obtaining medical and neurological evaluations, two EEG's with sleep tracings,[184] and other examinations, such as special audiometrics[141] when indicated. Special studies for metabolic and congenital syndromes frequently are necessary since they often overlap with the syndromes of autism and childhood schizophrenia,[161] and their etiological bases must be looked for independently (e.g., coexisting PKU and autism).

Special tactics for intellectual and cognitive assessments must be tailored for each patient.[89] They must be administered individually by an experienced examiner who is capable of eliciting maximum performance by the use of ancillary methods, such as those based on behavior therapy techniques.

Psychodiagnostic interviews are also necessary to determine each patient's level of ego development and specific personality strengths and weaknesses. This assessment is particularly helpful when selecting overall management strategies. Psychodynamic understanding of key family members is also necessary, as is an appraisal of the patient's social milieu and its resources.

The second strategy is to determine and coordinate symptomatic therapies. These include: (1) General family counseling.[88] (2) Specific psychotherapy—When family members have sufficient psychopathology to warrant referral for psychotherapy, it will need to be coordinated with the overall management program of the patient.

(3) Specific psychotherapy for patients—This frequently is helpful for patients at more advanced levels of ego development. Clinical experience indicates that such therapy is most helpful when it is of the supportive, educational, and integrative type (versus the uncovering, interpretive, and transference oriented type).[225] (4) Educational therapy—Several studies by Rutter and Sussenwein[198] and Flaharty[84] have documented that patients do best in highly structured, specifically designed educational programs.[177] (5) Behavior therapy programs—Extensive research over the past two decades has revealed that many children with the syndromes of autism and childhood schizophrenia can be "taught" specific skills in the areas of social adaptation and cognitive and motor skills.[86] At the present time, research indicates that such behavior therapy programs should be designed for individual children and carefully monitored so that modifications can be made as the patient's clinical state changes. Unfortunately, attempts to generalize specific behavior therapy treatments to groups of children have proved of little value.[140] (6) Medications and somatic therapies—Recent reviews by Campbell[39] are in agreement with the authors' clinical experience[69] that there is a place for psychotropic medication in managing specific symptoms. These included hyperactivity, aggressiveness, psychotic language, emotional lability, and sleep disorders. One must be careful to avoid excessive sedation when using psychotropic medications. This unwanted side-effect can reduce a patient's participation in other therapeutic programs, e.g., educational, behavioral, and psychotherapeutic. (7) Out of home placements—Respite care and residential treatment settings frequently are advisable for patients with severe behavior problems. The decision to hospitalize a child or use a foster home hinges on a careful assessment of the impact of the patient on the total situation. Not only the parents, but factors associated with the siblings must also be considered.

The third strategy provides for periodic reassessments and redirection of symptomatic treatments. For example, recent evidence from follow up studies indicates that many children with the syndromes of autism and childhood schizophrenia develop seizure disorders when they enter teen years. Often, they have provided no evidence of neurological dysfunction when younger.[197] Thus, serial EEG examinations and interval histories for seizures should be done on an annual basis. A reassessment of symptomatic therapies also should be made on an annual basis. Adjustments have to be made for changes due to the therapies as well as for changes caused by the natural history of the patient's illness. Such issues as a patient requiring hospital care in teen years, sterilization and/or hysterectomy for girls, and dealing with estate planning are now coming to reside within the province of the managing physician. Unfortunately, there is no systematic research available to augment one's clinical judgment in dealing with these problems.

REFERENCES

1. American Psychiatric Association, Committee on Nomenclature and Statistics, *Diagnostic and Statistical Manual of Mental Disorders*, 3rd ed., American Psychiatric Association, Washington, D.C., (in preparation), 1976.

2. American Psychiatric Association, Committee on Nomenclature and Statistics, *Diagnostic and Statistical Manual of Mental Disorders*, 1st ed., American Psychiatric Association, Washington, D.C., 1968.

3. American Psychiatric Association, Committee on Nomenclature and Statistics, *Diagnostic and Statistical Manual of Mental Disorders*, 1st ed., American Psychiatric Association, Washington, D.C., 1952.

4. ANNELL, A. L., "The Prognosis of Psychotic Syndromes in Children. A Follow-Up of 115 Cases," *Acta Psychiatrica Scandinavica, 39*:235–297, 1963.

5. ANTHONY, E. J., "An Aetiological Approach to the Diagnosis of Psychosis in Childhood," *Acta Paedopsychiatrica, 25*:89–96, 1958.

6. BALTAXE, C. A. M., and SIMMONS, J. Q., "Language in Childhood Psychosis: A Review," *Journal of Speech and Hearing Disorders, 40*:439–458, 1975.

7. BECK, S. J., *The Six Schizophrenias*, Research Monographs of the Orthopsychiatric Association, No. 6, American Orthopsychiatric Association, New York, 1954.

8. BENDA, C. E., *Developmental Disorders of Mentation and Cerebral Palsies*, Grune & Stratton, New York, 1952.

9. BENDER, L., "The Life Course of Schizophrenic Children," *Biological Psychiatry, 2*:165–172, 1970.

10. ———, "The Concept of Plasticity in Childhood Schizophrenia," in Hoch, P. H., and Zubin, J. (Eds.), *Psychopathology of Schizophrenia*, pp. 354–365, Grune & Stratton, New York, 1966.

11. ———, "A Twenty-Five Year View of Therapeutic Results," in Hoch, P. H., and Zubin, J. (Eds.), *The Evaluation of Psychiatric Treatment*, pp. 129–142, Grune & Stratton, New York, 1964.

12. ———, "Autism in Children with Mental Deficiency," *American Journal of Mental Deficiency, 64*:81–86, 1959.

13. ———, "The Concept of Pseudopsychopathic Schizophrenia in Adolescents," *American Journal of Orthopsychiatry, 29*:491–509, 1959.

14. ———, "Problems in Early Development," in Liebman, S., *Understanding Your Patient*, J. B. Lippincott, Philadelphia, 1957.

15. ———, *The Psychopathology of Children with Organic Brain Disorders*, Charles C Thomas, Springfield, Ill., 1956.

16. ———, "Schizophrenia in Childhood—Its Recognition, Description and Treatment," *American Journal of Orthopsychiatry, 26*:499–506, 1956.

17. ———, "Childhood Schizophrenia," *Psychiatric Quarterly, 27*:663–681, 1953.

18. ———, "Childhood Schizophrenia," *American Journal of Orthopsychiatry, 17*:40–56, 1947.

19. ———, "Childhood Schizophrenia," *Nervous Child, 1*:138–140, 1942.

20. ———, and FARETRA, G., "The Relationship Between Childhood Schizophrenia and Adult Schizophrenia," in Kaplan, A. R. (Ed.), *Genetic Factors in Schizophrenia*, pp. 28–64, Charles C Thomas, Springfield, Ill., 1972.

21. BENDER, L., and FREEDMAN, A. M., "A Study of the First Three Years in the Maturation of Schizophrenic Children," *Quarterly Journal of Child Behavior, 4*:245–272, 1952.

22. BENDER, L., and GRUGETT, A. E., "A Study of Certain Epidemiological Factors in a Group of Children with Childhood Schizophrenia," *American Journal of Orthopsychiatry, 26*:131–145, 1956.

23. BENDER, L., and HELME, W. H., "A Quantitative Test of Theory and Diagnostic Indicators of Childhood Schizophrenia," *American Medical Association Archives of Neurology and Psychiatry, 70*:413–427, 1953.

24. BENDER, L., et al., "Schizophrenia in Childhood, A Confirmation of the Diagnosis," *Transactions of the American Neurological Association, 77*:67–73, 1952.

25. BENNETT, S., and KLEIN, H. R., "Childhood Schizophrenia: 30 Years Later," *American Journal of Psychiatry, 122*:1121–1124, 1966.

26. BENTON, A. L., "Development of Finger Location Capacity in School Children," *Child Development, 26*:225–230, 1955.

27. BERGMAN, P., and ESCALONA, S. K., "Unusual Sensitivities in Very Young Children," in Eissler, R. S., et al. (Eds.), *The Psychoanalytic Study of the Child*, vol. 3–4, pp. 333–353, International Universities Press, New York, 1949.

28. BERNAL, M. E., and MILLER, W. H., "Electrodermal and Cardiac Responses of Schizophrenic Children to Sensory Stimuli," *Psychophysiology, 7*:155–168, 1970.

29. BIRCH, H. G., and WALKER, H. A., "Perceptual and Perceptual-Motor Dissociation. Studies in Schizophrenic and Brain-Damaged Psychotic Children," *Archives of General Psychiatry, 14*:113–118, 1966.

30. BOULLIN, D., COLEMAN, M., and O'BRIEN, A., "Abnormalities in Platelet 5-Hydroxytryptamine Efflux in Patients with Infantile Autism," *Nature, 226*:25, 1970.

31. BOULLIN, D., and O'BRIEN, A., "Uptake and Loss of L-Dopamine by Platelets From Children with Infantile Autism," *Journal of Autism and Childhood Schizophrenia, 2*:167–174, 1972.

32. ———, et al., "Laboratory Prediction of Infantile Autism Based on 5-Hydroxytryptamine Efflux From Blood Platelets and Their Correlation with the Rimland E-2 Score," *Journal of Autism and Childhood Schizophrenia, 1*:163–171, 1971.

33. BOWLBY, J., *Attachment and Loss*, Basic Books, New York, 1969.

34. BRADLEY, C., *Schizophrenia in Childhood*, Macmillan, New York, 1941.

35. BROWN, J. L., "Adolescent Development of Children with Infantile Psychosis," *Seminars in Psychiatry, 1*:79–89, 1969.

36. ———, "Follow-Up of Children with Atypical Development (Infantile Psychosis)," *American Journal of Orthopsychiatry, 33*:855–861, 1963.

37. ———, "Prognosis From Presenting Symptoms of Preschool Children with Atypical Development," *American Journal of Orthopsychiatry, 30*:382–390, 1960.

38. Bryson, C. Q., and Hingtgen, J. N., *Early Childhood Psychosis: Infantile Autism, Childhood Schizophrenia and Related Disorders. An Annotated Bibliography: 1964 to 1969*, National Institute of Mental Health, Rockville, Md., 1971.

39. Campbell, M., "Pharmacotherapy in Early Infantile Autism," *Biological Psychiatry*, 10:399–423, 1975.

40. ———, et al., "Blood Platelets Monoamine Oxidase Activity in Schizophrenic Children and Their Families: A Preliminary Study," *Neuropsychobiology*, 2:239–246, 1976.

41. ———, et al., "Levodopa and Levoamphetamine: A Crossover Study in Young Schizophrenic Children," *Current Therapeutic Research*, 19:70–86, 1976.

42. ———, et al., "Blood Serotonin in Schizophrenic Children," *International Pharmacopsychology*, 10:213–221, 1975.

43. ———, et al., "Blood Serotonin in Psychotic and Brain Damaged Children," *Journal of Autism and Childhood Schizophrenia*, 4:33–41, 1974.

44. Chess, S., "Autism in Children with Congenital Rubella," *Journal of Autism and Childhood Schizophrenia*, 1:33–47, 1971.

45. Cohen, D., Johnson, W., and Caparulo, B., "Pica and Elevated Blood Lead Level in Autistic and Atypical Children," *American Journal of Diseases of Children*, 130:47–48, 1976.

46. Cohen, D., and Young, G., "Neurochemistry and Child Psychiatry," *Journal of the American Academy of Child Psychiatry*, 16:353–411, 1977.

47. Cohen, D., et al., "Biogenic Amine in Autistic and Atypical Children: Cerebrospinal Fluid Measures of Homovanillic Acid and 5-Hydroxyindoleacetic Acid," *Archives of General Psychiatry*, 31:845–853, 1974.

48. Colbert, E. G., Koegler, R. R., and Markham, C. H., "Vestibular Dysfunction in Childhood Schizophrenia," *American Medical Association Archives of General Psychiatry*, 1:600–617, 1959.

49. Coleman, R. W., and Provence, S., "Environmental Retardation (Hospitalism) in Infants Living in Families," *Pediatrics*, 19:285–292, 1957.

50. Collins, W. E., "Manipulation of Arousal and Its Effects on Human Vestibular Nystagmus Induced by Caloric Irrigation and Angular Acceleration," *Aerospace Medicine*, 54:124–129, 1963.

51. Creak, M., "Childhood Psychosis: A Review of 100 Cases," *British Journal of Psychiatry*, 109:84–89, 1963.

52. ———, "Schizophrenic Syndrome in Childhood: Report of a Working Party," *British Medical Journal*, 2: 889–890, 1961.

53. ———, and Ini, S., "Families of Psychotic Children," *Journal of Child Psychology and Psychiatry*, 1: 156–175, 1960.

54. Creak, M., and Pampiglione, G., "Clinical and EEG Studies on a Group of 35 Psychotic Children," *Developmental Medicine and Child Neurology*, 11:218–227, 1969.

55. Dahl, V., "A Follow-Up Study of a Child Psychiatric Clientele with Special Regard to the Diagnosis of Psychosis," *Acta Psychiatrica Scandinavica*, 54:106–112, 1976.

56. DeMyer, M., Ward, S., and Lintzenich, J., "Comparison of Macronutrients in the Diets of Psychotic and Normal Children," *Archives of General Psychiatry*, 18: 584–590, 1968.

57. DeMyer, M., et al., "Free Fatty Acid Response to Insulin and Glucose Stimulation in Schizophrenic, Autistic and Emotionally Disturbed Children," *Journal of Autism and Childhood Schizophrenia*, 4:436–452, 1971.

58. DesLauriers, A., and Halpern, F., "Psychological Tests in Childhood Schizophrenia," *American Journal of Orthopsychiatry*, 17:57–69, 1947.

59. Despert, J. L., "Thinking and Motility Disorder in Schizophrenic Child," *Psychiatric Quarterly*, 15:522–536, 1941.

60. ———, "Schizophrenia in Children," *Psychiatric Quarterly*, 12:366–371, 1938.

61. Dutton, G., "The Growth Pattern of Psychotic Boys," *British Journal of Psychiatry*, 110:101–103, 1964.

62. Eisenberg, L., "The Course of Childhood Schizophrenia," *American Medical Association Archives of Neurology and Psychiatry*, 78:69–83, 1957.

63. Ekstein, R., *The Challenge: Despair and Hope in the Conquest of Inner Space*, Brunner-Mazel, New York, 1971.

64. ———, Bryant, K., and Friedman, S. W., "Childhood Schizophrenia and Allied Conditions," in Bellak, L., and Benedict, P. K. (Eds.), *Schizophrenia: A Review of the Syndrome*, pp. 555–693, Logos Press, New York, 1958.

65. Endicott, J., et al., "The Global Assessment Scale. A Procedure for Measuring Overall Severity of Psychiatric Disturbance," *Archives of General Psychiatry*, 33:766–771, 1976.

66. Fink, M., and Bender, M. B., "Perception of Simultaneous Tactile Stimuli in Normal Children," *Neurology*, 3:27–34, 1952.

67. Fish, B., "Neurobiologic Antecedents of Schizophrenia in Children: Evidence for an Inherited, Congenital Neurointegrative Defect," *Archives of General Psychiatry*, 34:1297–1313, 1977.

68. ———, "An Approach to Prevention in Infants at Risk for Schizophrenia: Developmental Deviations From Birth to 10 Years," *Journal of the American Academy of Child Psychiatry*, 15:62–82, 1976.

69. ———, "Pharmacotherapy for Autistic and Schizophrenic Children," in Ritvo, E. R. (Ed.), *Autism: Diagnosis, Current Research and Management*, Spectrum, New York, 1976.

70. ———, Unpublished analysis of data from Fish, et al., 1958, and the next 20 psychotic children admitted to the nursery, 1976.

71. ———, "Biologic Antecedents of Psychosis in Children," in Freedman, D. X. (Ed.), *The Biology of the Major Psychoses: A Comparative Analysis*, vol. 54, pp. 49–80, Association for Research in Nervous and Mental Disease, Raven Press, New York, 1975.

72. ———, "The 'One Child, One Drug' Myth of Stimulants in Hyperkinesis. Importance of Diagnostic Categories in Evaluating Treatment," *Archives of General Psychiatry*, 25:193–203, 1971.

73. ———, "The Maturation of Arousal and Attention in the First Months of Life: A Study of Variations in Ego Development," *Journal of the American Academy of Child Psychiatry*, 2:253–270, 1963.

74. ———, "The Study of Motor Development in Infancy and Its Relationship to Psychological Functioning," *American Journal of Psychiatry*, 117:1113–1118, 1961.

75. ———, "Involvement of the Central Nervous System in Infants with Schizophrenia," *Archives of Neurology*, 2:115–121, 1960.

76. ———, "Longitudinal Observations of Biological Deviations in a Schizophrenic Infant," *American Journal of Psychiatry*, 116:25–31, 1959.

77. ———, "The Detection of Schizophrenia in Infancy," *Journal of Nervous and Mental Disease*, 125:1–24, 1957.

78. ———, and Alpert, M., "Abnormal States of Consciousness and Muscle Tone in Infants Born to Schizophrenic Mothers," *American Journal of Psychiatry*, 119:439–445, 1962.

79. Fish, B., and Dixon, W. J., "Vestibular Hyporeactivity in Infants at Risk for Schizophrenia: Its Association with Critical Developmental Disorders," *Archives of General Psychiatry*, (in press).

80. Fish, B., and Hagin, R., "Visual-Motor Disorders in Infants at Risk for Schizophrenia," *Archives of General Psychiatry*, 28:900–904, 1973.

81. Fish, B., and Shapiro, T., "A Typology of Children's Psychiatric Disorders: I. Its Application to a Controlled Evaluation of Treatment," *Journal of the American Academy of Child Psychiatry*, 4:32–52, 1965.

82. ———, et al., "A Classification of Schizophrenic Children Under Five Years," *American Journal of Psychiatry, 124*:1415–1423, 1968.

83. ———, et al., "The Prediction of Schizophrenia in Infancy: III. A Ten-Year Follow-Up Report of Neurological and Psychological Development," *American Journal of Psychiatry, 121*:768–775, 1965.

84. FLAHARTY, R., "EPEC: Evaluation and Prescription for Exceptional Children," in Ritvo, E. R. (Ed.), *Autism: Diagnosis, Current Research and Management*, Spectrum, New York, 1976.

85. FOWLE, A., "Atypical Leukocyte Patterns of Schizophrenic Children," *Archives of General Psychiatry, 8*:666–680, 1968.

86. FRANKEL, F., TYMCHUK, A. J., and SIMMONS, J. Q., III, "Operant Analysis and Intervention with Autistic Children: Implications of Current Research," in Ritvo, E. R. (Ed.), *Autism: Diagnosis, Current Research and Management*, Spectrum, New York, 1976.

87. FREEDMAN, A. M., and BENDER, L., "When the Childhood Schizophrenic Grows Up," *American Journal of Orthopsychiatry, 27*:553–565, 1957.

88. FREEMAN, B. J., and RITVO, E. R., "Parents as Paraprofessionals," in Ritvo, E. R. (Ed.), *Autism: Diagnosis, Current Research and Management*, Spectrum, New York, 1976a.

89. ———, "Cognitive Assessment," in Ritvo, E. R. (Ed.), *Autism: Diagnosis, Current Research and Management*, Spectrum, New York, 1976b.

90. GESELL, A., and AMATRUDA, C. S., *Developmental Diagnosis*, Hoeber, New York, 1941.

91. GITTELMAN, M., and CLEEMAN, J., "Serum Magnesium Level in Psychotic and Normal Children," *Behavioral Neuropsychiatry, 8*:51–52, 1969.

92. GOLDFARB, W., "Childhood Psychosis," in Mussen, P. H. (Ed.), *Carmichael's Manual of Child Psychology*, 3rd ed., vol. 2, pp. 765–830, John Wiley, New York, 1970.

93. ———, "A Follow-Up Investigation of Schizophrenic Children Treated in Residence," *Psychosocial Process, 1*:1–64, 1970.

94. ———, "The Subclassification of Psychotic Children: Application to a Study of Longitudinal Change," in Rosenthal, D., and Kety, S. S. (Eds.), *The Transmission of Schizophrenia*, pp. 333–342, Pergamon Press, London, 1968.

95. ———, "Factors in the Development of Schizophrenic Children: An Approach to Subclassification," in Romano, J. (Ed.), *The Origins of Schizophrenia*, Excerpta Medica Foundation, New York, 1967.

96. ———, *Childhood Schizophrenia*, Harvard University Press, Cambridge, Mass., 1961.

97. ———, "Receptor Preferences in Schizophrenic Children," *American Medical Association Archives of Neurology and Psychiatry, 76*:643–652, 1956.

98. ———, "Rorschach Test Differences Between Family Reared, Institution-Reared, and Schizophrenic Children," *American Journal of Orthopsychiatry, 19*:624–633, 1949.

99. ———, BRAUNSTEIN, P., and LORGE, S., "Childhood Schizophrenia Symposium, 1955. A Study of Speech Patterns in a Group of Schizophrenic Children," *American Journal of Orthopsychiatry, 26*:544–555, 1956.

100. GOLDFARB, W., and DORSEN, M. M., *Annotated Bibliography of Childhood Schizophrenia and Related Disorders*, Basic Books, New York, 1956.

101. GOLDFARB, W., GOLDFARB, N., and POLLACK, R. C., "Changes in IQ of Schizophrenic Children During Residential Treatment," *Archives of General Psychiatry, 21*:673–690, 1969.

102. GOLDSTEIN, K., "Abnormal Mental Conditions in Infancy," *Journal of Nervous and Mental Disease, 128*:538–557, 1959.

103. GOODWIN, M., COWEN, M., and GOODWIN, T., "Malabsorption and Cerebral Dysfunction: A Multivariate and Comparative Study of Autistic Children," *Journal of Autism and Childhood Schizophrenia, 1*:148–162, 1971.

104. GOTTESMAN, I. I., and SHIELDS, J., *Schizophrenia and Genetics. A Twin Study Vantage Point*, Academic Press, New York, 1972.

105. Group for the Advancement of Psychiatry, Committee on Child Psychiatry, *Psychopathological Disorders in Childhood: Theoretical Considerations and a Proposed Classification*, vol. 6, Report No. 62, Group for the Advancement of Psychiatry, New York, 1966.

106. HANSON, D. R., and GOTTESMAN, I. I., "The Genetics, If Any, of Infantile Autism and Childhood Schizophrenia," *Journal of Autism and Childhood Schizophrenia, 6*:209–234, 1976.

107. HAUSER, S. L., DELONG, G. R., and ROSMAN, N. P., "Pneumographic Findings in the Infantile Autism Syndrome. A Correlation with Temporal Lobe Disease," *Brain, 98*:667–688, 1975.

108. HAVELKOVA, M., "Follow-Up Study of 71 Children Diagnosed as Psychotic in Preschool Age," *American Journal of Orthopsychiatry, 38*:846–857, 1968.

109. HEELEY, A., and ROBERTS, G., "Tryptophan Metabolism in Psychotic Children," *Developmental Medicine and Child Neurology, 7*:46–49, 1965.

110. HERMELIN, B., and O'CONNOR, N., *Psychological Experiments with Autistic Children*, Pergamon Press, Oxford, England, 1970.

111. ———, "Measures of the Occipital Alpha Rhythm in Normal, Subnormal and Autistic Children," *British Journal of Psychiatry, 114*:603–610, 1968.

112. HERTZIG, M. A., and BIRCH, M. G., "Neurologic Organization in Psychiatrically Disturbed Adolescents," *Archives of General Psychiatry, 19*:528–537, 1968.

113. HESTON, L. L., and DENNEY, D., "Interaction Between Early Life Experience and Biological Factors in Schizophrenia," in Rosenthal, D., and Kety, S. S. (Eds.), *The Transmission of Schizophrenia*, pp. 363–376, Pergamon Press, London, 1968.

114. HIMWICH, H., et al., "A Biochemical Study of Early Infantile Autism," *Journal of Autism and Childhood Schizophrenia, 2*:114–126, 1972.

115. HOBERMAN, S. E., and GOLDFARB, W., "Speech Reception Thresholds in Schizophrenic Children," *Journal of Speech and Hearing Research, 6*:101–106, 1963.

116. HUTT, C., FORREST, S. J., and RICHER, J., "Cardiac Arrhythmia and Behavior in Autistic Children," *Acta Psychiatrica Scandinavica, 19*:361–372, 1975.

117. HUTT, C., et al., "A Behavioural and Electroencephalographic Study of Autistic Children," *Journal of Psychiatric Research, 3*:181–197, 1965.

118. JØRGENSEN, S., MELLERUP, E., and RAFAELSEN, O., "Amino Acid Excretion in Urine of Children with Various Psychiatric Diseases: A Thin Layer Chromatographic Study," *Danish Medical Bulletin, 6*:166–170, 1970.

119. KALLMAN, F., and ROTH, B., "Genetic Aspects of Preadolescent Schizophrenia," *American Journal of Psychiatry, 112*:599–606, 1956.

120. KANNER, L., "Follow-Up Study of Eleven Autistic Children Originally Reported in 1943," in Kanner, L. (Ed.), *Childhood Psychosis: Initial Studies and New Insights*, pp. 161–187, John Wiley, New York, 1973.

121. ———, "To What Extent is Early Infantile Autism Determined by Constitutional Inadequacies?," in *Genetics and the Inheritance of Integrated Neurological Psychiatric Patterns*, Research Publications of the Association for Research in Nervous and Mental Disease, *33*:378–385, 1953.

122. ———, "Problems of Nosology and Psychodynamics of Early Infantile Autism," *American Journal of Orthopsychiatry, 19*:416–426, 1949.

123. ———, "Irrelevant and Metaphorical Language in Early Infantile Autism," *American Journal of Psychiatry, 103*:242–246, 1946.

124. ———, "Autistic Disturbances of Affective Contact," *Nervous Child, 2*:217–250, 1943.

125. ——, and Eisenberg, L., "Notes on the Follow-Up Studies of Autistic Children," in Hoch, P. H., and Zubin, J. (Eds.), *Psychopathology of Childhood*, pp. 227–239, Grune & Stratton, New York, 1955.

126. Kety, S. S., et al., "The Types and Prevalence of Mental Illness in the Biological and Adoptive Families of Adopted Schizophrenics," in Rosenthal, D., and Kety, S. S. (Eds.), *The Transmission of Schizophrenia*, pp. 345–362, Pergamon Press, London, 1968.

127. Knobloch, H., and Pasamanick, B., "Some Etiologic and Prognostic Factors in Early Infantile Autism and Psychosis," *Pediatrics*, 55:182–191, 1975.

128. Kohn, M. L., "Social Class and Schizophrenia: A Critical Review," in Rosenthal, D., and Kety, S. S. (Eds.), *The Transmission of Schizophrenia*, pp. 155–173, Pergamon Press, London, 1968.

129. Kolvin, I., Ounsted, C., and Roth, M., "Six Studies in the Childhood Psychoses. V. Cerebral Dysfunction and Childhood Psychoses," *British Journal of Psychiatry*, 118:407–414, 1971.

130. Kolvin, I., et al., "Six Studies in the Childhood Psychoses," *British Journal of Psychiatry*, 118:381–491, 1971.

131. Koppitz, E. M., *The Bender Gestalt Test for Young Children*, Grune & Stratton, New York, 1964.

132. Kramer, Y., Rabkin, R., and Spitzer, R. L., "Whirling as a Clinical Test in Childhood Schizophrenia," *Journal of Pediatrics*, 52(3):295–303, 1958.

133. Laufer, M. W., and Gair, D. S., "Childhood Schizophrenia," in Bellak, L., and Loeb, L. (Eds.), *The Schizophrenic Syndrome*, pp. 378–460, Grune & Stratton, New York, 1969.

134. Leitch, M., and Schafer, S., "A Study of the Thematic Apperception Tests of Psychotic Children," *American Journal of Orthopsychiatry*, 17:337–342, 1947.

135. Lelord, G., et al., "Comparative Study of Conditioning of Averaged Evoked Responses by Coupling Sound and Light in Normal and Autistic Children," *Psychophysiology*, 10:415–425, 1973.

136. Lockyer, L., and Rutter, M., "A Five- to Fifteen-Year Follow-Up Study of Infantile Psychosis: IV. Patterns of Cognitive Ability," *British Journal of Social and Clinical Psychology*, 9:152–163, 1970.

137. ——, "A Five- to Fifteen-Year Follow-Up Study of Infantile Psychosis—III. Psychological Aspects," *British Journal of Psychiatry*, 115:865–882, 1969.

138. Lotter, V., "Epidemiology of Autistic Conditions in Young Children. II. Some Characteristics of the Parents and Children," *Social Psychiatry*, 1:163–173, 1967.

139. ——, "Epidemiology of Autistic Conditions in Young Children. I. Prevalence," *Social Psychiatry*, 1:124–137, 1966.

140. Lovaas, O. I., et al., "Some Generalization and Follow-Up Measures on Autistic Children in Behavior Therapy," *Journal of Applied Behavior Analysis*, 6:131–166, 1973.

141. Lowell, M., "Audiological Assessment," in Ritvo, E. R. (Ed.), *Autism: Diagnosis, Current Research and Management*, Spectrum, New York, 1976.

142. Lucas, A., Krause, R., and Domino, E., "Biological Studies in Childhood Schizophrenia: Plasma and RBC Cholinesterase Activity," *Journal of Autism and Childhood Schizophrenia*, 1:172–181, 1971.

143. MacCulloch, M. J., Williams, C., and Davies, P., "Heart-Rate Variability in a Group of Cerebral Palsied Children," *Developmental Medicine and Child Neurology*, 13:645–650, 1971.

144. Mahler, M. S., *On Human Symbiosis and the Vicissitudes of Individuation. Vol. 1. Infantile Psychosis*, International Universities Press, New York, 1968.

145. ——, "On Child Psychosis and Schizophrenia. Autistic and Symbiotic Infantile Psychoses," in Eissler, R. S., et al. (Eds.), *The Psychoanalytic Study of the Child*, vol. 7, pp. 286–305, International Universities Press, New York, 1952.

146. ——, Ross, J. R., Jr., and DeFries, Z., "Clinical Studies in Benign and Malignant Cases of Childhood Psychosis (Schizophrenic-Like)," *American Journal of Orthopsychiatry*, 19:295–305, 1949.

147. Marcus, J., "Cerebral Functioning in Offspring of Schizophrenics. A Possible Genetic Factor," *International Journal of Mental Health*, 3:57–73, 1974.

148. Mednick, S. A., et al., "Perinatal Conditions and Infant Development in Children with Schizophrenic Parents," *Social Biology*, 18:S103–S113, 1971.

149. Meehl, P. E., "Schizotaxia, Schizotypy, Schizophrenia," *American Psychologist*, 17:827–838, 1962.

150. Meyers, D., and Goldfarb, W., "Psychiatric Appraisals of Parents and Siblings of Schizophrenic Children," *American Journal of Psychiatry*, 118:902–908, 1962.

151. Miller, W. H., and Bernal, M. E., "Measurement of the Cardiac Response in Schizophrenic and Normal Children," *Psychophysiology*, 8:533–537, 1971.

152. Narasimachari, N., and Himwich, H., "Biochemical Study in Early Infantile Autism," *Biological Psychiatry*, 10:425–432, 1975.

153. O'Neal, P., and Robins, L. N., "Childhood Patterns Predictive of Adult Schizophrenia: A 30-Year Follow-Up Study," *American Journal of Psychiatry*, 115:385–391, 1958.

154. Onheiber, P., et al., "Sleep and Dream Patterns of Child Schizophrenics," *Archives of General Psychiatry*, 12:568–571, 1965.

155. Ornitz, E. M., "Neurophysiologic Studies of Autistic Children," in Rutter, M., and Schopler, E. (Eds.), *Autism: A Reappraisal of Concepts*, Plenum Press, New York, (in press).

156. ——, "The Modulation of Sensory Input and Motor Output in Autistic Children," *Journal of Autism and Childhood Schizophrenia*, 4:197–215, 1974.

157. ——, "Childhood Autism. A Review of the Clinical and Experimental Literature (Medical Progress)," *California Medicine*, 118:21–47, 1973.

158. ——, "Development of Sleep Patterns in Autistic Children," in Clemente, C. D., Purpura, D., and Mayer, F. (Eds.), *Sleep and the Maturing Nervous System*, Academic Press, New York, 1972.

159. ——, "Disorders of Perception Common to Early Infantile Autism and Schizophrenia," *Comprehensive Psychiatry*, 10:259–274, 1969.

160. ——, and Ritvo, E. R., "Medical Assessment," in Ritvo, E. R. (Ed.), *Autism: Diagnosis, Current Research and Management*, Spectrum, New York, 1976.

161. ——, "The Syndrome of Autism: A Critical Review," *American Journal of Psychiatry*, 133:609–621, 1976.

162. ——, "Perceptual Inconstancy in Early Infantile Autism," *Archives of General Psychiatry*, 18:76–98, 1968.

163. ——, and Walter, R. D., "Dreaming Sleep in Autistic and Schizophrenic Children," *American Journal of Psychiatry*, 122:419–424, 1965.

164. ——, "Dreaming Sleep in Autistic Twins," *Archives of General Psychiatry*, 12:77–79, 1965.

165. Ornitz, E. M., et al., "The Recovery Cycle of the Averaged Auditory Evoked Response During Sleep in Autistic Children," *Electroencephalography and Clinical Neurophysiology*, 37:173–174, 1974.

166. ——, et al., "The EEG and Rapid Eye Movements During REM Sleep in Babies," *Electroencephalography and Clinical Neurophysiology*, 30:350–353, 1971.

167. ——, et al., "The Auditory Evoked Response in Normal and Autistic Children During Sleep," *Electroencephalography and Clinical Neurophysiology*, 25:221–230, 1968.

168. Paine, R. S., and Oppé, T. E., *Neurological Examination of Children*, Spastics Society Medical and Information Unit, Heinemann Medical, London, 1966.

169. PENDLETON, M. E., and PAINE, R. S., "Vestibular Nystagmus in Human Infants," *Neurology, 11:*450–458, 1961.

170. POLLACK, M., and KRIEGER, H. P., "Oculomotor and Postural Patterns in Schizophrenic Children," *Archives of Neurology and Psychiatry, 79:*720–726, 1958.

171. POTTER, H. W., "Schizophrenia in Children," *American Journal of Psychiatry, 12:*1253–1270, 1933.

172. PROVENCE, S., and LIPTON, R. D., *Infants in Institutions*, International Universities Press, New York, 1962.

173. QUITKIN, F., RIFKIN, A., and KLEIN, D. F., "Neurologic Soft Signs in Schizophrenia and Character Disorders. Organicity in Schizophrenia with Premorbid Associality and Emotionally Unstable Character Disorders," *Archives of General Psychiatry, 33:*845–853, 1976.

174. RACHMAN, S., and BERGER, M., "Whirling and Postural Control in Schizophrenic Children," *Journal of Child Psychology and Psychiatry, 4:*137–155, 1963.

175. RANK, B., "Intensive Study and Treatment of Preschool Children Who Show Marked Personality Deviations or 'Atypical Development,' and Their Parents," in Caplan, G. (Ed.), *Emotional Problems of Early Childhood*, pp. 491–501, Basic Books, New York, 1955.

176. REISER, D. E., and BROWN, J. L., "Patterns of Later Development in Children with Infantile Psychosis," *Journal of the American Academy of Child Psychiatry, 3(4):*650–667, 1964.

177. RICHEY, E., "The Language Program," in Ritvo, E. R. (Ed.), *Autism: Diagnosis, Current Research and Management*, Spectrum, New York, 1976.

178. RICKS, D. F., and BERRY, J. C., "Family and Symptom Patterns That Precede Schizophrenia," in Roff, M., and Ricks, D. F. (Eds.), *Life History Research in Psychopathology*, vol. 1, pp. 31–50, University of Minnesota Press, Minneapolis, 1970.

179. RICKS, D. F., and NAMECHE, G., "Symbiosis, Sacrifice and Schizophrenia," *Mental Hygiene, 50:*541–551, 1966.

180. RIEDER, R. O., BROMAN, S. H., and ROSENTHAL, D., "The Offspring of Schizophrenics II: Perinatal Factors and IQ," *Archives of General Psychiatry, 34:*789–799, 1977.

181. RITVO, S., and PROVENCE, S., "Form Perception and Imitation in Some Autistic Children: Diagnostic Findings and Their Contextual Interpretation," in Eissler, R. S., et al. (Eds.), *The Psychoanalytic Study of the Child*, vol. 8, pp. 155–161, International Universities Press, New York, 1953.

182. RITVO, E. R., et al., "Effects of L-Dopa in Autism," *Journal of Autism and Childhood Schizophrenia, 1:*190–205, 1971.

183. ———, et al., "Social Class Factors in Autism," *Journal of Autism and Childhood Schizophrenia, 1:*297–310, 1971.

184. ———, et al., "Correlation of Psychiatric Diagnoses and EEG Findings: A Double-Blind Study of 184 Hospitalized Children," *American Journal of Psychiatry, 126:*988–996, 1970.

185. ———, et al., "Increased Blood Serotonin and Platelets in Early Infantile Autism," *Archives of General Psychiatry, 23:*566–572, 1970.

186. ———, et al., "Decreased Postrotatory Nystagmus in Early Infantile Autism," *Neurology, 19:*653–658, 1969.

187. ROBINS, L. N., *Deviant Children Grown Up*, Williams & Wilkins, Baltimore, Md., 1966.

188. ROSENTHAL, D., *Genetic Theory and Abnormal Behavior*, McGraw-Hill, New York, 1970.

189. ———, et al., "Schizophrenics' Offspring Reared in Adoptive Homes," in Rosenthal, D., and Kety, S. S. (Eds.), *The Transmission of Schizophrenia*, pp. 377–391, Pergamon Press, London, 1968.

190. RUBENSTEIN, E. A., "Childhood Mental Disease in America: A Review of the Literature Before 1900," *American Journal of Orthopsychiatry, 18:*314–321, 1948.

191. RUTTER, M., "The Development of Infantile Autism," *Psychological Medicine, 4:*147–163, 1974.

192. ———, "Childhood Schizophrenia Reconsidered," *Journal of Autism and Childhood Schizophrenia, 2:*315–337, 1972.

193. ———, "Autistic Children—Infancy to Adulthood," *Seminars in Psychiatry, 2:*435–450, 1970.

194. ———, "Behavioral and Cognitive Characteristics of a Series of Psychotic Children," in Wing, J. K. (Ed.), *Early Childhood Autism: Clinical, Educational and Social Aspects*, Pergamon Press, London, 1966.

195. ———, "The Influence of Organic and Emotional Factors on the Origins, Nature and Outcome of Childhood Psychosis," *Developmental Medicine and Child Neurology, 7:*518–528, 1965.

196. ———, GREENFELD, D., and LOCKYER, L., "A Five to Fifteen Year Follow-Up Study of Infantile Psychosis. II. Social and Behavioural Outcome," *British Journal of Psychiatry, 113:*1183–1199, 1967.

197. RUTTER, M., and LOCKYER, L. "A Five to Fifteen Year Follow-Up Study of Infantile Psychosis. I. Description of the Sample," *British Journal of Psychiatry, 113:*1169–1182, 1967.

198. RUTTER, M., and SUSSENWEIN, F., "A Developmental and Behavioral Approach to the Treatment of Preschool Autistic Children," *Journal of Autism and Childhood Schizophrenia, 1:*376–397, 1971.

199. SALADINO, C., and SIVA-SANKAR, D., "Studies on Erythrocyte Magnesium and Potassium Levels in Childhood Schizophrenia and Growth," *Behavioral Neuropsychiatry, 10:*24–28, 1969.

200. SCHAIN, R., and FREEDMAN, D., "Studies on 5-Hydroxyindole Metabolism in Autistic and Other Mentally Retarded Children," *Journal of Pediatrics, 58:*315–320, 1961.

201. SCHAIN, R., and YANNET, H., "Infantile Autism: An Analysis of 50 Cases and a Consideration of Certain Relevant Neurophysiological Concepts," *Journal of Pediatrics, 57:*560–567, 1960.

202. SCHOPLER, E., "Visual Versus Tactual Receptor Preference in Normal and Schizophrenic Children," *Journal of Abnormal Psychology, 71:*108–114, 1966.

203. ———, "Early Infantile Autism and Receptor Processes," *Archives of General Psychiatry, 13:*327–335, 1965.

204. SHAPIRO, T., CHIARANDINI, I., and FISH, B., "Thirty Severely Disturbed Children. Evaluation of Their Language Development for Classification and Prognosis," *Archives of General Psychiatry, 30:*819–825, 1974.

205. SHAPIRO, T., and FISH, B., "A Method to Study Language Deviation as an Aspect of Ego Organization in Young Schizophrenic Children," *Journal of the American Academy of Child Psychiatry, 8:*36–56, 1969.

206. ———, and GINSBERG, G., "The Speech of a Schizophrenic Child From Two to Six," *American Journal of Psychiatry, 128:*1408–1413, 1972.

207. SHAPIRO, T., ROBERTS, A., and FISH, B., "Imitation and Echoing in Young Schizophrenic Children," *Journal of the American Academy of Child Psychiatry, 9:*548–567, 1970.

208. SHAW, C., LUCAS, J., and RABINOVITCH, R., "Metabolic Studies in Childhood Schizophrenia. Effects of Tryptophan Loading on Indole Excretion," *Archives of General Psychiatry, 1:*366–371, 1959.

209. SIMON, G. B., and GILLIES, S. M., "Some Physical Characteristics of a Group of Psychotic Children," *British Journal of Psychiatry, 110:*104–107, 1964.

210. SIVA-SANKAR, D., "Biogenic Amine Uptake by Blood Platelets and RBC in Childhood Schizophrenia," *Acta Paedopsychiatrica, 37:*174–182, 1970.

211. SLATER, E., and COWIE, V., *The Genetics of Mental Disorders*, Oxford University Press, London, 1971.

212. SMALL, J. G., "EEG and Neurophysiological Studies of Early Infantile Autism," *Biological Psychiatry, 10:*385–398, 1975.

213. ———, DeMyer, M. K., and Milstein, V., "CNV Responses of Autistic and Normal Children," *Journal of Autism and Childhood Schizophrenia, 1–2:*215–231, 1971.

214. Spitz, R. A., "Anaclitic Depression—An Inquiry Into the Genesis of Psychiatric Conditions in Early Childhood—I.," in Eissler, R. S., et al. (Eds.), *The Psychoanalytic Study of the Child,* vol. 2, pp. 313–342, International Universities Press, New York, 1946.

215. Spitzer, R. L., Endicott, J., and Robins, E., *Research Diagnostic Criteria for a Selected Group of Functional Disorders,* 1st ed., Biometrics Research, New York State Department of Mental Hygiene, New York, 1975.

216. Sutton, E., and Reed, J., "Abnormal Amino Acid Metabolism in a Case Suggesting Autism," *Journal of Diseases of Children, 96:*23–28, 1956.

217. Szurek, S. A., "Childhood Schizophrenia Symposium, 1955. Psychotic Episodes and Psychotic Maldevelopment," *American Journal of Orthopsychiatry, 25:* 519–543, 1956.

218. ———, and Berlin, I., "Elements of Psychotherapeutics with the Schizophrenic Child and His Parents," *Psychiatry, 19:*1–19, 1956.

219. Tanguay, P., "Clinical and Electrophysiological Research," in Ritvo, E. R. (Ed.), *Autism: Diagnosis, Current Research and Management,* Spectrum, New York, 1976.

220. Tilton, J. R., DeMyer, M. K., and Loew, L. H., *Annotated Bibliography on Childhood Schizophrenia: 1955–1964,* Grune & Stratton, New York, 1966.

221. Torrey, E. F., Hersh, S. P., and McCabe, K. D., "Early Childhood Psychosis and Bleeding During Pregnancy. A Prospective Study of Gravid Women and Their Offspring," *Journal of Autism and Childhood Schizophrenia, 5:*287–297, 1966.

222. Tucker, G. J., Campion, E. W., and Silberfarb, P. M., "Sensorimotor Functions and Cognitive Disturbance in Psychiatric Patients," *American Journal of Psychiatry, 132:*17–21, 1975.

223. Waldrop, M. F., and Halverson, C. F., "Minor Physical Anomalies and Hyperactive Behavior in Young Children," in Hellmuth, J. (Ed.), *Exceptional Infant, Studies in Abnormalities,* vol. 2, pp. 343–380, Brunner-Mazel, New York, 1971.

224. Walk, A., "The Pre-History of Child Psychiatry," *British Journal of Psychiatry, 110:*754–767, 1964.

225. Ward, A. J., "Early Infantile Autism—Diagnosis, Etiology, and Treatment," *Psychological Bulletin, 73:*350–362, 1970.

226. Watt, N. F., "Childhood and Adolescent Routes to Schizophrenia," in Ricks, D. F., Thomas, A., and Roff, M. (Eds.), *Life History Research in Psychopathology,* vol. 3, pp. 194–211, University of Minnesota Press, Minneapolis, 1974.

227 Wechsler, D., and Jaros, E., "Schizophrenic Patterns on the WISC," *Journal of Clinical Psychology, 21:*288–291, 1965.

228. Weil, A. P., "Clinical Data and Dynamic Considerations in Certain Cases of Childhood Schizophrenia," *American Journal of Orthopsychiatry, 23:*518–529, 1953.

229. Wender, P. H., et al., "Cross-Fostering: A Research Strategy for Clarifying the Role of Genetic and Experiential Factors in the Etiology of Schizophrenia," *Archives of General Psychiatry, 30:*121–128, 1974.

230. Werry, J., "Childhood Psychoses," in Quay, H. C., and Werry, J. (Eds.), *Psychopathological Disorders of Childhood,* John Wiley, New York, 1972.

231. Widelitz, M., and Feldman, W., "Pink Spot in Childhood Schizophrenia," *Behavioral Neuropsychiatry, 1:*29–30, 1964.

232. Woodruff, R. A., Goodwin, D. W., and Guze, S. B., *Psychiatric Diagnosis,* Oxford University Press, New York, 1974.

233. Yuwiler, A., et al., "Uptake and Efflux of Serotonin From Platelets of Autistic and Nonautistic Children," *Journal of Autism and Childhood Schizophrenia, 5:*83–98, 1975.

234. ———, et al., "Examination of Circadian-rhythmicity of Blood Serotonin and Platelets in Autistic and Non-Autistic Children," *Journal of Autism and Childhood Schizophrenia, 1:*421–435, 1971.

15 / The Borderline Child

Morton Chethik

Name of Syndrome, Alternative or Historical Name

Syndrome: The Borderline Child
Historical: The Borderline Psychotic Child

INTRODUCTORY NOTE

The term "borderline" describes a severe form of childhood psychopathology. In the last twenty years it has come into ever increasing use. Unfortunately, in clinical practice, it is a concept that is commonly misused and misunderstood. It is often regarded as a transitory state between psychosis and severe neurosis; children who give evidence of fleeting periods of psychosis, or of intense ego disruption are quickly diagnosed as "borderline syndrome."

In the last few years, there has been a progressive tendency in the literature to describe this syndrome as a form of pathology in its own right. This is a point of view that will be maintained here. It is assumed that particular levels of developmental arrest and specific forms of aberrant development have shaped ego development, object relations, and the sense of self into typical "borderline" form. These arrests promote fixed patterns which we can ultimately identify as belonging to this category. A major purpose of this chapter will be to delineate specifically the characteristic borderline genetic-dynamic factors, ego processes, pathology in object relations, and disturbances in the formation of the self.

Description of Syndrome Along With Some of Its Common Variants

What does the borderline child look like? The introduction suggested that a unity of genetic and dynamic concepts characterize the borderline child. At the same time, it is difficult to speak of prototypical borderline behavior and symptoms. A great many divergent phenomena including a considerable variety of different behaviors can stem from these underlying causes. Nonetheless, there are some characteristics that can be delineated in broad terms. Matthew, a youngster in residential treatment for a number of years, showed one particular kind of borderline adaptation.

"Cartoon boy," as Matthew was nicknamed by the other children in the residential treatment center, was ten years of age. Each day we found him, for long periods of time, engrossed in solitary play producing his shows and cartoons. His hero, Popeye, was represented by a little toy animal, who fought pursuing monsters and attacking tornadoes with great vigor and animation. When the demands of the day interrupted Matthew's cartooning, for example, when called to lunch, Matthew announced "intermission" and tentatively and fearfully joined his cottage mates in the dining room.

"Cartoon boy" didn't have any friends in the cottage. He felt very lonely, he told his therapist, and he wanted the boys to like him. He played "Sports Reel" in his sessions, in the course of which he vividly became a great baseball hero and football giant. He was cheered by huge throngs of imagined fans in the stands which surrounded him.

Often during the first year of his stay at the treatment center, Matthew would suddenly become furious. On one occasion a severe outburst came after a home visit. He was angry at the therapist and the furniture, threw toys and crafts around the office. On campus he seemed to direct his attacks toward younger girls, attempting at times to scratch and choke them. Following these open attacks, he would engage in self-abuse, such as throwing himself into the mud, banging his head against the wall, and asking to have his fingers cut off to keep from scratching. In his therapy hours Matthew was concerned that his "madness" was coming out. The madness came in the form of

dreams every night which filled the entire night—they involved tricking and killing his little sister in brutal ways. As he related these dreams, he pleaded with his therapist, "Please get me in control. If you get me in control, I'll control my dreams." Matthew's home visits aroused his intense jealousy toward the sister who remained at home.

"Cartoon boy" was also called "baby Matthew" because of his need to be unusually close to adult staff. At times he needed to be in their shadow, almost to touch them. He developed rituals in relation to his safe therapist. He visited the therapy building four times daily, always took the same path to go there, and sat in the same chair in the waiting room. The sameness gave a fixed reassuring quality to his contact with the therapist.

In order to cope with the chaos of the week, Matthew devised an early warning system which would help him be "on guard." He wanted lists of the kinds of events which could upset him (e.g., bigger boys, changes in schedule) and he developed charts to follow his mood swings. A graph followed the course of moods over the week and showed a range from the highest category "calmness" to the lowest category "blow-up." He wanted the charts hung on the bulletin board in a prominent position.

Descriptive Characteristics

ANXIETY

As a rule, borderline children are exceedingly anxious. Their anxiety is chronic, often diffuse and free floating. It is quickly evident that they have neither an adequate defensive system[15, 35] or adequate abilities to judge and appraise reality in a way which would help them bind their anxiety. They often evidence panic, their anxiety lacks the signal function that ordinarily triggers defense mechanisms, and that would help cope with frightening situations. Matthew, for example, limited himself to familiar surroundings, or fled into his cartoon fantasy because venturing out of the safe perimeters he had devised exposed him to this overwhelming anxiety.

Dangers from the outside are the most constant source of anxiety and act to induce fears of annihilation. In cartoon play, for example, Matthew attempted to master the tornadoes, hurricanes, etc. to which the real world could subject him. Borderline children also typically fear separation from objects. They tend to cling to adults who will protect them and often evidence much anxiety when their contact with the protective person is temporarily broken. They also often fear the strength of their impulses, as Matthew feared his "madness." They are menaced by the possibility of being overpowered by the strength of wishes or affects; at those moments they show intense fear. Allied with these feelings are fears of disorganization. Matthew urgently sought his therapist's help in "getting him in control" because of the fear of falling apart.

NEUROTIC SYMPTOMATOLOGY

Like many borderline children, Matthew manifested some neurotic symtomatology. He developed rituals and obsessions (daily invariable routines and procedures) that helped him cope with ever present fears. However, these obsessional features, were fragile and quickly came apart. While the borderline child does develop neurotic symptoms, they are typically fleeting and not fully structuralized. The obsessions are quickly replaced by multiple phobias or intense restrictions and inhibitions. Borderline youngsters often evidence a polysymptomatic neurosis that does not become fully established nor does it effectively bind their anxiety.

IMPULSIVITY

Their impulse expression is characterized by extremes. On the one hand, many borderline youngsters evidence chronic problems with impulse control. There is often a history of severe temper tantrums, and it is not unusual to see sequences of repetitive eruptions of aggression and rage. Matthew's "madness" was induced by rivalry with a sister whom he felt was favored; and at the treatment center his angry impulses were immediately discharged toward younger girls. However, there are also many borderline children who react globally to these potential eruptions. They avoid all social contacts (and thus establish severe forms of social isolation), or they develop intense fantasy involvement (and thus separate themselves totally from the frustrating and upsetting environment). In this way, major affective constriction and a total muting of impulses can sometimes ensue.

CHARACTER TRAITS

It is not unusual to see trends of severe character pathology in the personality of borderline children. Narcissistic features are often evident. In order to deal with his painfully low self-esteem, Matthew developed grandiose fantasies of baseball and football heroes, which he attempted to

live out. Masochistic elements can accompany borderline problems. Some of these children find relief from their anxiety by some form of self-mutilation. Matthew responded to his impulses to kill his sister by intense self-abusive reactions —he wanted his fingers cut off to keep from scratching little girls. In such cases the masochistic trends are often fueled by harsh superego precursors. At times paranoid aspects are also evident. The world may be misperceived as totally threatening and attacking. Oral dependent character features can be prominent. Many borderline children develop demanding, child-like, regressed relationships with "protecting" adults who symbolize safety and gratification. Like Matthew, they tend to become overattached, overinvolved and, at times, overidentified with specific characteristics of these adults in order to minimize any separation.

In the evaluation of the borderline child it is the whole gestalt which determines diagnosis, rather than single symptoms. Any of the characteristics described above should arouse the suspicion that borderline pathology may be present. Obviously, they do not in themselves determine the diagnosis. For example, chronic anxiety and persistent problems in impulse control may be expressive of a number of different conditions. However, if the majority of the above descriptive features are evident, they can suggest a borderline constellation. This would need to be corroborated by further metapsychological appraisal.

Chronic and conspicuous problems in ego development will tend to indicate the possibility of borderline problems, whereas neurotic children will show such developmental deviations only in minor degree. On the other hand, borderline children maintain their capacity to test reality and do not evidence the hallucinatory or delusional problems of childhood psychosis (autistic and symbiotic psychosis).

History of Its Identification, When, and By Whom?

In the late 1940s, as we gained greater knowledge of the developmental childhood psychoses (Autism[20] and Symbiosis[26]), another closely related disturbance immediately began to be reported in the literature. These children were recognized as a special group that were beyond neurosis, yet did not meet the criteria delineated for the childhood psychoses. In an article by Margaret Mahler[27] children were described who had "a certain kind of benign psychosis" that appeared neurosis-like. Annamarie Weil[37] described children who had not achieved emancipation from mother and showed similarities to Mahler's symbiotic cases without obvious psychosis. She called them "atypical, deviational children with fragmented egos." Others reported individual cases and used similar terms to describe these children who seemed to have "in-between" pathologies—Rank,[32] Harley,[18] Alpert,[1] Maenchen,[25] and Rochlin.[33] Two major foci were stressed in describing these children: the nature of their chronic and severe ego disturbances and the problems in object relations (particularly profound separation difficulties).

In the early and mid-1950s the term "borderline" began to be commonly and widely used to designate this child disturbance. Weil[36] drew parallels between these children and the "psychoneurotic schizophrenics and severe borderline states" that were described in the adult literature by Greenacre,[17] Deutsch,[4] and Polatin and Hoch.[31] In 1958, in an article entitled "Borderline States in Childhood and Adolescence," Elizabeth Geleerd reviewed this developmental syndrome and carefully separated it from childhood phychoses.[15] It was clear that this pathology was linked to arrests and fixations on a "higher" or more mature level than autism and symbiosis.

Since the mid-1950s several major clinical studies have been undertaken which sought to describe these disorders more completely and to develop theoretical formulations within which the resulting observations could best be understood. Ekstein, in discussing a group of children at the Menningers,[5] described another variety of ego disturbance they displayed. Rather than the chronic and relatively fixed ego deviance that most authors described, Ekstein saw many children in his study who showed markedly shifting levels of ego organization within the same child. These patients would oscillate quickly between primitive ego states and more advanced ego functioning. In their work at the Hampstead Clinic, Rosenfeld and Sprince[35] did a metapsychological "profile" analysis on a series of borderline children. They added a number of important concepts to understanding the phenomena of this pathology. They noted that there was a typical lack of phase dominance in psychosexual development and specifically explored the impact on the personality when there was an inability to utilize repression. They also felt that the central issue in borderline children was their struggle between primary identification with objects and object cathexis. Much of the borderline child's anxiety, they noted, was due to their fears of fusion.

In recent years (late 1960s to early 1970s) Frijling-Schreuder[14] has also completed a metapsychological analysis of a group of borderline youngsters differentiating psychotic, borderline, and neurotic processes. Chethik and Fast,[2, 7, 8] working with children in Ann Arbor, Michigan, have written a series of articles that attempt to describe the origin of the fixation and arrests. The authors have focused on the infantile period in which the child makes the transition out of narcissism, as the developmental source of their pathology.

The literature has addressed itself to three major themes. The descriptive boundaries of the pathology have slowly been delineated, differentiating it from neuroses and psychoses. Many articles have dealt with the clarification between borderline pathology and prepsychotic or latent psychotic conditions. The distinction has also been drawn between this pathology and that associated with regression from severe neurosis. Secondly, a number of authors have struggled with placing this pathology in a developmental framework. They have speculated on the kinds of fixations and arrests during infancy and early childhood that will produce this kind of problem. Thirdly, stemming from the inferences and hypotheses developed, treatment interventions have been described.

Clinical Course of the Syndrome Along With Associated Clinical Experience

The borderline syndrome is a form of severe developmental pathology; the signs of its presence and the functional difficulties are evident from infancy. At all levels of development, the child's progression is uneven and inadequate; often there is a major delay in achieving the milestones that mark the effective unfolding of personality. Commonly, there are peculiarities in the child's maturational patterning and physiological functioning as well as in the functioning of the psychological apparatus. In the very early histories of these children, it is at times difficult to distinguish between those that will emerge with psychotic features and those with borderline personality. Throughout their development, however, borderline children generally show greater object relatedness than do the overtly psychotic children. While there are no published studies of the incidence of borderline children (it is both unofficial and difficult to define), most clinics find that they appear with much greater frequency than do the cases of childhood psychoses.

INFANCY

Many authors discuss three primary factors that contribute to borderline pathology. The first involves hereditary and constitutional factors which may predispose these children, and place them at risk. The second refers to those severe developmental interferences (pain, illness) during the first year, particularly, which may also establish the foundation for a borderline sequence. And third, there has been a great deal of evidence to suggest that major problems in the infant-mother bond may be a primary source of this pathology. Combinations of the above are often evident.

Matthew, the youngster described earlier, seemed to evidence a constitutional vulnerability. His mother, a wholesome woman who cared very adequately for two older siblings, described a nightmare-like first year of development for this child. At first Matthew was unable to suck. He cried constantly during the day. Often his distress reached screaming intensity without any evident source of irritation or frustration. The parents finaly found that the only way to soothe him was to drive him endlessly in the family car. Even when he slept, Matthew was obviously fussy and troubled.

Throughout the first year, Matthew was tense and stiff when held in his mother's arms. He arched his back away from her, and she found herself unable to calm him. Mrs. L. had trouble with feeding. As the year progressed, Matthew refused to chew and would not take liquids other than milk and cocoa.

Tom, another borderline youngster, reflected the impact of pain and illness during his infancy and early childhood.

Tom underwent pyloric spasms during the first eighteen months of his life, and all medication seemed ineffective. His chronic pain was evident—he fought feedings, vomited frequently, suffered from diarrhea, and gained little weight during that period.

The mother-child interaction was not easy. Often in pain, Tom held onto his mother tenaciously, clutching her and digging his fingers into anything he could grasp on her person. Mother recalled no smiling during that first year. All toys and objects Tom found, he bit into. He developed his own unusual means of propulsion (rather than crawling, standing, and walking). Again, under the impact of pain, he dug his heels into the household carpeting while

lying on his back, and propelled himself backwards throughout the house with great momentum. On many occasions, he crashed into furniture.

As noted above, many of these children show deviant and erratic physiologic patterning in infancy. At times there was evidence of hypertonic states, erratic patterns of eating and sleeping, and vomiting and diarrhea without any evident causes. With many of these youngsters, one has the impression that they are overwhelmed by impulses from within or without (protective barrier concept, Freud, 1920[12]) and have intense difficulty in inhibiting stimuli. In contrast to the hyperactive picture illustrated by Matthew and Tom, the early histories of some borderline children evidence other drive deviations. Some are markedly apathetic and never cry or signal their needs.

The pre-stages of object relations are often problematic. A borderline infant may not respond to mother's face for months, may react negatively to cuddling, may mold poorly, and may fail to make anticipatory gestures when picked up. This poor foundation often disturbs later communication between mother and child, and the child will not develop an adequate system for signaling his needs to the environment.

Many of these children engage in excessive auto-erotic and auto-aggressive activity. They tend to evidence a greater degree of rubbing, rolling, head banging, and, at times, sucking and biting. These are forms of motor discharge, and may lead to later problems in motor development which are in turn expressed in peculiar gaits, unusual postures and rigidities, and a lack of modulation in speech.

CHILDHOOD

Beyond infancy, the maturational sequences continue to unfold in an unusual pattern. Problems of manageability are often prominent.

Mark, who later became a patient in residential treatment, was seen initially at age four. His mother described him as an "albatross around her neck." She could not limit him. At the supermarket he ran throughout the store pulling many items off the shelves and jumping and climbing over counters. Mother was unable to visit one when accompanied by Mark because he was restless and needed constant supervision.

At times Mark yelled and screamed in a very infantile way, and tantrums, produced by very minor frustrations, were an everyday affair. With Mark present, mother found it very difficult to share her attention. He seemed jealous and interfered with her when she was on the telephone. Mark also refused to do anything for himself—he refused to try to unbutton his jacket and waited for mother to take off his hat and coat.

In contrast to his usual wildness and distractibility, within the limits of his familiar room Mark could play for hours. He could sit and listen to his records over and over again and play with a group of plastic soldiers for long lengths of time. Mother experienced an uneasy feeling because at times, in the course of this play, Mark would let out a peculiar shriek for no apparent reason.

Mother also noted some of Mark's occasional efforts to restrain himself. He doubled up his fists and made squeezing noises as if to keep himself from breaking things.

During these childhood years the pregenital drives dominate (greedy, impatient, sloppy, dirty) the lives of many borderline children without the concomitant ego development usual for that age. Mark showed some beginning efforts to inhibit his destructive wishes (doubling up and squeezing), but this aspect of his development was very primitive and not well established. He showed a rather typical overload of anxiety and tension which was expressed in a driven restlessness, sleeplessness, and frequent inability to concentrate. Some borderline children become addicted to pretend play, which they are unable to stop. They have a greater tendency to get "lost" in their play and identify it as complete and real. Mark's mother's uneasiness regarding his shriek when he was engrossed with his toy soldiers reflected her awareness of his total absorption and his lack of a reality perspective.

Mark evidenced other usual borderline features in early childhood. We often note coercive behavior toward objects (Mark dominated his mother's attention) which forces parents to act as the child's omnipotent extension. Borderline toddlers and young children are often extremely anxious in new environments. They are terrified of separation and try to cope with this by constant efforts at domination and demands of the object which reassures them that they control their source of protection. In contrast to the coercive object tie that Mark evidenced, there are many borderline children who will show the opposite extremes of object detachment. They are withdrawn and aloof from their mothers and evidence a precocious independence. They may be indiscriminately outgoing to all strangers.

LATENCY

In normal latency there is a marked growth of ego development with many consolidations and beginning structuralization. Borderline youngsters in latency usually evidence a superficial structuralization. They struggle with their impulses and social expectations using their rather fragile ego resources to maintain an equilibrium. Their earlier aloofness may be superseded by a shallow, inadequately learned politeness and superficial conformity. Evidence of greater conflicts (newer superego demands) may be expressed in the form of neurotic symptoms described earlier. Intense primary identifications can be employed to counter the instinctual dangers which are pressing for expression. Aggression and rage may be handled by an increase in ritualistic and obsessional features; these then become very pronounced and absorb enormous amounts of energy. Precocious sublimations and intellectualizations can be brought into the service of control and the creation of order.

Matthew, an extremely intelligent youngster, was often overwhelmed in school. When frightened in this way, he tore at his books and cried, but then returned to struggle with his assignments. On many occasions we could get a glimpse of his intense anxieties, and the new coping processes he was developing. For example, when Matthew began learning about Paris in class, he became very frightened. When he grasped the fact that Paris and France were separated from America by a large body of water, "getting lost" worries were induced. It was as if learning about distant Paris reverberated with his own feelings of estrangement, and his anxiety was marked. In his therapy hours at this point, Matthew described some newfound solutions. He associated all of the foreign (dreaded) landmarks with familiar landmarks within the United States. The Champs Elysees was similar to a broad street in Detroit, the Arc de Triumphe was similar to the Washington Square Arch in New York, and the Eiffel Tower reminded him of the electrical transmitters he saw near his home.

The effect of these associations was to invest the foreign places with a kinship to more familiar places, and his separation anxiety seemed to abate. This very cumbersome system provided a view of the extraordinary amount of energy necessary for this child to cope with object loss; it was nonetheless a more effective pattern than his earlier method of attaching himself to his protecting teacher. By continuing to use this process of familiarizing associations, Matthew was presently able to move farther away from his home and immediate environment than had been possible for him earlier.

At this point in his development, Matthew began to display increased ritualistic and compulsive features. At times this made him appear like a youngster with a severe obsessional character structure. However, the quality of the structuralization in Matthew's latency and in that of many borderline youngsters betrays a continuing underlying deficit in personality organization.

Psychodynamic Factors

INTRODUCTION

A major contribution in understanding the genesis of the borderline syndrome stems from the theoretical work of Otto Kernberg in a series of articles from 1966 to 1975.[21, 22, 23, 24] It is his conception (also discussed by Pine,[30] Chethik and Fast[2]) that the prototype for borderline conditions emerge from problems in the transition out of narcissism.

In normal development, Freud[10] suggests that the move from the "pleasure ego" (narcissism) to the "reality ego" involves the recognition of a world of objects distinct from oneself. In the period of primary naricissism, all that is pleasurable is accepted as real, and there is no distinction between self and object. An undifferentiated omnipotent mother-child bond exists. The transition away from narcissism requires a commitment to the external world as the criterion of reality. Internal images are tested against that reality, and modified if they are discrepant from it. In order to accomplish this transition effectively (from pleasure principle to reality principle), two major tasks must be completed. Self and other differentiation must take place, and the "pain" aspects of reality must be synthesized with the "pleasure" aspects.

In the history of the severe childhood disturbances, the fate of aggression is critical. These children typically experience extreme frustration and intense aggressive arousal in the first few years of life. The origin may be due, as noted previously, to deprivation of poor maternal handling, constitutional or hereditary factors, or early developmental interference. Oral aggression, pregenital aggression, plays a critical role. In childhood psychosis, due to these intense early frustrations, the child is unable to transcend the narcissistic state. There is no differentiation between self and object, and major problems in reality testing develop and grow. Delusions and hallucinations become manifest where inner and outer experience cannot be separated. It is suggested that the borderline child makes a partial transition out of narcissism. In the borderline condition, self and object differentiation does take place, and fundamental problems in reality testing do not become evident. However, because of the early intensity of their frustration, borderline children lack the ability to synthesize and integrate their "good" and "bad" experiences, and good and bad aspects of self and object. The implications of this arrest and fixation are profound. Specifically, these factors shape and distort personality development. At the same time, these children experience the profound disturbances in reality testing that are fundamental to childhood psychosis.

What is the impact of the failure of synthesis of the aggressive and libidinal impulses and images? While reality testing is fundamentally preserved, reality remains threatening. All pregenital aggressive impulses are projected "outside," and the world is seen as a painful and frightening place. Borderline children tend to be aware of reality, what is expected from them, etc., but their sense of reality is distorted. They anticipate pain from the outside, and whatever sense of exhilaration, vividness, and lively gratification they experience is far more likely to derive from their fantasy world. However, their perception of objective reality remains intact, though their investment in it is limited. Borderline children do not, therefore, abandon the narcissistic pleasure world. They continue to search for early kinds of gratification; thus, they seek a fulfillment of their oral needs through an idealized mother-child relationship.

The impact of their splitting of pain and pleasure has other general implications. Due to the intensity of their projections, they experience the outside world as awesome. Generally there is a fundamental terror and sense of helplessness (helplessness of the ego) in relation to the real world. They live in a state of chronic trauma, and they are filled with anxiety and fears of being overwhelmed and annihilated. Since the splitting separates pain and pleasure, and the aggressive components of the self are warded off, the critical developmental process of fusion of libidinal and aggressive instincts is never accomplished. This failure has a profound impact on the unfolding of personality and promotes many problems in subsequent structuralization.

With these general comments, we will now turn to look more specifically at the nature of object relations, ego development, and the course of superego structuralization in the borderline child.

OBJECT RELATIONS

Separation of Self and Nonself: In the partially completed task of the transition out of narcissism, borderline children experience the objects as separate from the self. The object is "out there" and "other," and physically apart from the self. At the same time, the search for the all giving, all gratifying object is retained. In the face of this need, outer reality offers nothing but deprivation, it fills them with terror and makes them cling to earlier gratifications.

Sandra, a nine-year-old, developed her Cinderella story. In her therapy session, her "doctor" was given the role of fairy godmother. In the game, Cinderella and her protector were inseparable. When Cinderella went to bed, her fairy godmother tucked her in and sang to her. Each night as the Cinderella-child slept, her companion remained awake, never once shutting her eyes, scrubbing floors, sorting laundry, and drying dishes. Toward the early part of the morning, fairy godmother began to bake. As Cinderella awakened at dawn, she was immediately greeted by her godmother who hugged and kissed her and asked, "How many cookies do you want for breakfast?" At times Sandra reversed the roles in this repetitive game, but the format of the story—the separation in sleep, the godmother's nighttime activity and chores, the gentle reunion upon awakening—had to be repeated along exactly prescribed lines. Interventions, comments, and attempts by the therapist to understand were met with absolute fury or disregarded totally.

Self-Object: The therapist-fairy godmother is clearly a self-object, that is, a projection of the all-gratifying wished-for images of the earlier developmental period. Borderline children's object relations are often characterized by self-objects who serve as a prop for their projections. With many of these children, frustrating characteristics lodged in the real object are denied and made nonexistent. This denial has the function of avoiding contact with pain and frustration, but the effect is to make objects one-dimensional.

While the real characteristics of the object of the borderline child are often not perceived, the presence of this object is nonetheless critical.

At the start of hospitalization, Gary, aged eight, appealed to our ward staff. He had an unusually round and cherubic face and large, frightened eyes. He impressed the staff as a child much younger than his years, who seemed lost and overcome. He clung to staff, "shadowed" them on the ward, and it was evident that their aid and attention comforted him greatly. However, after about a month on the ward, staff experienced a sense of disillusionment and diminishing interest. While they continued to be necessary to Gary as protecting figures, it became clear that no one staff member mattered in any way more than any other. For Gary, they were interchangeable. He had little idea of the names, characteristics, or identities of the people on various shifts, and he increasingly evoked a sense of emptiness in those who dealt with him.

Reality Span: Like many borderline children, Gary experienced "object hunger" and dreaded all separations. Geleerd[15] discussed this imperative need to maintain contact, and described it as lack of "reality span." The need to hold onto the

object indicates difficulties in object constancy. When separate from the object, borderline children have difficulty in retaining the good internalized image of the object. Frustration creates a sense of terror, and the actual presence and continuing availability of the object (often physically) is the only source of soothing and calm. Since borderline children fear separation, they often act "coercively" toward the object; they seek to insure that they have complete control of any independent activity of the people they depend on. Mark, in an earlier example, became furious when his mother talked on the phone. When her attention was deflected from him in the slightest degree, he was immediately frightened that the union and tie could be severed. He then demanded her constant gaze and awareness.

Lack of Empathy: The prop and self-object components of the borderline relationship are often wearing and draining on the people who deal with these children. The real characteristics of these important people are often totally disregarded by the child; instead these objects are invested with projected, need-fulfilling characteristics. They must live out prescribed roles for the child. In this sense, the object relations of borderline children are characterized by an inability to develop empathy. Their projected needs dominate most interactions, and these youngsters are therefore unable to perceive and react to the needs of the object.

Unintegrated Self-Other Bonds: Kernberg[24] most clearly conceptualizes the myriad of unintegrated self-other bonds in adult borderline disturbances. He argues that primitive self-representations and primitive object relations are linked together as basic units of object relations, and that these units remain "non-metabolized" or dissociated from one another. Each self-other unit in therapy can represent a full-fledged transference paradigm. Gary illustrates this dissociation vividly.

Because we knew of Gary's longing and need for his parents, we were puzzled by his reaction to a projected five day visit home from the hospital. At first he was openly joyous at the prospect of being a boy at home with his parents "who cared." At the same time, increasing concerns about loss and desertion emerged sharply. His sessions were filled with the stories he acted out, such as one about a stray dog that was lost. The dog did many tricks to attract people, but all to no avail. As these themes developed, at times he became panic-stricken and glassy-eyed. It finally became clear that the growing anxiety and new sense of loss were related to the parents' hospital visits that were of great importance to Gary. The day and time that they were to pick him up coincided with that of their usual visit. Therefore, while Gary would indeed be going home with his parents, he would miss the time they spent together in reunion at the hospital. The image of the missed visit in the hospital, in the day room, with his parents, stimulated intense anxieties about the starved child whose parents have deserted. All this despite the fact that at that moment he would actually be snugly in the car riding home in the bosom of his family. Several sessions were spent trying to help him unite these images. Gary would have his parents; he would be together with them in his home, and there was therefore no need for his usual hour visit on the ward. To no avail. He suddenly became wildly exhilarated; he had a marvelous solution. They could have their visit in the hospital as usual and then take their trip home.

Gary illustrates the inability to integrate two separate self-other bonds with his parents: happy boy at home with loving parents, and frightened boy whose parents have deserted. Borderline children often evidence such dissociations, and the end this serves is to keep all "good" experiences apart from and uncontaminated by the "bad" experiences.

The Phenomenon of Merging: Rosenfeld and Sprince[35] quote Anna Freud as saying that the borderline child is constantly on the border between identification and object cathexis. The resultant fear of merging is an important aspect of borderline pathology There is much to suggest that the phenomenon of merging in borderline children is often misunderstood and misused. The most primitive form of merging is the fear that one's bodily characteristics will change to those of another. This phenomenon is characteristic of the symbiotic-psychotic child, and it involves a lack of self-other distinction. Borderline children often seek a form of union and oneness, but the critical factor here is that concerns with physical fusion are not characteristic of this pathology. Borderline children often try to see whether their parents' or therapist's experiences are identical to their own. They will insist that they read the same books, like the same music, have the same television set, etc. All tasks and belongings should correlate. This form of wanting to be one, however, relates primarily to controlling the independent life of the object, rather than to joining oneself to the object in a process of primitive merging. In fact, it is precisely the borderline child's ability to maintain a sense of separateness and self-integrity (particularly of physical boundaries) that distinguishes and differentiates him from the child with a psychotic disorder.

EGO DEVELOPMENT

The ego of the borderline child is often characterized as "weak," "helpless," "fragile." In defining "ego weakness," most authors refer to several levels of ego structure. Borderline children often evidence some problems in the early development of their ego functions (the foundation of the ego), and ultimately develop and solidify a primitive defensive system. We will discuss some ego functions that are often affected, and the specific defenses that are commonly developed. It is clear, however, that the maldevelopment of certain ego functions makes it much more difficult for the growing child to cope with and ultimately to integrate the aggressive drive derivatives. Without an adequate "ego foundation," the child finds it much more difficult to accomplish later developmental tasks, including the synthesis of "good" and "bad" aspects of the object and self. Further, it is also clear that a major mission of the primitive defenses that are erected is to contain the splitting off of the frightening aggressive images and maintain aspects of the "good" narcissistic world.

Ego Functions; Motoric Development: In infancy, many borderline children already evidence early deviant physiological functioning and erratic patterning. Subsequently, one often sees clearly motoric manifestations of early distress in the form of hyperactivity, body rigidities, and peculiar gaits or postures. Matthew, described earlier, discharged his intense distress into random motor behavior; there was little of the constructive kinds of motor adaptation that infants normally use to help arrest their distress. He was unable to establish a harmonious synchronization with his mother to modify his experiences of discomfort, and "soothing" came only with long car rides.

In the early histories of borderline children we often find a lack of physiological homeostasis; this may reach a point where it appears that the physical viability of the organism is threatened. Ordinarily, children who progress well show early motor skills (rudimentary ego skills); in conjunction with the object, these help them function more smoothly. For example, one can note purposive action in turning from a pillow which blocks breathing, or modifying one's sucking rate to modulate the flow of milk to a desired pace, etc. The inability of some children to modify early pain experiences (due either to defective physiology or inadequate care-taking) produces a number of fundamental problems. One notes an easy disruption in the normal functioning of physiological systems and the continued presence of a high level of primary anxiety. Another major effect is that the growing child "learns" that the outside world is painful and ungratifying, and that one can expect little pleasure from it.

Perceptual Development: In reviewing the function of perception, it is evident that there are many associated components that help the individual to receive and to order stimuli. Rosenfeld and Sprince[35] discuss the specific perceptual deficits that are found with some frequency in the early history of borderline children. At the Hampstead Clinic the borderline cases were observed to have difficulty in inhibiting stimuli. "They seemed to get swamped by them, and are unselective in their choice of what is relevant and what is irrelevant." This observation has also been made about a number of other borderline groups.[15,36]

As the child develops, the quality of perceptual function in infancy can later affect the function of reality discrimination. For example, difficulties in perception due to flooding of stimuli can promote difficulties in the ability to attend and discern the origin of stimuli. This in turn may create potential problems in distinguishing between inner and outer events. Similarly, such disturbances may lead to difficulties in perceiving the accuracy of the quality of the stimuli (e.g., anger or non-anger), or the accuracy of the intensity of stimuli. While the reality testing of borderline children is not markedly disturbed, there are evident reality testing problems in dealing with aggressive stimuli; the child cannot easily discern the source or origin of the aggressive impulses, nor can he readily assess their intensity (typically, aggressive impulses are markedly exaggerated). Early perceptual problems of the kind seen in a good number of borderline children may constitute important components of the disturbance in this critical affective area.

Control of Drive Activity: The descriptions of most borderline children discuss problems of impulse control (both libidinal and aggressive). There is often an ego systonicity to the expression of impulses during the time of eruptive behavior, and a repetitive quality to the lack of impulse control. With careful appraisal of the early histories of these children, one can often note problems in the first year of life which appear to relate to later impulse problems. As the normal infant grows, there is the expectation that he will develop an increasing ability to delay his tension release (e.g., the intensity of his crying, etc.) and that he will elaborate ever more controlled forms of tension release. In descriptions of these young disturbed children there is often an account of a lack of this ability to wait, to tolerate tension, or to inhibit. This growing ability to effect tension release is the foundation for later ego functions such as substituting thought for action, exercising control over one's self, and affecting the environment through action.

Thus, there are early impairments in delay mechanisms and perceptual and motoric processes. These indicate that in a number of borderline children physiologic immaturity and/or minimal brain damage may make an important contribution to the genesis of the syndrome. These rudimentary ego processes are the foundations for more complex ego functions, and early impairments will distort the later, more highly developed functions.

As the infant's ego grows, Freud[13] noted that a special form of energy must become available in order to promote adequate development. Through the process of neutralization (which Freud traces to a desexualization of libido, and Hartmann,[19] to a deaggressivization of the aggressive instinct) a modified form of energy emerges. This is the necessary ingredient for the effective development of ego functions. It is clear that in the early childhood of borderline youngsters, this critical modification of instinctual energy does not fully occur. Indeed, the ability to neutralize instinctual energy (particularly, aggression) appears to be lowered. This impairment in the process has a number of consequences. There is less energy available for ego building, a greater reservoir of energy remains attached to the primitive instincts, and later defense mechanisms are impoverished and primitive. The following clinical material (a detailed expansion of earlier clinical material) illustrates some of the problems in function that arise from the lack of adequate neutralization.

After Matthew (age ten) had been successful in controlling the cartoons (giving up a major defensive posture of withdrawal into fantasy), much more direct aggression appeared. In this post-cartoon period, Matthew often broke up the office. On campus, he seemed to direct his physical attacks toward younger girls, attempting at times to scratch and choke them. Following these open attacks, he would engage in intense self-abuse such as throwing himself against the wall, and asking to have his fingers cut off to keep him from scratching.

His theme in therapy was that his "madness" was coming out. The madness came in the form of dreams which filled the entire night every night and which he then had to relate fully in his therapy sessions. At first, in his dreams, little girls got hurt. They tripped, damaged their knees and had to go to the hospital for an operation. There was, however, a special rock near the hospital which became a rock monster; it rolled into the hospital and bashed and battered the little girls until they were all dead.

As this material poured forth, Matthew's anxiety mounted. He became more overtly agitated, and random aggressive and self-abusive behavior became a greater part of his total day. After awhile, in his fantasies, the little girls changed into one specific little girl—Matthew's sister Susie whom he described as having long blond hair. In his continuous dreams, Matthew tricked his sister into entering a rocket alone. His mother, sensing danger, tried in vain to stop him. The rocket flew into space, crashed into meteorites, broke apart, and Susie was killed. For long periods of time, as she rode into space, the wild flight made her scream and yell. There were variations in the dream. At times, Matthew was able to trick Mother into entering the rocket to take the fatal trip. In his sessions, he vigorously played out the rocket trip, smashing the rocket against the wall, mimicking the screams, and at some points stabbing Susie and Mother after the rocket had crashed.

Since Matthew's days were becoming almost as chaotic as the nights, he pleaded with his therapist for help. "Please get me in control. If you can control me, I'll conrtol my dreams, I'll control the rockets." On one occasion, as the therapist attempted to control the outflow of material (which he did by setting vigorous time limits to Matthew's agitated exposition) he used the word "mixed-up" feelings. Matthew seized upon the word "mixed-up"—it became special and sacred to him, uttered from the therapist's mouth. It was as though the therapist brought forth the word of God. On a number of occasions during the stormy period, Matthew seemed to use this word to calm down. Other interventions were utilized with Matthew which ultimately helped him restore order.

Among borderline children, pregenital instinctual material is all too available. It flows into consciousness directly from the original drive derivatives with little distortion, and it tends to overpower the helpless ego of the child. There is little neutralized energy at hand, and the quantitative energy balance lies heavily on the instinctual side. Often there is little direct progression, or phase-by-phase development of the instinctual material. Thus, while some more mature (oedipal or phallic) symbolism was evident in Matthew's material, it was in fact dominated by pregenital (sadistic) drive energy.

Synthetic Function: Nunberg[29] describes the synthetic function as the "ego's tendency to unite and bind," which "goes hand in hand with the tendency to simplify and generalize." Hartmann[19] felt that the synthetic function was a very basic mechanism, and an index of the ego's capacity to accept the reality principle and engage in rational thinking. Borderline individuals have fundamental problems with their synthetic function-

ing. Matthew, for example, would frequently show extremely warm, loving feelings toward his sister. At such moments she was regarded as a devoted person who never had a negative thought or feeling. However, when Matthew was dominated by his aggressive impulses, dismemberment and torture were to be her fate, and she became totally hated and despised. There was a failure in Matthew's ability to unite the libidinal and aggressive mental representations of his sister into a more realistic image of her as a person. This synthetic failure is characteristic of borderline functioning.

Thought Processes: The borderline child typically manifests much secondary process thinking. At the same time, he is quite capable of regression to the use of prelogical thought. Matthew expressed many of these characteristics when in the grip of his aggressive impulses. Primary process thinking then dominated his consciousness and poured out in a flood of primitive aggressive images, wishes, and fears. There was much evidence of magical thinking. Matthew overestimated the power of these wishes. He feared that his thoughts would have frightening effects on his family, and he sought immediate controls to ensure the safety of his mother and sister. Implicit, as well, was the omnipotence of thought. In keeping with this, he assigned the therapist incredible, god-like power to stop him from his destructive thinking-action. His thinking was typically concretistic, and the therapist's word "mixed-up" became the magical lever which could control his violence. Matthew did not relate to the idea the therapist was trying to convey; he insisted on hearing the specific word "mixed-up" as if those sounds had in and of themselves an intrinsic ability to control him. Throughout this chaotic period Matthew evidenced egocentric thinking, he viewed the world only in terms of his own drives, needs and fears.

Relation to Reality: Under the impact of intense aggressive impulses, reality testing becomes difficult for borderline children. Much of Matthew's anxiety in relation to his rage was his growing inability to distinguish his internal thoughts and ideas from his external perceptions. However, for the most part, reality testing remained intact. In this realm, the most marked disturbance of borderline children occurs in connection with their sense of reality. Matthew, for example, was very aware of reality; nontheless his earlier cartoon world absorbed him and was highly cathected. His sense of joy and pleasure (his libidinization) derived from his narcissistic fantasy world rather than from objective reality. This major investment with one's inner world is a common characteristic of borderline functioning. Mary, age ten, developed a pattern of play which became her central and all-consuming fantasy and expressed her attachment to the oral gratifying world.

During her second session with a new therapist, Mary found "Fluffy," a stuffed rabbit, in the toy closet. Fluffy became a critical figure in her developing play. Using Kleenex, Fluffy developed an even fluffier tail and a large nest. Slowly Fluffy was enveloped by a soft bed, a blanket, a supply of food, and a house (a desk drawer) where she would be safe. During many sessions, Mary became preoccupied with keys—was the desk drawer locked, and could she and the therapist hide the keys so that no one could disturb Fluffy in her castle? The therapist and Mary sewed, saved clothing for the rabbit, and bit by bit, additional soft animals gained entry to this safe, protected island. At points of separation (as hours came near their end) the Fluffies were equipped with many items (candies, thread, empty spools) to tide them over to the next meeting.

Defense Mechanisms: We have discussed at some length the problems of the borderline child in synthesizing positive and negative mental representations. We have also discussed the lack of neutralized energy which contributes to the failure in the developmental task of synthesis. This lack contributes as well to the impoverishment of the borderline child's defensive system. Without sufficient "deinstinctualized" energy, there is a failure in the ability to maintain the repression from which most "higher level" defenses develop. The individual's ability to repress is synonymous with his capacity to maintain a constant counter-cathectic force which keeps unconscious thoughts from becoming conscious. The energy to do this needs to be instinct-free; due to the impairment in the neutralization process, little of the necessary energy becomes available. Thus the defenses that are retained and reinforced, by and large, continue to be the early primitive mechanisms. Much of the function of these defenses is to maintain the division (all good—all bad) within the ego and to dissociate and expel the negative "all bad" impulses.

Generally speaking, the defenses of the borderline child are not as effective or as functional as those of the normal or neurotic youngster. Anxiety is not bound as effectively and erupts into consciousness. Over-compensation can occur; at times defenses are used so extensively and inflexibly that all affects are avoided (e.g., schizoid-like solution).

Splitting: Kernberg[23] describes splitting as an active process of keeping apart introjections and identifications of opposite quality. He considers this mechanism the fundamental defensive process in borderline personality organization, and other common defensive processes that occur take place in conjunction with such splitting. It is most commonly seen clinically in the division of objects into "all bad" and "all good."

Roger, an eight-year borderline youngster, was being driven to his therapy session by both his mother and father. He was carrying a bingo set and he announced his intention of playing the game with his therapist. His mother, evidently annoyed, told him angrily he should leave his set in the car so that he could get something accomplished in his session. Several minutes later Roger turned on his father in fury shouting, "You never let me do anything." This incident was typical of Roger. Regardless of the objective source of limits, admonishments, and frustrations, Roger regarded his poor father as the repository of all that was cruel and evil, and his mother as the source of all that was benign.

The most common clinical manifestation of splitting is the division of objects into entities that are "all good" and "all bad." This defense may also be expressed in alternate expressions of complementary sides of a conflict toward an object with a total lack of concern regarding the inherent contradictions. The following clinical material illustrates this along with a number of the other typical borderline defenses.

Tom came into treatment at age eleven for lifelong problems of "isolation." After a short period it was clear that he had made a schizoid-like adjustment. He had no friends, and his expressions of affect were minimal. On the weekend, he would watch TV endlessly and would rarley leave the perimeter of the land surrounding his home to adventure into the city (Ann Arbor, Michigan). He would drift off in school and didn't know what was said in class. He enjoyed his bedroom and liked to develop plans for arrangements that would keep his sleeping area hidden from the view from the doorway; it would be contained as a room within a room.

Ann Arbor was the city of pollution, he believed, and he couldn't stand the streets and shops. There was nothing good to buy in the shops. He told of worries that muggers were out to kidnap him for ransom, since he came from a wealthy family. While he knew it wasn't true, he nevertheless felt one could be assassinated on any street corner of the city. (He lived this fear out by not venturing into the city.) In contrast was the city of Sun Valley, Colorado, where he had spent his early years and many summers. Sun Valley was gorgeous, alive, vigorous, and healthy. He had constant fantasies of beautiful valleys—he lived there, in fantasy, in peace, within a small house, and he endlessly watched the wildlife, the vegetation, and beauty around him. There he would feel alive and breathe easily.

Tom's parents were divorced, and his father continued to live in Colorado. Periodically Tom would feel very "let down" by his father, who never sent birthday gifts, never acknowledged holidays, and didn't even call. For the most part, however, he felt his father was a unique genius, and there was an exceedingly strong bond between the two because they "thought exactly alike." Tom longed for his father; he "knew" that eventually there would be a total reunion and he would leave the "prison" of Ann Arbor. This wish was in marked contrast to the actual state of affairs in which he was totally disregarded by his father. He regarded his mother as totally worthless; she was weak, empty, and pathetic. He and his mother never had anything to talk about. Everybody took advantage of her, she was always physically ill, and she was addicted to alcohol. While some of these characterizations were partly true, Tom totalized his concept. His daily plan was to avoid any and all contact with her.

This clinical material further illustrates the use of splitting. Tom retains his "all good" affects in relation to his father and Sun Valley, while mother and Ann Arbor represent all that is negative and contaminated. He is unable to put together and to blend the positive and negative aspects of places and objects.

Denial: Borderline patients often resort to this mechanism. The most typical form is a "pushing away" any perceptions or thoughts that don't accord with the way the patient wishes to feel and experience the world. For example, Tom clearly knew of his father's rejection and disregard. Emotionally, however, he rejected these perceptions. They had no relevance for him because of his need to revere and worship his father. While this idealization of the absent parent is not uncommon in children of divorced parents, Tom's use of denial was unusual in degree. Similarly, he could not allow himself any good experience in Ann Arbor. Intellectually, he could describe a pleasant event or a nice day; emotionally his perception of the city was totally negative. This mechanism is closely linked with splitting.

Projection: Borderline children tend to externalize and expel all that they regard as bad. One effect of this extensive use of projection is the development of fears of retaliation from these outside objects. Tom, for example, was frightened to leave the safety of the island of his home. Pollution, muggers, kidnappers awaited him when he ventured from home. The hostile, aggressive, attacking impulses were separated from the self and infected the surrounding world. Tom then had to defend himself against this hostile environment. Projection and denial are typically associated with the phenomena of splitting.

Idealization and Devaluation: The phenomena of splitting fosters both these mechanisms. As perceptions and introjections are sorted into "all good" and "all bad," objects develop and retain total positive or negative characteristics for the borderline child. Thus Tom's mother became increasingly devalued and deplored, while his father assumed all of the virtues of the idealized savior, who provided constant resonance and empathy for his son.

Superego Development: Many of the difficulties recounted in the development of the ego of the borderline child apply as well to the development of the superego. Such ego functions as perception, reality testing, and synthesis participate as well in the development of the structure of the superego. When these building blocks are inadequately supplied, problems in superego development occur. In order to trace this process in the borderline child, it is helpful initially to review some aspects of normal development of the superego.

As the child grows, the prohibitions and standards of important love objects are imitated, identified with, and ultimately introjected. In the course of this introjection, there is a transfer of authority from the real object to its internal representation within the child. At first single, individual standards and prohibitions are introjected. However, under the impact of the oedipal complex, when love objects need to be given up directly because of intense psychic threat, major identifications and introjections occur. The prohibitions and ideals become a structure of their own, part of the self, and the child can then function somewhat autonomously from the parents. At this point, we can speak of an "internalized superego," a pattern of inner controls which can serve also as an important source of self-esteem for the child. Good feelings, for example, emerge when the youngster lives up to his own standards; with this, the growing child is less dependent on the object for narcissistic supplies.

An effective superego supports reasonable defenses against drives. Forbidden impulses promote "signal guilt" which will usually impede the expression of these wishes in behavior. When breakdowns do occur, guilt is experienced and anxiety and worry follow. The superego also aids in the establishment of aims and goals. An effective superego will set reasonable and attainable aims. Grandiose wishes, while not totally given up, become more and more relegated to the area of fantasy (pleasurable, but not realizable).

Problems in Structuralization: Borderline children tend to live in a frightening and hostile world. For example Tom, our schizoid-like youngster, was surrounded by muggers, kidnappers, and pollution, and he maintained a feeling of safety by isolating himself to the perimeter of his house. Matthew was concerned about tornadoes and killers, which his magic cartoon world sought to keep in check. There is often a paranoid aspect to much of the world surrounding the borderline child. With normal and neurotic children, as they develop, their controls tend to come more and more from within. In contrast to this, a great share of the inhibitions of the borderline child is maintained by their outside fears. For such youngsters, the prohibitions continue to be experienced in terms of frightening individuals or frightening places, rather than in terms of uncomfortable feelings arising from within.

The major reasons that sanctions remain projected are because the borderline youngster experiences great difficulty in the process of internalization, introjection, and identification. The difficulties with perception and reality testing distort his perceptions of the inhibiting model (parent). Typically, these mental representations of the parent model are filled with pregenital aggression and primitive sadistic components. These perceptions are frightening, and for the most part are split off and expelled from the self. The normal processes of identification and introjection are interfered with. Rather than taking in these perceptions, the more infantile mechanisms of reprojection are actively maintained to keep them as distant as possible. The result is that the process of building the internal prohibiting structures, the superego precursors, is at best less well developed or at worst often markedly impaired.

The superego remains in a preautonomous state for the borderline child. Many borderline children evidence marked dependency and a wish to maintain the gratification and pleasures of the narcissistic world. The problems in superego formation further reinforce object dependency and serve as an important stimulant for object hunger. The difficulties with internal controls create anxiety about being flooded by impulses. Borderline children then look outward for the stability and controls they lack within; in the nature of things they often turn to their most important objects. In addition they lack the good feelings regarding the self that come from meeting the superego goals, and this again drives them to turn to the object for self-esteem regulation. These "superego needs" are an important facet of the clinging behavior so often noted in borderline children.

Characteristics of Superego: Despite the many problems with the process of internalization, some prohibitions are introjected. For the most part, these are endowed with intense aggression and are therefore excessively severe. Matthew illustrates the presence of harsh superego reactions. After he struck and scratched little girls, he sought to have his fingers cut off, threw himself in the mud and banged his head against the mirror. The sadistic components of the drives become fuel for the child's superego. The superego is often terribly intolerant, hypercritical, and markedly self-depreciating, and the evidence suggests that the aggression is turned on the self. In addition, the superego of the borderline child will often appear inconsistent and there will often be breakthroughs of aggressive impulses. This inconsistency is due less to superego weakness than it is to the brittleness of the defensive structure and the power of the impulses themselves.

Specific Therapeutic Methods

INTRODUCTION

The most common therapeutic intervention described in the literature for the borderline child is individual psychotherapy. To employ this modality usefully, it is necessary to consider the goals, the problems and the techniques that direct treatment involves. In addition to therapy, many authors stress the management issues that arise in the course of the treatment of these children. Since such youngsters react intensely to frustration and change, it is essential that they live in an environment where stress is minimal, and their handicaps are understood. With borderline children who have severe impulse problems, institutional placement (residential treatment centers, hospitals, day treatment programs) is often necessary. In these settings one can best control the changes and frustrations of the day-to-day world. Where impulse control is not a major problem, the active work of the therapist with parents, school and any sources of significant "stress" is usually critical to the creation of an adequately benign and sympathetic surround.

What are the major goals of psychotherapy? There is controversy about what can be accomplished. Several authors imply that during childhood very significant structural change can occur in treatment. The Hampstead group[34] notes that there is a "later period of treatment when the borderline picture gradually changes, and internalized conflicts can become the center of treatment." Ekstein[5] also notes that "as regressive trends and as the neurotic aspects of the child's ego become stabilized, interpretations aim at giving insight, and thus eventually approximate those used with the neurotic child." This quality of change (from borderline to neurotic personality organization) described by Ekstein[5] and Rosenfeld and Sprince[34] during the course of psychotherapy is contrary to the experience of this author. Essentially it has been our experience through therapy that improvement in functioning may be profound, but borderline children nonetheless remain borderline children. The child's adaptation to the reality world may improve markedly; he may establish much better control of the severe regressive trends in his personality; and he may develop and maximize the healthier aspects of his defenses and his ego functioning. We have not experienced, through therapy, the marked changes in synthetic function, in the ability to neutralize energy, in the capacity for repression as a major defense, and in libidinal object relations that are necessary for the development of a neurotic personality structure.

THE PSYCHOTHERAPEUTIC PROCESS

What are major problems the therapist faces in the treatment of these children? Typically he is confronted by the child's attachment to the narcissistic fantasy world where he continues his attempts to deny the real world. The therapist is also confronted with the primitive level of object tie the child patient presents; this indeed begets a special form of transference which requires adequate handling. He must also attempt to deal with the enormous problems in structuralization and deficits in coping capacity that are evident in the borderline child's daily interaction with reality.

Narcissistic Fantasy World: As we have noted earlier, because of the impact of pregenital aggression (much of which is reprojected), the "outside" world remains a frightening and terrifying place. Typically, the borderline youngster is aware that the pleasurable island he builds for himself is fantasy, but he clings no less tenaciously to his narcissistic conception of the world. The mechanism of denial in fantasy is often a major adaptational device and represents an aversion to and a partial turning away from reality. Most authors recognize the formidable task of "reaching" a person whose primary source of pleasure lies within his fantasy preoccupations. The Hampstead group[34] noted that often, to the borderline patient, the "therapist can be like a stick of furniture;" they suggest that an early bridge can be established by judicious direct gratification with tangible supplies. They caution as well that borderline youngsters float in an overwhelming sea of fantasy material, and that the therapist should not elaborate this fantasy life since it can lead to flooding anxieties for the patient. They suggest techniques geared to facilitating repression and displacement.

In contrast, Ekstein[5] emphasizes the major technique in work with the borderline child as "interpretation within the metaphor." He comments that in order to communicate effectively with the borderline youngster, the therapist, in his interaction, must develop "a willing suspension of disbelief in the reality of the moment." It has been this author's experience that it is indeed critical to join with the child patient in his narcissistic world, since much of the child's cathexis (sense of pleasure, joy) remains attached to this illusory state. The therapist needs not only to join this world, but to become an indispensable member of it.

The following examples illustrate the early treatment stages in which the narcissistic world is gradually shared:

Gary, age nine, slowly developed an elaborate play called "the free house." With his therapist he found the house on Storybook Road in Ohio Free. There was a sign on the door that said "For Sale—Free," and Gary and the therapist moved in. The house was dirty and uncared for, and together they cleared the debris and rearranged furniture.

Gary and his therapist became inseparable within the fantasy. They took turns cooking and washing dishes, they cleaned and tidied up, played hide-an-seek within the house, built a fire and roasted marshmallows, ate in the living room and retired to their bed and slept together. In session after session the play was repeated, with Gary in tight control. Continuous gratification was the theme of each hour. Any attempt by the therapist to elaborate on the fantasy, however gently, to suggest possible sources of anxiety or meanings (like reactions to missing home), or even to contribute to the general format outlined by Gary, was met with rigid frantic avoidance. While the therapist's presence was desperately needed and became an invaluable part of the fantasy elaboration, the therapist served essentially as a puppet for Gary's self-created unfolding of the Free House saga.

In this narcissistic fantasy, Gary resurrected the Garden of Eden aspects of the narcissistic world. His therapist shared this pleasurable world where there was eternal gratification, no frustration, and no separation. Experience with borderline children indicates that once this libidinal tie is established in therapy, both the therapist and the fantasy become highly cathected, and the child's pleasure world is dependent on their simultaneous presence. The tie to the therapist, like the tie to the early mother, may be used to help the child move gradually from the total cathexis of illusion. The following description of the early stages of treatment with Matthew ("cartoon boy") illustrate the growing bond and the shift toward reality under the protective aura of the therapist.

As in the cottage, Matthew sat in the far corner of the therapist's office with his back to the therapist. Only roars, grimaces and screams were emitted as the course of the cartoon progressed. From his own extensive knowledge of cartoons, the therapist began identifying the specific characters, and slowly the idea of producing a written movie program of each session emerged. All the varied cartoons were listed in order of presentation, and, since Matthew had a vast variety of characters, he would pack in as many as twenty cartoons in a fifty-minute hour. The show's producer left the corner of the room, and in response to the therapist's interest, he unfolded the program on the therapist's desk.

After a long period, Matthew decided on a change. He would now include some full-length features. He particularly wanted to add an adventure serial, and the therapist was to play a prominent role. In the films the therapist was the big protector, as he and the little boy took on the frightening world. Together they faced spooky and haunted houses, high winds and hurricanes, and bad doctors who gave terrible shots.

After some time the therapist introduced his own variation into the program—the idea of a documentary. He insisted that this documentary contain the essential elements of a documentary, that is, it must reflect and record a true event. While Matthew eagerly agreed at first, he subtly fought the new rule and tested it out. For example, his first weather reports on a lovely spring day described deep snow, slipperly walking conditions, etc. Or he described the different fish he saw on a visit to the aquarium, but added wings to the fish and made them fly. The therapist pounded on the desk, noting that this was a violation of the documentary idea, and the weather and fish reports were not accepted until changed.

Presently, "true" documentary talks assumed a more prominent place in the sessions. They began to reflect many reality aspects of Matthew's life. He introduced sequences entitled "Homesick," "Home Sweet Home," "Hatred in the Cottage." In the course of these accounts, he described his feelings of loss of home, his present terrors, his questions about the treatment center. In addition, in his documentary "Hatred in the Cottage," "cartoon boy" noted he didn't have any friends, was lonely, wanted the boys to like him, and hated the name "cartoon boy."

Early in treatment, Matthew presented another aspect of his narcissistic world. He was struggling with the "split-off" terrors that he was unable to integrate. Like other borderline youngsters he experienced a state of continuous danger which he must attempt to master. To this end, he used the therapist as a narcissistic, omnipotent protector. Slowly, as a mother with a frightened toddler, and at a point where he felt the child could tolerate the anxiety, the therapist insisted that Matthew engage greater aspects of the real world. In the context of a strong libidinal tie, the therapist may help the borderline youngster modify major character patterns of flight from reality. This is only possible, however, after the therapist has accepted and become part of the gratifying narcissistic world of the borderline child, and after they have thoroughly explored it together. In a sense they must share a similar regression and metaphor.

The Nature of the Transference Tie: Earlier, in the section on object relations, an account was given of several aspects of the kind of relationship the borderline youngster establishes with important objects. As treatment unfolds, these typical relationships begin to include the therapist.. Early in the work, sometimes for protracted periods of time, borderline youngsters will use the therapist as a prop for projection, rather than as a person with his own individual characteristics. For example, Gary tightly controlled the Free Ohio Story, Matthew clearly and totally determined the therapist's protecting role in the adventure serials, and Sandra prescribed all the fairy godmother's lines in the Cinderella tale. The therapist's intrusions or deviations from the child's rigid rules either evoked fury or led to isolated play. Ekstein[5] describes the situation particularly well. Concerning a young adolescent patient, he says: "Unlike a hysterical patient . . . she projects the imaginary love relationships . . . [she is] in love with the introject of the therapist rather than [cathecting] the actual object." Modell[28] describes his borderline patients as having relationships to persons factually separate from themselves "but invested almost entirely with qualities emanating from the self." However, though the object may serve as little more than a prop for projection, the child's attachment to it is typically very intense. Without the attachment, without the therapist, there is often a fear of total loss of gratification.

What is the impact of this attachment on the therapist? It is not unusual for the therapist to feel manipulated and used by the patient for his private means. Under the impact of the patient's "coercion," therapists often feel helpless, bored, resentful, and in despair. They have no opportunity to feel real or that their insights or interventions are accepted. However, with an understanding of the inevitability of this kind of transference paradigm, many of these natural affects evoked by the borderline child can be better integrated.

Our present conception is that as the child begins to trust and feel greater security, the therapist may be allowed to function more independently within the fantasy, and he can then begin relating the fantasy elements to reality. Matthew slowly gave up some of the control of the adventure serial and allowed the therapist to make rules about documentaries. The therapist could then gradually broaden the illusory world and slowly integrate it with the real one.

The Problems of Structuralization: In the course of therapy, as the borderline children invest themselves ever more in reality, expose themselves to social interaction and to peer groups, and leave the protective aura of the narcissistic world, their anxiety increases. It is the task of the therapist to function as auxilliary ego, and to strengthen and develop coping skills.

Matthew sought out other children, and while his social relationships never reached intimacy, he had increasing associations with peers. He joined several clubs outside of the institution.

In his therapy sessions he developed an extensive evaluation system which he described as "charting." Charts were designed, for instance, for school progress, involvement in club activities and mood swings. The graph that followed the course of his moods over the week showed a range from the highest category "Calmness" to the lowest category "Blow-up," and he reacted with pleasure and received full praise when he managed a steady, placid week. Recognized achievement seemed to serve as a stimulating reward.

As he extended himself further, the need to anticipate potential upsets became singularly important. Matthew developed an early warning system, so that he could be on guard. When school was over, for example, he attempted to anticipate his summer fears. When camp began he worried about insect bites and poisoning, or his "getting lost" worry might return. Before travel vacations with his parents, he prepared himself for car accident thoughts, noise of the subway, reactions to tall buildings, and so forth. A heavy burden of homework, or a harsh comment from a cottage staff member would also put him "on guard."

He prepared for physical illnesses as well, since he knew that a stiff neck or sprained ankle would set him on edge, and he must be especially watchful at those times.

He used role play to help him cope with new situations. He played out how he would feel or how he would react when teased by peers he met in clubs; he simulated sitting through long synagogue services at home; and he practiced finding his way to classes and his locker room in a junior high school he began to attend.

During this "coping" period, the therapist's attempts to move beyond the systematizing, anticipating, and listing were met with intense resistance. In identifying internal conflicts, for example, the underlying severe masturbatory conflicts that Matthew's defenses were in part attempting to control, provoked terror in him, and the old Matthew would quickly reappear. Wild impulsive behavior emerged, self-disgust and self-punishment became prominent, moves toward isolation and flight into fantasy were resurrected. The tone of the hour would change quickly—the therapist became the feared devil, and Matthew began to avoid the sessions. In the face of these not-so-subtle cues, the therapist reversed himself and supported the systematizing and rehearsal behavior.

Experience suggests that as borderline children attempt to cope with reality, treatment techniques should be ego supportive, and interpretations should be related directly to building up defenses. During the developmental years, most of the borderline child's energy must be devoted primarily to mastery mechanisms. Matthew clearly extended his own form of signal anxiety (rather than the panic described earlier) and developed greater capacities for anxiety tolerance to more and more situations of reality frustration. This the therapist supported, and thus helped Matthew develop compulsive-like defensive systems which allowed him to master his environment for the first time.

ACKNOWLEDGMENT

Many of the ideas in this chapter have emerged during several years of collaborative work with Dr. Irene Fast, Professor of Psychology, University of Michigan.

REFERENCES

1. ALPERT, A., "Reversibility of Pathological Fixations Associated with Maternal Deprivation in Infancy," in Eissler, R. S., et al. (Eds.), *The Psychoanalytic Study of the Child*, vol. 14, pp. 169–185, International Universities Press, New York, 1959.

2. CHETHIK, M., and FAST, I., "A Function of Fantasy in the Borderline Child," *American Journal of Orthopsychiatry*, 40:756–765, 1970.

3. CHETHIK, M., and SPINDLER, E., "Techniques of Treatment and Management With the Borderline Child," in Mayer, M., and Blum, A. (Eds.), *Healing Through Living*, pp. 176–189, Charles C. Thomas, Springfield, Ill., 1971.

4. DEUTCH, H., "Some Forms of Emotional Disturbance and Their Relationship to Schizophrenia," *Psychoanalytic Quarterly*, 11:301–321, 1942.

5. EKSTEIN, R., *Children of Time and Space, of Action and Impulse*, Appleton-Century-Crofts, New York, 1966.

6. FAST, I., "The Function of Action in the Early

Development of Identity," *International Journal of Psychoanalysis, 51:*471–478, 1970.

7. ———, and CHETHIK, M., "Aspects of Depersonalization Experience in Children," *International Journal of Psychoanalysis,* (in press).

8. ———, "Some Aspects of Object Relations in Borderline Children," *International Journal of Psychoanalysis, 53:*479–484, 1972.

9. FREUD, S., "Instincts and Their Vicissitudes," *Collected Papers,* vol. 4, Basic Books, New York, 1959.

10. ———, "Negation," *Collected Papers,* vol. 5, Basic Books, New York, 1959.

11. ———, "On Narcissism: An Introduction," *Collected Papers,* vol. 4, Basic Books, New York, 1959.

12. ———, "Beyond the Pleasure Principle," *The Standard Edition of the Complete Psychological Works of Sigmund Freud* (hereafter, *Standard Edition*), vol. 18, Hogarth Press, London, 1955.

13. ———, "The Ego and the Id," *Standard Edition,* vol. 19, Hogarth Press, London, 1955.

14. FRIJLING-SCHREUDER, E. C. M., "Borderline States in Children," in Eissler, R. S., et al. (Eds.), *The Psychoanalytic Study of the Child,* vol. 24, pp. 307–327, International Universities Press, New York, 1970.

15. GELEERD, E., "Borderline States in Childhood and Adolescence," in Eissler, R. S., et al. (Eds.), *The Psychoanalytic Study of the Child,* vol. 13, pp. 279–295, International Universities Press, New York, 1958.

16. GREENACRE, P., "The Imposter," *Psychoanalytic Quarterly, 27:*359–382, 1958.

17. ———, "The Predisposition to Anxiety," parts 1 and 2, *Psychoanalytic Quarterly, 10:*66–94, 610–638, 1941.

18. HARLEY, M., "Analysis of a Severely Disturbed 3½ Year Old Boy," in Eissler, R. S., et al. (Eds.), *The Psychoanalytic Study of the Child,* vol. 6, pp. 206–234, International Universities Press, New York, 1951.

19. HARTMANN, H., "Notes on the Theory of Sublimation," *Essays on Ego Psychology,* International Universities Press, New York, 1974.

20. KANNER, L., "Autistic Disturbances of Affective Contact," *Nervous Child, 2:*217–250, 1943.

21. KERNBERG, O., *Borderline Conditions and Pathological Narcissism,* Jason Aronson, New York, 1975.

22. ———, "The Treatment of Patients With Borderline Personality Organization," *International Journal of Psychoanalysis, 49:*600–619, 1968.

23. ———, "Borderline Personality Organization," *Journal of the American Psychoanalytic Association, 15:*641–685, 1967.

24. ———, "Structural Derivatives of Object Relations, *International Journal of Psychoanalysis, 47:*236–253, 1966.

25. MAENCHEN, A., "Note on Early Ego Disturbances,"

in Eissler, R. S., et al. (Eds.), *The Psychoanalytic Study of the Child,* vol. 8, pp. 262–270, International Universities Press, New York, 1953.

26. MAHLER, M., "On Childhood Psychosis and Schizophrenia. Autistic and Symbiotic Infantile Psychosis," in Eissler, R. S., et al. (Eds.), *The Psychoanalytic Study of the Child,* vol. 7, pp. 286–305, International Universities Press, New York, 1952.

27. ———, "Clinical Studies in the Benign and Malignant Cases of Childhood Psychosis," *American Journal of Orthopsychiatry, 19:*295–305, 1948.

28. MODELL, A. H., "Primitive Object Relations and the Predisposition to Schizophrenia," *International Journal of Psychoanalysis, 44:*282–292, 1963.

29. NUNBERG, H., "The Synthetic Function of the Ego," *Practice and Theory of Psychoanalysis,* International Universities Press, New York, 1955.

30. PINE, F., "On the Concept 'Borderline' in Children: A Clinical Essay," in Eissler R. S., et al. (Eds.), *The Psychoanalytic Study of the Child,* vol. 29, pp. 341–367, International Universities Press, New York, 1974.

31. POLATIN, P., and HOCH, P., "Diagnostic Evaluation of Early Schizophrenia," *Journal of Nervous and Mental Disease, 105:*221–230, 1947.

32. RANK, B., "Aggression," in Eissler, R. S., et al. (Eds.), *The Psychoanalytic Study of the Child,* vols. 3/4, pp. 43–48, International Universities Press, New York, 1949.

33. ROCHLIN, G., "Loss and Restitution," in Eissler, R. S., et al. (Eds.), *The Psychoanalytic Study of the Child,* vol. 8, pp. 288–309, International Universities Press, New York, 1953.

34. ROSENFELD, S., and SPRINCE, M., "Some Thoughts on the Technical Handling of Borderline Children," in Eissler, R. S., et al. (Eds.), *The Psychoanalytic Study of the Child,* vol. 20 pp. 495–517, International Universities Press, New York, 1965.

35. ———, "An Attempt to Formulate the Meaning of the Concept 'Borderline,' " in Eissler, R. S., et al. (Eds.), *The Psychoanalytic Study of the Child,* vol. 18, pp. 603–635, International Universities Press, New York, 1963.

36. WEIL, A. P., "Some Evidence of Deviational Development in Infancy and Childhood," in Eissler, R. S., et al. (Eds.), *The Psychoanalytic Study of the Child,* vol. 11, pp. 292–299, International Universities Press, New York, 1956.

37. ———, "Certain Severe Disturbances of Ego Development in Children," in Eissler, R. S., et al. (Eds.), *The Psychoanalytic Study of the Child,* vol. 8, pp. 271–287, International Universities Press, New York, 1953.

---

16 / Affective Disorders

Leon Cytryn and Donald H. McKnew, Jr.

Introduction

Until the beginning of the twentieth century, affective disorders in childhood were completely disregarded as a clinical entity. It remained for writers and poets to portray depressed children and adolescents; these they presented in vivid fashion and usually as victims of depriving, unfavorable circumstances. At the beginning of the twentieth century, many seasoned clinicians described depressed children with great sensitivity and detail. Paradoxically, however, in the 1930s, with the advent of child psychiatry as an autonomous discipline, this modest but convincing accumulated clinical evidence was completely ignored. As a result, no major textbook of psychiatry or child psychiatry contained a chapter on childhood depression until the late 1960s. Both in America and in Europe, however, the interest in childhood affective illness started earlier in the wake of World War II.

Anthony, a pioneer in this area, stated that the picture of prepubertal depression includes, among other symptoms, "weeping bouts, some complaints, loss of appetite and energy, varying degrees of difficulty in school adjustment, and vacillation between clinging to and unreasonable hostility toward . . . (the) parent."[8] Anthony also postulated that some children are "predisposed to depression," although he did not suggest any possible origin for such a predisposition. In 1965, Sandler and Joffe[110] reported that the syndrome of childhood depression had several consistent features including sad affect, withdrawal, discontent, a feeling of being rejected or unloved, passivity, and insomnia.

Currently, a change in contemporary thinking about childhood depression is becoming evident. A 1967 report on Psychopathological Disorders in Childhood by the Group for the Advancement of Psychiatry[55] states: "Depression in children and even in adolescents may be manifested in ways somewhat different from those manifested by adults . . . The picture of depression may be much more clear and marked, particularly when precipitated by an actual, threatened, or symbolic loss of a parent or parent substitute . . . Psychomotor retardation is ordinarily less marked than in adults, and, except in young infants, the same is true of some of the other biologic signs of depression." (p. 236).

A paper describing the various clinical manifestations of childhood depression has been recently published by Poznanski and Zrull.[98] In another publication. Glaser[52] dealt with the problem of so-called masked depression in children in which the depressive affect is not a major component of the clinical picture.

Despite these favorable developments, there are still many workers in the behavioral sciences who do not accept the existence of affective disorders prior to adolescence. Some of their doubts center on theoretical issues such as the link between depressive illness and the time of the formation of the superego and ego ideal. Others feel that affec-

tive states in childhood are too evanescent to be given the status of a specific disease entity. Everyone in the field agrees that states of occasional sadness do occur in children, but many will fervently deny that this is any way related to a true psychopathological state. The best example of the lack of readiness on the part of the psychiatric community to give recognition to childhood depressive reaction is the failure of this syndrome to find mention in the DSM-II. The latter allows for some vague terms such as "withdrawal reaction" or "runaway reaction." Both of these, at best, reflect only some facets of the depressive syndrome; however, they do not allow for a proper and accurate diagnosis. The result is an unfortunate negative process by which the absence of a name for this entity in the DSM-II forces many professionals to misdiagnose their depressive patients. This, in turn, perpetuates the misconception that the condition does not exist. As this chapter unfolds, an attempt will be made to help the reader understand the reasons for this confusion and to present adequate support for an acceptance of the important clinical entity called childhood depressive reaction.

Historical Overview

Prior to Kraepelin's pioneering work in 1902,[71] almost all mental pathology was poorly understood. Kraepelin was a master classifier and broke entirely with the thinking contemporary to his day. His great conceptual breakthrough was to divide all serious mental disorders into two major categories: the episodic, nondeteriorating manic-depressive insanity, and the progressive, deteriorating dementia praecox.[70] This continues to be basic to all psychiatric nosology. Adolph Meyer thought of all affective disorders as variants of one disease. Kraepelin added that there were etiological factors in affective disorders and that "defective heredity is the most prominent."[92] Adolph Meyer was the first to consider a psychodynamic basis for the affective disorders; the same approach was followed by Freud and his school.

In 1911, Bleuler[19] published his famous monograph on schizophrenia. Bleuler's concept of primary and secondary symptoms was quickly accepted, and it became clear that a similar concept could apply to the affective disorders.

The last great debate concerned neurotic depression which Kraepelin had called congenital neurasthenia. This was the beginning of the debate over endogenous versus reactive depression which continues to this day. In 1952, Bellak[15] proposed a continuum extending from a minimum of external precipitating factors to a maximum. In 1971, Klerman[67] described the basic features of endogenous depression; he asserted that the patient could be expected to have a relatively stable and nonneurotic premorbid personality, and that the illness is less likely to be precipitated by life stresses. The typical configuration of signs and symptoms of endogenous depression consists of feelings of guilt, remorse and unworthiness, sleep disturbance, middle of the night insomnia, early morning awakening, psychomotor retardation, agitation, decreased libido, weight loss and loss of interest. In contrast to this, patients with reactive depression show a high degree of neuroticism and premorbid personality defect.

In 1957, Leonhard[76] introduced the concept of bipolar illness for manic-depressive conditions, and unipolar for depressive disorders . Winokur[134] introduced the concepts of primary affective disorder (characterized by the absence of psychopathology prior to the illness) and secondary affective disorder (in which the patient had suffered from a preexisting, nonaffective psychiatric illness). In most recent publications, the general position has been that bipolar and unipolar affective disorders fall into the category of primary affective disorder, while the neurotic depressive reaction is considered a secondary disorder.

Review of Analytic Literature

The first analyst to study depression was Carl Abraham. His basic notion was that a depressed person feels impoverished and unable to love, and that in trying to overcome this painful feeling, he represses to an oral stage of development.

In 1917, in *Mourning and Melancholia*, Freud[45] described the feelings of the depressed state as "profound painful dejection, abrogation of interest in the outside world, a loss of capacity to love, inhibition of all activity, and a lowering of self-regarding feelings." He then stated that "this loss could be of a loved person or the loss of some abstraction which has taken place, such as fatherland, liberty, an ideal, and so on." Freud also added that the sufferer need not have lost these things in reality, but merely have lost them in his imagination. Freud added that all persons who suffer losses incorporated that which was lost. When there was a lack of ambivalence, the incorporated lost object was slowly given up, and this was the process basic to normal mourning. However, when there was marked ambivalence towards this object, it was given up only with great suffering and pain, and what began as mourning could continue into a depression.

In 1924, Abraham[2] made the first psychodynamic distinction between neurotic and psychotic depression. He said that the psychotic patient regresses to the anal destructive phase of development and unconsciously expells the object that he had previously introjected; at the same time he becomes exceedingly depressed due to the psychic void thus created. The neurotic cannot tolerate such a loss and retains the object in his psyche. Abraham stresses five aspects in the psychogenesis of depression which may be important to an understanding of childhood depression. First, he felt that there was a constitutional overaccentuation of dependency needs. He observed that these people suffered early and repeated childhood disappointmnts in love. Next, he posited that many of these losses occurred in the pregenital period, before the child had resolved his oedipal wishes and had acquired the strength to withstand such losses. Lastly, he pointed out the compulsion to repeat a primary disappointment in later life, leading to a recurrence of these early overwhelming losses.

Sandor Rado[101] emphasized the importance of self-esteem in depression. Mabel Blake Cohen and her group at Chestnut Lodge first described the family situation of depressed patients. They felt that depression grew out of a continuously painful interpersonal environment.

Bibring[17] and Jacobson[58] (most especially the latter) began to turn in a new direction in order to understand affective disorders. Bibring[16, 17] stressed that depression is the result of the defense of the ego against the loss of self-esteem; there is a deprivation of the power to love rather than of a particular person. He then went on to say that this was a result of traumatic experiences in early childhood which brought about a painful state of helplessness and powerlessness; later in life this tended to recur easily under stress.

Edith Jacobson* is probably the major designer of the modern psychological view of depression. Her thoughts are based on a very sharp distinction between the ego and self,[59] the self standing for

---

* She gradually developed her concepts over the years. See references 55, 56, 57, 58, 59, and 60.

self-representation, and the ego standing for a set of psychological functions. She summarizes high self-esteem or lack of depression in the following way: if the self-representation is "highly energized," then self-esteem is said to be high. She sees two threats to this goal, much as David Levy had seen it back in the 1930s. On the one hand there is overgratification, with prolonged mother-child union, leading to a retarded development of independence and an unrealistic view of the world. On the other end of the scale, there is excessive frustration beyond the capacity of the developing ego to master, leading to feelings of inferiority and poor self-esteem. Edith Jacobson then summarizes all of her statements by saying that self-esteem is, in fact, an emotional expression of one's self-evaluation; it represents the degree of discrepancy or of harmony between the self-representation and the idealized concept of the self.

Child Analytic Literature

Like most of his predecessors, Sandler began with a heavy emphasis on self-esteem which he viewed as a "constant affective background to all our experiences."[109] In 1965, he and Joffe[110] wrote on depressive reaction in children. They made efforts to distinguish this condition from adult depressive reactions. In referring to this state in children as "as basic psycho-biological affective reaction," they view it as "an ultimate reaction to the experience of helplessness in the face of physical or psychological pain in one form or another." They point out that depression may occur even when there has been no actual object loss at all; an imagined loss of love and interest is enough. These authors also view depression as a signal on a par with anxiety. It may thus lead to a variety of defensive measures which may be more available to adults; this then may explain some of the differences between adult and childhood depression.

Melanie Klein[66] is the founder of the so-called "English School" and was its most influential member. She postulated that during the first year of life, every child went through a sequence of developmental stages. The paranoid stage occupied the first two months of life and was followed by a "depressive position" of three to four month's duration. This is the stage when good objects begin to be introjected along with the bad objects taken in during the earlier period. During this period, the child feels every loss of the good object as a frustration; a removal and absence of the mother is interpreted as being brought about by his own destructive fantasies; since at this stage projection is less available, these feelings are internalized and appear in the form of sadness, guilt, and regret. She believed that this feeling of loss and sorrow can occur only when the warmth of the relationship, or the loving whole person has already been experienced previously, and that there were many children who, throughout the remainder of their lives, never solidified good internalized objects.

Bowlby described in detail a child's reaction to the loss of its mother.* He thought the child's tie to the mother was instinctual and was not based on oral incorporative needs as described by previous writers. He divided the child's reaction to the loss of the mother into a sequence of three stages. The first stage is described as the period of protest and lasts from a few hours to a few weeks. In the course of this phase, the child experiences acute distress and appears to be attempting to get the mother back. This is followed by a stage of despair; the child manifests hopelessness, a depressed appearance, withdrawal and inertness. Finally, this is followed by the last stage, detachment. Here the child seems to accept the nurturance of other caretakers such as nurses but with a certain change in his own demeanor. He has adapted, but somewhere a price has been paid. If there then follows a series of lost mother figures, the child may gradually lose trust in other human beings and will assume an attitude of indifference to further human contact. Bowlby's views were based on ethological concepts of attachment; they were not immediately accepted by many analytic writers who saw primitive attachment as stemming from oral dependency needs rather than from primary instinctual needs. In this debate, Bowlby found an ally in Michael Balint[12] who agreed with him that there is, in infancy, a primary, primitive relationship hunger that is independent of any oral needs and is "a form of an object relationship that is not oral or genital, but is something on its own."

Margaret Mahler in 1961 expressed her belief that grief can begin to occur in children only after enough psychic structure has developed.[83] For this to be possible, the child must be able to experience mental images of the temporarily absent mother. In a later paper in 1966, she states more explicitly that the child's depressed mood may be

* See references 20, 21, 22, 23, 24, 25, 26.

caused predominantly by separation.[82] She believes, as does Bowlby, that these states create a basis for later depressive states.

René Spitz described 123 unselected infants whom he followed in a nursery.[124] He noted a number of them to develop weepy behavior, withdrawal, weight loss, psychomotor retardation, insomnia, and illness. This behavior which he called "anaclytic depression"[123] lasted up to three months and was sometimes followed by frozen, rigid posture. In all of the infants who developed these symptoms, the mother had been removed from the child somewhere between the sixth and eighth month, and the separation continued essentially without interruption for a period of three months. He felt that the differences between the child and adult pictures were due to the difference in psychic structure between adults and infants, along with the child's fewer psychological resources. In general, when the mother was returned to the child in less than three months, "they suddenly were friendly, gay, approachable, and the withdrawal, disinterest and rejection of the outside world, the sadness disappeared as if by magic." Without intervention, however, the picture of depression continued. Spitz was able to study children in a foundling home, where the love object was not restored. Here the picture of depression was clear cut but continued to a more advanced stage. In the worst cases, the clinical profile the children presented showed "stuporous, deteriorated catatonia, or in other cases, agitated idiocy." Most of these cases appeared to be irreversible, and, of the ninety-one childen that he observed, thirty-four died.

Wolfenstein views the process of mourning as it is seen in infancy, childhood, adolescence, and adulthood as a phenomenon which changes with the developmental stages of the person.[138] She comes to the conclusion that latency or young adolescent children deal with death through denial and dissocation of affect. There is often an expected magical return of the lost person. There were also periods of desperation, frustration, and rage. In summary, she says "we may consider that what is feared is the emergence of an unbearable panic state." She states that a successful adolescence is akin to the process of mourning in which the giving up of the initial objects forms the model for all future mourning operations.

Mahler[83, 84] points to the distinction between what happens to children who develop anaclytic depression versus those who become psychotic very early in life. She says that where there is sufficient love and proper objects for ego development, there is no psychosis, but, if there is a severe loss, the child is left with a potential for depression. She is amazed at the capacity shown by infants with anaclytic depression to recover despite the severity of their injury.

Engel and Reichsman described a famous patient, Monica, who at that time was fifteen to twenty-four months of age.[38] They reported that whenever the child experienced the loss of people she knew and was approached by strangers, she exhibited depression and withdrawal. The work of Engel and Reichsman clearly demonstrated that this young girl, showed marked effects of deprivation in care. Moreover, this was true not only in her bodily responses, but in her gastric responses as well. Interestingly, in her later adolescence she went on to make a very good adjustment; nonetheless, at appropriate times, she continued to show a mild version of the responses that she had displayed so many years earlier in her life. Engel and Reichsman introduced the concept of conservation-withdrawal to indicate that depressive behavior in infancy is primarily reactive and represents an attempt of the organism to preserve its integrity in response to an external stress. They have compared their concept with hybernation in animals. This comparison is supported by some recent data from animal work done by Reite and Kaufman.[104] They studied infant pig-tailed monkeys who showed severe psychomotor retardation, and a sad facial expression following separation from their mothers. During this phase, they exhibited a marked reduction in heart rate and body temperation as would be seen in hybernation. Of course, any extrapolation from animal models to human affective disorders has to be viewed with great caution. Sandler pointed to the tie between individuation and depression.[110] He says: "Mourning is associated with the pain of giving up the infantile ideal states of self." He feels that individuation requires repeated small stages of mourning for the former lost ideal states of self.

In contrast to the previous authors, there have been a number of prominent psychoanalytic writers who have not accepted the concept of childhood depression. Rochlin has been one of the most consistent critics.[107] He readily concedes that children do have periods of loss and mourning and deprivation that are extremely painful. However, he does not feel that the child maintains this sense of loss, but that he quickly passes it by "with a readiness to accept a substitute for the object that is lost." Despite his objections, he suggests that object loss and its discomfort are deeply imbedded in psychic development. However, he remarks that loss of self-esteem is able to appear only after some maturity of the ego has taken place. In essence, Rochlin is stating that very young children are capable of only brief rage reactions in response to loss, after which they substitute alternative love objects. Older children, on the other hand, acquire the ability to love objects in a relatively nonnarcissistic way, and it is when these objects are lost that the children then go through true depression, grief, and mourning. He points out that the two major affects in depression are helplessness and hopelessness. He defines helplessness as reflecting a loss of ego autonomy. Hopelessness, on the other hand, is the feeling of despair coming from the individual's awareness of his own inability to provide himself with gratification. He feels that there is quite a different time sequence for these two affects. He sees hopelessness as occurring in the first few months of life, resulting from feelings of deprivation and discomfort. By the sixth-tenth month of life, the young child is well differentiated from its mother and begins to fear the loss of the mother. This feeling becomes fully differentiated in the twelve to sixteen month period, when, as Piaget notes, the ego of the child is probably fully aware of its dependence on the external world for gratification, and it is when this gratification is not available that the child experiences helplessness.

Rie wrote the first survey of childhood depression in 1966.[106] For the most part, this article is critical; the author attempts to demonstrate, through logical reasoning and reliance on certain authority figures, that childhood depression could not exist. He dismisses Spitz's work on anaclytic depression, saying that "these children have a condition which evolves in early childhood into a disorder which is not reminiscent of depression at all." Rie then turns to Lehmann, who had described the syndrome as consisting of primary and secondary symptoms. In reviewing these symptoms, Rie concedes that Lehmann's primary symptoms did not require verbalization for assessment, but they consisted of a "sad, despairing mood, decreased motor productivity, retardation, or agitation in the field of expressive motor responses." However, Lehmann did later point out that many patients can be deceptive in appearance and will reveal their depression in the verbalization of their mood. The next chain in the logical argument grew out of the work of Rado, Freud, and, of course later, Bibring and Jacobson. They had all pointed out the importance in depression of low self-esteem. To obtain access to these feelings, however, would certainly require verbalization,

and, in this situation, not only verbalization, but also a certain awareness of one's self and one's idealized self. Rie, then turns to Rochlin who takes the most extreme position concerning depression. Rochlin insists that it exists only when there is a conflict between the superego and the ego, and that all depressions are characterized by guilt. He points out that depression requires a state of low self-esteem; hence, in order to be depressed, a child would have to have achieved a clear self-representation. He quotes Erikson who says that a child doesn't acquire a sense of ego identity until adolescence. Rie then summarizes by saying: "Chronically low self-esteem is regarded as a necessary condition for depression by all theorists," and then goes on to say depression cannot occur before adolescence.

Review of European Child Psychiatry

The European psychiatrists have more often adopted an adultomorphic view of childhood depression. In vivid clinical detail, they describe numerous cases of manic-depressive psychosis in children and attempt to group them into endogenous and exogenous forms. The division between the two forms seems arbitrary; it appears to be based on vague clinical impressions rather than on a solid scientific basis. Additional confusion stems from other artificial groupings, with the interrelationship among them remaining uncertain. One investigator, for instance, recognized no less than six "nosological" and six "diagnostic" syndromes. These include: psychogenic, constitutional, somatogenic, agitated, passive, and the more classifical manic-depressive states. Despite their often adultomorphic approach, most European authors stress that the depressive picture changes with age, i.e., the older the children, the more they resemble the adult affective disorder. Others stress the fact that even severe depressive manifestations during childhood do not necessarily evolve into manic-depressive illness in adulthood; instead they can result in a number of psychiatric disturbances, including psychotic and dissociative states.

In the 1950s many workers began to question the wisdom of a strict application of the classical criteria of adult manic-depressive illness to children. However, even those authors wrote about "affective psychoses of children" and drew a parallel to the dichotomy between childhood psychosis and schizophrenia. The most important leitmotif in the European description of childhood affective disorders was, and still is, the emotional and physiological lability, where the alternating, contrasting emotional states present a "cyclothymic" picture. This is considered to be a forerunner of the adult manic-depressive illness.

Clinical Picture

CLINICAL FEATURES

As is evident from the foregoing material, a reader is likely to become bewildered by the widely divergent clinical pictures, all subsumed under the heading of childhood depression. In this section, an attempt will therefore be made to identify and isolate the various types of childhood depression.

A review of the literature and analysis of the authors' own research material leads to the conclusion that, phenomenologically, depression in latency-age children may be divided into three distinct categories based on clinical manifestations. These clinical factors include family background, duration of illness, premorbid history, and precipitating events. Their grouping, in turn, gives rise to the categories, namely; masked depressive reaction of childhood, acute depressive reaction of childhood, and chronic depressive reaction of childhood.[32]

These three forms of childhood depression differ in several aspects, as described in the following case reports.

Case Reports

Case 1. Masked Depressive Reaction of Childhood. A. was a twelve-year-old boy who was referred by school authorities because of his disruptive behavior. He had a long history of school difficulties that included hyperactivity, aggressive behavior, poor scholastic performance, and marginal social adjustment. His behavior had led to several school suspensions in the past.

The home situation had always been very unstable. Due to her full-time work, the mother had been unavailable to the children; at one time she was investigated for child abuse. The father was a chronic alcoholic who frequently beat the patient and assumed no responsibility for his family. There was no history of overt depressive illness in the family.

In the interview situation the patient was in a very depressed mood; he was apathetic and sad throughout. He described himself as dumb and as the laughing-stock of his schoolmates; he expressed the belief that everyone was picking on him. On the fantasy level, the boy showed a strong preoccupation with themes of annihilation, violence, explosions, and death, invariably with a bad outcome for the main figures in those fantasies. From both verbal productions and figure drawings, it was also evident that the boy's body image was extremely defective. He viewed himself as inadequate and helpless, with very little initiative or autonomy.

The patient was hospitalized for a period of three weeks. During this interval, except for his sleeplessness, the overt signs of his depression gradually disappeared and gave way instead to aggressive and impulsive behavior.

The follow-up period of one and one-half years was very stormy. The boy continued to have serious school difficulties, leading finally to his suspension from school and admission to a residential setting for delinquent boys.

COMMENT

The child's acting-out behavior succeeded in masking his depression. This went unrecognized until his admission to the hospital, where it became clearly evident. The depth of his depression and the pain of his self-denigration, as revealed in the interview material, may help to explain his defensive use of aggressive and delinquent behavior. Although such a defense is self-destructive, it helps to ward off the unbearable feelings of despair.

Case 2. Acute Depressive Reaction of Childhood. B., a six-year-old girl, was referred by the pediatric clinic because of progressive withdrawal, depressed affect, sleep disturbance, lack of appetite, school failure, and separation anxiety of an extent sufficient to interfere with all social activities. These symptoms appeared after the rape of her seventeen-year-old sister three months prior to the referral. Before this incident the mother had been relatively unavailable due to full-time work, and the sister had served as a mother substitute to the patient. After the rape, however, the sister became withdrawn, preoccupied, and less attentive to the patient. Prior to the present illness, the paient never exhibited signs of depression and had a reasonably good social and scholastic record; she was, however, described by relatives and friends as stubborn and negativistic. There was no history of depression in other family members, but the father had been absent for many years and the mother was resentful of the burden she had to carry.

The girl was admitted to the hospital for a period of three weeks. At the time of admission her mood was markedly depressed. She evidenced a sad and tearful facial expression, slowness of movement, monotone voice, and verbal expressions indicating hopelessness and despair. On the ward, her clinical picture changed within several days. She became outgoing and started to eat and sleep regularly, her mood brightened, and she was sociable, active and alert.

Following her symptomatic improvement, the girl was discharged and followed for a period of two years. According to the mother's report, she maintained her gains and, during the follow-up period, she behaved very much as she had before the onset of the presenting complaints.

COMMENT

The patient had made a relatively good premorbid adjustment. The depressive signs and symptoms seem to have followed a traumatic event that resulted in a loss of a mother figure. The patient had suffered no such losses in the past, which may help to explain her quick and lasting recovery.

Case 3. Chronic Depressive Reaction of Childhood. C., a seven-year-old girl born out of wedlock, was referred on an emergency basis because of severe depression. For several months, she had had insomnia, anorexia, weight loss, and screaming episodes. She told the pediatric resident that she wanted to kill herself; according to the mother, she had made suicidal threats repeatedly, claiming that she was "a bad girl" and that nobody loved her. Ten months prior to this episode, she had been seen in the psychiatric crisis clinic because of persistent insomnia.

The girl's mother was an immature, helpless woman; she had a tendency toward frequent depressions and was overwhelmed by family responsibilities. She shared with her daughter a passive, helpless attitude toward life as well as poor self-esteem. There is some evidence that as a child the mother had been neglected by her own mother and had been exposed to frequent violence in her surroundings. She was hospitalized once with what seems to have been an agitated depression. Over the course of the contacts with her, she had at least one serious depressive episode during which she made suicidal threats. She had left home twice for several months, once when the patient was one and one-half years old and again when she was four. Her only marriage was stormy, and at the time of the contacts, the parents were separated, after the child's stepfather had beaten the child severely.

The father had a long history of delinquent behavior; following the child's birth, he had had little contact with either the girl or her mother. The paternal grandmother, however, kept the child during the day, while the maternal grandmother was maintaining a full-time job as a housekeeper. According to the child's mother, the paternal grandmother had been one of the most significant persons in the patient's life. This relationship, however, was abruptly interrupted when, at one year of age, the child was transferred to the care of a maternal aunt.

As the patient grew up she became shy and retiring, usually withdrawing from stressful situations. At the age of three she would punish herself (whenever she thought she had transgressed) by quitting her play or favorite toy and sitting quietly in the corner until she was told to resume her activities.

When first seen, C. wore a sad expression and appeared poorly nourished, very small for her age, and passive. The most striking features of her behavior were her withdrawal, apathy, lack of spontaneity, and psychomotor retardation. She was admitted to the hospital for a period of three weeks. At first she continued to be depressed, apathetic, and withdrawn; she refused most meals, and slept poorly. After two episodes of open expression of violent anger, however, steady improvement began, marked by more spontaneity, improved mood, appetite, and sleep, and increased social interaction. Along with the decrease of overt depression there was an increase in negativism, defiance, and, on occasion, even hostility.

After her discharge, there was much instability in the child's environment. Her mother went back to the stepfather, who in the past had been cruel to the girl. The patient thereupon again became depressed and developed abdominal cramps and diarrhea. When the mother again separated from the stepfather, these symptoms rapidly disappeared.

After three months of weekly follow-up visits, the team lost track of the patient because the mother did not keep appointments. During telephone conversations, the mother became depressed and threatened suicide; she asked for suggestions but did not follow through. She reported the patient to be doing well in school and at home, but the reliability of this information is doubtful.

COMMENT

The most striking features of this patient were the presence of depressed mood and behavior, including suicidal ideation very early in childhood, repeated separations from important maternal figures starting in infancy, and the presence of a chronic depression in the mother.

Depressive symptoms, especially sad affect in response to environmental trauma, are very common in children. Most of the time, however, they are only of short duration and do not interfere substantially with the child's thinking, functioning, and physical health. One thinks in terms of depressive illness rather than a depressive mood when such a state of mind is of long duration (of at least several months), when it is associated with severe impairment of the child's scholastic and social adjustment, and when vegetative disturbances are present, especially those of food intake and sleep. In more serious cases, the child's thinking is affected by feelings of despair and hopelessness, general retardation, and, not infrequently, by suicidal thoughts. In some cases, these children present a clearly identifiable depressive syndrome. This syndrome includes a persistent sad affect, social withdrawal, hopelessness, helplessness, psychomotor retardation, anxiety, school and social failures, sleep and feeding disturbances, and suicidal ideas and threats. Suicidal attempts are rare. The clinical picture is sometimes, but not always, preceded by a traumatic event; it usually takes at least two to three months before medical help is sought. The children with this clinical picture can be further subdivided into those with *acute depressive reactions* and those with *chronic depressive reactions*, based on precipitating factors and family history, as well as clinical course.

In children with acute depressive reactions, a precipitating cause could be found in all cases. This was either a severe trauma associated with the loss of an important person, or sometimes a more subtle form of withdrawal of interest or change in involvement on the part of important people, leading to a diminution of the love and care previously given. These families had considerable strength and cohesion and no clear-cut history of depressive illness. Because of the lack of any profound underlying family or personal psychopathology in these children, most of them recover from such a depressive episode in a few months time, and no serious sequelae have been noted.

In the patients with chronic depressive reactions, an immediate precipitating factor could not be found in most cases. In reviewing the background of these children, what did appear was a history of a series of many separations and losses of important people, usually beginning in early infancy and occurring repeatedly thereafter during the child's life. There has always been at least one parent (in most instances, the mother) with a history of recurrent depressive illness. The children often present a vicious cycle of low esteem leading to scholastic and social failure.

While studying the children with acute and chronic depressive reactions, it was noted that their dreams and fantasies—as displayed in play, storytelling, and drawings—regularly contained themes indicating frustration, despair, hopelessness, and helplessness. Being trapped, being lost or deserted, suicide and death were the most common occurrences, and were repeated with amazing regularity. When the authors became aware that the same fantasy material occurred in children who did not present a clear-cut depressive disorder, it was decided to study these children more thoroughly. This study led to the realization that many cases of childhood depression do not manifest themselves in a clearly recognizable form. Instead they present as a *masked depressive reaction*. The children thus afflicted may display the superficial appearance of a variety of emotional disorders, among them hyperactivity, aggressive behavior, psychosomatic illness, hypochrondriasis, and delinquency. Of course, these symptoms often manifest themselves in children without affective disorders and may be caused by a variety of organic or psychogenic factors. In cases of masked depression, one becomes alert to the *underlying* depression because of (1) periodic displays of a *purely* depressive picture, which would include sad affect, verbalization of depressive themes, and (2) the existence of depressive themes in dreams, drawings, and other fantasy material. In *masked depressive reactions* the investigators were unable to find a simple causative factor.

As stated in "Historical Review," European investigators frequently report psychotic affective illness in children. In contrast, our own experience, as well as that of other American investigators, shows that psychotic affective illness is virtually nonexistent prior to midadolescence. Thus, all the clinical phenomena discussed previously belong in the neurotic range of psychopathology.

Suicide

Many depressed children, express suicidal ideation and suicidal wishes, both on a conscious as well as on a fantasy level. However, under the age of fourteen, suicidal attempts, or even suicidal gestures, are very rare in these children. The occasional suicidal attempts in this age group are seen mostly in impulsive, angry children with a very low level of frustration tolerance who come from chaotic, disturbed, multi-problem families. In contrast to successful suicidal attempts which are more frequent in boys, suicidal gestures are far more prevalent in girls. Of those who were followed after an unsuccessful suicidal attempt or gesture, only very few developed depressive illness. As to the correlation between parental depression and childhood suicide, less than 5 percent of such children have a parent with a diagnosed affective disorder.

The frequency of successful and unsuccessful suicidal attempts increases dramatically after the age of fourteen, and suicide now ranks among the major causes of death in adolescence.[117] Even in this group, however, depressive illness is responsible probably for no more than 25 percent of the cases. The majority of suicidal attempts in adolescence are usually the expression of frustration, conflicts with parents, and lack of close relationships. Indeed, the most common precipitating event in these cases is the breakup of a boyfriend-girlfriend relationship.

Manic Disorders

In children, classic manic states, which include the characteristic persistent elation, grandiosity flight of ideas are very rare, although hypomanic states are found more often. In over eight years of research on affective illness in children, the authors encountered only one bona fide case of hypomania diagnosed in a nine-year-old boy.[91] Anthony and Scott,[11] who reviewed the world literature on manic states in children found only *three* cases which satisfied their very strict criteria for inclusion, such as: a bipolar clinical picture corresponding to the adult pathological state, "cyclothymic" personality, periodic recurrence of symptoms, absence of immediate precipitating factors and absence of schizophrenia or organic symptoms.

It is most likely that some psychiatrists confuse hyperactivity, hyperexcitability, occasional disorientation, and explosive behavior with manic states in children.

The rarity of manic disorders in childhood is supported by the authors' experience with the children of many adults with bipolar affective illness. In these children there was a strikingly low frequency of hypomanic features, and a total absence of manic state. The age-dependent emergence of manic symptoms needs further clarification.

Frequency and Prevalence

There is a marked paucity of prevalence studies of affective disorders in children in this country. As stated before, the available European data may not be applicable.

Maria Kovacs[69] and her colleagues at the University of Pennsylvania studied the incidence of depressive symptoms in: (1) thirty-nine children who were consecutively admitted to a psychiatric hospital for a random variety of psychopathology; and (2) twenty children with no current or prior psychiatric contact. The children in both groups were eight to thirteen and were matched for age.

Of the hospital sample, 14 percent were moderately to severely depressed, and an additional 24 percent showed mild depression. Among the control children, 5 percent showed mild depression and none showed the more severe types of symptoms.

We studied the occurence of affective disorders in the children of patients with unipolar and bipolar affective illness in order to determine whether they represent an at-risk group. These were fourteen adults who were hospitalized at NIMH because of a primary affective disorder. All of their thirty offspring were studied. The children ranged in age from five to fifteen. Seven of the thirty children were severely depressed and an additional nine were moderately so. The study supports the concept of a high frequency of depressive symptoms in the offspring of patients with primary affective disorders. Of course, it will remain for future research to determine whether this picture represents a genetic phenomenon or rather a reaction to living with an affectively disturbed parent.

The Changing Clinical Expression

of the Depressive Process

in Children

One of the most important reasons why depression in children has so long been unrecognized or misunderstood can probably be attributed to its age-related changing clinical expression, leading to frequent divergence from the common adult clinical pictures. In this section, an attempt will be made to clarify this phenomenon.

It was observed that the depressive process manifests itself in three different ways.

1. *Fantasy.* This category is based on the child's fantasy material as demonstrated in dreams or spontaneous play or as elicited by the use of projective techniques. These included the Thematic Apperception Test (TAT), Rorschach, Despert fables, dreams, associations to television, movies, and books, and free drawings accompanied by descriptive stories. Depressive themes in this category include mistreatment, thwarting, blame or criticism, loss and abandonment, personal injury, death and suicide.

2. *Verbal Expression.* This category is based entirely on the child's verbal content, spontaneous or elicited, and includes talk of hopelessness, helplessness, guilt, being unattractive, worthless, and unloved, as well as suicidal preoccupation.

3. *Mood and Behavior.* In this category are listed the manifestations of depressive affect that can be noticed by an observer without the need for verbal exchange. These manifestations in-

clude: psychomotor retardation, sadness evidenced through posture and facial expression, crying, disturbances in appetite and sleep, and such signs of masked depression as hyperactivity, aggressiveness, school failure, delinquency, and psychosomatic symptoms.

The data indicate further that the first category, depressive fantasy, is present almost all of the time in the children diagnosed as having a depressive reaction. The second category, verbal expression, exists less frequently in these same children. The third category, mood and behavior, is the least frequent and least stable finding. Furthermore, there were children in whom the gradual recession of depressive symptomatology could be closely observed. In those cases, the following predictable sequence of events was noted. The depressive mood and behavior disappeared first, usually followed by the disappearance of verbal expression. The fantasy material was the last to disappear, and usually did so only after the resolution of the depressive conflict.

PATTERN OF DEFENSES

These observations led the authors to formulate that a characteristic pattern of defenses helps many children to avoid experiencing or expressing depressive affect. On the first level, there is neither depressive mood and behavior nor verbalization of depressive content, but the fantasy material is rich in depressive themes. Many children with masked depressive reaction fall into this category. On the second level the defenses against depressive affect are less effective. There is no manifestation of depressive mood and behavior, but there is verbal expression of depressive content as seen in some children with receding chronic depressive reaction, and in most children with acute depressive reaction. On the third level, over prolonged periods of time, the defenses against depression fail. The child then manifests depressive mood and behavior, as seen in chronic depressive reaction as well as in early stages of acute depressive reaction.

At each level, most of the children make attempts to avoid the experience or awareness of depressive affect. On the first level (depressive fantasy), the defenses chiefly employed include denial, projection/introjection, acting out, avoidance, and splitting. At the second level (depressed talk), the predominant defenses are dissociation of affect and reaction formation. At the third level (mood and behavior), the preceding defenses against depression fail.

FACTORS INFLUENCING THE CHANGING CLINICAL PICTURE WITH AGE

There are many factors that singly or in combination reinforce the ability of the organism to defend against the depressive process. The child's maturation and growth promote a sense of optimism, exuberance, and hope, all of which help ward off any sense of despair or hopelessness. This may explain why, in adult terms, children's behavior so frequently appears to be mildly hypomanic. This emotional "push for growth" may have its counterpart in physiological mechanisms that counteract depression. When object constancy is not fully attained, the child has a greater ability to substitute a variety of love objects than do adults; this can militate against the full impact of object loss. Furthermore, the child's less developed ability to test reality favors the use of denial, projection/introjection, avoidance, splitting, and magical thinking, which ward off the perception of loss. Finally, the conscience of the young child is not as well developed, which tends to lessen the feelings of guilt and lowered self-esteem that are the basis of so many adult depressive states.

On the basis of the foregoing observations and deliberations, it is possible now to propose a framework that would clarify the uneven distribution of overt depressive symptomatology throughout the life cycle.

In infancy the child has only a limited repertoire of defense mechanisms available. The fantasy life is primitive and does not always allow for containment or discharge of depressive affect. Verbalization is unavailable either for abreacting depressive affect or for seeking solutions to depression-inducing situations. The combination of these factors can make an infant vulnerable to psychic flooding by depressive affect, manifesting itself in grossly depressed mood and behavior. However, the maturational push as well as the ability to substitute love objects with relative ease are factors that counteract the depressive process. This may explain why depression in infants is often short-lived except in situations where substitute love objects are unavailable, as in some institutions and hospitals.

In early childhood and latency, verbalization for the purpose of expression of feelings and problem solving is gradually increasing, although it remains relatively rudimentary. The push for growth, the tendency to translate affect into action, the increasing elaboration of the more primitive defenses, the still retained ability to substitute love objects, the increasingly rich fantasy life coupled with the yet immature reality testing, as well as a still not completely developed but often overly harsh conscience can together combine to contain the depressive process on the fantasy level. This constellation of factors helps to explain the relative frequency of masked depressive states as well as the rare appearance of depressive mood and behavior. The same constellation could also explain the evanescence of depressive symptomatology during this era of life.

With advancing age, the balance of the aforementioned forces increasingly shifts to favor a breakthrough of the depressive process into verbalization and overt mood and behavior. In late adolescence, the growth process gradually diminishes, and in adulthood, it stabilizes. Except in borderline and schizophrenic states, delayed object constancy is attained by this age, making substitution of love objects increasingly difficult. Maturing reality testing counteracts the tendency to use fantasy as an escape and forbids the free use of the more primitive defenses that were available earlier in life. In some individuals, the more developed conscience acts to exaggerate the development of guilt feelings and low self-esteem. The opposing forces include more mature defenses, the ability to verbalize feelings, and the capacity for problem solving. It is the combination of these factors which helps to explain the greater frequency of overt depression in adulthood, as opposed to childhood. However, where denial and other more primitive defenses and poor reality testing still prevail, one sees the adult counterpart of masked depression, e.g., depressive equivalents.

Etiological Considerations

ENVIRONMENTAL FACTORS

Frequent Separations: A recurrent theme in many of the patients' lives has been frequent separations for periods of several months from important love objects, particularly during the first few years of their lives. For many of these children, at some point in the child's maturing years, it was a grandparent, baby-sitter, or some distant relative who functioned as the major love object in addition to a parent. Frequently, episodes of reattachment to the original love object were followed by further separations. The child's substitute caretakers during the time of separation were frequently indifferent to the child or provided an unstable environment.

It is important to stress the fact that this was not the kind of deprivation in which there had never been an attachment to a significant love object or in which the significant object was withdrawn from the child's environment and no reattachment was ever allowed to occur. Such a sequence is often the case with chronically institutionalized children.

Sudden Loss: An experience common to many of these patients was the permanent loss of a crucial love object as a result of death, divorce, or a move away from the child's environment, with no further contact. The important factor here seems to be an excessive dependency on the particular loved one before the loss and the absence of any appropriate substitute after the loss. Until the loss of the love object, these children often functioned quite well.

Depreciation and Rejection: Many of the children studied have suffered rejection and depreciation by their parents or loved ones. This persisted either all during their lives or at least over a period of many years. Such rejection may take the form of blunt statements stressing the child's worthlessness or inadequacy, or it may be expressed more subtly through attitudes and actions that indicate a lack of respect, involvement, or caring. In some cases the parent has subjected the child to a constant barrage of criticism and humiliation. In other cases, there is no frank rejection or depreciation, but rather a void in the parent-child relationship. The parents may or may not be consciously aware of their behavior.

In some instances, this process of depreciation and rejection is related to an obvious characteristic of the child, such as a physical or mental handicap, or his sex, age, or position among his siblings. In other cases, the process is much less obvious and requires a good deal of extensive observation of the parent-child interaction in order to be understood.

Depreciation of the child can be shown through overprotection as well as through rejection; both attitudes convey the same basic message of the child's inadequacy and worthlessness. How much of the child's subsequent depressive outlook is caused by identification with this negative view of himself and how much is caused by a sense of alienation from important love objects is often hard to determine.

Loss of Involvement: In some situations a central figure in the child's life suddenly withdraws his interest in the child while maintaining a physically intimate presence. Here, one is not discussing a noxious interaction with the child (as in the category of depreciation and rejection), but rather the loss of a crucial positive relationship in the absence of alternative love objects. Such a loss of interest on the part of the adult is usually related to specific outside events such as illness, personal tragedy, a change in involvement with other people (as in the case of remarriage), or a new baby in the home.

Depression in Parents: In many of the cases at least one parent showed clinical evidence of depression. Some had been previously treated for depression. In some parents, however, the depression was manifested as a rather subtle mood disorder that never reached a clinical level requiring treatment.

Parental depression may affect the child either through the child's identification with the parent or through the parent's loss of involvement with the child as a result of his illness. Some children improved rapidly as soon as they were separated from their parents—a phenomenon that was frequently observed when a child was hospitalized. This may be attributed to a lack of internalization of the parent's depression. In such cases the child's chronically depressed mood improved within one or two days and recurred only during parental visits. On the other hand, those children in whom the process of internalization seemed to be already operating remained depressed while they were away from their parents. This was true for children as young as six years of age.

When there is a dramatic, clearly circumscribed event, such as death or divorce, the relationship between such an event and the affective disorder is more easily established. However, many subtle parental behaviors (for example, scapegoating, withdrawal of affection, transient depressive affect) are, in retrospect, irretrievable as historical events. They are blocked out by denial or repression of the behavior by the child or parent.

There is a finding that seems to favor the meaningful relationship between affective disorders and early childhood events. It turns out that each of the three types of childhood depression identified previously (and in the section "Clinical Picture") can be linked to a characteristic cluster of environmental factors.

Acute depression reaction always followed a sudden separation or a loss of involvement. On the other hand, every case of chronic depressive reaction was accompanied by clinically diagnosable depression in at least one parent. In the masked depressive reaction there was often an acute loss, or a loss of involvement, and almost always depreciation and rejection. Parental depression, however, was found only infrequently.

Family and Interpersonal Dynamics

The families of children with affective disorders present a broad range of clinical pictures. In acute depressive reaction, the family history usually reveals moderately neurotic problems in the parents but usually an absence of gross psychopathology. These families are, for the most part, intact and cohesive and show considerable strength, even when faced with a formidable stress. What is frequently missing, however, is the parent's awareness of the child's distress. This may go especially unrecognized when an object loss is of special importance to a particular child, but not to the rest of the family. In these children, one finds as a precipitating cause a severe trauma associated with an object loss. This is sometimes in the form of a death of the loved one. More often, however, it is in the more subtle form of withdrawal of interest or change of involvement on the part of a parent or a parental figure, because of remarriage, divorce, arrival of new siblings, or someone moving away. The child's emotional tie to the lost object is usually very strong and exclusive.

All of the children with chronic depressive reactions had at least one parent (in most instances, the mother) with a history of recurrent depressive illness (see previous section). An interesting phenomenon was noted in the treatment and follow up of these children. In some cases, the depression in the children and the parents started at about the same time. The parents were usually the first to exhibit depressive symptomatology, and the children, to use the words of Anna Freud, "produced the mother's mood in themselves."[42] However, in some cases the interaction between the parent's and the child's depression operated in a seesaw fashion; thus, whenever the patient improved, the parent would develop a depressive episode soon afterward.

In both acute and chronic depressive reactions, the family picture was similar in both lower-class and middle-class families. In the cases of masked depressive reaction, however, the picture differed sharply. In socially deprived children, the family members of the children with masked depressive reactions often presented a picture of disorganization and severe psychopatology, usually in the form of a character defect. Nonetheless, they gave no history of a clear-cut depressive illness. On the other hand, middle-class families of children with masked depressive reactions often presented a different profile. There the family structure was not unlike that seen in the families of children with acute or chronic depressive reactions. This included the presence of a depressed parent, a relatively stable home life and the absence of nonaffective psychopathology.

In all categories of affective disorders that could be observed directly in the course of family studies, two types of family interaction predominated. In the first one, the disturbed child was noted to be scapegoated and/or excluded from the interactions of family life. This was sometimes done by ignoring the child's efforts to communicate and to participate in family activities. This phenomenon of ignoring the child was vividly seen in two settings: (1) on the hospital ward, and (2) in family sessions. The pattern was one of active rejection of the child through depreciation, ridicule, or classical scapegoating maneuvers.

In some depressed children, a totally different family picture emerged. In these families, the distubed child was drawn into a tight bond with one of the parents (usually the sicker one). This almost symbiotic relationship promoted identification with parental pathology, induced guilt over the parent's illness, and prevented emotional growth and autonomy.

Depressed parents, in particular, are preoccupied with their own pathology. They are therefore unable to respond to the child's real needs to be loved and cared for, and to be given the freedom to mature in his own way. In the bipolar parent, there is an added hazard growing out of the shifting moods of the parent, leading to a sense of uncertainty and bewilderment on the part of the child.

In modern society, the presence of a depressed parent is especially hazardous because of the general absence of, or unavailability of, extended family. These are the people who normally could temporarily take over in loco parentis, in cases of object losses or breakdowns in the family's coping abilities. The extended family might help the depressed child by shoring up other important family members.

Biochemical Correlates of Affective Disorders

There has been a voluminous literature on the biochemical aspects of affective disorders in adults in an attempt to clarify the pathophysiology of these states. There has been little work done in this area with children.

Of the several theories proposed and studied, the so-called catecholamine theory of adult affective disorders assumes that levels of norepinephrine, a neurotransmitter, may be decreased in the brains of depressed patients at vital neuronal receptors, whereas mania might be associated with an excess of this amine. This theory has been the most widely accepted, although indolamines, steroids and electrolytes have also been extensively studied. Recently there has been a shift in emphasis from the presynaptic events to the study of the postsynaptic receptor mechanisms.

In the late 1960s, the authors[30] studied nine children aged six to twelve years, with affective disorders. The children were accepted in each case for a two- to three-week hospitalization. The urinary metabolites studied were norepinephrine, vanilmandelic acid, and 3-methoxy-4-hydroxy-phenylethyl glycol. Deviations from values in normal controls were found in all children; they were most apparent in those with chronic affective disorders.

These findings led to the following conclusions: changes in the excretion of urinary metabolites do occur in affectively disturbed children. These changes are most clear-cut in children with chronic affective disorders in contrast to those with acute or masked affective states. Finally, the patterns of these biochemical changes are not consistent, a phenomenon already found in adults with affective disorders.

In an unpublished follow-up study of eleven depressed children hospitalized for two weeks and nine hospitalized orthopedic control subjects, the following was found: The mean level of urinary 3-methoxy-4-hydroxyphenylethyl glycol (MHPG) was significantly higher in the depressed subjects than in controls. On the other hand, urinary norepinephrine (NE) and vanilmandelic acid (VMA) were lower in the depressed group. Urinary 3,5, adenosine-monophosphate (Cyclic AMP) was significantly lower in the depressed group.

The changes in MHPG may be of significance. MHPG is the only urinary metabolite of catecholamine of which a sizeable proportion comes from the brain rather than from peripheral catecholamine metabolism. The MHPG levels could reflect the activity level of the children, but this is unlikely since the values for NE and VMA did not parallel the changes in MHPG.

The authors' two studies suggest that clinical investigation of the biology of such childhood disorders may be as relevant for issues of cause and treatment as they have been in adult affective disorders.

Detection and Treatment

EARLY DETECTION

The pediatrician or family physician is in the most strategic position to detect early signs of childhood depression.[89] He frequently has information about the relationship between child and parent, is aware of critical events in the family life, knows something of parental attitudes toward the child, and can observe the child directly for any signs of depressive mood and behavior. His role may be especially invaluable in suspected cases of masked depression, in which the child is usually regarded by the family and school as delinquent or lazy. When a physician is consulted about such troublesome cases, he may elect to try to investigate the case himself through the use of simple playroom techniques, which will elicit fantasy material in drawings, dreams, or selected projective tests; or, he may prefer to refer the child to a psychiatrist. In either case, if the suspicion of a masked depressive reaction is confirmed, the all too frequent tragic mishandling of such cases can be avoided.

The finding that many depressed children have at least one depressed parent points to another avenue of early detection. Because children of depressed adults represent such a clearly at-risk group, it behooves any psychiatrist evaluating or treating such adults to inquire about the emotional status of the patients' children. The authors found that a screening family interview, including all family members, is particularly revealing. Conversely, all child psychiatrists who see depressed children should remain vigilant to the existence of a similar disorder in the siblings or parents.

A more subtle and difficult situation presents itself when attempting to detect masked depressive reaction. Experience indicates that parents of such children present either a variety of serious character disorders or a serious depressive illness. Simple history taking will often miss the masked depressive reaction that frequently occurs in some of the children of such families. The depression may be masked by behavior disorders, school difficulties, psychosomatic disorders, and even delinquency. However, there is much to suggest that in such cases careful and repeated interviewing will usually reveal the existence of occasional periods of unmistakable depression. The eliciting of such a history should prompt the psychiatrist to arrange for a thorough investigation of the child, which would include an exploration of fantasy material.

TREATMENT

After diagnosing childhood depression, the psychiatrist has at his disposal a number of therapeutic modalities, which are usually most useful in the earlier stages of the disorder. The most important of these is some form of family intervention. This can vary from intensive family psychotherapy, involving all family members, to periodic counseling of the parents without direct contact with the child. The choice of the type of family treatment will depend on the severity and duration of the depressive illness, the age of the child, and the parental motivation and adaptability. The younger the child, the more responsive he will be to environmental changes alone; in such instances, parental counseling is usually the treatment of choice. Where the child is older (past eight years), or when the illness is of long duration or great intensity, family therapy should include the affected child as well as other family members. In such cases, family therapy often has to be supplemented by individual work with the depressed child. The methods used in family therapy will depend on the family's psychological mindedness, intelligence and stability. Whenever possible, an interpretive, nondirective form of intervention is most efficacious in producing long term benefits; the insight developed in this way leads to more adaptive roles and defenses. However, many families respond better to direct guidance and emotional support. The latter may be true in families of children with masked depressive disorder. Of course, there are situations in which traditional psychiatric intervention of any kind is not feasible. In such cases, the psychiatrist may have to collaborate with community resources such as Juvenile Court, half-way houses, foster homes, and even the police.

Regardless of the type of therapy, family intervention would aim at decreasing depreciation and rejection of the child by an understanding of the process of "scapegoating;" the mere fact of starting family therapy will often result in increased family involvement which can further be fostered through an increased awareness of the child's needs. Where there has been a major object loss, the family needs help and guidance in providing adequate substitutes (either from its own ranks or from outside resources). Where there have been frequent early losses, the family is encouraged to help compensate by increased involvement with the child. However, one has to recognize that such early damage may be irreparable.

When it is recognized that the parent has a

depressive illness, it is of utmost importance to provide appropriate psychiatric help for him, both to improve the parent's functioning, as well as to provide the child with a nondepressed model for identification.

Experience demonstrates that family and parental treatment will suffice to handle many cases. However, where this intervention is not sufficient, individual treatment of the child is necessary. As a rule, a depressed child, like his adult counterpart, responds very favorably to psychotherapy. In play therapy, it is of importance diplomatically, to provide the child with opportunities for success. The therapist's interest in the child's successes outside of treatment provides another avenue for increasing self-esteem and ego strength. Once the depression begins to lift, one can employ more traditional methods of interpretation, which would fall on deaf ears in the initial stages of treatment. Later, group play therapy may be useful to help the child relate better to his peers.

All modalities are aimed at increasing the child's self-esteem, trust in adults, free expression of feelings, and a new model for identification; taken together, these should decrease hopelessness and helplessness.

One of the most fascinating results of the research to date was the relatively prompt and sustained improvement of even chronically depressed children when admitted to the Clinical Research Center for investigation. This was entirely unexpected since the authors anticipated a temporary worsening of the depression as a result of separation from home and family. This improvement happened despite the absence of any formal treatment program while in the hospital. Such improvement was almost universal in the acute depressive reactions; it was seen frequently in chronic depressive reaction; but it was almost not seen at all in the masked depressive reactions. It is suspected that this phenomenon is due to the removal of the child from one or more of the noxious environmental situations noted previously, coupled with the rallying of the family around the child who is labeled ill because of the hospitalization. In a five-year follow up, it turned out that many depressed children sustained the improvement initiated in the hospital, despite the fact that some patients did not avail themselves of follow-up therapy. This was most dramatically evident in several cases of chronic depressive reaction. This experience should encourage people to consider the possibility of brief hospitalization of depressed children as an effective form of crisis intervention.

Pharmacotherapy

In contrast to the adult affective disorders where a voluminous literature has been accumulating on the use of a wide variety of drugs, there is a paucity of similar information in the treatment of affective disorders in childhood. There are only scattered reports of clinical trials of antidepressant and antimanic drugs, mostly limited to one or several case histories.

Controlled, well designed studies, however, are conspicuous by their absence. Interestingly, in Europe where the concept of childhood affective disorder as an endogenous entity has been widely accepted, both antidepressant and antimanic drugs are frequently used and their administration is often strongly recommended. In the United States, on the other hand, the use of these drugs has been much more restrained; it is in fact curious that they have often been administered in nonaffective or even nonpsychiatric disorders.

MONOAMINE OXIDASE INHIBITORS

Because of their potential toxicity, these drugs are rather seldom employed in the United States, even for adults. Their use is much more frequent in Europe, where they are given to depressed children and adolescents, often in combination with minor tranquilizers such as chloriazepoxide. The use of monoamine oxidase inhibitors has also been reported to be of some benefit in autistic and schizophrenic children. The most widely used drugs in this class include phenelzine and nialamide, and the dosages prescribed vary widely. The most common side effects such as liver damage and hypertension have so far not been reported in children.

TRICYCLIC ANTIDEPRESSANTS

The most commonly used drugs in this class are: imipramine and amitriptyline, and their respective derivatives. Both have anticholingeric properties, and the latter also has a sedative effect. The daily dosage of the tricyclic drugs range from 20 to 100 mg daily. In several studies, where beneficial effects on the depressive symptoms have been reported, the groups were often diagnostically heterogeneous with mixed symptomatology. The results are consequently very difficult to assess. A notable exception has been the work of Puig-Antich and associates[99] who documented the beneficial effects of imipramine in severely depressed children who meet the Research Diagnostic Criteria for major affective disorders. Tricyclic drugs are widely used in children with enuresis, probably because of their anticholingeric properties. In addition, their use was reported in a variety of other psychiatric disorders such as autism, behavior disturbances and hyperactivity, all with ambiguous results. Of interest are recent reports of potentially harmful side effects of the use of tricyclic drugs in children, such as trachycardia and hypertension.

LITHIUM

As in the previously mentioned classes of drugs, lithium has been used for a whole gamut of childhood psychiatric disturbances and not necessarily only in manic disorders. In Europe it is often given to children with frequent mood swings which are regarded as forerunners of manic-depressive illness. A few typically hypomanic and manic children and adolescents have been reported to respond favorably to lithium. In addition, some investigators reported favorable results in children with a variety of symptoms which included: excitement, explosive anger, poor pulse control, and aggressive behavior. Lithium has also been tried in hyperactive children, but the only ones who responded favorably had parents with affective disorders who were also lithium responders. In the relatively new science of pharmacogenetics, the interesting possibility is discussed that the response to a drug may represent a hereditary trait not necessarily related to the type of psychiatric disorder.

The dosages used in children range widely from 50 mg to 1,800 mg daily. Most investigators strive for serum lithium levels of 0.5 meq/1.–1.5 meq/1., which represents the therapeutic range for adults. Because of superior renal clearance function in children, higher dosages per body weight than those used in adults are often needed to achieve and maintain the therapeutic serum levels. Again, probably because of the superior renal clearance, children are reported to tolerate high dosages of lithium very well, and side effects are very rarely reported.

In summary, one must conclude that more research of better quality than heretofore is needed before a rational use of antidepressant drugs and lithium can be recommended. The clinical impressions can hardly substitute for well designed, controlled studies. The diagnostic confusion has to give way to clearly defined clinical entities. The

potential of these drugs as an adjunct to other forms of therapy can be very significant. In the meantime, however, the often loose and sometimes promiscuous administration of these potentially dangerous drugs has to be deplored.

Epilogue

Despite the changing attitude in the last thirty years, there is still a lot of scepticism in professional circles about the existence of a clinical entity which may appropriately be called "childhood depression." Some of this scepticism is related to the diverse and manifold phenomena, subsumed under this heading by various investigators. It is, of course, a legitimate concern that such diversity may preclude the precise delineation of the concept and invite the danger of using the diagnosis of childhood depression loosely as a clinical waste basket, another variety of "the atypical child." The authors fully agree and suggest that it is necessary to continue to clarify the thinking about the various facets of childhood depression, such as its etiology, course, outcome, response to treatment and, above all, how it differs from other more traditional childhood diagnoses. The efforts of our research group, and those of others, have made some progress in this direction; obviously, however, much more basic research and conceptualization are needed. On the other hand, is it correct to disregard a clinical phenomenon, simply because one does not fully understand it? Such an attitude would be inconsistent with the medical history of most diseases, physical or psychiatric. They were often observed, described, and treated, long before all their aspects became well understood.

Finally, only future research will clarify the controversial issue of the relationship between adult and childhood depression. There are several possibilities.

1. Both adult and childhood depression are part of a limited spectrum of depressive disorders, the expression and the incidence of which are dependent on the given level of personality development.

2. Childhood depression leads to or predisposes toward depression in later life.

3. Despite clinical similarities, childhood and adult depressions, because of their disparity in etiology and course, can best be thought of as representing separate, independent entities.

REFERENCES

1. ABRAHAM, K., "The First Pregenital Stage of the Libido," in Abraham, K., *Selected Papers on Psychoanalysis*, pp. 248–279, Hogarth Press and The Institute of Psychoanalysis, London, 1927.

2. ———, "Notes on the Psychoanalytic Investigation and Treatment of Manic-Depressive Insanity and Allied Conditions," in Abraham, K., *Selected Papers on Psychoanalysis*, pp. 137–156, Hogarth Press and The Institute of Psychoanalysis, London, 1927.

3. ———, "A Short Study of the Development of the Libido, Viewed in the Light of Mental Disorders," in Abraham, K., *Selected Papers on Psychoanalysis*, pp. 418–502, Hogarth Press and The Institute of Psychoanalysis, London, 1927.

4. AJURIAGUERRA, J. D., *Manuel de Psychiatrie de L'Enfant*, Masson, Paris, 1971.

5. ANNELL, A. L. (Ed.), *Depressive States in Childhood and Adolescence*, Halsted Press, New York, 1972.

6. ———, "Lithium in the Treatment of Children and Adolescence," *Acta Psychiatrica Scandinavica, Supplement 207:*19–33, 1969.

7. ———, "Manic-Depressive Illness in Children and Effect of Treatment with Lithium Carbonate," *Acta Paedopsychiatrica, 39:*292–310, 1969.

8. ANTHONY, E. J., "Childhood Depression," in Anthony, E. J., and Benedek, T. (Eds.), *Depression and Human Existence*, Little, Brown, Boston, 1975.

9. ———, "The Influence of a Manic-Depressive Environment on the Developing Child," in Anthony, E. J., and Benedek, T. (Eds.), *Depression and Human Existence*, Little, Brown, Boston, 1975.

10. ———, "Psychoneurotic Disorders," in Freedman, A. M., and Kaplan, H. I. (Eds.), *Comprehensive Textbook of Psychiatry*, Williams & Wilkins, Baltimore, Md., 1967.

11. ———, and SCOTT, P., "Manic-Depressive Psychosis in Childhood," *Child Psychology anl Psychiatry, 1:*53–72, 1960.

12. BALINT, M., "Early Developmental States of the Ego. Primary Object Love," *International Journal of Psycho-analysis, 30:*265–273, 1949.

13. BARTON, H. M., "Our Present Knowledge About Manic-Depressive States in Childhood," *Nervous Child, 9:*319ff., 1952.

14. BECK, A. T., "Depressive Neurosis," in Arieti, S. (Ed.), *American Handbook of Psychiatry*, 2nd ed., pp. 61–98, Basic Books, New York, 1974.

15. BELLAK, L., *Manic-Depressive Psychosis and Allied Conditions*, Grune & Stratton, New York, 1952.

16. BIBRING, E., "The Development and Problems of the Theory of Instincts," *International Journal of Psychoanalysis, 22:*102–131; also *International Journal of Psychoanalysis, 50:*293–308, 1969.

17. ———, "The Mechanism of Depression," in Greenacre, P. (Ed.), *Affective Disorders*, International Universities Press, New York, 1953.

18. BIERMAN, J., SILVERSTEIN, A., and FINESINGER, J., "A Depression in a Six-Year Old Boy with Acute Poliomyelitis," in Eissler, R. S., et al. (Eds.), *The Psychoanalytic Study of the Child*, vol. 13, pp. 430–450, International Universities Press, New York, 1958.

19. BLEULER, E., *Dementia Praecox or the Group of Schizophrenias*, International Universities Press, New York, 1950.

20. BOWLBY, J., *Attachment and Loss, II: Separation*, Basic Books, New York, 1973.

21. ———, *Attachment and Loss, I: Attachment*, Basic Books, New York, 1969.

22. ———, "Pathological Mourning and Childhood Mourning," *Journal of the American Psychoanalytic Association, 11:*500–541, 1963.

23. ———, "Process of Mourning," *International Journal of Psycho-analysis, 42:*317–340, 1961b.

24. ———, "Separation Anxiety: A Critical Review of the Literature," *Journal of Child Psychology and Psychiatry, 1:*251–269, 1961a.

25. ———, "Grief and Mourning in Infancy and Early Childhood," in Eissler, R. S., et al. (Eds.), *The Psychoanalytic Study of the Child*, vol. 15, pp. 9–52, International Universities Press, New York, 1960.

26. ———, "Separation Anxiety," *International Journal of Psychoanalysis, 41:*89–113, 1960.

27. BROWN, F., "Childhood Bereavement and Subsequent Psychiatric Disorder," *British Journal of Psychiatry, 112:*1035ff., 1966.

28. CAMPBELL, J. D., "Manic-Depressive Psychosis in Children," *Journal of Nervous and Mental Disease, 166:*424–439, 1952.

29. CONNERS, C. K., "Child Psychiatry: Organic Therapies," in Freedman, A. M., Kaplan, H. I., and Sadock, B. J. (Eds.), *Comprehensive Textbook of Psychiatry II*, 2nd ed., pp. 2240–2246, Williams & Wilkins, Baltimore, Md., 1975.

30. CYTRYN, L., et al., "Biochemical Correlates of Affective Disorders," *Archives of General Psychiatry, 31:*659–661, 1974.

31. ———, and McKNEW, D. H., JR., "Factors Influencing the Changing Clinical Expression of the Depressive Process in Children," *American Journal of Psychiatry, 131:*879–881, 1974.

32. ———, "Proposed Classification of Childhood Depression," *American Journal of Psychiatry, 129:*149–155, 1972.

33. DE NEGRI, M., "Quelques Aspects des Depressions Infantiles," *Acta Paedopsychiatrica, 38:*182–190, 1971.

34. DIZMANG, L. H., "Loss, Bereavement and Depression in Childhood," *International Psychiatric Clinic, 6:*175–195, 1969.

35. DURELL, J., and SCHILDKRAUT, J. J., "Biochemical Studies of the Schizophrenic and Affective Disorders," in Arieti, S. (Ed.), *American Handbook of Psychiatry*, Basic Books, New York, 1966.

36. DYSON, W. L., and BARCAI, A., "Treatment of Children of Lithium-Responding Parents," *Current Therapeutic Research, 12:*286–290, 1970.

37. ENGEL, G. L., "Anxiety and Depression Withdrawal: The Primary Affects of Unpleasure," *International Journal of Psychoanalysis, 43:*89–97, 1962.

38. ———, and REICHSMAN, F., "Spontaneous and Experimentally Induced Depression in an Infant With Gastric Fistula," *Journal of the American Psychoanalytic Association, 4:*428–452, 1956.

39. EWALT, J. R., and FARNSWORTH, D. L., *Textbook of Psychiatry*, McGraw-Hill, New York, 1963.

40. FEINSTEIN, S. C., "Adolescent Depression," in Anthony, E. J., and Benedek, T. (Eds.), *Depression and Human Existence*, Little, Brown, Boston, 1975.

41. FISH, B., "Drug Use in Psychiatric Disorders of Children," *American Journal of Psychiatry, 124:*31–36 (Supplement), 1968.

42. FREUD, A., *Normality and Pathology in Childhood*, International Universities Press, New York, 1965.

43. FREUD, S., "An Outline of Psychoanalysis," in *The Standard Edition of the Complete Psychological Works of Sigmund Freud* (hereafter: *The Standard Edition*), vol. 23, pp. 141–207, Hogarth Press, London, 1964.

44. ———, "Instincts and Their Vicissitudes," in *The Standard Edition*, vol. 14, pp. 117–140, Hogarth Press, London, 1963.

45. ———, "Mourning and Melancholia," in *The Standard Edition*, vol. 14, pp. 243–258, Hogarth Press, London, 1957.

46. ———, "On Narcissism: An Introduction," in *The Standard Edition*, vol. 14, pp. 73–102, Hogarth Press, London, 1957.

47. FROMMER, E. A., "Depressive Illness in Childhood," in Coppen and Walk (Eds.), *Recent Developments in Affective Disorders: A Symposium*, Headley Brothers, Ashford, 1968.

48. ———, "Treatment of Childhood Depression with Antidepressant Drugs," *British Medical Journal, 1:*729–732, 1967.

49. GERSHON, E. S., DUNNER, D. L., and GOODWIN, F. K., "Toward a Biology of Affective Disorders," *Archives of General Psychiatry, 25:*1–15, 1971.

50. GILLESPIE, R. D., "The Clinical Differentiation of Types of Depression," *Guy's Hospital Reports, 79:*306–344, 1930.

51. GITTELMAN-KLEIN, R., and KLEIN, D. F., "School Phobia: Diagnostic Considerations in the Light of Imipramine Effects," in Klein, D. F., and Gittelman-Klein, R. (Eds.), *Progress in Psychiatric Drug Treatment*, Brunner-Mazel, New York, 1975.

52. GLASER, K., "Masked Depression in Children and Adolescents," *American Journal of Psychotherapy, 21:*565–574, 1967.

53. GREENBERG, L. M., and YELLIN, A. M., "Blood Pressure and Pulse Changes in Hyperactive Children Treated with Imipramine and Methylphenidate," *American Journal of Psychiatry, 132:*1325–1326, 1975.

54. GRINKER, R., SR., et al., *The Phenomenon of Depression*, Harper & Row, New York, 1961.

55. Group for the Advancement of Psychiatry, Committee on Child Psychiatry, *Psychopathological Disorders in Childhood: Theoretical Considerations and a Proposed Classification*, Report No. 62, Group for the Advancement of Psychiatry, New York, 1967.

56. JACOBS, J., *Adolescent Suicide*, John Wiley, New York, 1971.

57. JACOBSON, E., "The Depressive Personality," *International Journal of Psychiatry, 11:*218–221, 1973.

58. ———, *Depression*, International Universities Press, New York, 1971.

59. ———, *The Self and the Object World*, International Universities Press, New York, 1964.

60. ———, "On Normal and Pathological Moods," in Eissler, R. S., et al. (Eds.), *The Psychoanalytic Study of the Child*, vol. 12, pp. 73–113, International Universities Press, New York, 1957.

61. ———, "The Self and the Object World: Vicissitudes of Their Infantile Cathexes and Their Influences on Ideational and Affective Development," in Eissler, R. S., et al. (Eds.), *The Psychoanalytic Study of the Child*, vol. 9, pp. 75–127, International Universities Press, New York, 1954.

62. ———, "Contribution to the Metapsychology of Cyclothymic Depression," in Greenacre, P. (Ed.), *Affective Disorders*, International Universities Press, New York, 1953.

63. ———, "The Effect of Disappointment on Ego and Superego Formation in Normal and Depressive Development," *Psychoanalytic Review, 33:*129–147, 1946.

64. KLEIN, M., "Mourning and Its Relation to Manic-Depressive States," *International Journal of Psycho-Analysis, 21:*125–153, 1940.

65. ———, "A Contribution to the Psychogenesis of Manic-Depressive States," *International Journal of Psycho-Analysis, 29:*114–174, 1935.

66. ———, *The Psychoanalysis of Children*, Hogarth Press and The Institute of Psychoanalysis, London, 1932.

67. KLERMAN, G. L., "Clinical Research in Depression," *Archives of General Psychiatry, 24:*305–319, 1971.

68. KOHLER, C., and BERUARD, F., "Les Etats Depressifs chez L'Enfant," in Annell, A. L. (Ed.), *Depressive States in Childhood and Adolescence*, Halsted Press, New York, 1972.

69. KOVACS, M., Personal communication, 1977.

70. KRAEPELIN, E., *Psychiatrie: Ein Lehrbuch für Studierende und Artze: II. Klinische Psychiatrie*, Barth, Leipzig, 1913.

71. ———, *Clinical Psychiatry*, Macmillan, New York, 1902.

72. KUHN, R., "Über Kindliche Depressionen und Ihre Behandlung," *Schweizerische Medizinische Wochenschrift, 93:*86ff., 1963.

73. KUHN, V., and KUHN, R., "Drug Therapy for Depression in Children. Indication and Methods," in Annell, A. L. (Ed.), *Depressive States in Childhood and Adolescence*, Halsted Press, New York, 1972.

74. LEBOVICI, S., "Contribution Psychoanalytique a la Connaissance de la Depression chez L'Enfant," in Annell, A. L. (Ed.), *Depressive States in Childhood and Adolescence*, Halsted Press, New York, 1972.

75. LEHMANN, H. E., "Psychiatric Concepts of Depression: Nomenclature and Classification," *Canadian Psychiatric Association Journal, 4(Supplement):*1–12, 1959.

76. LEONHARD, K., *Aufteilung der Endogenen Psychosen*, 1st ed., Akademie Verlag, Berlin, 1957.

77. LIEBERMAN, D., "Suicide Among Adolescents," in Wolff, K. (Ed.), *Patterns of Self-Destruction: Depression and Suicide*, Charles C. Thomas, Springfield, Ill., 1970.

78. LUCAS, A. R., "Treatment of Depressive States," in Wiener, J. M. (Ed.), *Psychopharmacology in Childhood and Adolescence*, (in press).

79. ———, LOCKETT, H. J., and GRIMM, F., "Amitriptyline in Childhood Depressions," *Diseases of the Nervous System, 26:*105–110, 1965.

80. MAAS, J. W., FAWCETT, J., and DEKERMENJAN, H., "3-Methoxy-4-Hydroxy-phenylglycol (MHPG) Excretion in Depressive States," *Archives of General Psychiatry, 19:*129–134, 1968.

81. MAAS, J. W., and LANDIS, D. H., "In Vivo Studies of the Metabolism of Norepinephrine in the Central Nervous System," *Journal of Pharmacology and Experimental Therapeutics, 163:*147–161, 1968.

82. MAHLER, M. G., "Notes on the Development of Basic Moods: The Depressive Affect," in Loewenstein, R. M., et al. (Eds.), *Psychoanalysis—A General Psychology*, pp. 152–168, International Universities Press, New York, 1966.

83. ———, "On Sadness and Grief in Infancy and Childhood Loss and Restoration of the Symbiotic Love Object," in Eissler, R. S., et al. (Eds.), *The Psychoanalytic Study of the Child*, vol. 16, pp. 332–351, International Universities Press, New York, 1961.

84. ———, "Sadness and Grief in Childhood," in Eissler, R. S., et al. (Eds.), *The Psychoanalytic Study of the Child*, vol. 16, pp. 332–351, International Universities Press, New York, 1961.

85. MALMQUIST, C. P., "Depressions in Childhood and Adolescence I," *New England Journal of Medicine, 284:*887–893, 1971.

86. ———, "Depressions in Childhood and Adolescence II," *New England Journal of Medicine, 284:*955–961, 1971.

87. McHARG, J. F., "Mania in Childhood," *Archives of Neurology and Psychiatry, 72:*531–539, 1954.

88. McKNEW, D. H., JR., and CYTRYN, L., *Offspring of Patients with Affective Disorders*, Paper read at the meeting of the American Psychiatric Association, Miami, Fla., 1976.

89. ———, *Detection and Treatment of Childhood Depression*, Paper read at the meeting of the American Psychiatric Association, Anaheim, Calif., 1975.

90. ———, "Historical Background in Children with Affective Disorders," *American Journal of Psychiatry, 130:*1278–1279, 1973.

91. ———, and WHITE, I., "Clinical and Biochemical Correlates of Hypomania in a Child," *Journal of the American Academy of Child Psychiatry, 13:*576–585, 1974.

92. MEYER, A., "Construction Formulation of Schizo-

phrenia," in *The Collected Papers of Adolf Meyer, II*, Johns Hopkins Press, Baltimore, Md., 1951.

93. Moebius, P. J., *Diagnostik der Nervenkrankheiten*, Vogel-Verlag, Leipzig, 1894.

94. Nissen, G., *Das Depressive Syndrome im Kindes und Jugendalter*, Springer, Berlin, 1971.

95. Noyes, A. P., *Modern Clinical Psychiatry*, W. B. Saunders, Philadelphia, Pa., 1948.

96. Penot, B., "Contribution a L'Etude des Depressions Infantiles," *Psychiatrie de L'Enfant*, 16:301–380, 1974.

97. ———, "Caracteristiques et Devenir des Depressions de la Deuxieme Enfance," in Annell, A. L. (Ed.), *Depressive States in Childhood and Adolescence*, Halsted Press, New York, 1972.

98. Poznanski, E., and Zrull, J. P., "Childhood Depression," *Archives of General Psychiatry*, 23:8–15, 1970.

99. Puig-Antich, J., et al., "Prepubertal Major Depressive Disorder," *Journal of the American Academy of Child Psychiatry*, (in press), 1978.

100. Rado, S., "Psychodynamics of Depression from the Etiologic Point of View," *Psychosomatic Medicine*, 13:51–55, 1951.

101. ———, "The Problem of Melancholia," *International Journal of Psychoanalysis*, 9:420–438, 1928.

102. Rapoport, J. L., "Psychopharmacology of Childhood Depression," in Klein, D. F., and Gittelman-Klein, R. (Eds.), *Progress in Psychiatric Drug Treatment II*, Brunner-Mazel, New York, 1976.

103. ———, et al., "Imipramine and Methylphenidate Treatments of Hyperactive Boys," *Archives of General Psychiatry*, 30:789–793, 1974.

104. Reite, M., et al., "Depression in Infant Monkeys: Physiological Correlates," *Psychosomatic Medicine*, 36: 363–367, 1974.

105. Remschmidt, H., et al., "Kinder Endogen-Depressiven," in Fortschr. E. (Ed.), *Neurology-Psychiatry*, 41: 326–340, 1973.

106. Rie, H. E., "Depression in Childhood: A Survey of Some Pertinent Contributions," *Journal of the American Academy of Chi.d Psychiatry*, 5:653–685, 1966.

107. Rochlin, G., "The Loss Complex," *Journal of the American Psychoanalytic Association*, 7:299–316, 1959.

108. Rosenthal, S. H., and Gudeman, J. E., "The Endogenous Depressive Pattern," *Archives of General Psychiatry*, 16:241–249, 1967.

109. Sandler, J., "The Background of Safety," *International Journal of Psychoanalysis*, 41:352–356, 1960a.

110. ———, and Joffe, W. G., "Notes on Childhood Depression," *International Journal of Psychoanalysis*, 46:88–96, 1965.

111. Sandler, J., Holder, A., and Meers, D., "The Ego Ideal and the Ideal Self," in Eissler, R. S., et al. (Eds.), *The Psychoanalytic Study of the Child*, vol. 18, pp. 139–158, International Universities Press, New York, 1963.

112. Schachter, M., "Etude des Depressions et des Episodes Depressifs chez L'Enfant et L'Aolescent," *Acta Paedopyschiatrica*, 38:191–201, 1971.

113. ———, "The Cyclothymic States in the Prepubescent Child," *Nervous Child*, 9:357–362, 1952.

114. Schildkraut, J. J., "Biogenic Amine Metabolism in Depressive Illness," in Williams, T. A., Katz, M. M., and Shield, J. A. (Eds.), *Recent Advances of the Psychobiology of the Depressive Illness*, Department of Health, Education and Welfare, Washington, D.C., 1972.

115. ———, *Neuropsychopharmacology and the Affective Disorders*, Little, Brown, Boston, 1970.

116. Schou, M., "Lithium in Psychiatric Therapy and Prophylaxis," in Annell, A. L. (Ed.), *Depressive States in Childhood and Adolescence*, Halsted Press, New York, 1972.

117. Seiden, R. H., *Suicide Among Youth: A Review of the Literature 1900–1967*, Public Health Service Publica-tion No. 1971, U.S. Government Printing Office, Washington, D.C., 1969.

118. Shaw, C. R., and Lucas, A. R., "Psychoneurosis," in Shaw, C. R., and Lucas, A. R. (Eds), *The Psychiatric Disorders of Childhood*, 2nd ed., Appleton-Century-Crofts, New York, 1970.

119. Shneidman, E. S., "Suicide," in Freedman, A. M., Kaplan, H. I., and Saddock, B. J. (Eds.), *Comprehensive Textbook of Psychiatry*, 2nd ed., Williams & Wilkins, Baltimore, 1975.

120. Soblen, R., and Saunders, J. C., "Monamino Oxidase Inhibitor Therapy in Adolescent Psychiatry," *Diseases of the Nervous System*, 2:96–100, 1961.

121. Spiel, W. A., "Studien uber den Verlauf und die Erscheinungsformen der Kindlichen and Juvenilen Manisch Depressive Psychosis," in Annell, A. L. (Ed.), *Depressive States in Childhood and Adolescence*, Halsted Press, New York, 1972.

122. Spiel, W., *Die Endogenen Psychosen des Kindes und Jugendalters*, S. Karger, New York, 1961.

123. Spitz, R. A., "Anaclitic Depression: An Inquiry into the Genesis of Psychiatric Conditions in Early Childhood, II," in Eissler, R. S., et al. (Eds.), *The Psychoanalytic Study of the Child*, vol. 2, pp. 312–342, International Universities Press, New York, 1946.

124. ———, "Hospitalism: An Inquiry into the Genesis of Psychiatric Conditions in Early Childhood, I," in Eissler, R. S., et al. (Eds.), *The Psychoanalytic Study of the Child*, vol. 1, pp. 53–74, International Universities Press, New York, 1945.

125. Strauss, E. G., *Proceedings of the Royal Society of Medicine*, 23:894–895, 1930.

126. Stutte, H., "Psychosen des Kindesalers," in Opitz, H., and Schmid, F. (Eds.), *Handbuch der Kinderheilkunde*, Springer, Berlin, 1969.

127. ———, "Kinderpsychiatrie und Jugendpsychiatrie," in Gruhle, H. W., et al. (Eds.), *Psychiatrie der Gegenwart*, Springer, Berlin, 1960.

128. Toolan, J. M., "Suicide in Childhood and Adolescence," in Resnick, H. L. P. (Ed.), *Suicidal Behaviors: Diagnosis and Management*, Little, Brown, Boston, 1968.

129. ———, "Depression in Children and Adolescents," *American Journal of Orthopsychiatry*, 32:404–415, 1962.

130. Ulf, O., "Suicidal Attempts in Childhood and Adolescence—A Follow-up Study," in Annell, A. L. (Ed.), *Depressive States in Childhood and Adolescence*, Halsted Press, New York, 1972.

131. Van Krevelen, A. A., "La Mania Fantastique des Enfants," *Revue de Neuropsychiatric Infantile*, 10:133–138, 1962.

132. Van Krevelen, D. A., "Zyklothymien in Kindesalter," *Acta Paedopsychiatrica*, 38:202–210, 1961.

133. Winokur, G., "Heredity in the Affective Disorders," in Anthony, E. J., and Benedek, T. (Eds.), *Depression and Human Existence*, Little, Brown, Boston, 1975.

134. ———, "Depression Spectrum Disease: Description and Family Study," *Comprehensive Psychiatry*, 13:3–8, 1972.

135. ———, and Clayton, P., "Family History Studies: I. Two Types of Affective Disorders Separated According to Genetic and Clinical Factors," in Wortis, J. (Ed.), *Recent Advances in Biological Psychiatry*, vol. 9, Plenum Press, New York, 1967.

136. Winokur, G., and Pitts, F. N., Jr., "Affective Disorder: V. The Diagnostic Validity of Depressive Reactions," *Psychiatric Quarterly*, 39:727–728, 1965.

137. ———, "Affective Disorder: I. Is Reactive Depression an Entity?" *Journal of Nervous and Mental Disorders*, 138:541–547, 1964.

138. Wolfenstein, M., "How is Mourning Possible?" in Eissler, R. S., et al. (Eds.), *The Psychoanalytic Study of the Child*, vol. 21, pp. 93–123, International Universities Press, New York, 1966.

17 / Psychophysiologic Disorders

James G. Kavanaugh, Jr., and Åke Mattsson

Psychophysiologic Disorders in Childhood

This chapter will focus on the psychophysiologic disorders of childhood. In general, the current DSM-II classification and the suggested 1966 GAP classification of psychophysiologic disorders will be followed.[11, 63] The authors adhere to the psychosomatic viewpoint; this stipulates that in any evaluation and treatment planning for a physically ill child a biopsychosocial approach should be used. However, there are some diseases of childhood in which psychogenic mechanisms are major etiologic factors justifying the diagnosis of psychophysiologic disorder.

In the ordering of the material there is an initial brief review of the evolving concepts of psychophysiologic mechanisms as they pertain to childhood illness. This is followed by a selected presentation of the common entities of childhood psychophysiologic illness. Finally, a review of the principles of therapeutic management will stress the involvement of the child psychiatrist as an integral part of the health care team attending the child with such a disorder.

Early Theories of Disease

One might anticipate that a retrospective view of medical practice would disclose more diversity than order. If, however, one takes a close look at the ways in which man has coped with disease over time, certain basic issues emerge. These have persisted since prehistory. Some of these issues, such as the respective roles of healer and patient, are specific to the treatment situation; others involve more general considerations. These would include how people living in past epochs and different parts of the world conceptualized the workings of the universe; to what belief systems they gave allegiance; and what goals they sought.

One perennial question concerns the source of illness or dysfunction. When a man falls ill, is he the victim of a malign spirit? Or has his previously healthy body undergone sudden attack by some organism or agent? Is there something in his personality or behavior that may be implicated? Even the ability to articulate such questions and to attempt answers tells much about any period or culture. More than that, the manner of dealing with such considerations determines in a number of practical ways how, where, when, and by whom the sick are treated.

The idea that the "whole man" influences the health or disease of his body is not new. Indeed, it is expressed in early Greek medicine, the chief exponent of which, Hippocrates, is credited with saying: "The man who has the disease is as important as the disease the man has." Parallel with and complementary to this holistic notion, however, is one asserting that disease is altogether the consequence of malfunction or impairment of some specific body organ or system.

The modern schools of cellular pathology and infectious disease control have achieved many extraordinary successes. These have contributed significantly to the emergence of modern concepts of psychosomatic medicine. As the epidemics and scourges man had suffered throughout history were brought under control, medicine found itself faced, not with the millennium that had been confidently expected but with a new set of problems. The body is obviously vulnerable to invading organisms and deficits over which it has no control. But it has become clear that emotions too can be an agent of sickness.

Bodily Regulation

As the human body evolved, it became an organism of ever greater complexity and specialization. Of necessity, the degree of unconscious internal regulation necessary for the operation of all of its diverse parts and systems increased, and susceptibility to malfunction was correspondingly heightened. This whole is greater than the sum of its parts; the personality or "self," perceiving, knowing, and willing, crowns the assembly of bodily systems. This hierarchical ordering of functions exists in the living human being. This state of affairs is, in fact, the source of the current difficulties in pinpointing the moment of death. There is growing acceptance of the notion that "life" is more than specific organ systems functioning adequately. It is difficult to accept anyone as still living if he has lost self-awareness and any capacity, however slight, for voluntary action. A generally acceptable definition of the point at which life passes into death has yet to emerge. There are many tentative solutions which weigh the degree and quality of central nervous system functioning. Although the basic question may readily be put into words, it continues to elude any easy or simple solution.

Many highly important bodily functions do not require constant conscious monitoring; under ordinary conditions, they are best left to an almost automatic, low-level control. In the absence of conscious monitoring, however, a change in one set of physiological variables can become the cue to activate another; ultimately the response may take place in the central nervous system at a higher functional level.

The Mind-Body Problem

What has come to be identified as *the mind-body problem* was given its most definitive statement by the French philosopher and mathematician Descartes. His seventeenth century writings conveyed to posterity what has since been known as the theory of Cartesian dualism. His theory was an attempt to deal with the fact that the universe contains both matter, the so-called *res extensa*, and mind, the *res cogitans*. It was easy to accept that matter is subject to forces such as the law of gravity, and that it occupies space. It was, however, impossible to remain unaware of a coexistent mental entity expressed in emotions, feelings, and motives. This was perceived as being quite separate from matter proper and different in properties and function. The interaction of these two entities was hard to understand, and traditional philosophic attempts to explain it produced three different theories: that of psychophysical parallelism; of interactions; and of identities.

The theory of psychophysical parallelism speaks for the simultaneous occurrence of two separate trains of events that have no demonstrable interaction with one another. This theory is unwilling to acknowledge that what goes on in the mental realm can have any consequences in the physical universe. It is, indeed, able to explain how physical events come about without making any reference whatever to a mental realm or even tacitly acknowledging its existence.

The theory of interactions accepts the occasional influential intrusion of mind into matter, and the reciprocal possibility that matter enters mind; but it offers no clear-cut explanation of *how* the former, more difficult, invasion comes about. Thus, it remains more descriptive than explanatory.

The theory of identities grants that reality includes not only mental and physical events taken separately, but their reactive product as well. This view, however, considers only the kind of mental activity that takes place in conscious awareness. So much of what happens in the physical universe is altogether exterior to and unperceived by the mind of man, and much of what does go on in the mind is outside of conscious awareness. The failure of this theory to take unconscious mental processes into account causes it to create more problems than it solves. Such an explanation is made all the more difficult by its beginning with Cartesian dualism and attempting solution in Cartesian terms.

There are other more fruitful possibilities. Certainly, the data currently available offer more explanations of biological function than were known to seventeenth century science; that era was, in any case, uncritical of mechanistic views. God was regarded as the great artificer according to whose design all events in the universe proceeded in linear fashion from a known cause to a predictable result. This led to the view of man as an object—complicated, to be sure, but still an object moved by forces outside himself along a predetermined path. Ludwig von Bertalanffy[21] gives a thoughtful and thought-provoking review of the impact new data have had on this old problem. Among the important newly available insights is an increased understanding of how the individual develops his perceptions of himself and his surrounding world.

There are stages in the way an infant becomes aware of the distinction between himself and the world around him. In the beginning, the child experiences sensation without any clear distinction between the self and others; only gradually, and by trial and error, do external representations take on meaning and stability. Indeed, one of the most devastating of all developmental disabilities is that of the autistic child. Such a youngster is unable to construct a world peopled by others in which he can recognize beings outside himself and interact with them. This tragic condition only emphasizes the usual and predictable course of growth. Usually, the child becomes increasingly aware of his own physical separateness from others and is then able to identify the feelings he entertains toward events that take place in his surroundings.

However these processes are defined, it is clear that during his early years, the infant makes those vital first steps in the direction that will ultimately lead him to be a differentiated human adult. Only as the ability to observe and to measure human behavior increased was it possible to appreciate properly the complex problems the infant faces and solves. Heretofore it has been all too easy to view this helpless, inarticulate, and weak being as a dormant organism, one who slept most of his days away and who interacted little with his surroundings. The difficulty was not that the infant was an unpromising subject for study; rather, as in so many kinds of investigation, the methods chosen for his study were inappropriate. Before they considered the problems of infancy and childhood unusual enough to merit a special discipline of pediatrics, medical men had systematized the study and treatment of adult patients. As a result, the theoretical concepts of medicine were based largely on what was seen in the adult patient. It was some time before prevailing theories were adapted to recognizing the needs of the young patient. In the interim, he was often as poorly served by hand-me-down theories based on the situation of his elders as he would have been wearing their cast-off and over-sized clothing.

Psychosomatic Theorists

The basic data from which current concepts of psychophysiologic disorders derive, came, appropriately, from physiologic research. The Greeks explained dysfunction by hypothesizing a system of bodily fluids/humors; these accounted for personality differences by the relative proportions of each in any given individual. Their terminology has largely passed from the medical to the lay vocabulary. However, the persistence of the term "melancholic" in psychiatric descriptive nomenclature, as well as the evocative literary use of *choleric, phlegmatic*, and *sanguine*, indicate a kind of universality in the early descriptions, a quality

that lends them broad and general usefulness. Nevertheless, even the most astute and descriptive clinical observation falls short of the mark. The achievement of further advance awaited the results of the scientific, anatomic, and functional studies begun in the Renaissance. The limitations of even careful early anatomic research are indicated by the relatively late discovery of the circulation of the blood. This was not made by Harvey until the early seventeenth century.

The understanding of physiology and cellular pathology grew along with specialized examination of organs and organ system functions. Unfortunately the data continued to be based on an intellectual dissection of a whole functioning individual into various component subsystems. As a result therapeutic insights derived from that knowledge contributed little to the development of psychosomatic theory.

Claude Bernard[19] achieved something approaching the necessary synthesis with his elaboration of the theory of the *milieu internal*, which began to adumbrate an understanding of integrated body functioning. It is tempting to focus exclusively on one or another of the many bypaths that were identified; this would certainly provide a more detailed view of cardiovascular, renal, or hepatic functioning. Such a limited focus, however, would tend to neglect the simultaneous functioning of all of the other systems that run parallel with one another.

The work of Walter Cannon,[29] particularly his studies on bodily changes in fear, rage, and hunger, had greater immediate applicability to psychosomatic theory. This was reinforced by the success of his laboratory investigations. In his studies of states of emotional arousal, he was able to demonstrate their changing and measurable physiologic parameters. Work such as his animal studies made it clear that these principles of physiologic response are not unique to man; they operate throughout the natural world.

Such advances in psychophysiological research made possible ever greater precision in the investigation and reporting of physical phenomena. At the same time, psychiatric thought was progressing rapidly. Sigmund Freud had furthered his medical training with special studies in neurology with Charcot in France. He thus had an early interest in the interaction of emotional states and bodily function. His initial case reports[22] were studies of such interactions. Given the knowledge and the perspective of his times, it was not an easy matter to apply psychiatric theory to the differentiation of hysterical or conversion symptoms from disorders that were still considered organic conditions. Alfred Adler[1] contributed the concept of a constitutional type of organ inferiority that would predispose to a particular symptom picture. Felix Deutsch,[36] another Freudian theorist, suggested that previously diseased organs might be particularly susceptible to subsequent dysfunction under stress. As the Freudian position elaborated, physical symptoms appearing in organs innervated by the autonomic nervous system were given special attention. Deutsch[35] was among those who viewed these disturbances as symbolic manifestations.

It remained for Franz Alexander[7, 8] to present a basic theoretical position in regard to the effects of emotion on body functioning. His widely accepted theory made it possible to classify the somatic accompaniments of psychic disturbance into two categories.

The first, that of hysterical or conversion neurosis, was limited to disorders in which cortically controlled body structures, i.e., striated musculature, were affected. In these cases, the attendant defects had demonstrable symbolic meaning. Moreover, in the usual case, no structural damage occurs to the involved body part. For example, the impaired limb of a patient with hysterical paralysis is capable of its usual functions once the hysterical condition is relieved.

The second category included a group of physical conditions which Alexander termed psychosomatic. In these, the affected organ or system was innervated primarily by the autonomic nervous system. In these instances, however, the dysfunction was without symbolic meaning for the patient, it could lead to permanent structural alteration or damage, and it could even be fatal.

The contrast between these two categories is heightened by the usual failure of hysterical conversion symptoms to parallel any recognizable disease state. Since they are symbolic, they represent a bodily solution to an emotional problem unique to the individual patient. Here symptom formation relates more closely to the individual's problem and its solution than to any normal anatomic or physiologic correlation with the symptoms. On the other hand, prolonged emotional stress leads to disturbances which are expressed through symptoms. These take the form of exaggerations or inhibitions of normal functioning of organs regulated by the autonomic nervous system. For example, gastric hyperacidity represents overproduction of gastric acid, the excessive activation of a function normal to the gastric mucosa. What is etiologically unique about psychophysiologic

disorders is not their symptom picture (there are only limited forms of either normal or abnormal function possible for any given organ system) but the contribution of the patient's emotional state. This allows for new mechanisms that can be held theoretically accountable for the activation of target organs.

Flanders Dunbar devoted a productive and busy career to the study of psychosomatic disease and phenomena. Her contributions range from an early and exhaustive review of the extant literature[42] to the development of personality profiles by which the constellation of genetic factors, personality, and life experience thought to lead to specific diseases could be identified.[41] Her anamnestic studies suggested a high correlation between these theoretical constructs and the actual presence of the predicted organic disease. Other investigators, such as Grinker,[61] have been unable to reproduce such high statistical correlation and have not found these specific profiles to be helpful.

Autonomic Nervous System

In all theoretical thinking about psychophysiologic functions, the autonomic nervous system has played a prominent role. This is true for its anatomic and functional aspects, the role of neurotransmitters, and some recent work on learning theory where the effort is directed to modifying its regulatory functions.

Increased understanding of the structure of the autonomic nervous system has clarified the afferent and efferent innervation of body viscera and glands. This stands in striking opposition to the structure and functioning of the voluntary striated body musculature. Russian clinicians and investigators prefer the term "cortico-visceral," to the more common Western descriptive term of psychosomatic.

Beyond a difference in the end-organs of the voluntary and autonomic nervous systems, they differ in structural arrangement as well. The most striking functional differentiations of these subsystems were indicated by the names *autonomic* as opposed to *voluntary*. Cannon[30] was the investigator initially responsible for clarifying the specialization of function of the autonomic nervous system. Two subdivisions emerged which came to be called the *sympathetic* and the *parasympathetic*. The latter division is formed by the cranio-sacral roots as opposed to the thoraco-lumbar origins of the sympathetic nervous system. Cannon's early work emphasized that the coordinated functioning of the sympathetic portion of the autonomic nervous system is arousal for immediate and violent physical activity, or, as he characterized it, a reaction of "fight or flight." Such responses require heightened body activity, e.g., an increase in peripheral blood flow. These are opposed to functions used by an organism in a resting, restoring, and digesting phase. These latter functions belong to the parasympathetic division of the autonomic nervous system. Recognition of this divided function led to a heuristic but somewhat simplistic view of such dual innervation of most body viscera and glands. It was regarded as a balanced but oppositional set of controls. While this view is not true in all particulars, it is accurate enough to make such a concept useful as a first approximation.

Of greater importance for the constructs of psychosomatic theory is the existence of a general regulating neural network throughout the body. As is often the case, the increasing sophistication of the questions asked and the investigative techniques applied have greatly expanded the earlier views of the self-regulative character of the autonomic nervous system.

The degree of reciprocal interaction between hypothalamic and pituitary centers on the one hand, and the voluntary and autonomic nervous system on the other, adds to the complexity of this situation.

DISEASES OF THE ANTONOMIC NERVOUS SYSTEM

With increased knowledge about the anatomy and physiology of the body, symptom complexes were related to specific sites and to types of dysfunction. Allbutt[9] reported on fifteen cases of severe enteralgia for which he suggested the diagnosis of *visceral neurosis*. None of these patients, eight men and seven women, showed evidence of irritation of the bowel, constipation, lead poisoning, reflex changes, or other organic problems. Thus, Allbutt related the extremely debilitating and disruptive complaints to the personality types of his patients, and to their life situations. In each case, these were characterized by "cares and sorrows," making it difficult to bring about any improvement.

In 1909 Eppinger postulated that a relative imbalance between parasympathetic and sympathetic innervation of the visceral organs might account for such dysfunctions.[48] Clinical cases were classified as vagotonic or sympatheticotonic, according to the reaction of parasympathetic or sympathetic

nerves. This altered activity could be limited to a portion of the autonomic nervous system, or could involve the whole. It was further recognized that an increased circulation of stimulating substances rather than the exclusive response of nerves might account for the high reactive level demonstrated.

Familial Dysautonomia

Acute clinical observation coupled with a knowledge of normal body function is often a primary factor in advancing medical knowledge. It recognizes that some deviation, slight in itself, can be caused by significant but hitherto unsuspected pathophysiology. This was the case with the syndrome first described by Riley[132] as "central autonomic dysfunction with defective lacrimation." This report identified five children who cried without tears; in addition, they reacted to even mild anxiety with extreme transient elevations of blood pressure, excessive sweating, and hypersalivation. Their skin also blotched symmetrically and bilaterally; this pattern tended to recur in the same configurations. As additional cases were reported, diagnostic criteria were sharpened and the clinical picture was broadened. By 1966 Riley[131] was able to add that abnormal responses to norepinephrine infusion, including tachycardia and a sharp rise in systolic blood pressure, had been seen in patients with familial dysautonomia but not in normal controls. Many of those suffering from the disorder lack fungiform papillae on the tongue; there is no agreement as to whether this is a *sine qua non* for the diagnosis, but normal papillae contraindicate it. Geltzer[59] reported a nonfamilial case diagnosed in a day old neonate. There is yet no generally accepted etiology for the diverse abnormal findings. However, it has been established that familial dysautonomy is of autosomal recessive nature, predominantly found among Jewish people. Siggers[143] noted a highly significant increase in the serum antigen levels of the Beta nerve-growth factor. The question remains as to whether this abnormality is etiological or of secondary importance. Furthermore, in reviewing these findings, Levi-Montalcini[89] is unable to establish their significance.

The thirty-year history of familial dysautonomy would be fascinating if it showed no more than the progress of knowledge about its nature. The astute observation of a few infants crying in an unusual way led to the further observation of accompanying transient hypertension and manifestations on the skin; this in turn led to the discovery of abnormal physiologic responses to specific chemicals. Further, the serum of these patients is beginning to reveal some abnormal components when advanced micro-assay techniques are applied. Such a sequence should remind the field that to an acute clinician, the patient himself has much to disclose. This is true however remote from the patient some of the investigation may be and however refined some of the analysis. The key to understanding the patient's disease itself may come from the laboratory, but the disease itself must still be dealt with by the child and his family.

Because of the variety of disruptions it causes, this genetic disease forces the professional to consider the subtly interrelated complexity of harmonious responses that accompany the normal functioning of the autonomic nervous system. This system responds to its own normal feedback control systems and to the disruptions of such disease states as familial dysautonomia. More than that, its functioning can be altered in other ways as well. These include suggestion, hypnosis, biofeedback, and yoga.

A number of experiments reported by Fenz[50] demonstrate that what an individual perceives can alter his autonomic functioning. The subjects of one study were amateur parachutists presented with word lists and pictures carefully graded in respect to their connection with jumping from airplanes. Their responses were correlated with the evocative character of the stimuli. Respiratory pattern, heart rate, and galvanic skin response were recorded during the testing session, practice periods, and in the prejump period of flight. Novices and experienced jumpers were grouped separately, and the tests were repeated at intervals from weeks before the actual jump up to the moment of jumping. The novices reacted strongly to all stimuli symbolic of jumping, while the experienced jumpers showed less reactivity. As one might expect, in-flight testing showed that the respiration, heart rates, and galvanic skin responses of the novices increased as the moment for jumping approached, peaking just before jump-off. Although experienced jumpers registered high values at take-off, these tapered off, and, by the time of the jump, they nearly reached baseline.

Such an experiment demonstrates certain physiological responses to a situation of real danger. It also reveals the reduction of fear as technical mastery is achieved. An exercise such as this allows repeated measurements and is conducted on an established time-table. Such studies demonstrate the impact of mental processes on autonomic functioning; they are applicable to a variety of stressful situations.

The word lists and stimulus pictures used in Fenz's experiments were not in themselves dangerous, as the subjects were certainly cognitively aware. Nevertheless, the meanings attached to these stimuli reflected a threatening future event, and it was this perception that evoked responses in subjects facing the actual event. These physiological variations can be quantified by means of controlled stimuli and measured responses; they indicate that an event perceived as dangerous can produce end-organ responses mediated by the autonomic nervous system. Similar responses are evoked by frightening perceptions that are imagined, dreamed, or hallucinated. Although all the sequential mechanisms involved are not known, it is clear that a high level of response may be evoked from the autonomic nervous system by events that are purely mental.

Yoga

The tenets of Indian yoga are supported by tradition and folk belief. It offers the oldest still practiced type of voluntary control over what are normally involuntarily operated body functions. Through mental discipline, exercise, and conscious control of breathing, practitioners of yoga claim to lower their body temperature and substantially reduce oxygen intake. Some report an ability to "stop" their heart function. This latter claim has been most carefully investigated[155, 156] in studies that confirmed that breath-holding and raised intra-abdominal pressure retarded venous return to the heart. According to EKG tracings the heart did not actually stop, although cardiac and radial pulse sounds were greatly reduced. In agreement with other investigators, Wenger[155] feels that many yogis developed a striking ability to control their autonomic nervous system and thus modify their body responses. Although the means may not be clear, the phenomena deserve further investigation.

Hypnosis

In the late eighteenth century, Mesmer demonstrated the variety of responses that could be induced in a subject during hypnotic trance. Since that time, hypnosis has offered the experimenter a unique possibility for influencing bodily functioning. Proponents of this controversial activity maintain that through hypnosis physiologic changes can be achieved that are beyond the subject's ability to effect by himself. Its opponents challenge this; they point to the lack of controls in many of the reported cases and assert that the responses might have been brought about by direct suggestion without the necessity of placing the subject in a hypnotic state. Paul[116] presented a careful and critical review of relevant case reports; he pointed to the appearance of blisters due to hypnotic suggestion alone. Of the twenty-one reports he examined, he felt that in terms of methodology, procedure, and controls, only fourteen offered proof of hypnotic effect that could be considered satisfactory. The doubtful cases were examined further. With the closest scrutiny given to any possibility of mechanical injury, self-mutilation, unusual skin sensitivity, or atopic dermatitis, three of these could still be classified as definite skin anomalies that were apparently produced by suggestion.

Barber[15] surveyed an area that is as broad as the focus on specific skin lesion is narrow. He presented a critical review of those studies which reported the relief from pain through hypnosis. At best, the perception and reporting of pain are a complex matter. They are specially so in a social experiential setting. Nonetheless, Barber felt that in some instances, pain relief suggested in a hypnotic trance leads to a reduction in the usual physiologic concomitants of noxious stimuli. This was evident in a reduction in the need for pain-relieving medication. In some cases, however, it would seem that the subject either denied his pain or was reluctant to report it to the hypnotist. Some reports compare the effect of having the subjects imagine pleasant experiences while experiencing noxious stimuli. The outcome was altogether favorable, with effects equal to hypnotically suggested analgesia.

McLean[97] reported on the use of hypnotic techniques as the specific treatment for some psychophysiological disorders. In work with young patients suffering from early-onset asthma, he was able to bring about an immediate marked improvement by using direct suggestion under hypnosis. In most instances, the improvement lasted for many years. Similar treatment of several patients with skin disease showed equally long-lasting results; on the other hand, some cases of congenital skin disorder failed to respond. McLean also reported temporary remission in two cases of ulcerative colitis. He cautioned against the use of hypnotic techniques in this disorder, since occasionally they bring about emotional responses that may result in a rapid exacerbation of symptoms.

Under various sets of circumstances, hypnosis reportedy produces alterations of tissue, influences general physiologic responses such as pain, and improves the course of some chronic psychophysiologic disease states. Although the autonomic nervous system is clearly involved in this process, higher cognitive, affective, and symbolic functions, are also involved.

Biofeedback

In nature, the use of feedback to control the functioning of organ systems is common enough. The clinician who would assess the effect of lowered red cell volume on bone marrow makes a reticulocyte count; when he does this, he is merely collecting information relating to an activated biologic control loop. Similar principles govern the design of sophisticated machines where continuous regulation is provided by analysis of performance data. Wiener[158] coined the most widely used term for this field, cybernetics, and his work provides much of the theoretical background.

Biofeedback refers to the control mechanisms that appear in biologic systems. More specifically, it is used to denote the communication of information to the organism about its physiologic activity, information that normally is transferred outside its conscious awareness. In the study of the possibilities of such communication, laboratory work with animals parallels work with man. Work with animals is more rigorously controlled than is possible with man. Reward systems can be employed that are suitable only for animal subjects, such as the implantation of brain electrodes for self-administered electric stimulation, and the withholding of water until thirst dictates performance. Nevertheless, the yield of some animal work is transferable to human subjects and reveals much about the specific functioning of such structures as the autonomic nervous system. Miller,[37] whose findings have been largely substantiated by other experimenters, is generally recognized as a pioneer in this new field. One of his most striking discoveries is that animals can be "taught" to control physiologic responses assumed to be outside conscious awareness, e.g., changes in blood pressure, heart rate, and urine production. A growing body of such work has demonstrated not only that "teaching" can be done in a general way, but that it can achieve an unanticipated specificity in autonomic response. In the most astonishing experiment, a rat increases the blood flow to one of his ears while at the same time the blood flow in the other remains unaffected. It had long been thought that operant conditioning was more or less exclusively applicable to activity of the striated muscles. Such work has now made it quite clear that these techniques can be applied to the functioning of the autonomic nervous ssytem. Evidently, an animal has the ability to alter bodily functions beyond its immediate awareness as the result of sensory input and rewards related to physiologic change. This presents challenging new considerations to the clinician who deals with human disease and malfunction.

It was but a short step from the animal laboratory to the design of procedures by which a human could consciously participate in changing a specific variable toward a therapeutic goal. Such functions as the alteration of blood pressure and heart rate, the reduction of muscular tension, and the aborting of a potential seizure have been effected through the use of suitable instrumentation. The *sine qua non* for such results is some method of making the subject ongoingly aware of any change that takes place within one of those variable body systems that is ordinarily beyond conscious control. Notification may be given to the subject by visual, auditory, or tactile cues from a monitoring instrument. Their increasing popularity is evident in the coverage given this subject in the popular press and by the advertising of such devices as those that measure the brain's alpha wave activity. To date such methods have had limited therapeutic success. In any case, they offer no panacea, and obviously they might easily be oversold or misapplied.

The theories of such researchers as Miller are not notable for any demonstrated general clinical efficacy. They do provide striking and persuasive evidence that visceral physiologic functions, whether mediated by the autonomic nervous system or influenced by the higher central nervous system, can be modified to bring immediate (and in some cases, lasting) change to end-organ response.

Neurotransmitters

The highly sensitive measurement techniques now available have made possible increasing precision in the study of the functioning of the autonomic nervous system. A review by Knowles[84] of the modern discoveries about neurosecretion goes back no further than two decades. In his summary of the current thought about neurotransmitters, Axelrod[14] indicates that each new discovery raises further questions and suggests additional research.

Current work on neurotransmitters is by no means limited to the study of catecholamines (see Lefkowitz[82] for data about the function of dopaminergic mechanisms as a third type of adrenergic response). At the same time, the greatest amount of research data concerns the catecholamines, norepinephrine, and epinephrine. Their widespread physiologic effects throughout the body have long been recognized; in emergency responses to flight-or-fight situations, epinephrine functions by stimulating the heart, mobilizing glucose, and dilating the arterioles of skeletal muscles; norepinephrine on the other hand exerts more marked effects on vascular functioning by dilating coronary vessels and effecting general vasoconstriction throughout the body with resultant increase in both systolic and diastolic blood pressure. The increasing recognition of the sites of action of these substances and their modes of action underlies the development of some of the most effective pharmacologic agents. These deal not only with such conditions as hypo- and hypertension, but, even more specifically, with such a primary emotional disorder as depression.

Pheochromocytoma offers a disease model in which abnormally high production of naturally occurring bodily neurotransmitters can cause a diversified and fluctuating symptom picture in which the symptom complex can be related to the varying proportions of epinephrine and norepinephrine being produced.

Many studies report on the measurement of catecholamine levels in plasma as well as in urine; the latter can also be assayed for urinary metabolites. The range of normal measurements, as well as their diurnal variations, have been established by studies in normal situations and in situations of contrived as well as naturally occurring stress.

Frankenhaeuser[52] has reviewed the current status of studies relating catecholamine excretion in children to their behavior. The data on epinephrine, besides being more consistent than those for norepinephrine, indicate its importance in the successful coping behaviors of healthy children. Besides its traditional effectiveness in facilitating flight-or-fight reactions, it helps them face psychosocial stress and intellectual challenges. What specific mechanisms operate to bring about epinephrine effects within the central nervous system remain obscure.

Psychosomatic versus

Psychophysiological

Diagnostic manuals have always distinguished between these two terms; nevertheless, they are sometimes used in an overlapping and potentially confusing way. In the *Diagnostic and Statistical Manual I*[10] the section on "Psychophysiologic autonomic and visceral disorders" opened with the explanation: "This term is used in preference to 'psychosomatic disorders,' since the latter term refers to a point of view on the discipline of medicine as a whole rather than a certain specified condition. It is preferred to the term 'somatization reactions,' which term implies that these disorders are simply another form of psychoneurotic reactions." In order to encourage more accurate gathering of data concerning their etiology, course, and relationship to other mental disorders, the disorders in question were grouped separately as neither *psychotic* nor *psychoneurotic* reactions. Such grouping permits the useful differentiation of those identifiable disease states due primarily to emotional disturbance from those in which biosocial and psychosocial factors contribute significantly without being the specific and only cause. The general heading "Psychophysiologic disorders" was employed in both the 1968 DSM II and the 1966 GAP Manual.

The larger area of *psychosomatic* medicine continues to be the topic of much research activity; it encompasses much that contributes toward greater understanding of the pathogenesis and therapeutic management of specifically psychophysiologic disorders. It is inevitable that every person's past experiences and future expectations determine to some extent his awareness of and reaction to his specific illness or disability. Thus, all diseases are in a very real sense psychosomatic events. This concept was emphasized by Alexander,[6] who pointed out the fundamental difference in the response to trouble on the part of a complicated machine and of a self-aware human being: although a machine could be programmed to register "awareness" of its running out of fuel, there is no possibility of its being designed to "care" about the event or to "worry" about its consequences.

Psychosomatic theory can be viewed as that area of medicine in which the mind/body controversy is argued. It is, however, well to remember that the term psychosomatic has been widely used for a long time. As a result, it has lost some of the precision sought for by the early formulators of the concept. More than that, it has, inevitably, acquired different meanings through usage by different investigators. Confusion may arise because diagnostic lists often indicate that "some" cases of a specific disease entity arise from causes that are primarily emotional. This qualification can readily lead to misunderstanding and disagreement; it seems to imply that other instances of the same condition have no emotional components whatever.

For the physician who adheres closely to the linear cause-and-effect model of health and illness, the possibility that the patient's emotions are contributing to his illness will receive small consideration. A static view of health and of disease is apt to disregard the dynamic nature of the equilibrium within cells and organ systems. The endless flux within the individual and in groups of individuals will be readily overlooked, as will the concomitant possibility that even a slight alteration can result in disequilibrium. It is always more difficult to deal with the complexity of multiple variables than with the elegant simplicity of the cause-and-effect model, but it is often necessary for the clinician to embrace the multiple complexities of a problem. In the case of infectious disease, for example, this seems initially to involve little beyond the host's susceptibility to the infecting organism. However, it is a fact that some people exposed to a given infectious disease do contract it and some do not. Friedman[55] points compellingly, if not conclusively, to possible psychological determinants.

A pathogenic influence can, thus, include a factor as difficult to identify as mental symbolization. The classification of the resultant disturbance is necessarily not very precise; it is considerably less so than one in which microbiological or parasitological examination can bring the offending agent into a visual field. Nevertheless, the quality of anyone's mental life is cogently reflected in his general condition. Memory holds tightly to everything that has been experienced, and much of this cumulative record is stored in the unconscious; its effects are consequently as elusive as they are illogical. It is tacitly assumed that with the stimulus-response model, variable results are precisely correlated with measurable increases or decreases in the strength or amount of the stimulus. It takes time to realize that similar stimulation may elicit different responses from differently poised organisms. A propensity to deal in equations may lead to important errors in two significant ways: a failure to consider not only that the life experience of each person differs in reality from that of others, but also that it is further differentiated in many cases by idiosyncratic meanings attached to past events.

In a survey article on psychosomatic medicine, Galdston[56] attempts to define what falls within the purview of this specialty. He points out that its identification does not depend on its practitioners' unique skill, as do radiology and surgery; it is not limited to a specific organ system as are ophthalmology and gastroentreology; it is not age-specific, like pediatrics or geriatrics; nor is it oriented to diagnostic specialization in quite the same way as is oncology. He sees it, rather, as relating to a theory of causation that involves a distinctive pathological dynamism. A possible drawback to this viewpoint is that it may seem all too simply the reverse of the somewhat more readily understood view that somatic events affect the psyche. It is not enough to adhere either to the view that body influences mind, or to the belief that mind influences body; any attempt to deal with the diversity of clinical material by the exclusive use of one or the other does violence to an holistic concept of health and disease. It is fortunate that the field is not restricted to a straight-line cause-and-effect model, but may use an open-systems model, which is a more nearly adequate tool.

Biologic Models

Men have often had to deal with highly complex data, even some where the presence of interacting variables is postulated but not definitively established. In the face of such problems, they tend to construct an explanatory model. Model-building has been such an effective and productive method in the physical sciences, e.g., biochemistry and neurophysiology, that one is tempted to use it even in biologic and social systems that are more diffuse. Researchers are well aware of the dangers as they steer between the Scylla of unjustified and unsupportable precision and predictability, and the Charybdis of inexactness, incompleteness, and inapplicability. A good recent summary of the affirmative view of model-building has been written by Yates.[166] In their discussions, Waggoner[154] and Tsetlin[152] cover the drawbacks and limitations of biological models.

The linear model is perhaps the simplest, yet it is widely used to explain not only normal physiologic function, but the course of disease processes.

In this type of model, antecedent events are seen linked causally to predictable outcomes by means of intervening variables.

The *linear model* of psychosomatic relationship and psychophysiologic relationship links the person's internal and external life situations to his state of emotional arousal and to possible physical illness. This model provides a conceptualization of how psychologic stress leads to emotional arousal and the activation of psychological defenses; this in turn causes physiological arousal within the central nervous system. This arousal state spreads via cortical-limbic-hypothlmic pathways and may reach any of the three effector systems of the brain: the endocrine system, the autonomic nervous system, and the skeletal-muscular nervous system.[100] Sustained effector system input then flows into the target organs responsive to these effector systems. Changes in cellular functions thereupon follow and can lead to pathophysiologic conditions. This may take the form of, for instance, increased hormonal secretion or increased neurotransmitter activity of long duration.

The linear model permits the examination of any current situation for antecedent causes; such an introduction of a "cause" is expected to lead in a linked, straight-line movement toward an anticipated outcome. It may give highly accurate results when applied to the perfectly elastic collisions of billiard balls directed by a cue, or even to the millions of collisions between gas molecules in a closed container. The movement of the billiard ball does not depend on whether it had been struck with force on the previous day—or not moved at all. If, however, one seeks to predict what a human being will do in a specific situation, one must know something about what has happened to him in the recent (and, perhaps, even in the remote) past. Since man is influenced in his behavior today by what he remembers from the past and anticipates for the future, the best linear model cannot accurately predict how he will respond to the current situation. It can only indicate incomplete and inexact outlines of what he is likely to do.

Furthermore, the linear model cannot deal with the complexities of the interactional field which surround any individual, healthy or diseased.

An *open system model* presents a closer approximation of this actual human situation. Such a model, with its multiple interacting forces, directs attention to the variety of events that determine the pattern of behavior. Minuchin and associates[111] use such a model to explain why a given child

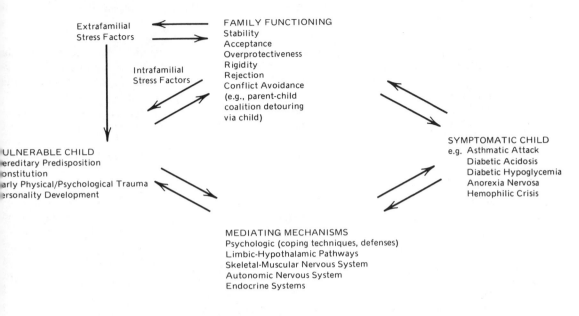

FIGURE 17–1
Open Systems Model of Psychosomatic Relationships

in a given setting develops a psychosomatic illness. A similar model could be applied to any instance of internal dynamic equilibrium. In particular, it would describe an organism in whose neural and hormonal functioning a variety of opposed or synergistic forces brings about physiologic change demonstrable by measurement. In terms of childhood psychophysiologic disorders, there was early recognition of how important the family context is in understanding the multiple causes of the child's illness.

In the past decade more emphasis has been given to the social environment and the multiple feedback loops that operate around persons living in groups. Such a model facilitates an understanding of the overdetermination of psychosomatic events, in their healthy as well as their pathological aspects.[101, 111, 118] The open systems model proposes multiple biopsychosocial interactions in and around the sick child (Figure 17–1). On the one hand, there are the sources of stress, physiologic psychologic, extrafamilial or intrafamilial; and on the other, there is the child who is constitutionally or hereditably vulnerable. The impact of the one upon the other finds expression as a specific psychophysiological disorder. The precipitating stressful situations engage mediating mechanisms in the child; these include psychologic events which cause physiologic central nervous system arousal mediated through limbic-hypothalamic

pathways. Further activation may involve any of the three effector systems: the endocrine system, the autonomic nervous system, and the skeletal-muscular nervous system. Through the action of these mediating mechanisms, physical signs and symptoms may appear.

Such psychophysiologic symptoms are common and all too well known. They include such events as: an asthmatic attack, an exacerbation of ulcerative colitis, a diabetic crisis, an attack of migraine, a "spontaneous" hemorrhage in a hemophiliac.

Such experiences bring about changes and reverberations in the child as well as within his family.

It is well known that the onset of asthmatic wheezing often evokes anxiety and panic in the child. This engages his nervous and endocrine systems to an even greater degree and may intensify his symptoms into a full-blown asthmatic episode. His environment, especially his family members, tend to react to the symptoms with various degrees of apprehension, protective behavior, anger, increased affection, and other similar attitudes. Even when he is symptom free, a large number of parents and siblings become overprotective and infantilizing toward the psychophysiologically ill child. The attention of the whole family may center around protection and concern for the ill child;[111] paradoxically, he in turn may feel responsible for maintaining this pathological homeostasis of his family. This experience may become a major reinforcement for his psychophysiologic symptoms.[101, 103, 111] Such overprotectiveness on the part of the family often jeopardizes psychosocial development of the physically ill child. Another possible maladaptive pattern that is characteristic is the rigid family where change and growth are made difficult. Any issues of the ill child or other family members that imply change in the family homeostasis create anxiety, especially for the parents. When the child reaches adolescence, he generally begins to express needs for independence, for an increased role in decision making, and for the right to his own friends and activities. Some of these are associated with medical risks, and all in all this is an especially critical time. Rigid parents run the risk of precipitating rebellious and risk-taking behavior in their chronically ill adolescent child.

Some parents unconsciously use such a child as a conflict-avoidance tool,[111] i.e., the child has become the means by which the parents hide emotional conflicts between themselves, as well as conflicts between them and their other children. Less frequently, the physically ill child has to cope with underprotective parents who are rejecting, angry, and negligent. Such parental attitudes often antedate the onset of the psychophysiologic disorder. The child may have been unwanted, there were marked social problems present, or serious parental pathology may have existed.

These are examples of negative family interaction around a physically ill child. They show how the child's illness can reverberate within the family systems and lead to secondary gains or paradoxical rewards for the child and other family members. In other words, where the family unconsciously reinforces the psychophysiologic symptoms, the illness may bring about a maladaptive learning process. The family systems model stresses the importance of multidisciplinary investigative work. This involves studies of precipitating factors, elements that make for predisposition or vulnerability within the child; the psychologic and physiologic mediating mechanisms behind disease exacerbations and remissions; biologic and psychotherapeutic approaches to the symptomatic child, and family counseling and family therapy. Later, there will be a discussion of the important implications of the family open systems model for the comprehensive therapeutic approach to the child with a psychophysiologic disorder.

Childhood Specifics

A great deal is known about the common growth pattern an infant follows into adulthood, and how this pattern can be interrupted or distorted by disease or by other hardship. However, in several important respects childhood is a unique state. One must, therefore, take care to avoid measuring childhood conditions by the same yardstick with which one measures health, normality, and disease among adults.

The child is significantly more dependent on others than is the adult. His caretakers appear not only as components of his external reality (mental objects) but actually control what happens to him. Robinson Crusoe, solitary and self-sustaining, survived as a castaway. The abandonment of small children, however, leads to their death, as was well understood by societies who exposed unwanted infants. One should also remember the child's limitations in assessing and communicating the onset of an illness or any other change in his condition. It is up to the caretaking adult to note when her (or, less usually, his) charge becomes symptomatic or alters behavior in a way that suggests trouble. Since the discrimination of pathological from normal conditions in a child will depend on the criteria the observer employs, it is important to establish theoretical constructs of what a normally healthy childhood state really is. It is also well to realize that, for better or for worse, the adults involved with a child are constantly interacting with him, and that they may contribute to the appearance of his problem, or to the continuation of a problem in which they have played no causative role. The reciprocal nature of this ongoing interaction is treated more fully under open systems. Suffice it to say here that when Anna Freud[53] tried to employ the psychoanalytic methods efficacious for adults in the treatment of children, she found it necessary to adjust her techniques. The young children were moving through periods of change and development the adult long ago had left behind, and their needs were different. Although many adults retain a potential for continued growth and change, they have completed the infancy-to-adulthood cycle and have achieved a reasonably healthy state. If they become sick or start malfunctioning, appropriate therapeutic measures can hope to return them to their state of health. It is, however, not enough to return the child patient to the competence he enjoyed during an earlier state of development, since he is passing through stages of increasing complexity. He strives toward mastery over self and environment, a goal already reached by most adults. A return to the past may lead the child into either permanent regression or fixation at an infantile level.

In the fetus and young infant, practical as well as ethical considerations influence the gathering of data about physiologic functions. Even the passive participation of an infant in experimental studies of his physiology is difficult. Nonetheless, serial measurements of such variables as sleep, wakefulness, temperature, excretion, and galvanic skin response have made possible the recognition of circadian rhythm in the newborn. It has also been possible to demonstrate the selective appearance of its aspects.* There is a specific time interval required for the establishment of statistically significant patterns of day/night variations of these functions. This ranges from one week (for galvanic skin response) to from sixteen to twenty months (for creatinine excretion).[137] Suggestive but less definitive data have been gathered[87] about the synchronization of maternal/infant functions —even in the prenatal period. The adult world observes a pattern of daytime work and nighttime rest. The infant is faced with more than the coordination of his physiologic variables to the demands, expectations, and convenience of this adult milieu. There is evidence that the infant's acquaintance with his own sensory modalities comes from putting them to use. This is evident from the contribution of visual stimulation to the development of adequate visual competence. Merskey[108] presented arguments for the learning of a sense of pain. With the exception of the rare child with analgia, he believes that the recognition and location of painful sensation is a process that children learn. The importance of this notion for the study of physiological disorder is not only that it might account for variability in pain threshold, but that it suggests the possibility of therapeutic conditioning.

Nosologic Entities

The presentation of psychophysiologic diseases in childhood will be divided into the customary units, Organ Systems, and follows the specifics of

* See references 12, 83, 90, 110, and 150.

the GAP "Psychopathological Disorders in Childhood: Theoretical Considerations and a Proposed Classification."[63] Of necessity the focus of this presentation cannot be inclusive. It will cover those conditions that the practicing child psychiatrists evaluate and treat, most often in consultation and collaboration with referring medical colleagues.

Psychophysiologic Skin Disorder

This category includes certain cases of the following: neurodermatitis; hyperhidrosis; seborrheic dermatitis; psoriasis; certain types of alopecia; certain atopic reactions such as eczema, urticaria, and angioneurotic edema; and certain types of verruca vulgaris, herpes simplex, and acne.[63]

SKIN

In many ways the skin is unique among the organ systems. Developmentally, it shares a common ectodermal origin with the central nervous system, and it provides vital protection in regulating body temperature, maintaining fluid balance, and opposing a barrier to traumatic injury and infection. It marks the limits of the body and separates it from its immediate surroundings. More than that, it envelops the body in a network of specialized sense-organ endings which receive impulses of pressure, heat and cold, and pain. A rudimentary involuntary muscular system of pyloerectors is attached to hair follicles, and an extensive capillary network subject to the autonomic nervous system may cause rapid and extensive vasodilation and vasoconstriction which give rise to readily observable blanching or flushing. The commonly used psychophysiologic measurement of galvanic skin response is merely a way of measuring with instruments these changes in sudation that accompany changes in emotional state. Meerloo[106] described how skin may act as an archaic system of communication that humans developmentally share with many animals. In a more total sense, the skin has been a medium of communication since mankind's archetypical parents, Adam and Eve, knew that they were naked and covered themselves. The judgment that someone looks "well" or "sickly" is generally based on how his skin is perceived. From birth on this most extensive and most visible portion of the body image is continually bombarded with stimulation.

The appearance of a baby's skin within one minute of his birth is one of the scoring signs on the Apgar Scale; the score of zero (pale blue) is strikingly different in meaning and appearance from the score of two given to the baby whose skin is altogether pink. Thus from the moment of birth, the skin is a reliable guide to the person's general physiologic condition.

Tactile impressions monitored through the skin contribute to the newborn infant's earliest perception of environmentally provided comfort or discomfort. In this earliest sensory world, the baby's awareness of such external stimuli as dampness, temperature change, and caresses competes with gastrointestinal and respiratory sensations which arise within the body. Anyone trying to soothe a young child checks for something irritating to his skin such as a soiled diaper and, at the same time, almost automatically communicates concern and tenderness by cuddling, patting, and stroking. Although one cannot be certain that this almost unconscious universal ritual teaches the impressionable infant to anticipate handling, the notion has heuristic appeal. Of equal appeal is the suggestion that idiosyncratic responses to cutaneous stimulation have their origin in this early caretaking. It is evident that response to cutaneous stimulation remains a complicated matter; thus, a person is unable to tickle himself, however well he imitates the actions of someone who tickles him.

Dermatologists generally agree that emotions may play a role in disorders of the skin but differ in their assessment of the importance of this factor to skin health. Thus, Norins[114] grants that emotions do influence skin disease but does not see them as a primary cause. Holter[68] proposes a classification in which emotional factors may be rated as primary, secondary, or collaborative influences on skin disorder.

ATOPIC DERMATITIS

Wittkower[162] has reviewed the psychological aspects of dermatitis among children. On the basis of published studies, he considers atopic dermatitis to be the most common emotionally mediated skin problem of childhood.

Since dermatitis may appear as early as the first weeks of life, prior investigators[157] resisted the idea that it was related to emotions and sought an organic explanation. More recent research has focused on the many mutually interactive factors that could play an etiologic role. In considering possible precipitating causes, particular attention has been given to patterns of mother-child interaction, the basic personality pattern of the child, and environmental stresses. A hostile-dependent parent-child relationship may develop in which the child cannot openly express the anger he feels. This may lead to intense conflicted emotions, particularly when the stability of the relationship, unsatisfactory as it is, is threatened. These emotions are assumed to find a channel for discharge through autonomic nervous system mediated skin changes.

The itching sensation of dermatitis can be relieved by the child's own efforts. Indeed, the immediate gratification afforded by scratching is often prolonged into excessive scratching, leading to pain and bleeding. This is often suggestive of self-punishment. The postulation of such a sequence of conscious and unconscious mechanisms as responsible for the appearance and perpetuation of a puzzling dermatitis does not minimize the need to consider the etiologic force of infection, contact dermatoses, and autosensitization.

The younger the patient, the more difficult it is to assess the part played by emotions in the emergence of this condition. The child is unable to express himself directly; the type of probing inquiry possible with adults is out of the question; and the attitudes and performances of those responsible for the child's care must be inferred from limited contact under special conditions. Current studies that allow for these difficulties support the importance of the role played by emotions. Brown[25] studied eighty-two patients ranging in age from eighteen to sixty-five, some of whom had suffered from dermatitis for as long as three years. His data documented the importance of emotional precipitants. Ironside[73] strongly supports the notion that emotional disturbance can cause skin disease and recommends treatment that combines psychiatry with dermatology.

Psychophysiologic Musculoskeletal Disorder

This category includes certain cases of the following: low back pain; rheumatoid arthritis; tension headaches, and other myalgias; various types of muscle cramps; bruxism and several types of dental malocclusion (both these latter may involve conversion components).[63]

MUSCULOSKELETAL

A major task of early childhood is the increasing mastery of the voluntary muscular system. Human expressive and interactive functions range all the way from the happy wriggling and gurgling of the infant to the degree of coordinated precision exhibited by the concert pianist. The largest portion of these actions is effected through the centrally controlled and modulated activity of this system. Its normal functioning is taken for granted, and the usual situation involves smooth transition from early fumbling attempts to mature mastery. Malfunctions and improper control may arise from a wide variety of causes; these range from birth injuries or later traumata to a wide variety of defects in function. They cover the spectrum from the cerebral motor strip through all the nerve pathways which finally activate the myoneural junction. But, setting aside all the many organic causes of neuromuscular disease, the clinician who deals with the effects of emotion on bodily function finds this a particularly challenging area in which to work.

The usual definition of a conversion symptom relates it to the voluntary musculature. There is thus a system overlap in this realm between conversion reactions and musculoskeletal psychophysiologic reactions. As an end organ of final response, muscle is limited in its reactions; it can contract and it can relax. It may contract upon receipt of a stimulus arriving via the appropriate motor nerve whether that stimulus is the result of a blow from a reflex hammer, or because the person has made a reasoned decision. It is evident that emotional causes of faulty musculoskeletal functioning stem from events which take place within the central nervous system. As symbolic solutions of neurotic conflict, conversion reactions seldom present in the same way or share the course of organic disease pictures. Within the musculoskeletal system, as in all others, there is significant overlap between disease pictures originating from a variety of causes. With such a universal and nonspecific reaction as pain occupying a major place in the manifestation of these disorders it could be scarcely be otherwise.

RHEUMATOID ARTHRITIS

Children comprise about 5 percent of the population of arthritics. This illness occurs as early as two years of age and is more common in girls than in boys.[58]

Because of the age distribution of the disease, most studies of rheumatoid arthritis involve retrospective work with adults. Robinson[135] reported on ten patients whose treatment for this disease had begun no longer than six months before they were studied. The personality variables in his cases were compared with those of long-term arthritic patients. He also studied these variables in newly diagnosed and chronic cases of diabetes mellitus, tuberculosis, and hypertension. It turned out that the different disease groups responded somewhat similarly to some of the items in the instrument used (16 Personality Factors Questionnaire). However, only among those with rheumatoid arthritis was there significant correlation (p<.001) between the test profiles of new and longstanding cases. Although this cross-sectional study indicated a similarity in personality test responses between the two arthritic groups, it could not establish whether the characteristics studied predispose to this disease or result from it.

A number of personality traits have been considered to be prodromal for rheumatoid arthritics. The commonality of anxiety, depression, obsessive-compulsive tendencies, introversion, shyness, and difficulty in the control and expression of aggression, precludes their specificity as etiologic agents in any single disease. Retrospective studies conducted with adequate controls are lacking and would be difficult to organize.

Among life situations which may possibly be contributory, early separation from (or loss of) a parent has been considered; in fact, this is a common finding among patients with rheumatoid arthritis. Robb[133] made a social survey of a sample of the population of Rotorua, New Zealand, examining the effects of early deprivation of maternal care. The population of Europeans and native Maoris there gave results from two different cultures. Although there were differences between the two populations in the incidence of rheumatic disease, in neither case did they correlate with deprivation of maternal care. At the same time, investigators note the very real problem of arriving at a valid and reproducible definition of early separation. McAnarney[94] compared forty-two chronic juvenile arthritics as a group aged six to seventeen with a control group in order to determine the impact of arthritic symptoms on child adaptation. As was anticipated, as a group, the arthritic children had more difficulties than the normal children. An unexpected finding, however, was that those least handicapped by arthritis had more psychological difficulties than those more seriously handicapped. It was suggested that when the handicap was severe and clearly evident, teachers and fellow students expected less of the arthritic youngsters and had a high degree of tolerance for their poor performance. The more mildly affected children, however, were expected to approximate normal performance and were criticized when they did not. This is a reminder of how the expectations and perceptions of others become important variables in the course of a chronic disease process.

Psychophysiologic Respiratory Disorder

This category includes certain cases of the following: bronchial asthma; allergic rhinitis; certain types of chronic sinusitis; some cases of hiccoughs and breath-holding spells. Hyperventilation syndromes and sighing respirations appear most often to partake of predominantly voluntary innervated mechanisms. If the appropriate psychodynamic factors are present, they may be classified under conversion reactions.[63]

From the very beginning of life, respiratory functions significantly contribute to the early bonding between the infant and the parenting persons. In the delivery room, the attendants watch for and help to elicit the infant's first spontaneous breathing and healthy cry. Loud, nonverbal respiratory behaviors involving the vocal organs are powerful ways for the infant to signal distress to his environment; this is usually the signal to which the mother responds. Soon she learns to distinguish between her child's cry of hunger, cry for attention, and cry of feeling uncomfortable. Other respiratory behaviors that assist in shaping the early mother-infant relationship are the child's sucking, his smelling, and his occasional coughing and sneezing.

Breath-holding spells have long been viewed as one of the earliest and most dramatic expressions of discomfort in infants and young children. In older children, anxiety states are often accompanied by wheezing or hyperventilation. Persistent cough without underlying organic causes can be used by children to convey their need for parental affecton. Some bouts of hiccoughs and sneezing, less common in children than in adults, may also represent a psychophysiologic expression of emotional frustration. Finally, the common role of emotional factors in precipitating and aggravating asthmatic attacks are well known to physicians and families caring for a child with asthma.

BREATH-HOLDING SPELLS

Breath-holding spells usually occur during the first three to four years of life; they are seen less commonly nowadays than one generation ago. A breath-holding spell is characterized by an interruption of respiration during the expiratory phase; it usually occurs in a child who is crying violently and seemingly angry. During the temporary laryngeal spasm and cessation of breathing, the child often becomes cyanotic, especially around his lips. At times, this is followed by unconsciousness and a localized or generalized seizure due to an hypoxic state. In most instances precipitating factors can be identified which produce fright or anger related to injury or frustration. Many authors have viewed breath-holding spells as an early form of temper tantrums before a child has the verbal ability to express his frustration.[78] During the spell, it is difficult for the caring persons to communicate with the child, a problem similar to that of a child in the midst of a temper tantrum. Breath-holding spells rarely continue after the first four years of life.

The earliest reference to breath-holding spells[14] mentioned that it was difficult to differentiate "the suppression of breathing with accompanying suffocated inspiration that presents itself frequently in angry children from spasm of the glottis." Early American authors, such as Meigs[107] and Bull,[27] suggested that breath-holding spells could be differentiated from laryngeal stridor and tetany and ascribed the condition to states of "fright, pain, or crying." Wile[159] suggested that the breath-holding spell represented the outcome of a conflict between a desire for "uninhibited physical movement" and "social pressure for quietness and inactivity"; he felt that this conflict caused strong negativism in the child. The breath-holding spell was an "aggressive physic response to social demand or restraint." This is in line with Kanner's[77] observation that breath-holding is "usually one of several signals of a disturbed parent-child relationship," a form of behavior that is often found among children with oversolicitous parents.

In terms of differential diagnosis, a careful history usually reveals that the onset of the breath-holding spell is preceded by crying, pallor, possibly with cyanosis, and, at times, stiffening, unconsciousness, a seizure, relaxation, and a return to fairly normal behavior. Congenital laryngeal stridor occurs during sleep as well as during waking hours. Laryngeal spasm related to low serum calcium is associated with latent tetany and such signs as Chvostek's, Erb's, and Trousseau's. Obviously, epilepsy must be carefully considered in those cases of breath-holding spells that are associated with twitching or convulsions. Most epileptic seizures are not associated with emotional tension, and they seldom occur in the midst of crying. The convulsions associated with breath-holding spells are usually mild. In severe cases of breath-holding spells, an EEG and careful neurologic examination are sometimes necessary to rule out epilepsy.

The treatment of the child with breath-holding spells must center on resolution of the parent-child conflicts. The first step is to reassure the parents about the nonorganic nature of the spells. Secondly, the parents have to be helped to identify those stressful situations that seem to precipitate the spells. They need help to remove possible sources of conflict, which often relate to rigid, coercive attitudes in raising the child. The parents should be instructed to handle their upset, angry, and fitful child with consistency and firm kindness. The prognosis for breath-holding spells is good. Their cessation can be accelerated by assisting the child in verbalizing his angry or upset feelings.

VOCAL NODULES

There is a group of children who abuse their respiratory system to express deep anger and frustration; these are patients with vocal nodules. It has been estimated that about 1 percent of school-age children, mostly boys, have vocal nodules, often causing hoarseness.[151] The primary cause of the nodules seems to be vocal abuse or misuse, such as in screaming. Many of these children have been described as hyperkinetic, aggressive, and impulsive. Therapeutic intervention includes speech therapy, parental counseling, and often direct therapy of the child.

HYPERVENTILATION

States of emotional arousal associated with anxiety or excitement are often accompanied by subjective complaints of difficulties in breathing. The individual may sigh deeply stating he cannot get enough air. Prolonged excessive deep breathing may result in a hyperventilation syndrome; this is characterized by multiple symptoms, such as light-headedness, feelings of unreality, numbness, tingling sensations, palpitation, chest pain, dyspnea, headaches, and even fainting. The syndrome is not uncommon among anxiety-prone adolescents

and increases among young adults. The physiologic basis of some of the symptoms is the respiratory alkalosis caused by sustained hyperventilation. Prolonged respiratory alkalosis reduces the plasma concentration of ionized calcium, leading to increased nerve excitability manifested by parasthesias, muscle tremors, and, in rare instances, even local spasm and tetany. This alkalosis also causes deficient oxygenation of the brain and reduction in consciousness associated with giddiness, faintness, and blurring of vision. At times, a careful history taking will reveal precipitating events of psychologic significance. In terms of differential diagnosis, one must consider other conditions such as external temperature, hypoparathyroidism, and brain lesions. A replication of the symptoms can be obtained by asking the patient to hyperventilate. This often clarifies the diagnosis and also reassures the patient about the benign nature of the syndrome and its causation. At times, instruction in relaxation is of value in helping the patient control his breathing. Psychotherapy might be indicated for those patients who continue to experience frequent anxiety states.

ASTHMA

Bronchial asthma is the most common chronic physical illness in childhood with a prevalance of at least 2 percent. It is defined as a diffuse, obstructive narrowing of the airways, usually leading to temporary impairment of respiration, primarily in expiration. Asthmatic symptoms involve wheezing, dyspnea, and cough. The symptoms are related to mucus membrane edema, increased secretion, and spasm of the bronchial musculature. Despite improved medical treatment, death due to status asthmaticus is not uncommon among children. Childhood asthma commonly interferes with the child's emotional development, family adjustment, peer relationships, and schooling. Recent epidemiologic studies report that psychiatric disorders, including learning problems, are almost twice as common in school age asthmatic children as in the general population.[101]

Presently, most allergists recognize two major groups of asthma: (1) The extrinsic type; here the symptoms are immunologic in nature due to reaginic sensitization to pollens, molds, epidermals, house dust, and, rarely, foods. This condition requires infrequent medication, shows positive skin tests, and there is frequently an elevated serum IgE. (2) The perennial, intrinsic type; the frequent attacks of this form of asthma cannot be linked to an immunologic cause and often seem to be precipitated by infection or physical exertion.

Asthma can thus have multiple hereditary, allergic, infectious, and other causes. In addition, most allergists and pediatricians agree that in many patients psychologic factors often seem to precipitate or aggravate asthmatic attacks. To be sure, there are emotional determinants in asthma as well as psychological complications for the asthmatic child and his family. Before turning to them, however, it is worth noting that from the mid 1930s until recently many psychiatrists made poorly substantiated claims regarding central emotional conflicts in asthma patients. In particular, these were related to unresolved dependency on the mother with the asthmatic attack viewed as equivalent to a repressed cry for the lost mother. Furthermore, proponents for a variety of psychiatric treatments have claimed great success with selected cases of asthma without attention to careful methodology and follow ups. It is important to note that patients suffering from psychophysiologic disorders who are seen by mental health specialists constitute a highly select sample. The child with intractable asthma who has failed to respond to medical management and who is referred to a psychiatrist as a last resort, or the mildly asthmatic child referred because of unrelated behavior problems, do not yield data which can be generalized to all children with asthma. Caution is also necessary in interpreting the findings of psychosocial evaluations and treatment data derived from asthmatic children who reside in special treatment centers.

There have been some recent long-term studies on unselected groups of children with asthma, followed over long periods of time. These have shown convincingly that there are no characteristic personality features among asthmatic children. In addition, these studies found no correlation between adequacy of family adjustment on the one hand and degree of severity of asthma and treatment response on the other. Only children with severe, continuing asthma showed a significantly greater prevalence of behavioral disturbance than healthy controls.[40, 98, 99] These studies also report that a majority of unselected children with asthma seem to adapt well to their chronic disorder. The severity of the asthma is not a valid criterion for psychiatric intervention but rather to the presence of emotional problems in the child or the family. Many times such difficulties seem to be secondary to illness rather than causative. Obviously, emotional factors can trigger or maintain some attacks of asthma.

An open systems model (see Figure 17-1) is helpful in presenting the current views on the contribution of psychosocial factors to the cause of childhood asthma. The model proposes that there can be extrafamilial or intrafamilial precipitants of an allergic, infectious, physically exhausting or psychological nature. Alone, or often enough in combination, these act upon a child who is somatically vulnerable due to bronchial hyperreactivity. Airway obstruction may occur via mediating psychophysiologic mechanisms; the result is the characteristic symptoms of asthma. The attack often leads to marked psychophysiologic repercussions upon the ill child and the family; the degree of the child's respiratory distress and the attendant anxiety of both the patient and others may arise and compound the crisis.

There is a currently favored theory upon which the suggested open systems model is based. It asserts that the fundamental vulnerability factor in asthma, i.e., the hyperreactivity of the bronchial tree, is due to a diminished responsiveness of the beta adrenergic receptors in the patient's airways and other tissues. This autonomic imbalance results in reduced production of smooth-muscle relaxing cyclic AMP. This leaves the cholinergic broncho-constrictive reflexes relatively unopposed to the bronchial stimuli that arise from immunologic, infectious, chemical, physical, and psychic sources.[109, 112]

In terms of those stimuli which provoke asthma or aggravate it, only psychologic factors will be mentioned here. A series of well-documented reports from the Children's Asthma Research Institute and Hospital in Denver have highlighted common emotional states that often seem to precipitate asthma.[125, 126] This is especially likely to occur in the nonallergic, nonsteroid-dependent patients who frequently show rapid remission of their symptoms when they are hospitalized or away from home. In contrast to steroid-dependent patients, among these children psychologic factors assume greater importance in precipitating symptoms than do allergic and infectious stimuli. Common emotional precipitants, pleasurable, or unpleasurable, include anger, anxiety, sadness, and excitement. Purcell and Weiss[126] have provided suggestions for taking a history which can help in identifying emotional precipitants. They emphasize careful reporting by the parents and, whenever possible, by the child about the emotional antecedents of wheezing and their time relationship to its onset. The clinician may also inquire whether separations from the child's family promptly improves his asthma. For instance, such improvements may occur when one or both parents are away from home or when the child enters the emergency room.

In regard to the mediating mechanisms, emotional arousal states are modified in the child's mind through psychologic operations, including various cognitive defense mechanisms. The physiologic arousal associated with these psychologic experiences is mediated in this way: percepts and thoughts send impulses via limbic-hypothalamic pathways to reach the autonomic nervous system. This system, acting through vagal and other stimulation in the vulnerable child initiates airway obstruction and wheezing. Another suggested route involves the hypothalamic-pituitary mediation of psychophysiologic arousal; this in turn may affect the child's adrenal cortical activity and his asthmatic symptoms. Some respiratory behaviors, like crying, laughing, coughing, and hyperventilation, which commonly accompany strong emotions, may also cause airway narrowing through mechanical and reflex means.

In the medical management of asthmatic children, extra care must be exercised in the use of sedatives and tranquilizers, because these agents pose a potential danger in depressing respiratory function and bronchial reflexes. For a symptomatic patient, if sedation should become necessary, chloral hydrate remains the safest drug.

Turning to the asthmatic child and the family situation: In general, the child in respiratory distress commonly experiences anxiety, sadness, irritability, and occasionally also fears of suffocation and dying. On a more long-term basis, the child with asthma must cope with the many emotional stress factors common to any serious physical illness. There are the uncertainties about future attacks, emergency hospital admissions, repeated, often painful medical procedures, and the interference his condition causes with schooling, family life, leisure time, and vocational training. The short- and long-term adaptation of the asthmatic child is closely dependent on his family's acceptance of his disorder. In regard to this factor, the parents' ability to master their natural feelings of fear, helplessness, anger, and self-blame, and their ability to control their tendency to overprotect their child have repeatedly been recognized in the literature. In addition, the parents are faced with handling frequent frightening attacks of asthma in their child, they must often pay for expensive medical care, and they are also expected to promote as normal a life as possible for their ill child without neglecting the needs of the other family members.[103]

Many parents of asthmatic children become overly attentive and infantilizing; this pattern persists even when the child is symptom free. The child of such oversolicitous, fearful parents often becomes fearful himself. He lacks self-confidence and age appropriate peer relationships. Although this is seen less frequently, some parents of asthmatic children become rejecting, angry, and negligent. In most of these families, there is evidence that the parental nonaccepting attitudes antedated the onset of the child's asthma.

At times, persons close to the asthmatic child child claim that the child seems to manipulate his environment. In an attempt to gain special attention, or to avoid certain duties, he deliberately begins to wheeze or hyperventilate. Some asthmatic children profess to have the power of controlling their symptoms. One occasionally encounters a child with asthma who consciously uses his respiratory symptoms to manipulate his environment. However, the majority of young patients who claim to be able to induce and control their attacks may be trying to master their anxiety about their asthma through these assertions. Some learning theorists have proposed that for certain children an asthmatic attack becomes conditioned to environmental and emotional stimuli.[80, 81] Consequently, some attacks are precipitated or aggravated by events which previously occurred with some consistency in temporal relation to asthmatic episodes. Thus, certain asthma attacks can be conceptualized as being learned in an operant conditioning manner. In such instances, the attacks carry with them certain gains for the child; they may bring him closer to his parent or, alternatively, lead to his separation from an unsuitable home environment. Such maladaptive learning processes probably occur among many children with the intrinsic, nonallergic type of asthma; they involve environmental reinforcement of the respiratory symptoms. Such a view, however, does not presuppose conscious awareness on the part of the child.

MANAGEMENT

Where psychosocial factors contribute significantly to the course of the illness, the long-range management of childhood asthma requires a close working relationship between the primary care physician, the allergist, and the psychiatrist or other mental health worker. The optimal collaboration of these caregivers helps them to establish a mutually trusting relationship with the child's parents; they become important therapeutic allies in the ongoing program.

The child mental health specialist is in a good position to teach his nonpsychiatric colleagues about the psychophysiologic nature of asthma. He can explain the potential importance of emotional and family interactional factors in precipitating or aggravating some attacks as well as in influencing the family's overall adjustment to the chronic illness. (See "General Therapeutic Principles" at the end of this chapter.) The child psychiatrist may also want to suggest teaching some asthmatic children and their parents systematic muscle relaxation combined with deep breathing exercises; these are to be employed at the first signs of wheezing. Many attacks of asthma can be avoided in this manner; one reason is that the child and his parents are together engaged in a constructive, anxiety-reducing activity. Several recent studies have been conducted in residential centers for children with asthma. The investigators have concluded that systematic relaxation training, with or without facilitation by biofeedback apparatus, results in a reduction in airway resistance.[5, 34] The long-term effects of relaxation training and lessened emotional arousal on the course of childhood asthma have yet to be firmly assessed.

In the following situations, direct involvement of the child mental health team with the family of an asthmatic child seems indicated: (1) children in whom emotional factors appear to be of a precipitating and aggravating importance; (2) children whose chronic illness perpetuates individual and family maladaptation; (3) behavioral problems in the child seemingly unrelated to the asthma. It should be noted again that in the treatment of bronchial asthma, practically every psychotherapeutic modality has claimed a measure of success. Most of these claims have been based on poorly-designed studies. In terms of the attempted psychologic interventions with childhood asthma, systematic long-term evaluations of effectiveness are still lacking. In general, psychiatric treatment aims at prevention of emotionally triggered and aggravated symptoms, modification of the child's and the family's attitudes towards the illness, and alleviation of any concurrent behavior disorder. Often, all three goals are pursued together. Individual psychotherapy, usually complemented by work with other family members, allows the child to vent feelings, memories, and fantasies associated with his chronic illness and disturbed family equilibrium. In general, it is imperative to involve the child's significant caretakers and other important people in his close environment in any psychotherapeutic work. In many instances, the family tends to be overinvolved with the ill child, leading to overprotective or, less frequently, to nonaccepting attitudes. Due to the great concern over the asthma situation, many psychologic conflicts between the parents and the siblings get diffused. In effect, the asthmatic child serves as a "conflict avoidance" tool[101, 111] and a protection for other family members. Whenever significant family maladaptation is present, the child psychiatrist is likely to suggest family psychotherapy as part of the total management of the patient. There is a small group of children with severe asthma who are resistant to all available medical and psychologic interventions in the home setting. For such cases, there continues to be a need for placement in residential treatment centers or specially chosen foster homes. Before such placement occurs, careful preparation of the child and his parents is necessary. This is equally true for concomitant work with the family while the child remains separated from his home.

Psychophysiologic Cardiovascular Disorder

"This category may overlap somewhat with respiratory disorders; it includes certain cases of paroxysmal tachycardia; certain types of peripheral vascular spasm, such as Raynaud's disease and central angiospastic retinopathy; migraine; erythromelalgia; causalgia; vasodepressor (as distinguished from conversion) syncope; certain types of epistaxis; essential hypertension; some cases of hypotension, and, in adolescents and adults, eclampsia." (p. 260)[68]

CARDIOVASCULAR

From the embryonic state onward, the development and growth of the human organism depend on the effective functioning of the cardiovascular system. Health depends on it throughout life. Krovetz[85] points out how early in life the heart is shaped and formed as a functioning organ; between the third and seventh weeks of gestation it completes its development; at that time, its 3 mms. of attained length is pulsating within an embryo which is only 25 mm. long. It is the first organ of the body to achieve an actual state of function. It is not only the adequate functioning of the circulatory apparatus, however, that is crucial for the continuing development of embryo and foetus. Salk[138] demonstrated that, pre- and postnatally, the maternal heartbeat rhythm is a stimulus for the infant's behavioral patterns. His experimental design included the exposure of newborns and children sixteen to thirty-seven months of age to various auditory stimuli. The newborns in the nursery were exposed day and night to seventy-two paired beats of a normal heart sound at a level of 85 decibels. A control group received identical care without the recorded heart sounds. On occasion, a gallop rhythm or a rate of 128 beats a minute was substituted for the normal heart sounds. The infants rapidly responded to the abnormal sound and rate patterns by increased crying and restlessness. They consistently showed the least anxiety when listening to the pattern of sound that most closely resembled the normal heartsounds.

The English language recognizes that the heart is involved in emotional states. Those with courage are spoken of as "stout-hearted" or having "the heart of a lion," and someone overcome by sadness and dejection over an unrequited love is "broken-hearted." When one speaks of thinking with the head and feeling with the heart, this acknowledges a division well-established in popular thought, one that echoes the attempt to categorize the perception of systemic body functioning. However much it defies reply, the question: "Tell me where is fancy bred./In the heart or in the head?" is still germane.

Medical practitioners have long recognized a connection between an individual's emotional state and his cardiac function, but the evidence for this has been generally anecdotal. Increasing knowledge of neurotransmitter function, and the identification of specific receptor sites have begun to clarify the situation. There are a number of factors believed to be predictive of coronary heart disease. Currently, an attempt is being made to relate these to certain behavioral patterns and their attendant emotional states. The result is the formulation of coronary-prone Type A behavior. Even "voodoo death" can now be seen as an extreme example of the fatal effect of parasympathetic discharges on cardiac rhythms, rather than an event of magical causation. Keegan[79] reviews the interaction of emotional states and cardiovascular disorders. He considers the contribution of emotional and personality variables to the causation of heart dysfunction, to the quality of the postoperative course following cardiac surgery, and to the vicissitudes of convalescence from heart attack.

HYPERTENSION

Hypertension in the adult is widely accepted as a serious health problem, but the majority of identified cases—those with essential hypertension—are usually untreated. The 1 percent with hypertension secondary to confirmed renal, vascular, or endocrine disorder are more likely to receive medical care because of the presumed specificity of treatment. Indeed, there is controversy as to whether essential hypertension is a disease state or simply an inherited physical trait like height or coloring. Oldham[115] reviewed evidence for both points of view while declining to classify blood pressure levels as categorically normal or abnormal.

A number of factors contribute to the present interest in early detection and long-term treatment of essential hypertension. One was the discovery of a variety of pharmacologic agents that combined effectiveness with a relative absence of side-effects. The availability of efficacious treatment led to research with control groups, with demonstrable reduction of serious complications among those who had received treatment. The mass screening programs then undertaken documented not only the extent of the problem, but the absence of effective treatment for many of those identified as hypertensive. Stamier,[146] reporting on a survey from 1,171 screening sites operating from 1973 through 1975 and screening more than a million persons, found that 247 out of 1,000 had diastolic readings higher than 90, and 116, higher than 95. Like other large scale investigations, this indicated that the pressure level is higher in men than in women, and more commonly higher in blacks than in white. There were increases in all groups as age advances to fifty. Of the detected hypertensives, 27 percent had not been previously identified as hypertensive. Ten percent were untreated although they had been previously diagnosed, and 16 percent were uncontrolled in spite of treatment. Thus, more than 50 percent of those identified as hypertensive were not receiving effective treatment.

Most of what is known about the incidence of hypertension and the efficacy of its treatment was learned from adult patients. It was more or less taken for granted that the condition was rare in adolescence; when it was detected, it was assumed to be secondary to other causes. Kilcoyne[82] reported that hypertension among adolescents is more common than previously thought. Although less usual and less serious than later in life, it should be of concern to those responsible for the health care of young people. Kilcoyne emphasizes that there is considerable danger in rigidly applying the criteria used for screening adults to adolescents. This is true because (1) pressure levels have a lower range among young people than among adults; (2) female adolescents have lower systolic pressures than males; (3) there is no racial differential at this age; and (4) there is no stable pattern for progression from childhood levels to those of adulthood. What is necessary is to allow for the greater lability of pressures in the young and at the same time to recognize those changes in an individual child's blood pressure which can be evaluated in terms of standard deviation. There should be enough appropriate serial measurements taken to smooth out any transient extremes that would compromise the accuracy of the basal pattern.

Surprisingly little attention has been paid to blood pressure among pediatric patients. A survey of three pediatric teaching hospitals made by Pazdral[117] indicated that blood pressure was measured in only .3 percent of 1,156 patients visit in walk-in or emergency clinics. When it was, there was little on the record to indicate the condition under which it was taken, e.g.: neither the child's physical position nor the cuff size was noted. The older patient groups showed a higher incidence of hypertension; the figures varied from a low of 0.4 percent for those under one year to a high of 15 percent among those ten or older. House officers recorded pressures more often than did attending physicians. The investigator concluded that this valuable diagnostic procedure was underused, and that without routine and widespread gathering of relevant data, too little will be learned about the incidence of pathologically high pressures. In addition, there will continue to be a lack of data about what constitutes a normal sequence of pressure changes as an individual moves toward adult life.

Psychophysiologic Hemic and Lymphatic Disorder

Numerous physiologic concomitants of anxiety are seen in relation to this system, including variations in the blood level of leukocytes, lymphocytes, eosinophiles, glutathione values, relative blood viscosity, clotting time, hematocrit, and sedimentation rate. These ordinarily are reversible; chronic or recurrent states of leukocytosis of lymphocytosis may occur, however, as may alterations in other physiologic values which may be classified under this heading. Leukemia and lymphoma, as well as some cases of pernicious anemia, apparently may be precipitated by physiologic and interpersonal stimuli; these should be

classified under existing headings of predominantly physical disease with a secondary personality diagnosis, for example, "reactive disorder or depressive type." (p. 261)[63]

The influence of psychological stress on human clotting mechanisms is only a suggested one. Many attempts have been made to draw comparisons between humans and animals. Research on dogs, for instance, has shown that stress in the form of trauma, hemorrhage, cortisone administration, and induced anesthesia causes elevation of blood fibrinogen levels; this results in hypercoagulability of the blood. Such a state can result in disseminated intravascular coagulation leading to renal damage, venus thrombosis, and other lesions. It has also been suggested that psychologic and physiologic stress can bring about an elevation of other clotting factors of the blood. It seems likely that many of these stress factors at least increase the fibrinogen level through stimulation of the pituitary-adrenal cortical axis.

Many anecdotal reports and poorly designed studies have sought to link psychologic stress factors with the onset of certain hemic and lymphatic disorders in childhood and young adulthood. In this chapter, two groups of blood disorders will be described in which emotional factors seem to be important determinants in the development of hemorrhagic symptoms. First, the syndrome of psychogenic purpura or autoerythrocyte sensitization and, secondly, hemophilia due to factor 8 and 9 deficiency. Several of the studies of young patients with these disorders fulfill strict scientific criteria. They thus provide the child psychiatrist with practical models of how psychosocial influences might exacerbate bleeding tendencies in vulnerable patients. This can be of material assistance in consulting with colleagues in hematology and general pediatrics.

AUTOERYTHROCYTE SENSITIZATION

Autoerythrocyte sensitization, or psychogenic purpura, is an intermittent purpuric state. It is seen in adolescent and adult females and is manifested by episodes of painful, spontaneous bruising. The bruises or ecchymoses usually appear rapidly following sudden pain and swelling. Characteristically, no trauma is reported to precede the lesions. The earlier suggestion that these patients have become sensitive to their own red blood cells has been questioned by investigators such as Ratnoff and Agle.[127] In a series of carefully documented studies, the latter concluded that many of these women patients did not show clotting defects, and that psychological factors appear important in the production of the eccymotic lesions. Hysterical and masochistic character traits were commonly seen in addition to problems in dealing with hostility. In many patients, the skin test for autoerythrocyte sensitization could be influenced by hypnotic suggestion, and new bruises appeared at sites suggested under hypnosis. In terms of the physiologic mechanisms responsible for the extravasation of blood in these women, Ratnoff and Agle suggested that the patients' blood vessels might become permeable to erythrocytes. This was thought to be due to the action of bradykinin-like agents serving as humoral mediators between the central nervous system and the local tissue reaction. This type of spontaneous purpura has been observed in young adolescent girls; typically, they report a history of physical or sexual abuse often involving a sado-masochistic relationship with a parent.

There are specific personality characteristics and psychological factors that often seem to trigger the appearance of spontaneous ecchymoses in women and female adolescents with spontaneous purpura. These are suggestive of the mechanisms of conversion reaction. Following Alexander's lead, many writers have attempted to limit the concept of conversion symptoms to events mediated through the voluntary nervous system. They maintain that structural changes resulting from involvement of the autonomic nervous system should be classified as psychophysiologic reactions. More recent authors such as Nemiah[113] and Engel[45] have reported, however, that structural lesions may occur as a complication of conversion reactions. Consequently, Agle, Ratnoff, and Wasman[3] have suggested that in patients with spontaneous purpura, the lesion production itself is a complication of the conversion, a difficulty which takes the form of inflammation or bruising. In these patients, the true conversion symptoms would be the experience of painful sensation, and the physical location determined by such psychological factors as identification, sado-masochistic gratification, and unconscious punishment to deal with guilt. As a result of these processes, the effector system of the autonomic nervous system becomes engaged; it releases the proposed bradykinin-like substances in the subcutaneous tissues. These induce vasodilation and increased vascular permeability, and the overall results are the ecchymosis.

These studies on spontaneous purpura are reminiscent of cases of religious stigmatization. A recent report[43] describes a ten-and-one-half-year-old Baptist girl who manifested religious stigmata periodically over a three-week period. This suggests a psychophysiologic route of bleeding similar in nature to the mechanisms described by Ratnoff and Agle.

HEMOPHILIA

In certain cases of hemophilia, so-called "spontaneous" bleeding episodes and cycles of increased bleeding tendency have been related to emotionally stressful situations.[104] This has been described in connection with hemophilia related to factor 8 and factor 9 deficiency, and many hematologists, pediatricians, as well as families of the boys have attested to such events. Curiously, the emotional triggers are often of a positive nature, such as anticipation of a pleasant event, a holiday, a birthday, or a camp meeting. Often the parents would then describe the boys as "overenthusiastic" and "excited" in anticipating the happening. In particular, these spontaneous bleeding episodes have been observed in pre-adolescent hemophiliacs and no discernible changes in their activities are reported that otherwise explain the cycles of increased bleeding. In other words, there is evidence that in hemophiliacs, emotional arousal might be related to episodes of an increased bleeding tendency. There is, however, no evidence of significant changes in levels of the antihemophilic factors at times of stress. Some authors have, therefore, suggested that variations in the integrity of the capillary wall, occurring as an autonomic response to stress, may be responsible for certain periods of increased bleeding.[2] On the other hand, in evaluating spontaneous bleeding episodes and the possible influence of emotional factors, one must be cautious about the difficulty of ruling out possible undetected minor physical trauma. Nonetheless, the likelihood remains that psychosocial stress factors may precipitate or aggravate bleeding in hemophilic patients (Mattsson, 1975). This possibility should be clearly stated to the patient, his family, and the physician responsible for his care.

Psychophysiologic Gastrointestinal Disorder

This category includes: certain cases of peptic ulcer; chronic gastritis; ulcerative colitis; cardiospasm; mucous colitis; spastic or irritable colon;

certain types of constipation; certain types of nonspecific diarrhea; certain cases of regional enteritis; some types of "heartburn"; and gastric hyperacidity; pseudopeptic ulcer syndrome; certain types of pylorospasm; anorexia nervosa; megacolon (nonganglionic type); idiopathic celiac disease and nontropical sprue; certain types of polydipsia; reactive obesity; certain types of marasmus or failure to thrive; persistent colic; certain types of recurrent vomiting without significant symbolic components; certain disorders in salivation; and some types of periodontal disease.[63]

GASTROINTESTINAL

Some of the classic investigations of body structure and function were made on subjects who had sustained injury. Beaumont was the first to study gastric function systematically. He was able to do so because the fistula Alexis St. Martin developed after being shot in the abdomen in 1822 permitted the actual sighting of gastric changes. Wolf[163] availed himself of the opportunity to study the function of his patient Tom, for whom a permanent gastric fistula had become necessary after the burning and scarring of his esophagus. These studies, among others, identified two basic patterns of gastric activity: the first, a riddance pattern, involving the cessation of gastric digestion and ejection, often with nausea and vomiting; in the second, gastric hyperfunction appears to be caused by feeding behavior.

It was not, however, until Engel[46, 47] reported studies of the infant Monica that it was established that the patterns identified in adults also appear in the very young. Moreover, in their cases, these changes are also associated with emotional states. Since behavioral research is more readily accomplished with adult subjects, it is possible to be misled about the precursors of any dysfunction that is first noted in adult life. The stage of life in which a behavioral manifestation or physiologic mechanism appears is not necessarily the stage of its inception.

The gastrointestinal system is a vegetative and visceral system par excellence. It is of the greatest importance to the human being in earliest infancy, not only as the conduit for body-building nourishment but also as one of the earliest modalities available to him by any means of which he can establish and maintain contact with the world around him. Gastrointestinal function is, indeed, vital to health throughout life, even in the later stages after maximum growth has been achieved.

The infant finds oral and nutritive functions gratifying or frustrating. The intensity of these reactions contributes not only to the earliest stage of personality formation, but exerts a lifelong influence. Even intrauterine events may, in fact, be influential in the infant's postnatal functioning. Dodge[38] presents evidence to suggest that the excess occurrence of pyloric stenosis among firstborn infants may be influenced by the mother's emotional stress during pregnancy. He believes that some maternal humoral agent, possibly gastrin, conveyed transplacentally, may be responsible.

A. Freud[53] reviews the psychoanalytic position on the primacy of need-satisfaction that is subserved by early experiences of eating. She notes the vital contribution this first pleasure makes to personality formation. It is asserted that ample and ready satisfaction of hunger is of critical importance. Perhaps the strongest argument for this is given by cases in which the basic nurturant needs are not met. Spitz[145] has written about the devastating effects of what he calls "hospitalism"; if specific proof were required that man does not live by bread alone, it is supplied by clinical examples of his study. His work furnishes dramatic evidence that children require more than physical nutrition for their very survival. And the child who does manage to survive physically in a world only minimally responsive to his needs, does so as a rule at the cost of his developmental potential. Provence and Lipton[123] carefully documented this principle in a study of the early development of children raised in an institutional setting. They charged this environment with unique responsibility for the many deficits the children presently exhibited.

Even children cared for at home may fail to thrive due to disturbances in the mother-child relationship. In the earliest months of life, the preverbal child is just beginning to adapt to his specific physical and emotional milieu. The subtler shapings of emotional states develop later, as does the language to describe them, yet the smallest infant is more or less comfortable, more or less happy or upset, more or less pleased or angry. He has neither the vocabulary to express his reactions nor the neuromuscular apparatus with which to communicate even the most intense feelings. Explicitly, instead, he seems to respond largely through changes in his visceral systems.

As personality is developed, the focus of control and mastery is no longer the receptive and incorporative mouth. Toward the end of the first year, the anal end of the gastrointestinal system, with its potential for retaining or expelling body waste, increases in importance. At the same time, more body functions are subject to emotional interference. An extreme example, fecal retention related to emotional conflict, is to be seen in children with nonaganglionic megacolon. This condition must be differentiated from true Hirschsprung disease in which the pathologic bowel function is a direct result of the anatomic absence of ganglia. Based upon a series of thirty cases of psychogenic megacolon, Pinkerton[119] offers a theory to account for them and recommends a treatment approach which involves both the parents and the children in an effort to restructure faulty interactional patterns. Less severe than that seen in megacolon is common and often relates to a struggle over issues of bowel control.

The hyperfunctioning bowel can offer a clinical problem as severe as that which hypofunctions. The most serious disease entity in this category is ulcerative colitis. In this disease, the intestinal tract (particularly the terminal portion of the large colon) is not only hypermotile but can also become hyperemic. Mucosal vulnerability to mechanical trauma then appears. These pathophysiological changes may cause severe diarrhea, bleeding, and even that most dangerous complication, perforation of the bowel. Although ulcerative colitis in adults was recognized and reported as early as the late nineteenth century, Helmholz[66] was the first to describe its appearance among young people. Until that time, the few cases of ulcerative colitis were not differentiated from the more commonly occurring diarrheas of young children. Platt[120] reports on sixty-two cases in which the most common age of onset was eight years; in fact, 11 percent of these cases were symptomatic during the first year of life. The usual clinical course involves remissions and exacerbations; it is rare for the disease to have a fulminating terminal course. Steroids are often helpful in the clinical management of ulcerative colitis, but if the disease is severe and progressive, surgical intervention may be necessary. McDermott[95] studied forty-nine child patients and found that emotional illness played a significant part in their problem. He recommended that the treatment team combine medical and psychiatric skills, with surgical intervention when indicated. He found that the emotional improvements associated with psychotherapy were not necessarily correlated with an improvement in the diseased bowel, or a reversal in the course of the illness. This would be in line with the currently held view that ulcerative colitis has an auto-immune basis. The nature of the illness often correlates with significant emotions and stress factors. The specificity model which sought to relate personality type as well as specific emotional conflicts in this disease has not been verified.

ABDOMINAL PAIN

Pain is one of the most common accompaniments of organic malfunction. The colicky infant is in obvious distress, but the distress is a common occurrence for which no single cause has been found. It seems evident that emotional factors contribute to the condition, whether to initiate or to simply sustain it. Or it may reflect a mutually unsatisfactory parent-child relationship. It is most common in infants under three months of age. The treatments are largley empiric, and the passage of time usually seems to do as much for the sufferer as any particular remedy.[153] It is striking how greatly the malfunction of an infant's gastrointestinal system can upset the day-to-day parent-child relationship. The child's digestion is not only a sensitive barometer of his emotional state, but any impairment of digestion from whatever cause brings distress—not only to the child but to his caretakers as well.

In his monograph on the abdominal pain of children, Apley[13] reported that more than 10 percent of a random sample of school children had recurrent abdominal pain. Girls were more commonly affected than boys, 12 percent of them reporting such pain, compared to 9 percent of the boys. Apley[13] is a practicing pediatrician and stated in his preface that his initial interest in this problem was the identification and relief of organic causes of such pain. His subsequent experiences, however, convinced him that an emotional etiology was most common. The autonomic nervous system is implicated as the likely mediating agency. Pupillary size, as a readily available measure of autonomic nervous reactivity, has been studied in children with recurrent abdominal pains.[136] Preliminary data support the view that such children have large pupils than unaffected controls; this is presumptive evidence for increased reactivity of their autonomic nervous systems.

CYCLIC VOMITING

The difficulty in differential diagnosis of children with abdominal pain is further complicated when the pain is associated with vomiting and fever. Gee[57] described recurrent vomiting in terms recognizable to any current practitioner. Although recurrent vomiting has long been recognized as an entity, attempts have been made to relate it to epilepsy as well as to migraine. Follow-up studies of adults who had recurrent vomiting as children are inconclusive as to its precise etiology.[64, 130]

RUMINATION (MERYCISM)

Infants can develop a voluntary regurgitation of previously ingested food, some of which is re-chewed and swallowed and some of which is spit out. A rare disorder, most commonly having its onset in the second half of the first year, this infant behavior is a pathologic response to a severely disturbed maternal relationship. Misdiagnosed or inadequately treated cases can progress to death. Therapy is directed toward establishing appropriate emotional supports and stimulation for the child and to improving maternal-infant relationships. Flanagan[51] reviews current psychiatric thinking relative to this condition.

PEPTIC ULCER

Abdominal pain is the commonest presenting symptom of peptic ulcer, since such pain is commonest among children; for a long time peptic ulcer was not identified as a significant disease entity in childhood nor was it thought to contribute even rarely to childhood mortality. Another factor that made it difficult to identify peptic ulcer in children is related to its usual location in the duodenum, a more difficult site for x-ray examination. Goldberg,[60] a British surgeon, noted that, after the staff had become especially interested in this condition, many more cases of peptic ulcer were diagnosed in his hospital. Within a five-year period there were twenty children between the ages of seven and fifteen who were diagnosed as having peptic ulcer; of these, two perforated and required surgery, but the rest responded well to medical management. This experience was consistent with that of Cameron,[28] who surveyed the American literature through 1953, and found only thirteen reported cases of surgical treatment of children's peptic ulcer.

The etiological significance of emotional factors in childhood ulcer has been a matter of speculation. The earliest case reports by surgeons, pediatricians, and pathologists dealt almost entirely with the organic examination, and indicated no study of the patient's familial or social circumstances. Later reports, of which that of Taboroff[149] is typical, have tried to fit the current psycho-

somatic thinking about causation in adults to cases in children, with only minimum success.

More recent studies have utilized epidemiologic methods, with interesting results.[148] A higher than anticipated incidence (and one that seems to be increasing) has been documented; a rate of 0.5 per 100,000 children was recorded in the 1947–1949 period; by 1956–1958 it had increased to 3.9. A challenging finding was the marked increase in incidence among fifteen-year-olds, who were almost exclusively males. It was felt that the young people studied (in Erie County, New York) were responding to the stressed characteristic of modern urban society, and further, that in the upper socio-economic segment, the high number of mixed marriages and the occurrence of peptic ulcer among parents were additional risk factors for the development of childhood peptic ulcer.

Psychophysiologic Genitourinary Disorder

This category includes: certain cases of menstrual disturbances, such as dysmenorrhea, amenorrhea, and premenstrual tension; certain types of functional uterine bleeding; certain types of leukorrhea; certain types of polyuria and dysuria; certain types of vesical paralysis; certain types of urethral and vaginal discharges; and some instances of persistent glycosuria without diabetes. Habitual abortion, male and female infertility, and other disorders may occur in older adolescents and adults. Disturbance in the sexual function of the genital organs in older adolescents (as in vaginismus, frigidity, frequent erections, dyspareunia, priapism) often involve conversion disorders of the voluntarily innervated musculature; certain cases, however, may include psychophysiologic components (pp. 261–262).[63]

There is probably no body system wreathed about with greater symbolic importance than the genitourinary. This is true both of the appearance and function of its several elements. From birth onwards it elicits the interest and concern of the individual child and everyone about him. This includes the parents and extended family, and as he grows older, the peer group. The initial assignment of anatomic sex type at the moment of birth not only answers the question so vital to parents, "Is it a little girl or a little boy?" but has immediate, fundamental, and lifelong impact for the infant concerned. A myriad of ideas and expectations are activated in the environment; these become the continuing warp and woof upon which the developing child forms the picture which becomes, for better or worse, both his inner self and outer active and interacting persona.

The importance of form and function in the genitourinary system transcends the on-going role it plays in excretion and, later, its more specific role in somatic growth and change at puberty. To some degree, self-approval and peer group acceptance are dependent on one's adequate approximation to prevailing group standards; far beyond this, however, is the issue of fertility. It is evident that comfortable function for the individual includes an acceptable gender role. The questions of delayed or absent puberty, however, with possible infertility, while of the most immediate and agonizing urgency for the pre-adolescent or adolescent, at the same time are also issues of the greatest importance for the family. Thus, throughout the developmental cycle, from gender assignment at birth to increasing sense of self and ultimate adult social and sexual partner selection, the genitourinary system retains its potential for causing and perpetuating emotional conflicts. In their importance and effects, the resulting personal problems can exceed the impact of any accompanying organic dysfunction. Further, the social importance of secondary sexual characteristics, and sexual functioning in general, can fill the teenager with anxiety, shame, and guilt. The evaluation and treatment of such problems demand careful coordination between primary physicians, urologists, gynecologists, and a consulting child psychiatrist. Therapy, whether individual, conjoint, or family, must also be conducted with an awareness of what fears and fantasies may be aroused by problems affecting genital and sexual functioning.

DYSMENORRHEA

The establishment of a regular menstrual cycle is a complex event in a young girl's life in which the full range of bio-psycho-social factors interact. Even the age of onset of menarche varies in relation to genetic, social, nutritional, climatic, and personality variables. Sloan[144] found dysfunctional menses or "painful periods" to be the leading cause of pelvic pain in the young female. Dysmenorrhea has been reported to be the largest cause of work and school absenteeism in the United States.

As might be expected from a complaint so widespread and occurring throughout female reproductive life, no single cause will explain dysmenorrhea nor will any single treatment relieve it. For those occurrences for which a specific underlying organic pathology can be established, e.g., endometriosis or pelvic inflammatory disease, the accepted terminology designates the condition as secondary. All remaining cases are classified as primary. For any age group, primary cases far outnumber the secondary ones; among adolescents this difference is greater still.

Thus, in adolescent dysmenorrhea, the majority of cases is without organic findings. Having eliminated biologic causes, the usual adequate work-up brings the therapist face to face with the patient's psychosocial issues. The physician thus must be responsive to a multitude of social factors and to their meaning for the individual patient. The adolescent girl's concerns tend to cluster around general areas such as body image, role satisfaction, ideas about cleanliness, and acceptance of sexual feelings. Many girls figd it difficult to share and examine these topics; they perceive these subjects as threatening and shameful but at the same time as exciting and stimulating. In many cases the therapist's own sex role can be a complication. For most cases, it is enough to be a respectful, sympathetic listener who, upon request, offers accurate professional advice. Especially intransigent, prolonged cases warrant attention from a psychiatrist.

AMENORRHEA

Any discussion of amenorrhea must differentiate between primary and secondary cases, i.e., those cases where menarche has not occurred (primary) and those in which menses, having begun, do not continue (secondary). The distinction, while clearcut as stated, can on occasion be difficult to establish. Early cycles, in addition to being anovulatory as a rule, can be irregular and vary widely in timing. Slight staining in a young girl resulting from irritation or trauma can be erroneously perceived as menarche.

Primary amenorrhea requires an evaluation of genetic, anatomic, and endocrine factors as well as an awareness of the appropriateness of the concerns that led the girl and her family to seek a professional opinion. The rare case in which a psychiatric explanation might be forthcoming, e.g., anorexia nervosa, will present with the other findings of the condition. In primary amenorrhea the commonest findings are either an organic condition or a faulty understanding on the part of the girl and/or her family of the normal variations in the timing of menarche.

Any investigator should include pregnancy as a possible cause; if it does exist, abortion, if desired, is much simpler in early pregnancy. Pseudocyesis is covered under psychophysiological endocrine disorder.

Grodin[62] presents a useful classification of the varied etiologies to be considered in cases of seconary amenorrhea in adolescence. He divides his list first into ovarian and nonovarian; psychogenic causes are then covered in the hypothalamic-pituitary subheading under nonovarian causes. The classification of psychogenic causes under hypothalamic-pituitary recognizes both the effect of hypothalamic releasing factors on the pituitary production of FSH and LH as well as the hierarchical ordering of the effects of central nervous system activities on organ systems. In amenorrhea, the target tissues are the ovary and the uterine endometrium.

ENURESIS

Enuresis can be defined as, "involuntary micturition after five years of age, either nocturnal, diurnal, or both."[96] The newborn empties his small capacity (30-60 ml) bladder from twelve to sixteen times per twenty-four hours as a reflex response to increased intravesical pressure. Sympathetic and parasympathetic innervations function without cortical input.

The norm for adolescence is to have attained a capacity of 250 to 550 ml as well as the ability to empty at will even a partially filled bladder, as well as inhibit micturition, especially throughout the sleep cycle. This range of control is achieved by stages; the toddler developing awareness of sensations of bladder fullness as afferent sensory nerves become myelinated, the three-year-old briefly delaying the emptying of a full bladder, and the four-year-old voluntarily emptying his partially filled bladder. Further developments include conscious cortical control replacing the earlier use of local musculature to delay voiding and, by six or seven years, the ability to void from an almost empty bladder.

The symptom of enuresis is evidence of some delay or disruption in this complex sequence. The proper functioning of the urinary system requires normal kidneys, bladder, and urethra and appropriate neural control. The initial pediatric study of an enuretic child, with careful attention to details of urinary function and dysfunction, will determine if there is a need for more specific urologic examinations. Routine physical evaluation and laboratory tests may furnish evidence for urinary tract infection, or chronic renal failure, or indicate the presence of such less common entities as nocturnal epilepsy, diabetes mellitus, or diabetes insipidus.

The goal of any evaluation, to establish a specific treatable etiology, is not often accomplished. This factor, as well as the number of enuretic children involved, have influenced the variety of treatment modalities employed. With an estimated 10 percent of children over age five being bed-wetters, parental demands for help run high. Medication, conditioning devices, training regiments, and psychotherapy all have their proponents, as does the school of benign neglect. The fact that a considerable, though undetermined, number of children do become asymptomatic under any treatment used, or even if none is used, makes the validity of outcome studies at least doubtful. In addition to determining whether enuresis is perceived as a problem, family attitudes will determine to a large extent the acceptability of a specific treatment plan. In respect to the general family attitude, it is often an important factor that three-quarters of enuretic children have a close relative who is, or was, enuretic.

Enuresis due to specific anatomic or physiologic pathology does not usually come to the psychiatrist for primary management. Nor do enuretics who present straightforward developmental delay or faulty and incomplete learning. In such cases, the primary care physician may provide adequate guidance and explanation for the child and his parents.

The psychiatrist may offer treatment in those cases in which enuresis is embedded in a more complex emotional situation. It would be fruitless to focus on it as a solitary symptom unrelated to the totality of the child's mental life. There are, of course, differences regarding the identification of such cases; some authors even question their existence. Bertalanffy,[20] for example, accepts the behavioral explanation for the etiology and treatment of bed-wetting. Winnicott,[161] on the other hand, supports the position that a child can "need" a symptom and that until that need is understood and met, symptom relief can be antitherapeutic in a broader context. His article presents a detailed and moving case history of a boy whose complaints included enuresis.

Esman[49] has summarized current concepts of primary nocturnal enuresis with an emphasis on neurophysiological maturational factors.

Psychophysiologic Endocrine Disorder

This category includes: certain cases of hyper-insulinism; certain types of growth disturbances; and, in adolescents and adults, pseudocyesis and certain disorders in lactation.[63]

The endocrine system is composed of the organs of internal secretion; it represents one of the organism's major regulating modalities. A unique property of the endocrine system is that both its regulation and its effects are mediated via the bloodstream. This fact has several important consequences. First, since the common circulation of the body effectively reaches all its cellular components, it is only by the development of highly specific receptors that organs activated by such a "master gland" as the anterior pituitary can respond appropriately to a chemical regulator directed toward them. At the same time, the potential exists for more general body responses. At the cell level, every organ can respond to changes in circulating hormones such as insulin, thyroxin, and somatotropin. Considered teleologically, however, this system is not one best adapted to rapid responses or adjustments. It is rather more likely to mediate functions of longer periodicity such as digestion or menstruation. These are patterns with daily or monthly fluctuations, or they can have even greater temporal extension such as the sequence of growth and development from birth toward adulthood.

GROWTH RETARDATION

The child of short stature does not escape notice. Normal growth results from the interplay of a number of variables. These include nutrition and the general healthy functioning of the mechanisms of digestion, absorption, and metabolism. They include, as well, the subtle chemical regulators of the processes involved, which operate under the influence of a general genetic predisposition to rate of growth. Some families exhibit short stature as a heritable characteristic. Powell[122] reported on a series of thirteen children whose growth retardation highlighted another variable in an already complex picture; the influence of psychosocial factors on pituitary function. The children, three females and ten males, were initially thought to exhibit growth failure due to idiopathic hypopituitarism. All were studied in detail in an inpatient hospital setting and subsequently followed in a convalescent hospital for periods of three and one-half to twelve months. Once they had entered their new environments, these children grew at rapid rates, and concurrently, their growth hormone levels returned to normal. It is this demonstrated ability to grow at a normal rate in one environment, contrasted with the marked delay in growth in their previous, emotionally unsettled settings that argues most persuasively that an emotional disturbance can suppress the centrally controlled release of growth hormone. Now this syndrome, often referred to as psycho-social dwarfism, has been identified and accepted as a not rare cause for growth failure in children.

An earlier study by Fried[54] also demonstrated the susceptibility of children to emotional upsets leading to failure to grow. He was reporting on children who, subsequent to admission to a carefully supervised therapeutic group living situation, showed an unexpected decline in their growth. Among his conclusions was that no matter how adequately a setting may provide nutrition, recreation, and medical supporting services, some children still fail to grow until such time as emotional conflicts are adequately resolved. At that point, there is often not only a resumption of growth, but even periods of accelerated growth that erase previous deficits.

PSEUDOCYESIS

The erroneous conviction that one is pregnant, together with some accompanying physical signs and changes, is a condition that has been recorded since the time of Hippocrates. While much less common than other disturbances of menstruation (see anorexia nervosa and amenorrhea which are classified respectively under gastrointestinal and genitourinary psychophysiological headings), the association of mental contents and thought processes with bodily changes makes pseudocyesis a quite straightforward psychophysiological entity. Not that the false beliefs are solely those of the affected females. Physicians have been misled along with the person's close associates; Selzer[142] has reported a case of pseudocyesis in a six-year-old girl. In this case, the investigation of the condition included exploratory abdominal surgery.

The reported incidence is linked to the broadness or narrowness with which pseudocyesis is defined. Criteria have varied from the existence of one or more somatic signs suggestive of pregnancy (e.g., amenorrhea, morning nausea and vomiting, abdominal distention) to the presence of any physical symptom related to an unconscious wish or fantasy coupled with a strong conscious belief in pregnancy.

Barglow and Brown[16] suggest a broad definition for pseudocyesis: ". . . psychic or somatic manifestations which upon psychiatric investigation, appear to originate from two intimately interconnected components:

1. The awareness of recent bodily change or disturbance, linked to

2. A conscious fantasy about some aspect of a pregnancy wish, fantasy or fear." They have found this definition useful in evaluating and treating a variety of cases among whom secondary amenorrhea was the most common presenting symptom.

Aldrich[4] reports an interesting historical speculation about Mary Tudor, Queen of Scots, and presents a persuasive account of how her two "pregnancies" were actually recurrent episodes of pseudocyesis. In any event, the occurrence is not limited to any social or economic group, but is more an expression of the patient's mental set as related to the solution of a problem, conscious or unconscious. It is this element of function of the higher brain centers, the reason and the emotions, that essentially differentiates human cases of pseudocyesis from the analogous condition studies in animals. Brown[26] included a summary of techniques and procedures used to induce pseudopregnancy in the dog, rat, and rabbit; he compares and contrasts this with his and Barglow's conjectural explanation relating central mental events in humans to a decreased production of biogenic amines. Reduced amine production in turn would affect the secretion of follicle stimulating hormone, lutenizing hormone and prolactin, resulting in amenorrhea and, less commonly, lactation. They suggest that the usual precipitating event is a depressive state.

The reduced libido more commonly seen with depression in both sexes would also be theoretically explainable by such a mechanism of centrally reduced biogenic amine production. Here, however, the symptom picture is more generalized than the rather striking one in pseudocyesis.

Just as careful physical and endocrinologic study can determine the presence or absence of pregnancy, so can a careful psychiatric examination elicit specific personal reasons why an individual develops and persists in maintaining a false interpretation of bodily changes.

Psychophysiologic Nervous System Disorder

This category includes certain cases of asthenic disorders, formerly called neurasthenia, although some may be classified as conversion disorders;

idiopathic epilepsy (including petit mal, psychomotor epilepsy, and other equivalents); narcolepsy; certain types of sleep disturbances; spasmus nutans; dizziness; vertigo; certain types of hyperactivity; motion sickness; and certain recurrent fevers.[55]

The quoted listing of psychophysiologic nervous system disorder in childhood was influenced by the 1952 edition of the American Psychiatric Association's Diagnostic and Statistical Manual (DSM-I).[11] This edition emphasized asthenic symptoms and cases of neurasthenia as the major psychophysiologic nervous system reactions. A significant change of the second edition[10] of this manual (DSM-II) was the elimination of the heading "Psychophysiologic nervous system reaction," primarily due to the new inclusion of "Neurasthenia" as one of the "Neurotic Disorders."

While sound nosological principles support the view that asthenic disorders are of neurotic origin, there still remain pediatric syndromes that best can be understood as nervous system psychophysiologic illness. The significant ones include idiopathic epilepsy and certain types of hyperactivity. On the basis of recent neurophysiologic studies of sleep, certain disorders such as narcolepsy, sleepwalking, pavor nocturnus, and primary nocturnal enuresis have been viewed as disorders of arousal due to lags in central nervous system maturation.[12, 24] Such a current formulation is a helpful reminder that a nosological schema, at best, represents a temporary fusion of clinical observations with available scientific thinking.

The concept that the central nervous system may contribute to its own malfunctioning seems to arouse more opposition than is the case with any other concept of body organ system. Albeit speculatively, mechanisms can be advanced to explain pathological functioning by organs whose paths of innervation are clearly delineated portions of the autonomic nervous system. The idea that mental representations can be perceived and responded to as threats and dangers with accompanying physiological arousal states is a powerful one and carries a certain heuristic appeal. But for whatever reason, the idea that the central nervous system itself can function in a way to create a symptom picture is less generally acceptable. Viewing the central nervous system as a coordinated group of functioning subunits helps clarify its dual role of initiator and target organ of emotionally determined disorders.

The problem of observing and quantifying the functioning of the central nervous system, particularly in its higher functions, present unusual difficulties to any scientific study. The results of thought, emotion, and volition are not too difficult to measure. Pavlov quite early described the technique for collecting saliva from his canine subjects, and assessed end-organ responses to centrally active stimuli. But actual attempts to enter "the black box" and study higher-order functions leave the observer with the less precise tools of subjective reporting, or the equally subjective attempts to equate a subject's performance with the observer's idea of what is taking place. For this kind of study, temperament and tools to supplement those of the laboratory scientist's are called for, and artists can best supply them. Dostoyevsky, an epileptic as well as a supremely gifted novelist, furnishes data about epilepsy and central nervous system functions that would appear on no electroencephalogram. In *The Brothers Karamazov*, he presented the servant Smerdyakov as a most petty and disagreeable person who could induce his epileptic attacks to serve his own dark ends. His character is to be contrasted with that of the epileptic Prince Myshkin, the hero of *The Idiot*, whom Dostoyevski consciously depicted as a "truly beautiful soul."

EPILEPSY

Epilepsy is one of the common chronic disabilities of childhood with an estimated prevalence of 5.4/1,000.[121] While 80 percent of childhood epilepsy is of the grand mal variety, petit mal seizures are the type usually limited to childhood. The appearance of this condition before age three, or its continuation after age fifteen is uncommon.[87]

The clinical picture presented in any type of seizure disorder results from a discharge of excessive, transient neuronal activity within the brain. The etiology, and the somatic and psychic components, vary widely. An aura or premonitory period of varying duration precedes many attacks and causes sensory, psychic, or physical symptoms. Psychic symptoms may include olfactory, auditory, or visual hallucinations, or nonspecific behavioral changes such as irritability, confusion, or restlessness. The seizure proper may have a motor component of a tonic or clonic nature— separately or associated. Loss of consciousness may be complete, partial, or absent. Postictal states range from immediately recovery with a clear sensorium to varying degrees of confusion,

fatigue, restlessness, and irritability, lasting hours or even days. Major seizures are usually followed by a period of complete amnesia.

A disorder of such protean manifestations, originating within a system susceptible to metabolic, circulatory, toxic, infectious, traumatic, and psychic influences, challenges the best efforts of any interdisciplinary health team. The challenge is not just that of differential diagnosis, complex as that task is.[39] The issues that arise in long-term work, especially with patients presenting complex partial seizure, are addressed by Rodin.[135]

HEADACHE AND MIGRAINE SYNDROME

Wolff in his monograph *Headache and Other Head Pains* notes,

It has been said that migraine headache is the commonest complaint of civilized people, though few reliable data exist concerning its frequency. Grimes found that "of 15,000 individuals examined in general practice with reference to migraine, 1200 or 8 per cent were afflicted." There are all graduations of the migraine complaint from the most severe and disabling illness to trifling symptoms, and it is safe to say that less than half the migraine victims ever consult a physician. (p. 255)[184]

It is quite common for migraine headaches to have their onset in childhood. Dalsgaard-Nielsen[33] stressed that determining the "age of onset" is subject to considerable error. Having stated this caveat, he reported that among his patients, 43 percent had had migraine attacks before puberty, and 14 percent at puberty. His literature review showed an average age of onset between five and eleven years, with the attacks generally occurring earlier in males. In specific cases, an individual attack may be provoked by any one of a number of factors, e.g., psychogenic, hormonal, hypnoclinostatic, or alergic, singly or in combinations. He reported, too, that the frequency of psychogenic factors was second only to that of idiopathic attacks, i.e., those in which an identifiable cause could not be assigned.

Rees[129] supports such findings: "Psychological factors play a role in precipitating some attacks of migraine in some patients." He further warns of the potential for error in drawing broad conclusions from the population that seeks and accepts medical management. It seems that an estimated one-half of all migraine subjects shun medical care, and the details of their illness picture are unavailable.

Psychophysiologic Disorders of Organs of Special Sense

"This category includes certain cases of glaucoma; asthenopia; keratitis; blepharospasm; Ménière's syndrome; certain types of amblyopia; and certain types of tinnitus and hyperacusis."[63]

Within the medical realm, one indication of the importance of sight and hearing is that each has a separate specialty to measure its normal functioning and to diagnose and treat the disease states that can arise. Test instruments and procedures of great sophistication and high precision are used in this work; indeed, the practice of modern ophthalmology or otology would be impossible without such instrumentation. But this increasing power to examine and measure specific functions carries with it the ever-present danger that the single organ or system will come to dominate the entire field of study. The examiner may lose sight of the basic reality that these highly specialized tissues are nourished, innervated, hormonally regulated, and integrated within the total functioning of the body in ways not fundamentally different from any other organ system. This fact is acknowledged within the specialty areas themselves; it is perhaps a view more often expressed by experienced practitioners who have treated and followed a variety of patients over time. A certain number of these situations do not fit the most straight-forward organic disease explanations. Hoople,[69] drawing on forty years of experience in otolaryngology, presents case material which, while admittedly not "scientific," had been such an important part of his practice that he felt compelled to present a paper on his experiences with psychosomatic otolaryngology. In a similar vein, Schlaegel[140] wrote an extensive review article entitled "Psychosomatics: The Second Face of Ophthalmology."

VISION

The normal development of the sense of sight is a compelling example of practice making perfect. And conversely, the lack of early practice, i.e., input stimuli, has a detrimental effect on all subsequent performance of the system. And it is a most intricate system that sequentially develops. Even the perception of a single, upright, colored picture, in depth, and with smooth response to position changes requires the closest coordination of intrinsic and extrinsic musculature and central nervous system coding and processing.

The eyes are not merely the crucial entry points for an individual's major sensor link with the surrounding environment; throughout life they furnish a means by which people reveal themselves to one another. From the infant who fixates on the concentric circles of his mother's eyes in preference to a random pattern[75] to the adult male who responds erotically to a female's widened pupils (formerly elicited by the application of belladonna ["Beautiful Woman"]),[67] the appearance of the eyes is revealing of an individual's emotional state.

The lacrimal apparatus affords another avenue by which emotional states are translated into a language which is easily read by others. Even a state near tears or silent weeping can be detected, and there is concern that "dry-eyed grief" somehow does not afford the emotional release of crying. No one challenges the existence of a correlation between internal emotional states such as grief and sorrow and the resultant tears and reddened corneas. The involvement of the visual apparatus in other instances of emotional arousal does not meet such ready acceptance.

In myth, and later in more formal literature, the eye has always functioned as a powerful symbol. From the dreaded evil eye of antiquity, still believed in to some degree by many people, to the popular juvenile hero, Superman, with his "x-ray vision," the tendency to elaborate the ability to see into an act filled with magical power and force is a constant human theme.

Literature develops and refines this idea. Classical Greek writers gave the fundamental human emotions universal recognizability and appeal. Prominent among their fictional characters was Oedipus, a character caught in the web of an eternal dilemma. From his anguished self-mutilation at the conclusion of Sophocles' Theban Trilogy comes the term oedipism to describe self-inflicted injury to the eyes.

Self-injury may be deliberate and for conscious cause. It may also be a response to unconscious guilt and the implacable demands of a primitive superego. The "Talon Law" forms a natural part of a child's earliest moral thinking; more than that, it is later reinforced by such injunctions as the biblical warning, "and if thy right eye offend thee, pluck it out, and cast it from thee." Schlaegel[141] studied the records of 218 children through age fifteen years hospitalized for eye injuries. There were 171 boys and 47 girls. A control group of children with other-than-eye injuries was used for comparison. Two principal findings were reported. First, the frequency of eye injuries among the girls did not vary with age; secondly, the boys showed a greater frequency of eye injuries at ages four through six and ten through twelve. This frequency distribution was not found among boys with other injuries. The study was designed to eliminate the effects of, "an increase in general activity, clumsiness, or play involving danger to the eye." The authors suggested that the observed differences were due to variations in psychosexual development.

In a large ophthalmology clinic population, Kalthoff[76] found psychogenic amblyopia five times as common in patients under fifteen years of age as in those over fifteen. While these younger patients comprised only 25 percent of the total clinic population (6,705 patients), they presented five cases of amblyopia that, after complete medical evaluation, were felt to be due to psychiatric causes. Correspondingly, the clinic population over age fifteen had only three such cases.

Throughout a long career in ophthalmology, Inman[70] maintained an active interest in relating emotional factors to disorders of the visual apparatus. His clinical reports, while lacking control cases, showed this intriguing recurrent association: "Styes are almost invariably associated with preceding thoughts about birth (Inman, 1935, 1946), whilst corneal lesions seem to follow stresses connected with thoughts about loss of virginity and its natural sequel, birth." His material shows no breakdown by ages, but the case vignettes included patients in mid-adolescence.

HEARING

Hearing loss and deafness are among the common chronic disabilities of childhood. The estimated prevalence for hearing loss is 9/1,000; for deafness 1.2/1,000.[121] Despite the numbers involved, in the literature on this subject there are seldom any references to possible psychological factors. Lucente[93] has surveyed a broad range of psychiatric issues that can complicate the work of the otolaryngologist. He believes that, "numerous symptoms which patients present to the otolaryngologist may reflect on underlying psychologic disturbance which either constitutes or modifies the etiology. Among these symptoms are hearing loss, dizziness, tinnitus, dyspnea, stuffy nose, dysphagia, hoarseness, headache, defective speech, and pain in the head and neck—virtually the entire spectrum of otolaryngologic complaints."

Ménière disease, or syndrome, as some would wish to designate it, is a condition affecting children as well as adults. Clinicians, however, differ markedly as to the etiologic significance of psychological factors. Williamson[160] strongly states the case for frequent psychological etiology. Pulec[124] has edited a monograph in which the consideration of psychological issues is striking only by its absence. Harrison[65] further widens the diagnostic field when he writes, "vertiginous attacks with a similar symptom complex occur in children but are seldom serious and usually disappear before puberty; this condition may be termed pseudo-Ménière's disease of childhood."

Tinnitus as a solitary symptomatic complaint was related by Leventon[88] to palatal myoclonus. The myoclonus was compared to a psychogenic tic which warrants psychiatric evaluation and followup. Two of the five patients reported were teenagers.

Obesity

Excessive body weight is a common problem, especially among people living in the developed countries. Since the norms for classifying people as overweight are not uniform, however, it is difficult to establish figures on its prevalence.

Johnson and his colleagues[74] found that according to the Wetzel Grid, more than 10 percent of the school children in the Boston area could be classified as "overweight." One-third of the overweight girls and almost half of the boys exhibited "persistent obesity," i.e., they were overweight throughout the school period under study. However, only 12 percent of the overweight girls and more than a third of the overweight boys showed "late obesity," i.e., they became overweight during the latter half of the same period. Wolff and Lloyd[165] cite data demonstrating that one-third of a sample of 200 infants exceeded what they were expected to weigh (according to their height) by more than 20 percent. There is increasing evidence that childhood obesity is often a precursor of obesity in adult life.[31] Child health workers are concerned with the problem on two counts: first, because of the psychological consequences to the child of being overweight—and these are serious enough; and second, because of the need to take preventive measures against a condition significantly implicated in adult morbidity and mortality.

It is obvious that for the neonate birth brings about a radical and abrupt change in his way of obtaining nourishment. While in utero, the fetus receives a largely carbohydrate nourishment which allows him to add fat to the body as he approaches term; this comes to him, of course, as predigested nutriment which is almost continuously supplied directly into his circulatory system. Once a neonate, however, the baby's diet is largely fat. Thus, birth brings with it a radical alteration in chemical composition of his food supply. More than that, he must now make oral efforts to obtain this food, and he must digest what he obtains by means of his own metabolic processes. Such a massive change in a vital life-sustaining function requires many adaptations; it thus affords many opportunities for faulty learning to take place.

It would be natural to suppose that one's ideas about eating, including the recognition of hunger and satiety, stem from childhood experience. In fact, however, the available data about faulty perceptions of gastric functions and its requirements have been obtained chiefly in clinical and experimental work with adults. Bruch[32] has hypothesized that obesity and even anorexia nervosa may be the consequence of faulty learning of "gastric perceptivity." She has observed the presence of erroneous monitoring of feeding cues, and she regards the persistence of this tendency as reflecting unsuccessful interaction between the infant and his nurturing caretaker, usually the mother. The assumption is that the latter failed to provide the infant with the normal range of experiences in interpreting his sensations of hunger and satiety. This causes him to confuse these stimuli with other, unrelated emotional states such as anger and fear. Such confusion can lead to one's eating as an emotional response to situations in which eating is quite inappropriate.

In order to observe the effects of gastric motility on the perception and reporting of hunger pangs, Stunkard[147] studied seventeen obese and eighteen nonobese women. Since contractions of the empty stomach are believed to account for the sensation of hunger, these subjects had inflatable gastric balloons placed in their stomachs. After an overnight fast, kymographic tracings of pressure variations were recorded for four hours. The subjects had been selected to differ solely with respect to obesity or nonobesity, and there was little recorded difference in gastric motility for the two groups. Nonetheless, the nonobese women reported sensations of hunger associated with stomach contractions significantly more often (at the 1 percent level) than did the obese women.

Schacter[139] has summarized a number of studies directed toward differentiating the eating be-

havior of obese and normal subjects. A consistent picture emerges. It seems that the obese individual, unlike the more normally weighted person, has no reliable internal cues with which to monitor food intake. The subjects were placed in surroundings devoid of social or behavioral cues but whose nutritive liquid was available on a self-demand basis. Under these conditions, the caloric intake of the obese dropped significantly, while the intake of persons of normal weight was essentially unchanged. Clearly, there was a marked responsiveness to external situational cues on the part of the obese. This suggests that such an individual is prone to eat whenever food is available in attractive surroundings or impinges on his awareness by sight or smell. This differentiation in responsiveness was even seen to hold under nonexperimental conditions, e.g., the ratio of obese and nonobese Columbia undergraduates who cancelled membership in a cafeteria prepayment food plan. The majority of those cancelling the plan, the obese, were those to whom the situation of eating and the various stimuli other than hunger were most important. In the main, the normally weighted, to whom nutritional intake was most closely related to bodily need, stayed in the plan.

It seems unlikely that a single cause can account for a condition as common as obesity, which occurs in both sexes, among all classes, at all ages. In addition, there is actually no clear-cut distinction between the presence or absence of identifiable obesity; there is, rather, a transition from normal weight through all stages to extreme obesity. A comprehensive review of the subject by Mayer[105] covers in detail the genetic, traumatic, and environmental factors of etiologic importance. He makes it clear that although, in any particular case, one factor may predominate, it is more usual for a number of factors to contribute in varying proportions to the plight of the badly overweight individual.

Recent studies, based on the examination of adipose tissue, stress the importance of early eating habits throughout life. Brook[23] reported on fifty-four obese children and twenty-five obese adults, all without known endocrine disorder. The former weighed 20 percent more than expected for their height, and their triceps and subscapular skinfold thickness measurements exceeded the 90th percentile. Adults were assessed by skinfold measurements only, all exceeding the 95th percentile. Control data came from a study of sixty-four children and seventeen adults scheduled for elective surgery. Based on the criterion of skinfold thickness, these people were not obese. All the obese subjects had adipose cells that were larger than average in size. But a larger than average number of adipose cells was found only among children who had been obese at the age of one year, and among adults obese since childhood.

There are studies demonstrating that mice over-fed during the first weeks of life are heavier than littermates fed lightly; these have been replicated with human beings. Charney[31] compared adult weight to the weight recorded during the first six months of a subject's life. A retrospective study of 366 subjects between twenty and thirty years of age determined that 36 percent of those whose weight as infants had exceeded the 90th percentile were overweight as adults. Weight over the 75th percentile in infancy correlated significantly ($p < .001$) with obesity in adult life. Although this study does not try to determine what makes infants overweight, it does connect the weight status of an infant with the weight status of the same person while in the third decade of life. A simple measurement, weighing, can be used to identify the infant who is at a higher than average risk of becoming an obese adult.

Ravelli[128] explores the question from the viewpoint of deficient maternal and infant nutrition. Three hundred thousand nineteen-year-old men who had been exposed to the Dutch famine of 1944–45 were examined, and the results related to the time when they had lived under famine conditions. It was found that those whose starvation occurred during the last trimester of prenatal life were significantly less obese ($p < .005$) than the others. This was seen as consistent with deprivation of the fetus at a period critical for his development of adipose-tissue cellularity. Those subjects whose mothers had been undernourished only during the first half of their pregnancy had significantly higher ($p < .0005$) obesity rates. The authors suggest that this reflects an interference with normal development of hypothalamic centers regulating food intake and growth.

This material supports a multicausal view of etiologic factors in obesity. Influences operating as early as the intrauterine period or the effects of the earliest feeding experiences can find expression as obesity in later life.

It is thus evident that a large number of the obese represent the outcome of determinants which impact on development quite early. At the same time, there remain children who are vulnerable to developing obesity as a response to a later life stress or crisis. Some advance the view that such an occurrence would be a simple reactive event, i.e., in terms of energy balance, caloric intake exceeds caloric expenditure. The corresponding emotional equation, however, is not that simple. A vulnerable child, exhibiting an obesity response, represents the additive effects of predisposition, stress, and food and nurture in all their symbolic dimensions. Further, in many cases, the emotional state, e.g., depression, significantly lowers the activity level. Only a bio-psycho-social approach is adequate to identify and deal with such an array of multiple and interacting factors.

Conclusion

The foregoing material deals with specific psychophysiologic disease entities which find symptomatic expression through various organ systems. Potentially, such symptoms can be as diverse as the structures and functions of the components of any system in the body. Certain theoretical principles, however, underlie this seeming complexity and give it order and clarity sufficient to justify a view of psychophysiologic disease as a diagnostic entity.

Foremost among these principles are the postulated mechanisms whereby conscious and unconscious mental events, acting via central nervous system mediating systems, alter the performance of major body systems. Currently, these explanatory schemes are broad in concept and proposed application. On-going investigations continue to generate relevant data; these support, in general, the principle that for some organic disease states emotional vectors are among the primary etiologic factors. Any physician who intends to effect more than symptomatic relief for his patients, needs to be conversant with these general propositions.

Specific treatment modalities, such as the psychotherapies and psychopharmacology, have demonstrated a considerable degree of effectiveness in working with emotional disorders. These are treated in detail elsewhere.

THERAPEUTIC CONSIDERATIONS

Primary care physicians, such as pediatricians and family physicians, are responsible for the long-term management of most children with psychophysiologic disorders. In this role, the primary care physician usually has to serve as the "ombudsman" or advocate for the chronically ill child; this requires that he pay continued attention to the psychosocial adjustment of that child and his family.[18, 103] The emphasis should be on promoting the youngster's normal personality development. This becomes possible only if the health workers can establish a trusting relationship with the child and his parents who are the crucial therapeutic allies in the on-going medical management. Such a close working relationship often includes a psychiatrist or other mental health worker in the role of consultant. The various health professionals assist the parents in learning to accept the child's illness; this can happen when the parents are able to master their conflicting emotions about the various aspects of their child's disease.

The child psychiatrist is in a unique position. He can help his primary care colleague learn to elicit and to listen for the expression of all the family's conflicted feelings about the ill child. He can encourage him to instruct the parents to have their child develop an increasing responsibility for self-care and independence. It is essential for the child and adolescent with a chronic illness to have regular schooling and to be guided toward age appropriate activities. The parents should pay attention to their healthy children; all the care given to their sick sibling often leaves them feeling resentful and left out. The health team should also call attention to parental attitudes of overprotection, lenient discipline, rejection, or neglect; these may endanger the child's personality development as well as his physical condition. The physician and his team colleagues often have to initiate vocational guidance; this should take into account the patient's intellectual and scholastic achievement levels, along with his physical limitations and personality characteristics. The psychiatrist is aware of how important it is to give repeated, age appropriate information regarding the illness and its management to the patient and his family members; he is in a good position to emphasize this to the physician in charge. All treatment procedures must be explained without trying to withhold information about the negative aspects. When the child with a psychophysiologic illness approaches adolescence, he should be expected to assume major responsibility for his treatment program. At that point he can begin to see his physician alone, and to talk about the illness, and his future.

There are many situations where individual and family problems clearly aggravate a psychophysiologic condition. Ideally, in such instances, the psychiatrist will collaborate with the primary care physician. Usually he will suggest family counseling. While that is often centered around the ill child, it will focus upon the pathological interaction within the family. This approach aims at removing the patient from the role of the sole concern, or the symptom bearer for the family. Throughout, the psychiatrist stresses the biopsycho-social viewpoint of the psychophysiologic disorder as conceptualized within an open systems model. This is true of his work with the family, just as it is of his work with primary care physicians or subspecialist. Family therapists have worked with malfunctioning families of children with many syndromes. These include severe asthma, labile or brittle diabetes (psychologically triggered recurrent ketoacidosis), and anorexia nervosa.[103, 111] Encouraging treatment results have been reported with such conditions. The family therapy approach must often be combined with individual psychotherapy with the ill child. In rare instances, family and social pathology necessitates a temporary removal of the child from his home. Such a drastic recommendation requires considerable preparation of both the child and his family. With the youngster placed in a foster home or institution, on-going work with the key family members is essential to facilitate the child's eventual return to his original setting. The field has come a long way from the old concept of "parentectomy." This involved a "cure" of the child's physical symptoms while away from home, but frequent recurrence of his symptomatology upon returning to the unchanged maladaptive home setting.

Nothing can be more rewarding to the child psychiatrist than the rehabilitation and continued guidance of a child with a psychophysiologic illness. It involves working with his nonpsychiatric colleagues and their team in a collective biopsycho-social approach. The success of such liaison work depends upon a good deal of trust and continuous communication between the mental health worker and the primary care team. In the course of this, each member recognizes his special contributions to the care of the child. Where interdisciplinary approaches to children and families with a psychophysiologic disorder function well, they present good learning opportunities for medical students and other health care trainees. The importance of such an approach was recently stressed by George Engel[44] in a thoughtful article on "The Need for a New Medical Model: A Challenge for Biomedicine." He observes that only a "biopsychosocial model provides a blueprint for research, a framework for teaching and a design for action in the real world of health care."

An interdisciplinary approach to the management of a psychophysiologic illness offers benefits to all concerned. From the beginning students to the experienced teachers, physicians must strive to comprehend sick individuals with the totality of their life situations. Each time they do this, their scientific professionalism becomes tempered with humanism. Like art and science, medicine is the richer for these endeavors. Most important of all, in the course of this effort, primary care workers, pediatric and surgical specialists, and psychiatrists direct their knowledge toward a common problem. This collaboration focuses where of necessity it began, on the multiple needs created each and every time that a child is sick.

REFERENCES

1. ADLER, A., *The Practice and Theory of Individual Psychology*, Harcourt, Brace, New York, 1924.

2. AGLE, D. P., "Psychiatric Studies of Patients with Hemophilia and Related States," *Archives of Internal Medicine, 114:*76–82, 1964.

3. ——, RATNOFF, O. D., and WASMAN, M., "Conversion Reactions in Autoerythrocyte Sensitization," *Archives of General Psychiatry, 20:*438–447, 1969.

4. ALDRICH, C. K., "A Case of Recurrent Pseudocyesis," *Perspectives in Biology and Medicine, 16:*11–21, 1972.

5. ALEXANDER, A. B., MIKLICH, D. R., and HERSHKOFF, H., "The Immediate Effects of Systematic Relaxation Training on Peak Expiratory Flow Rates in Asthmatic Children," *Psychosomatic Medicine, 34(5):*355–394, 1972.

6. ALEXANDER, F., "Preface," in Adler, A., Mortimer, J., and McGill, V. J. (Eds.), *Biology, Psychology, and Medicine*, p. V, Encyclopaedia Britannica, Chicago, 1963.

7. ——, *Psychosomatic Medicine*, W. W. Norton, New York, 1950.

8. ——, *The Medical Value of Psychoanalysis*, W. W. Norton, New York, 1936.

9. ALLBUTT, C. T., "Neuroses of the Viscera," *Lancet, 1:*601–606, 1884.

10. American Psychiatric Association, Committee on Nomenclature and Statistics, *Diagnostic and Statistical Manual of Mental Disorders*, (DSM-I), American Psychiatric Association, Washington, D.C., 1952.

11. American Psychiatric Association, Committee on Nomenclature and Statistics, *Diagnostic and Statistical Manual of Mental Disorders*, 2nd Ed. (DSM-II), American Psychiatric Association, Washington, D.C., 1968.

12. ANDERS, T. F., and WEINSTEIN, P., "Sleep and Its Disorders in Infants and Children: A Review," *Pediatrics, 50:*312–324, 1972.

13. APLEY, J., *The Child with Abdominal Pains*, Blackwell Scientific Publications, Oxford, 1975.

14. AXELROD, J., "Neurotransmitters," *Scientific American, 230:*59–71, 1974.

15. BARBER, T. X., "The Effects of 'Hypnosis' on Pain: A Critical Review of Experimental and Clinical Findings," *Psychosomatic Medicine, 25:*303–333, 1963.

16. BARGLOW, P., and BROWN, E., "Pseudocyesis to Be and Not to Be Pregnant: A Psychosomatic Question," in Howells, J. G., *Modern Perspectives in Psycho-Obstetrics*, p. 59, Brunner-Mazel, New York, 1972.

17. BARTHEZ, E., and RILLIET, F., *Traite des Maladies des Enfants*, Hagen, E. R. (trans.), p. 620, C. E. Kollman, Leipzig, 1855.

18. BATTLE, C. U., "The Role of the Pediatrician as Ombudsman in the Health Care of the Young Handicapped Child," *Pediatrics, 50:*916–922, 1972.

19. BERNARD, C., *An Introduction to the Study of Experimental Medicine*, Henry Schuman, New York, 1949.

20. BERTALANFFY, L. von, "The Unified Theory for Psychiatry and the Behavioral Sciences," in Feinstein, S. C., and Giovacchini, P. L. (Eds.), *Adolescent Psychiatry*, vol. 3, p. 45, Basic Books, New York, 1974.

21. ——, "The Mind-Body Problem: A New View," *Psychosomatic Medicine, 26:*29–45, 1964.

22. BREUER, J., and FREUD, S., "Studies on Hysteria" in *The Standard Edition of the Complete Psychological Works of Sigmund Freud*, vol. 2, Hogarth Press, London, 1968.

23. BROOK, C. G. D., LLOYD, J. K., and WOLF, O. H., "Relation Between Age of Onset of Obesity and Size and Number of Adipose Cells," *British Medical Journal, 2:*25–27, 1972.

24. BROUGHTON, R. J., "Sleep Disorders: Disorders of Arousal?" *Science, 159:*1070–1078, 1968.

25. BROWN, D. G., "Stress as a Precipitant Factor of Eczema," *Journal of Psychosomatic Research, 16:*321–327, 1972.

26. BROWN, E., and BARGLOW, P., "Pseudocyesis—A Paradigm for Psychophysiological Interactions," *Archives of General Psychiatry, 24:*221–229, 1971.

27. BULL, T., *The Maternal Management of Children in Health and Disease*, 2nd ed., pp. 246–247, Blakiston, Philalelphia, 1853.

28. CAMERON, A. L., "Surgical Aspects of Chronic Duodenal Ulcers of Childhood," *Archives of Surgery, 66:*827–845, 1953.

29. CANNON, W. B., *Bodily Changes in Pain, Hunger, Fear and Rage*, rev. ed., Appleton-Century, New York, 1929.

30. ——, "The Emergency Function of the Adrenal Medulla in Pain and the Major Emotions," *American Journal of Physiology, 33:*356–372, 1914.

31. CHARNEY, E., et al., "Childhood Antecedents of Adult Obesity," *New England Journal of Medicine, 295:*6–9, 1976.

32. CODDINGTON, R. D., and BRUCH, H., "Gastric Perception in Normal, Obese and Schizophrenic Subjects," *Psychosomatics, 11:*571–579, 1970.

33. DALSGAARD-NIELSEN, T., "Some Aspects of the Epidemiology of Migraine in Denmark," in Cochrane, A. L. (Ed.), *Background to Migraine*, Third Migraine Symposium, pp. 11–17, Springer-Verlag, New York, 1969.

34. DAVIS, M. H., et al., "Relaxation Training Facilitated by Biofeedback Apparatus as a Supplemental Treatment in Bronchial Asthma," *Journal of Psychosomatic Research, 17:*121–128, 1973.

35. DEUTSCH, F., "Thus Speaks the Body. I. An Analysis of Postural Behavior," New York Academy of Science, series 2, *12:*2, 1949.

36. ——, "Der Gesunde und Der Kranke Körper in Psychoanalytischer Betrachtung," *Internationale Zeitschrift fuer Psychoanalyse, 8:*290, 1922.

37. DiCARA, L. V., and MILLER, N. F., "Instrumental Learning of Vasomotor Responses by Rats: Learning to Respond Differentially in the Two Ears," *Science, 159:*1485–1486, 1968.

38. DODGE, J. A., "Psychosomatic Aspects of Infantile Pyloric Stenosis," *Journal of Psychosomatic Research, 16:*1–5, 1972.

39. Dreifuss, F. E., "The Differential Diagnosis of Partial Seizures with Complex Symptomatology," in Penry, J. K., and Daly, D. (Eds.), *Advances in Neurology*, vol. II, chapter 22, Raven Press, New York, 1975.

40. Dubo, S., et al., "A Study of Relationships Between Family Situation, Bronchial Asthma, and Personal Adjustment in Children," *Journal of Pediatrics, 59:*402–414, 1961.

41. Dunbar, F., *Psychosomatic Diagnosis*, Hoeber, New York, 1943.

42. ———, *Emotions and Bodily Changes*, Columbia University Press, New York, 1935.

43. Early, L. F., and Lifschutz, J. E., "A Case of Stigmata," *Archives of General Psychiatry, 30:*197–200, 1974.

44. Engel, G. L., "The Need for a New Medical Model: A Challenge for Biomedicine," *Science, 196:* 129–135, 1977.

45. ———, "A Reconsideration of the Role of Conversion in Somatic Disease," *Comprehensive Psychiatry, 9:* 316–326, 1968.

46. ———, and Reichsman, F., "Spontaneous and Experimentally Induced Depressions in an Infant with a Gastric Fistula," *Journal of the American Psychoanalytic Association, 4:*428–452, 1956.

47. ———, and Segal, H. L., "A Study of an Infant with a Gastric Fistula," *Psychosomatic Medicine, 18:*374–398, 1956.

48. Eppinger, H., and Hess, L., "Zur Pathologie Des Vegetativen Nervensystems," *Zeitschrift Für Klinische Medizin, 66:*345–351; and *68:*205–230, 1909.

49. Esman, A. H., "Nocturnal Enuresis: Some Current Concepts," *Journal of the American Academy of Child Psychiatry, 16:*150–158, 1977.

50. Fenz, W. D., "Strategies for Coping with Stress," in Sarason, I. G., and Spielberger, C. D. (Eds.), *Stress and Anxiety*, vol. 2, pp. 305–317, John Wiley, New York, 1975.

51. Flanagan, C. H., "Rumination in Infancy—Past and Present," *Journal of the American Academy of Child Psychiatry, 16:*140–149, 1977.

52. Frankenhaeuser, M., and Johansson, G., "Behavior and Catecholamines in Children," in Levi, L. (ed.), *Society, Stress and Disease*, vol. 2, pp. 118–126, Oxford University Press, London, 1975.

53. Freud, A., *The Psycho-Analytical Treatment of Children*, pp. 40–42, Imago, London, 1946.

54. Fried, R. I., "Socio-Emotional Factors Accounting for Growth Failure in Children as Measured by the Wetzel Grid," in *Life Stress and Bodily Disease*, Williams & Wilkins, Baltimore, Md., 1950.

55. Friedman, S. B., and Glasgow, L. A., "Psychologic Factors and Resistance to Infectious Disease," *Pediatric Clinics of North America, 13:*315–335, 1966.

56. Galdston, I., *Psychiatry and the Human Condition*, pp. 128–142, Brunner-Mazel, New York, 1976.

57. Gee, S., "On Fitful or Recurrent Vomiting," *Saint Bartholomew's Hospital Reports, 18:*1–6, 1882.

58. Geist, H., *The Psychological Aspects of Rheumatoid Arthritis*, p. 82, Charles C Thomas, Springfield, Ill., 1966.

59. Geltzer, A. I., et al., "Familial Dysautonomia: Studies in a Newborn Infant," *New England Journal of Medicine, 271:*436–440, 1964.

60. Goldberg, H. M., "Duodenal Ulcers in Children," *British Medical Journal*, June 29: 1500–1502, 1957.

61. Grinker, R. R., *Psychosomatic Research*, pp. 31–33, W. W. Norton, New York, 1953.

62. Grodin, J., "Secondary Amenorrhea in The Adolescent," *Pediatric Clinics of North America, 19:* 619–630, 1972.

63. Group for the Advancement of Psychiatry, Committee on Child Psychiatry, *Psychopathological Disorders in Childhood: Theoretical Considerations and a Proposed Classification*, vol. 4, Report No. 62, Group for the Advancement of Psychiatry, New York, 1966.

64. Hammond, J., "The Late Sequelae of Recurrent Vomiting of Childhood," *Developmental Medicine and Child Neurology, 16:*15–22, 1974.

65. Harrison, M. S., and Naftalin, L., *Meniere's Disease Mechanism and Management*, p. 13, Charles C Thomas, Springfield, Ill., 1968.

66. Helmholz, H. F., "Chronic Ulcerative Colitis in Childhood," *American Journal of Disease in Children, 26:*418–430, 1923.

67. Hess, E. H., "Attitude and Pupil Size," *Scientific American, 212:*46–54, 1965.

68. Holter, F., and Burgoon, C. F., Jr., "Psychologic Considerations of the Skin in Childhood," in Burgoon, C. F., Jr. (Consulting Ed.), *Symposium on Pediatric Dermatology*, p. 722, Pediatric Clinics of North America, W. B. Saunders, Philadelphia, 1961.

69. Hoople, G., "A Neglected Subject," *Laryngoscope, 76:*1312–1317, 1966.

70. Inman, W. S., "Styes, Barley and Wedding Rings," *British Journal of Medical Psychology, 20:*331–338, 1965.

71. ———, "Emotional Factors in Diseases of the Cornea," *British Journal of Medical Psychology, 38:*277–287, 1965.

72. ———, "The Emotional Factor in Causation of Diseases of the Eyelids," *Medical Press, 196:*96–99, 1938.

73. Ironside, W., "Eczema, Darkly Mirror of the Mind," *Australian Journal of Dermatology, 15:*5–9, 1974.

74. Johnson, M. L., Burke, B. S., and Mayer, J., "The Prevalence and Incidence of Obesity in a Cross-Section of Elementary and Secondary School Children," *American Journal of Clinical Nutrition, 4:*231–238, 1956.

75. Kagan, J., "The Distribution of Attention in Infancy," in Hamburg, D. A., et al. (Eds.), *Perception and Its Disorders*, Research Publications, Association for Research in Nervous and Mental Disease, vol. 48, p. 216, Williams & Wilkins, Baltimore, Md., 1970.

76. Kalthoff, H., "Psychogene Amblyopie Bei Kindern," *Medizinische Monatsschrift, 22:*255–258, 1968.

77. Kanner, L., *Child Psychiatry*, pp. 377, Charles C Thomas, Springfield Ill., 1972.

78. Katan, A., "Some Thoughts About the Role of Verbalization in Early Childhood," in Eissler, R. S., et al. (Eds.), *Psychoanalytic Study of the Child*, vol. 16, pp. 184–188, International Universities Press, New York, 1961.

79. Keegan, D. L., "Psychosomatics: Toward An Understanding of Cardiovascular Disorders," *Psychosomatics, 14:*321–325, 1973.

80. Khan, A. U., "Present Status of Psychosomatic Aspects of Asthma," *Psychosomatics, 14:*195–200, 1973.

81. ———, Staerk, M., and Bonk, C., "Role of Counter-Conditioning in the Treatment of Asthma," *Journal of Psychosomatic Research, 18:*89–92, 1974.

82. Kilcoyne, M. M., "Adolescent Hypertension," *The American Journal of Medicine, 58:*735–739, 1975.

83. Kleitman, N., "Development of Circadian Rhythm in the Infant," in Fomon, S. J. (Ed.), *Circadian Systems: Report of the Thirty-Ninth Ross Conference on Pediatric Research*, pp. 35–37, Ross Laboratories, Columbus, Ohio, 1961.

84. Knowles, F., "Twenty Years of Neurosecretion," in Knowles, F., and Vollrath, L. (Eds.), *Neurosecretion—The Final Neurendocrine Pathway*, pp. 3–11, Springer-Verlag, New York, 1974.

85. Krovetz, J. L., Gessner, I. H., and Schieber, G. L., *Handbook of Pediatric Cardiology*, pp. 9–10, Hoeber, Hagerstown, Md., 1969.

86. Lefkowitz, R. J., "B-Adrenergic Receptors: Recognition and Regulation," *New England Journal of Medicine, 295:*325–328, 1976.

87. Lester, B., cited in Luce, G. G., *Biological Rhythms in Psychiatry and Medicine*, p. 37, U.S. Department of Health, Education, and Welfare, National Institute of Mental Health, U.S. Government Printing Office, Washington, D.C., 1970.

88. LEVENTON, G., et al., "Isolated Psychogenic Palatal Myoclonus as a Cause of Objective Tinnitus," *Acta Oto-Laryngologica, 65*:391–396, 1968.

89. LEVI-MONTALCINI, R., "Nerve-Growth Factor in Familial Dysautonomia," *The New England Journal of Medicine, 295*:671–672, 1976.

90. LIPTON, E. L., and STEINSCHNEIGER, A., "Studies on the Psychophysiology of Infants," in Sigel, I. E. (Ed.), *Selected Papers on Current Research in Infant Development, Merrill-Palmer Quarterly, 10*:103–117, 1964.

91. LIVINGSTON, S., *Comprehensive Management of Epilepsy in Infancy, Childhood and Adolescence*, pp. 52–55, Charles C Thomas, Springfield, Ill., 1972.

92. LUCE, G. G., *Biological Rhythms in Psychiatry and Medicine*, Public Health Service Publication No. 2088, p. 37, National Institute of Mental Health, Chevy Chase, Md., 1970.

93. LUCENTE, F. E., "Psychiatric Problems in Otolaryngology," *Annals of Otology, Rhinology, and Laryngology, 82*:340–346, 1973.

94. McANARNEY, E. R., "Psychological Problems of Children with Chronic Juvenile Arthritis," *Pediatrics, 53*:523–528, 1974.

95. McDERMOTT, J. F., JR., and FINCH, S. M., "Ulcerating Colitis in Children, Reassessment of A Dilemma," *Journal of the American Academy of Child Psychiatry, 6*:512–525, 1967.

96. McKENDRY, J. B. J., and STEWART, O. A., "Enuresis," *Pediatric Clinics of North America, 21*:1019–1028, 1974.

97. McLEAN, A. F., "Hypnosis in 'Psychosomatic' Illness," *British Journal of Medical Psychology, 38*:211–230, 1965.

98. McLEAN, J. A., and CHING, A. Y. T., "Follow-up Study of Relationships Between Family Situation and Bronchial Asthma in Children," *Journal of the American Academy of Child Psychiatry, 12*:142–161, 1973.

99. McNICHOL, K. N., et al., "Spectrum of Asthma in Children—III, Psychological and Social Components," *British Medical Journal, 4*:16–20, 1973.

100. MASON, J. W., "Strategy in Psychosomatic Research," *Psychosomatic Medicine, 32(4)*:427–439, 1970.

101. MATTSSON, A., "Psychologic Aspects of Childhood Asthma," *Pediatric Clinics of North America, 22(1)*:77–88, 1975.

102. ———, "Psychophysiological Study of Bleeding and Adaptation in Young Hemophiliacs," in Anthony, E. J. (Ed.), *Explorations in Child Psychiatry*, pp. 227–246, Plenum Press, New York, 1975.

103. ———, "Long-Term Physical Illness in Children: A Challenge to Psychosocial Adaptation," *Pediatrics, 50*:801–811, 1972.

104. ———, and GROSS, S., "Social and Behavioral Studies on Hemophilic Children and Their Families", *Journal of Pediatrics, 68*:952–964, 1966.

105. MAYER, J., "Genetic, Traumatic and Environmental Factors in the Etiology of Obesity," *Physiological Review, 33*:472–508, 1953.

106. MEERLOO, J. A. M., "Human Camouflage and Identification with the Environment," *Psychosomatic Medicine, 19*:89–98, 1957.

107. MEIGS, J. F., *Practical Treatise on the Diseases of Children*, pp. 417–448, Lindsay & Blakiston, Philadelphia, 1848.

108. MERSKY, H., "On the Development of Pain," *Headache, 10*:116–123, 1970.

109. MIDDLETON, E., "Autonomic Imbalance in Asthma with Special Reference to Beta Adrenergic Blockade," *Advances in Internal Medicine, 18*:117–197, 1972.

110. MILLS, J. N., "Development of Circadian Rhythms in Infancy," *Chronobiologia, 2*:363–371, 1975.

111. MINUCHIN, S., et al., "A Conceptual Model of Psychosomatic Illness in Children," *Archives of General Psychiatry, 32*:1021–1038, 1975.

112. NELSON, H. S., "The Beta Adrenergic Theory of Bronchial Asthma," *Pediatric Clinics of North America, 22(1)*:53–61, 1975.

113. NEMIAH, J. C., "Conversion Reaction," in Freedman, A. M., and Kaplan, H. I. (Eds.), *Comprehensive Textbook of Psychiatry*, pp. 870–885, Williams & Wilkins, Baltimore, Md., 1967.

114. NORINS, A. L., "Atopic Dermatitis," in *Symposium on Pediatric Dermatology*, p. 803, Pediatric Clinics of North America, W. B. Saunders, Philadelphia, 1971.

115. OLDHAM, P. D., et al., "The Nature of Essential Hypertension," *Lancet, 1*:1085–1093, May 1960.

116. PAUL, G. L., "The Production of Blisters by Hypnotic Suggestion: Another Look," *Psychosomatic Medicine, 25*:233–244, 1963.

117. PAZDRAL, P. T., "Awareness of Pediatric Hypertension," *Journal of the American Medical Association, 235*:2320–2322, 1976.

118. PINKERTON, P., "Childhood Asthma," *British Journal of Hospital Medicine, 6*:331–338, 1971.

119. ———, "Psychogenic Megacolon in Children: The Implications of Bowel Negativism," *Archives of Disease in Childhood, 33*:371–380, 1958.

120. PLATT, J. W., SCHLESINGER, B. E., and BENSON, P. F., "Ulcerative Colitis in Childhood, A Study of Its Natural History," *Quarterly Journal of Medicine, 29*:257–277, 1960.

121. PLESS, J. B., "Teaching of Chronic Illness in Childhood and Adolescence," in Clark, D. W., and Williams, T. E. (Eds.), *Teaching of Chronic Illness and Aging*, p. 71, Department of Health, Education, and Welfare, Publication No. 75–876, National Institute of Health, U.S. Government Printing Office, Washington, D.C., 1973.

122. POWELL, G. F., BRASEL, S. A., and BLIZZARD, R. M., "Emotional Deprivation and Growth Retardation, Simulating Idiopathic Hypopituitarism. I. Clinical Evaluation of the Syndrome. II. Endocrinologic Evaluation of the Syndrome," *New England Journal of Medicine, 276*:1271–1283, 1967.

123. PROVENCE, S., and LIPTON, R. C., *Infants in Institutions*, International Universities Press, New York, 1962.

124. PULEC, J. L. (Ed.), "Symposium on Ménière's Disease," *Otolaryngologic Clinics of North America*, pp. 715, W. B. Saunders, Philadelphia, 1968.

125. PURCELL, K., and WEISS, J. H., "Asthma," in Costell, C. G. (Ed.), *Symptoms of Psychopathology*, pp. 597–623, John Wiley, New York, 1970.

126. PURCELL, K., et al., "The Effect of Asthma in Children on Experimental Separation from the Family," *Psychosomatic Medicine, 31*:144–164, 1969.

127. RATNOFF, O. D., and AGLE, D. P., "Psychogenic Purpura: A Re-Evaluation of the Syndrome of Auto-erythrocyte Sensitization," *Medicine, 47(8)*:475–500, 1968.

128. RAVELLI, G. P., "Obesity in Young Men After Famine Exposure in Utero and Early Infancy," *The New England Journal of Medicine, 295*:249–353, 1976.

129. REES, W. L., "Psychiatric and Psychological Aspects of Migraine," in Cumings, J. N. (Ed.), *Background to Migraine*, p. 53, Fourth Migraine Symposium, Springer-Verlag, New York, 1970.

130. REINHART, J. B., EVANS, S. L., and McFADDEN, D. L., "Cyclic Vomiting in Children: Seen Through the Psychiatrist's Eye," *Pediatrics, 59*:371–377, 1977.

131. RILEY, C. M., and MOORE, R. H., "Familial Dysautonomia Differentiated From Related Disorders," *Pediatrics, 37*:435–446, 1966.

132. RILEY, C. M., et al., "Central Autonomic Dysfunction with Defective Lacrimation," *Pediatrics, 3*:468–478, 1949.

133. ROBB, J. H., and ROSE, B. S., "Rheumatoid Arthritis and Maternal Deprivation: A Case Study in the Use of a Social Survey," *British Journal of Medical Psychology, 38*:147–159, 1965.

134. ROBINSON, H., KIRK, R. F., JR., and FRYE, R. L.,

"A Psychological Study of Rheumatoid Arthritis and Selected Disease," *Journal of Chronic Disease, 23:*791–801, 1971.

135. RODIN, E. A., "Psychosocial Management of Patients with Complex Partial Seizures," in Penry, J. K., and Daly, D. (Ed.), *Advances in Neurology*, vol. 2, chapter 9, Raven Press, New York, 1975.

136. RUBIN, L., BARBERO, G., and SIBINGA, M. S., "Pupillary Reactivity in Children with Recurrent Abdominal Pain," *Psychosomatic Medicine, 29:*111–120, 1967.

137. RUTENFRANZ, J., "The Development of Circadian System Functions During Infancy and Childhood," in Fomon, S. J. (Ed.), *Circadian Systems: Report of the Thirty-Ninth Ross Conference on Pediatric Research*, pp. 38–41, Ross Laboratories, Columbus, Ohio, 1961.

138. SALK, L., "The Importance of the Heartbeat Rhythm to Human Nature: Theoretical, Clinical, and Experimental Observations," in *World Congress of Psychiatry* (3rd), Proceedings vol. 1., pp. 740–746, University of Toronto Press, Montreal, 1961.

139. SCHACTER, S., "Obesity and Eating," *Science, 161:* 751–756, 1968.

140. SCHLAEGEL, T. F., "Psychosomatics: The Second Face of Ophthalmology," in Gordon, D. M. (Ed.), *The Eye in Systemic Disease, II*, pp. 409–485, International Ophthalmology Clinics, vol. 8, no. 2, Little, Brown, Boston, 1968.

141. ——, and SEITZ, P. F. D., "Age and Sex in Eye Injuries of Children," *Psychosomatic Medicine, 15:*349–353, 1953.

142. SELZER, J. G., "Pseudocyesis in a Six-Year-Old Girl," *Journal of the American Academy of Child Psychiatry, 7:*693–720, 1968.

143. SIGGERS, D. C., et al., "Increased Nerve-Growth-Factor B-Chain Cross-Reacting Material in Familial Dysautonomia," *The New England Journal of Medicine, 295:*629, 1976.

144. SLOAN, D., "Pelvic Pain and Dysmenorrhea," *Pediatric Clinics of North America, 19:*669–680, 1972.

145. SPITZ, R. A., "Hospitalism, An Inquiry into the Genesis of Psychiatric Conditions in Early Childhood," in Eissler, R. S., et al. (Eds.), *The Psychoanalytic Study of the Child*, vol. 1, pp. 53–74, International Universities Press, New York, 1945.

146. STAMIER, J., "Hypertension Screening of One Million Americans," *Journal of the American Medical Association, 235:*2299–2306, 1976.

147. STUNKARD, A. J., and WOLFF, H. G., "Pathogenesis in Human Obesity," *Psychosomatic Medicine, 20:*17–29, 1958.

148. SULTZ, H. A., et al., "The Epidemiology of Peptic Ulcer in Childhood," *American Journal of Public Health, 60:*492–498, 1970.

149. TABOROFF, L. H., and BROWN, W. H., "A Study of the Personality Patterns of Children and Adolescents with the Peptic Ulcer Syndrome," *American Journal of Orthopsychiatry, 24:*602–610, 1954.

150. TENNES, K., and CARTER, D., "Plasma Cortisol Levels and Behavioral State in Early Infancy," *Psychosomatic Medicine, 35(2):*121–128, 1973.

151. TOOHILL, R. J., "The Psychosomatic Aspects of Children with Vocal Nodules," *Archives of Otolaryngology, 101:*591–595, 1975.

152. TSTELIN, M. L., *Automation Theory and Modeling of Biological Systems*, pp. 131–132, Academic Press, New York, 1973.

153. VAUGHAN, V. C., III, McKAY, R. J., and NELSON, W. E., *Nelson Textbook of Pediatrics*, 10th ed., p. 180, W. B. Saunders, Philadelphia, 1975.

154. WAGGONER, P. E., "Idols of the Model or Bringing Home the Bacon," in Vernberg, J. F. (Ed.), *Physiological Adaptation to the Environment*, pp. 547–557, Text Education Publishers, New York, 1975.

155. WENGER, M. A., and BAGCHI, B. K., "Studies of Autonomic Functions in Practitioners of Yoga in India," *Behavioral Science, 6:*312–323, 1961.

156. ——, and ANAND, B. K., "Experiments in India on 'Voluntary' Control of the Heart and Pulse," *Circulation, 24:*1319–1325, 161.

157. WHITE, P. J., "The Relation Between Colic and Eczema in Early Infancy," *American Journal of Diseases of Children, 38:*935–942, 1929.

158. WIENER, N., *Cybernetics or Control and Communication in the Animal and the Machine*, 2nd Ed., p. 11, Massachusetts Institute of Technology Press, Cambridge, Mass., 1961.

159. WILE, I. S., "Physio-Pathology in Child Guidance," in Harms, E. (Ed.), *Handbook of Child Guidance*, p. 153, Child Care Publications, New York, 1947.

160. WILLIAMSON, O. G., and GIFFORD, F., "Psychosomatic Aspects of Ménière's Disease," *Acta Oto-Laryngology, 72:*118–120, 1971.

161. WINNICOTT, D. W., "Symptom Tolerance in Paediatrics," *Proceedings of the Royal Society of Medicine, 46:*675–684, 1953.

162. WITTKOWER, E. D., and HUNT, B. R., "Psychological Aspects of Atopic Dermatitis in Children," *Canadian Medical Association Journal*, pp. 810–817, Nov. 15, 1958.

163. WOLF, S., and GLASS, G. B. J., "Correlation of Conscious and Unconscious Conflicts with Changes in Gastric Function and Structure. Observations on the Relation of the Constituents of Gastric Juice to the Integrity of the Mucous Membrane," in *Life Stress and Bodily Disease*, pp. 665–676, Williams & Wilkins, Baltimore, Md., 1950.

164. WOLFF, H. G., *Headache and Other Head Pains*, p. 255, Oxford University Press, New York, 1948.

165. WOLFF, O. H., and LLOYD, J. K., "Childhood Obesity," *Proceedings of the Nutrition Society, 32:*195–198, 1973.

166. YATES, E. F., "On the Mathematical Modeling of Biological Systems: A Qualified 'Pro,'" in Vernberg, J. R. (Ed.), *Physiological Adaptation to the Environment*, pp. 539–546, Text Education Publishers, New York, 1975.

18 / Acute and Chronic Brain Syndromes

Maurice W. Laufer and Taranath Shetty

In clinical syndromes suggesting nervous system involvement, one may not always be able to find evidence for structural or biochemical alterations in the neurons, their processes, or the supporting and surrounding cells. A separation of "functional" syndromes from "organic" syndromes by clinical methods is often difficult; some degree of overlap seems invariably to exist.

During the past few years, more and more experimental evidence has been brought forth showing that biochemical alterations in the brain are often present in schizophrenic syndromes as well as in affective disorders. However, it is not known whether these biochemical findings have etiological significance or are epiphenomena. If future research proves these biochemical differences are primary and causative, future editions of this section would have to include a large number of psychiatric syndromes, so far not marshalled under the rubric: organic brain syndromes.

The DSM-II defines "Organic Brain Syndromes" as "Disorders caused by or associated with impairment of brain tissue function."[5] Impairment or alteration of cerebral function often leads to certain characteristic clinical phenomena which, when they occur as a group, help in distinguishing the "organic brain syndromes" from the wide variety of patients referred for psychiatric care. The clinical manifestations of this group of disorders are these:

1. Impairment of orientation to time, place, and person.
2. Impairment of remote as well as recent memory. Confabulation may ensue as a secondary phenomenon.
3. Decreased attention—this can be discerned by testing digit span. Secondary confusion may be present.
4. Impaired ability to manipulate and abstract acquired knowledge—this can be ascertained by testing calculation and ability to interpret proverbs.
5. Impairment of judgment and insight.
6. Impairment of speech and praxis.
7. Impaired ability in construction (figure drawing).
8. Lability and shallowness of affect.

If, in addition, a physical examination provides evidence for alteration of any motor, sensory, or coordinating functions, it becomes easier to make the diagnosis.

There may be alterations from normality in ancillary studies. There are many. They include the skull x-ray, electroencephalogram, ventriculogram, echogram, radiologic and isotope studies, computerized axial tomography, as well as changes in spinal fluid chemistry or dynamics. Any abnormalities of this kind help confirm the organic nature of the clinical syndrome.

However, they too have their "grey" areas. There is a good deal of uncertainty about whether "soft" neurological signs, nonspecific EEG abnormalities, and a history of perinatal abnormality (all of which may be found in association with certain types of child psychiatric disorders) can be equated with structural or functional brain disease, and, if they can, whether the relationship is a causal one.

The GAP classification[48] notes that while organic brain syndromes are produced by diffuse impairment of brain tissue, particularly in the cerebral cortex, and are characterized by impairment of orientation, judgment, discriminations, learning, memory, and other cognitive functions; associated personality disturbances are common. There may be manifestations of psychosis, neurotic symptoms, or disturbances in behavior. They further note that these associated disorders are not necessarily proportionate in severity to the degree of the brain tissue dysfunction or the degree of brain damage. Instead they may vary with the predisposing personality patterns, current emotional conflicts, the child's level of development, the character of familial interpersonal relationships, as much as with the nature of the precipitating brain disorder. The meaning of the dysfunction to child and parents introduces a further important factor. The GAP classification notes too that artificial separation between totally organic and completely functional problems in this area are particularly inappropriate, conceptually as well as clinically. In a growing brain, compensation can follow after an insult; or, there may be interference with as yet undeveloped cognitive functions.

The terms "acute" and "chronic" refer primarily to reversibility of brain pathology and to the accompanying brain syndromes. The same etiology may produce either temporary or permanent brain damage. However, a brain disorder which initially appears acute, and hence reversible, may later prove to be a chronic brain syndrome with permanent damage.

Acute Brain Syndromes

The GAP classification notes:

Under the heading should be classified those types of acute brain disorders associated with intracranial infection, systemic infection, drug or poison intoxication, alcohol intoxication, trauma, circulatory disturbances, certain types of convulsive disorder, metabolic disturbances, and certain disorders of unknown etiology.[48]

In general, these disorders produce a delirium characterized by agitated or confused behavior and altered sensory experiences; the latter illusions arising from misperception of stimuli in the environment or true hallucinations. Such disturbances may also be subclinical, with subtle shifts in awareness, mildly stuporous states, withdrawn behavior, or irrational fears. Even in the absence of persistent brain damage, after apparent clinical recovery, perceptual motor difficulties may persist for some time. This may render the child more vulnerable to learning difficulties. Where preexisting or underlying psychotic, psychoneurotic, or personality disorders have been present, they may become more manifest after such insults to the central nervous system. Reactive disorders or later developmental deviations may follow from the insult as indeed they may from any traumatic sequence.

DELIRIUM

Delirium is a toxic confusional state, often transitory, and commonly occuring during the peak of a febrile episode in childhood.

DSM-II (294:2) says of "Psychosis with Systemic Infection:"

This category includes disorders caused by severe general systemic infections such as pneumonia, typhoid fever, malaria and acute rheumatic fever. Care must be taken to distinguish these reactions from other disorders, particularly manic depressive illness and schizophrenia which may be precipitated by even a mild attack of infectious disease. (p. 30)[48]

The child with delirium manifests altered consciousness, inappropriate behavior, partial or total lack of orientation, attention deficit, impaired ability to lay down new memories, and disturbed recognition, along with visual and auditory illusions and hallucinations. While fever is the most common cause of this state in children, a similar clinical picture is seen at times after head trauma. It is also encountered in children waking up from anesthesia (particularly when ketamine is the anesthetic) and in adolescents after drug abuse.

Dementia is differentiated from delirium by the fact that it presents a decline in intellectual powers without accessory symptoms such as impairment of consciousness, hallucinations, or disorientation. Further, delirium has an acute onset and is reversible.

Mild to moderate generalized EEG slowing accompanies delirium and is reversible, as the underlying condition resolves. It helps in differential diagnosis from focal brain disease which may present initially as a delirous state, or from hysterical fugue states.[76, 88]

No structural or biochemical alteration has been demonstrated within the brain during a febrile delirium. The most likely explanation seems to be a transient derangement of neuronal function secondary to the "toxic" state. The nature of this derangement remains to be elucidated.

Therapy consists of treatment of the basic infection, a lighted room, avoidance of unnecessary stimulation, and mild chemical sedation.

EPILEPTIC DELIRIUM

The clinical picture has the usual characteristics of a delirium—a hallucinatory confusional state with an altered level of consciousness. The patients are often active, hypomanic with acceleration of their thought processes; delusions are seen, often ecstatic or expansive in type, and compulsive behavior. Landolt[63] observed a diminution or disappearance of the epileptic EEG activity during these episodes and termed the phenomenon "forced normalization." The notorious "furor epilepticus," described by Ey,[28] can properly be included with epileptic delirium. During this state, murders may sometimes be committed.

Epileptic delirium requires differentiation from night terrors (pavor nocturnus). These are more common in preschool children than in older children and adults. These occur after the individual has been sleeping. The child suddenly sits up in bed, stares, screams in apparent terror, has physiological concomitants appropriate to this, such as extreme tachycardia. The child may be disoriented, show sleep walking and sleep talking, is hard to get back to sleep, and is usually amnesic for the attack on next waking.

EEG studies generally do not show consistent or significant abnormalities between episodes, but the sleep polygraph reveals that the attack itself is a disorder of arousal. It occurs when the sleeper is coming out of deep NREM sleep ("slow wave sleep," "delta sleep," "Stage ¾ sleep") toward Stages 2 and 1 and REM sleep. These episodes apparently may be triggered by external stimuli or by internal psychic conflict. If severe and frequent, they may respond to the use of diazepam.

Differentiation is aided by the fact that the delirium occurs in patients with epilepsy, whose EEG's are apt to show characteristic abnormalities, and in whom the episodes are not always associated with sleep.

Instructive discussions are provided by Anders and Weinstein[6] and by Fisher and associates.[31]

STATES OF DRUG OR POISON INTOXICTAION

DSM-II (294:3)—An organic brain syndrome due to past or current "drug" abuse is currently all too common in the adolescent of either sex. In this group the incidence of drug abuse has exceeded alcoholic intoxication. This subject is dealt with in greater detail in chapter 33 of this volume.

The acute picture differs with the kind of drug used, with age, and with previous experiences with these drugs. The usual acute picture consists of restlessness, confusion, lethargy, and visual hallucinations. Users who develop the chronic syndrome display intellectual deterioration with impairment of orientation and memory.

Marijuana: Brief use of cannabis is widespread in the teenage population. The most common effect is a "dreamy" state with euphoria, hilarity, and a feeling of well being. Memory and judgment tend to be impaired and speech is rapid. Impulsive behavior, eccentric responses, and disturbed perception are common. Higher doses may produce hallucinations and delusions. The issue of whether or not chronic marijuana use produces permanent effects on the brain remains controversial. In experienced drug users the feeling of being "high" is correlated with increases in alpha rhythms and decreases in beta rhythms in the EEG.[106]

Amphetamines: These are usually taken orally but may be taken intravenously. A similarity between amphetamine psychosis and acute paranoid schizophrenia has recently been shown.[100] The amphetamines may cause two possible types of psychotic reaction in nonpsychotic individuals. There are both "normal" (nonspecific) toxic psychosis (usually delirious) and a "genuine" (specific) amphetamine-induced psychosis: a paranoid syndrome with ideas of reference, auditory hallucinations, paranoid delirium, and no clouding of consciousness (in some cases consciousness may be even unusually clear). This type occurs after administration of large parenteral doses of amphetamine. There are three indications that dopaminergic hyperstimulation plays a role in this.

1. Agents blocking dopaminergic transmission (neuroleptics) produce a favorable effect, remarkably quickly, in amphetamine induced psychosis.[25]

2. L-amphetamine and d-amphetamine are equally effective in their ability to provoke psychosis.

3. Cocaine can provoke a psychosis that closely resembles a "genuine" amphetamine induced psychosis. It is possible that both result from similar mechanisms, because cocaine, too, increases central dopaminergic action by inhibiting reuptake of catecholamines.

The Hallucinogens (LSD and Mescaline): The effects usually last eight to twelve hours. Visual and auditory hallucinations are basic parts of the experience along with distortions of perception and body image. The mechanism of action again most probably involves alteration of dopaminergic systems within the brain. LSD has been shown to be a dopamine agonist in low doses and to block dopamine receptors in high doses. A little understood sequelum is the periodic recurrence ("flashback") of subjective aspects of the drug experience during abstinent periods for as long as three years afterwards. A psychotic reaction may develop after drug use.[55] A transient rise in serum creatine phosphokinase has been shown in psychosis produced by LSD.[52] However, a rise in spinal fluid creatine kinase in 30 percent of patients with acute evolution of all forms of psychosis has been also shown.[104]

Opiates: The clinical syndromes of intoxication consist of obtundation, decreased physiologic and psychologic "drive," and a sense of inner well being. Clinically, the usual features of intoxication are lethargy, flushing, itching, constricted pupils, decreased rate and depth of respiration, decreased blood pressure, temperature, and slow pulse. Physical dependence and abstinence syndromes occur.[69]

Initial treatment of the acute intoxication requires hospitalization and supportive care; in some cases substitution drugs are appropriate. Definitive treatment consists of identifying the psychologic disturbances and providing long term follow up and rehabilitation.

Sedative Type: Barbiturates are commonly abused. The intoxication syndrome consists of feelings of relaxation and euphoria, increasing dysarthria and ataxia, and decreasing mental alertness.

Intoxication Inhalants: Gasoline and "Airplane Glue" may be inhaled by children for their intoxicating effect. A motor polyneuropathy has recently been described in "glue sniffers"—the main toxin has been identified to be N-Hexane.[44]

NARCOTIC WITHDRAWAL SYNDROME

An acute organic brain syndrome often seen in newborns is the narcotic withdrawal syndrome. The classical syndrome seen when the mother has abused narcotics during pregnancy is also seen when the mother has been on a substitution drug such as methadone. The manifestation of withdrawal in the infant, untreated, are similar to those of the "cold-turkey" treatment of the adult. Marked tremors, irritability, hypertonicity, vomiting, high pitched cry, respiratory distress, and fever are the most frequent signs. Severe cases may go on to myoclonic twitching, seizures, and even death. Methadone addiction in mother produces more severe withdrawal reaction in the infant than heroin. Drugs used in treatment have been chlorpromazine, paregoric, phenobarbital, and diazepam. Chlorpromazine is generally considered to be the most efficient drug available. The effective dosage is 2.2 mg per kilogram bodyweight per twenty-four hours, given in four divided doses either by mouth or by injection. As the symptoms decrease, dosage is gradually tapered and discontinued. Phenobarbital is also effective in reducing symptoms but does not suppress vomiting. No prolonged follow up of these infants has, as yet, been done.[115]

Adverse Neurological Reactions to Medical Treatment

DSM-II (309:1)—Nonpsychotic organic brain syndrome with drug, poison, or systemic intoxication: Several drugs used in medical therapy can produce side effects referable to the neural system.

Diphenylhydantoin, a very commonly used anticonvulsant may at times produce psychologic aberrations in the absence of clinical neurotoxicity and even when the serum levels are in the accepted therapeutic range of 10 to 20 micrograms per ml.[110] A progressive encephalopathy has been also described as secondary to diphenylhydantoin. On discontinuing therapy, the encephalopathy stops progressing and in 50 percent, repairs itself entirely. In addition to cerebellar signs, there is also a dementia, which may even be severe enough to warrant an otherwise normally intellectual child being admitted to an institution for the mentally retarded.[105] When toxic blood levels are present, diphenylhydantoin can produce asterixis and multifocal myoclonus[78] and sometimes choreoathetosis.[70] Epileptics who display psychomotor slowing, intellectual deterioration, new or increased psychiatric illness or personality changes often have higher diphenlhydantoin and/or phenobarbital levels than those without such symptoms. It seems likely that these mental changes are related to elevated anticonvulsant levels; this is particularly so in brain damaged, mentally retarded patients.[87]

Clonazepam, a new anticonvulsant for refractory petit mal seizures, produces undesirable side effects in 50 percent of patients. These are: irritability, irrational, antisocial behavior, and outbursts of aggressive rage.[15] Behavioral side effects in children due to primidone (Mysoline) and the exacerbation or precipitation of the hyperkinetic reaction of childhood by phenobarbital are well known.

Ethosuccinimide, the most effective anticonvulsant for treatment of petit mal, may produce feelings of anxiety, insomnia, hallucinations, lassitude and mild paranoid symptoms. The state of consciousness varies from normality to mental confusion. It is speculated that this is in some way associated with reduction of epileptic EEG activity and equivalent to the "forced normalization" postulated for "epileptic delirium."[32]

Treatment of schizophrenia with psychotropic drugs and anticholinergic, antiparkinsonian drugs may produce a "central anticholinergic syndrome." This consists of hallucinations, anxiety, short term memory loss, disorientation, and agitation. This syndrome is identified by dramatic improvement with intramuscular physostigmine.[27] Similarly, physostigmine can reverse tricyclic antidepressant induced coma, choreoathetosis and myoclonus.[17, 99] Methyldopa, even in "normal" dosage, can cause difficulty in concentration and amnesia-like episodes; this is quickly reversed when the drug is withdrawn.[1] Methyldopa is also known to intensify schizophrenia and may sometimes induce a psychosis. Acute psychosis associated with massive steroid therapy is also well known.

Neuroleptic drugs like phenothiazines and butyrophenones may produce several differing neurologic syndromes, which most likely are determined by the state of the dopaminergic receptors in the striatum. The commonest clinical picture is one of akinesia or bradykinesia, with mental apathy. The syndrome of akathisia (motor restlessness and insomnia) is less common. Phenothiazines are commonly employed by the practicing pediatrician in the treatment of a variety of illnesses characterized by vomiting. In some children, even a simple dose can produce a dramatic dystonia and/or oeulogyric crises. The picture is so dramatic that tetanus is sometimes suspected. This form of dystonia is always reversible, and testing the urine for phenothiazines makes diagnosis easy. Treatment consists of withdrawal of drug and parenteral injection of an anticholinergic drug like diphenylhydramine hydrochloride. Tardive dyskinesias persist for many years after cessation of the drug therapy and are probably secondary to permanent injury and hypersensitivity of dopamnergic receptors induced by these receptor blocking drugs.[22]

A combination of lithium carbonate and high doses of haloperidol given to acutely agitated patients may result in lethargy, tremulousness, confusion, extrapyramidal and cerebellar dysfunction. In some cases severe brain damage and/or dyskinesia may persist.[19]

Even though vincristine has often been reported to produce mental changes and convulsions, so far a sensorimotor neuropathy is the only clear neurological complication.[89]

Chronic Brain Syndromes

The GAP terminology reads "These disorders result from relatively permanent, more or less, irreversible diffuse impairment of cerebral function." This classification notes that while the effects may be permanent, remarkable compensation may occur during development. It further points out that there is one particular syndrome frequently seen in preschool and young school children characterized by impulsivity, distractibility, and hyperactivity. It is thought to result from cerebral insult at birth or in very early childhood. However, it is stated, significant psychological disturb-

ance in young children may also present difficulties in impulse control, distractibility, and hyperactivity, together with delayed perceptual motor development and dysrhythmic electroencephalographic patterns.

Children with frank CNS disturbances constitute only a small proportion of the child psychiatric population. In the Isle of Wight Study,[93] fewer than 5 percent of disturbed ten-to-eleven-year-olds had a detectable abnormality of the central nervous system.

CAUSES OF CHRONIC BRAIN SYNDROME IN CHILDHOOD

There are a group of major etiological agents that operate before, at or soon after birth to provide chronic brain syndromes. These include developmental malformations of the brain, perinatal, ischemic, hypoxic, or traumatic insult to brain or effects of major metabolic aberrations in the immediate newborn period. In the postnatal period, trauma, infection, and genetically determined dystrophies of the central nervous system are major causes.

The developmental malformations may be confined to the brain or may occur in conjunction with other somatic malformations, making diagnosis easier. Gross developmental anomalies such as anencephaly (incompatible with survival beyond a few hours) may be recognized by an elevation of alpha-feto-protein in the amniotic fluid. This is detectable by the eighth week of gestation; it can be found in the maternal serum by the second trimester. Others, associated with a chromosomal anomaly, as in Down's syndrome, Holoprosencephaly or the Cri Du Chat syndrome, may be recognized even prior to birth by a chromosomal count in the amniotic fluid cells. Still others associated with a distinctive facies may be recognized at birth as the Cornellia de Lange syndrome or cretinism. Athyrotic cretinism is often difficult to recognize at birth but the characteristic somatic features appear by three to six weeks of age. If a goiter is present at birth, cretinism can be recognized and treated in the neonate. Most instances of such thyroid deficiency are secondary to inherited disorders in thyroxine synthesis; some may be due to maternal ingestion of vitamin preparations containing cobalt. Porencephaly or an agenesis of the Corpus Callosium or an aqueductal stenosis may present with an enlarging head in early infancy; an air encephalogram would make the diagnosis certain. Developmental malformation may produce mental retardation without an abnormality in the brain that is evident either by inspection or by routine histologic methods. Purpura,[85] using Golgi studies, has shown a dendritic spine "dysgenesis" as a common feature in profound mental retardation of unknown etiology.

Prenatal infections with cytomegalic inclusion virus, rubella virus, or with the protozoan parasite toxoplasma gondi, form another major group. They produce diffuse encephalopathies that may sometimes continue to progress for years after birth. Hypoxia or ischemia secondary to difficulties in labor, abnormalities of presentation or accidents of labor are common causes of chronic brain syndromes. Prematurity often results in hypoxic injury and in intraventricular bleeding secondary to the typoxia. At times maternal medications may produce a "drugged" newborn with hypoxia. Immunological incompatibility resulting in bilirubin toxicity used to leave many children injured, but effective preventive and therapeutic measures now available have made this unusual.

Metabolic derangements in calcium and glucose are very common in the newborn period and may cause seizures. An exclusive diet of phosphorous-cow's milk, for example, may bring this about. If unrecognized and untreated, these may lead to permanent brain injury. Recent experimental work in rats seems to indicate that repeated seizures in the newborn period may result in impaired brain growth, even if anoxia is prevented.[107] Some clinical data supporting this idea have also been reported.[2]

Postmaturity itself may be associated with impaired brain functions. This may be due to intrauterine asphyxia secondary to placental insufficiency.

Head trauma occuring in postnatal life is another major cause of neurologic impairment. Infections involving the meninges often involve the brain as well, and primary viral infections of the brain parenchyma are also common in childhood. Degenerative diseases and neoplasms may have an insidious onset; a family history is often present in the former.

Intoxication, particularly with lead, is another major cause of brain damage.

An insult of any of the aforementioned has a greater impact on a brain that is still developing, than it does on a fully mature adult brain. There are probably critical periods for development of various functional skills. If an insult occuring at a certain stage in development interferes with a skill, adequate acquisition of the skill may never occur. Moreover, since developmental progress occurs segmentally, as well as sequentially, early interference may secondarily distort later development as well.

At the same time, to a remarkable extent, the developing brain has the capability of compensating for lost functions. While the exact mechanisms by which this occurs are not well understood, it seems likely that adjacent synaptic areas increase in size and take over some functions. The classic example is where early insult occurs to the dominant hemisphere, interfering with development of speech. The other hemisphere takes up this function and speech always develops, even though at times, it is slightly delayed. However, in the process of taking over this function other functions may suffer, thus it has been our observation that acquisition of speech occurs at the expense of "intellect." When such switching of speech from one hemisphere to the other takes place, IQ scores drop even when measured only by nonverbal methods.

Interaction of Psychodynamic and Psychophysiologic Concepts

In the field of child psychiatry, as in other realms of psychiatry, the past twenty-five to thirty years has been marked by controversy between "organic" and "psychodynamic" modes of thinking and treatment. There has been much acrimony and little collaboration. Therapists seemed to require of their patients and themselves, a whole hearted and total commitment to the tenets of one faith or the other. In retrospect, this was inimical to the interests of patients. It also reflected rigidities which contradicted the implications of truly dynamic thinking, on the one hand; and on the other, it challenged the willingness of the true scientist to explore, test out and evaluate alternatives to his current "position."

This era of blind dogmatism seems to have come to an end. Much of this is summarized in the publication *Pharmacotherapy and Psychotherapy: Paradoxes, Problems and Progress.*[49]

Known Psychiatric Sequelae to Central Nervous System Disease

A review of pertinent clinical observations with reflections upon their significance is given by Shaffer.[95]

There was some evidence that cerebral trauma and infection in early life predisposed to behavioral disturbance, but without showing the usual predominance of boys. It appeared that involvement of left temporal, left parietal, or either frontal lobe would incline toward such a result. However, there was even stronger evidence to indicate that a generalized disturbance affecting cerebral function rather than deforming structure is more likely to induce behavioral consequences.

There was no satisfactory statistical evidence of a relationship between perinatal complications and subsequent psychiatric disorder. The same could be said of generalized metabolic disease and infection.

The Isle of Wight Study, however, showed a rate of psychiatric disorder, which was seven times greater amongst children with hydrocephalus and cerebral palsy than among the general population. This does not contradict the previous reference (p. 385) to the Isle of Wight Study, which reported that among children with psychiatric impairment, relatively few showed frank cerebral abnormality.

The reviewer felt there was no satisfactory significant relationship established between hyperkinesis and brain injury. As for infantile psychosis, evidence of abnormalities of central nervous system function have been noted in many autistics, but by no means in all. There was some question, but no satisfactory conclusion, as to whether phenylketonuria and maternal rubella were particularly likely to induce infantile autism.

In children with head injury, problems of anger control, overactivity, and distractibility were noted in a significant proportion of children (boys more than girls) during the year following injury.

It was noteworthy that family and social variables were quite as potent for the development of psychiatric disorders within this group of children with central nervous system abnormalities as in those without such evident organic problems. The evidence suggested a summing of the effects of these psychosocial components with those of the central nervous system dysfunction.

Intellectual retardation had a very potent effect in evoking psychiatric disorders.

(Several of the chronic brain syndromes such as mental retardation, speech disorder and Gilles de la Tourette's syndrome are treated elsewhere in this text and will not be dealt with in detail here.)

Epilepsy

An alteration in the state of consciousness and in the ability to control one's behavior is common to all forms of seizures. Both aspects have psycho-logic implications for the patient and for those around him.

In most forms of epilepsy, there is a distortion of body image and self-concept. This is true even in cases where there has not as yet been a clinical diagnosis of epilepsy. The child may have a conviction that something is wrong in his head. He may respond with aggressiveness, withdrawal, difficulty in learning, and a vast variety of other behaviors that either act out or deny these distorted views of himself.

Brain injured or epileptic children tend to have psychiatric disturbances five times more often than normal children, and three times more often than children with physical disorders which do not involve the CNS.[92] Psychiatric disorder is particularly common in children with temporal lobe epilepsy.[3] It is likely that in focal epilepsy the behavior disorder derives from a generalized disturbance of cortical function rather than from a loss of function in the damaged area. In the Isle of Wight Study, psychiatric disorder in children with structural damage was increased when the damage was associated with fits, and children with idiopathic epilepsy showed more psychiatric disorder than nonepileptic children.[92]

Gottschalk[45] earlier reported on effects of psychotherapy in two epileptic children and one epileptic adolescent. No consistent, characteristic fantasies were elicited and no single specific conflictual drive could be identified as the constant psychologic precipitant for seizures.

Rather, it was felt that seizures were apt to be activated by a chain of events which consistently included the blocking of any drive or strong emotion from gratification or expression by either an internal factor or external agent or situation. There was some reason to believe that psychotherapy could diminish the impact of such situations.

In hemiplegic children removal of the damaged hemisphere may result in improvement of behavior.[111] This is probably due to normalization of electrical activity in the unaffected hemisphere. In one study[69] improvement in intellectual functions after hemispherectomy was greater in children who showed such normalization.

When a child has repeated generalized seizures one of the common parental reactions is to overprotect him. The parents limit the child's range of activities in all spheres. This confirms the child's view of himself as someone different and interferes with the processes of socialization and internalization of controls. The end result is a distortion of psychologic development.

Psychic phenomena are particularly common in

temporal lobe epilepsy. These include: (1) hallucinations, generally in the form of reliving an emotionally charged experience; (2) perceptual illusions, temporary distortions of subjective relationships with surroundings; (3) change of emotional tone, most often fear, terror, or dread; (4) disorders of thought or language, arrest of thinking processes, aphasia, forced thoughts or words; and (5) automatisms, repetitive actions that vary from the very simple to the extremely complex.

Children with behavioral disorders often show a temporal or occipital spike focus without any overt evidence of seizures. These children may show a hyperkinetic picture or oscillations in behavior, difficulty in relating to others, withdrawal or hostile aggressive attacks, enuresis or nightmares, or poor school work and paroxysmal headaches. (Our unpublished work showed that such spike foci can be made to disappear with intravenous dextroamphetamine injections, and to reappear as the effect of the drug wears off.)

Contrasted with this is the description by Goldensohn and Gold[43] of prolonged episodes of behavioral disturbance, which seemed similar to temporal lobe epilepsy. The EEG tracing, however, showed only generalized disturbance without specific temporal lobe abnormalities. These episodes lasted as long as seventy-two hours. They persisted with or without automatisms but with apparent retention of consciousness along with confusion, hostility, negativism and withdrawal.

STRESS SEIZURES

Occasionally a seizure occurs following severe stress without a previous individual or family history of epilepsy. This is found particularly in males with a family history of febrile seizures; lack of sleep is the dominant stress factor. Anticonvulsants do not prevent recurrence of stress convulsions and the EEG is of no value in diagnosis or prognosis.[35]

PSYCHOSIS IN EPILEPSY

Psychotic states in epileptics may be brief or prolonged. Differentiation from "twilight" states is important. The twilight states are usually due to absence status or psychomotor status and are associated with a disturbance of consciousness. The short lasting psychotic episodes may appear as epileptic delirium (which was considered under acute brain syndromes) or as brief periods of mania or depression. Paranoid syndromes are the commonest of all forms of chronic epileptic

psychoses. A frequently mentioned characteristic of epileptic delusions is their mystical, religious quality.[98] Psychic regression to a primitive, often infantile, form is another type that resembles a chronic exacerbation of an epileptic personality disorder. The boundaries between these two are not clearly defined but the term "psychosis" can certainly be applied if there are hallucinatory experiences or delusions. Psychosis with thought disorder and disturbance of affect, reminiscent of schizophrenia also occurs.[98] Manic-depressive psychosis is also occasionally noted in epileptics.

The psychotic states are predominantly seen in temporal lobe epilepsy.[98] Risk of psychosis in temporal lobe epilepsy seems to be greater if the dominant hemisphere is involved.[33] It has been suggested that a correlation exists between schizophrenic psychosis and left temporal lesions, and manic-depressive psychosis and right temporal lesions. There seems to be some correlation between duration of epilepsy and onset of psychosis.

Landolt[63] has reported a normalization of EEG during psychotic episodes, but this finding has been questioned.[42]

EPILEPTIC PERSONALITY

The epileptic personality between seizure episodes has been variously described as egocentric, sensitive, irritable, rigid, resistive, suspicious, and hostile. Many studies with depth intracerebral electrodes have shown that there may be abnormal subcortical electrical activity, even when the scalp or direct cortical electroencephalogram shows no abnormality whatsoever.[113] Conceivably the behavior of an epileptic between overt seizures may reflect the effects of subclinical seizure activity. In addition, there is the contribution to the epileptic's behavior of his own adversely altered self-image and his reactions to the real or fantasied depreciation visited on him by others.

Some small part of what has been considered the epileptic personality may derive from the frequent concomitant presence of hyperkinetic impulse disorder. If barbiturates are used to treat the epilepsy, they will tend to accentuate, to intensify or even to precipitate the appearance of hyperkinetic impulse disorder. They may also unfavorably alter other behavioral characteristics, obtund the individual, or make him more irritable, depressed, or suspicious. All of this may then contribute to the stereotype of the epileptic personality.

In one group of epileptic children behavior disorder was most common in those having minor seizures. Aggressive behavior, on the other hand, was more strongly related to family disruption than to EEG or neurological diagnosis. Emotional and depressive symptoms occured most commonly in children with high IQ; they were less frequent in children with generalized brain damage.[7] Hartlage and associates[54] measured dependent behavior in matched groups of children with epilepsy and cystic fibrosis and among patients admitted to the hospital for tonsillectomy. The epileptic children were significantly more dependent, but within the epileptic group, excessive dependency did not relate to type or frequency of seizures nor to nature of EEG abnormality. However, other studies have shown a relation to frequency of seizures.[56] Environmental factors probably play a role. Gruenberg and Pond[50] found that epileptic children with a conduct disorder came from more deviant families than those without psychiatric disturbance. The Isle of Wight Study showed that epileptic children who had their fits at night and at home were more likely to be disturbed than children who had fits at school. The rate of disturbance among epileptic children was unrelated to whether or not the teacher knew of the child's disease.[92]

Although the aggressive behavior and psychosis seen in temporal lobe epilepsy improve with temporal lobectomy, the effects are not very striking.[29] Amygdalotomy has also been reported to benefit the aggressive behavior noted in certain epileptic patients.[110]

Gibbs and Low noted the frequent occurence of 14 and 6 per second positive spiking in the sleeping EEG's of young adolescents with antisocial behavior; they referred to the disorder as "Hypothalamic and Thalamic Epilepsy."[39] However, several recent studies have shown that 14 and 6 per second positive spiking is seen in the drowsing state in nearly 50 percent of normal school children and adolescents.

Electroencephalographic abnormalities, epileptic fits, poor motor coordination, and histories of abnormalities of pregnancy and delivery have been noted in a large proportion of children showing autistic behavior.[61]

INTELLECTUAL EFFECTS

Brenda Milner[73] found that epileptogenic lesions involving the left temporal lobe caused a specific deficit in verbal learning and retention. However, when the lesion was predominantly right temporal, there was a consistent impairment of rapid visual identification and picture comprehension.

These deficits increase, rather than decrease, when the epileptogenic area is excised. This is the case even in those cases where a postoperative increase in IQ occurs, and seizures cease completely. Certainly some patients with unusually active electroencephalographic foci before operation do show general intellectual impairment. This is probably due to widespread interference with cortical functioning rather than to the temporal lobe lesions specifically. Unlike the specific deficits, this more general intellectual inefficiency is apt to disappear after removal of the epileptogenic area.

For epilepsy to manifest, it seems that some biological, physiochemical abnormality or predisposition must be present. Given this, stress, generalized or specific, may precipitate a particular seizure. In a person who does not have the epileptic predisposition, a similar constellation of emotional stresses will not produce a seizure. Some other means of expression will no doubt be resorted to, but not that one.

This factor was studied methodically by Luborsky and associates.[68] They carried out an intensive exploration of the preseizure mental content of three patients with petit mal. One of these showed characteristic psychologic antecedents, generally negative affects, such as feeling depressed or blocked prior to seizure.

MODIFICATION OF SEIZURES BY BEHAVIORAL TECHNIQUES

If seizures are considered as a terminal link in a behavioral chain, identifying and modifying behavior that precedes a seizure climax might prevent a seizure. The fact that autonomic functions can be controlled by operant conditioning lends credence to the belief that this might be possible. Lennox[64] has reported interruption of seizures before the climax, most commonly in reflex seizures, by methods as diverse as mustard applications and stimulation. There are isolated single case reports in the literature of elimination of reflex epilepsies by using systematic desensitization. The first application of operant conditioning for control of seizures was used by Gardner.[50] He abolished psychogenic seizures in a ten-year-old girl by differential reinforcement, i.e., extinction contingent upon seizure occurence and reinforcement for incompatible behavior, such as appropriate play with siblings. A more recent[117] effort at predicting and modifying reliable preseizure behaviors confirmed previous studies and suggested that nonprofessionals and parents can be employed successfully as therapists.

Behavioral Syndromes Secondary to Altered Body Image

A child's developing body image begins with his own narcissistic investment in his body. It includes as well his perceptions of the views of significant others (parents, siblings, and peers) in relationship to his body. Furthermore there is a self-image to correlate with the body image. Indeed basic to all ego development and functioning is the original body ego. Since ego functions evolve against a background of body and self-image, disfigurement (and depreciating views of the self) are bound to have an effect on ego functions. The methods of assessment and understanding the psychodynamics is dealt with in detail in a recent review by Woods.[114]

He observes and quotes others as reporting there are pathological attempts at restitution through psychic economic shifts in which libido is withdrawn from the object world and focused on the body ego, perhaps as an attempt to restore fantasied narcissistic perfection prior to the injury. He found denial or undoing to be a most frequent reaction, serving to put the defect out of existence. Many children were provocative, arrogant and belligerent, along with having fantasies of possessing special powers and strengths. One child, who had a clawlike hand as a residual of a cerebral vascular accident, recurrently attacked his parents and also fantasied himself as an attacking eagle. Woods points out that often, as time goes on, the unresolved injury remains a continuing source of rage.

The therapist needs to help the child to accept his limitations and to recognize that he is made up of more than his defect. He needs to help the child express his feelings over the defect or injury, to lead the child to give up the exclusive focus on the lost or damaged image, and encourage the child to create a productive and satisfying social existence in which the healthy aspects of the body structure are accepted as the basis for a new body image. Work with the parents is particularly necessary, as is an awareness of and dealing with the therapist's own counter-transference.

However, the Isle of Wight Study suggested that a physical handicap without an associated brain injury did not increase incidence of psychiatric disturbance.[93] It may be, then, that a disturbance in social perception produced by the brain injury may in some way distort the child's pattern of social interactions.

Brain Trauma

After a head injury, a delayed posttraumatic syndrome is common in children, just as it is in adults. It consists largely of headaches, poor school work, fatigability, emotional instability, and vertigo. A retrograde as well as an anterograde amnesia may remain, and it probably represents a temporal lobe contusion. Sleep disturbances are common along with anxiety dreams in which the circumstances of the accident are recapitulated again and again. Some children generate a tremendous amount of anxiety following head trauma.

Black and associates[13] found that 31 percent of children without previous psychiatric disturbances develop behavioral problems following head trauma. The most common symptoms were deficient control of anger and hyperactivity. The posttraumatic somatic complaints like headache and dizziness, so common among adults, were seen less often in children. Boys were more likely to develop symptoms than girls.

Brain injury itself may certainly produce psychiatric sequelae; but the same familial and social factor's that create psychiatric disorder in normal children have an even greater influence in brain injured children.[93] Broken homes, emotional upset in mother and poor socioeconomic status were more frequent in brain injured children with conduct disorder than in those without. The Isle of Wight Study also showed that these factors are more prone to induce psychiatric disorders in brain injured children than in children with physical handicaps not involving CNS.

The relation between perinatal brain trauma and psychiatric disorders in children is not certain. Both perinatal complications and psychiatric disorders are particularly common in families of low socioeconomic status, but whether the one causes the other is by no means established. Graham and associates[46] studied 350 children with neonatal asphyxia. When compared to controls at age three and one-half, the asphyxia children showed cognitive deficiencies but no personality differences.

A comparison of the behavior of brain injured and noninjured retarded children[37] showed that brain injured children were more demanding and less able to defer gratification. A differential effect may be seen depending on side of injury. Right-sided brain injury has been associated with deficits in nonverbal expression of creative thinking and spatial visualization as well as in the appearance of behavior characterized by impatience and disrespect; whereas those with left-sided brain injury tend to have lower verbal intelligence. "Misoplegia," a morbid dislike directed toward offending hemiplegia is more often seen in a left hemiplegia.[20]

Psychiatric disturbance is particularly likely to occur when manifest signs of brain injury coincide with an abnormal perinatal history.

It has been suggested[24] that the conduct disorder in brain damaged children does not respond well to psychotherapy as the prime treatment agent. This, however, does not preclude the usefulness of psychotherapy for associated emotional disturbance. Also, behavior modification techniques may have a particular usefulness for dealing with important target symptoms in this condition.[90]

Cerebral Palsy

This condition in many ways represents a paradigm for consideration of how handicapping physical conditions may psychologically affect the child, the parents, their interactions, and those of the siblings, and help to determine functional outcome.

In brief review, there are many possible causes for and contributions to the causation of this entity. They include genetic and other prenatal factors—poor implantation of the ovum, maternal illness, malnutrition, emotional stress. In addition, there are the manifold components which may stem from the birth process itself. A perfectly normal delivery, especially in a primipara, imposes physical stresses upon the infant brain. Deviations of all kinds—premature labor, postmature labor, prolonged labor, excessive sedation, artificial induction of labor, instrumental or operative intervention, immunologic incompatibilities—all may play a role.

From these various causes may stem, among a variety of other consequences, the condition known as cerebral palsy. In early infancy this can manifest itself as deviations in infant responsiveness and development. From the toddler era on, specific subcategories may be apparent, such as the: spastic, ataxic, athetoid, and mixed forms. These children often also may have other handicaps, such as mental retardation, epilepsy, and hyperkinetic impulse disorder. In addition, those with the spastic type may develop a variety of secondary crippling conditions, and the therapy

for these (medication, braces, operations, involved and demanding forms of physiotherapy) may be tremendous sources of stress for child and family.

When the infant is unresponsive, irritable, or unsatisfiable, mothers frequently view this as an indication that they are in some way deficient and that the deviant child is clear evidence of their failure as a mothering woman. The impact upon them of such feeling may be accentuated by their fatigue from trying to meet the needs of such infants.

Feelings of responsibility lead to feelings of guilt which may mobilize a retrospective search for those errors, feelings, etc. upon which may be placed the blame for this dread outcome. Attempts to evade the responsibility may lead to a search for incriminating contributions on the part of the marital partner or family thereof.

Father, too, must deal with the same feelings and has the same possible repertoire of disruptive responses.

For both parents, the child, being an extension of themselves, may represent more and more of an indictment, the more the disability develops. This may lead to a variety of reactions, including genuine pity and a wish to spare the child further disability and pain. There also may be rejection and hostility, not only because the child symbolizes imperfection in the parents, but also because the child cannot fulfill parental expectations and, furthermore, is a source of emotional demand and drain of energy and money.

For some parents, especially the mother, the intensity and prolongation of the child's dependence may fulfill a need to be "needed." For others, father as well as mother, the demands and drains of this special child may evoke hostilities which are sometimes openly expressed but more often appear as overprotectiveness with an underlying hostile component.

The parent or parents may demand of the child that he or she prove a basic competence by struggling to achieve—or, truly, overachieve—in the areas in which they are obviously deficient. Or, to compensate for this by achievement, or overachievement, in other areas.

Parents may deny the existence of a disability and/or attack those who diagnose it and propose means of overcoming it. They may pass through stages of, or oscillate among phases of denial, depression, and anger.

These and similar feelings and reactions may precipitate or accentuate marital tensions. The presence of the cerebral palsied child in the family and the parental reactions may present great stresses for the siblings who must deal with this situation in addition to handling the usual aspects of sibling rivalry and their own relationship with their parents.

For the child who is the patient, there are suggestions that the cerebral abnormality itself may lead to a different mode of intellectual functioning (such as a more primitive level; lessened ability to abstract; diminished fantasy) and impairment of psychosexual development, beginning with increased primary narcissism. Both distractibility and perseveration are often noted.

In addition to these handicaps, the child must deal with normal developmental tasks and must deal with the impact of the varying and often variable parental and sibling feelings and the ways in which these are manifested. These feelings and behaviors interact with the child's awareness of his or her own weaknesses and strengths to help determine body image and modes of coping.

An on-going need in regard both to these children and their parents is for continuing evaluation and monitoring of their intellectual, educational, physical, innerpersonal and interpersonal current capacities and potentials for same. This allows for the setting of current, steadily changing goals, for long-range expectations, for the selection of modes to achieve what can be done and for constructive acceptance of what it is unrealistic to expect. Both child and family may need help in setting reasonable expectations as to what child should contribute to family life.

In the context of the needs and difficulties which have been described, it seems reasonable and efficient to emphasize the family approach as early as possible and also the utilization of groups, both of parents and patients. Both have the potential for maximizing the constructive tendencies present within patient and family members. Also, the utilization of groups should diminish tendencies toward dependency upon professionals and needs to act out against them. This does not gainsay the fact that there will be situations in which individual psychotherapy and casework will be needed.

There are two areas of prominent concern which are inadequately handled. The first is vocational, linked with education. It is often difficult to ascertain what would be a realistic and practical vocational goal for the given child and even more difficult for child and parent to accept and adapt to the recommendation offered.

The other major problem area, so often poorly handled (and, not infrequently, ignored) is the sexual, linked with social, maturation as a person, potential for function as a marital partner, and as a parent. Arbitrary conclusions may be drawn: that such a child has no sexual drives, interests, needs; will never want to or be capable of sexual relations with others, or of marrying, or of parenting.

Just what the possibilities are, in regard to these latter two, are actually highly variable, partly dependent upon many other factors (such as degree of intellectual, emotional and social maturation, capacity for "independent living") and need to be evaluated for each person. All, however, have the need and right to receive sexual information appropriate to their stage of development and capacities, to have an opportunity to communicate and to learn to accept their feelings. Many of these aspects are well reviewed and discussed by Freeman.[34]

Most of this discussion has concentrated on potential for disturbance in development, on parental turmoil, and family dysharmony. These are by no means the necessary outcome. Pediatricians are more likely than child psychiatrists to see and attest to the existence of families in which these stresses call forth healthy, reparative, and compensatory responses with a strengthening of bonds and enrichment and maturation of the personalities of those involved.

In contrast to this is a report by Kogan, Tyler and Turner[60] in which they observed interaction patterns between ten young cerebral palsied children and their mothers over a two-year period. It was noted that, over this time, both therapists and mothers showed progressively decreasing expressions of affection and positive acceptance. For the mothers, this was especially so where children were not walking by the end of the study. It was considered that this reflected a focus by both staff and parents on physical handicaps, with relative inattention to intellectual, social, emotional factors.

Infection of Brain as a Cause of Organic Brain Syndome

A variety of viruses can produce an acute encephalitis. In the acute phase this produces an alteration of behavior, confusion, delirium, lethargy leading to stupor and often seizures. Sequelae may consist of intellectual deficits, hyperactive behavior and motor paresis or sensory deficits.

Such sequelae are most common when the infection occurs during the first two years of life.[30] Arthropod borne viruses are common and of these, Eastern equine encephalitis is the most severe. Herpes simplex virus is responsible for 10 percent of all cases of encephalitis and produces a very characteristic clinical picture consisting of behavioral and speech abnormalities preceding motor signs. Since this virus particularly affects the temporal lobes, severe cases that recover have a close resemblance to the "Kluver-Bucy Syndrome" seen in Rhesus monkeys after bilateral removal of temporal lobes and of the rhinencephelon.[59] This syndrome consists of visual agnosia, an urge to examine all objects by mouth, irresistible impulse to touch every object in sight, increased sexual behavior, and changes in emotional behavior.

J. G. a six-year old, white male started with a febrile illness and a behavioral alteration which progressed over a period of a week to produce coma, multiple seizures, and a right hemiparesis. When signs of brain stem herniation began to appear he was transferred to a teaching hospital where the disease was immediately recognized to be a herpes encephalitis and the increased intracranial pressure was vigorously treated with osmotic agents, steroids, hyperventilation through a respirator and, finally, bilateral subtemporal surgical decompression. Herpes simplex virus Type I was demonstrated in the brain biopsy and also grew in tissue culture of the brain. He needed respirator care for four weeks. One year following the illness he was able to walk and run but with a hemiplegic gait. Speech was limited to a few words and comprehension of speech was poor. However, he could repeat well and recite brief nursery rhymes that were taught to him. He did not seem to recognize the use of common objects. He put everything within reach into his mouth, was very impulsive, and engaged in constant masturbation. Seizures were frequent and resistant to therapy. EEG's showed bilateral temporal slow waves and spike foci.

SLOW VIRUS INFECTIONS

Measles virus is known to produce a chronic encephalitis (subacute sclerosing panencephalitis) characterized by slowly progressive dementia and myoclonic seizures. There is a characteristic "periodic" EEG and elevation of spinal fluid gamma globulin and measles antibody titre. A typical hemorrhagic miaculopathy is often present, and clinical diagnosis is frequently possible.

Very recently, a few patients have been reported in whom congenital rubella produced a progressive illness in the second decade of life characterized by spasticity, ataxia, intellectual deterioration and seizures. Increased cerebrospinal fluid protein and gamma globulin and elevated serum and spinal fluid rubella antibody titres were found. Rubella virus has been isolated from the brain of one such patient.[101, 108] The characteristic "periodic" EEG seen in subacute sclerosing panencephalitis due to measles virus is not seen in this disease.

The common sequelae of congenital rubella infection, however, are microcephaly and intellectual retardation, together with deafness, cataracts, and cardiac deficits. Cytomegalovirus also may produce a congenital infection resulting in intellectual retardation, seizures, and microcephaly. Autistic behavior is disproportionately common in rubella embryopathy and also in association with toxoplasmosis and syphilis.

A. P. a twelve-year-old Yugoslavian born male emigrated to the United States in late 1972. His parents had arrived several years earlier, and he was being brought up in Iceland by an aunt until the time he reached here. The initial language difficulty was overcome, but six months after starting school in this country, school performance started falling. The poor school performance was attributed to emotional difficulties and "culture shock;" counseling and psychotherapeutic medication were started. Despite this form of therapy, his intellectual abilities continued to regress over the next six months and a neurologic opinion was sought. A "periodic" EEG, myoclonic spasms, dementia, and retinal findings offered a clear-cut clinical diagnosis. The measles titre in spinal fluid confirmed this. Over the next three years, his disease progressed and produced a severe dementia, spasacity with multiple contractures in flexion, and frequent myoclonic seizures.

BACTERIAL INFECTIONS

Purulent menigitis is common in childhood with severe meningical involvement, some cerebral parenchynal involvement usually occurs as well. Cerebral abscess may develop by contigous spread or as a metastatic infection. These diseases are more apt to produce neurologic and intellectual defects than significant psychiatric residuals.

Pertussis infection, as well as pertussis vaccine, may produce a toxic encephalopathy. While hyperactive behavior is a common sequela, there may also be a disturbance of relationships and reality testing severe enough to be classed as prepsychotic or psychotic.

Congenital syphilis is rare today. Juvenile general paresis produces a progressive dementia with apathy, forgetfulness, irritability, restlessness, night terrors, temper tantrums, and impulsive behavior. The euphoria, expansiveness, delusions, and hallucinations, so often seen in the adult form, are much less common in the juvenile form.

393

PARASITIC INFECTIONS

The most common parasitic congenital infection is produced by the protozoan parasite Toxoplasma gondi. Usual sequelae are intellectual retardation and microcephaly and skull X-rays show a characteristic pattern of intracranial calification.

POST-INFECTIOUS ENCEPHALOMYELITIS

A variety of the common exanthematous fevers as well as mumps can produce a monophasic illness with involvement of the CNS at multiple sites. This is likely to begin about two weeks after onset of the systemic illness. Nonspecific upper respiratory viral infections are sometimes the only antecedent infections. Varicella often produces a cerebellar syndrome while the others produce a disseminated encephalomyelitis. One suggested cause has been an alteration in the antigenicity of central myelin basic protein secondary to the viral infections. A clinical and pathological similarity to experimental allergic encephalitis in animals supports this view. It is produced by injection of central myelin basic protein with an adjuvant. Vaccination for protection against smallpox and rabies sometimes produces a very similar post-vaccinial encephalomyelitis. Spontaneous recovery is the rule with these forms of encephalomyelitis and residuals are rare.

Toxins

LEAD POISONING IN CHILDREN

Childhood plumbism generally occurs as an accidental poisoning; while in adults it is usually an occupational hazard. Although peeling lead paint in old houses has been implicated as the major source of severe exposure among children, the source of poisoning in many cases remains undetermined.[65]

Lead poisoning caused by paint ingestion in infants and children was reported in the Australian literature around the turn of the century,[40] and gradually gained recognition in the United States as a public health problem in the 1920s when pica was linked to its occurrence.[14] In the late 1960s it was suddenly realized that lead was taking a high toll among children in many areas.[91] A recent survey of twenty-one screening programs that tested a total of 344,657 children revealed that 26.1 percent had levels of 40/mg per 100 ml or more, indicative of undue lead absorption.[41] In this survey 7.6 percent had levels of 80/mg per 100 ml or more—levels designated by the United States Surgeon General as constituting "unequivocal cases of lead poisoning." More and more reports are being published suggesting that this problem is not limited to the "inner cities" but is seen in children from white middle-class and upper-middle-class homes in rural areas.

Sources of lead in the environment vary from lead based paint, dust and dirt, ambient air, newspapers and children's books with ink of high lead content; lead in pencils, toothpaste with high lead content, and also some canned infant food and evaporated milk.

Pica: Pica, a perverted appetite for nonfood items, occurs commonly in preschool children and is most prevalent among those eighteen to twenty-four months old. Most surveys indicate a higher prevalence in black clinic patients compared to white private patients. The prevalence drops sharply in both groups after three years of age. However, one study[9] found the condition in 18.5 percent of 439 chiidren, and no relation to race, sex, size and social position of the family was found. In several studies 70 to 90 percent of children suffering from lead poisoning have a history of pica and 30 percent of children with such a history have lead poisoning.[65]

The variety of items consumed by children with pica is limitless. Selectivity for particular items may develop later, taking on a symbolic meaning, and appears to increase with age.

While pica has a most important role in causing excessive lead intake in children, normal oral exploration and hand to mouth activity is to be expected in young children. The ages of the highest incidence of pica overlaps that of lead poisoning: between eighteen and thirty months. Since it is established that three to six months of fairly steady lead ingestion generally precedes the appearance of clinical manifestation of lead poisoning,[65] it appears that some children who present clinical evidence of toxicity at twelve to twenty-four months may have begun consuming hazardous amounts of lead even before pica developed. Barltrop[9] reported thumb sucking in 18 to 28 percent of children one to six years old whose parents were interviewed and nail biting in 2 percent of those between one to two, and 17 percent of those between four to six years of age. Among those surveyed by mail, finger sucking occurred in 65 percent of the group from one to two and in 30 percent of the group six to seven years old. The studies of lead content of dust found on the hands of inner city children lend support to the belief that a substantial amount of lead might be introduced into the body through hand to mouth activity.

Studies of absorption of lead indicate that children are better able to absorb and retain lead. Studies in lower amounts have suggested that nutritional inadequacies may potentiate the toxic effects of lead. These findings are of particular importance since children at risk for lead poisoning are also at risk for inadequate nutrition. It seems likely that deficiency of iron, protein, and calcium contribute to the occurrence of acute lead encephalopathy.

There seems to be increasing evidence that many children who have undue lead absorption but never overt lead poisoning later give evidence of "minimal brain injury" seen as perceptual handicaps, hyperactivity and impaired fine motor coordination.[84] (This subject is also discussed under the secton on "Hyperkinetic Impulse Disorder of Childhood").

Excessive lead exposure of women during pregnancy is known to result in neurologically damaged infants with intrauterine and postnatal growth retardation.[80]

Acute lead encephalopathy presents with altered sensorium, proceeding to coma if untreated, seizures, and clinical signs of increasing brain swelling. Death ensues rapidly unless treatment directed towards reducing the brain swelling, controlling the seizures, and chelation of lead is started immediately. A history of pica aids in the diagnosis. Presence of an iron deficiency anemia, evidence of renal involvement, elevation of spinal fluid pressure and protein, and bilateral nonfocal showing of the electroencephotogram are other pointers to diagnosis. Treatment consists of maintenance of hydration and nutrition, control of seizures with parenterol anticonvulsants, measures to reduce increased introcranial pressure and chelation of lead with parenterol BAL and Ca EDTA.

Neuropsychologic sequelae are common in those who survive an acute lead encephalopathy.[18] A follow-up study of twenty children after recovery from lead poisoning showed that all but one was failing in school and that a high percentage were impulsive, had short attention spans, and were having difficulty with spatial tasks. Visual motor disturbances were found in twelve of eighteen children treated for lead encephalopathy by Bradley and Baumgartner.[16]

Degenerative Diseases

Most degenerations of brain present regression in behavior and loss of functional skills. Development of neurologic deficits make the distinction from a psychiatric disorder fairly easy. The leukodystrophies produce an elevation in spinal fluid protein and show diminished nerve conduction values. Pelizaeus-Merzbacher disease is a very slow progressive leukodystrophy that combines characteristic shaking of head and movement of eyes with, most often, a progressive dementia.[102]

Degenerative diseases involving the basal ganglia do occur in childhood, and at the outset they often simulate functional diseases. Wilson's disease may initially present psychiatric symptoms but the easily available biochemical measures make distinction easy. In Hallervorden-Spatz disease, an iron containing pigment is deposited in the basal ganglia and a characteristic picture of parkinsonian rigidity is seen in the second decade of life. Most of the reported cases with this disease were diagnosed as catatonic schizophrenia in the first year or two of their illness. When it occurs in childhood, Huntington's Chorea is characterized by spasticity and seizures in addition to dementia; an autosomal dominant inheritance makes diagnosis easy. Torsion dystonia is a fairly common disorder of childhood and is often misdiagnosed as hysteria. This disease may be inherited in an autosomal dominant or autosomal recessive fashion or be secondary to perinatal brain injury. The inherited forms have a normal intellect (a superior intellect in the recessive form) and the brain is normal on gross and microscopic examination. Recent reports have suggested that the enzyme dopamine B-hydroxylase is elevated in the serum in affected members and families of one type of this disorder (Autosomal dominant—non-Jewish).

W. G. a seven-year-old white male was initially evaluated at age three years for developmental and speech delay. Perinatal history did suggest that some cerebral hypoxic insult might have occurred. Minor choreic movements were noted during initial examination. Family pathology was suspected, counseling was provided to the family and the boy, and the boy was put on tranquilizing medications. Educational help was also provided in school. By age seven his movement disorder has progressed and he started to have frequent torsion spasms; primarily of the trunk and the proximal limb muscles. A pneumoencephalogram showed lateral ventricular dilatation primarily on the left without obstruction and without cortical atrophy and with normal caudate shadows.

This suggests that the patient did not have Wilson's disease but had basal ganglia injury resulting from the perinatal complications.

Storage Disorders

Mucopolysaccharidosis result in storage of muco-polysaccharides in the visceral organs as well as in neuronal cells. Characteristic somatic features are always present as well as retardation and seizures.

Neurologic problems are most often seen in those who excrete excess quantities of heparitin sulphate in urine. Recently a correlation has been shown between the levels of heparitin sulphate in spinal fluid and the degree of retardation.

Closely related sphingolipidosis involves pathological lipid storage within the brain. Some types have characteristic macular findings and the enzyme deficiency may be demonstrated in cells in some. The late onset, slowly progressive form (Spielmeyer-Vogt) often presents as a personality disorder in the initial stage. It has not infrequently been confused with childhood schizophrenia.

A continuum between the mucopolysaccharidosis and sphingolipidosis has recently been demonstrated and two disorders (metachromatic leukodystrophy and Krabbe's disease) formerly classified as degenerative diseases of brain have recently been recognized to be lipid storage diseases. Hence, a common classification is provided.

LIPIDOSIS INVOLVING THE CENTRAL NERVOUS SYSTEM

1. Cerebroside—Gaucher's disease. Infantile, juvenile, and adult forms are present and a ganglioside is present in abnormal quantities in visceral organs as well as the CNS.
2. Sphingomyelin — Niemann - Pick's disease. Several forms are present with age of onset varying from infancy to adulthood. Missing enzyme—sphingomyelinase. The sphingolipid is stored in viscera as well as the brain in the classical form. The brain is not involved in the "visceral form" subtype and in the "Nova Scotia" subgroup.
3. Ganglioside—Two major subtypes are present depending on the kind of ganglioside stored: GM_1 (β galactosidase deficiency) or GM_2 (Hemoxaminidase deficiency). The Amaurotic family idiocies constitute this group—Gangliosidosis; Tay Sach's; Landing's; Sandhoff's; the late infantile form (Jansky-Bielchwosky); the juvenile

form (Batten-Spielmeyer-Vogt) and the adult form (Kuf's).

A cherry red spot is a common clinical feature in the above three categories of lipidoses.

4. The Mucopolysaccharidosis—Visceral and neuronal storage of GM_1, GM_2 and GM_3 occurs as a result of deficiency of thermolabile β-galactosidase isozymes.
5. Sulphatide—Metachromatic leukodystrophy. Diagnosis is easily made by detecting deficiency of arylsulphatase in urine. Infantile and adult forms are present.
6. Ceramide Trihexoside—Febry's disease. Characterized by skin and kidney involvement, corneal opacities and premature cerebrovascular accidents due to ceramide trihexosidase deficiency.
7. Tetramethylhexadiczmic acid — Refsum's disease. Primarily manifests as a polyneuropathy with elevation of spinal fluid protein and decrease in serum phytanic acid.
8. Sterols—The cerebrotendinous xanthomatosis—(Wolman's and Farber's disease) and Hand Schuller-Christian disease.
9. Miscellaneous—Krabbe's (infantile and adult forms. Due to galactocerebroside-β-galactosidase deficiency). Diminished nerve conduction valves and elevation of spinal fluid protein are common in this entity as well as metachromatic leukodystrophy. Alexander's disease and Canavan's disease are two other leukodystrophies occurring in childhood and are characterized by distinctive neuropathologic features (Rosenthal fibres in the former and spongy degeneration in the latter), but the exact Merzbacher's is another leukodystrophy beginning in adolescence and having a slow course with distinctive (tigroid dysmyelination) pathologic features.

Schilder's disease (diffuse cerebral sclerosis of inflammatory type) or leukoencephalitis periaxialis diffusa produces a large continuous cerebral demyelinating lesion and in some cases is associated with adrenocortical atrophy (Bronze Schilder's disease). The latter variety is inherited in a sex-linked recessive fashion.

Alper's disease, a poliodystrophy of childhood, is another degenerative disease of the nervous system without an established etiology at this time.

Metabolic Disorders

Several inherited disorders of the metabolism of amino acids, carbohydrates or lipids can result in intellectual retardation and seizures as well as behavior disorders.

Emotional instability and anxiety are common in thyrotoxicosis, whereas apathy and lack of interest are common in hypothyrodism. In the latter where onset was congenital, characteristic somatic features help in recognition. Behavioral abnormalities secondary to episodes of hypoglycemia are common in poorly regulated juvenile diabetes. Idiopathic hypoglycemia can often masquerade as a behavior disorder, with or without a seizure disorder.

Behavior disorders are particularly common in phenylketonuric children, even in those without significant retardation. They may have a dull, expressionless face, be negativistic and apprehensive. Even psychotic behavior, manifested by withdrawal from reality, failure to relate to people, catatonic posturing, and echolalia is sometimes seen. Loosening of association and a distorted process of thinking may be present. A higher rate of psychiatric disorder was found in a group treated from infancy as compared to an untreated group.[51] It is also possible that the psychiatric disturbance in phenylketonuria is at least partly due to the stress imposed on the child and the family by the vigorous feeding regime given as treatment.[10] Autistic behavior has been reported to be disproportionately common in phenylketonuria and has also been found in galactosemia.

Galastosemic children are also characteristically withdrawn, depressed and hostile.[62]

Of special interest to child psychiatrists, self-mutilation has been found to be a characteristic behavioral abnormality in the Lesch-Nyhan syndrome. In addition to this behavior, it is also characterized by mental retardation, choreoathetosis, and hyperuricemia due to an inherited deficiency of the enzyme hypoxanthine quanine ribosyl transferase. Porphyria is uncommon in childhood. During an acute episode it may produce a confusional state.

Malnutrition, Brain and Behavior

Kwashiorkor is due to protein calorie malnutrition and is seen primarily in tropical underdeveloped poor countries. Classical clinical features are edema of feet, dyspigmentation of hair and skin, dermatitis, and hepatomegaly. The commonest age of onset is the second year of life. Apathy is the most constant and earliest neurologic feature and is invariably present in children with this syndrome whose weight is less than 40 percent of average value.[103]

Psychologic manifestations include cognitive inadequacies resulting in delay in learning, particularly reading and writing.[23] About one-fifth become drowsy within three to four days after being started on a normal diet. Often this encephalopathy is self limited but occasionally is accompanied by asterexis and may progress to coma with a fatal outcome.[8] The nature of this encephalopathy is unknown but may reflect hepatic failure resulting from a sudden load of protein.

Malnutrition beginning in early infancy has been demonstrated to result in brains small for chronological age with decreased number of neurons, degree of myelination, and total cerebral lipid content.[12, 26, 112]

When malnutrition is present from birth, it has been shown to affect brain weight and intellectual growth.[66] Accompanying behavioral disturbances include apathy and irritability.[71, 86] Thiamine deficiency, as in beriberi, and niacin deficiency in pellagra also lead to organic mental syndromes, but these are today found only in some very underdeveloped countries. Environmental deprivation also has been observed to retard cognitive and emotional growth. Experimental evidence has now been added to this observation in that rats raised in "complex" environments have more dendritic branching in their frontotemporal and temporal cortex than those reared "socially" or in isolation.[47]

However, the human data presented thus far is controversial, and it is quite possible that the intellectual inadequacy which is a residuum of malnutrition in early life may not be the result of protein calorie malnutrition alone but also may result from a defective nervous system present from birth with poor ability to feed and interact with the mother.

Chromosomal Disorders

An increased incidence of XXY syndrome (Klinefelter's syndrome) has been reported in prisons and penal institutions and a definitive correlation suggested between aggressive antisocial behavior, tall stature, and XYY genotype. However, a recent study[79] concluded that while this syndrome was associated with an increase in height and a psychological set in which there was an "inability to integrate aggression normally into their perception of reality" subnormal intelligence and criminality were not parts of this syndrome. Girls with Turner's syndrome may exhibit space-form dysgnosia, directional dysgnosia, and mild-numerical disability, that suggests a developmental parietal lobe anomaly.[74] A review of literature seems to indicate there is no evidence that children with Down's syndrome are more friendly, outgoing, and musical than other children.[92] However, they do exhibit less antisocial behavior.

Brain Tumors

Personality changes are more common with supratentorial tumors and vary depending on whether the frontal, temporal, parietal, or occipital lobe is primarily involved. Increased intracranial pressure due to an intracranial tumor can in itself produce behavioral changes regardless of the location of the lesion.

The general consensus is that nothing really specific defines a child's reaction to intracranial tumor. Emotional instability, irritability, anxiety, withdrawal, regressive tendencies, and learning difficulties seem to reflect the fact that cerebral function is impaired. This interferes with the child's ability to deal with the already present emotional stresses.

Specific Learning Disability

This subject is dealt with in greater detail elsewhere in this book but is mentioned here primarily because of its frequent association with the hyperkinetic impulse disorder. Specific learning disability refers to an impairment in ability to learn scholastically up to a level appropriate to the individuals intellectual endowment, as a result of some form of disturbance in information processing. Presumably it is due to some disorder of cerebral function.

One particular variety of specific learning disability referred to as the developmental Gerstmann syndrome deserves mention. The Gerstmann syndrome consists of finger agnosia, acalculia, and agraphia (without alexia), and disturbed right-left discrimination. Constructional apraxia is also often present. This syndrome is due to a parietal lesion of the dominant hemisphere. Among children with learning disabilities a few cases have been recognized in whom the same syndrome may be present in whole or in part; presumably this is due to a developmental abnormality of the dominant parietal lobe.

D. G., a fourteen-year-old white male, was referred for a neurologic evaluation because of poor school performance despite a full scale IQ of 130 on the WISC. Parents reported that he had always had difficulty managing his body and he never learned to swim or dive. He never did adequate work in art and spelling. Neurologic examination showed a severe difficulty with abstract calculation and in writing. There was right-left confusion and finger agnosia. This school performance had improved to a remarkable extent since he had been provided with a pocket calculator and writing assignments have been diminished.

The Anatomic Basis of Certain Emotional States in Organic Brain Syndromes

It is hard to determine the locus of brain injury or malfunction responsible for a particular element within an organic brain syndrome. In most instances the symptoms are multiple and intermingle with each other, and the brain injury, bilateral and diffuse.

However, where primary emotional disturbances have been present in their pure form in organic brain disease, cliniocopathologic studies have pointed to the limbic system as the primary seat of disease.

Only a few selected emotional states will be considered here.

AGGRESSIVE BEHAVIOR

Aggressiveness is part of social behavior. Pathologic rage is differentiated from aggressive behavior by virtue of the fact that it can be elicited by nonspecific stimuli, it is disproportionate, its course is aimless, it cannot be stopped, and it does not fatigue. Such pathologic rage is seen in temporal lobe epilepsy, as well as in rabies where encephalitic lesions occur primarily in the two Ammon's horns. Rage attacks have also been seen in tumors of midline centering on the septum pellucidum,[116] the hypothalamus,[4] and temporal lobes.[11] The specific areas involved in reported cases have been the olfactory tubercle, tuberal region, anterior thalamus, pre-optic area, septum pellucidum, hippocampus, and the amygdaloid nucleus. The temporal lobe lesions are bilateral in typical cases.

PLACIDITY

This term refers to a decrease or loss not only of aggressive behavior but also of affective response in general. Placidity is observed primarily after bilateral temporal lobectomy or in deep bilateral temporal lesions. In addition, bilateral lesions of the cingulate gyrus can decrease drive and affective reactions to the point of akinetic mutism.[109] Fulton[36] has pointed out that the tranquilizing effect of prefrontal leucotomy is due to interruption of projections from the anterior cingulate gyrus to the prefrontal lobe.

ANXIETY AND FEAR

These are usually seen as ictal phenomena in temporal lobe epilepsy. Periodic or paroxysmal anxiety also occurs in rabies. Experimentally, electrical stimulation of the anterior half of temporal lobe; the insula; the outflow of the hippocampal gyrus and the fornix elicit anxiety and fear.[77]

DEPRESSION

Depressive states occur in tumors of the temporal lobe and can occur at times as ictal phenomena.

The consideration of the anatomic relationships does support the hypothesis proposed by Papez[81] of closed functional loops in the nervous system, the intactness of which is necessary for balanced emotional feelings and behavior. Recent data on the dopaminergic and serotonergic systems within the brain and their alteration in behavioral disease suggest that as yet poorly understood biochemical pathways play a primary role in disorders of emotion.

ENVOI

Brief mention was earlier made of "Learning Disabilities." If a handbook such as this one were to have been contemplated fifteen years ago, it might have had to choose between a series of publications from one center asserting that, without question, learning disabilities were invariably due to inner psychic conflict, while another was asserting that they reflected problems in information-processing.

Fortunately, affairs have changed. This is illustrated by Schechter.[94] In one article he conceptualizes learning disabilities as due to psychosocial causes, or to organic causes, or to both and procedes to illustrate how diagnosis and treatment may call upon analytic theory, psychotherapeutic techniques, a knowledge of neurology and neurophysiology, the use of medications, a tremendous respect for people, and all the areas of training and knowledge which should characterize a physician.

The same indication of a return to and an honest use of our training and background as physicians is indicated in a recent GAP report.[49]

It is time, indeed.

REFERENCES

1. ADLER, S., "Methyldopa Induced Decrease in Mental Activity," *Journal of the American Medical Association*, 230:1428, 1974.

2. AICARDI, J., and CHEVRIE, J. J., "Convulsive Status Epilepticus in Infants and Children," *Epilepsia*, 2:187, 1971.

3. AIRD, R., and YAMOMOTO, T., "Behavior Disorders of Childhood," *Electroencephalography and Clinical Neurophysiology*, 21:148, 1966.

4. ALPERS, B. J., "Personality and Emotional Disorder Associated with Hypothalamic Lesions," *Research Publications of the Association of Nervous and Mental Disease*, 20:725, 1939.

5. American Psychiatric Association, Committee on Nomenclature and Statistics, *Diagnostic and Statistical Manual of Mental Disorders*, 2nd ed. (DSM-II), American Psychiatric Association, Washington, D.C., 1968.

6. ANDERS, T. F., and WEINSTEIN, P., "Sleep and Its Disorders in Infants and Children: A Review," *Pediatrics*, 50:312, 1972.

7. BAGLEY, C., "Social, Psychological and Neurological Factors and Behavior Disorders in Epileptic Children," *Acta Paedopsychiatrica*, 38:78, 1971.

8. BALMER, S., HOWELS, G., and WHITEMARSH, B., "The Acute Encephalopathy of Kwashiorkor," *Developmental Medicine and Child Neurology*, 10:766, 1968.

9. BARLTROP, D., "The Prevention of Pica," *American Journal of Diseases of Children*, 112:116, 1966.

10. BENTOVIM, A., "Continual Observations of Phenylketonuric Children On and During Withdrawal from Low Phenylalanine Diet," *Archives of Diseases in Childhood*, 43:745, 1968.

11. BINGLEY, T., "Mental Symptoms in Temporal Lobe Epilepsy and Temporal Lobe Gliomas," *Acta Psychiatrica Scandinavica*, 33: Supplement 120, 1958.

12. BIRCH, H. G., et al., "Relation of Kwashiorkor in Early Childhood and Intelligence at School Age," *Pediatric Research*, 5:579, 1971.

13. BLACK, P., et al., "The Posttraumatic Syndromes in Children," in Walker, A. E., Caveness, W. E., and Critchley, M. (Eds.), *The Late Effects of Head Injury*, p. 142, Charles C Thomas, Springfield, Ill., 1969.

14. BLACKFAN, K. D., "Lead Poisoning in Children With Special Reference to Lead as a Cause of Convulsions," *American Journal of Medical Science*, 153:877, 1917.

15. BLADIN, J. F., "The Use of Clonazepam as an

Anticonvulsant—Clinical Evaluation," *Medical Journal of Australia*, 1:688, 1973.

16. BRADLEY, J. E., and BAUMGARTNER, R. J., "Subsequent Mental Development of Children with Lead Encephalopathy as Related to Type of Treatment," *Journal of Pediatrics*, 53:311, 1958.

17. BURKS, J. S., et al., "Tricyclic Antidepressant Poisoning Reversal of Coma, Choreoathetosis and Myoclonus by Physostigmine," *Journal of the American Medical Association*, 230:1405, 1974.

18. BYERS, R. K., and LORD, E. E., "Late Effects of Lead Poisoning on Mental Development," *American Journal of Diseases of Children*, 66:471, 1943.

19. COHEN, W. J., and COHEN, N. H., "Lithium Carbonate, Haloperidol and Irreversible Brain Damage," *Journal of the American Medical Association*, 230:1283, 1974.

20. CRITCHLEY, M., "Misoplegia or Hatred of Hemiplegia, *Mount Sinai Journal of Medicine*, 41:82, 1974.

21. DAVIS, G., "Effect of Central Excitant and Depressive Drugs on Locomotor Activity in the Monkey," *American Journal of Physiology*, 188:619, 1957.

22. DELAY, J., and DENIKER, P., "Drug Induced Extrapyramidal Syndromes," in Vinken, P. J., and Bruyn, G. W. (Eds.), *Handbook of Clinical Neurology*, vol. 6, p. 248, Elsevier, Amsterdam, 1973.

23. EICHENWALD, H. F., and FRY, P. D., "Nutrition and Learning," *Science*, 163:644, 1969.

24. EISENBERG, L., "Psychiatric Implications of Brain Damage in Children," *Psychiatric Quarterly*, 31:72, 1957.

25. ELLINWOOD, E. H., SUDILOVSKY, A., and NELSON, L. M., "Evolving Behavior in the Clinical and Experimental Amphetamine (Model) Psychosis," *American Journal of Psychiatry*, 130:1088, 1973.

26. ELLIOT, K., and KNIGHTS, J. (Eds.), "Lipids, Malnutrition and Developing Brain," *CIBA Foundation Symposium*, Churchill, London, 1972.

27. EL YOUSEF, M. K., et al., "Reversal of Antiparkinsonian Drug Toxicity by Physostigmine: A Controlled Study," *American Journal of Psychiatry*, 130:141, 1973.

28. EY, H., *Etudes Psychiatriques*, vol. 3, Desclee de Brouwer, Paris, 1954.

29. FALCONER, M., "Reversibility by Temporal Lobe Resection of the Behavior Abnormalities of Temporal Lobe Epilepsy," *New England Journal of Medicine*, 289:451, 1973.

30. FINLEY, K. H., et al., "Western Encephalitis and Cerebral Ontogenesis," *Archives of Neurology*, 16:140, 1967.

31. FISHER, C., et al., "A Psychophysiological Study of Nightmares and Night Terrors, I. Physiological Aspects of the Stage 4 Night Terror," *Journal of Nervous and Mental Disease*, 157:75, 1973.

32. FISHER, M., KORSKA JAER, G., and PEDERSEN, E., "Psychotic Episodes in Zarontin Treatment," *Epilepsia*, 6:325, 1965.

33. FLOR, H. P., "Psychosis and Temporal Lobe Epilepsy," *Epilepsia*, 10:363, 1969.

34. FREEMAN, R. D., "Psychiatric Problems in Adolescents with Cerebral Palsy," *Developmental Medicine and Child Neurology*, 12:64, 1970.

35. FRIIS, M. L., and LUND, M., "Stress Convulsions," *Archives of Neurology*, 31:15, 1974.

36. FULTON, J. F., *Frontal Lobotomy and Affective Behavior*, W. W. Norton, New York, 1951.

37. GALLAGHER, J. J., *A Comparison of Birth Injured and Non-Birth Injured Mentally Retarded Children on Several Psychological Variables*, Society for Research in Child Development Monographs, vol. 22, 1957.

38. GARDNER, J., "Behavior Treatment Approach to a Psychogenic Seizure Case," *Journal of Consulting Psychology*, 31:209, 1967.

39. GIBBS, F., and LOW, N., "EEG in Children," *Pediatric Clinics of North America*, 2:291, 1955.

40. GIBSON, J. L., "A Plea for Painted Railings and Painted Walls of Rooms as the Source of Lead Poisoning Among Queensland Children," *Australian Medical Gazette*, 23:149, 1904.

41. GILSINN, J., *Estimates of the Nature and Extent of Lead Paint Poisoning in the United States*, Department of Commerce, National Bureau of Standards, NBS TN-746, Washington, D.C., 1972.

42. GLASER, G. H., "The Problem of Psychosis in Psychomotor Temporal Lobe Epileptics," *Epilepsia*, 5:272, 1964.

43. GOLDENSOHN, E. S., and GOLD, A. P., "Prolonged Behavioral Disturbance as Ictal Phenomena," *Neurology*, 10:1, 1960.

44. GOTO, I., et al., "Toxic Polyneuropathy Due to Glue Sniffing," *Journal of Neurology, Neurosurgery and Psychiatry*, 37:848, 1974.

45. GOTTSCHALK, L., "Effects of Intensive Psychotherapy on Epileptic Children," *Archives of Neurology and Psychiatry*, 70:361, 1953.

46. GRAHAM, F. K., et al., "Development Three Years After Perinatal Anoxia and Other Potentially Damaging Newborn Experiences," *Psychology Monographs*, 76:1, 1962.

47. GREENOUGH, W. T., VOLKMAN, F. R., and JURASKA, J. M., "Effects of Rearing Complexity on Dendritic Branching in Frontotemporal Cortex of Rat," *Experimental Neurology*, 41:371, 1973.

48. Group for the Advancement of Psychiatry, Committee on Child Psychiatry, *Psychopathological Disorders in Childhood: Theoretical Considerations and a Proposed Classification*, vol. 6, Report No. 62, Group for the Advancement of Psychiatry, New York, 1966.

49. Group for the Advancement of Psychiatry, Committee on Research, *Pharmacotherapy and Psychotherapy: Paradoxes, Problems, and Progress*, vol. 9, Report No. 93, Group for the Advancement of Psychiatry, New York, 1975.

50. GRUENBERG, R., and POND, D. A., "Conduct Disorders in Epileptic Children," *Journal of Neurology, Neurosurgery and Psychiatry*, 20:65, 1957.

51. HACKNEY, I. M., et al., "Phenylketonuria, Mental Development, Behavior and Termination of Low Phenylalanine Diet," *Journal of Pediatrics*, 40:373, 1968.

52. HARDING, T., "The Effect of LSD on Serum Creatine Kinase Levels," *Psychopharmacologia*, 40:177, 1974.

53. HARPER, R. G., et al., "The Effect of a Methadone Treatment Program Upon Pregnant Heroin Addicts and Their New Born Infants," *Pediatrics*, 54:300, 1974.

54. HARTLAGE, L. C., GREEN, J. B., and OFFUTT, L., "Dependency in Epileptic Children," *Epilepsia*, 13:27–30, 1972.

55. HATRICK, J., and DEWHURST, K., "Delayed Psychosis Due to LSD," *Lancet*, 2:742, 1970.

56. HOLDSWORTH, L., and WHITEMARSH, K., "A Study of Children with Epilepsy Attending Ordinary Schools," *Developmental Medicine and Child Neurology*, 16:746, 1974.

57. KAHN, E., and COHEN, L. H., "Organic Driveness—A Brain Stem Syndrome and an Experience," *The New England Journal of Medicine*, 210:748, 1934.

58. KILOH, L. G., et al., "Sterotactic Amygdalotomy for Aggressive Behavior," *Journal of Neurology, Neurosurgery and Psychiatry*, 37:437, 1974.

59. KLUVER, H., and BUCY, P. C., "Psychic Blindness and Other Symptoms Following Bilateral Temporal Lobectomy in Rhesus Monkeys," *American Journal of Physiology*, 119:352, 1937.

60. KOGAN, K., TYLER, N., and TURNER, P., "The Process of Interpersonal Adaptation Between Mothers and Their Cerebral Palsied Children," *Developmental Medicine and Child Neurology*, 16:518, 1974.

61. KOLVIN, I., "Psychosis in Childhood—A Comparative Study," in Rutter, M. (Ed.), *Infantile Autism: Concepts, Characteristics and Treatment*, p. 7, Churchill-Livingston, Edinburgh, 1971.

62. KOMROWER, G. M., and LEE, D. H., "Long-term Follow Up of Galactosemia," *Archives of Diseases in Childhood, 45:*367, 1970.

63. LANDOLT, H., "Serial EEG Investigation During Psychotic Episodes in Epileptic Patients and During Schizophrenic Attacks," in de Haas, L. (Ed.), *Lectures on Epilepsy*, p. 91, Elsevier, Amsterdam, 1958.

64. LENNOX, W., *Epilepsy and Related Disorders*, Little, Brown, Boston, 1960.

65. LINTON, J. S., "Vulnerability of Children to Lead Exposure and Toxicity," *The New England Journal of Medicine, 289:*1229, 1973.

66. LLOYD STILL, J. D., et al., "Intellectual Development After Severe Malnutrition in Infancy," *Pediatrics, 54:*306, 1974.

67. LOMBROSCO, C. T., et al., "Ctenoid in Healthy Youth: A Controlled Study of 14 and 6 per Second Spiking," *Neurology, 16:*1152, 1966.

68. LUBORSKY, L., et al., "A Content Analysis of Psychologic States Prior to Petit Mal Episodes," *Journal of Nervous and Mental Disease, 160:*282, 1975.

69. McFIE, J., "The Effects of Hemispherectomy on Intellectual Functioning in Cases of Infantile Hemiplegia," *Journal of Neurology, Neurosurgery and Psychiatry, 24:* 240, 1961.

70. McLELLAN, D. L., and SWASH, M., "Choreoathetosis and Encephalopathy Induced by Phenytoin," *British Journal of Medicine, 2:*204, 1974.

71. MANCKEBERG, R., "Malnutrition and Human Behavior," *Nutritional Review, 27:*191, 1969.

72. MAURER, D. V., and BOGEL, S. H., *Narcotics and Narcotic Addiction*, Charles C Thomas, Springfield, Ill., 1970.

73. MILNER, B., "Psychological Effects Produced by Temporal Lobe Excision," in Solomon, H. C., Cobb, S., and Penfield, W. (Eds.), *The Brain and Human Behavior: Proceedings of the Association for Research in Nervous and Mental Disease, Dec. 7–8, 1956*, Williams & Wilkins, Baltimore, Md., 1958.

74. MONEY, J., "Turner's Syndrome and Parietal Lobe Functions," *Cortex, 9:*387, 1973.

75. MONTCRIEF, A. A., et al. "Lead Poisoning in Children," *Archives of Diseases in Childhood, 39:*1, 1964.

76. MORSE, R. M., and LITIN, E. M., "The Anatomy of Delirium," *American Journal of Psychiatry, 128:*111, 1971.

77. MULLAN, S., and PENFIELD, W., "Illusions of Comparative Interpretation and Emotion," *Archives of Neurology and Psychiatry, 81:*269, 1959.

78. MURPHY, M. J., and GOLDSTEIN, M. N., "Diphenyl Hydantoin Induced Asterexis, A Clinical Study," *Journal of the American Medical Association, 229:*538, 1974.

79. NOEL, B., et al., "The XYY Syndrome—Reality or Myth," *Clinical Genetics, 5:*387, 1975.

80. PALINSANO, P. A., SNEED, R. C., and CASSADY, G., "Untaxed Whiskey and Fetal Lead Exposure," *Journal of Pediatrics, 75:*869, 1969.

81. PAPEZ, J. W., "A Proposed Mechanism of Emotion," *Archives of Neurology and Psychiatry, 38:*725, 1937.

82. PASAMANICK, B., and KNOBLOCH, H., "Brain Damage and Reproductive Casualty," *American Journal of Orthopsychiatry, 30:*298, 1960.

83. PERLSTEIN, M. A., and ATTALA, R., "Neurologic Sequelae of Plumbism in Childhood," *Clinical Pediatrics, 5:*292, 1966.

84. PUESCHEL, S. M., KOPITO, L., and SCHWACHMAN, H., "Children With an Increased Lead Burden—A Screening and Follow-Up Study," *Journal of the American Medical Association, 222:*462, 1972.

85. PURPURA, D. A., "Dendritic Spine Dysgenesis and Mental Retardation," *Science, 186:*1126, 1974.

86. RANDT, C. T., and DERBY, B. M., "Behavioral and Brain Correlations in Early Life Nutritional Deprivation," *Archives of Neurology, 28:*167, 1973.

87. REYNOLDS, E., and TRAVERS, R., "Serum Anticonvulsant Concentrations in Epileptic Patients with Mental Symptoms: A Preliminary Report," *British Journal of Psychiatry, 124:*440–445, 1974.

88. ROMANO, J., and ENGEL, G. L., "Delirium, I. EEG Data," *Archives of Neurology and Psychiatry, 51:*356, 1944.

89. ROSENTHAL, S., and KAUFMAN, S., "Vincristine Neurotoxicity," *Annals of Internal Medicine, 80:*733, 1974.

90. ROSS, A. O., "Behavior Therapy," in Quay, H. C., and Werry, J. S. (Eds.), *Psychopathological Disorders of Childhood*, p. 273, John Wiley, New York, 1972.

91. ROTHSCHILD, E. O., "Lead Poisoning—The Silent Epidemic," *The New England Journal of Medicine, 283:* 704, 1970.

92. RUTTER, M., *Psychiatry in Mental Retardation: An Annual Review*, vol. 13, p. 186, Grune & Stratton, New York, 1971.

93. ———, GRAHAM, P. J., and ULE, W., "A Neuropsychiatric Study in Childhood," *Clinics in Developmental Medicine*, No. 35/36, Heinemann, London, 1970.

94. SCHECHTER, M. D., "Bridge Over Troubled Water: An Interventive Method in Cases of Maternal Deprivation," *Australian and New Zealand Journal of Psychiatry, 5:*191–198, 1971.

95. SHAFFER, D., "Psychiatric Aspects of Brain Injury in Childhood: A Review," *Developmental Medicine and Child Neurology, 15:*11, 1973.

96. SILBERGILD, E. K., and GOLDBERG, A. M., "Lead Induced Behavioral Dysfunction: An Animal Model of Hyperactivity," *Experimental Neurology, 42:*146, 1974.

97. SKLAR, B., HANLEY, J., and SIMMONS, W., "An EEG Experiment Aimed Towards Identifying Dyslexic Children," *Nature, 240:*414, 1972.

98. SLATER, E., BEARD, E., and GLITHERO, E., "The Schizophrenia-Like Psychosis in Epilepsy," *British Journal of Psychiatry, 109:*95, 1963.

99. SNYDER, B. D., BLONDE, L., and McWHIRTER, W. R., "Reversal of Amitriptyline Intoxication by Physostigmine," *Journal of the American Medical Association, 230:*1433, 1974.

100. SNYDER, S. H., "Catecholamines in the Brain as Mediators of Amphetamine Psychosis," *Archives of General Psychiatry, 27:*169, 1972.

101. TOWNSEND, J. J., et al., "Progressive Rubella Panencephalitis," *The New England Journal of Medicine, 292:*990, 1975.

102. TYLER, H. R., "Pelizaeus-Merzbacher Disease," *Archives of Neurology and Psychiatry, 80:*162, 1958.

103. UDANI, P. M., "Neurologic Manifestations in Kwashiorkor," *Indian Journal of Child Health, 9:*103, 1960.

104. VALE, S., et al., "Creatine Phosphokinase," *Archives of Neurology, 30:*103, 1974.

105. VALLARTA, J. M., BELL, D. B., and REICHERT, A., "Progressive Encephalopathy Due to Chronic Hydantoin Intoxication," *American Journal of Diseases of Children, 128:*27, 1974.

106. VALVAKA, J., et al., "EEG Heart Rate, and Mood Change ("High") After Cannabis," *Psychopharmacologia, 32:*11, 1973.

107. WASTERLAIN, C. G., "Inhibition of Cerebral Protein Synthesis by Epileptic Seizures Without Motor Activity," *Neurology, 24:*175, 1974.

108. WEIL, M. L., et al., "Chronic Progressive Panencephalitis Due to Rubella Virus Simulating Subacute Sclerosing Panencephalitis," *The New England Journal of Medicine, 292:*994, 1974.

109. WHITTEY, C. W. M., "Effects of Anterior Cingulectomy in Man," *Proceedings of the Royal Society of Medicine, 48:*463, 1955.

110. WILDER, B. J., and RAMSEY, R. E., "Psychological

Abberations Associated with Antiepileptic Drugs," *Clinical Electroencephalography, 5:*199, 1974.

111. Wilson, P. J. E., "Cerebral Hemispherectomy for Infantile Hemiplegia: A Report of 50 Cases," *Brain, 93:* 147–180, 1970.

112. Winik, M., "Malnutrition and Brain Development," *Journal of Pediatrics, 74:*667, 1969.

113. Woodruff, M. W., "Subconvulsive Epileptic Discharge and Behavioral Impairment," *Behavioral Biology, 11:*431, 1974.

114. Woods, T. L., "Comments on the Dynamics and Treatment of Disfigured Children," *Clinical Social Work Journal, 3:*16, 1975.

115. Zelson, C., "Infant of the Addicted Mother," *The New England Journal of Medicine, 288:*1393, 1973.

116. Zeman, W., and King, F. A., "Tumors of the Septum Pellucidum and Adjacent Structures with Abnormal Affective Behavior: An Anterior Midline Structure Syndrome," *Journal of Nervous and Mental Disease, 127:* 490, 1958.

117. Zlutnick, S., Mayville, W. J., and Moffat, S., "Modification of Seizure Disorders: The Interruption of Behavioral Chains," *Journal of Applied Behavior Analysis, 8(1):*1–12, 1975.

19 / Mental Retardation

Henry H. Work

Classification

Mental retardation (mental deficiency, feeblemindedness, subnormality of intelligence, intellectual defect, stupidity, etc.) occupies the lead section of DSM-II.[5] Under that heading, with its attendant subcategories, mental retardation is defined as referring to "subnormal general intellectual functioning which originates during the developmental period and is associated with impairment of either learning and social adjustment or maturation, or both." The more recent definition from the American Association on Mental Deficiency modifies this by adding the word "significantly" to make the definition read "Mental retardation refers to a significantly subaverage general intellectual functioning existing concurrently with deficits in adaptive behavior and manifested during the developmental period."[4]

The GAP classification is based largely on etiology and includes a group of biological disorders, an environmental group, and an intermediate group.[21] This categorization notes the variability of the pictures shown by children with mental retardation: those associated with the intellectual limitations, and those related to the individual's awareness of the defect. The description also points out that psychotic, neurotic, or other personality disorders may occur.

The ninth revision of the International Classification of Disease[52] has recommended that "for each patient, the following four types of information would be recorded: (1) degree of mental handicap, (2) etiological or associated biological or organic factors, (3) associated psychiatric disorder, and (4) psychosocial factors. For each patent, all four types of information would be routinely reported, instead of only the degree of mental handicap.

All of these categories suggest a very wide range of the syndrome of individuals with defects in intellect. They also emphasize that not only is the syndrome characterized by intellectual deficiencies, but also by varying degrees of adaptation to life. All of these levels of defect relate to the lower end of a continuum of normal intelligence. The various subcategories defined in DSM-II spell this out clearly.[5] Borderline mental retardation, a group comprising individuals with an IQ of 68–85, approaches the capacity of a large number of individuals who are functioning adequately in society. Below that, the category of mild mental retardation with an IQ of 52–67 also includes many individuals who are not labeled as retarded unless they are faced with the complexities of learning which will be described below. The moderately, the severely, and the profoundly retarded, all of whose IQ's fall under the level of 50 demand more intensive care, adapt less well, and, at the lowest level, are usually cared for in an institutional or other sheltered setting.

Description and Variants

Many of the categories of severe retardation occur in relation to biologic syndromes that involve and disfigure the entire body. These range from hydrocephalics through microcephalics with a host of intermediate somatic conditions. On the other hand, as one goes up the intellectual ladder, the appearance of the individual is not necessarily distinguished from the population at large. Function then becomes of greater importance, both in the capacity to pass intellectual tests and in the capacity to adapt to the society in which one lives. Since the critical aspect of mental retardation is related to development, a true appreciation of the defect depends on a knowledge of the expectations of society at various levels of development.

As the GAP category implies, in recent years it has been appreciated that the bulk of the retardates can be separated into two relatively distinct groups with an intermediate category.[21] The first of these constitute the "clinical" types and those of the second, the "sociocultural" or environmental, retarded.

An example of a child in the first grouping is a one-month-old female with multiple birth defects including myelomeningocele, hydrocephalus and imperforate anus. The child was born at term to a twenty-nine-year-old mother after six hours of very difficult labor. Although the child weighed seven pounds and eight ounces, it was apparent on inspection that the multiple defects precluded normal development. While it was possible to repair the imperforate anus, the other existing conditions pointed to a projection of severe disability with intelligence around the 10–20 IQ range.

Characteristically, the clinical group includes children on whom a diagnosis can be made early and in whom the intellectual defect is either severe or profound. Most of these children need considerable care. The diagnosis tends to be fixed and unchanging throughout the life of the individual. Development as suggested by the intellectual level is profoundly delayed. This type of retardation is not related to social class.

That form of retardation labeled sociocultural or environmental by the GAP classification comprises approximately 75 percent of the total group of retardates.

A characteristic child is Margery. The second child in a lower-middle-class family, she was a planned birth with a normal pregnancy and delivery. The child was approximately three weeks premature, but the only outstanding characteristic following birth was that she was considered to be a poor eater. She was late in turning over and did not sit until she was between eight and nine months old. She walked at approximately eighteen months, but was an appealing child and was the focus of considerable family attention. Her own personality was somewhat obsessive, with great concern about becoming dirty, but otherwise she had normal habits of eating and sleeping. She was well into the first grade in school when the teachers became concerned at her inability to understand numbers and letters and brought this to the attention of the parents. It became obvious that she functioned in the category of mild mental retardation, and it was necessary to plan a special schooling program for her.

Another variant of this category is seen in Peter, the third son in a black ghetto family. Peter was the product of a normal pregnancy and delivery and was in no way considered different from his siblings. None of them had been advanced in development and when Peter did not sit until seven months and did not walk until fifteen months he was not considered unusual. The environment was notable for the families' poverty and marked by inadequate parent-child relationships. What communication existed was mostly related to anger at the child's behavior, his awkwardness, or his seeming inability to understand. When Peter entered school, it became apparent within a short time that he was incapable of understanding and learning simple first-grade academic tasks. Testing showed that he achieved a level of 63 with a considerable scatter in his IQ scores.

This environmental group is characterized by the lateness of the diagnosis, the individual's normal appearance, the surfacing of problems in a school setting, and by the fact that more children of this category are found in the lower socioeconomic levels of society. These children are often not diagnosed as retarded until they face the tasks of school, and because no demonstrable physical signs are present, this phenomenon has been described as "six-hour retardation." Many of these children cease to be considered as retarded once they have finished schooling and merge into the general population.

Parents of children who manifest severe clinical retardation seek help early. Occasionally, help is forced upon them by relatives or other agents of society. Families of the larger environmental group, however, generally do not observe any major difference between their child and other members of the family or the neighborhood children, and therefore the diagnosis is often imposed on these families from without.

The first category (described as the "clinical" group) includes a host of subcategories. The DSM-II[5] lists these types of retardation as those (1) following infection and intoxication, (2) following trauma or physical agent, (3) with disorders of metabolism, growth or nutrition, (4) with chromosal abnormality, and (5) of complications associated with prematurity (pp. 15–22).

The larger group described as "with psychosocial (environmental) deprivation" includes two subgroups. The subgroup termed "cultural-familial retardation" requires that evidence of retardation be found in at least one of the parents and one or more of the siblings, suggesting that this is a multifactorial genetic familial retardation. The second subgroup is that associated with environmental deprivation such as described earlier. Those individuals who fall into the clinical category not only may be usually diagnosed at birth, but with increasing diagnostic skills, the diagnosis may even be suggested during pregnancy. The host of syndromes which relate to genetic origin of intellectual defect grows daily.

History

Like the poor, the dull have been with us always. Too often the poor and the dull are the same. The authors of the Old Testament wrote of foolish people, but by and large when they called someone a fool, they meant someone who willfully did not seem to understand his tasks.

For centuries life spans were short for all but the most wealthy and protected. Large segments of the population died of either neglect or infection. The early deaths of many retarded individuals probably explains why the concept of special care for backward children remained unorganized from a social viewpoint until recently.

For many years the retarded were viewed by some as holy, by others as the only innocents. However, they were often ultimately responsible for their own fates. A few probably did simple jobs, a few were kept at home, many found their way into workhouses and parish institutions. During the Industrial Revolution, it was not uncommon for an employer to buy a batch of three or four hundred orphans from such institutions and among this number he was obliged to take some of the idiot children. The mind of the idiot, like that of the infant, was still connected with the idea of the animal soul.

During the last two centuries we have looked at human beings in a more scientific fashion. This has made it possible to separate out various categories of etiologies and degrees of adaptation and accommodation, even though medical and pedagogic classification has been, and still continues to be at times, a very confusing thing.

Itard found his wild boy in 1800. By that time, however, he was prepared by his own studies of teaching methods to begin the training of a mental defective. Within a few decades, his pupil, Seguin, proposed newer methods of teaching of individuals of subnormal intellect and by the middle of the nineteenth century, his message had spread to the United States.[28] The first school for retardates, which later became the Fernald School, opened in Massachusetts under the leadership of Howe. Seguin himself had established a variety of teaching methods as well as institutions, one of which, founded in New York about 1878, bore the rather unique name of the "Physiological School for Weak-minded and Weak-bodied Children."

It waited, however, on this century for improved testing methodology to sort out individuals of less than normal intelligence and to begin to apply the many teaching methods, retraining procedures and opportunities for care that exist today. Kanner states that progress in every science depends on dissatisfaction, curiosity, and caution.[28] To paraphrase him, it is these qualities that have led devoted and serious students and caretakers to ameliorate the stresses of the retarded individual as well as the distress of the families in which they live.

Retardation: Frequency, Incidence, Prevalence and Distribution

The entire subject of prevalence and incidence of mental retardation has been under considerable review in recent years. If one were to survey the total population in a search for individuals of all ages having intelligence quotients below 70, approximately 3 percent of the population would be included. If one surveys the school age population, such a correlation can readily be found. It is essential to be aware that testing procedures vary rather widely and that there has been much criticism of a lack of cultural relationship in testing procedures for wide segments of the population. A stormy debate rages as to whether the standardized tests which are used are appropriate and applicable to minority groups as well as to poverty groups. A proper consideration of these factors is important in understanding the prevalence of this disorder. From the point of view of the psychiatrist, the proper testing of any one individual becomes a matter of clinical concern.

As we have noted above, the number of individuals who are suspected of being retarded changes with development and with the tasks imposed by society. Therefore, that proportion of the population which is actually *labeled* as retarded, probably does not include more than 1 percent of the population, or roughly some 2 million in the United States. Other diagnostic errors probably add to the disproportion of males labeled as mental retardates. One biological explanation for this phenomenon is based on the X chromosome and the advantage of the female in relationship to that chromosome. There is no question, however, as is demonstrated in other psychological conditions, that the demands on males are different and therefore society, by its expectations, is more likely to find the retarded male and label him for his defect.

Of equal importance in recent years has been the clearer description of sociocultural group in relationship to socioeconomic conditions. This category (sociocultural retardation) is more commonly used in the United States than in other countries. In a group of articles concerned with the classification of mental retardation issued as a supplement to the *American Journal of Psychiatry* in May 1972, there are a host of observations on this particular category.[8, 49] From a time when such retardation was called undifferentiated, until it became labeled familial, the field has moved into two major groupings, cultural-familial (psychosocial, sociocultural), and environmental deprivation. As noted above, these instances of retardation comprise over 75 percent of the total groupings. The retardation is usually of a mild degree with IQ's in the range of 50–70, very frequently it is the kind that falls into the "six hour" category or is seen especially in the six- to eighteen-year-old groups since the children are primarily identified at school. These children also demonstrate a capacity for adaptive functioning that makes their deficit apparent chiefly when confronted with a highly organized learning situation such as posed by the tasks of school.

The normal appearance of these children and their otherwise usual life style mean that such retardates are not identified until a specific task of learning is applied. Many of them come from economically, socially, and educationally underprivileged backgrounds. Tarjan[47, 49] has pointed out that the risk of mild retardation, including sociocultural retardation, is at a level fifteen times higher for impoverished urban and rural children than those of middle-class suburban origin.

What is most apparent is that these children are products of a series of potentially clinically important hazards, frequently having been born to mothers who were undernourished and whose pregnancies were ill-cared for, with a resultant high prematurity rate. Mothers, as well as the children, are often unprotected by customary public health measures and suffer from inadequate nutrition. Severe forms of malnutrition lead to the more definitive kinds of retardation, but milder forms may add just one more handicap to the growth of these children. In addition, the stimuli which would form the normal curriculum of existence are missing. Pavenstedt, who has very clearly described these children, notes that they come from chaotic homes where language and speech are inadequate or absent and the exposure to the normal tactile sensations of life are missing.[38] Eisenberg and others have described a causal model of such environmental deprivation.[17] Most notably the children who suffer from this type of disability come from situations where there is a lifelong causality based on deficit. Pregnancy, birth, infancy, nutrition—all of these become hazards which continue to produce this type of deprived and nonfunctioning retardation. Rutter[43] has proposed a model for the interaction of these various forces tending to produce the mild type of retardation with a high prevalence in impoverished population groups. Mercer has described it more clearly in her Riverside studies.[36] What is critical for psychiatrists is the large number of these children who, with their school failures, develop emotional disabilities and behavioral problems that ultimately focus the attention of the professionals on this particular group.

There is another group of children where the primary source of the disability appears to be of a psychogenic nature. Children with childhood psychosis, autism, and mild or minimal brain dysfunctions fall into this category. The term pseudoretardation has been used to describe some of these children. More specifically, this label should apply to those patients where mental retardation is a concomitant of psychosis, severe emotional disturbance, neurotic disorder, or other types of major personality disorders during infancy and early childhood. One of the unfortunate aspects of the treatment of children with severe autism and childhood psychosis is that the effort to treat them sometimes results in improved behavior patterns with an underlying intellectual deficit. In such instances, this becomes part of the hazard of therapy.

Clinical Course of the Condition

It is obvious from the material presented that not only must mental retardation be viewed and diagnosed as a developmental disorder, but the professional approach to it must consider the level of the individual's intelligence, his capacity for adaptation, the environment in which he is living, and very importantly, the reaction of his parents to the situation.

It is equally important to be aware that psychiatrists, including the child psychiatrist, are rarely the primary professionals who make the diagnosis and confront the parents with a prognosis. In the case of the biological disorders, the obstetrician or pediatrician is usually the first one to appraise the parents of the situation and either to make predictions or to give advice in management. In the case of the mildly retarded, the diagnosis is frequently made in an educational setting. It is communicated to a physician only if there is a need for a more clear diagnostic approach or for management of the family and/or the behavioral and personality problems of the child.

It is therefore worth noting at the outset that the role of the psychiatrist may very well be one of coordination or management as well as the usual psychotherapeutic functions. There are many individuals outside the psychiatric and medical profession who are involved in the care of retarded individuals. Indeed, educators see the whole problem in the light of their experience, and it is quite true that the educational programs for the retarded may comprise the individual's major contacts with professionals. It is important, therefore, to describe the various reactions of families, professionals, and others to the presence of retardation.

Family as well as professional dynamics are most clearly observed in those instances where severe retardation is diagnosed early. Utilizing the example of the child with a massive meningocoele and complete paralysis of the lower limbs, it is possible to discuss the dynamics of the parents in relationship to this disability. Over the first few weeks and months it was very apparent that in terms of normal development no progress was being made. The child was unresponsive except in a vegetative sense, and it was obvious to everyone except the parents that this was a severely damaged child.

The critical situation which confronts the parents of the retarded occurs at the time that they become aware consciously or unconsciously of the diagnosis of the child's situation. Over the years, a great deal of concern has been expressed over the role of the professional in assisting the parents to "accept" the diagnosis and all it means. Somehow there is the impression that this is a quick and immediate situation based on the professional's evaluation of what confronts them. For the parents, however, such a critical choice is rarely quick and certainly never easy. It is very obvious that confrontation with a diagnosis that suggests a long-time difficulty and periods of adjustment cannot come easily for anyone.

With all parents there is an expectation of reward in their children. Children are to be born bright and intelligent, they are to achieve, and through their performance they are to requite their parents for all of their care. One of the distressing aspects of the internal relationships of a retarded individual and his family is that the rewards are not there. Growth and development occur slowly. Speech comes late. Learning is difficult. In every way, the child balks the parents' desire for their due reward, and instead demands care far beyond that needed by most children.

Thus it is that the caretaker, particularly the physician, must meet people at their immediate temporal and emotional levels. Rarely are the parents ready to accept the diagnosis—most are far from doing so, and others postpone such an acceptance endlessly.

Most commonly, the initial reaction of a parent or parents is to avoid the fact that there is a difficulty. Their reaction is to ignore or deny the obvious differences in their child. Subsequently they deny the fact that progress may not occur. The "he will grow out of it" concept applies particularly to the slow-to-develop child and often stands in the way of a rational approach.

As recognition of the concept of the developmental disability grows in the parents, they begin to experience guilt. Then comes blame, first of the clinical situation and then of themselves. The mother may start by becoming concerned about her pregnancy, her obstetrician, her hospitalization, the birth, etc. If it becomes impossible to project blame onto others, there is always the genetic situation or the other parent's family. The problem may be attributed to the other because of the family background, or "bad habits." The projection may be to impersonal events occurring during the pregnancy such as intercurrent infections.

In dealing with the parents of the retarded, one can assume that there are always some guilt feelings and that the mother, aware of her unique role in the pregnancy, will bear a major burden of responsibility about the conception, the birth, and the irregularities that have occurred. Physicians and other caretakers may be the recipients of this guilt and the hostility that goes with it.

As the child grows older, the burden of care often increases. It is then that stronger feelings about the child become either evident or latent. The parents of a very young baby may see him as hopelessly deformed and physically incapable of self-help; nonetheless it is rare to hear them express the wish that the child would not survive. More commonly, these feelings are kept hidden and erupt later in other forms.

It is important to realize that parental burdens vary with the degree of damage. The more seriously retarded the individual, the greater the demands upon the parents. Thus it is neither unusual nor abnormal for them to wish that the problem, and even the child, did not exist. The nature of conscience suggests that such thoughts will be felt as unacceptable—they must be warded off. Reaction formations develop.

The parents of such children frequently spend much time in caring for medical ills of a seemingly trivial nature. The excessive care, protection, and concern that develops often seems inexplicable, even to professionals. The parent not only demonstrates close protectiveness, but sees the outside world as callous and hostile. Even those who are offering service are seen as antagonists to the parental concept of the particular needs of this child. Other members of the family complicate the process; at times they seem to be adversaries of the parents, and at other times they themselves assume the overprotective role.

If the concept of having a retarded child, particularly a severely retarded one, is unacceptable, it is not surprising that parents desperately go looking for help. The phenomenon of "shopping" is a serious one and will be considered subsequently in the light of the professional's reaction. It is important, however, to realize that the parental concerns that lead to shopping pose tremendous demands on all the caretaking professions, both clinical and pedagogical.

An important aspect of parental reactions to the fact of having a retarded offspring, especially a severely retarded one, lies in their very acute sense of a lack of support from society as a whole. If parents feel beleaguered by unfriendly relatives and their own concept of a calloused physician, it merely mirrors the fact that this may be the attitude of society as a whole. In an age where progress is demanded, where performance is critical and where excellence is a byword, the parents of a retarded child feel pushed out of the normal societal situation. The following case is illustrative.

Joan was seen at the age of seven as a part of a preliminary screening for a special schooling program for retarded children. Joan was the third of four children. It had been apparent at birth that she had all of the characteristics of Down's Syndrome.

In describing the family, the mother stated that the other children were quite normal and that her pregnancy with Joan was equally normal. At birth it was apparent that there was something different about the child, but the mother was not immediately aware of the situation. She was, however, told about the condition within the first forty-eight hours and a rough prognosis was given to her at that time. It was her understanding that the child would not develop as rapidly as the rest of her children, that the symptom picture, which presented with characteristic eyes, hands, skin, etc. was clear, and that she should not expect much progress from this child.

At the time that Joan was first seen, the mother was still bland about the entire situation. She said that once the prognosis had been described to her, there seemed to be no further need for concern, but she felt that she should rear the child in a way appropriate to the possibility of her not succeeding as well as her other children had.

At that time the mother was quite comfortable in stating that Joan had progressed to somewhat less than a three-year-old level, but it was equally obvious that the mother was intrigued with this child and felt happy and comfortable with what progress had been made. Joan was indeed functioning at a roughly three-year-old level. She had a rudimentary form of speech which was partially understood by the family although quite incomprehensible to others. She was a happy, vivacious child and was a considerable show-off. When she was presented to a group of students, she was pleased to stand on a chair, to babble away and to respond to their amusement with a showmanshiplike enjoyment.

Down's Syndrome, the most common of the genetic disorders, is also unique in the panoply of retardation. Whereas many of these children died earlier of infectious diseases, they are now alive and well. They continue to grow, and live into young adulthood. It is their disposition; friendly, at times histrionic, that makes them stand out from the general category of retarded individuals. Whereas it has often been suggested that families utilize retarded individuals as "pets," this is particularly true with the Down's Syndrome group. Despite their Mongoloid appearance, the children appear cherubic to many families and are treated thus. They tend to be seen as the comedians of the retarded group.

Within the Mongoloid category, there is an amazingly wide range of intelligence. It has been stated that some have gone on to college and certainly some have completed high school. On the other hand, some of the most severely retarded are also suffering from Down's Syndrome. As with any child, predictions about their progress have to be made on the basis of early developmental observation. The fact that the diagnosis can be made, as an obstretician would put it "as the head comes over the pelvis" does not define the outcome. Within the organic category, the Mongoloid child stands out as the most common severe form of retardation. As a type, they are also so appealing and so attractive that the care of these children tends to be more comfortable and more agreeable than that afforded most retardates.

It is worth pointing out that the range of intelligence is such that a child with normal intelligence living in a family of brilliant individuals may appear retarded.

Jane was a classical example of this situation. She was a fourth child. Both of her parents were professionals—the father a physicist, the mother an artist. She seemed like an ordinary baby except for her slowness in development. Because of the family's intellectual drive, she was expected to attend the highly progressive and very active school in which her siblings were doing well. Her inability to perform along with other outstandingly intelligent children caused considerable distress. Testing showed her to be of average intelligence. She would have functioned quite well had the parents not demanded superior performance at all times. In effect, then, she was a relative retardate despite her normal intelligence. The parents felt ashamed of her, but also pushed and blamed her for her inability to keep up with her siblings.

The parents of a severely retarded child feel not only shamed but condemned by society for their contribution to the community at large. In some instances, this leads to a walling off and a total isolation of parents and child from society. Obviously it has also led to the development of institutions where a child can be placed away from the world and hidden from everyone including the parents themselves.

For the parents, placement of a child, even one who is severely retarded, is not a simple process. The overprotectiveness that characterizes their reaction is manifest by clinging and cloying relationships between the parents and the child. Out of their own sense of protection, they feel it is impossible for any other agency of society to care for their child. When the professional suggests such placement, there is usually horror and concern.

Subsequently, there often occurs a paradoxical response to this. Once the parents have made the break and moved the child from the family, either to foster care or institutional surroundings, it becomes apparent that their overprotectiveness was due largely to guilt and concern. Once placed, visits diminish in frequency and, in the eyes of the institutional staff, such parents often seem to abandon the child.

CLINICAL COURSE OF THE SOCIOCULTURAL GROUP

As noted, the massive educational system with its great emphasis on learning, particularly learning to read, imposes a strain on all individuals who fall below the normal level of intellect. School can therefore be looked upon as a screening mechanism that filters out large numbers of mildly and moderately retarded from other functioning children. The customary tasks of learning cannot easily be coped with by individuals with IQ's from 50–70, and pose hardships for those in the borderline category, 70–85. A large number of these fall into the category of familial retardation, wherein one or more members of the family are of the same intellectual level. It has been suggested that there is a "normal curriculum" in the middle-class family which leads children to learn a great deal about their society and their environment by largely unconscious processes. This has called attention to the fact that there are many families where this kind of learning does not occur. The writings of Pavenstedt portray most graphically the severe aspects of this type of environment for child rearing.[38] She describes families that are chaotic in organization, unpredictable in action and uncommunicative in styles of relation. The children grow up, therefore, with an unpredictable view of society, often frightened and fearful of any actions of adults, and unable to cope with the normal routines that are imposed from without. In consequence, these children have a very difficult time, not only in day care and nursery school, but particularly when they encounter the academic level of school.

Other children whose defects are less well noted and whose home may be less chaotic appear at school with inability to comprehend the classical tasks of learning, particularly reading. These children fail to accommodate to cognitive tasks and therefore are marked by the school for failure, a situation which grows worse during the school years. The intellectual section of society sets standards that everyone must try to meet. Since these are children who come from levels of society where demands are not as great, it is only when they come into contact with the usual institutional settings that the situation becomes critical. Of special note in this area are Mercer's Riverside, California studies. These emphasized the concept of the six-hour retardate, pointing out the number of such individuals who are not suspected of being retarded before coming to school and who cease to be so regarded after they leave.[36]

This has been supported by Edgerton's writings in which he pointed out that in "nontechnological cultures" such as the Navajo, and in some insular cultures such as the Hutterites, parents do not respond to the mentally retarded "with the same degree of antagonism that is seen in the middle-class American culture." In fact, in a more positive vein, the mild and borderline retardates could be seen as unused resources.[15]

In this group of mild and borderline individuals, there are gross discrepancies in function. Not only does the IQ not give a clear picture of capacity and adaptability, but it does not describe clearly the differentials in speech, performance, and language recognition that occur. Yet the presence of these individuals in society exposes them to all the demands of society. How society treats them modifies their capacity to perform. In those parts of society where deprivation and lack of the common curriculum of development are the rule, these children fall further back. How they react to adolescence and adulthood will be discussed in the next section.

Specific Therapeutic Methods for the Sociocultural Syndrome

The socioeconomic range of incidence of this disorder matched against demands for mental health care suggests that psychiatric help is initially more likely to be sought by parents in the middle- and upper-class groups. They seek relief for their own anxieties about the situation. The psychiatrist may thus be confronted by problems related to a developmental sequence.

There is a group of parents, usually referred by an obstetrician or pediatrician, who are concerned about the failure in development of their very young child. These parents may or may not be facing the difficulties relative to care outside the home, but this problem frequently arises. As noted, in considering the developmental problems

of parents, the anger, frustration, and anxiety about the lack of reward stands out in this particular group. The management of these parents' anxieties vis-à-vis placement of various kinds, as well as genetic counselling for the future, are of prime concern.

Anxiety may also be induced in those parents whose child has entered school, is discovered to be slow in learning and has begun either to act-out in the school situation or to experience failure. This type of reaction occurring in children of even normal intelligence where the rest of the family is of high intellectual capacity has been described. In such a family, the discrepancy makes a normally functioning child seem retarded. The behavior of the child is one index of the difficulty. The other is the actual report card, which may be seized on by the parents as evidence of their failure as well as that of the child. Except in degree, the reactions of these parents are not dissimilar from those of parents of the severely retarded when the discovery is made earlier, nor are they different from the reactions of parents whose child is acting-out in school for neurotic reasons.

EMOTIONAL AND BEHAVIORAL DISTURBANCES IN ADOLESCENTS

One must be aware that in America today as well as in European countries, there is an increasing amount of sheltered care, usually in educational settings, for children with milder degrees of retardation. Much of this sheltered care ceases when the child comes into adolescence and is continuing to perform below the customary level. In some communities, sheltered workshops have been utilized to help individuals prepare for vocational tasks. All of these caretaking procedures cease at some point in time. Whenever that moment is reached, certain common casualties occur among the moderate and mildly retarded.

A typical example is Eileen, a plain girl of nineteen whose parents sought help because of mutual frustration. She had early been diagnosed as suffering from moderate retardation and from ages eight to sixteen had been in a variety of private and public schools. When schooling stopped at age sixteen, she found herself totally unprepared, unable to travel in her neighborhood because of the protectiveness of her mother, and completely frustrated at home. The event which precipitated seeking help was a one-day absence from home. She spent the day at the house of a girlfriend while her parents frantically combed the neighborhood seeking her and fearing for her safety—they envisioned her as kidnapped and sexually assaulted.

Because of her lowered intelligence, she had been unable to achieve beyond a fourth grade level. Her home situation was complicated because her father felt that she was merely feigning ignorance; he couldn't understand why she didn't read the paper and pay attention to news programs on television.

It is not impossible to find facilities for further training of such a girl. Indeed, there was a sheltered workshop not far from her neighborhood, but one which did require bus transportation. It was extremely difficult to get the mother to accept the reality of utilizing such transport to get her to the sheltered workshop. On the one hand it was apparent that once she had arrived at the agency, she herself was more content. She had the capacity to learn and she was able to be with other individuals and have a more comfortable time. At the same time, there was a psychotherapeutic problem in terms of her fears and anxieties about her capacity to learn. She had been dependent for too long and did not feel that she could accomplish anything, including getting to and from the school. It required not only some practical help in getting her adjusted to the work situation and capable of getting there, but also some careful therapy in listening to her, taking account of her personal anxieties and fears, and treating her as one would any neurotic sufferer.

This case demonstrates clearly how extremely apprehensive parents are about the general conduct of their retarded children as well as the worries parents have about sexual behavior. The usual parental anxieties related to independence and maturation are greatly exaggerated in this group of children. Without the training that other growing individuals have had, the moderate and mildly retarded child may indeed lack the judgmental capacity to cope with the fact of increasing sexual desire.

The lack of judgment is a critical aspect of the development of problems in this group. Because of their almost normal capacities, they are expected to perform in the outside world and to take their place in society. Their desires are not dissimilar from those of their otherwise more normal peers. Since they have less contact with peers and diminished outlets for recreational or vocational choice, they are often confined to home and therefore increasingly frustrated. The isolation which they suffer becomes exaggerated. A lack of ordinary psychological resources makes the situation even more intolerable. The repressive and restrictive activities of the parents lead to a greater fear, but at the same time, tempt the child to make sexual explorations without the judgment and the controls available to other children. They thus become vulnerable and prey to anyone who wishes to take advantage of a nubile girl or a sexually competent boy. Over the

years there has been a shibboleth that these individuals have greater prowess in sexual activity. There is no current scientific evidence that this is the case.

A clear delineation of the psychologic problems of the retarded has been given by Philips.[40] He points out three common misconceptions about their maladaptive behavior. The first concerns the frequent sense that all problems of the child are a function of the retardation rather than those of interpersonal relations. Second, there is a general assumption that emotional disorders in the retarded are different from those in the normal child. A third misconception is that many of the causes of their behavioral difficulties come from organic brain damage.

Such misconceptions not only die hard, but interfere with an approach to therapy. The problem for the psychiatrist and others working on the psychologic problems of the retarded is not only to assess the intelligence and capacity of the child, but as in any clinical appraisal, to assess the neuroticism, the anxiety, or the behavioral problems with equal diligence. If these can be seen as problems of interpersonal relationship with parents and others, if the behavior can be seen as responses to frustration and fear, they can be more sensibly coped with.

As Lott notes, "the retarded are just as human as normal people. They have the same varied emotional quirks, similar inhibitions, frustrations, guilt feelings, conflicts, and erroneous self-concepts as do others."[32]

A critical factor in assessing the anxiety associated with the behavioral disorders of the retarded is the fact that the scope of their imagination and ability to organize experiences is probably considerably less than that of their normal peers. This demands, therefore, that the approach of the therapist be consonant with the past experiences of the individual. At the same time, he must be aware that the anxieties and psychological impetus for disturbed behavior may be identical with those seen in children with normal intellect. All of the customary techniques which reduce anxiety and promote more healthy relationships are valid tools. If irrational fear can be reduced, if guilt can be assuaged, it is as important to do so here as it would be in any patient. Generally speaking, while the need for continuity in the care of the retarded is paramount, long-term therapy is probably not as productive as short-term therapy focusing on relatively immediate goals. As Menolascino makes clear in his comprehensive overview of the situation,[32]

The necessity for high intellectual endowment has been overemphasized as a prerequisite for psychotherapy. Psychotherapeutic efforts with mentally retarded children must often focus heavily on play therapy, with emphasis on nonverbal techniques. Accordingly, both the attitudinal and methodological treatment issues in psychotherapy with the mentally retarded must be reviewed. Inasmuch as the strong bond that exists between the parent and child has been built up not only over the years, but in the framework of considering the child inadequate, much of the therapeutic problems of the retarded relate to the working out of familial difficulties.

Retardates grow older as does everyone. The current capacity to keep individuals physically well increases the number of older retardates in our society. The problems which these individuals face are very much like those confronted by Eileen when the end of sheltering poses the stress of facing society on the outside. Many such individuals retreat from society. The clearest description of these difficulties is found in Edgerton's work, especially his brilliant description of married retardates. *The Cloak of Competence.*[15]

THE PROFESSIONAL ROLE

Unlike most patients that physicians and other professionals are called on to care for, the mentally retarded comprise a unique group. They are a part of society and yet they cannot accommodate to it nor cope with its everyday problems. They demand extra care and attention on a lifelong basis. They balk the therapeutic zeal of the physician and impose on the patient labors of the educator. They are a source of chronic dismay to their families. It is part of the task of the psychiatrist to view professional as well as parental roles in the care of such individuals. Inasmuch as the specific management and care of these children affects and is affected by those who must do the caring, it is appropriate to discuss the role of that caretaker. Unlike many other medical patients, the retarded seem to be caught up in a tug of war between parents and those who would normally minister to them and provide advice and care. The economic hazards of mental retardation seem to be complicated by the fact that parents of these children, particularly of those who are severely retarded, wander from clinic to clinic, from educational institution to educational institution, and, at times, from quack to quack, seeking an answer to their child's difficulty, an answer that never seems available.

Psychiatrists are as human as parents. On the one hand, they are often highly sympathetic toward the parents of such a child. At times, their sympathy even leads to being oversolicitous and, therefore, ineffective. Equally, however, they are frequently repulsed by the fact and appearance of a mentally retarded child. This is especially true for those severe mental retardates where the medical condition includes deformities. The average psychiatrist, who sees relatively few severely deformed retarded individuals, may be quite as shocked as the general public by the presence of such a child.

Any medical practice, however, may include a considerable number of relatively or mildly retarded individuals. With this group, the psychiatrist may have attitudes carried over from his own childhood and, possibly, from a lack of training. He shares common feelings about "dumb" and "stupid" individuals. Parents are hesitant to use such words, but society does readily enough, and the words of such less charitable people come quickly to the mind if not the mouth of the professional. It takes skill not to slip and make remarks which are in keeping with a fairly natural cynicism.

Many professionals, therefore, face mental retardation, especially severe retardation, with all the defensive reactions that have been elsewhere described for parents. They can easily deny the presence of the retardation. This can, at times, cloud and confuse the diagnosis. They can overreact by being overly solicitious or overly condemnatory of the parents who are trying to handle the problem. All caretakers may have a very strong wish to be rid of the problem, and of the parents who present it.

Such reactions toward the retardate can best be understood in the chronology which matches the defensive reactions of the parents. The shock and repulsion of parents to a damaged newborn may very well be matched by their physician; when he sees this unattractive child, his emotional responses may interfere with his normal objective approach to parents. At a time when he might be comforting, his own sense of concern about his feelings may lead him to be awkward and confused, as well as confusing. The awkwardness with which he approaches parents is compounded of his own sense of revulsion plus his general sense of inadequacy in trying to support parents at a time of crisis. And yet the parents must be supported. If they are not, they will react toward the physician very much as they have reacted toward their child.

To the professional, the parents' adoption of the concept of denial is an annoying and threatening experience. In their denial, the parents seem to be as stupid as the child that they cannot allow themselves to accept. The professional aligns his defensive reaction with the lack of intelligence that he perceives in the child. All of this makes him annoyed. He is bothered by their disbelief of his words. He is "turned off" when they go further and actually deny the presence of the retardation. It is not easy to see that parents who are stunned (even as the physician may himself be shaken) are hiding behind a strong barrier— the assertion that this could not have happened.

The next phase of the parents' reaction is the attempt to blame. Such blame often falls on physicians. The most logical and clear-thinking doctor may be quite confused by the parents' projection of blame onto him. He feels that he has tried to carry out his medical duties properly and adequately. He cannot understand the vehemence of this attack. In fact, doctors very often become quite defensive even when a parent criticizes a colleague whom they feel to be blameless. In their defensiveness, they may accuse parents and toss the blame back at them. They may accuse them of not having carried out orders, and thus increase the load of parental guilt. At times, physicians can be quite cruel in such a setting.

Professionals publicly talk as though the parents must accept the responsibility and reality of the situation. Since it is sometimes hard for doctors to accept this responsibility and reality, it is not surprising that the parents fail to do so. And it is very easy to say, "As soon as they accept the situation we can make adequate plans with them." It is very obvious that this is true, but it is equally obvious that parents cannot quickly accept the burden of retardation. As a result, a certain amount of planning may have to be done without their acceptance.

The phase in which the parent becomes overprotective of the child and begins to bring all kinds of minor maladies to medical attention evokes an equal kind of overreaction. Eventually, clinicians become bored, then annoyed, and finally angered at the parents' inability to see what is really going on and what they are doing. Since the parental inability to accept the idea of a poor mind (which can't be cured) leads to an overconcentration on the body (which they hope can be), it is not surprising that parents continue to pester.

This leads to a very important stage in the relationship between parent and professional. The parent becomes angered at the person who should be helping. He feels eventually that he would like to get rid of his doctor and his child. It seems likely that physicians and other caretakers may easily communicate this sense of rejection. It is customary to blame parents for "shopping." If one could see that the difficulty in "shopping" arises from the separate two and conflicting problems of the parents and the professionals, it might be more understandable. The parent is "shopping" for someone who will accept him or her as a person, and understand what it is that is so bothersome. Physicians tend to feel that parents go from physician to physician and clinic to clinic hoping for a good word or something that will allay their concerns about the child. The thing that leads them on seems entirely internal. It may well be, however, that each physician or clinic repudiates the parent in its own way. Each suggests that the parent has made a mistake in diagnosis, does not understand the child, does not understand the physician, and therefore, cannot be helped. It is this sense of not being able to be helped that contributes widely to the parents' quest.

Finally, the professional, plagued by the parent and unable to help the child, may also have very strong wishes to rid himself of the whole situation. Indeed, the extreme frustration of being unable to provide a medicine or a cure threatens his professional integrity in his relationship with both parent and child. The fact that the clinical armamentarium does not include magical cures makes doctors vulnerable, and they dislike that feeling intensely. Out of this, the wish to get rid of the child may become as strong in the physician as it is in the parent. At times, this leads to poor planning on the part of both. The clinician is likely to jump at the suggestion on the part of the parent that the child be placed in a school or institution. It seems to offer relief from his problem as much as it does that of the parent.

One should be very careful to sense this particular problem as one deals with the anxieties of the parents. The professional who can understand his own situation vis-à-vis both the child and the parent is in an excellent position to help. The focus should not necessarily be on the presenting problem—namely, the child. In fact, one of the major jobs is to carefully lead the parent away from an intense focus on the child's pathology to an understanding of the parents' own interests and concerns. Parental anxiety about the child leads to an avoidance of looking at themselves. When talking to others, they continue to put the child out in front both literally and figuratively.

Similar problems are often apparent in the approach to institutional placement. Professionals become annoyed because the parent cannot see usefulness or value in the placement. They forget that the strain of separation has much less to do with the child than it does with the parent. The latter abets this position by talking about how difficult it would be for the child to be away, how upset the child would be in a strange setting, and how worried the child would be about missing the parents. To face such a parent very directly and honestly with the meaning of the loss will very often resolve such a situation. If the parent can see that the guilt or anger that they feel against the child is what stands in the way of giving him up, then a new stage for discussion is reached. Parents react more effectively when, after presentation of a plan, they are asked, "Could you let him go at this time?" It puts the problem in a truer perspective.

THE ROLE OF THE PSYCHIATRIST VIS-A-VIS THE SCHOOL

It is very obvious that since the defect in mental retardation relates to learning, the problems of the care of children also relate largely to schools. In his approach to the retarded, a physician will have to adapt to the fact that others are doing things for the retarded child that he cannot do as well. However, there is a special role for him in helping parents and teachers to understand the true character of the intellectual functioning of the child and the aberrant adaptive reactions to it. Part of this is related to the therapy of the behavioral disorder.

Equally, however, the parent may very well be frustrated by a sense that the child is not in the proper school, or that the demands of the school are excessive. Somewhere in this relationship, the physician must take a management role and at times be a mediator between the various pulls and tugs that can result in a lack of care for the child. He must be aware that the problem of the child will continue over a long period of time, and that even as an adult, the reactions of the individual may be childlike.

The complexity of the causes of mental retardation and the wide range of intelligence produced by these various damaging conditions lead to difficulties in the long-range care of the affected individuals. Many states are beginning to pass laws which require that teaching be required for all individuals despite any limitations of their capacity. This poses considerable strain on school systems, but it also emphasizes the fact that, for the retarded, the job of accommodation to life includes adaptation to schooling or other forms of teaching.

In the case of the severely retarded, the learning problems are most commonly encountered in institutional settings. It is not within the scope of this chapter to describe teaching methods useful in institutional areas that are based primarily on behavioral modification. More important for the psychiatrist are the emotional consequences of adequate or stressful teaching confronted by the child with mild to moderate retardation. Children who have been slow in their development may already have experienced frustrating encounters with other children in play situations. The alertness demanded by children of their peers is sometimes very difficult for those with moderate intellectual defects. The fact that the physical growth of the child may continue when he is intellectually unable to compete with his age peers, adds to a pattern of self-isolation and to an avoidance of new, competitive tasks. When a child who is moderately retarded arrives at school age, classrooms either will not admit him or will place him in a separate category. There has been a whole wave of "special schooling" for these children and only recently have there been changes designed to adapt the school setting to the adequacy of the child. At any rate, the child may well feel like a segregated citizen, unworthy, and increasingly isolated. A special vulnerability characterizes the child who considers himself different, unwanted, and set apart. Other children are very quick to see his disability, and he may be shunned and teased by his peers, taunted, and made a "fall guy." Many such children become victims of other children's hostilities and also offer themselves as likely targets for trouble. A common phenomenon encountered outside the classroom is the child who volunteers himself as the perpetrator of gang delinquency. Where groups of children are commiting minor delinquent acts in a community, it is not infrequent for a dull child to volunteer that he is the cause in order to have a brief moment of notoriety in a community which otherwise may shun him.

The pressures of schooling are obviously more difficult for those children who are misdiagnosed and put in a regular classroom. It is not surprising that they become truant, develop psychosomatic conditions, and often end up as runaways to avoid the stress of the learning situation. During the past fifty years there have been a host of attempts to provide educational facilities for retarded individuals. Many of these facilities have a sheltered quality about them that increases and reinforces the dependency of the children. Just as the parents have been overprotective of them at home, the school situation, by its segregation and special treatment, reinforces the dependency situation. While school comes to an end in late adolescence, new problems arise, some of them from the very overprotection these individuals have had over the years.

The future role of psychiatrists in relationship to the overall syndrome of retardation is a function of the prospects for the care of such individuals by society generally. There are clinical problems that will change with the years as knowledge grows. In an exciting lecture, Tarjan makes certain predictions about the future treatment of the retarded.[47]

1. There will be a clearer separation of categories, particularly with a better understanding of the mild and moderately retarded individuals.

2. There will be better methods of measuring both intelligence and adaptation in order to assist this clearer separation. The concept of the IQ may very well give way to a profile of assets and deficiencies.

3. There will be better community programs related to the high incidence of mild to moderate retardation which will include preventive programs derived from better child-rearing practices.

4. The psychiatrist of the future may very well become primarily a consultant in this area.

The therapeutic needs will continue to be important, but the role of the psychiatrist in assisting others to care for needs may become progressively greater. There is evidence over the last ten years that psychiatrists have ceased to be as interested in mental retardation as they were, even a decade ago.

One of the major problems in the preparation of psychiatrists for dealing with the retarded is the absence of training programs focusing on the clinical situation. Constant efforts are being made to include the teaching of retardation in medical schools, but, as has been noted, the retarded do not attract interest. In fact, many individuals are repelled by the victims of the syndrome and the teaching is therefore fragmented. While many children suffering from retardation are brought to pediatric settings, they very often are handled more in terms of presenting symptom, be it heart or kidney or bone, than in terms of a child who is retarded and who has certain medical difficulties. Only by teaching in a setting which focuses on a totality of the growing individual's situation can concepts of retardation properly be taught. To enable psychiatrists to become consultants of the future, they must learn to appraise the syndrome, the effect of the disorder on families, the problems of schooling, and the difficulties that society faces in coping with these individuals.

REFERENCES

1. ABBOTT, J. M., and LADD, G. M., "Any Reason Why This Mentally Retarded Couple Should Not Be Joined Together . . .," *Mental Retardation, 21*:45–48, 1970.

2. ABRAMOWICZ, H. K., and RICHARDSON, S. A., "Epidemiology of Severe Mental Retardation in Children: Community Studies," *American Journal of Mental Deficiency, 80(1)*:18–39, July 1975.

3. American Academy of Pediatrics, Committee on Children with Handicaps, "The Pediatrician and the Child with Mental Retardation," American Academy of Pediatrics, Evanston, Ill., 1971.

4. American Association on Mental Deficiency, *Manual on Terminology and Classification in Mental Retardation*, Grossman, H. (Ed.), American Association on Mental Deficiency, Washington, D.C., 1977.

5. American Psychiatric Association, Committee on Nomenclature and Statistics, *Diagnostic and Statistical Manual of Mental Disorders*, 2nd ed. (DSM-II), American Psychiatric Association, Washington, D.C., 1968.

6. ANDERSON, K. A., and GARNER, A. M., "Mothers of Retarded Children: Satisfaction with Visits to Professional People," *Mental Retardation, 11*:36–39, 1973.

7. BEGAB, M. J. (Ed.), "Research Reports from the Mental Retardation Research Centers," *American Journal of Mental Deficiency, 77(5)*, 1973.

8. ———, and LA VECK, G. D. (Eds.), "Classification of Mental Retardation," *American Journal of Psychiatry, 128(11)*: Supplement, 1972.

9. BERNSTEIN, N. R., "Review of Human Sexuality and the Mentally Retarded," *Journal of Child Psychiatry, 13(4)*: 711ff., 1974.

10. BRANDWEIN, H., "The Battered Child: A Definite and Significant Factor in Mental Retardation," *Mental Retardation, 11(5)*:50–51, 1973.

11. BROWN, B., and COURTLESS, T. F., "The Mentally Retarded in Penal and Correctional Institutions," *American Journal of Psychiatry, 124(9)*:50–56, 1968.

12. DAVID, H. (Ed.), *Child Mental Health in International Perspective: Report of the Joint Commission on Mental Health of Children*, Harper & Row, New York, 1972.

13. DINGMAN, H. F., EYMAN, R. K., and WINDLE, C. D., "An Investigation of Some Child-Rearing Attitudes of Mothers with Retarded Children," *American Journal of Mental Deficiency, 67(6)*:899ff., 1963.

14. DWYBAN, G., "Psychiatry's Role in Mental Retardation," in Bernstein, N. (Ed.), *Diminished People*, Little, Brown, Boston, 1970.

15. EDGERTON, R. B., *The Cloak of Competence*, University of California Press, Berkeley, 1967.

16. ———, and DINGMAN, H. F., "Good Reasons for Bad Supervision: "Dating" in a Hospital for the Mentally Retarded," *Psychiatric Quarterly*, Supplement (2), State Hospital Press, Utica, N.Y., 1964.

17. EISENBERG, L., and EARLS, F. J., "Poverty, Social Depreciation, and Child Development," in Arieti, S.

(Ed.), *American Handbook of Psychiatry*, 2nd ed., vol. 6, pp. 275–291, Basic Books, New York, 1975.

18. ELKIND, D., "Infant Intelligence," *American Journal of Diseases of Children, 126:*143–144, 1973.

19. GABRIEL, H. G., and GLUCK, R., "Management of an Autistic Child Undergoing Open Heart Surgery," *Pediatrics, 51(2):*251–253, 1973.

20. Group for the Advancement of Psychiatry, Committee on Child Psychiatry, *Psychopathological Disorders in Childhood: Theoretical Considerations and a Proposed Classification,* vol. 6, Report No. 62, Group for the Advancement of Psychiatry, New York, 1966.

21. Group for the Advancement of Psychiatry, Committee on Mental Retardation, *Mild Mental Retardation: A Growing Challenge to the Physician,* Report No. 66, Group for the Advancement of Psychiatry, New York, 1967.

22. ———, *Mental Retardation: A Family Crisis—The Therapeutic Role of the Physician,* Report No. 56, Group for the Advancement of Psychiatry, New York, 1963.

23. ———, *Basic Considerations in Mental Retardation: A Preliminary Report,* Report No. 43, Group for the Advancement of Psychiatry, New York, 1959.

24. JOHNSON, G., "Psychological Characteristics of the Mentally Retarded," in Cruickshank, W. (Ed.), *Psychology of Exceptional Children and Youth,* 3rd ed., Prentice-Hall, Englewood Cliffs, N.J., 1971.

25. JORDAN, T. E., *The Mentally Retarded,* 3rd ed., Charles E. Merrill, Columbus, Oh., 1972.

26. JUSTICE, R. S., O'CONNOR, G., and WARREN, N., "Problems Reported by Parents of Mentally Retarded Children—Who Helps?", *American Journal of Mental Deficiency, 75(6):*685–691, 1971.

27. KANNER, L., "Childhood Psychosis: A Historical Overview," *Journal of Autism and Child Schizophrenia, 1(1):*14–19, 1971.

28. ———, "Early Infantile Autism Revisited," *Psychiatry Digest, 29:*17–28, 1968.

29. KNOBLOCK, H., and PASAMANICK, B., "Mental Subnormality," *The New England Journal of Medicine, 226 (20):*1045–1051, 1092–1096, 1962.

30. LOTT, G., "Psychotherapy of the Mentally Retarded: Values and Cautions," in Menolascino, F. (Ed.), *Psychiatric Approaches to Mental Retardation,* pp. 227–250, Basic Books, New York, 1970.

31. MARSH, R. L., FRIEL, C. M., and EISSLER, V., "The Adult Mentally Retarded in the Criminal Justice System," *Mental Retardation, 13(2):*21–25, 1975.

32. MENOLASCINO, F. J., *Psychiatric Aspects of the Diagnosis and Treatment of Mental Retardation,* Special Child Publications, Seattle, Wash., 1971.

33. ———, "Psychiatric Aspects of Mongolism," *American Journal of Mental Deficiency, 69(5):*653–660, 1965.

34. ———, and PEARSON, P. H. (Eds.), *Beyond the Limits: Innovations in Services for the Severely and Profoundly Retarded,* Special Child Publications, Seattle, Wash., 1974.

35. Mental Health Law Project, *Basic Rights of the Mentally Handicapped,* Mental Health Project Law, Washington, D.C., 1973.

36. MERCER, J. R., BUTLER, E. W., and DINGMAN, H. F.,

"The Relationship between Social Developmental Performance and Mental Ability," *American Journal of Mental Deficiency, 69:*195–203, 1964.

37. NIHIRA, L., and NIHIRA, K., "Normalized Behavior in Community Placement," *Mental Retardation, 13(2):* 9–13, 1975.

38. PAVENSTEDT, E., "A Comparison of the Child-Rearing Environment of Upper-Lower and Very Low-Lower Class Families," *American Journal of Orthopsychiatry, 35:*89–98, 1965.

39. PHILIPS, I., "Psychopathology and Mental Retardation," *American Journal of Psychiatry, 124(1):*67–73, 1967.

40. ——— (Ed.), *Prevention and Treatment of Mental Retardation,* Basic Books, New York, 1966.

41. ———, and WILLIAMS, N., "Psychopathology and Mental Retardation: A Study of 100 Mentally Retarded Children: Psychopathology," *American Journal of Psychiatry, 132(12):*1265ff., 1975.

42. RICHMOND, J. B., TARJAN, G., and MENDELSOHN, R. S. (Eds.), *Mental Retardation: A Handbook for the Primary Physician,* 2nd ed., American Medical Association, 1974.

43. RUTTER, M., "Why Are London Children So Disturbed," *Proceedings of the Royal Society of Medicine, 66:*1221–1225, 1973.

44. SARATA, B. P. V., "Employee Satisfactions in Agencies Serving Retarded Persons," *American Journal of Mental Deficiency, 79(4):*434–442, 1975.

45. TARJAN, G., "Mental Retardation and the Organization of Services," the D. G. McKerracher, M.D. In Memoriam Lecture, presented at the Second Interamerican Conference on Mental Health of Children and Youth, Mexico City, 1975.

46. ——— (Ed.), "Mental Retardation," Psychiatric Annals Reprint, New York, 1974.

47. ———, "Mental Retardation: A Brief Review," *Bulletin of the New York State District Branch of the American Psychiatric Association, 15(4):*7, 1972.

48. ———, and EISENBERG, L., "Some Thoughts on the Classification of Mental Retardation in the United States of America," *American Journal of Psychiatry, 128(Supplement):*14–18, 1972.

49. TARJAN, G., EYMAN, R., and MEYERS, C. E. (Eds.), *Sociobehavioral Studies in Mental Retardation: Papers in Honor of Harvey F. Dingman,* Monograph No. 1, American Association on Mental Deficiency, Washington, D.C., 1973.

50. ———, EYMAN, R. K., and MILLER, C. R., "Natural History of Mental Retardation in a State Hospital, Revisited," *American Journal of Diseases of Children, 117:* 609–620, 1969.

51. TAYLOR, J. T., and SCHENBACH, T. M., "Moral and Cognitive Development in Retarded and Non-Retarded Children," *American Journal of Mental Deficiency, 80(1):* 43–50, 1975.

52. WALLACE, P., "Complex Environments: Effects on Brain Development," *Science, 185:*1035–1037, 1974.

53. WORLD HEALTH ORGANIZATION, *International Classification of Diseases,* 9th ed., World Health Organization, Geneva, 1973.

20 / The Minimal Brain Dysfunction Syndrome

Larry B. Silver

Introduction

It is estimated that about 10 percent of most school populations have difficulty performing academically at an age-appropriate level. For some of these children the underlying problem is mental retardation; for others, the below-normal performance relates to primary emotional problems. A third group of children have difficulty with learning because of the way their nervous system performs. These children have specific deficits in their learning performance; at the same time they are sensorily intact and of average or above average intellectual ability. Many show other evidence of neurological dysfunction such as hyperactivity, distractibility, or perseveration.

Throughout this century, physicians, educators, psychologists, and other professionals have increasingly focused their attention upon this population of children. As each aspect of the problems was studied, and as each professional group viewed these children within the context of their own discipline, different descriptions and diagnostic labels were developed. Even now, the multiple approaches to viewing these children and the many diagnostic labels in use pose major problems in reviewing the literature or in understanding the data or claims about different treatment efforts or follow-up studies. Some professionals view the child with specific learning disabilities as a unique clinical entity; others focus on the child with hyperactivity as a separate clinical picture. It appears most likely that these cases do not comprise a single clinical condition, but that there are a cluster of findings often found together; that is, these children fit into a common syndrome.

Since no consensus on the clinical picture and the diagnostic label has yet been reached, different professionals often use different labels. A brief review of the history of this syndrome may clarify some of this confusion.

In the 1940s Alfred Strauss, a psychiatrist, and Heinz Werner, a psychologist, studied brain injured children.[99] They sought to account for divergent patterns of functioning in a population of mentally defective children. Based on background histories, they classified these children into two categories, those that did and those that did not have extrinsic damage to the nervous system. When they compared the cognitive and emotional behaviors of the two groups, they found there was considerable overlap. Despite this, however, the group with a history of perinatal or later childhood nervous system damage contained a larger proportion of hyperactive, emotionally labile, perceptually disordered, impulsive, distractible, and abnormally rigid and perseverative children than did the group with no such history. It was to the cases with these peculiar patternings of behavioral organization that the term "brain damaged" or "brain injured" came to be applied, and with it came the concept of "the brain-damaged child." Since most of these children showed no overt evidence of the major forms of brain damage, their condition was labeled, "minimal brain damage." Subsequent studies gave little support to the view that these children have tissue damage; nonetheless this label remains popular.

Later, as the condition of increasing numbers of these children was recognized and evaluated, evidence was found to suggest subtle functional disturbances of the central nervous system rather than definite brain damage. The emphasis then shifted from brain damage to the possibility of some form of dysfunction[23] or immaturity[1] of the central nervous system. Since the primary area of learning was considered to be the cerebral cortex, another diagnostic label applied was, "minimal cerebral dysfunction." Others referred to these children as cases of "minimal brain dysfunction." Clements,[23] in his monograph on terminology, recommended the term "minimal brain dysfunction syndrome," emphasizing that these children suffered combinations of learning disabilities, emotional problems, difficulty with attention, and impulsivity.

Many other investigators entered the field. They began to observe these children, to study them, and to conceptualize their observations and their diagnostic formulations in terms of their disciplines. Thus, the child with difficulty in reading had "dyslexia;" with difficulty in math or calculations, "dyscalcula;" with written language or graphics problems, "dysgraphia." Children with language and auditory disabilities were called cases of "congenital aphasia." Children who were distractible were referred to as suffering "distractibility" or "attentional deficit syndrome;" and children who were noted to be hyperactive were called "hyperactive" or "hyperkinetic" children. In the education literature these are often referred to as children with "learning disabilities" or "specific learning disabilities."[48, 54]

In the medical literature the term, minimal brain dysfunction (or *MBD* for short) is most common. The term minimal brain dysfunction syndrome is preferred for this term reflects the multiplicity of the clinical picture. These children may have multiple patterns of dysfunctional behavior. However, they all present similar groups of findings and thus their cases fit the same syndrome.

At the time this chapter was completed, a working draft of the third edition of the Diagnostic and Statistical Manual of Mental Disorders was available. If the categories in the January, 1978 draft become official, it will be difficult to classify individuals presenting this syndrome. One will have to classify each component separately. There is a category, "Attentional Deficit Disorders" with two subsections, "Attentional Deficit Disorder with Hyperactivity" and "Attentional Deficit Disorder without Hyperactivity." There is no reference for the individual who may be hyperactive but not distractible. Some of the learning disabilities can be classified under the category of "Specific Developmental Disorders." Examples are: "Specific Reading Disorder," "Specific Arithmetical Disorder," and "Developmental Language Disorder." There is no reference for motor or written language disorders.

Whichever label is used, the theme common to this syndrome is the presence of one or more types of specific learning disabilities. In addition many (about 40 percent) show other evidence of altered central nervous system functioning. Hyperactivity and/or distractibility with a short attention span are the most common findings. Some of these children are perseverative. Because of the frustrations and failures they experience, many develop secondary emotional problems. Thus, one can construct a schema as this:

1. Primary Finding: One or more areas of specific learning disability.
2. Secondary Finding: Hyperactivity and/or distractibility with a short attention span (approximately 40 percent).
3. Tertiary Finding: Many develop secondary emotional problems.

As is true in other syndromes, the clinical findings with these children are not homogeneous. As noted, the common factor is that most, if not all, cases have one or more specific types of learning disabilities; each child presenting with a different profile of learning strengths and disabilities. Of this whole group, about 40 percent are either hyperactive or distractible, or hyperactive and distractible; but by the same token, about 60 percent are not. Most are brought to the clinician with evidence of social and/or emotional difficulties; some few may not show this difficulty.

Because of the relatively recent recognition of this syndrome along with the multiplicity of confusing definitions used by researchers, it is difficult to establish the prevalence of this problem. Some studies are based on the presence of hyperactivity, others on the recognition of specific learning disabilities. Some studies are school-based populations, others use physician-referred cases; and still other studies use referrals to a child mental health setting as the population base. Stewart and associates[89] used a school population and noted approximately 4 percent had such difficulties. Huessy and associates[44] noted 10 percent.

The ratio of boys to girls appears to be between four to one[64] and nine to one.[100] No explanation is yet known for this difference.

The Minimal Brain Dysfunction Syndrome

SPECIFIC LEARNING DISABILITIES

It is useful to conceptualize the process at work in specific learning disabilities by using a cybernetics model. This provides a basis for observing the steps involved in the learning process. The first step in learning is *input*; that is, recording information in the brain. The second step is *integration*; the process of organizing and comprehending the information after it has been received. The third step is *memory*; the ability to store and later to retrieve the integrated material. The final step is *output*; the ability to communicate information from the brain to the environment or to someone in the environment.

INPUT

Information enters the brain through all the senses. In the learning process one is primarily concerned with visual and auditory inputs; however, the other input systems may also be used. Since input relates to how one sees, hears, or perceives the environment, the term *perception* is used. Thus, one has visual perception, auditory perception, and intrasensory perception (e.g., learning by listening to a teacher speak while writing material on the board).

Visual Perceptual Disability: A child with specific learning disabilities might have difficulties with one or more aspects of this function. For example, he or she may have trouble organizing the percept when it comes in, confusing left with right or top with bottom. The child may confuse "d" and "b" and "p" and "q"; for, each can be transposed to the other by rotating vertically or horizontally. The child might see the word "was" and read it as "saw," or see the word "dog" and read it as "god." This confusion with correct spatial positioning might also show up in copying geometric designs or in doing tasks with the hands that require guidance from the eyes (visual-motor tasks).

Another form of visual perceptual disability relates to the ability to organize oneself in space. Children with this problem might have difficulty with spatial relationships, confusing left and right or their position in space. Some, when placed in an open-spaced environment like a gym, become so spatially disoriented that they appear to be dizzy or off-balance.

A child might have a visual perceptual disability in the area of "figure-ground." When one looks at a visual field, he or she must know on which figure to focus and how to identify this as differentiated from all other figures (the background). Children with such a disability might have difficulty doing tasks because they can not identify the significant part of their visual field from the other stimuli.

Depth perception problems are another aspect of a visual perceptual disability. A child with this problem might misjudge distances, bump into things, or fall off a chair. Parents might complain that this child is clumsy at the meal table, for he or she often knocks over the glass. Possibly the child misjudged the distance to the glass and bumped into it before he thought he would.

A final aspect of a visual perceptual disability relates to tasks in which the eyes have to tell the hands what to do, such as catching a ball, doing puzzles, or using a hammer and nail. The eye has to focus on the object, perceive it correctly, and tell the hands exactly where to move or when to act. It is for this reason that coaches say to

"keep your eye on the ball." For the normal person, such tracking will direct the hands to the right place for the catch. Children with a disability in this area may misjudge the distance or speed; the hands will get there too soon or too late and the child will miss the ball. The same may be true in kicking, hitting, or throwing a ball. It is important to remember that the areas of the brain involved in visual perception matures in at about five and one-half years; thus, younger children would normally show such "difficulties."

Auditory Perceptual Disability: As with visual perception, a child might have difficulty with one or all aspects of auditory perception. He or she might have difficulty distinguishing subtle differences in sounds (phonemes) much as they might have had difficulty distinguishing subtle differences in shapes (letters). Because of this confusion, the child might misunderstand what is being said and respond incorrectly. Words such as "blue" and "blow," or "ball" and "bell" might be confused. Or, one might say to the child, "How are you?" and he or she answers, "I am eight years old." The "how" and the "you" were correctly received, but the "are" was heard as "old."

Figure-ground problems might be noted with auditory perceptual disabilities. One has to distinguish the significant sounds to attend to (e.g., a particular voice) from the other sounds (noise, other voices, etc.). A child with such a disability might have trouble attending the appropriate auditory inputs. A mother might speak to her child. She is into her fourth sentence before the child becomes aware and listens. She may describe him as inattentive or negative.

A final possible aspect of an auditory perceptual problem is referred to as auditory lag. When auditory inputs reach the brain, they have to be recorded. For some children, this recording process is slower than normal; they cannot process sound inputs as fast as normal children. Parents or teachers find that intuitively they speak slower to this child. If they say too much too fast, the child will not be able to handle the inputs.

Other Sensory Inputs: Less is understood about other sensory inputs. Some children appear to be dysfunctional with tactile perception. They have difficulty orienting to and interpreting touch. Such children may be tactilely defensive, perceiving touch as confusing or uncomfortable. Perhaps some of the children who appear to be awkward or to have gross motor or celebellar disabilities really have difficulty in interpreting proprioceptive inputs.

INTEGRATION DISABILITIES

All of the incoming sensory stimuli have to be put together in sequence and then interpreted. If this is not done, the perceptions are meaningless. For some children the problems fall in these areas.

One aspect of integration is *sequencing*, the ability to take the pieces of information coming in from the various senses and organize them in the correct sequence. Children may have difficulty with visual sequencing, auditory sequencing, and/or intrasensory sequencing. A child with such a disability might hear or see a story; but, in explaining it, may start in the middle, go to the beginning, then shift to the end, completely confusing the sequence. A child may see a number such as "23" and record it on the paper as "32." A child might be given the math problem, "2 + 3 = ?" and answer, "2 + 5 = 3." The child knew the answer was 5 but placed the numbers in the wrong sequence. Or, a child may spell incorrectly: all the letters are present but in the wrong sequence.

Another aspect of integration is *abstraction*. Once the information is recorded in the brain and placed in the correct sequence, the child has to be able to infer from the literal imprints of stimuli to a more general connotation or interpretation of the stimuli. An example for a child might be a classroom language arts exercise. The teacher has the children read a story about a policeman. He or she then begins a discussion on policemen in general, asking the children if they have policemen in their community and what they do. The child having difficulties with abstraction might be unable to go from the policemen in the story to policemen in general; he or she can only stick with the policemen in the story.

MEMORY DISABILITY

Once information is received in the brain and integrated, it has to be stored, later to be retrieved. There are two forms of memory, short-term and long-term. Short-term memory refers to data that one can retain as long as he or she continually attends to the information. Long-term memory refers to that information which has been stored and can later be retrieved at will. An example of short-term memory would be when one calls the information operator and gets a long distance phone number. One can hang up the phone, retain the ten digits in his or her head, and dial the phone number. However, if interrupted the information may be lost.

Children might have a short- or long-term memory disability relating primarily to visual, auditory, and/or intrasensory memory.

There are children with short-term memory disabilities who can go over a math exercise or a spelling list and grasp the material. However, when retested an hour later, they have lost it. If the child repeats the learning process often enough he may finally store it. Thereafter it will be available for recall an hour or a day later. Parents often note this inconsistency. Their child cannot remember things recently taught or discussed, but can recall places or experiences from two and three years ago. Such a history suggests that the child might have a short-term memory disability; but, that once the material is recorded, the long-term memory is adequate.

Long-term memory disabilities are less commonly found. This type of disability overwhelms the learning process to such an extent that the affected children are usually seen as retarded.

OUTPUT DISABILITIES

Information can leave the brain through words, *language output*, or through muscle activity (such as writing, drawing, or other muscle activities), *motor output*. A child might have a specific learning disability relating to language output, motor output, or both.

Language Output: There are two forms of language used in the service of communication, spontaneous language and demand language. Spontaneous language refers to situations when one initiates a conversation. In this situation one has the luxury of a fraction of a second to organize his or her thoughts and to find the correct words prior to speaking. In a demand language situation, one is asked to communicate verbally; for example, being asked to answer a question, or say what one did today or what a story was about. In this case, the individual does not have that fraction of a second to organize his or her thoughts or find the right words but, has simultaneously to organize, to find words, and to respond. Children with a specific language disability usually have no problem with spontaneous language but have difficulty with demand language. The inconsistency is often quite apparent. When such a child initiates a conversation, he or she sounds age-appropriate. However, in a demand language situation, the same child might respond by saying, "huh," "what," or "I don't know." Or, the child might ask to have the question repeated, primarily to allow more time to organize his or her thoughts.

If this child does respond, he or she might have difficulty finding a word and try to cover this up by using other words. After a short time the language may become so confusing or circumstantial that it is difficult to follow or to make sense out of it.

This inconsistency in language often confuses both parents and others. The contrast makes sense only when one remembers to differentiate between spontaneous and demand language situations. A teacher might say that a particular child was lazy because when he wanted to answer, he would raise his hand and answer; however, whenever the teacher called on him he would say he didn't know. The difference in these cases could be demand versus spontaneous language.

Motor Output: The child with a *gross motor* disability may be noted to be clumsy or to have difficulty with walking, running, or riding tricycles or bicycles.

The child with a *fine motor* disability may well have difficulty with puzzles, using a hammer and nail or assembling block designs, but he will be considered problematic primarily in the area of written language. He cannot get his hand to work as well or as fast as his head is thinking. The problem is similar to that of being forced to use one's nondominant hand to write. Since the automatic circuitry is not functioning for this hand, one has difficulty holding the pen or producing the letters. Shape, size, spacing, and positioning become labored and tedious. So it is with these children. They often have two choices: they can either write very slowly and fail to finish the assignment, or they can write as fast as possible but get a poor grade for penmanship. They have trouble with spelling, grammar, space and size of letters. The total problem is sometimes referred to as written language disability. Such a fine motor disability may also manifest itself with other tasks requiring the use of the hand.

If a child has both a visual perceptual and a fine motor disability, he will have difficulty with any tasks for which the eyes have to tell the hands what to do; for example, in hitting a nail, doing a puzzle, or doing a block design. This combined problem is referred to as a *visual-motor* disability.

There is another type of fine motor disability that is less commonly thought of as a motor disability, that is, speech production. It is easy to observe that about forty muscles in the hand must work as a team to produce written language. By the same token, intercostal and diaphragm muscles, the muscles controlling the vocal cords, plus muscles in the oral and nasal pharynx, mouth,

tongue, and lips must work as a team to produce speech. Children with this type of fine motor disability are said to have *dysarthria*. They have difficulty with articulation and speech production. Since the same muscles are involved in swallowing, they may have had difficulty with sucking and eating as an infant and may continue to drool.

The preceding cybernetics model describing the specific learning disabilities is simplistic. It is apparent that the learning process is much more complex. Each child will have his or her own profile of learning weaknesses and learning strengths. There is a certain trend for the disabilities to group themselves into one of two basic patterns. One pattern relates to disabilities in visual perception, visual integration, visual memory, fine motor, and/or visual-motor areas. Another group of children suffer disabilities in the auditory perceptual, auditory integration, auditory memory, language output areas. The groupings are variable; the important theme within this syndrome is that most children will have one or more types of learning disability. If one were to evaluate one hundred children with this condition, he or she might find thirty or forty different profiles of strengths and disabilities; however, each child still fits the definition of the syndrome.

HYPERACTIVITY AND/OR DISTRACTIBILITY

Of children with the minimal brain dysfunction syndrome, about 40 percent will be hyperactive and/or distractible. Those who are distractible will consequently have a short attention span. It is significant that about 60 percent of these children will demonstrate the specific characteristics of learning disabilities but will not be hyperactive and/or distractible.

Hyperactivity: These children's increased motor activity is physiologically-based; it is not an anxiety-based motor response. This is a differentiation of very considerable significance. With the child who utilizes an increase in motor activity as a means of coping with anxiety, the behavior usually relates to a specific life-space experience. The history will suggest that hyperactivity began during the first grade or that it happens only in school but not at home. With physiologically-based hyperactivity, there is usually a history of such activity since birth. In some cases, the parent might even report that the child kicked more than usual in utero prior to birth. He or she squirmed in his mother's arms, rolled in his crib, ran before he walked, has been in almost constant motion since birth. This motor hyperactivity does not relate to any specific events; it certainly is not limited to school hours; it occurs all the time and any place.

Distractibility: Some children with this syndrome have difficulty filtering sensory inputs; thus, most or all inputs reach the cortex and compete for full attention. For some children, the distractibility relates more to visual inputs; for others, auditory inputs; and for some, both.

The child with this disability might try to attend and work; but other visual and/or auditory inputs continue to distract. With each distraction, there is the need to reattend; thus, they have a short attention span.

The distractibility caused by external stimuli appears to be clinically different from a type of internal distractibility in which some children have difficulty inhibiting their thoughts. They are distracted because the internal thoughts are competing for their attention. I find it helpful to distinguish between distractibility and dysinhibition as a cause for the clinical behavior. The former, as will be discussed later, often improves with the use of psychostimulants; the latter will not.

SOCIAL AND EMOTIONAL PROBLEMS OF THE CHILD

Because of the specific learning disabilities as well as, with some, the hyperactivity and/or distractibility, these children become frustrated. They experience many failures and have difficulty coping in the family, neighborhood, and school. In time they are all too likely to develop social and emotional problems. Very often the learning disabilities are not recognized or treated, and the child continues to experience repeated frustrations and failures. If the child withdraws from learning and stops trying, he or she is likely to be sent to an educational resource such as tutoring or a special class. If his emotional stress takes the form of behavioral disorders, however, he is then likely to be referred for a psychiatric evaluation. To view such a child as suffering primary emotional difficulty or a character problem rather than a secondary emotional reaction to the unrecognized underlying syndrome is to miss a significant etiological factor and to plan an incomplete treatment approach.

These children have difficulty with all stages of psycho-social development.[36, 82] The learning disabilities, hyperactivity, or distractibility may interfere with mastery of many different developmental tasks. The child's difficulties in turn weigh heavily on the parents who may become frustrated, helpless, and dysfunctional.[35, 67, 83]

A child with this syndrome may develop many types of emotional disabilities as he or she tries to master the normal stages of psycho-social development and at the same time to cope with the frustrations and failures experienced in all aspects of life. To illustrate these difficulties quotes from the author's personal clinical cases will be used.

Some children deal with such frustrating life experiences by trying to avoid the stress. One might see a withdrawal reaction. The child avoids any potentially frustrating or uncertain situation by drawing back from it and becoming passive. He or she becomes unavailable for learning. Because of her unrecognized learning disabilities, an eight-year-old girl of superior intelligence had failed several grades and was currently in second grade. She was asked what she did in school when she couldn't do her work. "When I was younger I used to crumble up my paper and cry. . . . Then they teased me and called me a crybaby. . . . So . . . I decided that since school was no fun, I had to get away. . . . I couldn't leave so I sat and pretended that I was home in my room with my dolls. . . . I made up stories and had a good time." The teacher complained that this girl would "daydream the day away if I let her."

Others avoid stress by regressing to an earlier stage of psychological or social development. There is a recurrence of earlier behaviors or of immature or infantile interactions with peers or adults. The parents of a seven and one-half-year-old girl complained that their daughter had been happy and normal until she entered kindergarten. As mother explained it, at this point, "she had a change in personality. She had trouble keeping up with her work. In first grade she just didn't learn much and is now repeating first." Father added, "Home life is terrible, we yell at her all the time. Since school began this year, she's gone backwards, acting like a baby, talking like a baby. . . . It's impossible. . . . She won't listen and tunes me out. . . . She's begun to wet her bed for the first time since she was three. . . . She even eats with her fingers." At a therapy session, Debbie talked of school. "I have trouble because I don't understand the work, especially reading and math. . . . It's hard and I can't do it. . . . The teacher yells at me all the time. . . . Maybe I'm just not as smart as the other kids."

Children might try to avoid the stress, the conflicts, and the resulting feelings by displacing the focus. Some develop fear reactions. Their overall, school-related feelings seem to take on specific meaning. Rather than experiencing a general anxiety or depression whenever he or she is in school, the child develops a special fear of a particular child on the school bus who always teases him. Now he can make sense out of his feelings when he wakes up to go to school. He does not have to relate the feelings to incomprehensive and dismaying school failures. Some of these children displace the cause of their anxiety into bodily functions. The child may develop somatic complaints, stomachaches, lower abdominal cramps, headaches, diarrhea, or frequency of urination or bowel movements. The complaints are often present only in the morning of school days, never on weekends, holidays, or summers. These children have to leave the class to go to the school nurse or to go home. As with other somatic symptoms, the discomfort is real. The pain goes away when he or she is allowed to stay home, not necessarily because the child was faking, but because the stress was relieved. A seven-year-old girl once explained, "Sometimes I get into trouble because I forgot to do what the teacher said or I erase too much. . . . The teacher yells at me and I get scared. . . . Then my stomach starts to hurt and I have to go to the nurse." An eight-year-old awoke each school day with major stomach cramps and vomiting. His mother kept him home from school and the pains usually disappeared by noon. Complete medical studies were done and found to be normal. Joe must have guessed why he was to be seen. He greeted the evaluator with, "I know my stomach trouble is because I'm afraid of school. . . . Only it really does hurt, I'm not kidding."

Other children might focus their anxiety on their increasing awareness that something is wrong with their body. They have heard parents and professionals talk of his or her brain and have had many examinations and tests. Their hypochondria is reflected in complaints of bodily difficulties: "My back hurts" or "My head aches" or "My knee feels funny." Sometimes this concern with their body extends into a general concern with body integrity or body damage. At times the complaints become their rationalization for failures. "I can't help it if I made a mistake. My arms hurts today."

Children might avoid the stress by becoming paranoid and projecting their feelings and thoughts to others. Teachers, classmates, books, desks, all get blamed; everyone is out to get them or to show them up. A ten-year-old boy in a special class had frequent episodes of explosive behavior resulting in his hitting, yelling, or throwing things. His usual explanation was that someone was talking about him or making a face to try to get him into trouble. At home he refused to go out and play because the neighborhood children were always talking about him. A review of his school history revealed that two years earlier he was a withdrawn, sad boy. One year ago he was described as an angry child who continually criticized himself. Now he had moved into his latest attempt to cope: displacement, projection, and paranoia. It is significant that on examination he was not psychotic.

Another form of rationalization is seen with the child who uses his or her diagnosis as the excuse for the problems. They have heard various descriptions and labels used by parents and professionals. A child might say, "I'm brain damaged so I can't do that." He or she might generalize his disability and feel totally worthless. "I'm just no good; I can't read." A child who had been confronted by his teacher for an error on his math paper responded, "I can't do that; I'm a retard." A twelve-year-old boy explained why he didn't have friends; "I'm brain damaged so I can't catch a ball too good. . . . All the kids play ball; so, since I can't play, I don't have friends."

Some children with this syndrome are not successful in developing a competent defense system that allows them to avoid the stress with the resulting painful feelings and thoughts. They experience a true sense of depression. Because of the failures, feelings of inadequacy, and poor interactions with peers and significant adults, the child feels angry and devalued. Prelatency children are often unable to internalize the anger. He or she might express the depression by being irritable and aggressive toward everyone. With the older child the classic symptoms of depression may be seen. In some instances so much anger is turned inward that the children become self-destructive or suicidal. An eleven-year-old child with this syndrome and a long history of failures was referred for evaluation because of his overly polite, passive manner. During the evaluation he described himself as a "bad troublemaker who was stupid and couldn't do anything right." He added, "I get so mad with myself when I make a mistake I send myself to my room. . . . Sometimes I punish myself by making myself go to bed early or by picking my favorite TV show and then not letting myself see it. . . . Once I got so mad I slapped myself."

For some children their superego takes on a

punitive role and prevents them from accepting praise. If a teacher compliments a piece of work, the child might have to destroy it.

Often those children who internalize such conflicts develop a poor self-image. The child sees himself or herself as an inadequate, bad, worthless person who can't do anything right. Perhaps this self-image is based on outside feedback. One markedly depressed ten-year-old boy with such feelings had been hyperactive since birth. His mother reported that he was always all over the place. "All he ever heard from me was 'no' or 'don't' or 'bad boy.'" He was kicked out of nursery school for being a "monster." Kindergarten was a disaster, as was first and second grade. Still undiagnosed, he repeated second grade, started third, and was then suspended from school. He had never known himself to be other than bad, inadequate, or stupid. The fact that he was very bright but was hyperactive, distractible, and had multiple areas of learning disabilities, perhaps explained his problems. However, it didn't change his self-image. Usually these children cannot be talked out of their image; it is based on a body of real experiences. The self-image improves, however, when they experience changes, when they get the appropriate help, and begin to master learning and behavioral tasks. A twelve-year-old boy had been diagnosed at five as having this syndrome. He was placed on a psychostimulant, received several years of intensive special educational therapy, and was in psychotherapy. He was now in a regular sixth grade class and doing well. He reminisced, "Remember when I was at the special school and you kept telling me how smart I was. . . . I thought you just wanted to make me feel good because I couldn't read or do anything. . . . I almost gave up and felt that I would just never make it. . . . Then one day it clicked and I started to read. . . . I really read. . . . Then I started to do math. . . . Boy, I could really learn just like you told me. . . . I must have grown five years that first week I started to read."

A given child might have difficulty dealing with anger and might choose an indirect way of showing it. One such style is to be passive-aggressive. The behavior in and of itself is not aggressive; yet, people become angry with him or her. Dawdling is an example of this. The child might play with his or her clothes until a parent becomes furious. The child then might look up in bewilderment and say, "Why are you so mad? I didn't do anything." A special education teacher once described such a child in his class by saying, "He was so cooperative and helpful and sweet that I felt like bash-

ing him in the teeth." Other children might become passive-dependent. Initially the child might avoid failure and unpleasant feelings by avoiding situations that might result in failure; this passivity might expand into a veritable life style. He or she avoids taking the initiative and minimizes getting involved. Unlike the helpless child who creates feelings of sympathy or empathy in adults, this child's helpless dependency and passivity create feelings of anger.

Another common approach some of these children use in order to handle stress is clowning. Clowning serves several functions. With some children, clowning is a way of controlling feelings of inadequacy, and the child might clown to cover feelings of lack of worth and depression; an element of mastery may be present. By playing the role of clown or freak, it is as if the child were saying, "They call me a clown or freak but it is only because I have chosen to be one. I really can turn it off if I wanted to, but it's too much fun this way." If the child is successful at clowning, he or she will disrupt the lesson plan or be asked to leave the group, thus avoiding the academic work that perhaps produced the stress in the first place. Frequently this wins a certain measure of peer acceptance. Suddenly, the boy everyone teased is the class hero. The clowning becomes reinforced. In some schools, being sent to the principal's office is rewarded by no school work or by talking to a secretary, delivering messages, or playing with the typewriter. A thirteen-year-old boy, after four years of educational and psychiatric help, returned to public school and was doing well. He returned to visit his therapist and was asked to describe what he remembered about his previous school problems. At one point, he said, "Boy, were those teachers stupid. Anytime it was my turn to read or do anything I had trouble with, I would tease another boy or joke around. . . . It worked great. I got sent out of the room." He added, "Only you and the teachers got me to see that I was the stupid one. . . . You can't get help if you're not in class, and I sure didn't want to spend the rest of my life in a special school."

Children with this syndrome who are hyperactive and/or distractible are likely to develop an impulse disorder. The normal child learns with age to delay longer and longer between the initial impulse to act and the actual behavior, gradually building on past experiences to choose the appropriate behavior. Children with this disorder, however, might be explosive or aggressive, might have temper tantrums, or experience catastrophic reactions. Some may be emotionally labile, crying or yelling at the slightest frustration. Sometimes he or she will break something or hurt someone unintentionally, simply because he moved or acted too quickly and without thinking. Such impulse disorder children show other evidences of this problem: stealing, bedwetting, firesetting, hoarding of food, or excessive eating. An eight-year-old hyperactive girl continually broke things and had one tantrum after another. She was a bedwetter, hid food at home, stole money from her mother's pocketbook, and set fires. When asked about the firesetting, she reflected her own concern with impulsivity and impulse control as she explained that what she enjoyed the most was ". . . letting the fire get big and almost ready to burn everything up. . . . Then I would put it out before it exploded all over the place."

Occasionally such children will appear to be pseudo-mature for their age. Faced with the feelings and thoughts related to being different and inadequate, and fearful that no one will take care of him, a child might decide to grow up quickly. Often, this child needs to be in control and becomes upset if he cannot control all situations. He looks, acts, and relates like a serious young man. This behavior may pay off; adults compliment or spend more time with him. A seven-year-old boy was described by his parents as not needing anyone to take care of him. He was totally independent; in fact, he took care of everyone else in his family and class. He enjoyed most having discussions with his teacher. He had no sense of humor and was described as a perfect little man, completely self-sufficient. In a playroom diagnostic session, his fantasy and play reflected great concerns about dependency needs and a fear that they would not be met; thus, he had to take care of himself. The anger was denied; reaction-formation was actively used. All of his emotional energies were being used to maintain his protective façade.

Often these children appear to be socially immature, preferring to play with younger children. They cannot handle the interactions or do the activities of their age-appropriate peer group; so, they intuitively seek out an age group whose skills can be handled. As they overcome or compensate for their disabilities, they often relate to activities with age-appropriate peers.

By adolescence, many of these children, if not provided the necessary help, become school dropouts and possible delinquents. As adults they often continued to pay the price for their academic underachievement, emotional, and social difficulties.

SOCIAL AND EMOTIONAL PROBLEMS WITHIN THE FAMILY

When one member of a family suffers, everyone feels the pain and reacts. The parents and siblings of children with this syndrome need help understanding the child's problems as well as with understanding their own reactions to her or her disabilities.[35, 36, 67, 83] The usual pattern is for an individual or a member of a team to meet with his parents and interpret the clinical findings and conclusions. This may be provided in pieces with the educator or psychologists exploring one area, the physician another. Occasionally someone explains the clinical findings with the child. Rarely does anyone explain the impressions to the siblings. Yet, all need to know and understand.

The parents of these children may have to go through a grief reaction similar to the reaction parents have to loss from death, albeit of lesser intensity. They must "give up" a part of their child or a hoped for ambition that may never be realized. Initially, they experience denial, followed by phases of anger and self-blaming. Thus, when parents first learn that their child has a disability and deal with their loss, they may react in such a way to as to alienate their physician. In particular, they may be vulnerable to seeking out a quick cure or magic pill.

The initial phase of the grief-like reaction, as with other grief reactions, is often denial. "It can't be true. . . . He must be mistaken. . . . He only saw him for half an hour. . . . I don't believe it." A parent may doubt the professional's competence or castigate him. Frequently, another opinion is sought. Unfortunately, while getting other opinions is often useful, "doctor shopping" for someone who will tell the parent what he or she wants to hear is not. Another form of denial might be the cover-up reaction. One parent, usually the mother, will want to "protect" the other parent by not sharing the results of the studies or by minimizing the problems. Some parents successfully cover up special school programs for years. Sadly, the noninformed parent builds up unrealistic expectations or demands things of his or her child that the child cannot produce. The child often sees through this cover up and perceives the true reason: "They can't accept me as I am; they have to deny and pretend I'm different." He may feel anger or sadness and may have difficulty accepting himself if he does not feel that the parents can accept him.

The denial stage may be followed by a period of anger. The anger reaction is not uncommon. This anger might be directed inward or projected outward. On learning of a child's disability, it is normal to feel anger and such sentiments as, "Why me?" "How could God do this to me?" This initial reaction often reflects feelings of helplessness and frustration.

If the initial anger is turned inward, the attack is against the self and there ensues a feeling of depression. Associated with this reaction is a feeling of guilt—"It's all my fault." The parent might berate himself or herself with "God is punishing me because . . ." or "I didn't follow my doctor's advice," or "I've been given this extra burden to prove my worthiness."

If the depression is allowed to continue, the parent might withdraw from the child or the other parent at just the time that the child or other family members needs him or her the most. With some parents, the guilt feeling might be an attempt to establish control over a situation considered to be hopeless. By attributing the cause to himself, the parent puts into his own hands the power to understand the situation and to control it. The "logic" is that if he or she does not again practice the transgressions it will not happen again.

If the initial anger is displaced outward, the parent enters into a pattern of blaming or attributing the fault to someone else. Like the guilt reaction, it places responsibility in the hands of mankind and protects one against feelings of helplessness. The parent might blame the physician because "He didn't get to the hospital fast enough," or "I told him I was in labor, but he wouldn't believe me and I almost delivered in the car," or "If the pediatrician had come out to see him rather than prescribe over the phone he wouldn't have had that high fever." This reaction might generalize to all professionals who are then considered bunglers, incompetents, and charlatans: "It's the school's fault," or "She's just a young, inexperienced teacher," or "She's just an old, rigid teacher." The professional may never hear of the parents' complaints, but the child may never be allowed to forget them. Such reactions may undermine the child's faith in or respect for the very people he or she must turn to for help and for hope.

Some parents may attempt to suppress their feelings of guilt by overprotecting the child. The most normal thing to do when a child is hurting is to reach out and protect him. This is necessary and helpful. But, the goal is to protect him where he needs protecting and to encourage his growth where he does not need protecting. A blanket of overprotection covers the weaknesses but also blunts the strengths. Not only does this behavior keep the child immature or delay areas of growth; but, it also makes the child feel inadequate. He or she knows what's happening. When everyone else has a chore to do and he does not, when everyone takes turns clearing the table but he never has to, he might conclude "See, they agree with me. . . . I am inadequate."

Most parents of such handicapped children work through the early stages of denial, anger, and guilt. They might go through a stage similar to the hypercathexis prior to decathexis seen in the mourning process. During this time the parent may need to review the clinical findings again or might ask repeated questions about their child. It is as if they have to overinvest in the symptoms and treatment programs before they can accept them.

Some parents have difficulty working through these normal reactions. The initial attempts to handle feelings and thoughts might prolong and extend into a fixed, often dysfunctional, pattern of behavior.

Some parents cannot give up their denial. They must continue to "doctor shop" in a continuing search for the doctor with the magic cure or for someone who will say that nothing is wrong with their child. Such parents greet the newest professional with flattery and praise, depreciating the numerous professionals who have proceeded him. Ultimately, he or she too is rejected and attacked. As the frustration grows, they might go from one promised cure to another, often becoming the victim of people who capitalize on such parents. During this "shopping," the child may be deprived of valuable programs and therapy that he or she needs. There are other potentially serious consequences of a chronic denial reaction. Because each professional must be criticized and downgraded as the parent moves on to the next, the child may pick up the message that he cannot trust or have faith in professionals. He needs this trust and faith in order to have hope; in order to work toward overcoming this handicap. The child may also pick up another subtle but clear message from his parents: "We can't accept you as you are. . . . We must find someone who will tell us that you are not the way you are." He hears and may react with feelings of anger, shame, and inadequacy.

A parent might handle his or her unresolved guilt by becoming overly dedicated to this child; and is covetly furious about it. What comes across overtly is the dedication. No task, no trip, no expense is too great to help "my child." What comes across covertly may be the anger at having to do these things. Occasionally, a parent will become a professional martyr and never let anyone forget it. The surface behavior is to be admired, but somehow the child picks up a parallel message: "Look how much I do for you, you ungrateful good-for-nothing child. You are worthless to begin with and you show no appreciation."

If the initial anger is not handled, this feeling might continue to be felt or projected. Nothing can go well. Someone is always doing something wrong in the parent's mind: "After all the time and money, you haven't helped my child. . . . How come?" Such parents may become miserable and difficult to live or work with.

For some, the normal initial reaction of overprotecting the child might become a life style, both preventing growth and increasing the child's feelings of worthlessness. The child might be infantalized. Occasionally this reaction is an attempted cover up for feelings of inadequacy as a parent. A parent with low self-esteem and feelings of worthlessness may attain a feeling of being needed and wanted by deluding oneself that he or she is "all the child has in the world." The child's immaturity and feelings of incompetence lead to failure and a retreat back to the home. The overprotecting parent will see this and feel even more justified in moving in and protecting. A repetitive cycle ensues, the child repeatedly realizing that he is helpless without his parent and the parent reinforcing the notion that the child cannot survive without him.

A parent may handle unresolved guilt by withdrawing and totally dedicating himself to the child to the point where there is no energy left for further relationships with the other children in the family or the other parent. Taking care of the child's needs are so taxing and demanding that the parent is too weary for social or sexual relations with the spouse or for meeting the needs of the siblings. The result is a dysfunctional family. Often the anger is not expressed between the parents; instead, it may be displaced onto this child.

The siblings of children with this syndrome may react as well. In response to their feelings of anger, they might feel guilty. This is especially likely when the verbal or nonverbal message from the parent is, "He can't help it" or "It's not his fault." A brother or sister might feel guilt for having normal thoughts such as "I'm glad it's him and not me with the problem."

These feelings of anger or guilt might be acted out against the sibling with the disability. A brother or sister might provoke or scapegoat this child to encourage his misbehavior; as the handicapped child gets punished by his parents, the sibling feels revenged. Sometimes normal siblings will set the handicapped child up to look or act bad because they perceive that the worse he looks, the better they look.

Some siblings become worried and feel anxious. This is especially true in families where little is said. They ask, "What's wrong with Jimmy?" Their parents say, "Oh, nothing special. . . . It's O.K." Yet, they see the parents taking him from one place to another and they hear the parents talking. Occasionally they heard words like "brain damage" or "where are we going to get money for all of this?" They see mother upset, maybe in tears. With lack of truth and with an awareness that something is wrong, their fantasy will take over. Frequently, they fantasize worse situations than exists in reality. Then they worry. Brothers and sisters might say, "Will he live?" "Is he going to die?" "Will it happen to me?" "If it's not serious, then why all the whispers and secrets?" They need clear information at a level they can understand and to the degree that they need to know.

Siblings may become angry for other reasons, they might fight with the child who has problems or with the parents. They resent the double standard. "How come I've got to fix my bed and she doesn't?" or "He broke my toy and you did nothing." They may get angry with the amount of time and energy parents spend with the disabled child. Between taking him to the special tutoring, special programs, and doctors, there is little time for anyone else. The handicapped child might use up so much money that everyone has to do without or vacations may have to be compromised. Children at school might tease a brother or sister, "Hey, how's your retarded brother?" or "Your sister sure acts funny. . . . What's wrong with her . . . is she a mental case?" They are embarrassed by the comments or the behavior and get angry. This may happen at home also; a sibling might stop bringing friends home because he or she is embarrassed by his brother or sister's behavior.

The Diagnostic Process

The evaluation of a child with minimal brain dysfunction requires a team effort. Because there are so many areas of disturbance, the child psychiatrist must work with the family physician, neurologist, psychologist, social worker, special educator, speech pathologist, and others. Each contributes to the full understanding of the total child.

Frequently, the history obtained from the parents begins to suggest the syndrome. Descriptions of the child's behavior, inconsistencies in the child's performance, delays in motor or language development, or poor academic performance imply possible specific learning disabilities. Continuous increased motor activity speaks for hyperactivity; a short attention span might connote distractibility. If behavioral problems associated with poor academic performance began in the first year of school, this raises the possibility that the emotional difficulties might be related to this syndrome.

Observations during a playroom diagnostic session may be helpful as one notes the child's ability to understand, organize, and perform various types of interactions and activities.[80]

Once one suspects this syndrome, it is important to differentiate it from other clinical conditions. The presenting academic difficulties might initially be attributed to mental retardation. Children with maturational lag in motor or language development usually present with the same academic problems plus, possibly, hyperactivity and distractibility. The perceptual distortions and thinking disorders that occur in childhood schizophrenia might appear initially to be clinical evidence of a specific learning disability. It may not be until the clinical picture develops that the correct diagnosis becomes apparent. Some of these minimal brain dysfunction syndrome children at ages one to three resemble an autistic child. The underlying learning and language disabilities interfere with normal psycho-social development. Especially when they are under stress, these children appear to function as though they were in the early stages of establishing object constancy. By age three they usually achieve object constancy, but they remain psycho-socially immature. With children who have a degenerative disease of the central nervous system (such as Schilder's disease), the earliest clinical findings are often a loss of memory and cognitive skills. These clinical findings start in early latency. The associated academic problems may initially be diagnosed as the minimal brain dysfunction syndrome; the fuller picture of degeneration of the central nervous system only becoming apparent with time

Through a special educational evaluation, one can determine whether a child has any specific learning disabilities and, if so, which ones. An intellectual assessment can rule out mental retardation. With retardation the subtests of the intelligence tests are consistently low. The child with specific learning disabilities will do well on subtests that utilize his or her areas of learning strength but poorly on subtests that tap areas of learning weakness. This subtest scatter should in itself suggest this syndrome. As but one example, a child with visual perceptual, visual integrative, and visual motor disabilities might score below average on the subtests requiring such skills (e.g., WISC performances scores) but might score in the average range or above on other subtests (e.g., WISC verbal scores). The psychologist might also do specific visual motor tests. Projective tests might help to rule out a thought disorder. The speech pathologist could further differentiate hearing, speech, and language disabilities.

Clinical neurological evaluations are frequently useful in completing the diagnosis.[76, 92] However, it should be kept in mind that many of these children have no evidences of neurological deficits other than "soft signs"; i.e., signs suggestive of central nervous system dysfunction but not firm proof of such dysfunction. Usually there are no clear "hard signs" of organicity such as paresis, paralysis, anesthesia, or reflex changes. It is information from the educational and psychological test materials that suggest the brain is not functioning normally ("soft signs"). EEG evaluations may not be meaningful in establishing the diagnosis. Many pediatric neurologists will not order an EEG unless there is some evidence of a seizure disorder.

Etiology

The cause of this syndrome is not known. There are probably several etiologic factors that could lead to its multiple clinical aspects.

BRAIN DAMAGE

Some of these children may have brain damage.[49, 93] Circulatory, toxic, metabolic, or other forms of embarrassment to the fetal nervous system during a critical period of prenatal development; perinatal stresses or insults to the brain; or stress to the nervous system during the critical early years of life (trauma, fever, inflamation, etc.) may have resulted in subtle central nervous system damage. There may be a spectrum of disorders caused by pre-, peri-, and postnatal brain damage. Depending on location, extent of damage, time of life, and developmental stage at the time of damage, the stress might cause fetal or neonatal death, cerebral palsy, minimal cerebral palsy, epilepsy, or mental retardation. The less severe forms might produce a variety of learning and behavioral disorders.

MATURATIONAL LAG

A delay in the development of the central nervous system may be another cause.[1] For such children, the nervous system develops more slowly but finally reaches full maturation, often at about eight to nine years of age. During the lag period, however, they present as having findings of this syndrome.

Dr. L. Taft[91] has noted a familiar history from parents of children who later showed evidence of maturational lag and/or this syndrome. Such children reflect one or more characteristics at birth secondary to the continuation of perinatal reflexes that normally extinguish during the early hours of life. These behaviors often lead to difficulty with parenting and might be the first evidence of the syndrome interfering with child-parent relationships. With an insecure or ambivalent parent such negative interactions might lead to a life pattern of poor relationships with a child.

For some children, the tonic neck reflex persists for several weeks. The mother holds her child to her body and turns his head toward the bottle or nipple. As she does this the hand closest to the body pulls up. The mother might perceive this as the child pushing her away.

During the early days of life most infants overreact to reflex stimulation. They overextend or overflex. For some children, this reaction might persist. The mother places the baby over her arm to feed him. This pressure on his mid back causes his back to overextend. She perceives the child as pulling away. Parents who had infants with both of the aforementioned responses might report: "We didn't get along from the beginning. Every time I tried to feed him he pulled back and pushed me away."

A third possible evidence of an immature nervous system during early infancy is the child who is hypersensitive to touch. Touch is perceived as unpleasant or painful. A parent holds his or her child and the child cries. The more the parent holds or cuddles to comfort the child, the more the child cries. Some parents report that they intuitively learned to place the child on a pillow and then hold the pillow. Such hypersensitivity often extinguished by five to six weeks of life. Dr. Taft suggests that some cases of "milk allergies" might be secondary to this dermal hypersensitivity. It may not be that the particular type of milk tried at six to seven weeks of life finally works. It might be that the hypersensitivity extinguished and the child could relax. Any milk tried at that time would have worked.

A history from a parent suggesting one or all of the preceding clinical examples of an immature nervous system might add to the explanation of the poor parent-child relationship or to the history of colic or other evidences of infant stress. Explanations to the parents often relieve guilt and feelings of inadequacy and might lead to reexploring relationships.

GENETIC

The probability of a genetic basis for this syndrome has been studied. Silver[84] found that in as many as 40 percent of these children a familial pattern can be discerned with parents, siblings, and extended family having the same clinical picture. Morrison and Stewart[59] found a familial pattern in half of the cases; Cantwell[21] found slightly less. Matheny, Dolan, and Wilson[57] found that, in their longitudinal study of twins, identical pairs were more likely than fraternal pairs to be concordant both for academic difficulties and for such preschool behavioral difficulties as delay in language or motor development. These studies with others[62, 63] support the possibility that this is a heterogeneous syndrome and that in some, if not many, cases there is a genetic determinant. Since the preceding studies found affected relatives on both sides of the family, this inheritance is probably polygenic and not due to a simple dominant gene.

One study of karyotype analysis of lymphocytes from peripheral blood showed no evidence of a chromosomal abnormality.[95]

Several studies have explored the psychiatric status of parents of children with this syndrome. Their findings suggest a higher incidence of sociopathy among these parents than would be expected from a normal population of children.[20, 21, 61] However, these studies did not look into the possibility that the psychopathology noted in the parents was secondary in character. They may have been reacting to the frustrations and academic failures their children experienced because of their unrecognized and untreated learning disabilities and/or hyperactivity. Possibly these studies do not show evidence of a familial relationship between this syndrome and such sociopathy but measure some of the consequences of not fully treating this syndrome.

Adoption[60, 74] compared to studies of twins[57, 101] add further support to the possibility of a genetic pattern with this syndrome.

BIOCHEMICAL

In recent years evidence has accumulated which suggests a neurophysiological basis for the syndrome.[86, 98] It is possible that the hyperactivity and/or distractibility might be related to a pattern of deficiencies and/or altered homeostasis in the epinephrine-norepinephrine metabolism of the brain, probably in the ascending reticular activating system. This imbalance might relate to DOPA, dopamine, epinephrine or norepinephrine pathways within the brain.*

CORTICAL DYSFUNCTIONS

Studies in neuropsychology are helping to clarify higher cortical functions relating to learning. Luria, in particular, studied the multi-level function of each area of the cerebral cortex as well as the interaction between areas.[52, 53] Difference in functioning of each cerebral hemisphere[102] might relate to specific disabilities. Such data might someday shed light on the etiology of the specific learning disabilities.

ORTHOMOLECULAR DYSFUNCTIONS

Recent reports that attempted to relate the syndrome to deficiencies in specific vitamins, trace elements, or glucose have not been found to be valid.[6, 81] The reports on biophysiological reactions to food allergies[33, 66] have not yet been validated.

Feingold has proposed that this syndrome is related to ingestion of artificial food colors, flavors, and preservatives.[32,33] Several investigators are currently studying the validity of Feingold's concept.[25, 88, 90] The data to date suggest the possibility that he is correct about some children but not most. Further studies are in progress. These findings should help to clarify this theory.

In summary, it is probable that there are multiple etiologies for each aspect of this syndrome. The specific disabilities might be caused by subtle brain damage within the cerebral cor-

* See references 24, 56, 70, 86, 98.

tex, by dysfunctional physiology secondary to an inherited type of nervous system disturbance, perhaps an imbalance or deficiency of neurotransmitters. The hyperactivity and/or distractibility might be caused by neurohumoral or other biochemical imbalances or might arise from other physiological difficulties within the ascending reticular activating system or other brain sites. The interrelationships between the cortex and the brain stem in this syndrome have not yet been clarified. The emotional problems are a result of the stress and altered ego-function produced by the syndrome.

The clinical picture appears to be the resultant of the interactions among the compromised central nervous system functions produced by the specific etiologic pattern.

Pathogenesis of the Syndrome

Studies of the natural history of these children often are not easy to follow. As with other aspects of this syndrome, the confusion relates to terminology and to definition of terms. If one focuses on one aspect of the syndrome, treating only these symptoms, then follow up studies are inconclusive.

Some investigations report follow up studies of hyperactive children on psychostimulants, concluding that they do not improve academically. But, then, the psychostimulants do not treat the learning disabilities only the hyperactivity. The wrong outcome variable is being measured. This finding does not suggest that the psychostimulants are not effective in improving the hyperactivity, only that the psychostimulants do not treat the learning disabilities. Medication without special education intervention will not overcome the learning disabilities.

This concept of treating the total syndrome is so important that several follow up studies will be discussed to illustrate the point. Weiss, Minde, Werry, and associates[97] followed the progress of sixty-four hyperactive children for five years; they noted that they became less hyperactive, yet their learning disabilities persisted with chronic and severe underachievement in school despite the maintenance of normal or superior intelligence. No reference was made to special educational intervention. Laufer[50] followed twenty hyperactive children on medication. He concluded that the only characteristic common to all was poor school performance despite adequate intelligence. There was no reference to the presence of or treatment for the learning disabilities. Ambrosino and Del Fonte[4] followed thirty hyperactive children. This study focused on the activity level; yet, they were forced to note on follow up that, "although none of the children had been referred for their learning difficulties, almost all of them required remediation." Gittelman-Klein and Klein[38] followed sixty-one children on placebo and methylphenidate. They noted improvement in classroom behavior but not in academic performance. Rie, Rie, Stewart, and Ambuel[73] concluded after their study that methylphenidate (Ritalin) improved behavior but did not enhance learning. Any follow up study that does not identify and treat all aspects of the syndrome will not provide a complete picture of progress.

Follow up studies that focus on the parents of hyperactive children also might reflect the problem of not focusing on all aspects of the syndrome. If an adult who was known or suspected to have been hyperactive as a child is sociopathic or functioning at a low socioeconomic position, are these findings due to residual behavioral aspects of the hyperactivity or to the unrecognized and untreated learning disabilities? Either is possible; however, unless both possibilities are considered no one conclusion can be reached. Borland and Heckman[18] did a twenty-five-year follow up study of hyperactive boys and their brothers. They observed that nearly one-half of the hyperactive children when adults had psychiatric problems and had not achieved socioeconomically as well as their nonhyperactive brothers, even though they were of normal IQ. No reference was made to learning disabilities; although, they observed that none of the hyperactive children did as well in school as their normal brothers. One must question whether the findings as adults were due to the hyperactivity or to the unrecognized and untreated learning disabilities. The same concern with finding possible causative relationships for follow up findings when all aspects of the syndrome are not looked for or followed is present with other studies.[20, 21, 60, 61]

There probably are multiple determinants for this syndrome. Several different etiologic factors can result in the clinical findings. The outcome may be based on the etiologic factors as well as on the types of clinical interventions.

The specific learning disabilities improve with special educational intervention. Without help, they compound as the child gets older and further behind. Children with learning disabilities due to maturational lag appear to need special educational help until about age eight; then, often the disabilities minimize or are no longer noted. Children with learning disabilities due to an inherited, dysfunctional central nervous system need to develop learning pathways and to develop compensation skills; they often need special help for four to five years and may need additional support for longer. Some of these disabilities, especially the fine motor ones, may persist throughout life. When structural brain damage results in learning disabilities, special educational help may be needed throughout the child's education. Residual findings usually persist as adults.

The hyperactivity and/or distractibility usually will improve on the psychostimulants. Most children will need such medication until puberty. Perhaps as many as 20 percent will continue to need this medication throughout adolescence and young adulthood.

The increased interest in and study of minimal brain dysfunction in children has resulted in an awareness that it may not disappear at puberty. Evidence of this syndrome and its sequelae can be found in adolescents[2, 3, 58] as well as in adults.* For some the learning disabilities, hyperactivity, or distractibility persists into adult life. If unrecognized or not treated when young, the adults show the academic, emotional, and social consequences of these handicaps.

Thus, without total treatment of the total child for the total syndrome, the emotional problems that develop might result in major psychiatric problems as adolescents and adults. No studies have yet documented the percentage of school dropouts, delinquents, or adolescent psychiatric hospital admissions for whom this behavior is secondary to unrecognized and untreated learning disabilities and/or hyperactivity. The author's clinical experience suggests that such studies would find as much as 30 to 40 percent of such individuals might fit this picture.

Treatment

As with other types of handicaps, the basic approach is to correct or compensate for weaknesses while utilizing strengths. This is a chronic syndrome. It is not just a school disability but effects all aspects of the child or adolescent's life. Total intervention is needed in order to minimize the handicaps and the secondary complications.

* See references 10, 16, 41, 55, 68, 78, 103.

THE SPECIFIC LEARNING DISABILITIES

In this area special education is the treatment of choice. The special educator might use environmental techniques to minimize the hyperactivity, distractibility, or short attention span when these are present. The specific areas of intervention, however, are with the learning disabilities. The basic theme is to build on the learning strengths while strengthening (or compensating for) the areas of learning weakness. This is an on-going process that may well take several years. As noted earlier, some children appear to overcome their handicaps and move ahead at a rapid pace while others progress at a slower rate.

Once the specific areas of learning or language disabilities are clarified, a prescriptive teaching program is designed. For example, if a child has input problems in the auditory perceptual area, the special educator might teach reading by building on visual and tactile input strengths (e.g., looking at wooden letters covered with sandpaper while moving one's finger over the letters) while working on the weakness (auditory perceptual training). Knowing what not to do is an essential part of the educational process; thus, if a child has auditory perceptual difficulties, the educator should not subject him or her to a phonics method in order to teach him to read.

HYPERACTIVITY-DISTRACTIBILITY

Children with physiologically based hyperactivity or distractibility usually respond to the psychostimulants with a decrease in motor activity and an increase in attention span.

Bradley was the first to describe the effect of amphetamine sulfate (Benzedrine), a psychostimulant drug on these children.[19] Since Bradley's work, numerous papers have reported on the value of such psychostimulants as dextroamphetamine (Dexedrine) and methylphenidate (Ritalin). Other psychostimulants such as caffeine may be used.[37, 72, 77] Pemoline (Cylert) is also effective.[26] Imipramine will decrease the hyperactivity or distractibility with some children.[45, 69, 83, 86]

These drugs have a common effect on neurotransmitters. D-amphetamine releases dopamine and norepinephrine from their presynaptic axon terminals as well as inhibits the cellular reuptake of these catecholamines.[11, 86, 98] Methylphenidate is a more specific agent, releasing only dopamine from cerebral dopamine neurons.[34, 51] Imipramine, a tricyclic antidepressant, blocks the neuronal uptake of norepinephrine and serotonin primarily but also inhibits dopamine reuptake.[40, 87] Pemoline is also a specific dopamine agonist.[31]

Consideration of the pharmacological activity of these agents suggests that alternations in the activity of dopamine and perhaps other monoamines is linked to the pathogenesis of the hyperactivity and distractibility aspects of this syndrome.[55, 81, 98]

The reason for the effect of such stimulants is still unclear. One theory is that the ascending reticular activating system in these children is immature or dysfunctional.[86, 98] Thus, the sensory filtering processes are not effective, resulting in distractibility and a short attention span. At the same time, the motor inhibitory processes are not effective, resulting in the motor hyperactivity. The neurochemical site of function for the psychostimulants is the ascending reticular activating system. Such medication stimulates or "strengthens" this dysfunctional area, thus improving the sensory filtering and the motor inhibiting process. By the same token psychodepressants which sedate this area of the brain may act to increase the dysfunction, thus the deficits; the result of such medication is a higher level of hyperactivity and distractibility. Another theory suggests that the neocortex is hyposensitive and thus requires increased bombardment with stimuli in order to respond.[75] Current neurophysiological and pharmacological data support the former dysinhibition theory.

It is unclear if the clinical evidence with these children of a calming effect with psychostimulants and a stimulating effect with psychodepressants is a true paradoxical effect. Rapoport and associates found, for example, that dextroamphetamine produced a calming effect in normal prepubertal boys.[71]

All children with learning disabilities are not hyperactive and/or distractible; however, most children who are hyperactive and/or distractible have learning disabilities. It is important to note that the psychostimulants improve only the hyperactivity and/or distractibility. They do not affect the specific learning disabilities. In effect, they only make the child more available for learning. Thus, it is important to have an educational evaluation done on children who respond positively to such medication. To make a child less active or less distractible helps; but the learning disabilities still exist, and the child still needs special educational therapy.

It is also important to differentiate between physiologically based hyperactivity and increased motor activity that is anxiety-based.[80] The former often responds to the psychostimulants; the latter may respond to a minor tranquilizer, but will not respond to the psychostimulant. A child whose aggressive or agitated behavior reflects an underlying depression might also respond to a psychostimulant (mood lifter) with an improvement in behavior. Here, too, the history and description of the behavior offer clues in the differential diagnosis. For reasons not yet understood, the physiologically based hyperactivity and/or distractibility may disappear at puberty; children who have been on medication throughout latency may no longer need such medication after age thirteen to fourteen. Clinical observations suggest that some individuals may need this medication throughout adolescence and young adulthood.

MEDICATION MANAGEMENT

Dextroamphetamine is available both as an elixir and in tablets. The elixir may be less effective than the tablets, perhaps because alcohol is used as the vehicle and acts as a central nervous system depressant. This counteracts some of the effect of the stimulant. A combination of dextroamphetamine and amobarbital is less effective than dextroamphetamine alone; again, perhaps the barbiturate counteracts some of the effects of the stimulant. Once a dosage for dextroamphetamine has been established, the twelve-hour timed-release capsules can be considered. If a child needs 5 mg three times a day, one 15 mg timed-released capsule in the morning might be substituted. This eliminates the problem of supervising the noon dose for the child in school. In addition, the even discharge of medication sometimes decreases the up-and-down shifts in the effectiveness of the tablets. One study suggested that excretion of dextroamphetamine may be more rapid in some children than in others.[30] This difference in excretion rates might explain the varied effectiveness of the drug. Even so, when a daily dosage of 30 mg is reached, either a rethinking of the diagnosis or an alternative medication should be considered.

Methylphenidate (Ritalin) is available in 5 mg, 10 mg, and 20 mg tablets. Up to 20 mg three times a day may be used. As with dextroamphetamine, when more is needed the possibility of giving a different drug should be considered. Over a period of years, some children can be shifted from one drug to another as tolerance is developed.

If neither psychostimulant has been successful, it is helpful to determine whether: (1) the medication is being given as prescribed; (2) the child is truly taking the medication; (3) the hyperactivity is anxiety-based rather than psyiologically-based; or (4) the family or school situation is so stressful that medication alone cannot produce the desired effects.

The hyperactivity and/or distractibility are not only educational disabilities; they are life disabilities. Such behaviors interfere with family activities and peer activities. Thus, if a child responds positively to such medication he or she should be on medication all day everyday, not just during school hours. It is just as important for a child to sit calmly and attend at the dinner table or while playing a game with friends as it is to behave well in class. This is an important point, for many physicians still feel that the child should be on medication only during school hours. This model leaves the child off of medication during after school and evening hours, weekends, and summers. The hyperactive and/or distractible child who responds positively to medication needs the medication to help function better during all hours; not just during school hours. He or she must be on medication during times when it is important to relax, relate, and function (dinner with family, TV with siblings, Cub Scouts, Sunday School, summer camp, etc.).

The parents should be informed about the effects and duration of the medication. The psychostimulants work for about four hours with minimal or no residual effects. Knowing this, a parent can add or subtract from the usual dosage pattern to fit the activity. The child may be scheduled to take his or her last pill in the middle of the afternoon; however, if company is coming or if a Scout meeting or other activity is planned, he or she may need an extra dose at 6:00 or 7:00 P.M.

The idiosyncrasies and toxic effect of the psychostimulant drugs are described in the drug manufacturers' literature. There are a few clinical side effects which can usually be managed.[85] The psychostimulants may produce a loss of appetite. This effect usually decreases or disappears within a month and the parents should be encouraged to continue the treatment program. If the anorexia persists and weight loss ensues, the drug may have to be discontinued. It is the loss of weight that is the critical issue, not the loss of appetite. The medication decreases the child's appetite so that he or she may become more selective about what he eats. Thus, a given child may not eat his meals but will eat candy and other snacks. Controlling the sweets might result in better meal intakes.

Some children will have difficulty falling asleep while on these drugs and may lie in bed restlessly for three or four hours. Like anorexia, this effect may disappear during the first month. With some children, the sleeplessness is a legitimate result of the psychostimulant, and it becomes necessary to discontinue the mid- or late-afternoon dose. With other children, the sleeplessness is not due to the medication but due to the rebound effect of being off of the medication. That is, a child on a three times a day schedule is under the effect of the medication from morning until about four hours after the last dose. When the medication wears off, at 8:00 or 9:00 P.M., the child rebounds to his usual level of activity (or higher). The result is increased hyperactivity and restlessness at bedtime. He or she is put to sleep at 9:00 or 9:30 but can't unwind. For this child, an additional dose of the stimulant at about 8:00 P.M. may eliminate his difficulty with sleep. Stopping the afternoon dose does help in some cases; adding a bedtime dose helps in others. The two possible causes for sleeplessness are difficult to differentiate and often a trial dose at bedtime is necessary to clarify the issue.

Parents may report that their child is clinically improved on the medication but that he or she now talks constantly or breaks into tears or explodes at the slightest frustration. It is not clear how much of this emotional lability is a result of the medication and how much is functional. Because the medication lessens the motor activity, the child may be better able to interact and communicate; thus, a quiet child may become more verbal. It is also possible that, because the medication allows the child to sit still and be available for learning, he is forced to deal with his learning problems and thus becomes frustrated and more anxious. The increased anxiety might explain an increase in verbiage or in emotional lability. If reassurance to the parents and special educational help for the child do not minimize the emotional lability, the drug dosage might be decreased. If this does not help, stopping the medication might have to be considered.

Other Medications: Major tranquilizers such as the phenothiazines have been used to decrease hyperactivity. They seem to work best with children whose thinking is disorganized or who display other psychotic features. With children having this syndrome, any decrease in their hyperactivity on such medication is likely to be the result of drowsiness or of extrapyramidal signs rather than a true physiological shift toward normal activity levels. Children with anxiety-based hyperactivity on the other hand might respond favorably. Some of the children who are distractible due to internal dysinhibition might respond to the major tranquilizers.

Minor tranquilizers have been tried. These medications work best for the child with anxiety-based hyperactivity but do not help those with the neurologically-based symptom picture. With some children, anticonvulsants like diphenylhydantoin (Dilantin) and primidone (Mysoline) have been reported to lessen the behavioral difficulties. There have been no studies that show in a clear way just how effective these drugs are for children with this syndrome. Lithium carbonate has been tried and found to be ineffective in handling the hyperactivity or the distractibility.[39]

Emotional Problems

As discussed earlier, when an emotional difficulty is found, it is important to differentiate between a primary emotional problem and an emotional problem which is secondary to the learning disabilities. Because of the frustrations and failures experienced by these children, many do develop emotional difficulties. In this case, the emotional problems arise because of the learning disability and are not themselves the cause of the disability. However, such secondary emotional problems compound and add to the child's unavailability for learning.

Psychotherapy will help the child cope and will make him or her more available for learning. However, such help will be minimal when a child is experiencing frustration and failure all week long at school. It is difficult to help a child rethink a poor self-image when he or she experiences daily failure in school. Unless the child is in the appropriate educational program, the effects of psychotherapy may be quickly negated.

Many of the treatment approaches that have been advanced to help children and adolescents with this syndrome are, to say the least, controversial.[79, 81] One group of such efforts relates to the concept of neurophysiological retraining. The basic premise is that by stimulating specific sensory inputs or exercising specific motor patterns one can retrain, recircuit, or in some way improve the functioning of a part of the central nervous system. Three such approaches are in use today: (1) patterning, as developed by Doman and Delacato; (2) optometric therapy; and (3) the sensory-integrative therapy described by A. Jean Ayres.

PATTERNING

The "patterning" theory and techniques was initially developed by Robert Doman and Carl Delacato[28] following the principle that ontogeny recapitulates phylogeny. They postulated that failure to pass properly through a certain sequence of developmental stages in modality, language, and competence in the manual, visual, auditory, and tactile areas reflected poor neurological organization and may indicate brain damage.[46] As described by Doman and Delacato patterning reaches ". . . the brain itself by pouring into the afferent sensory system . . . all of the stimuli normally provided by his environment but with such intensity and frequency as to draw, ultimately a response from the corresponding motor systems."[46] In the more severe cases of brain damage, patterns of passive movement are imposed with the goal of producing normal activities which would have been the product of the injured brain level had it not been injured.[29] In addition to the aforementioned methods of manipulation, other techniques used include sensory stimulation, rebreathing of expired air with a plastic face mask (alleged to increase vital capacity and to stimulate cerebral blood flow), and restriction of fluid, salt, and sugar intake (alleged to decrease cerebrospinal fluid production and cortical irritability).[46] The American Academy of Pediatrics,[8] the American Academy of Cerebral Palsy,[5] the United Cerebral Palsy Association of Texas,[94] and the Canadian Association for Retarded Children[46] have published statements expressing concern about the effectiveness of this form of therapy.

OPTOMETRIC THERAPY

There are two general views held by optometrists on the roles they should play with children who have learning problems. Most optometrists evaluate the child's visual abilities and may prescribe lenses or the use of conventional visual training or orthoptic techniques, if indicated. There is, however, a particular group of optometrists who use a developmental vision approach and who see a broader role for the optometrist in learning problems.[22] This group feels that learning in general and reading in particular are primary tasks in visual perception. They point out that visual perception processes are also related to the child's sensory motor coordination and employ a wide diversity of educational and sensory-motor-perceptual training techniques in an attempt to correct educational problems in children.

It is the second group of optometrists who have been active with children with learning disabilities. The American Academy of Pediatrics, the American Academy of Ophthalmology and Otolaryngology, and the American Association of Ophthalmology issued a joint organizational statement critical of this approach.[7] This joint communique emphasizes the need for a multidisciplinary approach to such children. It cautions that there are no peripheral eye defects which can produce dyslexia and associated learning disabilities. It minimizes the effect of visual or neurological organizational training as used by optometrists. It states that glasses have no value in treating learning problems except where there is a refracting problem. And, it concludes that the treatment of learning disabilities is primarily for the special educator. This controversy between ophthalmologists and optometrists often catches the parents in the middle, as they try to decide what is best for their child.

SENSORY INTEGRATIVE THERAPY

A. Jean Ayres feels that the capacity of the neocortex to react to auditory and visual processes is dependent on the brain stem's ability to organize auditory and visual processes; thus, if the brain stem is inadequate to organize such sensory integrative processes the individual may have learning disabilities.[14, 15] Her research data suggest that there are disorders which are consistently observed in learning disability children. These problems can be accounted for in terms of inadequate sensory integration in the brain stem. These include immature postural reactions, poor extracurricular muscle control, poorly developed visual orientation to environmental space, difficulty in the processing of sound into percepts, and a tendency toward distractibility.[14]

She proposes that carefully controlled sensory input can be introduced through vestibular and somatosensory systems. Such graded stimulation enhances the capacity of the brain for intersensory integration. This allows for improved interconnections between these sensory modalities and the visual and auditory inputs.[12] She further hypothesizes that the normalization of postural mechanisms organized in the midbrain would enable better cortical interhemispheral communication, upon which reading must in fact be dependent.[12] In the models of therapy based on these concepts, vestibular stimulation is seen as improving auditory processes, thus helping with the auditory-language disorders of learning-disability children.[13] This vestibular stimulation might also improve visual perceptual functioning via the intersensory effect of multisensory or convergent neurons and nuclei.[13]

A second group of controversial approaches to helping children and adolescents with this syndrome relates to the concept of Orthomolecular Medicine. Linus Pauling defines Orthomolecular Medicine as the treatment of mental disorders by the provision of the optimum molecular environment for the mind, especially the optimum concentrations of substances normally present in the human body.[65] The use of megavitamins, trace elements, and other molecules has been suggested.

Megavitamins: The use of massive doses of vitamins to treat emotional or cognitive disorders began with the treatment of schizophrenia. Osmond and Smythies formulated the hypothesis that schizophrenia was the result of stress-induced anxiety and a failure of metabolism resulting in highly toxic mescaline-type compounds. Hoffer, Osmond, and Smythies[43] proposed that adrenochrome, a psychotoxic oxidation production of epinephrine was this mescaline-like substance. Its production was thought to be the result of the increased phenolase (oxidase) activity of schizophrenic serum. Hoffer and Osmond[42] proposed the use of nicotinic acid and nicotinamide in the treatment of schizophrenia. They reasoned that nicotinic acid as a strong methyl group accepter would compete for methyl groups and prevent the conversion of norephinephrine to epinephrine. Diminution of epinephrine would diminish the quantities of adrenochrome and adrenolutin formed. Initially they used Nicin (nicotinic acid); later they added vitamins C and B_6 (pyridoxine) to the treatment regime.

To date, no biochemical studies on schizophrenic patients have documented Hoffer and Osmond's proposed theory on schizophrenia. A five-year study carried out by the Board of Directors of the Canadian Mental Health Association[17] strongly suggests no therapeutic effect from nicotinic acid treatment. The American Psychiatric Association published a task force report, *Megavitamin and Orthomolecular Therapy in Psychiatry*.[9] After reviewing the history and literature relating to this subject, the members of this Task Force concluded that there was no valid basis for the use of megavitamins in the treatment of mental disorders. As noted earlier, the American Academy of Pediatrics also reports there is no validity to this concept.[6]

The first paper to suggest megavitamin treatment for children with learning disabilities was written in 1971 by Dr. Allan Cott.[27] The theoretical basis for his theory (those of Hoffer and Osmond) do not appear to be valid. The 500 cases used in the study were for the most part autistic and schizophrenic children; they were not children with minimal brain dysfunction. His conclusion that megavitamins can help these children has not been confirmed by others. Despite these negative data, this approach remains popular; Dr. Cott's paper remains the primary reference.

Trace Elements: Trace elements including copper, zinc, magnesium, manganese, and chromium along with more common elements such as calcium, potassium, sodium, and iron are necessary nutrients. Their presence is essential for the maintenance of normal physiological function. No one to date has published data supporting the theory that deficiencies in one or more of these elements is a cause of the minimal brain dysfunction syndrome. Yet, in many parts of the United States children are treated with such replacement therapy. In the paper by Cott,[27] discussed earlier, he spoke of the possibility of such deficiencies. He presented no research data to support this view nor has any subsequent data supported this theory. In particular, there has been no report of observed clinical improvement with such treatment.

Hypoglycemia: Another orthomolecular approach to treating children with this syndrome regards the symptoms as secondary to hypoglycemia. The treatment is, therefore, to place the child on a hypoglycemia diet. The possible relationship of hypoglycemia to such children was reported in the same paper by Dr. Cott.[27] Again, however, no data were presented to support this view. It is indeed possible for children to suffer from hypoglycemia and to need such a special treatment program. Currently, there is no clinical evidence to show any relationship between hypoglycemia and this syndrome. Before concluding that the etiology is hypoglycemia, a full five- to seven-hour glucose tolerance study should be done.

ALLERGIC REACTIONS

Philpott, Mandell, and Von Hilsheimer[66] suggest that some types of learning disabilities are the result of an allergic sensitivity of the central nervous system to specific foods. They discuss specific test procedures for establishing this possible etiologic factor. To date, the relationship between food allergies and this syndrome is not yet clear.

FOOD ADDITIVES AND PRESERVATIVES

As noted earlier, Feingold[32, 33] suggests that certain food additives (artificial coloring, flavors, and preservatives) in foods and beverages might cause this syndrome. Children are treated by placing them on diets free of such additives. If parents want to try this treatment approach they should be made aware that evidence supporting this concept is not yet established.[25, 88, 90]

Conclusions

The child with the minimal brain dysfunction syndrome does not have just a school disability—he or she has a total life disability. The same group of learning disabilities that interfere with the normal learning processes also impinge on self-concept, self-image, peer relationships, family relationships, and social interactions. The same hyperactivity or distractibility that affects the child's abilities in the classroom interfere with his adaptation to home and neighborhood.

Such a child often does not develop normally or begins to develop secondary social and/or emotional problems and is referred to the child psychiatrist for evaluation. In doing the evaluation it is important to observe clues that might suggest this syndrome. It is extremely important to differentiate between the emotional problems that reflect the stresses caused by this syndrome and those that are a primary cause of the presenting symptoms.

If the emotional difficulties are secondary to the learning disabilities' aspect of this syndrome, psychotherapy alone will not succeed. Indeed, it may add to the child's burden by giving credence to the belief that the academic problems are emotionally based. If special educational programs and appropriate medication are not included along with the psychotherapeutic intervention, it is difficult for the child to overcome the problems.

Properly recognized, diagnosed, and treated, the child with this syndrome has the potential of a reasonably successful future. Without help, the disabilities can become incapacitating and function as a major handicap in all aspects of life.

Perhaps the price an individual and society may pay if this syndrome is not identified and treated early is best reflected in a reported episode of a nineteen-year-old who admitted killing a seventeen-year-old and, later, two police officers.

The psychiatric report was discussed in a newspaper story.[96] He was described as a "non-achiever in an achieving family." "He suffered repeated failures—academic, social, and in mechanical school. . . . He thought of himself as stupid and worthless, and developed intense anger at himself and the world."

His mother reported that he was identified as dyslexic when he was about twelve. The report commented, "perhaps too late to reverse the feelings of stupidity engendered by his inability to learn, too late to hold back the overwhelming boredom that was engulfing him." Later in the report it noted," he became convinced that he was dumb." In another part, "Every time he struggled helplessly with a math problem, every time he stumbled over a sentence from his first reader, every time his brother beat him in a fight . . .[he] grew a little more hostile, a little more withdrawn, a little more convinced of his worthlessness."

This boy became rebellious, defiant, and a frequent truant. He dropped out of school in tenth grade. A school dropout or school pushout? How many delinquent adolescents or disturbed adults show clear evidence of the price paid by not identifying or treating this syndrome?

The confusing feature of this syndrome is the multiple types of clinical pictures such children can present. All aspects of this minimal brain dysfunction syndrome must be considered in understanding the child, planning a treatment program, and advising the family and schools. Any approach which does not see this syndrome as a serious total life disability which affects both the total child and his family is not likely to be successful.

REFERENCES

1. ABRAMS, A. L., "Delayed and Irregular Maturation Versus Minimal Brain Injury. Recommendations for a Change in Current Nomenclature," *Clinical Pediatrics, 7:* 344–349, 1968.
2. ACKERMAN, P. T., DYKMAN, R. A., and PETERS, J. E., "Learning Disability Boys as Adolescents: Cognitive Factors and Achievement," *Journal of the American Academy of Child Psychiatry,* 16:296–313, 1977.

3. ———, "Teenage Status of Hyperactive Learning Disabled Boys," *American Journal of Orthopsychiatry,* 47:577–596, 1977.
4. AMBROSINO, S., and DEL FONTE, T., "A Psycho-educational Study of the Hyperkinetic Syndrome," *Psychosomatics,* 14:207–213, 1973.
5. American Academy of Cerebral Palsy, *Statement of the Executive Committee,* February 15, 1965.

6. American Academy of Pediatrics, Committee on Nutrition, "Megavitamin Therapy for Childhood Psychoses and Learning Disabilities," *Pediatrics, 58:*910–911, 1976.

7. American Academy of Pediatrics, Joint Organizational Statement, "The Eye and Learning Disabilities," *Pediatrics, 49:*454–455, 1972.

8. American Academy of Pediatrics, Statement of the Executive Board, *American Academy of Pediatrics Newsletter, 16:*1, 1965.

9. American Psychiatric Association Task Force on Vitamin Therapy in Psychiatry, *Megavitamin and Orthomolecular Therapy in Psychiatry*, American Psychiatric Association, Washington, D.C., 1973.

10. ARNOLD, L. E., STROBEL, D., and WEISENBERG, A., "Hyperactive Adult: Study of the 'Paradoxical' Amphetamine Response," *Journal of the American Medical Association, 222:*693–694, 1972.

11. AXELROD, J., "Amphetamine: Metabolism, Pharmacological Disposition and Its Effect on Catecholamine Storage," in Costa, E., and Garattini, S. (Eds.), *Amphetamines and Related Compounds*, pp. 207–216, Raven Press, New York, 1970.

12. AYRES, A. J., "Improving Academic Scores Through Sensory Integration," *Journal of Learning Disabilities, 5:*338–343, 1972.

13. ———, "Sensory Integration Dysfunction," Read before the Ninth International Conference of the Association for Children with Learning Disabilities, Atlantic City, New Jersey, February 1972.

14. ———, "Deficits in Sensory Integration in Educationally Handicapped Children," *Journal of Learning Disabilities, 2:*160–168, 1969.

15. ———, "Patterns of Perceptual-Motor Dysfunction in Children: A Factory Analytic Study," *Perceptual and Motor Skills, 20:*335–368, 1965.

16. BELLAK, L., "Psychiatric States in Adults with Minimal Brain Dysfunction," *Psychiatric Annals, 7:*58–76, November 1977.

17. Board of Directors of the Canadian Mental Health Association, quoted in Ban, T. A., "The Niacin Controversy: The Possibility of Negative Effects," *Psychiatric Opinion, 10:*19–23, 1973.

18. BORLAND, B. L., and HECKMAN, H. I., "Hyperactive Boys and Their Brothers: A 25-Year Follow-Up Study," *Archives of General Psychiatry, 33:*669–675, 1976.

19. BRADLEY, C., "The Behavior of Children Receiving Benzedrine," *American Journal of Psychiatry, 94:*577–584, 1937.

20. CANTWELL, D. P., "Genetic Studies of Hyperactive Children," in Fiere, R., Rosenthal, D., and Brill, H. (Eds.), *Genetic Research in Psychiatry*, pp. 273–280, Johns Hopkins University Press, Baltimore, 1975.

21. ———, "Psychiatric Illness in the Families of Hyperactive Children," *Archives of General Psychiatry, 27:*414–417, 1972.

22. CARLSON, P. V., and GREENSPOON, N. K., "The Uses and Abuses of Visual Training for Children with Perceptual-Motor Learning Problems," *American Journal of Optometry, 45:*161–169, 1968.

23. CLEMENTS, S., *Minimal Brain Dysfunction in Children*, National Institute of Neurological Diseases and Blindness, Monograph No. 3, Department of Health, Education, and Welfare, Washington, D.C., 1966.

24. COLEMAN, M., "Serotonin Concentrations in Whole Blood of Hyperactive Children," *Journal of Pediatrics, 78:*985–990, 1971.

25. CONNERS, C. K., et al., "Food Additives and Hyperkinesis: A Controlled Double-Blind Experiment," *Pediatrics, 58:*154–166, 1976.

26. ———, et al., "Magnesium Pemoline and Dextroamphetamine: A Controlled Study in Children with Minimal Brain Dysfunction," *Psychopharmacologia, 26:*321–336, 1972.

27. COTT, A., "Orthomolecular Approach to the Treatment of Learning Disabilities," *Schizophrenia, 3:*95–107, 1971.

28. DOMAN, G., and DELACATO, C., "Doman-Delacato Philosophy," *Human Potential, 1:*113–116, 1968.

29. DOMAN, R. J., et al., "Children with Severe Brain Injuries: Neurological Organization in Terms of Mobility," *Journal of the American Medical Association, 17:*257–261, 1960.

30. EPSTEIN, L., et al., "Correlation of Dextroamphetamine Excretion and Drug Response in Hyperkinetic Children," *Journal of Nervous and Mental Disease, 146:*136–146, 1968.

31. EVERETT, F., "A Unique Dopaminergic: Pemoline (abs)," *The Pharmacologist, 17:*227, 1975.

32. FEINGOLD, B. F., "Hyperkinesis and Learning Disabilities Linked to the Ingestion of Artificial Food Colors and Flavors," *Journal of Learning Disorders, 9:*19–27, 1976.

33. ———, *Why Your Child is Hyperactive*, Random House, New York, 1975.

34. FERRIS, R., TANG, F., and MAXWELL, R., "A Comparison of the Capacities of Isomers of Amphetamine, Deoxypipradiol and Methylphenidate to Inhibit the Uptake of Tritiated Catecholamines into Rat Cerebral Cortex Slices, Synaptosomal Preparations of Rat Cerebral Cortex, Hypothalamus, and Striatum and into Abrenergic Nerves of Rabbit Aorta," *Journal of Pharmacology and Experimental Therapeutics, 181:*407–416, 1972.

35. GARDNER, R. A., "The Guilt Reaction of Parents of Children with Severe Physical Disease," *American Journal of Psychiatry, 126:*636–644, 1969.

36. ———, "Psychological Problems of Brain-Injured Children and Their Parents," *Journal of the American Academy of Child Psychiatry, 7:*471–491, 1968.

37. GARFINKEL, B., WEBSTER, C., and SLOMAN, L., "Methylphenidate and Caffeine in the Treatment of Children with Minimal Brain Dysfunction," *American Journal of Psychiatry, 132:*723–728, 1975.

38. GITTELMAN-KLEIN, R., and KLEIN, D. F., "Methylphenidate Effects in Learning Disabilities: Psychometric Changes," *Archives of General Psychiatry, 33:*655–664, 1976.

39. GREENHILL, L. L., et al., "Lithium Carbonate in the Treatment of Hyperactive Children," *Archives of General Psychiatry, 28:*636–640, 1973.

40. HALARIS, A. E., and FREEDMAN, D. X., "Psychotropic Drugs and Dopamine Uptake Inhibition," in Freedman, D. X. (Ed.), *Biology of the Major Psychoses*, pp. 247–258, Raven Press, New York, 1975.

41. HARTOCOLLIS, P., "The Syndrome of Minimal Brain Dysfunction in Young Adult Patients," *Bulletin of the Menninger Clinic, 32:*102–114, 1968.

42. HOFFER, A., and OSMOND, H., *The Chemical Bases of Clinical Psychiatry*, Charles C Thomas, Springfield, Ill., 1960.

43. ———, and SMYTHIES, J., "Schizophrenia: A New Approach: II. Results of a Year's Research," *Journal of Mental Science, 100:*29–54, 1954.

44. HUESSY, H. R., "Study of the Prevalence and Therapy of the Choreatiform Syndrome or Hyperkinesis in Vermont," *Acta Paedopsychiatrica, 34:*130–135, 1967.

45. ———, and WRIGHT, A. L., "Use of Imipramine in Children's Behavior Disorders." Read before the 122nd annual meeting of the American Psychiatric Association, Bal Harbor, Fla., May 7, 1969.

46. Institutes for the Achievement of Human Potential, *Mental Retardation*, p. 27, Institutes for the Achievement of Human Potential, 1965.

47. Institutes for the Achievement of Human Potential, *A Summary of Concepts, Procedures and Organizations*, Institutes for the Achievement of Human Potential, Philadelphia, 1968.

48. JOHNSON, D. J., and MYKLEBUST, H. R., *Learning Disabilities. Educational Principles and Practices*, Grune & Stratton, New York, 1964.

49. KNOBLOCH, H., and PASAMANICK, B., "The Syndrome of Minimal Cerebral Damage in Infancy," *Journal of the American Medical Association, 70:*1384–1387, 1959.

50. LAUFER, M., "Long-term Management and Some Follow-up Findings on the Use of Drugs with Minimal Cerebral Syndromes," *Journal of Learning Disabilities, 4:*519–522, 1971.

51. LEWANDER, T., "Discussion," in Sjoquist, F., and Tottie, M. (Eds.), *Abuse of Central Nervous Stimulants*, pp. 435–443, Raven Press, New York, 1969.

52. LURIA, A. R., *The Working Brain. An Introduction to Neuropsychology*, Basic Books, New York, 1973.

53. ———, *Higher Cortical Functions in Man*, Basic Books, New York, 1966.

54. MANN, H. B., and GREENSPAN, S. L., "The Identification and Treatment of Adult Brain Dysfunction," *American Journal of Psychiatry, 133:*1013–1017, 1976.

55. MARGOLIN, D. I., "The Hyperkinetic Child Syndrome and Brain Monamines: Pharmacology and Therapeutic Implications," *Journal of Clinical Psychiatry, 39(2):* 120–130, 1977.

56. MATHENY, A. P., JR., DOLAN, A. B., and WILSON, R. S., "Twins with Academic Learning Problems: Antecedent Characteristics," *American Journal of Orthopsychiatry, 46(3):*464–469, 1976.

57. MCCARTY, J. J., and MCCARTY, D. J., *Learning Disabilities*, Allyn and Bacon, Boston, 1969.

58. MENDELSON, W., JOHNSON, N., and STEWART, M., "Hyperactive Boys as Teenagers: A Follow-up Study," *Journal of Nervous and Mental Disabilities, 153:*273–279, 1971.

59. MORRISON, J. R., and STEWART, M. A., "A Family Study of the Hyperactive Child Syndrome," *Biological Psychiatry, 3:*189–195, 1971.

60. ———, "The Psychiatric Status of the Legal Families of Adopted Hyperactive Children," *Archives of General Psychiatry, 28:*888–891, 1973.

61. ———, "Bilateral Inheritance as Evidence for Polygenicity in the Hyperactive Child Syndrome," *Journal of Nervous and Mental Disease, 158:*226–228, 1974.

62. OMENN, G. S., "Genetic Issues in the Syndrome of Minimal Brain Dysfunction," in Walzer, S., and Wolff, P. H. (Eds.), *Minimal Cerebral Dysfunction in Children*, Grune & Stratton, New York, 1973.

63. OWEN, F. W., et al., *Learning Disorders in Children: Sibling Studies*, Monographs of the Society for Research in Child Development, Serial No. 144, Vol. 36, No. 4, November 1971.

64. PAINE, R. S., WERRY, J. S., and QUAY, H. C., "A Study of Minimal Cerebral Dysfunction," *Developmental Medicine and Child Neurology, 10:*505–520, 1968.

65. PAULING, L., "Orthomolecular Psychiatry," *Science, 160:*265–271, 1968.

66. PHILPOTT, W. H., MANDELL, M., and VON HILSHEIMER, G., "Allergic Toxic and Chemically Defective States as Causes and/or Facilitating Factors of Emotional Reactions, Dyslexia, Hyperkinesis, and Learning Problems," in Ansara, A. (Ed.), *Selected Papers on Learning Disabilities. Our Challenge: The Right to Know*, Association for Children with Learning Disabilities, Pittsburgh, 1975.

67. POZNANSKI, E., "Psychiatric Difficulties in Siblings of Handicapped Children," *Clinical Pediatrics, 8:*232–234, 1969.

68. QUITKIN, F., and KLEIN, D. F., "Two Behavioral Syndromes in Young Adults Related to Possible Minimal Brain Dysfunction," *Journal of Psychiatric Research, 7:* 131–142, 1969.

69. RAPOPORT, J. L., "Childhood Behavior and Learning Problems Treated with Imipramine," *International Journal of Neuropsychiatry, 1:*635–642, 1965.

70. ———, et al., "Dextroamphetamine: Cognitive and Behavior Effects in Normal Prepubertal Boys," *Science, 199:*560–563, 1978.

71. ———, QUINN, P. O., and LAMPRECHT, F., "Minor Physical Anomalies Plasma Dopamin-B-Hydroxylase in Hyperactive Boys," *American Journal of Psychiatry, 131:* 386–390, 1974.

72. RICHARD, C. C., and ELDER, S. T., "The Effects of Caffeine on Reaction Time in Hyperkinetic and Normal Children," *American Journal of Psychiatry, 134:*144–148, 1977.

73. RIE, H. E., et al., "Effects of Ritalin on Underachieving Children. A Replication," *American Journal of Orthopsychiatry, 46:*313, 322, 1976.

74. SAFER, D. J., "A Familial Factor in Minimal Brain Dysfunction," *Behavior Genetics, 3:*175–187, 1973.

75. SATTERFIELD, J. H., CANTWELL, D. P., and SATTERFIELD, B. J., "Pathophysiology of the Hyperactive Child Syndrome," *Archives of General Psychiatry, 31:*839–844, 1974.

76. SCHAIN, R. J., *Neurology of Childhood Learning Disorders*, Williams & Wilkins, Baltimore, 1972.

77. SCHNACKENBERG, R., "Caffeine as a Substitute for Schedule II Stimulants in Hyperkinetic Children," *American Journal of Psychiatry, 130:*796–798, 1973.

78. SHELLEY, E. M., and RIESTER, A., "Syndrome of Minimal Brain Damage in Adults," *Diseases of the Nervous System, 33:*335–338, 1972.

79. SHRAG, P., and DIVOKY, D., *The Myth of the Hyperactive Child*, Curtis Brown, New York, 1975.

80. SILVER, L. B., "Playroom Diagnostic Evaluation of Children with Neurologically Based Learning Disabilities," *Journal of the American Academy of Child Psychiatry, 15:*240–256, Spring 1976.

81. ———, "Acceptable and Controversial Approaches to Treating the Child with Learning Disabilities," *Pediatrics, 55:*406–415, 1975.

82. ———, "Emotional and Social Problems of Children with Developmental Disabilities," in Weber, R. E. (Ed.), *Handbook on Learning Disabilities*, Prentice-Hall, Englewood Cliffs, N.J., 1974.

83. ———, "Emotional and Social Problems of the Families with a Child who Has Developmental Disabilities," in Weber, R. E. (Ed.), *Handbook on Learning Disabilities*, Prentice-Hall, Englewood Cliffs, N.J., 1974.

84. ———, "Familial Patterns in Children with Neurologically-Based Learning Disabilities," *Journal of Learning Disabilities, 4:*349–358, 1971.

85. ———, "The Neurological Learning Disability Syndrome," *American Family Physician, 4:*95–102, 1971.

86. ———, "A Proposed View on the Etiology of the Neurological Learning Disability Syndrome," *Journal of Learning Disabilities, 4:*123–133, 1971.

87. SNYDER, S. H., et al., "The Role of Brain Dopamine in Behavioral Regulation and the Action of Psychotrophic Drugs," in Ellinwood, E. H., and Cohen, S. (Eds.), *Current Concepts on Amphetamine Abuse*, U.S. Government Printing Office, Washington, D.C., 1972.

88. SPRING, C., and SANDOVAL, J., "Food Additives and Hyperkinesis: A Critical Evaluation of the Evidence," *Journal of Learning Disabilities, 9:*28–37, 1976.

89. STEWART, M. A., et al., "The Hyperactive Child Syndrome," *American Journal of Orthopsychiatry, 36:* 861–867, 1966.

90. STINE, J. J., "Symptom Alleviation in the Hyperactive Child by Dietary Modification: A Report of Two Cases," *American Journal of Orthopsychiatry, 46:*637–645, 1976.

91. TAFT, L., Personal communication, March, 1975.

92. TOUWEN, B. C. L., and PRECHTL, H. F. R., *The Neurological Examination of the Child with Minor Nervous Dysfunction*, Clinics in Developmental Medicine, No. 38, Spastics International Medical Publications, London, 1970.

93. TOWBIN, A., "Organic Causes of Minimal Brain Dysfunction. Perinatal Origin of Minimal Cerebral Lesions," *Journal of the American Medical Association, 217:*1207–1209, August 30, 1971.

94. United Cerebral Palsy Association of Texas, "The

Doman-Delacato Treatment of Neurologically Handicapped Children," *Information Bulletin*, United Cerebral Palsy Association of Texas.

95. WARREN, R. J., et al., "The Hyperactive Child Syndrome: Normal Chromosome Findings," *Archives of General Psychiatry, 24*:161–162, 1971.

96. *The Washington Post*, Washington, D.C., p. 1, cont. on p. 14, August 8, 1976.

97. WEISS, G., et al., "Studies on the Hyperactive Child. VIII. Five Year Follow Up," *Archives of General Psychiatry, 24*:409–414, 1971.

98. WENDER, P. H., *Minimal Brain Dysfunction in Children*, pp. 163–191, Wiley-Interscience, New York, 1971.

99. WERNER, H., and STRAUSS, A. A., "Pathology of Figure-Background Relation in the Child," *Journal of Abnormal Social Psychology, 36*:236–248, 1941.

100. WERRY, J. S., "Studies on the Hyperactive Child: An Empirical Analysis of the Minimal Brain Dysfunction Syndrome," *Archives of General Psychiatry, 19*:9–16, 1968.

101. WILLERMAN, L., "Activity Level and Hyperactivity in Twins," *Child Development, 44*:288–294, 1973.

102. WITELSON, S. F., "Developmental Dyslexia: Two Right Hemispheres and None Left," *Science, 195*:309–311, January 21, 1977.

103. WOOD, D., et al., "Diagnosis and Treatment of MBD in Adults," *Archives of General Psychiatry, 33*:1453–1460, 1976.

21 / Hyperkinetic Reactions

Leon Eisenberg

Terminology

According to the *Diagnostic and Statistical Manual of Mental Disorders*, 2d edition, (DSM-II),[2] the hyperkinetic reaction of childhood or adolescence (308.0) is "characterized by overactivity, restlessness, distractibility and short attention span, especially in young children; the behavior usually diminishes in adulthood." The instructions include the notation that: "If the behavior is caused by organic brain damage, it should be diagnosed under the appropriate nonpsychotic organic brain syndrome." Under the latter category (309), DSM-II states: "In children, mild brain damage often manifests itself by hyperactivity, short attention span, easy distractibility and impulsiveness . . . If the organic handicap is the major etiologic factor and the child is not psychotic, the case should be classified here." (pp. 31–32)[23] Thus, in APA diagnostic nomenclature, hyperkinetic behavior disorder is defined by the *presence* of a clinical syndrome and the *absence* of brain damage. However, the criteria for the diagnosis of "mild brain damage," also known as "minimal brain dysfunction" or "minimal cerebral dysfunction," are far less clear than this dichotomous allocation requires, if reliable differentiation is to be made.

A different scheme has been suggested by the World Health Organization Seminar on Psychiatric Disorders in Childhood,[71] in preparation for the forthcoming revision of the International Classification of Diseases (ICD) in 1979. That Seminar proposed a tri-axial classification of mental disorders in childhood. The first axis specifies the clinical psychiatric syndrome, the second, the intellectual level of the patient and the third, associated or etiologic factors thought to be related to the psychiatric syndrome. This proposal is an attempt to rectify the inherent illogic of the APA classification which is partially based on cause (the group of acute and chronic brain syndromes), partially based on intellectual level (since mental retardation is separated out as a unique diagnostic category) and partially based on clinical-descriptive categories. The WHO proposal requires the psychiatrist first to rate psychiatric status on a series of categories from normal variation through definable clinical syndromes; secondly, to evaluate intellectual level; and thirdly, to specify, where possible, associated or etiologic factors. In this classification, the hyperkinetic syndrome

should be used for disorders in which poorly organized and poorly regulated extreme overactivity, distractability, short attention span and impulsiveness, are the chief characteristics and in which the disorder is clearly *not* secondary to any other *psychiatric* syndrome. Marked mood fluctuations and aggression are also common symptoms of the disorder.[71]

The diagnosis is applicable whether or not the patient is thought to have minimal brain damage; if a brain syndrome is present, it would be specified on the third axis.

Thus, under the rules of DSM-II, the clinician must choose between hyperkinetic reaction and nonpsychotic organic brain syndrome. Under the rules proposed for ICD, the term hyperkinetic syndrome would apply to both groups of cases but the latter would be indicated by listing, on the third axis, "disease or disorder of the central nervous system" further specified by cause where known.

The problem is further confused by the use of the term hyperkinetic or overactive in clinical settings, to characterize pathological conditions. This stands in contrast to its use in child development studies where the investigator may separate out for study children whose activity level is in the upper quartile of the population distribution, without implying a judgment that the behavior is necessarily abnormal. It is rare for the child to complain of overactivity; it is usually parents and teachers who are troubled when such an individual is brought for clinical evaluation. This gives cogency to Werry's definition of hyperactivity as a chronic, sustained, excessive level of motor activity which is the cause of significant complaint both at home and at school.[95]

In this chapter, the term hyperkinetic reaction will be used to describe the clinical syndrome in children who do not have a clearly diagnosable neurologic disease or mental deficiency, in conformity with DSM-II. However, many of these patients have a history of developmental delay, so-called soft neurologic signs, nonspecific EEG abnormalities, learning problems, and deviant psychometric test performance, the presence of which leads some clinicians to employ the term "minimal cerebral dysfunction." This concept is based on an inference about underlying CNS status in the absence of demonstrable brain pathology.[95] Both terms are in contemporary use for the same group of patients; in consequence, the literature cited in the "References" will be drawn from both sources. The distinction between them is terminologic rather than empiric.

NOTE ADDED IN PROOF

In the draft version of DSM-III, a new and much superior term, Attention Deficit Disorders, has been introduced to replace "hyperkinetic reaction of childhood." This category is further subdivided into Attention Deficit Disorder with Hyperactivity and Attention Deficit Disorder without Hyperactivity, on the basis of the presence or absence of motor symptoms. The virtue of the new proposal is the emphasis on the attention disorder,

which is the aspect of psychopathology most disruptive of learning, the principal task of the school-aged child. The new classification allows the clinical recognition of the child who is impaired in the ability to concentrate but is able to sit still and does not exhibit excessive gross motor movements. Some such children are in fact underactive despite the presence of a short attention span. Academic difficulties are as common in the latter group but behavior problems are less prominent because of the absence of hyperkinesis. Such children are readily overlooked and may not receive the academic and therapeutic assistance they require. Because this chapter was written before the new classification was introduced, it is focused on what now would be called Attention Deficit Disorder with Hyperactivity.

Description of the Syndrome

The most frequent clinical presentation is that of a distraught mother who complains of an "impossible" son of elementary school age who is constantly on the go, unable to sit still, fingering, touching and mouthing objects.[28] She reports distress at school about his restlessness, inattentiveness, failure to conform to classroom discipline, and poor academic record. The child may be described as destructive; careful inquiry usually establishes that he breaks things because of his impulsive and poorly controlled movements and his constant touching and fiddling with objects not intended for manipulation. In the physician's waiting room, the child may have left behind him a shambles of scattered toys and magazines and an exasperated receptionist.

Parallel to the movement disorder are short attention span and marked distractibility.[33] Such youngsters seem at the mercy of every extraneous sight or sound. Their interest flits from object to object in the environment, resting for only a very brief period on each. This leads to considerable difficulty in school. The inability to exclude irrelevant sensory impressions makes the task of learning highly problematic. Sequences requiring sustained application are often failed This occurs often enough because any one of the individual operations, as well as the ordering of the ensemble migh be beyond the child's grasp. Even when he is able to perform them, his failure to stay with the problem until its completion and his tendency to blurt out an answer without reflection will mar his efforts.

Many such children display marked lability of mood. Their frustration threshold is reduced and outbursts of angry behavior are frequent. Unprovoked frenzies of rage, in which for no apparent reason the child strikes out blindly at all about him, are often noted. When these attacks terminate, the child may be bewildered by what he has done and genuinely apologetic for it—only to undergo another uncontrollable crisis not long afterward. The mother may comment that she can tell what kind of a day it's going to be by the way her son awakens. The reasons for this variability remain unknown.

In many instances, parents report that the child was restless and irritable as an infant and "began to run" as soon as he could walk; because of his combination of boundless energy and poor judgment, parents become fatigued by the necessity for constant supervision to avoid accidents and injury. Referrals to the pediatrician or child psychiatrist in the preschool years are uncommon; when they do occur, they imply a severe degree of hyperkinesis. Some time after the child begins day care, kindergarten, or public school, parents usually begin to apply for help. The child has proven unmanageable and/or fails to learn. Referals are more common during the winter season, both because of pressure from the school, and because the child is more often under foot when inclement weather keeps him indoors after school. A degree of overactivity, which is intolerable at home or school, evokes far less notice on the playground or in the countryside. In such loci, a high activity level is both commonplace and less troublesome to others.

Secondary or Associated Hyperkinesis

The clinical syndrome of hyperkinesis may occur in association with a variety of other psychiatric and neurological disorders. For example, in epidemiologic studies of elementary school populations, the syndrome is more frequent among those with cerebral palsy, epilepsy, and other neurological syndromes than in physically healthy children.[70] It is more frequent in special schools and institutions for mentally defective children and in children with lead poisoning. It may be manifest in childhood psychosis.[69] In such instances, the prognosis is heavily influenced by the primary disorder which should be listed as the preferred diagnosis; nonetheless, clinical attention

to the hyperkinetic syndrome may be essential in developing an effective therapeutic program.

Overactivity may be a manifestation of hypoglycemia. This is one reason for the greater frequency of overactive behavior in schools serving lower-class neighborhoods where children may often come to the morning session without breakfast.[30] Motor behavior may quiet noticeably after milk and cookies have been served to the children.

The most difficult problem in differential diagnosis is presented by overactivity secondary to anxiety. The distinction is suggested when the child has multiple fears and worries, difficulty sleeping, complaints of frequent nightmares, and a morbid preoccupation with impending catastrophe. The anxiety may be provoked by an acute situation at school or at home; careful inquiry is essential to elicit the situational factors. The recognition of acute and chronic family pathology will suggest the diagnosis; obviously, a hyperkinetic child may also come from a disturbed family; sensible clinical judgment is required to assess the degree to which the symptoms are secondary to family stress rather than independent of, or even responsible for, the family disequilibrium. Indeed, despite our inability to modify the family situation substantially, symptom remission may follow drug or other treatment directed at the hyperkinetic syndrome. This can occur even when these symptoms are secondary.

The History of the Syndrome

The behavior complex was first described among the sequelae to post-encephalitic and posttraumatic central nervous system injury.[8, 9] The clinical syndrome was labeled "organic drivenness" by Kahn and Cohen.[44] It was further elucidated by the work of Strauss and Werner[88] and Strauss and Lehtinen.[87] In these initial contexts, the behavior syndrome was related to overt or presumptive damage to the brain. When Bradley first employed amphetamines in the treatment of childhood behavior disorders,[10] he was astute enough to notice that among the patient population, a subgroup with hyperkinesis and distractibility responded in a "paradoxical" manner by becoming quieter, more attentive, and better able to learn. Bradley's work, in children without manifest central nervous system damage, led to the recognition of a clinical syndrome that responded to pharmacologic treatment.[10] The subsequent work of Laufer, Denhoff, and Solomons,[50] demonstrating a low threshold to photometrazol EEG activation in these children and its "normalization" by amphetamines, was a major step in establishing the existence of a physiologic component in a childhood behavior disorder at a time when the emphasis on psychogenic factors in child psychiatry preempted clinical interest.

Prevalence

Epidemiologists distinguish between incidence (the number of new cases of a disorder appearing in a defined population during a given period of time) and prevalence(the number of cases of a disorder detectable in a population survey at a point in time). With a relatively chronic disorder like the hyperkinetic syndrome, prevalence is necessarily very much greater than incidence. We have no data on incidence; such data would be extremely difficult to obtain because the specification of time of onset of a case is problematic. Available prevalence data show great variability. Stewart and associates,[86] in a study of elementary school children in St. Louis, obtained a prevalence of approximately 4 percent. Huessy and associates,[41] in an informal study in Vermont, arrived at a figure of 10 percent. In the most recent study, Gorin and Kramer[36] in Connecticut estimated prevalence from teacher responses to questionnaires on second grade students. Forms were returned for approximately 14,000 children (only 27 percent of the total enrolled, because the larger school systems in the state chose not to participate in the study). Of the children evaluated by their teachers, 4.95 percent were identified as displaying the hyperkinetic behavior syndrome. The male-female ratio was approximately 6 to 1 (in accord with other estimates that have varied from 4 to 1 to 10 to 1). In teacher reports, Spanish-surnamed and black children were almost twice as likely to be described as hyperkinetic than whites. There was also an excess of urban as compared with rural children. If teacher identification is accepted as valid, it is noteworthy that only one-quarter of the 685 hyperkinetic children had been "previously diagnosed" and less than one-sixth were in care for their disorder.

Clinicians are widely agreed that hyperkinesis tends to diminish with age; prevalence data for the later years of elementary and junior high school would be expected to show much lower figures. This may be, in part, the explanation for the very low rate reported by Rutter and his associates in eleven-year olds on the Isle of Wight,[70] although it is also likely that the criteria for the diagnosis were more rigorous than in the other studies described. Follow-up reports, to be detailed later in this chapter, confirm the clinical impression that hyperkinesis diminishes with age, but they also reveal that many of the children continue to show marked academic, conduct, and self-image problems; the symptom pattern changes, but the disorder does not remit.

The hyperkinetic behavior syndrome appears to occur far more frequently among American school children than in other populations. Our English colleagues express surprise at our experience with referrals for this disorder. Yet, the syndrome itself is recognized in almost all countries, as is revealed by the agreement among child psychiatrists from many countries at the WHO Seminar on the necessity for this clinical category.[71] It has been suggested that the relatively greater freedom for self-expression and the lower expectations for self-control by parents and teachers in the United States may be factors in the difference in activity levels from other cultures. American visitors to the People's Republic of China, for example, comment on the remarkable orderliness of children's behavior in nursery schools as well as in elementary schools.[16] Whether dietary, toxic, genetic, or other factors that differ among countries may play a role, remains purely speculative.

Clinical and Diagnostic Considerations

NEUROPSYCHIATRIC EXAMINATION

In the office or playroom, the child may manifest the characteristic overactivity and distractibility. Offered a set of play materials, he may move from one to another without sustained attention to any.[67] He is likely to fidget in the chair, to finger and touch things, and to be difficult to engage in continuous conversation on a single topic. His concerns are likely to be projections of his own difficulties; he may claim that the teacher picks on him, that other children fight with him, and that his parents constantly blame him, all the time protesting his own innocence against all charges. Rarely does he recognize that his own behavior provokes the responses that trouble him. Occasionally children will acknowledge "bad" behavior and may even tear-up as they describe their own inability to stop doing the things that lead them to be ostracized. Poor self-esteem characterizes the older children. However, in a significant number of these children, the observed behavior will be unremarkable despite steady complaints from home and school. Symptomatic behavior is more manifest in group than in individual situations and is particularly evident when demands are placed upon the child; this contrasts with the one-to-one interview situation with a sympathetic adult who does not have to press the child to perform. Failure to exhibit symptoms during the psychiatric interview does not exclude the diagnosis, though it does point to the importance of reexamining home and school circumstances to determine whether the environment is unduly stressful.

Many hyperkinetic children exhibit minor or "soft" neurological signs.[96] Although choreiform movements are common in children with behavior and learning problems, they do not discriminate those with hyperkinesis, contrary to earlier reports.[100] Waldrop and associates[90] have reported a significant association between overactivity and a constellation of minor development anomalies, pointing to dysembryogenesis in intrauterine development. On a systematic examination, such as the Lincoln-Oretsky Motor Performance Test, these children perform poorly as a group but the great variability in performance limits the utility of test findings in the individual case. Neurologic and behavioral assessment of hyperkinetic children reinforces the concept of what may be variously termed "maturation lag" or "cerebral dysfunction."[89]

Clinical diagnosis rests upon the ensemble of findings rather than on any single abnormality. Perhaps the most appropriate analogy is to the role of the white count in the diagnosis of appendicitis. If the count corresponds with the clinician's judgment, it is used as further vertification of the diagnosis. But if the rest of the clinical picture does not suggest appendicitis, the experienced clinician will simply ignore the discrepant finding.

PSYCHOMETRIC FINDINGS

Hyperkinesis can occur in children at almost any test level of intelligence. Most clinical reports have, by definition, excluded children with IQs lower than 80. Nonetheless, patients in the normal range of intelligence exhibit wide subtest scatter on the WISC, do poorly on tests which purport to measure perceptual-motor function and

attain scholastic achievement scores below expectation for age and grade.[25] However, none of these findings is pathognomonic, and some children perform at superior levels.

Conners[20] has demonstrated a significant improvement in Porteus Maze "IQ" following stimulant drug treatment. Palkes and associates[61] were able to obtain similar gains on the Porteus by training the child in self-directed verbal commands designed to inhibit impulsive responses. A well-designed study by Campbell and associates[14] demonstrated that hyperactive children were "more impulsive, more field dependent, more constricted in ability to control attention, and slower on measures of automatization than the control group." Methylphenidate diminished impulsiveness and improved ability to inhibit incorrect responses. In a subsequent study of these children as adolescents, Cohen and associates[18] reported that the former patients "took less time to reflect over a problem solution when a number of alternative solutions were possible and had greater difficulty isolating a simple figure hidden in a complex background." Whatever the role played by problems in perceptual motor performance, major contributions to the academic difficulties exhibited by these children stem from distractibility and impulsivity. The utility of careful psychometric evaluation lies in the specification of the functional impairments in a particular child as an initial step to planning an effective remediation program.

ELECTROENCEPHALOGRAPHIC STUDIES

From the time of Jasper's 1938 report of EEG studies in behavior problem children,[43] electroencephalographers have reported higher than expected percentages of *nonspecific* abnormalities in various categories of child psychiatric patients. Identical "abnormalities" may be seen in normal children, though somewhat less frequently; there is poor correlation between symptom pattern and EEG characteristics; rarely have the EEG studies on the patient and control groups been done with the rater blind to the source of the record. The voluminous literature on the hyperkinetic syndrome is replete with similar findings, but there is little evidence that the EEG study contributes significantly either to diagnosis or management of the individual patient. A recent report by Kenny and associates[45] exemplifies the problem. Of seventy-eight children "referred for hyperactivity," thirty-eight had normal EEGs, twenty-five "abnormal," and fifteen had "fourteen and/or six per second positive spike complexes." However, the distribution of EEG findings bore no relationship to concurrent neurological examination or to the final diagnosis. Kenny and associates conclude: "The decision to prescribe psychotrophic medication for hyperactivity should, therefore, be made on behavioral rather than on neurologic or electroencephalographic evidence."

On the other hand, special studies employing sophisticated EEG techniques have been instructive in establishing central nervous system dysfunctions in groups of hyperkinetic children. Laufer, Denhoff, and Solomons,[50] utilizing Gastaut's method for photometrazol activation of the EEG, demonstrated a significantly lower activation threshold in hyperkinetic as compared to nonhyperkinetic disturbed children. Furthermore, they found that the threshold for activation was raised into the normal range by the administration of amphetamines. In a recent extension of this work, Shetty[77] reported that intravenous injection of stimulant drugs decreased photic driving responses and photomyoclonic responses in hyperkinetic children. Analyzing EEG power alpha range (8–12 Hz), Shetty[76] noted that enhancement of alpha by intravenous stimulants predicted successful response to oral treatment with these drugs. Shetty concluded:

The basic neurologic defect in hyperkinesis of childhood seems to be a disorder of inhibitory mechanisms in the central nervous system such that irrelevant stimuli are not filtered out and the child is at the mercy of all the stimuli in his environment. Central nervous stimulant drugs seem to be able to activate or strengthen these inhibitory mechanisms.

Investigators at the University of Freiburg,[39] employing EEG measures in neurologically normal hyperactive children, reported a lower state of EEG arousal, slower development of amplitude reduction to tone, and shorter arousal responses to light stimulus, together with longer latencies of reaction time. Small and associates[81] studied sleep patterns in hyperactive children on and off medication. Baseline sleep patterns did not differ from that of age-matched controls. Stimulants prolonged sleep latency and delayed the onset of the first REM period but did not affect total sleep time or the constituent EEG stages. There was no evidence of REM "rebound" after cessation of medication. These findings differ sharply from those reported for adults. Buchsbaum and Wender[13] studied visual and auditory average evoked responses (AERs) in twenty-four children with "minimal brain dysfunction" and age and sex matched controls. The patients exhibited AERs like those of relatively normal younger

children. More immature responses were characteristic of the patient subgroup who profited from amphetamine treatment. Buchsbaum and Wender conclude that their findings are compatible with the existence of "maturational lag" in such patients.

Thus, while EEG studies contribute little to diagnosis or management in the individual case (unless there is reason to suspect epilepsy), special methods of study indicate that there are physiologic differences between hyperkinetic disturbed children, nonhyperkinetic disturbed children and normal controls.

Natural History of the Syndrome

The clinical observation that hyperkinesis diminishes with age led initially to optimism about prognosis; the therapeutic task was envisaged as supporting the patient and his family through the difficult elementary school years with the expectation that deviance would no longer be a problem by the time of adolescence. This belief was challenged by the report of Menkes and associates[54] on fourteen patients twenty-five years after clinical evaluation at Johns Hopkins; four were in mental hospitals diagnosed as psychotic, two were retarded, and, of the eight who were self-supporting, three had had periods of institutionalization for antisocial behavior. Weiss and her colleagues[92] followed sixty-four youngsters at a mean age of thirteen five years after initial diagnosis. Although overactivity had indeed diminished, the patients were still more active than matched controls. Distractibility remained a major source of difficulty. Poor academic adjustment characterized 80 percent of the sample, 70 percent were rated as having significant psychopathology and 25 percent had a history of antisocial behavior (with court action in 15 percent of the cases). Mendelson and associates[53] studied eighty-three hyperkinetic children as adolescents two to five years later. Although about half of the group were reported to be improved, Mendelson commented: "The symptoms of restlessness, distractibility, impulsiveness, excitability and aggressiveness seemed to persist in most of the children and were associated with poor performance in school and low self-esteem." Huessy and associates,[42] in an eight- to ten-year follow-up study of eighty-four children, found eighteen institutionalized in either mental hospitals or correctional facilities. These follow-up studies make it clear that the hyperkinetic syndrome carries with it the potential for serious consequences in personality development and thus make imperative careful and continuous medical supervision.

In addition to these longitudinal studies, a number of reports have appeared describing psychiatric problems in adults whose history warrants a retrospective diagnosis of hyperkinetic reaction. Quitkin and Klein[63] described nineteen young adults with destructive-impulsive behavior, low frustration tolerance, apparently endogenous mood swings, overreactive emotionality, and temper tantrums. Twelve of these patients had a history of childhood overactivity. Shelley and Riester[78] reported sixteen patients referred because of difficulty in meeting the requirements for military training at an Air Force base. They had difficulty in spatial orientation and in learning new motor tasks and symptoms of irritability, anxiety, self-depreciation, and emotional lability. Twelve of the sixteen subjects had a childhood history compatible with hyperkinetic behavior syndrome. More recently, Morrison and Minkoff,[55] on the basis of three case reports, propose the thesis that explosive personality, included in DSM-II, is a sequel to the hyperkinetic syndrome in childhood. All three patients showed marked improvement on tricyclic antidepressant medication. There are other similar reports of adults with sequelae of the hyperkinetic syndrome.[40] Although these follow-up and adult studies focus primarily on personality disorders, Robins[68] has documented adult schizophrenia as one outcome of aggressive and antisocial behavior in childhood, an all too common accompaniment of the hyperkinetic syndrome. Present data are too fragmentary to permit quantitative estimates of the frequency with which psychopathology may be anticipated in the adult years of ineffectively treated hyperkinetic children.

The Search for Causes

GENETIC

It is a common clinical experience to obtain a history that the father of a hyperkinetic son had the same symptoms himself in childhood. Indeed, this not infrequently results in delay in bringing the child for care, because the behavior may be interpreted as "all boy," "running in the family,"

and in any event a pattern that will be outgrown. In a case-control study, Morrison and Stewart[57] reported that 20 percent of hyperactive children had a parent who had been hyperactive in contrast to 5 percent of control children. Safer[72] studied the records of siblings and half-siblings of seventeen children with "minimal brain dysfunction" who were in foster care. There was a significantly higher occurrence of the signs and symptoms in full sibs than in half-sibs, a result compatible with a hereditary diathesis. For example, seven out of nine sibs were found to be hyperactive as compared to two of fourteen half-sibs; short attention span was found in nine of nineteen sibling combinations and three of twenty-two half-siblings. Willerman[97] studied activity level in twins of the same sex. Intraclass correlations for activity level were considerably higher for monozygotic than dizygotic twins. Among those twin sets where at least one member scored in the hyperactive range (that is, the upper 20 percent of the sample), MZ twins showed a high correlation for activity level whereas DZ twins showed no correlation. Willerman concluded that the heritability component was .71.

Morrison and Stewart, in the study previously cited, found a significantly higher prevalence of sociopathy, hysteria, and alcoholism in the mothers and fathers of the hyperactive children. Similar results were obtained by Cantwell[15] in a case-control comparison in a population of military dependents. In contrast, when Morrison and Stewart[56] interviewed the legal parents of thirty-five adopted hyperactive children, there was no such prevalence of psychiatric disorder nor of a childhood history of hyperactivity. Finally, Stewart and Morrison contrasted the families of biological and adoptive relatives of hyperactive children and of a matched group of controls.[85] They searched in particular for a history of affective disorder in view of the crude similarities between hyperkinesis in children and mania in adults. They found no significant differences between the three populations, a finding which takes on particular importance because of the hypothesis that hyperkinesis may be a "depressive equivalent" in children in view of its responsiveness to stimulant and antidepressive medication.

Since chromosome anomalies are sometimes associated with abnormal behavior, Warren and associates[91] reported karyotype analysis on lymphocytes from peripheral blood on twenty-three patients. No evidence of X chromosome aneuploidy or other chromosome anomalty was found.

In sum, there is strong evidence for a hereditary

component in the pathogenesis of the hyperkinetic reaction, although the mode and mechanism of transmission is obscure.

THE ROLE OF BIOGENIC AMINES IN HYPERKINESIS

Wender has formulated the hypothesis that hyperkinetic children (for whom he prefers the designation minimal brain dysfunction) suffer from an abnormality in the metabolism of one or more of the monoamaines: serotonin, norepinephrine, or dopamine. The biochemical abnormality in turn leads to functional derangement in two brain systems: the reward mechanism and the activating system. These derangements, he believes, account for the decreased experience of pleasure and pain (anhedonia), a generally high and poorly modulated level of activation, and extroversion, three features which he proposes as the "primary" psychological defects in this reaction pattern.[93]

The therapeutic effectiveness of stimulant drugs provides indirect support for this hypothesis, since stimulants affect reuptake of transmitters at central synapses. Direct test of the hypothesis is difficult; blood levels of the transmitters, their metabolites, and the enzymes that control their concentration may not reflect levels of these substances at the central nuclei where they act; measurements of urine output are even more remote; both blood and urine levels are influenced by outputs from the peripheral nervous system.

Employing the blood platelet as a "model" for the serotonergic neurone, Coleman[19] reported low concentrations of platelet serotonin in 88 percent of twenty-five children with symptoms of hyperactivity. With her coworkers,[6] she subsequently determined the levels of serotonin and pyridoxal phosphate (PLP) in eleven hyperactive children and eleven controls. The patients had lower serotonin values but normal PLP. Nonetheless, when four of the patients with normal PLP values were placed on oral doses of vitamin B_6 (pyridoxine hyrochloride), there was "an appreciable increase in the serotonin content" in the blood. The authors are in the process of studying whether B_6 administration can be shown to influence clinical status in hyperkinetic children.

Rapoport and Quinn[64] have studied, in hyperkinetic children, plasma dopamine-beta-hydroxylase (DBH), the terminal enzyme in the biosynthesis of norepinephrine. In a subgroup of patients with an increased incidence of minor physical anomalies,[90] approximately one-third of the eighty-one patients in the study, plasma DBH correlated significantly with a weighted score based on the number of anomalies present. This finding takes on additional interest in view of the observation that stimulant drugs increase plasma DBH activity,[65] though in no relationship to clinical change.

These findings add support for the hypothesis of a biochemical basis for the hyperkinetic reaction. However, they are not yet at a stage which permits clinical utility in patient management nor has the theory been fully established.

SUBCLINICAL LEAD POISONING: AN ANIMAL MODEL OF HYPERKINESIS

Silbergeld and Goldberg[79] have produced a hyperkinetic syndrome in mice which simulates the clinical condition, particularly its responsiveness to stimulant drugs. Sublethal lead exposure was produced by substituting solutions of lead acetate for the drinking water of mice twelve hours after parturition. In addition to retarded growth and development, the lead-treated offspring exhibited three times the activity level of control mice. D- and l-amphetamines and methylphenidate increased activity in *control* mice; phenobarbital depressed it. Yet both isomers of amphetamine as well as methylphenidate *decreased* activity in the lead-treated animals and phenobarbital paradoxically increased their already high levels of activity, very much as the clinical treatment of hyperkinetic children.[31] D-amphetamine was about four times more effective in suppressing activity in the experimental animals than l-amphetamine, a finding divergent from their relatively similar effectiveness in patients.[3]

In addition to the intrinsic interest of this animal model as a basis for studying pharmacodynamics, its relevance is enhanced by the report of David and associates[23] that, when compared to a control group, hyperactive children had somewhat higher blood lead levels and higher postpenicillamine urine lead levels. However, Lansdown and coworkers at the Hospital for Sick Children in London, studying a population of children living in a working-class area exposed to undue amounts of lead, were unable to discover a relationship between blood lead levels, general intelligence, reading ability, or rate of behavior disorder.[48] Nonetheless, in the clinical evaluation of patients, it would be prudent to make careful inquiry into the history of exposure to environmental lead and to undertake an appropriate evaluation for lead intoxication if there is clinical evidence to suggest this possibility. The larger question of lead as an environmental toxin which is harmful at levels lower than those conventionally regarded as encephalopathic remains open; Needleman[58] has reviewed the evidence and argues persuasively for this thesis.

PSYCHOSOCIAL FACTORS

Lower-class children are at increased risk for the hyperkinetic reaction; such factors as complications of pregnancy and parturition,[46] malnutrition,[7] and exposure to environmental toxins[58] are associated with poor socioeconomic conditions and greater likelihood of CNS damage.[94] Further, disrupted and disorganized homes are less likely to provide the stimuli that promote the maturation of attention span: regular and organized meal times, sedentary games, being read to, exposure to the rules of play under adult supervision, and the like. Thus, activity levels in classrooms serving slum neighborhoods are considerably higher than those in suburban schools. This does not necessarily lead to higher referral rates; it is the child who stands out against the "norm" of his reference group who is noticed by the teacher; moreover, clinical services are far more readily available in affluent neighborhoods; the hyperkinetic child in the ghetto is more often regarded as a disciplinary than as a psychiatric problem.

Idiosyncratic family factors may play an important role in determining patienthood. Once designated by his parents as a trouble-maker, the youngster may respond as much to what is expected of him (i.e., to be difficult) as to any internal drive state. Parents may displace onto a child chosen for the role of scapegoat the tensions between them. In such situations, parents may report no benefit (or even worsening) after treatment at the same time that the teacher notes considerable gains. Such discrepancies should alert the clinician to the urgency of conjoint family therapy if progress is to be made.

Although the evidence summarized in this chapter points to physiological defects as primary in the genesis of hyperkinesis, the secondary problems, which appear in the older child: poor self-esteem, antisocial behavior, and personality disorders, are almost certainly psychogenic in origin. The experience of being blamed, the labeling as deviant, the ostracism at school and in the neighborhood, and the repeated encounters with failure result in alienation and development attrition.[27] The child comes to view himself as inadequate or evil—and sometimes as both. In his search for acceptance and affection, he turns to other rejected children at the fringes of the social group. His academic difficulties lead to giving up on school and seeking alternative ways of being noticed and admired. It is this spiraling course leading to social deviance that constitutes the most serious consequences of the hyperkinetic syndrome.

ALLERGY AS A CAUSAL ELEMENT

Feingold[34] has reported a series of clinical observations on hyperkinetic children whose symptoms responded to a diet designed to eliminate artificial food colors and flavorings, which he incriminates as an important cause of this syndrome. Currently, several controlled studies are under way to evaluate the efficacy of this treatment and the hypothesis on which it is based.

MULTIPLE CAUSALITY

There is little reason to suppose that a clinical-descriptive syndrome such as the hyperkinetic reaction, which is so variable in its manifestations, is a single entity. Some cases may result from hereditary, some from intrauterine, others from perinatal, and still others from post-natal causes —and some from the conjunction of several factors. Indeed, present evidence makes this the most likely supposition.

Treatment

FAMILY COUNSELING

A thorough diagnostic evaluation is the first and crucial step in the treatment process. By the time the parents apply for help, they are likely to be overwhelmed by the problem, confused at the multiplicity of explanations they have been offered, and guilty at their own inability to manage the child's behavior. Sensitive and sympathetic listening to their travails, willingess to order a complete and careful neuropsychiatric and psychometric evaluation, and time spent in pulling together the findings into a coherent and understandable presentation set the stage for effective treatment. The formulation that the child suffers from a physiological disorder (whether this is presented as "constitutional," "maturation lag," "developmental delay" or "minimal cerebral dysfunction") helps to shift the focus from parental inadequacy (and hence guilt) to a medical condition that requires special methods of assistance. The point is to be stressed that parental management *does* matter, and matter greatly, but that the very approaches which might be adequate for an average child do not suffice for the patient.[31]

Parents are well-advised to avoid situations that predictably provoke difficult behavior; that is, those associated with large groups and high levels of stimulation: supermarkets, department stores, parties, and the like. Discipline needs to be prompt, unambiguous, and immediately related to the behavior it is intended to discourage. When early signs of an impending tantrum are detected, immediate steps to remove the child from the situation and offer him alternative distractions can abort the episode. Once an explosion has occurred, there is nothing to be done but to wait it out, making sure that the child does not harm himself, and that he does not gain his aim as a bribe to end the episode. The nuisance value of the symptoms put the parents at risk of paying attention to the child primarily when he is misbehaving and thus inadvertently reinforcing him in this behavior. Instruction in the principles of operant conditioning[5] may be particularly useful to parents; this approach lends itself to group counseling.[84]

Whether the parents need counseling directed at their own problems as a couple, in addition to guidance on child rearing, will obviously depend on the extent and severity of intrafamilial pathology. Hyperkinetic children, precisely because of their poor response to ordinary parenting practices, are likely to be swept into the center of family discord, with each parent blaming the other for failure to manage the child properly. It is imperative that such issues be identified and brought into the open in order that they be resolved. Whether the primary focus of the sessions with the parents is educational or psychotherapeutic, sustained and continuous treatment is required in view of the potential for long run academic and psychiatric difficulties. Parents should be told at the outset of treatment that, although symptomatic improvement can be expected confidently, continuing care will be necessary in order to promote healthy development. Too frequently, parents and clinicians alike settle for only occasional oversight after the most troublesome symptoms remit.

REMEDIAL EDUCATION

Most hyperkinetic children exhibit academic problems by the time of first referral, problems likely to be the more severe the older the child when seen. Psychiatric treatment, when successful, can do no more than enhance the patient's readiness to respond to learning. Scholastic achievement will depend on the teacher's ability to capitalize on that opportunity. Close working relations between the clinician and the teacher are essential. Indeed, the teacher is a major and valuable source of information by which the child's response to treatment can be gauged. Conners[21] has developed a symptom check list for classroom use that provides a semiquantitative measure of problem status. In addition, regular reports on academic progress are an essential part of clinical management. It is beyond the scope of this chapter to discuss techniques of remedial education.

DRUG THERAPY

Since the initial clinical paper by Bradley, it has been abundantly demonstrated that stimulant drugs bring about symptomatic improvement.[30] The initial optimism that they would suffice has been considerably dampened by the follow-up studies already described. What is to be condemned is the all-too-common medical practice of prescribing drugs with little or no attention to parent guidance, remedial education, and continuous clinical surveillance.[82] It cannot be too frequently emphasized that drugs are a useful adjunct to care but only the beginning to treatment rather than a total plan of care.

Amphetamines: Bradley initially employed racemic amphetamines (Benzedrine) but as the pure d-isomer became available, it became the preferred agent. It induces a pharmacologic response within thirty minutes and remains active for four to six hours. The usual clinical practice is to begin with a dose of five mg. given at breakfast and to increase at several day intervals by five milligram increments to a maximum of twenty mg. in a single dose until clinical benefit appears.[28] If the patient should become more active or irritable (as may occur in 5 percent to 10 percent of patients), the drug should be discontinued. If the patient shows a good response to the morning dose but reverts to hyperkinetic behavior during the afternoon school session, a second dose (starting with the smallest amount) should be added at lunch time, to a total *daily* maximum of forty mgm. The second dose should not be given later than noon to minimize the probability of troublesome anorexia.

It is good practice to discontinue the drug during vacation periods—and perhaps as well over weekends unless home problems are severe. Since the drug suppresses symptoms, whose time course is difficult to predict, it is difficult to know when drug treatment is no longer essential. Many clinicians interrupt treatment periodically to determine when the child is able to manage without them. Since drug concentrations are not cumulative, it is safe to stop them totally (unlike anticonvulsants); if they are still needed, hyperkinesis will manifest itself promptly. The most effective way to make this determination is to employ identical-appearing placebos so that neither parent, child, nor teacher is aware of the change; in this way, effects due to placebo-dependence are minimized.[80]

Recently, trials with l-amphetamine have been reported.[3] Results were generally similar to those with the d-isomer, but there are children who appear to benefit preferentially from this agent.

Methylphenidate: The indications for and the modes of prescribing methylphenidate are similar to those for the amphetamines, except that ten milligrams of methylphenidate is used in place of five milligrams of amphetamines.[28] Results are very much the same. For reasons that are unclear, some children who fail to respond to one will do well with the second. Which is used initially will depend on the clinician's preferences and familiarities, as well as considerations of relative pricing and availability. Because of public apprehension about the dangers of "speed," some parents will object to d-amphetamine but be willing to accept methylphenidate, despite the pharmacologic similarity between the drugs.

Magnesium Pemoline: A recent multiclinic trial of magnesium pemoline[60] demonstrated roughly similar effectiveness to the other stimulant drugs. Dosage ranged from 2 to 4.5 mgm/kg/day, prescribed in individual doses of 18.75 mgm (to a maximum of 112.5 mgm/day). It is given in a single morning dose, thus avoiding the need for lunchtime administration, a problem if no school nurse is available or the child does not come home at noon. Its disadvantage is its longer mode of onset of action (no effect may be evident for two to three weeks). No serious side effects were noted in treatment up to seventy-seven weeks in duration.

Its recency of introduction, and thus the limited experience with its use, suggest a need for caution in employing it until further evidence is accumulated. For the moment, it remains an agent to be kept in reserve for the patient who does not do well on amphetamine or methylphenidate.[22]

Imipramine: The tricyclic antidepressant, imipramine, has been shown to be an effective drug for suppressing hyperkinesis.[66] The dose employed varied from 50 to 150 mgm, and the results were comparable to, though somewhat less impressive than, those obtained with methylphenidate. Again, caution is indicated because of uncertainties about toxicity, discussed later in this section.

Other Drugs: Caffeine[35] and lithium carbonate[37] have been found to be ineffective. Chlorpromazine and other phenothiazines do decrease hyperkinesis but frequently at the expense of excessive sedation. The so-called minor tranquillizers (chlordiazepoxide and diazepam), anticonvulsants (diphenylhydantoin) and diphenhydramine are sometimes useful, but much less reliable and dramatic than the stimulants and anti-depressants. Barbiturates are contraindicated; they are likely to produce paradoxical excitation.[31]

Drug Toxicity: Complaints of anorexia and insomnia are common at the outset of stimulant drug therapy but usually remit within a few weeks or if dosage is diminished. Less common are complaints of abdominal discomfort, dizziness, headache, and drowsiness. Occasional children exhibit episodes of unprovoked crying and depressed feelings. It is rare that treatment has to be discontinued because of these side effects; they tend to be self-limited. Ney[59] has reported one case of psychosis associated with amphetamines, and Lucas and Weiss,[51] three cases with methylphenidate. In each instance, symptoms remitted when the drug was stopped. The paucity of case reports, in contrast to the large number of children treated, attests to the rarity of psychosis as a complication of therapy.

More serious questions have been raised about growth suppression. Safer and Allen[73] have reported slower growth rates among treated children when compared with hyperkinetic cases not receiving drugs. Further, growth rebound was noted upon cessation of drug treatment.[74] Similar short-term effects have been noticed with the use of magnesium pemoline[60] during the first few months of treatment; by three to six months, the patient group did not differ significantly from population growth norms. Beck and his colleagues[4] reexamined thirty adolescents (mean age seventeen) who had had at least six months of drug treatment but were not in treatment at the time of the study. They were compared with a control group of thirty patients selected from medical and surgical wards. There were no differences in height between the two groups and no evidence of permanent stunting of stature. Safer's findings establish the importance of monitoring height and weight in children under drug treatment. However, placed in perspective, the available studies indicate that stimulants can be used safely if careful clinical control is maintained. Unfortunately, too many physicians prescribe with little more than telephone follow up.[82]

Side effects from imipramine are common and include: dry mouth, difficulty falling asleep, anorexia, drowsiness, and headaches; most are mild. Cardiotoxic effects from the use of large doses of imipramine have been reported by several authors,[12, 99] including one case fatality.[75] On the other hand, electrocardiographic monitoring of a group of enuretic children receiving doses in the 25–75 milligram range revealed no significant ECG changes.[52] These studies caution against high dosage treatment but indicate that low and moderate dosage can be safely tolerated.

Public and professional concern has been expressed that sustained drug treatment may encourage the development of a drug-taking habit.[38] This belief persists despite the lack of clinical or epidemiologic evidence to support it. Laufer's parent survey[49] and Beck's follow up[4] both failed to identify any increase in drug use among late adolescents and young adults who had been treated with stimulant drugs during childhood. Neither of these studies settles the question unequivocally, but such evidence we have is against the supposition that addiction is promoted. It is nonetheless clear that a final answer would require additional long-term studies.

There would appear to be a distinct difference in the social implications to the child between being under medically prescribed treatment for an identified disorder, on the one hand, and peer socialization into drug use in search of peak experiences, on the other. There is no evidence that children with other chronic disorders treated by medication (epilepsy, diabetes) are more vulnerable to street drug addiction by virtue of their medical introduction to sustained drug use. Furthermore, very few children under treatment report subjective euphoria, the main self-reinforcement for drug use among addicted adolescents.[29]

Despite the journalistic furor which alleges a degree of overprescription of stimulant drugs for children, approaching epidemic levels, the data available indicate rates of use that are well below estimates of prevalence for hyperkinesis. Sprague and Sleator,[83] from a survey of prescribing practices of Chicago physicians, estimated that about 2 percent of elementary school children were receiving stimulant drugs in the 1970–1971 period. Krager and Safer[47] obtained reports from school nurses serving public and parochial schools in Baltimore County. The percentage of elementary

school children receiving medication for hyperkinesis was 1.73 percent in the public schools and 0.62 percent in the parochial schools in 1973. More than four-fifths were receiving stimulant drugs (methylphenidate two times more often than dextroamphetamine). It is of interest that children in the more affluent areas of the county, in both public and parochial schools, were more likely to receive medication than their less advantaged peers.

BEHAVIOR THERAPY

The methods of operant conditioning, applied consistently in the classroom, can diminish the manifestations of hyperkinesis and distractability.[1, 24, 26, 62] There is some evidence that stimulant drugs can potentiate behavior therapy.[17] Behavior modification methods can be taught to parents and employed at home.[84] They are clearly effective in symptom suppression; they obviate problems of drug toxicity. But competent personnel are not available in many communities and whether it is simply control that is attained or whether academic achievement is facilitated has been questioned.[98]

PSYCHOTHERAPY

Comparative studies have demonstrated the superiority of stimulant drug treatment over brief psychotherapy plus placebo administration in attaining symptom relief.[29] When drug benefit is dramatic both the patient and his parents may experience a rapid transformation from self-defeating to self-enhancing modes of interrelating. For many families, however, particularly those with older children, individual and/or family psychotherapy will be essential if there is to be any hope of reversing overlearned pathological attitudes and relationships. Drug (or behavioral) treatment remains essential to remove the disruptive consequences of the hyperkinetic symptoms, but only sustained psychotherapeutic intervention will enable family members to establish constructive interactions and help the patient to overcome low self-esteem and pathological personality trends.

THE NEED FOR COMPREHENSIVE AND CONTINUOUS CARE

The poor outcome in adolescence and early childhood described earlier in this chapter, in contrast to the many reports of symptomatic benefit from drug and behavior therapy over the short run, emphasizes the importance of psychiatric care that is comprehensive (an appropriate mix of family counseling, remedial education, medication, behavior modification, and psychotherapy) as well as continuous (responsible surveillance of the patient's progress from the time of consultation through adolescence or until a normal developmental pattern has been established). Unfortunately, customary experimental paradigms and the urge for prompt publication have resulted in therapeutic trials averaging three months in length and only occasionally extending for as long as a year. There are as yet no reports of the outcome of systematic treatment monitored continuously by a single clinical group throughout the years of risk. That the investment is warranted is indicated by the natural course of the hyperkinetic reaction; that continuous care is likely to be useful is suggested by the immediate benefit yielded by appropriate interventions. In the light of current evidence, it is clear that the hyperkinetic reaction must be reconceptualized as a *chronic* disorder, analogous to epilepsy, requiring long-term medical care if the patient is to attain his full developmental potential.

REFERENCES

1. ALLEN, K. E., et al., "Control of Hyperactivity by Reinforcement of Attending Behavior," *Journal of Educational Psychology, 58*:231–237, 1967.
2. American Psychiatric Association, Committee on Nomenclature and Statistics, *Diagnostic and Statistical Manual of Mental Disorders*, 2nd ed. (DSM-II), American Psychiatric Association, Washington, D.C., 1968.
3. ARNOLD, L. E., et al., "Levoamphetamine and Dextroamphetamine: Comparative Efficacy in the Hyperkinetic Syndrome," *Archives of General Psychiatry, 27:* 816–822, 1972.
4. BECK, L., et al., "Childhood Chemotherapy and Later Drug Abuse and Growth Curve: A Follow-up Study of 30 Adolescents," *American Journal of Psychiatry, 132*:436–438, 1975.
5. BERKOWITZ, B. T., and GRAZIANO, A. M., "Training Parents as Behavior Therapists: A Review," *Behavior Research and Therapy, 10*:297–317, 1972.
6. BHAGAVAN, H. N., COLEMAN, M., and COURSIN, D. B., "The Effect of Pyridoxane Hydrochloride on Blood Serotonin and Pyridoxal Phosphate Contents in Hyperactive Children," *Pediatrics, 55*:437–441, 1975.
7. BIRCH, H. G., and GUSSOW, J. D., *Disadvantaged Children*, Grune & Stratton, New York, 1970.
8. BLAU, A., "Mental Changes Following Head Trauma in Child," *Archives of Neurology and Psychiatry, 35:* 723–769, 1936.
9. BOND, E. D., and SMITH, L. H., "Post-Encephalitic Behavior Disorders: A Ten-Year Review of the Franklin School," *American Journal of Psychiatry, 92*:17–31, 1935.
10. BRADLEY, C., "Benzedrine and Dexedrine in the Treatment of Children's Behavior Disorders," *Pediatrics, 5*:24–36, 1950.
11. ———, "The Behavior of Children Receiving Benzedrine," *American Journal of Psychiatry, 94*:577–585, 1937.
12. BROWN, D., et al., "Imipramine Therapy and Seizures: Three Children Treated for Hyperactive Behavior Disorders," *American Journal of Psychiatry, 130:* 210–212, 1973.
13. BUCHSBAUM, M., and WENDER, P., "Average Evoked Responses in Normal and Minimally Brain-Dysfunctioned Children Treated with Amphetamine," *Archives of General Psychiatry, 29*:764–770, 1973.
14. CAMPBELL, S. B., DOUGLAS, V. I., and MORGANSTERN, G., "Cognitive Styles in Hyperactive Children and the Effect of Methylphenidate," *Journal of Child Psychology and Psychiatry, 12*:55–67, 1971.
15. CANTWELL, D. P., "Psychiatric Illness in the Families of Hyperactive Children," *Archives of General Psychiatry, 27*:414–417, 1972.

16. CHAN, I., "New People in New China: As Reflected Through Education and Child Rearing," Presented at the Biennial Meeting of the Society for Research in Child Development, Denver, April 11, 1975.
17. CHRISTENSEN, D. E., and SPRAGUE, R. L., "Reduction of Hyperactive Behaviors by Conditioning Procedures Alone and in Combination with Methylphenidate," *Behavior Research and Therapy, 11*:331–334, 1973.
18. COHEN, N. J., WEISS, G., and MINDE, K., "Cognitive Styles in Adolescents Previously Diagnosed as Hyperactive," *Journal of Child Psychology and Psychiatry, 13*:203–209, 1972.
19. COLEMAN, M., "Serotonin Concentrations in Whole Blood of Hyperactive Children," *Journal of Pediatrics, 78*:985–990, 1971.
20. CONNERS, C. K., "Recent Drug Studies with Hyperkinetic Children," *Journal of Learning Disabilities, 4*:476–483, 1971.
21. ———, "A Teacher Rating Scale for Use in Drug Studies with Children," *American Journal of Psychiatry, 126*:884–888, 1969.
22. ———, et al., "Magnesium Pemoline and Dextroamphetamine: A Controlled Study in Children with Minimal Brain Dysfunction," *Psychopharmacologia, 26:* 321–336, 1972.
23. DAVID, O., CLARK, J., and VOELLER, K., "Lead and Hyperactivity," *Lancet, 2*:900–903, 1972.
24. DOUBROS, S. G., and DANIELS, G. J., "An Experimental Approach to the Reduction of Overactive Behavior," *Behavior Research and Therapy, 4*:251–258, 1966.
25. DOUGLAS, V. I., "Differences between Normal and Hyperkinetic Children," in Conners, C. K. (Ed.), *Clinical Use of Stimulant Drugs in Children*, Excerpta Medica, Amsterdam, The Netherlands, 1974.
26. EDELSON, R. I., and SPRAGUE, R. L., "Conditioning of Activity Level in a Classroom with Institutionalized Retarded Boys," *American Journal of Mental Deficiency, 78*:384–388, 1974.
27. EISENBERG, L., "Primary Prevention and Early Detection in Mental Illness," *Bulletin of the New York Academy of Medicine, 51*:118–129, 1975.
28. ———, "The Overactive Child," *Hospital Practice, 8*:151–160, 1973.
29. ———, "The Clinical Use of Stimulant Drugs in Children," *Pediatrics, 49*:709–715, 1972.
30. ———, "Principles of Drug Therapy in Child Psychiatry with Special Reference to Stimulant Drugs," *American Journal of Orthopsychiatry, 41*:371–379, 1971.
31. ———, "The Management of the Hyperkinetic Child," *Developmental Medicine and Child Neurology, 8*:593–598, 1966.

32. ———, "Behavioral Manifestations of Cerebral Damage in Childhood," in Birch, H. G. (Ed.), *Brain Damage in Children*, pp. 61–72, Williams & Wilkins, Baltimore, Md., 1964.

33. ———, "Psychiatric Implications of Brain Damage in Children," *Psychiatric Quarterly, 31:*72–92, 1957.

34. FEINGOLD, B. F., *Why Your Chld is Hyperactive*, Random House, New York, 1975.

35. GARFINKEL, B. D., WEBSTER, C. D., and SLOMAN, L., "Methylphenidate and Caffeine in the Treatment of Children with Minimal Brain Dysfunction," *American Journal of Psychiatry, 132:*723–728, 1975.

36. GORIN, T., and KRAMER, R. A., "The Hyperkinetic Behavior Syndrome," *Connecticut Medicine, 37:*559–563, 1973.

37. GREENHILL, L. L., et al., "Lithium Carbonate in the Treatment of Hyperactive Children," *Archives of General Psychiatry, 28:*636–640, 1973.

38. GRINSPOON, L., and SINGER, S. B., "Amphetamines in the Treatment of Hyperkinetic Children," *Harvard Educational Review, 45:*515–555, 1973.

39. GRUNEWALD-ZUBERIER, E., GRUNEWALD, G., and RASCHE, A., "Hyperactive Behavior and EEG Arousal Reactions in Children," *Electroencephalography and Clinical Neurophysiology, 38:*149–159, 1975.

40. HUESSY, H. R., "The Adult Hyperkinetic," *American Journal of Psychiatry, 131:*724–725, 1974.

41. ———, "Study of the Prevalence and Therapy of the Choreatiform Syndrome or Hyperkinesis in Rural Vermont," *Acta Paedopsychiatrica, 34:*130–135, 1967.

42. ———, METOYER, M., and TOWNSEND, M., "8–10 Year Follow-up of 84 Children Treated for Behavior Disorder in Rural Vermont," *Acta Paedopsychiatrica, 40:*230–235, 1974.

43. JASPER, H. H., SOLOMON, P., and BRADLEY, C., "Electroencephalographic Analyses of Behavior Problem Children," *American Journal of Psychiatry, 95:*641–659, 1938.

44. KAHN, E., and COHEN, L. H., "Organic Drivenness: A Brain Stem Syndrome and an Experience," *New England Journal of Medicine, 210:*748–756, 1934.

45. KENNY, T. J., et al., "Characteristics of Children Referred Because of Hyperactivity," *Journal of Pediatrics, 79:*618–622, 1971.

46. KNOBLOCH, H., and PASAMANICK, B., "Prospective Studies on the Epidemiology of Reproductive Casualty," *Merrill-Palmer Quarterly of Behavior and Development, 12:*27–43, 1966.

47. KRAGER, J. M., and SAFER, D. J., "Type and Prevalence of Medications Used in the Treatment of Hyperactive Children," *New England Journal of Medicine, 291:*1118–1120, 1974.

48. LANSDOWN, R. G., et al., "Blood-lead Levels, Behavior and Intelligence: A Population Study," *Lancet, 1:*538–541, 1974.

49. LAUFER, M. W., "Long-term Management and Some Follow-up Findings on the Use of Drugs with Minimal Cerebral Syndromes," *Journal of Learning Disabilities, 4:*518–522, 1971.

50. ———, DENHOFF, E., and SOLOMONS, G., "Hyperkinetic Impulse Disorder in Children's Behavior Problems," *Psychosomatic Medicine, 19:*38–49, 1957.

51. LUCAS, A. R., and WEISS, M., "Methylphenidate Hallucinosis," *Journal of the American Medical Association, 217:*1079–1081, 1971.

52. MARTIN, G. I., and ZANG, P. J., "Electrocardiographic Monitoring of Enuretic Children Receiving Therapeutic Doses of Imipramine," *American Journal of Psychiatry, 132:*540–542, 1975.

53. MENDELSON, W., JOHNSON, N., and STEWART, M. A., "Hyperactive Children as Teenagers: A Follow-up Study," *Journal of Nervous and Mental Disease, 153:*273–279, 1971.

54. MENKES, M. M., ROWE, J. S., and MENKES, J. H., "A 25-Year Follow-up Study on the Hyperkinetic Child with Minimal Brain Dysfunction," *Pediatrics, 39:*393–399, 1967.

55. MORRISON, J. R., and MINKOFF, K., "Explosive Personality as a Sequel to the Hyperactive-Child Syndrome," *Comprehensive Psychiatry, 16:*343–348, 1975.

56. MORRISON, J. R., and STEWART, M. A., "The Psychiatric Status of the Legal Families of Adopted Hyperactive Children," *Archives of General Psychiatry, 28:*888–891, 1973.

57. ———, "A Family Study of the Hyperactive Child Syndrome," *Biological Psychiatry, 3:*189–195, 1971.

58. NEEDLEMAN, H. L., "Lead Poisoning in Children: Neurologic Implications of Widespread Subclinical Intoxication," *Seminars in Psychiatry, 5:*47–54, 1973.

59. NEY, P. G., "Psychosis in a Child Associated with Amphetamine Administration," *Canadian Medical Association Journal, 97:*1026–1029, 1967.

60. PAGE, J. G., et al., "A Multiclinic Trial of Pemoline in Childhood Hyperkinesis," in Conners, C. K. (Ed.), *Clinical Use of Stimulant Drugs in Children*, pp. 98–124, Excerpta Medica, Amsterdam, The Netherlands, 1974.

61. PALKES, H., STEWART, M., and KAHANA, B., "Porteus Maze Performance of Hyperactive Boys after Training in Self-directed Verbal Commands," *Child Development, 39:*817–826, 1968.

62. PATTERSON, C. R., et al., "A Behavior Modification Technique for the Hyperactive Child," *Behavior Research and Therapy, 2:*217–226, 1965.

63. QUITKIN, F., and KLEIN, D. F., "Two Behavioral Syndromes in Young Adults Related to Possible Minimal Brain Dysfunction," *Journal of Psychiatric Research, 7:*131–142, 1969.

64. RAPOPORT, J. L., and QUINN, P. O., "Multiple Minor Physical Anomalies (Stigmata) and Elevated Plasma DBH: A Major Biologic Subgroup of Hyperactive Children," Presented at The Conference on Psychiatric Problems of Childhood, New York City, January 31–February 2, 1974.

65. ———, and LAMPRECHT, F., "Minor Physical Anomalies and Plasma Dopamine-B-Hydroxylase in Hyperactive Boys," *American Journal of Psychiatry, 131:*386–390, 1974.

66. ———, et al., "Imipramine and Methylphenidate Treatments of Hyperactive Boys," *Archives of General Psychiatry, 30:*789–793, 1974.

67. ———, et al., "Playroom Observations of Hyperactive Children on Medication," *Journal of the American Academy of Child Psychiatry, 10:*524–534, 1971.

68. ROBINS, L., *Deviant Children Grown Up*, Williams & Wilkins, Baltimore, 1966.

69. RUTTER, M., and LOCKYER, L., "A Five to Fifteen Year Follow-up Study of Infantile Psychosis: I. Description of Sample," *British Journal of Psychiatry, 113:*1169–1182, 1967.

70. RUTTER, M., TIZARD, J., and WHITMORE, K., *Education, Health and Behaviour*, Longman, London, 1970.

71. ———, et al., "A Triaxial Classification of Mental Disorders in Childhood: An International Study," *Journal of Child Psychology and Psychiatry, 10:*41–61, 1969.

72. SAFER, D. J., "A Familial Factor in Minimal Brain Dysfunction," *Behavior Genetics, 3:*175–186, 1973.

73. ———, and ALLEN, R. P., "Factors Influencing the Suppressant Effects of Two Stimulant Drugs on the Growth of Children," *Pediatrics, 51:*660–667, 1973.

74. ———, and BARR, E., "Growth Rebound after Termination of Stimulant Drugs," *Journal of Pediatrics, 86:*113–116, 1975.

75. SARAF, K. R., et al., "Imipramine Side-effects in Children," *Psychopharmacologia, 37:*265–274, 1974.

76. SHELLEY, E. M., and REISTER, A., "Syndrome of Minimal Brain Damage in Adults," *Diseases of the Nervous System, 33:*335–338, 1972.

77. SHETTY, T., "Alpha Rhythms in the Hyperkinetic Child," *Nature, 234:*476, 1971.

78. ———, "Photic Responses in Hyperkinesis of Childhood," *Science, 174*:1356–1357, 1971.

79. SILBERGELD, E. K., and GOLDBERG, A. M., "Lead-induced Behavioral Dysfunction: An Animal Model of Hyperactivity," *Experimental Neurology, 42*:146–157, 1974.

80. SLEATOR, E. K., VON NEUMANN, A., and SPRAGUE, R. L., "Hyperactive Children: A Continuous Long-term Placebo-controlled Follow-up," *Journal of the American Medical Association, 229:* 316–317, 1974.

81. SMALL, A., HIBI, S., and FEINBERG, I., "Effects of Dextroamphetamine Sulfate on EEG Sleep Patterns of Hyperactive Children," *Archives of General Psychiatry, 25*:369–380, 1971.

82. SOLOMONS, G., "Drug Therapy, Initiation and Follow-up," Presented at The Conference on Minimal Brain Dysfunction, New York Academy of Sciences, New York, March 22, 1972.

83. SPRAGUE, R. L., and SLEATOR, E. K., "Effects of Pharmacologic Agents on Learning Disorders," *Pediatric Clinics of North America,20*:719–735, 1973.

84. SROUFE, L. A., and STEWART, M. A., "Treating Problem Children with Stimulant Drugs," *New England Journal of Medicine, 289*:407–413, 1973.

85. STEWART, M. A., and MORRISON, J. R., "Affective Disorder Among the Relatives of Hyperactive Children," *Journal of Child Psychology and Psychiatry, 14*:209–212, 1973.

86. ———, et al., "The Hyperactive Child Syndrome," *American Journal of Orthopsychiatry, 36*:861–867, 1966.

87. STRAUSS, A. A., and LEHTINEN, L., *Psychopathology and Education of the Brain-Injured Child*, Grune & Stratton, New York, 1950.

88. ———, and WERNER, H., "Disorders of Conceptual Thinking in the Brain-injured Child," *Journal of Nervous and Mental Disease, 96*:153–172, 1942.

89. TOUWEN, B. C. L., and KALVEBOER, A. F., "Neurologic and Behavioral Assessment of Children with Minimal Brain Dysfunction," *Seminars in Psychiatry, 5:* 79–94, 1973.

90. WALDROP, M., PEDERSON, F. A., and BELL, R. Q., "Minor Physical Anomalies and Behavior in Preschool Children," *Child Development, 39*:391–400, 1968.

91. WARREN, R. J., et al., "The Hyperactive Child Syndrome: Normal Chromosome Findings," *Archives of General Psychiatry, 24*:161–162, 1971.

92. WEISS, G., et al., "Studies on the Hyperactive Child. VIII: Five Year Follow-up," *Archives of General Psychiatry, 24*:409–414, 1971.

93. WENDER. P. H., *Minimal Brain Dysfunction in Children*, Wiley-Interscience, New York, 1971.

94. WERNER, E., et al., "Reproductive and Environmental Casualties," *Pediatrics, 42*:112–127, 1968.

95. WERRY, J. S., "Developmental Hyperactivity," *Pediatric Clinics of North America, 15*:581–598, 1968.

96. ———, et al., "Studies on the Hyperactive Child. VII: Neurologic Status Compared with Neurotic and Normal Children," *American Journal of Orthopsychiatry, 42*:441–451, 1972.

97. WILLERMAN, L., "Activity Level and Hyperactivity in Twins," *Child Development, 44*:288–293, 1973.

98. WINNET, R. A., and WIKLER, R. C., "Current Behavior Modification in the Classroom: Be Still, Be Quiet, Be Docile," *Journal of Applied Behavior Analysis, 5*:499–504, 1972.

99. WINSBERG, B. D., et al., "Imipramine and Electrocardiographic Abnormalities in Hyperactive Children," *American Journal of Psychiatry, 132*:542–545, 1975.

100. WOLFF, P. H., and HURWITZ, I., "Functional Implications of the Minimal Brain Damage Syndrome," *Seminars in Psychiatry, 5*:105–115, 1973.

22 / School Phobia

John C. Coolidge

School phobia is the generally accepted name for this syndrome. It is also referred to as school resistance, school refusal, or separation anxiety. It was formerly included under the general term, truancy—DSM-II: (300.2) Phobic neurosis characterized by fear of school. GAP terminology: (4b.) Psychoneurotic Disorder, Phobic Type, manifested by fear of school.

Description of Syndrome

PRIMARY SYNDROME

School Phobia is characterized by a strong reluctance to go to school as a result of morbid dread of some aspect of the school situation. The specific fear may be of a teacher, another child, the janitor, toilet, eating in the dining hall, or almost any aspect of the school. As the time for departure from home to school approaches, anxiety rapidly rises to massive proportions and is invariably accompanied by somatic symptoms, usually nausea and vomiting, less seldom headaches, elevated temperature, sore throat, or leg pains. If there is parental coercion and insistence that the child proceed to school, the boy or girl becomes desperate and panicky and may physically resist attempts to propel him to the bus or car. When such attempts are abandoned and the child is allowed to remain at home, the anxiety rapidly abates, the somatic symptoms melt away, and the child returns to a seemingly contented and cheerful state.

Particularly among the younger children, on

superficial observation, it may appear that the child is developing normally were it not for the problems regarding school. Under closer scrutiny, however, this will be found not to be so.

SECONDARY TO OTHER DISTURBANCES

As a symptomatic expression of other underlying conditions, school phobic-like symptoms can occur in children at times of acute stress at home such as following the birth of a sibling. There may be a transient reluctance to return to school, but, unlike the primary disorder, such a child does not demonstrate the intense fear of school but quite consciously is preoccupied and troubled with the situation at home, and does not manifest the phobic quality of true school phobia. The school-phobic symptom can occur as a precursor to an impending psychotic break, especially in adolescence. It can be part of a reaction to an associated physical illness, such as a child with acute social problems caused by his epilepsy. Children with asthma, colitis, and other psychosomatic illnesses may have an undercurrent of the same phobic attitudes toward school which are largely masked by their primary disorder. Asthmatic children, for instance, frequently have attacks on Monday mornings, especially after vacations.

History of School Phobia Identification

ORIGINAL FORMULATION OF SYNDROME

Until the 1940s, school phobia was not widely recognized as a discrete, neurotic disturbance. It was frequently mistaken for, confused with, and treated as truancy. In 1941, Adelaide Johnson and her coworkers[9] coined the term "school phobia" and identified the roots of the disorder as beginning at home and emanating from a poorly resolved hostile-independent relationship between mother and child with resultant fear of separation. The central conflict is externalized and displaced to some aspect of school. In 1957, Johnson stated that "school phobia was a misnomer and should, in fact, be labeled as separation anxiety."[8] Others have challenged the validity of the name, but the original name has now become entrenched and widely used. It is actually not inaccurate, as there are true phobic aspects and mechanisms which are aimed at the school.

REVIEW OF LITERATURE

Waldfogel, Coolidge, Hahn and associates[15] at the Judge Baker Guidance Center studied the disorder intensively in the 1950s and in a series of papers replicated the findings of Johnson and associates, augmented the understanding of the psychodynamics placing emphasis on the importance of magical thinking in addition to the triad of phobic defenses—externalization, displacement, and projection. They outlined treatment techniques for both younger and older children in a child guidance center. Waldfogel and associates[14] outlined a model of cooperation between clinic and school.

Studies were made of the differences and similarities between school phobia in latency and in adolescence.[4, 6] The subclinical and acute clinical episodes of young children were found to yield quickly to proper treatment and to represent a discrete, neurotic episode in marked contrast to the disorder in adolescence, which usually has had a long insidious and unrecognized origin. By the time of the clinical eruption, the phobic qualities are already deeply entrenched, secondary elaboration is more extensive and treatment is more difficult. Focus on the vicissitudes of aggression[5] in school phobia led the observers to postulate that unresolved early emotional problems of the mother are rearoused in the early object relationship with her child. The mother tends to project upon the child her own thwarted oral needs, then views the child as the insatiable part of herself which has to be fended off lest she be consumed by its devouring needs. She handles the child in an overcompensatory manner to alleviate her guilt and to deny her hostility.

Sperling[13] speaks of the basic conviction of these children (and their parents) that separation unconsciously signifies death of the mother and in turn of the child. The events which precipitate the phobia are always interpreted unconsciously by the child as a danger to his mother's life and therefore to his own. Sperling[12] offers a classification of school phobias. "Common" school phobia, which may be acute or chronic, erupts after a traumatic event and resembles a traumatic neurosis. In the "induced" school phobia, the traumatization is insidious and results from induction of pathology in the child through the relationship with a disturbed parent. This type may also be either acute or chronic. The papers by Sperling are lucid and incisive.

Coolidge and associates[3] reported a ten-year follow-up study of school-phobic children. Forty-seven of forty-nine had been able to return to and remain in school. Thirteen children demonstrated no limitations, twenty were moderately limited, and fourteen were severely limited in their activities. There was widespread evidence of phobic character structure causing personality constriction and cautiousness, even among many of their adolescents who, from general behavioral indications, seemed to be developing normally. It was also noted that there was some blunting of the expected mood swings and divergent polarities of ordinary adolescent behavior.

Coolidge and Brodie[2] reported their findings on the mothers of these same children. The mothers were divided into three groups. Group one included mothers who were able to make great use of their psychiatric casework and who were able to define and alter their role in the hostile dependent relationship. Group two earnestly cooperated with the clinic, made use in a dependent way of their casework but were much less able to define and understand their roles in the child's disorder. Group three were those who were defensive, uncooperative, or who were unable to use the help that was offered. Comparing these findings showed a marked correlation with improvement in the children from group one to group three. The degree of depth of the psychotherapy with the children did not appear to be as significant in the final outcome of the child's development as the effectiveness of the work accomplished with the mothers. This underscores again the enormous significance of unconscious forces acting on the parents in the dynamics of this syndrome.

Frequency of School Phobia

Episodes of school phobia probably occur in every school, either in its acute, dramatic form, in transient episodes, or in a chronic and subclinical state in which the child manages to continue to attend school but with a greater or lesser degree of discomfiture and with frequent absences often totaling twenty to thirty during one school year.

DISTRIBUTION ACCORDING TO GENDER

It has frequently been stated that there is a higher incidence of school phobia among girls than boys, but in a case finding survey by Waldfogel and associates[14] among primary grade students, the sex incidence from kindergarten through the sixth grade was identical.

SOCIOECONOMIC AND CULTURAL DATA

Socioeconomic questions do suggest that the incidence is higher (or more recognizable) in upward striving and upper economic categories in which enormous concern and value is placed on education and achievement. The concerns of the marginal and lowest economic classes are different, and the emotional troubles of their children appear in other areas.

School phobia also occurs in a number of families in which there has been rapid social and economic upward shift in the generation between the parents and the grandparents, some of whom emigrated to this country. Such parents often experience alienation from their childhood culture, and some guilt and sadness that they have left their parents behind. They, in turn, cling to their own children fearing a similar abandonment by them when the children grow up.

This phenomenon has also been reported in the Southwest among Mexican-American families.

The syndrome occurs in the countries in Western Europe. Also it is reported that in the Republic of China, a child's refusal to attend school is not tolerated.[11] The same type of conflict is expressed by headache, but the child continues to comply to the expectation that he must remain in school.

AGE OF ONSET AND INCIDENCE

The disorder is clearly evident in nursery schools. Frequently the school suggests that the seemingly immature child be withdrawn, or the parents themselves may spontaneously do so. Since by law, the child does not have to attend school, the issue is often dropped only to occur again later when the child attends kindergarten or first grade. The highest incidence occurs in kindergarten and grades one through three. From the fourth grade on, it tapers off. However, it does occur in every grade through high school and even in college, either for the first time or as a recurrence of previous episodes. Rate of occurrence in schools is not really known. The figures depend enormously upon the level of awareness among school personnel regarding the true emotional nature of the syndrome. In a suburb of Boston of approximately 90,000 people, from largely middle- to upper-class families, the counseling service of this very good school system believed that three to five cases ocurred each year. A clinical team from the Judge Baker Guidance Center, working in conjunction with the counseling service, offered consultation services for all cases of school phobia from kindergarten through grade six. As the teachers became increasingly aware of the existence of the disorder, the number of valid referrals increased enormously. In one three-and-one-half-month period, twenty-four valid cases of school phobia were referred.[15] In this study, 51 percent of the children were five to seven years of age, 36 percent were eight to ten, and 13 percent were eleven years of age and older.

DISTRIBUTION WITHIN SIBLING PATTERN

There is no clear-cut ordinal incidence among siblings, other than an impression that oldest and youngest children are slightly more afflicted. Occasionally, more than one child experiences the disturbance, either concurrently or in sequence.

Clinical Course of the Syndrome

CHARACTERISTIC FEATURES AT EACH LEVEL OF CHILD DEVELOPMENT

Although the underlying disorder is the same in all stages of childhood development, the picture does vary to some degree with age. By definition, disturbances in separation before the child attends school can scarcely be called "school phobia." Problems regarding separation can begin before the first year of life. Many of the parents of the later school-phobic children reported their own anxiety at each step of separation in the growth of their children. The pathetic child clinging to its mother at a birthday party for two-year-olds or crying frantically at the threat of being left may not experience somatic symptoms. He is not as torn by the internal conflict between the desire to remain versus the panic of being left as is the same child later at school. At this age, and often in the three-year-olds and four-year-olds at nursery school, the child is withdrawn from the situation and often the disturbance is considered an "insecurity" or a social anxiety that will be outgrown by the following year.

Once the child has started in school proper, the situation has changed. Child, parent, and school alike are convinced the child must remain in school, not only because of the law but because of the basic tenets of our society and the hard reality that without education there is little that a human being can achieve in this world. Separation from home is considered mandatory and is no longer a choice. Attendance at school seems to symbolize for the child and his parents the acceptance of latency and the relinquishment of the special privileges and omnipotence of early childhood. Normally, children sense the reality aspects of schooling and look forward to attending school albeit with some trepidation. Once enrolled, they are proud of the sense of mastery and gain pleasure from the learning. They experience shame if they cannot live up to the standards set by themselves, their families, and society. By consensus, however, the very same forces which propel a child to school also hold that illness is the only legitimate reason for failing to attend, and this is a powerful factor in the somatization of the school-phobic child.

In the lower grades, the absent child will play happily with playmates after they return when school is out. In older children, embarrassment and shame about nonattendance becomes stronger. Wishing to avoid questions and taunts from their fellows, they may shun old playmates and withdraw more and more to the bastion of their homes. This agoraphobic spread of the school phobia also protects against self-recrimination, which is projected onto peers.

In pre-adolescence and adolescence proper, the unabashed tears and wailings of the youngest children are replaced by attempts to conceal the anxiety. Truculance, defiance, rationalizations with strong emphasis on "dislikes" rather than fear are manifest. But the massive anxiety is easily recognized and the pale face and nausea may be obvious. The younger children with acute episodes usually respond to treatment quickly and demonstrate essentially intact personality structures. In the adolescent group, more deeply embedded problems are encountered. They yield much more slowly to treatment and the prognosis is graver. In reviewing their life histories, almost invariably there were earlier episodes of either a subclinical or overt, but transient, symptomatology which subsided spontaneously or diminished to a chronic state of discomfiture regarding school attendance. Attendance waxed or waned depending upon personalities of teachers and chance experiences at school. In some of the children the symptomatology disappeared in the later latency years only to recur in adolescence. Upon examination of their earlier interfamily relationships, there appears a striking parallel to the pattern that is found in the younger children with acute school phobias.

It is not an inaccurate approximation to state that a child with a sounder ego and a more vigorous personality structure can generate a more definitive symptom which forces the problem regarding separation into the open. In this case, the disorder can be recognized and dealt with. In many of the adolescent cases, however, such strong overt symptomatology had not previously appeared. Accommodation by all concerned helped the child adapt to the chronic level of subclinical or manageable symptomatology. At home, there was often an implicit emotional agreement that "real" separation would never be expected. Then came adolescence with its built-in thrust toward self-definition and separation, which is diametrically opposite to the direction of the latent school phobic process. When these children break down with school phobia, there appears a more general collapse of functioning, and what is revealed is a much more serious intrinsic disturbance of general adjustment.

OTHER VARIETIES OF SCHOOL REFUSAL
AND DIFFERENTIAL DIAGNOSIS

It is important to distinguish school refusal as a phobic process from other types of reluctance to attend school, because the therapeutic regimen and the handling of the situation will vary accordingly.

Truancy: In truancy, there is no conscious manifest anxiety regarding separation. In contrast to the school-phobic child, who invariably pursues the quickest route home when running from school, the truant, usually older, avoids both school and home. Again in contrast to the school-phobic child, who desires to learn, the truant is bored with and dislikes school and has little or no internal conflict about his avoidance actions. The truant child is usually older and waits impatiently for the day he is legally released from obligatory attendance. There are usually moderate to severe learning disabilities, and the character structure is more delinquent. Some truants have experienced school-phobic episodes in early latency. Others have not.

Realistic Fears: A child coping with a realistic threat to his physical safety as a result from attacks of older, marauding students or a child who has been tormented by a vindictive or sadistic teacher may respond with panic similar to that of the school-phobic child. This child differs from the school-phobic child, however, in that there is not the presence of the typical phobic, defensive maneuvers in which the parents are also embroiled or with underlying problems regarding separation. Proper protection, change in school, or transfer to the classroom of a different teacher will remove the source of fear and the difficulties clear up.

Learning Difficulties and School Avoidance: Children with chronic learning difficulties who have experienced repeated failure may begin to fear school and wish to avoid it. Here, the motive is to avoid the loss of self-esteem from the expected learning failure.

"Normal" School Refusal: Many a younger child, while coping with some inner conflict or with some episode of stress at home or following an illness, may show a transient reluctance to attend school yet has not previously demonstrated such concerns and is not a child who has demonstrated problems regarding separation. Ordinarily, parents not caught up with the hostile-dependent struggles and intense ambivalences so characteristic of school phobia will not feel threatened by such a situation. Seeing it for what it is, a temporary crisis in the child's growth, they can easily manage the episode by comfortable firmness and giving the child help in resolving his concerns and overriding his own regressive wish. If necessary, they can allow the child to stay home for a day or so knowing that when he is ready (his batteries recharged) he will willingly return to school. Pediatricians, consulted at such a time, must decide whether the child's reluctance is a signal of a childhood neurosis that requires referring the child for proper treatment, or whether this is part of the ebb and flow of normal growth. The key to the situation is frequently the quality of the parents' reaction to the child's distress. If the parents show the desperate panicky uncertainty so typical of parents of school-phobic children, the chances are that the child's distress augers more than meets the eye, and the pediatrician should think in terms of a possible school phobia.

Organic Etiological Factors

No endogenous factors are considered as being of major or primary consideration in the genesis of school phobia. The children are usually robust and physically healthy with no measurable genetic, neurological, biochemical, endocrinological, or physiological substrata. A child with a physical defect, a neurological, metabolic, or other chronic illness, and especially psychosomatic illness, may become school phobic and weave aspects of his illness into his rationalization about his fear of attending school. The primary disturbance, however, will still be the unconscious fantasies regarding separation.

Among exogenous factors, any event such as an acute illness or toxic state in, accident or other trauma, which consciously or unconsciously is experienced by the child as a narrow escape from death, can precipitate a school-phobic episode. Although theoretically this could happen to any child, in all probability the occurrence takes place when there is already an underlying phobic proclivity.[12]

Psychodynamic Factors

INDIVIDUAL

Psychic Trauma: School phobia is a true neurosis, and the symptomatology expresses a compromise solution of intense internal fantasies and conflicts, both conscious and unconscious. The traumatizing events which precipitate a large number of cases can be traced back to experiencing or witnessing some event at school which consciously is experienced as loss of control or threat of loss of control and has the meaning of a threat to life of the child, his parents or both. Although the event itself may be viewed by adult observers (and frequently is so) as of significant, frightening, or shaming dimensions sufficient to explain the panic in and of itself, this is not the case. The child will not return to school comfortably until the unconscious significance of the event is uncovered and interpreted.

Becky, age eight, accidentally wet her pants while on the stage in a class play. For this she was ridiculed by some of her peers. This caused her intense mortification, and Becky could not return to school the next day for fear she would not be able to reach the bathroom in time and would wet again. The parents believed completely that Becky's concern was an appropriate fear that could, therefore, be mastered by support and reassurance. Only after three weeks had passed with no school return was clinical referral acceptable to her parents, who still staunchly believed that this was only a reaction to an unfortunate incident. Treatment of the family revealed a high degree of open exhibitionistic behavior on the part of both parents which had led to direct sexual games between father and daughter. This had aroused an enormous oedipal preoccupation on a conscious but covert level in Becky. As soon as the parents were able to contain their exhibitionistic behavior and gently but firmly avoid the sexualized games, Becky's anxiety lessened and she could accept to some degree the unconscious exhibitionistic aspect of her "accident." With reduction of her feeling of guilt and shame about her sexual thoughts, she was able to return to school.

Fixation: As with phobias in general, there is fixation midway between the obsessive-compulsive and hysterical neuroses, but closer to the former, with regression from oedipal and postoedipal levels to the anal sadistic level of pregenital organization, with its intense ambivalence, reliance and belief in magical thinking, and powerful needs for internal control and controlling struggles with the parents.

Defenses Characteristically Associated with the Syndrome: Externalization, displacement, and projection are the defenses heavily relied upon to maintain repression. By externalization, the ego, fearing an internal instinct, denies its internal nature and experiences it as originating in the world outside. It can then be avoided as an external danger. By displacement, real or imagined, conflict is split off from ambivalently loved parents at home to teachers or other personnel at school. Parents are then experienced only as good and protecting objects and the teacher as the bad, punitive, therefore, dangerous object. As a result, the child can live in harmony at home believing "it is the teacher I fear, not my mother." By projection, there is reversal of subject and object regarding the aim of the child's unacceptable, destructive, or sexual wishes. They are now experienced as not emanating from him but from the displaced objects toward him.

The Nature of Associated Ego Disturbances: In the younger children with acute school phobia, the neurosis is more clear-cut without pathological spread to other areas of ego functioning and organization. In those children who have remained untreated or who have for years been struggling with insipient school phobia, there can be marked blunting of ego development, regression, or both. In such children, there is a spreading from discrete phobic symptoms to generalized phobic character traits. The children develop tentativeness and cautiousness in many or all areas of their behavior and develop a life style governed by the need to avoid situations which would arouse anxiety. The child's normal assertiveness is restricted. This takes its toll among the boys, a high percentage of whom during adolescence show an essentially passive orientation toward life.[3] The adolescent girls with such widespread phobic traits can hide their high degree of dependency and need for obligatory companionship by planning an early marriage and, as this is socially acceptable, simply transfer their phobic attachment from parent figures to husbands.

School-phobic symptoms may be the presenting symptom of an underlying schizophrenic disorder in which the refusal to attend school is only part of a profound withdrawal from the world of reality of which school is a specific part. It can occur before there is a manifest appearance of thought disorder or can appear concurrently with this development. The underlying impending psychosis may be masked or may be readily apparent upon clinical examination. A contrary situation may exist in children of chronically psychotic parents. Such a child, although not himself psychotic, has to choose between his parents' psychotic "world" and the other "world" as portrayed by the school. He may become school phobic and renounce the school "world" in order to remain true to his parents.

Richard, age ten, was brought to the clinic by his ambulatory, schizophrenic, and actively deluded mother. He had been out of school for a month. His mother had led the public school officials to believe that the boy had been enrolled in a private school, while the director of the latter was unaware that the boy had not returned to the public school. She openly wanted her son to remain at home. When this state of affairs was finally discovered, the family doctor applied pressure for a clinic referral. Richard was a puzzled and depressed boy, not knowing whom or what to believe. He was not psychotic and was able to return to school within a few weeks after the peculiarities of his family were made clear. Fortunately what thread of reality was left in the mother responded to our encouragement and to our expectation that she, in turn, would require that Richard return to school. The following year, his sixteen-year-old sister also became school phobic. She, however, was hovering on the edge of a psychosis and was developing many ideas of reference, believing that people were laughing at her and observing her. She made progress in psychotherapy and was able to return to school. Her mother terminated the treatment, and the following year, the girl became violent and homicidal, believing her mother had poisoned her. She had to be hospitalized.

Associated Narcissistic Disturbances: The very nature of the interpersonal relationships with parents of children with this syndrome augments and perpetuates the grandiose self, inflated omnipotence, and sense of entitlement of infantile narcissism. This is expressed by the child's magical thinking, control over parents, and the undiluted expectation that the parents "should" cater to every need. In the more severely disturbed adolescents, concurrent with the narcissistic disturbance, there is marked failure of development of self-esteem regulating mechanisms. In a twenty-two-year follow-up study of school-phobic children currently being conducted, we have been struck by the high incidence of this type of difficulty. Some of the now adults show marked narcissistic personality disorders that are clearly traceable to the quality of parental relationship we witnessed in the same individuals as young children and as adolescents.

Involvement of Character Organization: The major task of adolescence is the child's ultimate separation from his infantile frame of reference with final revival and resolution of pregenital and oedipal factors. It leads ultimately to discarding of primitive superego forces and early parental introjects as regulatory mechanisms which the ego fears and to which it submits. Such a change is necessary for the resolution of contests with authority, the assumption of assertive drives, and definitive sexual identification. It is imperative for the growth of the ego ideal as the governing agency of the ego, and for the regulation of self-esteem. This process, so important for definitive character formation, is the antithesis of the school-phobic process which is essentially symptomatic of the pregenital hostile-dependent fixation. It is no wonder, then, that if school phobia is not successfully treated there will be severe compromises in the adolescent and young adult task of character formation. Reference has been made previously to the extensive phobic character traits and retention of early narcissistic elements in our former patients in whom psychological separation had not been successfully completed. In our ten-year follow-up study, we observed that in adolescence many of our subjects showed an even course of constriction and inhibition with few attenuated mood swings. Despite their chronological age, many of them psychologically seemed to be in latency. In their interviews, they lacked spontaneity and humor. Challenges to authority were the exception rather than the rule, and, to many of them, heterosexuality was of minimum interest. In our present twenty-two-year follow-up study, there is much evidence of severe character pathology and tenaciously lingering unresolved conflicts with authority. There is also sexual inhibition.

Dynamics of Symptom Formation: The dynamics of the child's symptom formation cannot be explained without some clarification of the premorbid relationship to his parents, usually the mother, sometimes the father, often both. The stereotypical mother is a woman of many strengths and deep concern for the energetic growth of her children but who, through the years, has more or less successfully concealed her own phobic qualities and an unresolved oral dependency upon her own mother. Confused and conflicted by the reawakening of her own oral needs following the birth of her child, she cannot experience the ordinary needs of her infant in quantitative proportions and tends to fear its needs as insatiable —the projection of her own unfulfillment. She experiences any frustration, anger, or demandingness on the part of her child as being as dangerous as her own anger toward her mother and also her mother's anger toward her. Her infant's cry is heard as an accusation that she has not been a good enough mother. It is this which propels her overcompensatory care and her effort to keep the child's tension at the lowest possible level, a goal which cannot be achieved. With such overprotection, of course, the child cannot learn to master the usual frustrations, to temper his needs, and to tolerate ordinary levels of tension. Management and limit setting become difficult when to the mother firmness means "I'm hurting my child" and his hostile response means "He hates me." This, in turn, reaffirms to the child the magical dangers of his easily aroused, vengeful feelings when frustrated. To manage the built-up resentment, both parent and child rely increasingly on the phobic triad of defenses to perpetuate repression of their hostility in the mutually dependent tie. The rupture of this precarious equilibrium, leading to the acute phobia, frequently follows two important events—one for the child and one for the parent. For the child, it may be the birth of a sibling, a death, an illness, which to him significes a threat of abandonment. This arouses rage at the caring person for "causing" the danger. The rage is magically feared as possibly leading to destruction of the object, thereby producing the feared abandonment. In the parent, the stress may be a marital problem, an illness in the mother's mother, or some similar tension, which is equally feared as abandonment. In each, the aroused anger is consciously felt as anxiety. It is then that some event at school is interpreted as symbolic of the dreaded expectation, and anxiety turns to panic. One mother, whose young daughter suddenly became school phobic, had recently lost her own mother, and described her daughter's school as "like a dank, dark basement" and felt as if she were "leading a lamb to slaughter" each day when taking her frightened child to school.

Panic in child begets panic in parent. The rapidly generated anger is held in check by mutual surveillance but inevitably breaks through in each, followed by rise in guilt, greater clinging, rapid undoing, and apologies. The fantasy of magical control over life and death is shared by both mother and child and is expressed in each by the intense need and struggle for control over the other and over external situations. The phobia in the child is literally experienced as lifesaving for both partners, and it expresses the child's identification with that pathogenic part of its parent. One eight-year-old girl, as the crisis subsided and she could again return to school, agreed to do so only if her mother acquiesced to her command to remain in the house "and not even go out on the back porch to empty the garbage." With her mother controlled, her fear that she would be killed abated and she trudged off to school.

Most school-phobic children wish to be able to return to school. To learn and often to excel is deeply desired. If return to school is accomplished quickly, secondary gain for the child does not become an important factor. When school absence drags on, however, the child becomes bored, falls behind in school work, and gradually feels the effects of his mother's and his own irritability regarding his absence from school. As self-esteem is corroded, he attempts to find secondary compensation in his regressed behavior at home rationalizing that he really does not care about his friends anyway or about his favorite activities at school, which is now viewed as an "awful" place. The involved parent receives secondary gain by becoming the child's "protector." By taking this active position, the parent is able to some degree to contain aroused anger within and to prevent a more total regression in him as a result of the onslaught of his own difficulties.

FAMILIAL AND INTERPERSONAL DYNAMICS

Family Structure: By and large, the parents of school-phobic children are upward striving, often determined to provide more for their children than they had received themselves. Both are often strongly child-oriented, yet uncertain regarding child-rearing practices, especially in the areas of gratification and discipline. Among these parents there tends to be much soul-searching and intellectual scrutiny, which detracts from easy and spontaneous interactions with the child. At time of stress, this intellectual control breaks down. The parents lash out irritably and punitively at the child, then, feeling great guilt over their attack and loss of control, attempt to undo the transgression, leaving the child confused. The majority of the fathers actively participate in the child's rearing, some competing with their wives, trying to be "better mothers." Other fathers are energetic only at their work. At home, they are passive and dependent, leaving all the household and child-rearing practices to the mothers. Preoccupation with the child's welfare often starts at birth and fear of entrusting infants to baby-sitters enslaves them to the child's care. This anxious overconcern often contains a concomitant element of resentment at feeling enslaved. The subtle, phobic qualities in one or both parents are quite easily recognized.

Sibling Factors: There is some indication that oldest and youngest children are more prone to school phobia, and it is probably not coincidence that these two ordinant positions among the siblings have the greatest meaning to parents regarding immediate and eventual separation. Difficulties in renunciation and in sharing with siblings are common. There is frequent displacement of angry resentments and oedipal struggles from parents to siblings. This is often subtly (or not so subtly) encouraged by the parents. In marked contrast to the usually compliant behavior toward the parents, there may be open, chronic, and fiercely demonstrated anger and outspoken jealousy toward the siblings. In her attempts to control or to contain this fighting, the mother frequently sounds like a sibling herself.

Models of Identification: Strong identifications are felt frequently by both parents with the child in his period of stress, often with a paralytic type of sympathy that renders the parents helpless: "I felt so badly for him; I could do nothing except cry inside. I remember so vividly feeling like that myself," said one father who quickly added, "When I'm at work and don't see him suffering, then I'm furious and want to be tough and tell him, 'I have to go to work every day whether I like it or not, why can't you go to school.' " The children sense this identification and it frightens them. In retrospect, some have stated they could not see their parents as competent models for identification.

Assigned Role Within Parental Relationship: A subtle, neurotic cooperation between parents can and often does assign roles to the school-phobic child. In families with withdrawn, passive fathers, the school-phobic boy may be idealized by the mother who considers him her "little man." She infantilizes him, and viewing him as being younger than he is, may allow quite sexualized behavior to take place, saying, "He is only a child" and gains considerable physical and emotional satisfaction from his continued clinging and need for affection from her. The father may not interfere as it allows him his continued remoteness, knowing his wife's needs have been met. Similar situations occur among the girls. The parents often are not aware of the sexualized aspects of their behavior and the resultant anxiety that is generated in the child, usually because the gratification experienced by the parent is actually of a pregental nature.

Associated Disturbances in Family Communication: The use made of the child for gratification of parents' needs takes place when there is parental (therefore family) inability to make needs known or to discuss the barriers between them. One mother, sitting alone and lonely in the living room, repeatedly heard her daughter and her husband giggling and chatting in the parental bed but felt absolutely helpless to interfere or to initiate a discussion with her husband about the impropriety of such behavior. Neither were able to face or to discuss their own sexual problems.

Family History and Role of Extended Family: Since lingering childhood conflicts and old parental images are so prevalent in the parents, it is no wonder that the parents feel literally sandwiched between their own parents and their children. The effects of generational change have been touched upon previously in this chapter. Grandparents, aunts, and uncles, acting as surrogate parents, may be very much in the immediate background and are heavily relied upon as sources of authoritative truths for advice and strength. This is particularly true regarding the grandmothers—albeit with strong ambivalence.

Treatment Methods

An acute school phobia is one of the severe emergencies of childhood and should be treated without delay. The family coming for the initial interview is often exhausted and distraught and the child is terrified. There is a sense of enormous urgency, and pressure is put on the therapist to "do something," usually meaning to "get the child back to school." The generally accepted treatment of choice is psychoanalytically oriented psychotherapy. As inevitably there is parental involvement in the child's neurotic episode, the parents must be incorporated in any treatment plan. Sometimes with the very youngest children, work with the parents alone and airing of the basic conflicts can suffice, and the child can be released from the neurotic constriction. The therapist must staunchly adhere to the principle that the internal conflict is more important than the symptom and should resist pressures put upon him to focus solely upon school return. Naturally, it is important to the child to return to school as soon as practicable, but this can be accomplished better by unraveling the sources of the neurotic fear than by some manipulation.

Melita Sperling summarizes succinctly the basic tenets of treatment:

In our treatment of phobic children we reconstruct in as much detail as possible the events immediately preceding and dynamically related to the onset of the phobic behavior. In most cases, both the child and his parents offer numerous rationalizations and overlook the significant events which have to be discovered by specific questioning. This phenomenon appears to be the result of a selective repressive tendency aimed at keeping vague those events that touch upon the repressed conflict of the child. The pathological effect of seemingly innocuous events results from their unconscious association with the child's basic conflict which is thus activated. After establishing the unconscious significance of these events and their specific connections with the subsequent phobia and if possible with earlier phobic episodes, we interpret these connections and meanings convincingly to the child on the basis of the evidence obtained directly and from the mother.[13]

From the reconstruction of the traumatic incident, it can be demonstrated to the child how his fears about his mother's safety, illness, or death had been augmented and how he, in turn, had sensed her uncertainty regarding his safety. Careful review can be made of the resentments and hostile wishes that were stirred up toward mother for her behaviors, which were interpreted by him as not protecting him. Direct explanations are made of the child's fear of the possible magical power of his hostile thoughts with the concomitant reassurance that wishes to hurt by themselves cannot harm or kill anyone. It is also important to clarify that the conflict itself is within the child and not with the school, where in fact he really wants to go. It may be remarkable in fresh cases how quickly the child is able to return to school. Once the child returns, the parents frequently wish to withdraw, usually to avoid resolution of the underlying pathological tie. Continued work with the child, but especially with the parents, is of paramount importance to uncover and work

through the powerful forces that entrapped the child in the first place. A combination of exploration of the genetics underlying the seductive and overprotective controlling tendencies of the parents, accompanied by explanations of the unrecognized effects of these upon the child, can be most helpful to the parents. The lasting value of therapy, however, comes from the working through of the parents' childhood neurotic residuals, which are reawakened and reenacted with the child.

In cases of longer standing or where the influence of the parents is more pervasive, the child will not be able to return to school quickly. There are times, in fact, when the child is himself ready to go back to school, but the parents are not ready to have him do so. Home tutoring may be necessary even for months before there is sufficient therapeutic progress for the child to be able to return. Meeting and cooperation with school personnel in the planning for the child's continued education is of paramount importance. There are times when a psychiatrist may actually recommend that the child not return to school at a particular moment because to do so may clearly be seen as resistance to the treatment, which has become a threat to the pathological relationship. This has to be explained to the school in order that the school does not unwittingly become partners in resistance to the treatment.

In treatment of adolescent cases, meeting with the parents may be contraindicated by the patient's therapist, and they should then be referred to another therapist.

Progress is usually much slower because of the entrenchment of defenses, the characterological spread, and the added burden to the child of the arousal of adolescent forces which are in opposition to but can cause vast augmentation of the school-phobic process.

Learning and behavior theory has been applied to school phobia, and reports of its effectiveness in reduction of anxiety with resultant capacity of the child to return to school have been published.[7] In this theoretical framework "losing mother" becomes a danger signal producing a fear response which becomes associated with the neutral stimulus—"school." "School" then becomes a conditioned stimulus producing the conditioned response—the physiological response of fear connected with "loss of mother." Desensitization can be accomplished by mastering a cue weak in producing anxiety (proximity to school), and by coupling this cue with a stronger cue producing a positive response—the presence of the therapist. By gradual steps on subsequent days taken closer to the classroom, increasingly anxiety is mastered until the child, anxiety-free, can again enter his classroom. There is no question that in many cases the child can be relieved of his symptom at least temporarily. This author is aware of the positive response in many school-phobic children to the presence of a caring person who is deeply interested in the child, especially if the parents are also receiving simultaneous support. This may often break up the regressive pathological vortex enmeshing parent and child. However, what such a return to school does not accomplish is the resolution of the underlying pathology which may spread to other areas, for instance, to difficulties in beginning learning and more ominously to later characterological difficulties.

Residential treatment in intracable cases has been recommended.[16] The milieu provided by the institution blocks the pattern of avoidance at which the children are so adept and simultaneously separates the children from the vortex of the chronic home pathology. The institution provides ego supportive experiences and by confrontation helps the child to understand the sources of the anxiety as it is being generated.

Family therapy is rapidly becoming an important therapeutic tool and can be exceedingly useful in cases of school phobia where there are strong indications of extensive family pathology. Malmquist[10] states:

The need for focusing on the family dynamics is stressed when a given child happens to be the first person in a family to appeal for psychiatric treatment because of failure to attend school. This will obviate symptom focusing and viewing one member of the family as "sick," but will rather alert psychiatrist to the "phobogenic" family. In turn, it is felt that the opposite omission of emphasizing the family but ignoring the internalized conflict of the child and the parents will not occur.

In cases particularly of adolescent school phobia, which prove intractable to traditional clinic treatment, family therapy can be most helpful.

A sixteen-year-old, very articulate girl finally stated after two years of psychotherapy that she understood the conflict within herself but was powerless to change until the family as a whole could effect certain shifts. In family therapy, both parents, unhappy in their marriage, revealed an enormous fear of being left to themselves when their children would eventually grow up and leave them. Intense fighting between the parents embroiled the children and served to bind them to the home to avoid that dreaded day. As the real issues behind the parental fighting surfaced, their daughter was able to return to school.

In summary, school phobia can lead to profound and lifelong ego constriction and pathological adaptation. Diligent therapy usually results in a more effective return to school, a happier child back in the mainstream of life, and often prevents subsequent profound pathology.

REFERENCES

1. COOLIDGE, J. C., and BRODIE, R. D., "A 22-year Follow-Up Study of 66 School-Phobic Children," Presented at the annual meeting of the American Academy of Child Psychiatry, St. Louis, Mo., 1975.

2. ———, "Observations of Mothers of 49 School-Phobic Children Evaluated in a 10-Year Follow-Up Study," *Journal of the American Academy of Child Psychiatry*, 13:275–285, 1974.

3. ———, and FEENEY, B., "A Ten-Year Follow-Up Study of Sixty-Six School-Phobic Children," *American Journal of Orthopsychiatry*, 34:675–684, 1964.

4. COOLIDGE, J. C., HAHN, P. B., and PECK, A. L., "School Phobia: Neurotic Crisis or Way of Life," *American Journal of Orthopsychiatry*, 27:296–306, 1957.

5. ———, et al., "Patterns of Aggression in School Phobia," in Eissler, R. S., et al. (Eds.), *The Psychoanalytic Study of the Child*, vol. 17, pp. 319–333, International Universities Press, New York, 1962.

6. ———, et al., "School Phobia in Adolescence: A Manifestation of Severe Character Disturbance," *American Journal of Orthopsychiatry*, 30:599–607, 1960.

7. GARVEY, W. P., and HEGRENES, J. R., "Desensitization Techniques in the Treatment of School Phobia," *American Journal of Orthopsychiatry*, 36:147–152, 1966.

8. JOHNSON, A. M., "School Phobia Workshop, Discussion," *American Journal of Orthopsychiatry*, 27:307–309, 1957.

9. ———, et al., "School Phobia," *American Journal of Orthopsychiatry*, 11:702–711, 1941.

10. MALMQUIST, C. P., "School Phobia: A Problem in Family Neurosis," *Journal of the American Academy of Child Psychiatry*, 4:293–319, 1965.

11. SHUN, C. C., Personal communication, 1959.

12. SPERLING, M., "School Phobias: Classification, Dynamics, and Treatment," in Eissler, R. S., et al. (Eds.), *The Psychoanalytic Study of the Child*, vol. 22, pp. 375–401, International Universities Press, New York, 1967.

13. ———, "Analytic First Aid in School Phobias," *Psychoanalytic Quarterly*, 30:504–518, 1961.

14. WALDFOGEL, S., TESSMAN, E., and HAHN, P. B., "A Program for Early Intervention in School Phobia," *American Journal of Orthopsychiatry*, 29:324–332, 1959.

15. WALDFOGEL, S., COOLIDGE, J. C., and HAHN, P. B., "The Development, Meaning and Management of School Phobia," *American Journal of Orthopsychiatry*, 27:754–776, 1957.

16. WEISS, M., and CAIN, B., "The Residential Treatment of Children and Adolescents with School Phobia," *American Journal of Orthopsychiatry*, 34:103–112, 1964.

23 / Disorders of Speech

Clyde L. Rousey

DSM-II and GAP Report (1966) Classification

Disorders of speech are generally viewed as problems in sound and language production which are only secondarily related to the usual diagnosis and treatment provided by a psychiatrist. DSM-II classifies speech disorders (306.0) as psychopathology which is manifested by a single and specific symptom. As such, it falls within the category reserved for such behaviors as tics, enuresis, learning disturbances, and encopresis. No differentiation is made of the varying speech or language disorders. Further, the influence of hearing on these disturbances is not indicated. In contrast the GAP Report, "Psychopathological Disorders in Childhood,"[23] is quite specific in noting possible variations in speech sound and language symptomatology. Further, some minimal consideration is given to relating disorders of hearing to speech and language production. Variations in verbal communication are seen in this GAP Report as developmental deviations.

Description of the Disorder

In the present chapter, the term speech, unless otherwise noted, will refer to individual sounds* which when combined in varying orders will produce a spoken language† which is peculiar to a given culture or nationality. Both speech and language are independent forms of behavior.

Speech disorders are usually described in terms of phonetic variations which occur in words (called articulation disorders*), variations in phonation and resonance (called voice disorders*), and variations in fluency (called stuttering†). Language disorders are described in terms of variations in formal language production and understanding such as seen in aphasia, and the varying grammatical and semantic variations seen in differing stages of childhood or among and between differing racial or cultural subgroups. Delayed onset of spoken language is also included in the category of language disorders.

Historical Roots

Most child psychiatrists conceive of speech and language as autonomous ego functions which have a potential for being secondarily infiltrated by psychopathology. This position stems from the theoretical positions and writings of analysts such as Hartmann[26] and neurologists such as Head[27] and Goldstein.[21] When these writers took this position, the data were not yet available which would show (1) the independence between speech and language; (2) the presence of a speech disorder without demonstrable organic insult; and (3) the primary psychological meanings of sound production.

Attention to disorders of verbal communication has been paid by such varying groups as psychiatrists, neurologists, laryngologists, phoneticians, linguists, psychologists, and, most recently, speech pathologists and audiologists. The field of speech pathology and audiology, while initially borrowing heavily from many of the disciplines just noted, has developed a substantive scientific literature of its own as well as an independent national association called The American Speech and Hearing Association. Within the past ten years, Rousey and Moriarty[55] and Rousey[50] have proposed a

---

* Carrell and Tiffany[9] list sixteen vowels and twenty-five consonants as phonemes of American speech. Vowels are thought of as providing the energy and consonants the structure of spoken language.

† Spoken language is usually studied in terms of grammar and syntax.[8] The content of spoken language has both cognitive and affective meanings.

‡ Included in this group are sound substitutions (e.g., the person says *wed* for *red*); sound omissions (e.g., the person says *back* for *black*); and sound distortions (e.g., the listener cannot distinguish what sound is produced).

* Included in this group are such voice quality disturbances as hoarseness, breathiness, nasality, etc.

† This disorder includes sound, syllable, word, or phrase repetition or prolongation, silent stoppages of sound and accessory body movements accompanying the above behavior. The term stuttering is preferred over stammering in the United States.

theory which conceptually relates the discipline of speech pathology and audiology to the disciplines of child and adolescent psychiatry. This position in essence holds that while the organic status of an individual must be carefully considered in any speech disorder, it is both clinically and theoretically more productive to understand individual speech sounds as primary reflections of a person's emotional life. In contrast spoken language seems a primary reflection of a person's cognitive state.

Incidence

Studies of the rate of occurrence of speech disorders have generally been few in number. Extant literature as summarized by Milisen[42] indicates that from 7 to 10 percent of all school children have one of the previously described speech and language disorders.* Estimates of speech disorders in the early part of elementary school are around three times greater than found when all ages are considered. Study of incidence in the middle and late school years has received scant attention. Boys, by roughly a two-to-one ratio, have more speech disorders than girls. More articulation problems are found among lower socioeconomic levels, among blacks, and among the retarded. Of importance is the fact that among all the foregoing groups, levels of intelligence, neurological status, and emotional health were not described or taken into account. Articulation problems are reportedly found in 70 percent of cerebral palsy children. Milisen's foregoing review of the literature did not cite Rousey and Toussieng's[56] study, which indicated that, at a minimum, at least 60 percent of psychiatric patients (all ages combined) have speech problems. Recently, Gordon[22] has reported three times as many speech disorders in the early school years among military dependents as is found in the usual public schools.

There are further problems in evaluating the meaning of estimates made of the incidence of specific difficulties such as articulation problems, stuttering, voice disorders, or language disorders. For example, if one views sound production as a developmental phenomenon, some sounds which are not produced correctly may not be adjudged

an error by a given investigator.[64] Further, since sound deviations are not always present in every word containing similar sounds,[39] the tester may inadvertently sample material which does not elicit an error. What does emerge from this clouded situation with some degree of stability is the finding that articulation problems apparently decrease in number with advancing chronological age.

Van Riper's[68] summary of studies of the incidence of stuttering is the most extensive to date. He indicates that roughly 1 percent of the school age population appears to stutter. In the preschool years, Van Riper suggests the figure may be as high as 4 percent. Most stuttering seems to have its onset prior to age five. There is some evidence which seems to suggest extreme competitiveness and upward social mobility increase the probability of stuttering being present in children. The incidence of stuttering seems unusually great among retarded children in general and mongoloid children in particular. Males appear to stutter more often than females with the ratio being about four to one. Although there is a familial tendency for stuttering, no evidence has as yet been presented which demonstrates genetic factors. Stuttering is found with greater frequency in twins and occurs more often in monozygotic than dizygotic twins. Among persons having epilepsy or cerebral palsy, there is also an unusually high incidence of stuttering. However, in the case of the congenitally deaf, the diabetic, and the psychotic patient found in state mental hospitals, there is a disproportionately small number of persons who stutter. Follow-up studies after childhood of persons who began stuttering are sparse. Sheehan[59] cites work with a colleague (Martyn) which suggests that about 80 percent of all persons who begin stuttering eventually stop on a spontaneous basis.

When voice problems (e.g., hoarseness, breathiness, etc.) and language disorders (e.g. delayed onset of talking, aphasia, etc.) are considered in terms of their frequency of occurrence, considerably less data are available. Examination of the previously cited work of Milisen suggests the incidence of voice disorders to be from .5 to 2 percent of the general population. The factors of age and sex have not been demonstrated as related to the general category of voice disorders. In the case of language disturbance approximately .6 percent of the child and adolescent population probably manifest delayed onset of talking and/or childhood aphasia. Such an estimate does not take into account modern day interest in grammatical and semantic variations among children of varying ethnic, racial, and geographic distributions.

---

* This overall incidence of speech disorders is remarkably similar to studies cited by Bower[6] of the prevalence of emotional difficulties in a school-age population.

Clinical Course

ARTICULATION PROBLEMS

Correct articulation of sounds appears to vary considerably among children. At one point it was a generally accepted notion among speech pathologists that mastery of correct sound production was a developmental phenomenon which was mastered parallel with the increasing motoric skill of the growing child. The findings by Hall[24] and Healey[28] that many children use sounds perfectly,* from the time they begin speaking argues against the notion of sound being a developmental learning task or a function of motoric skill.

By the time a child reaches one year of age, he has produced all of the vowels and consonants which he will later use.[32, 33] The majority of sounds present in the first six months of life are vowels. By the end of the first year all consonant and vowel sounds have emerged. Other vowel and consonant sounds not found in usual spoken English appear for a short time and then seem to disappear. Omission of sounds by a child above five years is atypical. Whether or not the child receives speech therapy for articulation defects, there is a strong likelihood of a decrease in the occurrence of the errors. Just why this occurs is explained by some writers as "learning" having taken place.

From a psychiatric standpoint it may also represent an instance of symptom substitution. The concept of symptom substitution has attracted relatively scant attention from psychiatrists because of the difficulty in demonstrating the phenomenon in other than psychosomatic problems. However, Rousey and Diedrich[52] were able to demonstrate in school age children receiving speech therapy that there was a significant increase of new speech symptoms as compared to what occurred in a control sample of children not receiving speech therapy. The phenomenon of symptom change in the control sample was also present but to a significantly less degree. These data suggest that both "normal" and "reactive" variations in emotional life can be traced through study of speech behavior. By testing speech behavior periodically, the psychological system may be monitored in a way similar to monitoring the physiological system through recording a person's

* The only exception is the likelihood that below age five years, it is common for a child to omit at least one sound in a word which contains two or more consonants in sequence. Thus, the word *smile* might be said as *mile*.

temperature, pulse, and respiration. Rousey and Diedrich's study appears to offer the first empirical demonstration of the clinical phenomenon of symptom substitution. Kernberg and Rousey[34] reported on the clinical course of articulation and other speech disorders in a child psychiatric patient. In the present context, it is of interest to note that changes in articulation behavior paralleled intrapsychic changes noted by the therapist.

Changes in the articulation pattern which are obviously related to changes in the physical status of the speech mechanism is sometimes, but not invariably, seen in such clinical states as cleft palate. However, missing teeth, size and movement of the tongue or lip mobility, all have little influence on articulation ability. With reference to hearing loss, the popular conception is that speech difficulties are not only found in hard of hearing children but are also a function of the nature of the hearing loss. Hence, in those patients with high frequency components, voiceless sounds (e.g., *s* as in *s*un and the voiceless *th* as in *th*ank) would be most affected. The thesis that we speak to the extent that we hear is usually accepted. However, Smith[61] was unable to demonstrate any pattern of articulatory errors specific to residual hearing. Further, Hudgins' and Numbers'[31] seminal work on intelligibility of speech in the deaf emphasized the necessity of good rate and rhythm over good articulation.

STUTTERING

Stuttering usually has its onset around age three. Van Riper[68] feels that sound, syllable, or word repetitions are the first indications of stuttering. Only an infinitesimal number of individuals begin their stuttering by prolonging sounds. In the beginning, there is usually little other associated body tension or movements. However, the child who stutters often either fiures out for himself or takes the advice of well-meaning parents that he should take a deep breath or move his head or mouth or some extremeity in order to break his blockage in talking. These behaviors, labeled as secondary symptoms, are what create the rather bizarre appearance often associated with stuttering. Generally, the more the person feels under pressure to talk, the greater the probable number of distracting behaviors which are superimposed on the basic pattern of stuttering (i.e., repetition or prolongation of sounds, syllables, words, or phrases). A form of stuttering which is not as apparent as the ones previously described occurs when the person who stutters is afraid to say one word and substitutes another for it. Some reading problems of children may well reflect this disability.

VOICE PROBLEMS

With the exception of hoarseness and breathiness, there appear to be no developmental time periods where the onset of phonation or resonance (voice quality) problems are likely. Even the onset of these two variations is not an invariant event. Clinically, hoarseness often begins in boys in late preschool years while breathiness often has its onset in girls in early adolescence. Instances of aphonia or dysphonia are, in many instances, related to personality issues; but a laryngeal examination is indicated in all voice disorders to rule out any disease process. Left unattended and assuming no organic pathology can be detected, problems with breathiness or hoarseness may resolve themselves spontaneously, although the potential exists for continued damage to the vocal cords through misuse.

Nasality in the voice usually, but not always, implies problems with velopharyngeal closure. This condition when organically caused does not change without proper surgical intervention or use of a dental prosthesis and may result in secondary emotional reactions as time passes. Where nasality reflects characterological problems with aggression, little change in the symptom occurs without psychotherapy. As might be expected, this nasality is found in adolescence rather than childhood. Its anlage in childhood is manifested by a persistent whiny voice.

Problems with harshness are usually not a part of voice problems in childhood and adolescence. A voice problem resulting from obvious disease or external trauma to the larynx is an essentially stable behavior although secondary emotional complications may exacerbate the vocal symptomatology.

An abnormally high or low pitch in boys and girls may represent a major organic disease or significant psychological problems. The common belief that voice breaks are "normal" in boys at puberty has little basis. Many boys go through this time without losing control of phonation. Instances of voice breaks, in the absence of obvious organic pathology, may be clinically understood as the struggle to assume the appropriate masculine role. The appearance in adolescent girls of breathiness appears to be the vocal counterpart to voice breaks in boys. The psychological meaning appears related to struggles over assuming an appropriate feminine role. In the congenital deaf, voice quality may be described as flat. This distortion relates to loss of the monitoring function and has been empirically confirmed through acoustic studies completed by Angelocci, Kopp and Holbrook.[2]

LANGUAGE DISORDERS

Disorders of language have a clinical course which is primarily determined by etiology. Thus, an accurate diagnosis is a necessity. Delayed onset of talking in the child resulting from mental retardation will resolve itself primarily in relation to the final mental age obtained. Emotional reactions of parents to the retardation may cause a functional delay in onset of talking which is superimposed on the basic limitations resulting from the retardation.

In the instance of delayed onset of talking related to brain dysfunction, the course of development is uncertain and essentially unpredictable. It is a clinical observation that until around age seven or eight some spontaneous improvement in language can be expected even in obvious instances of brain dysfunction. Presumably, this phenomenon is related to transfer of functions in the brain. However, such an hypothesis is at present unproved. The reacquisition of language is more likely in the case of brain insults which occur after the child has already begun to talk. Further, since the left hemisphere is the dominant language area in about 95 percent of the population, damage to that area may more likely affect the course of language development.

Language development is also a function of both peripheral and central hearing loss. Other things being equal, only one ear with normal hearing is necessary for monitoring one's environment and acquiring normal spoken language. Predictably, a bilateral, congenital, and severe loss of hearing can be expected to delay normal acquisition of language. In the past, because of problems in measurement of hearing, such severe losses often went essentially undetected until after the child's first birthday and even beyond. Such problems in detection can now be overcome as a result of the development of indirect physiological measures of peripheral auditory functioning.[7] Of further importance is the fact that without adequate amplification, the child with a bilateral, profound loss of hearing loses the significant affective and cognitive contact with the world which is transmitted by sound. Providing profoundly deaf children with amplification and alternate means of communication (e.g., signs, gestures, finger spelling) helps but does not do away with basic differences in academic functioning. These differences grow more pronounced as the years pass. This is in spite of the fact that performance tests of intelligence among the deaf demonstrate comparable functioning to that found in hearing children. Secondary emotional reactions to the deafness may occur as a result of the child's response to parental feelings, attitudes, and behaviors.[51] Guidance at the time of the initial diagnosis by personnel who are psychologically sophisticated can materially affect the extent of language acquisition. Services of this kind are offered by such institutions as Saint Elizabeth's Hospital in Washington, D.C. The role of psychiatry in this area has been described by Ranier and Altshuler.[48] Lasting impairment in language function is less likely or pronounced if deafness occurs after the child has begun talking.

In contrast, delayed onset of language due to emotional factors characteristically has a different course. Filippi and Rousey[17] have described this process in detail elsewhere. Basically, the problem seems related to a high negative valence placed on sound production by the parents. This often is connected to parental discord and displacement onto the child of maternal anger towards the child's father. The infants' early sound productions (which as in any child contain both demanding, irritating, and soothing elements) seemingly remind her of her husband and arouse the anger she has toward him. The child responds in an adaptive sense by becoming quiet and not making sounds or using spoken language. Important in this clinical entity is the normal capacity of the child to understand spoken language. Such children are the ones who often seem to "outgrow" their not talking and probably form the basis for many parents' delay in getting an early diagnosis and appropriate treatment.

Study of language variation in children as it is related to varying psychopathologies has received only passing interest until the last few years. A general summary by de Hirsch[14] is typical of what is found in psychiatric literature, while Hick's[30] summary is typical of the publications in speech pathology. Neither of the aforementioned authors approach the problem at the theoretical level found in the work of Steingart and Freedman.[62] While the latter authors focus on adult psychiatric patients, their presentation of the course and variation of language disturbance in the emotionally disturbed adult offers a paradigm for clinicians and researchers working with children and adolescents.

Etiological Factors

ENDOGENOUS ORGANIC FACTORS

There is little evidence of endogenous influences on specific speech and language behavior. However, central nervous system difficulties such as seen in cerebral palsy or childhood aphasics, the embryological failures common to the condition of cleft palate and the various inherited and congenital hearing problems[35] grossly affect communication ability in proportion to their severity.

EXOGENOUS ORGANIC FACTORS

Probably the most comprehensive discussion of these factors is provided by Luchsinger and Arnold.[38] Such obvious factors as traumas secondary to accidents or impairment of central nervous system function because of disease are noted. Although there is a general lack of specificity of the speech disorder in terms of the disease involved, Hecker and Kreul,[29] Friedman and Rosenman,[20] and Rousey[49] have made preliminary studies which indicate possible vocal reflections of such physical states as coronary problems, laryngeal tumor, and cerebral vascular attacks. Toxic reaction to various drugs may cause hearing loss with its subsequent effect on communication.

Psychodynamic Factors

SPEECH BEHAVIOR

Understanding both normal and abnormal speech and language usage from a psychodynamic viewpoint is both theoretically and clinically productive. With reference to speech, this author[50] has presented elsewhere in detail the theory and supporting studies which tie both normal and abnormal speech behavior to personality viewed within the context of psychoanalytic theory. Speech behavior is seen as a primary indicator of emotional states rather than an autonomous ego function which may only secondarily be infiltrated by psychological difficulties. Such a position has significant meaning to the child psychiatrist for it allows indications of emotional illness in children to be recognized and subsequently treated earlier than is usually possible. Delays in diagnosis often occur because of difficulties in un-equivocal diagnosis of emotional problems in a child who is impaired in speaking. Viewing speech behavior in this way also gives the traditional psychiatric team (psychiatrist, psychologist, and social worker) a separate discipline, which can independently assess psychological functioning both in a diagnostic sense and as a result of treatment.

The theory proposed by Rousey assumes that vowel sounds are expressions of libidinal and aggressive drives, while consonant sounds reflect ego development and object relationships. Because of these assumptions, deviations in sound production, when considered within known features of child and adolescent development and the various kinds of psychopathology, can lead to meaningful psychological inferences. Under this theory any deviation in sound production from the usual acoustic productions is understood as reflecting some unusual degree of psychological stress or developmental failure. Or in other words, no child should ever produce sound variations which deviate from the usual and customary production heard in a given country. In the case of the United States, the three large speech areas accepted by most phoneticians are General American Speech, Eastern Speech, and Southern Speech. The phonetic variations grossly associated with these regions are relatively few in number. The meaning of even these variations within the theory proposed by Rousey will be discussed later.

All other variations are considered indications that the child, adolescent, or adult is struggling with significant and conflictual emotional dilemmas. Such an apparent extreme position results in strong reactions by persons who are reluctant to see emotional problems in children or by linguists who are committed to the view that sound production is a cognitive act which at most can be influenced by environmentarl factors or ethnic or racial background. Rousey's position is often criticized as failing to take into account the principle of multiple determination. Such a principle is valid primarily for symbolic language behavior whether spoken, printed, or transmitted through body movement. As already noted, such behavior is not the same as speech production. Further, both Hartmann[25] and Anna Freud[19] have suggested that some forms of behavior can have very specific meanings. Thus, the principle of multiple determination need not be considered as a fixed psychological reality. Further, the position that explains speech behavior as primarily cog-

nitive and environmental cannot so parsimoniously cope with all the individual variations seen, even with a tightly defined racial or geographic unit. Thus, the need exists for a theoretical position which is more generally applicable.

The "normal" variance in speech (sound) production between cultures occurs primarily on vowels as opposed to consonants and is understandable in terms of drive expression among differing national personalities. For example, a defensible stereotype of the speech of persons from England is that their sounds are clipped. In general, this means the duration of the vowels is shortened. If the stereotype of the English as affectively constricted and inhibited is correct, and vowel sounds as posited by Rousey are the primary way of discharge for aggression and sexual drives, then the sound pattern of individuals from England is not surprising. A similar argument, although on the other end of the affect discharge continuum, can be made for speakers of Spanish. That is, the greater emphasis on vowels as compared with speakers of general American speech appears to be related to the "freer" discharge of drives in Spanish cultures. The preceding examples do not imply that such characteristics are common to all persons from England or Latin American countries, but rather that the role of culture in shaping of emotions is observable in a general way through a person's speech patterns. Examination of phonemic characteristics of other nationalities (e.g., German, Chinese, etc.) should reflect distinctive patterns of drive expression. Labov[36] attempted to equate sound variation (especially vowels) to differences in social structure. His data can also be interpreted as reflecting cultural variations in drive expression. For example, he noted ". . . that high centralization of (ay) and (aw) is closely correlated with expressions of strong resistance to the incursions of summer people" (p. 28).* Finally, the person who moves to a new geographical area does, indeed, often suffer greater than usual emotional stresses, and the maintenance of dialect is seen as suggestive of failure to make a complete emotional as well as physical move.

It will be recalled that earlier in this chapter more articulation problems (presumably in consonant sounds) were noted in lower socioeconomic classes and in black children. Such findings are not seen as contradicting the thesis of Rousey but rather as reflecting the emotional stresses of dis-

---

* He is talking about the effect of tourists on the stable population of Martha's Vineyard in Massachusetts.

rupted object relationships and emotional deprivation often experienced in our society by such groups. These findings do not mean that a person with better economic means or social class has fewer or different emotional problems, but rather that emotional symptomatology may be expressed in different aspects of speech behavior than have to date been studied. For example, such psychiatric factors as depression, thought organization, etc., are displayed in other forms of speech behavior such as voice quality and pitch.

Within the present chapter it is not feasible to present the total data and theory which relate speech sounds to both normal and psychopathological emotional development. It is possible to provide some basic tenets of the theory and to note some of the relevant studies completed with children. Basic to understanding how consonants reflect both psychological conflicts and object relationships is a specific psychological reference point for each consonant sound. Although less emphasis is currently attached to psychosexual development by some psychoanalytic writers, Rousey made the following assumptions:

Using Erikson's (1950) discussion of infantile sexuality, the sound "m," "p," "w," "h," "y" as in yellow, "l," "n," and "t" are hypothesized as belonging to the oral respiratory-sensory stage, while "b," "f," "k," "g," and "d" are hypothesized as reflecting the oral-biting stage. The "ch" as in church and the "j" as in judge are felt associated with the anal-expulsive stage, while the "s," "r," "sh" and "z" as in azure are theorized as reflecting the anal-retentive stage. In conclusion, the voiceless "th" as in thanks, the "v," the voiced "th" as in them, and the "z" as in zoo are sounds believed associated with the phallic period. (p. 8)[50]

Using these assumptions, Kernberg and Rousey[34] have reported in detail the relation between speech and psychological behavior of an eight and one-half-year-old white male over the course of psychotherapy. One speech error of this child consisted of the child substituting the *f* for the voiceless *th* sound. Thus, the child would say *bof* instead of *both*. Elsewhere Rousey[50] posits this error as being related to conflict between the child (gender of the patient is not a factor) and father. The conflict is further specified as related to a deprivation in early father-child psychological interaction with a resulting confusion over sexual identity and role. Study of the initial social history and psychological tests of the case in question supports the psychological distance and probable deprivation in interaction by the father as well as problems with sexual identity. The father reported not only being uncomfortable about having a son, but also stated openly he would have been more comfortable with a girl. In addition, he feared his son would take his wife away from him and played the role of a son with his wife. Projective material gathered from analysis of human figure drawings of the patient clearly demonstrated confusion over his own sexual identity. When his speech behavior was studied at the end of psychotherapy, the substitution of *f* for the voiceless *th* sound had disappeared. His therapist noted that the patient now felt very much like a growing young man. He was able to demonstrate his differentiation of male-female roles.

Of importance to a therapist is the finding that not only positive psychological changes are reflected in speech behavior, but also one can ascertain psychological work which remains to be done. In the case of the aforementioned patient the final speech examination also revealed a propensity toward somatization. This inference was based on an auditory test which is a part of the standard speech examination[50] and allows the examiner to discover various defenses. The inferred use of somatization was confirmed by the therapist in her final discharge summary which was written without knowledge of the speech test.

The possibility for speech behavior to be interpreted in terms of emotional status may well be of crucial importance as an increased need develops for independent evaluation of psychiatric intervention. Another dimension of use for this approach is in evaluation of the chances for a successful therapeutic process. Success in psychotherapy is a difficult concept to define to everyone's satisfaction. However, Rousey and Levy[54] have demonstrated, in a group of twenty patients judged by the therapist as profiting from therapy and twenty patients judged by the therapist as not profiting from therapy, that it is possible to make a highly accurate prediction of how the therapist will judge the outcome of a treatment process if the initial psychiatric diagnostic impression is compared with a psychiatric diagnosis compatible with data from the speech examination. For example, if a psychiatric diagnosis of obsessive-compulsive neurosis is made and there are no articulation errors consonant with such a diagnosis, then there is about a 90 percent chance of the therapist conceiving of the treatment as a failure. Conversely, if the speech data contain errors supportive of a diagnosis of obsessive-compulsive neurosis, then there is about a 90 percent chance that the therapist will conceive of the treatment as a success. Similar examples can be given for other psychiatric diagnoses. The therapist apparently treats a patient on the basis of diagnosis to a closer degree than most clinicians imagine. Although there are many possible explanations of this striking finding, a parsimonious one would hold that, as in other branches of medicine, an accurate diagnosis is a prime requirement for successful treatment.

In the foregoing examples, attention has been paid primarily to consonant production and its psychodynamic meaning. Attending to how the patient produces vowels is equally rewarding from a diagnostic and prognostic sense. Earlier it was noted that vowels are believed to reflect both aggressive and libidinal drives. Thus, the angry roar of a crowd at an athletic contest when an official makes an obviously incorrect call is a straightforward expression of aggression. The dominant acoustic sound in such a situation can best be categorized as a vowel. Similarly, the contented cooing of an infant or the lullaby of a mother (both expressive of a love relationship) are also basically vowel sounds. Both of the foregoing examples represent experiences of drive discharge common to many persons.

It becomes possible to infer psychopathology when vowel sounds are substituted and proper allowance is made for the cultural norms of the individual. Thus, if a male adolescent were to consistently substitute the vowel *e* as in the word *sell* for the vowel *a* as in the word *sale*, we would have an expression of psychopathology which would predate the kinds of conflict which have earlier been inferred when consonant substitutions occur. In this instance, because we know that adolescent males struggle with drive expression, it is possible to infer the likelihood the person would have committed a sexual and aggressive attack. If such an adolescent had speech difficulties suggestive of conflict with only maternal figures, the further inference would be made that such an attack would be made on females. Vowel difficulties are also apparent through such voice disorders as hoarseness, breathiness, and the like. For example, in the case of hoarseness with no basis due to an active disease process, it is readily demonstrable that there is almost invariably an inappropriate hyper-masculine and aggressive stance in relationships with others.

Use of speech in making a psychiatric diagnosis of a child should also assist in understanding the psychiatric status of the parents. Indeed, the findings should be complementary since the emotional life of the child reflects the early psychological interaction with the parents, and the psychological functioning of the parents largely determines how they will interact with their children. Analysis of the speech behavior of the parents should also allow one to ascertain with reasonable certainty the probable state of internalized objects of the child. Understanding speech behavior in such a dynamic way offers potential help to the psychiatric social worker.

Many therapists are accustomed to attending to their own countertransference responses exhibited either through words or behavior. A therapist who is in tune not only with the foregoing but also his own speech sounds has another cue to use. Thus, where the therapist hears a sharp whistle suddenly developing on his sibilant sounds, he needs to be aware of rapidly developing anxiety. If such a whistle is not usually present, the anxiety is probably reactive in nature. Contrary to popular belief, interdental spacing does not cause whistling sibilants. If the therapist hears other sound substitutions by himself, it is possible to spot and hopefully analyze the arousal of old, unresolved conflicts.

The dynamic meanings of speech sounds may also be used in the diagnosis and treatment of stuttering. Assuming a thorough neurological and physical examination has ruled out organic factors, study of where stuttering occurs may be clinically helpful. Where psychogenic factors are prominent, clinical observation of the present writer suggests stuttering may occur mostly on sounds and syllables. Study of the specific sounds involved will help specify the genetic level of the conflict. In word or phrase repetitions, the clinical picture is often, but not exclusively, suggestive of a neurological dysfunction of a subtle nature.

Numerous clinical research studies have been completed investigating speech behavior and psychological functioning. In addition to the studies already mentioned, Filippi and Rousey[18] describe how children's speech behavior can be used to study not only object relations but also affect and impulse expression. Decker and Rousey[13] describe detection of minimal brain dysfunction through speech behavior. Mehrhof and Rousey[41] discuss recognition of self-destructive potential through speech behavior. Norris[45] gives a clinical example of how sound omissions are related to intelligence. Of particular importance is the use of changes in speech behavior as an independent indicator of psychological change not only during psychotherapy but also as a result of treatment in a therapeutic nursery school[69] and as a result of a group process.[16] Sehdev and Rousey[57] have also demonstrated how underachievement is identified through sound variations and how the procedure can be used to facilitate the diagnostic process either in an established child guidance program or in community mental health work.[58] The close relationship of hearing to psychopathology (as a function of both dynamic and neurological causes) is emphasized in material of Switzer and Rousey[63] and Rousey and Goetzinger.[53] The foregoing material can be integrated within the usual psychiatric examination by use of the classification and diagnostic schema proposed by Morrow.[44] Deviations in speech and language may be viewed both developmentally and as manifestations of intrapsychic, environmental, developmental, structural, and dynamic factors.

LANGUAGE BEHAVIOR

Probably the most extensive exposition of the dynamic meanings of individual words has been provided by Thass-Theineman.[65, 66] His work does not focus specifically on children but rather on language and its etymology. In contrast Steingart and Freedman,[62] using more conventional psycholinguistic terms, are able to examine self-object representation through language in varying clinical states. They summarize the work of numerous researchers with regard to elements of grammar found in varying clinical states. While this work is concerned for the most part with older patients, the findings have relevance for child psychiatry. For example, research suggests neurotic patients show more use of substantives, adjectives, prepositions, conjunctions, and articles than normals. Obsessive patients use more "qualifying" adverbs and adjectives with the converse being true in conversion hysterics. Other research noted by Steingart and Freedman indicates less use of the personal pronoun *I* and more use of the pro-he, she, we and you among patients who are improving.

In their own work Steingart and Freedman contend ". . . language behavior variation in the selective use of syntactic competence to provide relational information is mediated by the degree of differentiation between self- and object-representation. . . ." [p. 166][62]

The importance of Steingart and Freedman's efforts centers around the bridge they began to build between psychoanalytic theory and psycholinguistics. It is important to note that psycholinguistics in its current focus attends largely to cognitive meanings of words while psychiatry and psychoanalysis attend largely to the emotional component of language. If it develops that cooperation is possible between varying disciplines

through Steingart and Freedman's efforts, the way will be open for significant gains in understanding both the cognitive and pschodynamic meanings of language.

Bradford[7] has reviewed in the most comprehensive fashion to date the psychodynamic factors which affect hearing. He makes a refined differentiation of impairment of hearing as a function of hysteria as opposed to impaired hearing which binds a psychotic or borderline personality organization state. The effect on language is dependent upon the time of fusion of the psychiatric state and the psychogenic deafness.

LEARNING AND BEHAVIOR THEORY

The role of learning and behavior theory in the understanding of speech disorders can be most efficiently discussed by considering speech and language separately. Basic to such consideration are the underlying assumptions that both speech and language development can be modified by a cognitive structure which is externally imposed, and that emotions play at most a secondary role. This position is derived from the early observations of neurologists, the later work of ego-psychology and the current interests of psycholinguists.

In terms of sound development, Chomsky and Halle's[10] publication, explaining the distinctive features of the sounds of English, must be considered a basic reference. McReynolds and Huston[40] have used such concepts in developing a treatment program based on learning principles. Chomsky's influence is also evident in Brown's recent volume[8] on language. In brief, it is Brown's position that the primary determinants of how language is progressively acquired are reflected in a cumulative way by both semantic and grammatical factors. Further, he concludes that while the order of acquisition is similar across children learning the same language, the reason which impels the child to improve is still unknown. He feels that earlier linguistic assumptions about telegraphic and pivot grammar in the beginning stages of language are currently untenable. Throughout his and Chomsky's entire approach there is an omission of affective factors as a parameter involved in language acquisition and growth.

NEUROLOGICAL AND BIOLOGICAL THEORY

There has always been a strong disposition to see speech and language as a reflection of a neurological and physical state. This reflects the early interests of physicians in the treatment and diagnosis of language disturbances following cerebral vascular attacks. Lenneberg's[37] position relating language primarily to a person's biological characteristics appears to express the assumption of many current psycholinguists. In 1967 Millikan and Darley[43] edited a volume describing the state of neurological theory with reference to language. The pioneer studies of Penfield and Roberts[46] have already mapped out the essential cortical areas of language. The contributors to Millikan and Darley's volume considered in greater detail such topics as the contribution of the various cortical areas to speech and language functions, the relationship between cross-modal effects and language, and hemispheric connections and language. Speech disorders from a neurological standpoint are usually placed under the rubric of dysarthria. Darley further defines dysarthria: "Originally, it simply referred to an affectation of articulation, but nowadays we extend it to include neurogenic problems in all the basic aspects of execution of the speech act: respiration, phonation, articulation, resonance and prosody." [p. 237][12]

Therapy

The treatment of communication disorders largely reflects the theory used. This statement is illustrated nowhere more clearly than when one examines the range of treatment for articulation disorders. The point of view which maintains that speech behavior reflects drives and object relations necessarily dictates its treatment by psychotherapy.[50] In their summary of treatment of articulation disorders, Weston and Rampp[71] describe phonetic placement based on the assumption there are standard ways to adjust the tongue, lips, etc., and the moto-kinesthetic method which assumes that by correct movement of the articulators the child will develop a proper kinesthetic pattern. Both of these approaches are tied closely to a neurological understanding of speech production. With the advent of learning theory the patient was taught to hear the correct and incorrect sound production (called Ear Training). Interpersonal assumptions led to the use of group interaction in facilitating articulation development.[3] Most recently, Weston and Irwin have

developed a technique called paired-stimulus which is based on Skinner's assumptions. They write:

Skinner's (1957) basic paradigm—discriminatory stimulus, response, and contingent reinforcer—is exemplified in the paired-stimulus approach. The stimulus is the picture-presentation situation; the response is the articulation of a selected phoneme; the reinforcer is a value-ratio token, whose acceleration of desired behavior is empirically determined. (p. 947)[70]

Treatment of voice disorders, following proper laryngeal diagnosis, again follows naturally from the conceptual understanding of the problem. Apart from psychotherapeutic intervention which is based on an understanding of the conflict expressed by the vocal symptom, there are manipulative techniques which stem from assuming a habit disorder with the resultant need for learning new skills. The works of Boone,[5] Cooper,[11] and Perkins[47] adequately describe this approach. In instances of laryngectomy, where the patient must learn esophageal speech, learning approaches combined with psychotherapy are useful.

The state of treatment of stuttering is similar to the problems well known to psychiatrists in the treatment of such psychiatric problems as schizophrenia. Thus, while the symptomatology may be straightforward, almost every conceivable form of treatment has been attempted with no clear-cut advantage being apparent in any form of therapy.[67] Part of the treatment problem undoubtedly rests in treating the symptom of stuttering as if it were indicative of a single etiology.

In the case of language disorders caused by organic insult, a careful diagnosis has to be made to determine whether receptive language is intact and whether there is significant motor impairment of the speech articulators. Assuming good receptive language, recovery of expressive language is generally, but not universally, excellent. This is probably so regardless of the stimulation techniques used by the speech pathologist or clinician. If receptive language is impaired because of central nervous system damage, the prognosis for recovery becomes poorer, although spontaneous recovery in children seems to occur up until about age seven or eight years. The teaching of language to remediate problems with syntax and acquisition is a recent undertaking by speech pathologists, and independent judgments of its value and success are not yet crystallized. Treatment of communication disorders caused by hearing loss is usually necessary only with sensorineural losses. If there are no complications such as speech discrimination difficulties, impaired intelligence, or significant neurological involvement of the peripheral speech mechanism, etc., a hearing aid may be indicated, and its use usually brings about improvements in speech and language.

The finding that psychotherapeutic changes are reflected by speech behavior suggests that most professional workers who treat children or ado-

lescents have been providing excellent care for speech disorders. The task in the years ahead is for interdisciplinary efforts between speech pathologists and the usual psychiatric team, so that knowledge common to the various professions involved can be shared with a resulting improved care for the child or adolescent.

REFERENCES

1. American Psychiatric Association, *Diagnostic and Statistical Manual of Mental Disorders* (DSM-II), 2nd ed., American Psychiatric Association, Washington, D.C., 1968.

2. ANGELOCCI, A., KOPP, G., and HOLBROOK, A., "The Vowel Formants of Deaf and Normal-Hearing Eleven- to Fourteen-Year-Old Boys," *Journal of Speech and Hearing Disorders, 29:*156–170, 1964.

3. BACKUS, O., and BEASLEY, J., *Speech Therapy with Children,* Houghton Mifflin, Boston, 1951.

4. BERG, F., "Educational Audiology," in Berg, F., and Fletcher, S. (Eds.), *The Hard of Hearing Child,* pp. 275–318, Grune & Stratton, New York, 1970.

5. BOONE, D., *The Voice and Voice Therapy,* Prentice-Hall, Englewood Cliffs, N.J., 1971.

6. BOWER, E., *Early Identification of Emotionally Handicapped Children in School,* 2nd ed., Charles C Thomas, Springfield, Ill., 1969.

7. BRADFORD, L. (Ed.), *Physiological Measures of the Audio-Vestibular System,* Academic Press, New York, 1975.

8. BROWN, R., *A First Language,* Harvard University Press, Cambridge, Mass., 1973.

9. CARRELL, J., and TIFFANY, W., *Phonetics: Theory and Application to Speech Improvement,* McGraw-Hill Book Company, New York, 1960.

10. CHOMSKY, N., and HALLE, M., *The Sound Pattern of English,* Harper & Row, New York, 1968.

11. COOPER, M., *Modern Techniques of Vocal Rehabilitation,* Charles C Thomas, Springfield, Ill., 1973.

12. DARLEY, F., "Lacunae and Research, Approaches to Them-IV," in Millikan, C., and Darley, F. (Eds.), *Brain Mechanisms Underlying Speech and Language,* pp. 236–240, Grune & Stratton, New York, 1967.

13. DECKER, L., and ROUSEY, C., "Speech Indicators of Neurological Dysfunction," in Rousey, C. (Ed.), *Psychiatric Assessment by Speech and Hearing Behavior,* pp. 291–302, Charles C Thomas, Springfield, Ill., 1974.

14. DE HIRSCH, K., "Language Disturbances," in Freedman, A., and Kaplan, H. (Eds.), *Comprehensive Textbook of Psychiatry,* pp. 1376–1380, Williams & Wilkins, Baltimore, Md., 1967.

15. ERIKSON, E., *Childhood and Society,* W. W. Norton, New York, 1950.

16. FAGUNDES, J., "A Study on Training Groups with Student Nurses," Graduation Thesis, Menninger School of Psychiatry, Topeka, Kansas, 1974.

17. FILIPPI, R., and ROUSEY, C., "Delay in Onset of Talking: A Symptom of Interpersonal Disturbance," *Journal of the Academy of Child Psychiatry, 17(2):*316–329, 1968.

18. ———, "Positive Carriers of Violence Among Children: Detection by Speech Deviations," *Mental Hygiene, 55(2):*157–161, 1971.

19. FREUD, A., "Links Between Hartmann's Ego Psychology and the Child Analyst's Thinking," in Loewenstein, R. M., et al. (Eds.), *Psychoanalysis—A General Psychology,* pp. 16–27, International Universities Press, New York, 1966.

20. FRIEDMAN, M., and ROSENMAN, R., *Type A Behavior and Your Heart,* Knopf, New York, 1974.

21. GOLDSTEIN, K., *Language and Language Disturbances,* Grune & Stratton, New York, 1948.

22. GORDON, D., *Survey of Speech Articulation Disorders Among Military Dependent Children,* Office of Education, U.S. Department of Health, Education and Welfare, 1972.

23. Group for the Advancement of Psychiatry, Committee on Child Psychiatry, *Psychopathological Disorders in Childhood: Theoretical Considerations and a Proposed Classification,* vol. 6, Report no. 62, Group for the Advancement of Psychiatry, New York, 1966.

24. HALL, W. F., "A Study of the Articulation Skills of Children from Three to Six Years of Age," Unpublished doctoral dissertation, University of Missouri, 1962.

25. HARTMANN, H., "Psychoanalysis and Developmental Psychology," in his *Essays on Ego Psychology,* pp. 99–112, International Universities Press, New York, 1964.

26. ———, "Ego Psychology and the Problem of Adaptation," in Rapoport, D. (Ed.), *Organization and Pathology of Thought,* Columbia University Press, New York, 1951.

27. HEAD, H., *Aphasia and Kindred Disorders of Speech,* Macmillan, New York, 1926.

28. HEALEY, W. C., "A Study of the Articulatory Skills of Children from Six to Nine Years of Age," Unpublished doctoral dissertation, University of Missouri, 1963.

29. HECKER, M. H. L., and KREUL, E. J., *Research on Speech Changes Related to Disease,* SRI Project 7742, 8853, Stanford Research Institute, Menlo Park, Calif., 1974.

30. HICK, J. S., "Language Disabilities of Hearing Impaired Children," in Irwin, J., and Marge, M. (Eds.), *Principles of Childhood Language Disabilities,* pp. 137–158, Appleton-Century-Crofts, New York, 1972.

31. HUDGINS, C., and NUMBERS, C., *An Investigation of the Intelligibility of the Speech of the Deaf,* Genetic Psychology Monographs, 25, 1942.

32. IRWIN, O. C., "Infant Speech: Consonantal Sounds According to Place of Articulation," *Journal of Speech and Hearing Disorders, 12:*397–401, 1947.

33. ———, "Infant Speech: Development of Vowel Sounds," *Journal of Speech and Hearing Disorders, 13:* 31–34, 1948.

34. KERNBERG, P., and ROUSEY, C., "Variations in Speech Sounds During Psychotherapy: An Independent Indicator of Change," *American Academy of Child Psychiatry, 9(4):*762–777, 1970.

35. KONIGSMARK, B., "Hereditary Deafness in Man," *New England Journal of Medicine, 281:*713–720, 774–778, 827–832, 1969.

36. LABOV, W., *Sociolinguistic Patterns,* University of Pennsylvania Press, Philadelphia, 1972.

37. LENNEBERG, E., *Biological Foundations of Language,* John Wiley, New York, 1967.

38. LUCHSINGER, R., and ARNOLD, G., *Voice-Speech-Language,* Wadsworth Publishing, Belmont, Calif., 1965.

39. McDONALD, E., *Articulation Testing and Treatment:*

A Sensory-Motor Approach, Stanwik House, Pittsburgh, 1964.

40. McReynolds, L., and Huston, K., "A Distinctive Feature Analysis of Children's Misarticulations," *Journal of Speech and Hearing Disorders, 36(2):*155–166, 1971.

41. Mehrhof, E., and Rousey, C., "Speech Difficulties Symptomatic of Destructive Behavior Toward Self or Others," *Journal of Nervous and Mental Disease, 152(1):* 63–67, 1971.

42. Milisen, R., "The Incidence of Speech Disorders," in Travis, L. E. (Ed.), *Handbook of Speech Pathology and Audiology*, pp. 619–633, Appleton-Century-Crofts, New York, 1971.

43. Millikan, C., and Darley, F. (Eds.), *Brain Mechanisms Underlying Speech and Language*, Grune & Stratton, New York, 1967.

44. Morrow, J. T., Jr., "Factors of Classification in Diagnosis and Treatment Planning," in Rousey, C. L. (Ed.), *Psychiatric Assessment by Speech and Hearing Behavior*, pp. 24–54, Charles C Thomas, Springfield, Ill., 1974.

45. Norris, V., "Speech Disturbances and the Assessment of Mental Retardation in Children," in Rousey, C. L. (Ed.), *Psychiatric Assessment by Speech and Hearing Behavior*, pp. 211–227, Charles C Thomas, Springfield, Ill., 1974.

46. Penfield, W., and Roberts, L., *Speech and Brain Mechanisms*, Princeton University Press, Princeton, N.J., 1959.

47. Perkins, W., "Vocal Function: Assessment and Therapy," in Travis, L. (Ed.), *Handbook of Speech Pathology and Audiology*, pp. 505–534, Appleton-Century-Crofts, New York, 1971.

48. Ranier, J., and Altshuler, K. (Eds.), *Psychiatry and the Deaf*, U.S. Government Printing Office, Washington, D.C., 1968.

49. Rousey, Carol, "Voice Analysis of Coronary Heart Disease, High Risk and Normal Control Individuals," Unpublished Ph.D. Dissertation, University of Kansas, 1975.

50. Rousey, C. (Ed.), *Psychiatric Assessment by Speech and Hearing Behavior*, Charles C Thomas, Springfield, Ill., 1974.

51. ———, "Psychological Reactions to Hearing Loss," *Journal of Speech and Hearing Disorders, 36(3):*382–389, 1971.

52. ———, and Diedrich, W., "Tracing Symptom Change," Unpublished manuscript, 1975.

53. ———, and Goetzinger, C. P., "Auditory Dysfunction in Schizophrenic Patients," *Journal of Auditory Research, 10(2):*180–184, 1970.

54. ———, and Levy, E., "Predicting Outcome of Psychotherapy," Unpublished manuscript, 1975.

55. ———, Moriarty, A., *Diagnostic Implications of Speech Sounds*, Charles C Thomas, Springfield, Ill., 1965.

56. ———, and Toussieng, P., "Contributions of a Speech Pathologist to the Psychiatric Examination of Children," *Mental Hygiene, 48(4):*566–575, 1964.

57. Sehdev, H., and Rousey, C., "Speech Deviation: Indicator of Underachievement," in Rousey, C. (Ed.), *Psychiatric Assessment by Speech and Hearing Behavior*, pp. 328–336, Charles C Thomas, Springfield, Ill., 1974.

58. ———, "Delivery of Mental Health Services: A New Approach," in Rousey, C. (Ed.), *Psychiatric Assessment by Speech and Hearing Behavior*, pp. 170–178, Charles C Thomas, Springfield, Ill., 1974.

59. Sheehan, J., *Stuttering: Research and Therapy*, Harper & Row, New York, 1970.

60. Skinner, B. F., *Verbal Behavior*, Appleton-Century-Crofts, New York, 1957.

61. Smith, C., "Residual Hearing and Speech Production in Deaf Children," Unpublished Ph.D. dissertation, City College of New York, 1972.

62. Steingart, I., and Freedman, N., "A Language Construction Approach for the Examination of Self/Object Representation in Varying Clinical States," in Holt, R., and Peterfreund, E. (Eds.), *Psychoanalysis and Contemporary Science*, pp. 132–178, Macmillan, New York, 1972.

63. Switzer, R., and Rousey, C., "Audiological Assessment of the Child Psychiatric Patient: A Case Example," in Rousey, C. (Ed.), *Psychiatric Assessment by Speech and Hearing Behavior*, pp. 277–283, Charles C Thomas, Springfield, Ill., 1974.

64. Templin, M., *Certain Language Skills in Children*, Institute of Child Welfare Monograph Series, No. 26, University of Minnesota Press, Minneapolis, 1957.

65. Thass-Theineman, T., *Symbolic Behavior*, Washington Square Press, New York, 1968.

66. ———, *The Subconscious Language*, Washington Square Press, New York, 1967.

67. Van Riper, C., *The Treatment of Stuttering*, Prentice-Hall, Englewood Cliffs, N.J., 1973.

68. ———, *The Nature of Stuttering*, Prentice-Hall, Englewood Cliffs, N.J., 1971.

69. Ware, L., and Rousey, C., "Assessment of Change in a Therapeutic Preschool Program," Unpublished paper, 1975.

70. Weston, A., and Irwin, J., "Use of Paired Stimuli in Modification of Articulation," *Perceptual and Motor Skills, 32:*947–957, 1971.

71. ———, and Rampp, D., "Articulation Intervention," in Wingo, J. W., and Holloway, G. (Eds.), *An Appraisal of Speech Pathology and Audiology*, pp. 96–114, Charles C Thomas, Springfield, Ill., 1973.

24 / Elective Mutism

Paul C. Laybourne, Jr.

The disorder known today as elective mutism was first described as aphasia voluntaria. Some authors have referred to it as selective mutism. The current DSM-II diagnosis is: "withdrawing reaction of childhood" (308.1).[1] In the GAP (Group for Advancement of Psychiatry) classification the syndrome is properly designated as: "overly inhibited personality, elective mutism."[7]

Description of the Syndrome

PRIMARY ELECTIVE MUTISM

Children who manifest elective mutism characteristically refuse to speak in school and to strangers. However, they can, and do, speak to specific people, usually one or both parents. Sometimes they speak to peers, or to certain peers, and they nearly always speak to their siblings. Although they tend to be shy and somewhat withdrawn, many of these children function effectively on a nonverbal level. They are characteristically immature. Most of them have average or above average intelligence, and, in general, they display no evidence of any organic disorder.

SECONDARY FORMS OF THE DISORDER

There are a number of other conditions in which failure to speak is part of the symptomotology. This may occur in cases of hearing loss, schizophrenia, hysterical aphonia, and aphasia. In none of these is the mutism elective in the same sense as in the primary form, and they should not be given this designation.

Review of the Literature

The earliest descriptions of elective mutism are found in the German literature. Von Misch[19] reported that in 1877, Kussmaul had used the term aphasia voluntaria to describe mentally sound persons who forced themselves into mutism for purposes they refused to disclose. Tramer,[18] in 1934, coined the term elective mutism to describe children who were silent in all of their interpersonal contacts with the exception of a small circle of intimate friends and relatives. In 1945, he interpreted the infantile shyness of mute children in the presence of strangers as "an archaic defense reflex retained abnormally long." Von Misch observed that: (1) environmental factors may precipitate mutism; (2) mutism often occurred upon the child's separation from the family, especially at the time of his entry into school; (3) while heredity and intelligence may play some part, the disorder was basically psychogenic; (4) all cases demonstrated excessive ties to the mother; and (5) the selection of mutism as a symptom was perhaps related to a traumatic experience at the time the child was developing speech.

In 1963, Browne, Wilson, and Laybourne[4] emphasized the use of the symptom to punish a parent. They were particularly impressed with the neurotic split in the families of these children. The mute child characteristically identified with one of the parents. He or she would side with that parent against the other and refuse to speak in order to punish him or her.

Cultural and Hereditary Factors

Little is known about the natural history, frequency, and distribution of elective mutism. In talking with teachers of latency age children, one gets the impression that it is not an uncommon disorder in the school age child. At the same time, the diagnosis is only rarely recorded by child psychiatric clinics. School personnel tend to deal with it by benign neglect on the assumption that the child is shy and that the problem will go away. This assumption is not necessarily correct. The author's case series, as well as those reported in the literature, contain patients who were referred for the first time as young adolescents.

It is difficult to establish the frequency of the disorder in the population, as well as to ascertain whether there is any difference between the numbers of boys and girls who do not speak. The literature suggests that girls are more likely to suffer from elective mutism than boys, but the numbers reported are so small that they probably lack statistical significance.

There are some families in which more than one child is mute, but this appears to be more a product of the so-called "twinning reaction" than of any genetic predisposition. There are a few accounts of mute twins in the literature, but again the numbers are too small to allow for valid conclusions. In those families where there are two electively mute children, the children appear to be very dependent upon each other. More than that, they tend to support and reinforce the symptom in one another.

Clinical Course and Associated Clinical Experience

Young children are frequently shy and reticent around strangers, and it is not uncommon for the preschool child to fall silent when spoken to by a stranger. Within such a context, even if the mother encourages the small child to talk, he may not only remain mute but actually attempt to hide behind his parent. This behavior is probably related to the fear seen in eighth-month anxiety. Phylogenetically, it may have served a primitive race preservative function, since most small, herd mammals will go to the parent and remain silent in the presence of danger. This reticence persists in many children up to the time they enter school. Many kindergarten and first-grade teachers have had children in their classes who were mute the first few days of school, and who began to speak only after they became accustomed to the teachers and other children. Elective mutes, however, are those children who do not spontaneously abandon this behavior. They may maintain their stubborn silence in the school setting for years. The long-range outcome of the untreated elective mute is unknown. Since the syndrome is not described in the adult psychiatric literature, it can be assumed that they eventually talk enough to cease to be identified as "electively mute." Follow-up studies of these children indicate that they do not all begin speaking in school. This may hold true even though they were treated in a hospital setting and they changed to a different school upon discharge.

Despite the fact that most authors define elective mutism as beginning in the early preschool years and manifesting itself upon entry into school, Kaplan and Escoll[9] have described a form of adolescent elective mutism which has its onset after the age of twelve years. This variety differs from the early onset form in that the patients do not talk to their family nor to strangers. Moreover, in these cases the chief complaint was not failure to talk but "stealing, conversion reaction, and suicide attempts." The authors postulate different dynamics for this disorder. In the cases that they present, the failure to talk seems to be only one symptom of a more global disturbance than that associated with the childhood form. Reed[15] has proposed that the syndrome be split into two categories on the basis of function of the symptom, which he feels can represent: (1) a normal learned behavior used as an attention getting mechanism; or (2) a fear-reducing device. The latter formulation is that proposed by most authors and presumably applies in the majority of cases. Clinical experience does confirm, however, that some of the children are not particularly sensitive and shy; indeed, they rather enjoy the attention that their behavior attracts. The following case is illustrative of such a child.

Richard was brought to a university Division of Child Psychiatry at the age of five, because he would talk only to family members and close friends of the family. His mother said the problem started when Richard was three years old. At first, when he would turn and walk away from strangers who spoke to him, she thought it was "cute."

At the time of his initial evaluation, he was enrolled in preschool but spoke to no one at school. With the encouragement of their pediatrician, the parents decided to seek help before he entered regular school. The first time that he was brought to the clinic, he spoke openly to his mother in the waiting room. During the evaluation, however, he did not speak to the psychiatrist. Instead, he barked like a dog and made numerous sounds in a manner not at all typical of the behavior seen in a frightened, reticent child. During the evaluation of the parents, it became evident that neither had loved the other at the time of their marriage. They both acknowledged that Richard was neither planned for, nor wanted. The father complained that the mother "nuzzled, kissed, overindulged Richard." One month after the initial interview, the mother called and asked the therapist to see her and her husband because they were getting a divorce. This had not been revealed during the evaluation. A few weeks later, the father divorced the mother and left the country with a new bride. The mother found the situation difficult to accept. When the father returned to the area a few months later, she was pleased to note that Richard refused to speak to the father's new wife. The therapist tried to discourage the mother from infantilizing Richard. Nonetheless, she continued to treat him like a baby, even wiping him after a bowel movement (although by this time he was six years old and quite capable of caring for himself). Parallel with her overindulging behavior, she continued to complain of her son's immature behavior and temper tantrums. Despite the fact that she had been seen for nine months on a weekly basis, the mother had never told Richard that she expected him to talk in school. Since that was considered a critical communication between the child and his mother, it was finally suggested to her that if she could not change her ways and expect age-appropriate behavior from Richard, perhaps, residential treatment should be considered. Faced with the threat of separation from her child, and one year and one month after the beginning of treatment, she finally told him that he must talk in school. Much to the surprise and delight of the teachers and other children, Richard thereupon spoke in class. A short time later he was speaking to everyone except his therapist. Since it was felt to be unimportant whether he ever spoke to his therapist or not, he was terminated and considered successfully treated. A five-year follow-up showed no problem in the area of communication, but he was showing some disciplinary disturbances in that he was obeying the teacher and his mother rather poorly.

This case was treated before behavior modification became a well-known form of therapeutic intervention. Currently, in the view of the author, this form of elective mutism responds best to the techniques of behavior modification. It was hypothesized that Richard's symptom probably developed because early in life his parents thought that his mute behavior was cute and reinforced it. Later, the mother was pleased when the child punished his father by refusing to talk to his stepmother and continued to encourage the preservation of the symptom. The symptom finally disappeared when the mother was told she would have to change the way she related to the child. In effect, the message was: either she must give up her symbiotic relationship with him, or he would be placed in residential treatment. She responded to this contingency by telling him for the first time that he must talk to people. It was at this point that he began to talk to the teacher and the children at school. Once verbal communication was underway, he demonstrated his good intelligence (IQ 120) and his ability to read as well as the other children in his class. His good school achievement is typical of many elective mutes who obtain credit each year on the basis of their written work. The family structure showed classical neurotic splitting: the mother and child formed an immature, symbiotic unit which was allied against the father. The symptom grew out of this mother-child unity and was employed to punish the father.

At the other end of the spectrum is the shy, inhibited, schizoid child. It is obvious that family pathology can never be ignored in the production of this symptom, yet in this group, the mutism seems rather determined by temperament than by family pathology.

Judy, a thirteen-year-old female, was referred to a university division of child psychiatry for a combination of failure to talk in school and extreme negativism. She had been evaluated at the age of six for the same symptoms, but the parents had not followed through with the recommended treatment. This may well have been because her mother was admitted to the inpatient section of the department for treatment of her own severe depression. At that time, the history revealed that Judy did not speak unless she was alone with her family. This had started after her brother had lacerated her head with a Coca-Cola bottle when she was four. Since the family did not follow through with the psychotherapeutic intervention recommended at age six, Judy spent the next seven years in several different schools, manifesting an unbroken record of mutism. For at least the last three years before her second referral, she was under the direction of an experienced and capable principal, who exercised great ingenuity in setting up situations to trap her into talking, all without success. Virtually every school counselor and speech therapist who encountered her had enthusiastically attacked Judy's problem for a while and had then given up.

At the time of her second evaluation, Judy was just thirteen years old. She was physically normal except for being chronically dirty and unkempt. The second of six children, she lived in a culturally and economically deprived neighborhood. Such conversation as occurred among family members was the minimum necessary for coexistence. The parents tended to ignore the children until they became too disruptive, whereupon they punished them physically and with little explanation. Intellectual evaluation revealed that Judy's WISC score was 89 and that she was about three years below national norms in scholastic achievement. This was not uncommon in the school she attended. Judy's father was a semiskilled laborer, who was shy and hesitant in speaking. When not directly addressed, he had a strong tendency to sit huddled and gaze into space. He stated that as a youth he had lived on a farm and had not talked much. He began normal speech behavior only when he left the farm and entered the military. Judy's mother was in psychiatric treatment at the time of the evaluation and was described by a psychiatrist on the staff as "severely incapacitated by her own lack of communication with her husband and other children. She was also severely lacking in insight, very unobservant and insensitive to events and circumstances around her." The mother's physical appearance was that of an obese, untidy woman.

At thirteen years three months, Judy was hospitalized for thirty hours and given an amobarbital (Amytal) interview in an attempt to break through her mutism. Neither amobarbital (Amytal) nor methamphetamine (Desoxyn) had any impact on her stubborn silence. During ten months of outpatient therapy, Judy sat with her head covered with a coat, sucking her thumb, and remaining mute. It was then decided to give a trainee in child psychology an opportunity to institute a behavior modification program with her. He first tried to get Judy to speak to her father, asking the father to reinforce this behavior with money or candy. The psychologist hoped to approach Judy while she was talking to her father. Unfortunately, in the experimental setting, Judy refused to speak to her father. The father's response to her refusal was to beat her, striking her on the face and body with his hand, a ruler, and his belt. In one instance when she was moaning loudly, he struck her hard and said, "Shut your mouth" as the belt landed.

Next the method of successive approximation was attempted. She was given pennies and candy for the initiation of any of thirty motor responses. In spite of this, she would never imitate mouth sounds. Since none of these techniques worked, she was finally hospitalized on the pediatric ward to "gain control over her food intake." For seven days her food was to be given to her by a speech pathologist familiar with operant conditioning procedures. Judy was to be shaped for motor responses through coughing, sticking out her tongue, and mouthing words to whispering. However, by this time, Judy had formed so negative a relationship with the psychologist attempting to carry out the behavior modification that she would not accept free food from him. On the sixth day, he decided to play the role of villain, while the speech pathologist took the role of defender and savior. In the course of this role assumption, the psychologist threatened to remove even the bed from Judy's already drab room unless she got to work on her speech lessons. During the following session, Judy began whispering to her speech therapist. It could have been attributed to the behavior modification except for the fact that on the eighth day of Judy's hospitalization the floor nurse reported that Judy had been speaking in full voice to the night maid in Judy's room.

The maid was promptly interviewed, and once she understood that the staff was interested in how she got Judy to speak, she cheerfully reported as follows: She was temporarily assigned to the ward. Since her job was to clean up, no one had instructed her about policies in regard to patients. If she felt like it, she gave them candy. In particular, no one had instructed her about Judy so she gave her candy and gum upon meeting her. Judy had been speaking to her since the second day of hospitalization. It turned out that the maid had been electively mute herself until adolescence. Moreover, she had an electively mute sister, in many respects very similar to Judy. She recognized the behavior and teased and wheedled speech from Judy as she had done with her sister, alternately cajoling, giving bribes, and firmly threatening not to return because her feelings would really be hurt if Judy did not talk to her.

It was obvious that Judy had not responded to the behavior modification techniques which seemed only to increase her negativism. She had begun to speak because of the positive, warm, therapeutic relationship she formed with the floor maid. Once she knew that it had been discovered that she spoke to the maid, she spoke to the nursing staff and other personnel in Child Psychiatry.

After discharge from the hospital, she returned to her home and gradually relapsed into her silence at school and in the outpatient setting. At this point, residential treatment was recommended, but the parents did not follow through with it. A seven-year follow up revealed that Judy remained silent, speaking only to her parents, and then only when they insisted that she answer them. She dropped out of school in the ninth grade and sat around home doing very little. At about the age of twenty, she began to speak at church and in other situations, but remained very shy, reticent, and inhibited.

It is obvious that this type of child responds poorly to the mechanistic manipulations of behavior modification, and that therapeutic change should be credited more to: (1) the removal from the home, which placed her in a new environment and removed her from the punitive, frightening qualities of her home environment; and (2) to the warm, empathic interpersonal relationship that she developed with the maid. Eventually this permeated all her interpersonal relationships with the exception of that with the clinical psychologist. Dynamically this appeared to recreate her hostile, frightened relationship with her father and she was silent.

Specific Therapeutic Methods

These case vignettes were not meant to be examples of the treatment to be utilized with electively mute children. They were intended rather to indicate that different children with the same syndrome are silent for different reasons and need individually developed therapeutic programs. The exclusive utilization of psychoanalytic techniques or behavior modification techninques will result in a high percentage of failures, since some children seem to respond better to the one, and some to the other.

The fact is that widely disparate methods have been utilized successfully, and each therapist has offered theoretical explanations to account for why his approach worked. Those of the psychoanalytic school reject the behavior modification techniques as mechanistic and not dealing with the real problem, while behavior modifiers complain that clinicians are unscientific and cannot document and replicate their work. However, certain facts do seem to emerge as a result of a review of the treatment processes used in working with these children.

Psychodynamic Approaches

The literature regarding speech and language development in children offers a plethora of articles regarding the cognitive aspects, but very little organized research has been done concerning the affective aspects of talking and not talking at various ages. Baltaxe and Simmons[3] have reported the importance of the mother-child interaction in the development of speech and language. The quality of this relationship seems to have a marked effect on how the child speaks and may perhaps determine whether or not he will speak at all.

In view of the fact that research has demonstrated the close relationship between mutism and the quality of the mother-child interaction, it is not surprising that clinicians have reported early disturbances and fixations at preoedipal levels. As the author has previously reported, Glanzmann felt that elective mutes were "anal sulkers" and demonstrated a syndrome of: (1) mutism, total or elective; (2) urinary retention; and (3) voluntary retention of stools.

Kubie and Israel[10] reported the case of a five-year-old girl who became mute when her father, in a sudden explosion of anger, spanked her. During her treatment she indicated that she "thought of duty and that children like to put it in their mouths." She began to speak when a number of people at a teaching conference were able to respond to her by saying "I am sorry." The authors felt that during the early phases of her illness, she was severely regressed and that the link between her inner world of "I" and her outer world of "non I" was severed. She showed numerous obsessions and compulsions, as did the children described by Pustrom and Speers.[14]

All these observations indicate that there is a fixation at the anal stage of development, but other developmental tasks are also involved. Separation individuation issues are important problems for these children, as are family secrets which lead the children to fear that they will be abandoned if they aggressively reveal the secrets.

Kaplan and Escoll[9] emphasize that elective mutism may occur in adolescents and that they have the same central preoedipal conflicts as other elective mutes, i.e., dependency, separation-individuation, and anality, but that they also have additional problems which explain their silence. Silence for these adolescents solved the "problem of separation, the problem of prohibition against the expression of anger, and the problem of excess stimulation of sexual feeling toward the parent of the opposite sex."

In some cases, the disorder seems to be a true "speech phobia." One of the author's patients was required to give a speech in school. She recorded it on tape at home, brought the tape recorder to school, turned it on, and fled from the classroom.

There is some evidence to indicate that these children may experience a traumatic event at the time speech is forming which is, theoretically, a critical phase of speech development. One child was hospitalized with acute giant urticaria at the age of twenty-two months, and it was after this event that his tendency to speak to fewer and fewer people developed. Another child at two and one-half years of age frequently grabbed at her mother, who was pregnant at the time; her father scolded her severely for the action. She immediately ceased talking to her father and did not speak to him until the time of her psychiatric evaluation nine years later.

The author has been impressed with the importance of identification in the production of the symptom, as have Kaplan and Escoll.[9] Frequently, one or the other parent will use silence as punishment or a method of winning a power struggle.

A number of authors have reported the treatment of these children by the use of psychoanalytically oriented psychotherapy. Pustrom and Speers[14] conceptualized the symptom as an expression of family conflict, and they treated the mothers with frequent interviews. The fathers were seen as well, but only infrequently. The child was encouraged to draw, fingerpaint, and make up stories utilizing the typewriter. The child was not pressed early or directly to talk. Instead, interpretations were offered which focused on the aggressive aspects of talking and the child's demands for a dependency relationship with the mother. All three of their cases eventually talked to everyone but the therapist. Chethik[5] utilized a similar approach in describing the treatment of Amy over a two-year period. Amy seemed to have a number of neurotic symptoms, in addition to the mutism. In time, she also spoke to nearly everyone except the therapist, and follow up indicated no regression. Ruzicka and Sackin[16] have addressed the countertransference problems the therapist faces in treating a silent patient; a conflict each therapist should keep in mind if he undertakes to treat these children.

Learning and Behavior Approaches

For approximately fifteen years, a group of therapists have been utilizing a learning theory approach to the treatment of childhood disorders. Their methods are quite different from those of the dynamically oriented therapist. They conceptualize the "symptom" as the basic problem and do not hesitate to attack it directly, utilizing various degrees of coercion if necessary. Halpern[8] presents two cases treated by behavior modification. In the first case the child was given a choice. When he had completed a test, he could either communicate verbally or tap his teacher's hand. Once this was accomplished, he was required to say "go," before leaving the room with his classmates. He was informed of this contingency in class and received much praise from the teacher and classmates when, with some difficulty, he was able to comply. From this point on, his speech production spread to other areas, and his shy, withdrawn behavior improved markedly. Halpern also reported a case of electively mute twins who were successfully treated by behavior modification.

The literature does not contain any specific references to undesirable results of treatment in elective mutism, but Pfeffer,[13] in a personal communication, reported a three-year-old girl, electively mute, who also displayed temper tantrums and tended to interrupt her mother's telephone conversations. The mother complained of the tantrums and interruptions but did not mention the mutism to the personnel of the Well-Baby

Clinic, where she brought the child. A behavior modification program was initiated, whereupon the child became totally mute.

The use of technical instruments has been described by a number of authors. Norman and Broman[12] used visual feedback from the volume level meter of a tape recorder to induce sounds and raise volume in an electively mute boy. Straughan[17] reported using a light and buzzer, as well as a class party, to reinforce speech from a fourteen-year-old boy. This child, however, did not meet the criteria for elective mutism as defined earlier in this chapter.

It is likely that the most effective modality available to the therapist is removal of the child from the home and placement in a hospital. Arajarvi[2] reported twelve cases of hospitalized children studied at the University of Helsinki. He provided a good follow-up report, but it is unclear how the children were treated in the hospital and what happened subsequent to their discharge.

His data do suggest that changing schools, the use of foster homes, and continued treatment do in fact help. Elson and associates[6] described the inpatient treatment of four children and their follow-up studies. The children were treated from four to twelve months on an inpatient basis and, at follow up, three of the four were speaking in school. The treatment consisted of interpretive and supportive psychotherapy, plus milieu therapy in one case. Miller and Laybourne[11] have reported how the removal of a child from his home and placement in the hospital bring about many changes. The child must relate to a whole new set of circumstances. In the face of this, symptoms of long duration often respond to treatment for the first time. When the elective mute is hospitalized, all of the previously described treatment techniques are available to the treatment team on a twenty-four-hour basis. In this setting, the most stubborn elective mute will usually start to talk. It should be emphasized at this point that the author's experience and the experience of others indicate that once the child has started talking to teachers, classmates, neighbors, etc., it is not necessary for him to talk to his therapist. This seems to have no effect on the long-term prognosis. A review of the available cases indicates that many children have been treated for long periods of time after the talking had generalized to everyone except the therapist, and this extended period of treatment was probably neither necessary nor desirable.

REFERENCES

1. American Psychiatric Association, *Diagnostic and Statistical Manual of Mental Disorders*, 2nd ed. (DSM-II), American Psychiatric Association, Washington, D.C., 1968.
2. ARAJARVI, T. "Elective Mutism in Children," *Annales Paediatriae Fenniae*, 2:46–52, 1965.
3. BALTAXE, C., and SIMMONS, J. Q., III, "Language in Childhood Psychosis: A Review," *Journal of Speech and Hearing Disorders*, 40:439–458, 1975.
4. BROWNE, E., WILSON, V., and LAYBOURNE, P. C., "Diagnosis and Treatment of Elective Mutism in Children," *Journal of the American Academy of Child Psychiatry*, 2(4):605–617, 1963.
5. CHETHIK, M., "Amy: The Intensive Treatment of an Elective Mute," *Journal of the American Academy of Child Psychiatry*, 12(3):482–498, 1973.
6. ELSON, A., et al., "Follow-up Study of Childhood Elective Mutism," *Archives of General Psychiatry*, 13: 182–187, 1965.
7. Group for the Advancement of Psychiatry, Committee on Child Psychiatry, *Psychopathological Disorders in Childhood: Theoretical Considerations and a Proposed Classification*, Jason Aronson, New York, 1974.
8. HALPERN, W. I., HAMMOND, J., and COHEN, R., "A Therapeutic Approach to Speech Phobia—Elective Mutism Reexamined," *Journal of the American Academy of Child Psychiatry*, 10(1):95–105, 1971.
9. KAPLAN, S. I., and ESCOLL, P., "Treatment of Two Silent Adolescent Girls," *Journal of the American Academy of Child Psychiatry*, 12(1):59–71, 1973.
10. KUBIE, L. S., and ISRAEL, H. A., in Eissler, R. S., et al. (Eds), *The Psychoanalytic Study of the Child: Clinical Presentations*, vol 10, pp. 289–299, International Universities Press, New York, 1955.
11. MILLER, H. C., and LAYBOURNE, P. C., "Pediatric Hospitalization of Psychiatric Patients: Diagnostic and Therapeutic Implications," *The American Journal of Orthopsychiatry*, 32(4):596–603, 1962.
12. NORMAN, A., and BROMAN, H. J., "Volume Feedback and Generalization Techniques in Shaping Speech of an Electively Mute Boy: A Case Study," *Perceptual and Motor Skills*, 31:463–470, 1970.
13. PFEFFER, J., Personal communication, 1975.
14. PUSTROM, E., and SPEERS, R. W., "Elective Mutism in Children," *The Journal of the American Academy of Child Psychiatry*, 3:287–297, 1964.
15. REED, C. F., "Elective Mutism in Children: A Reappraisal," *Journal of Child Psychology and Psychiatry*, 4:99–107, 1963.
16. RUZICKA, B., and SACKIN, H. D., "Elective Mutism: The Impact of the Patient's Silent Detachment Upon the Therapist," *Journal of the American Academy of Child Psychiatry*, 13(3):551–560, 1974.
17. STRAUGHAN, J. H., POTTER, W. K., JR., and HAMILTON, S. H., JR., "The Behavioral Treatment of an Elective Mute," *Journal of Child Psychology and Psychiatry*, 6: 125–130, 1965.
18. TRAMER, M., "Elektiver Mutismus bei Kindern," *Zeitschrift fuer Kinderpsychiatrie*, 1:30–35, 1934.
19. VON MISCH, A., "Elektiver Mutisimus im Kindersalter," *Zeitschrift fuer Kinderpsychiatrie*, 19:49–87, 1952.

25 / Behavioral and Antisocial Disorders

John E. Meeks

Introduction

This chapter will consider a broad range of behaviors. They include stealing, running away, vandalism, cruelty to animals, sexual assault, lying, firesetting, outbursts of rage and violence, provocative behavior, defiance and disobedience, and manipulative behavior. These are frequently brought to the attention of the child psychiatrist for evaluation and treatment. Obviously, they cannot all be contained within any single diagnostic category. Some are seen regularly in the course of normal development, while others may appear as symptomatic expressions of a variety of pathological conditions.

According to DMS-II, these symptomatic behaviors may be important manifestations of a variety of diagnostic categories. They may appear as relatively normal behaviors in response to transient situational disturbances or become manifest in the course of illnesses as severe as the psychoses. However, those youngsters whose difficulties are expressed primarily through their behavior tend to be diagnosed either as suffering from behavior disorders or personality disorders. This will be true unless there is evidence that the behavior results from central nervous system damage of a toxic, infectious, or traumatic etiology.

The DSM-II classification of behavior disorders is controversial. Many clinicians feel that the categories were devised on the basis of a single population which has not proved to be representative of other patient groups. For example, only three of the behavior disorders (the runaway reaction of childhood and adolescence, the unsocialized aggressive reaction of adolescence and childhood, and the group delinquent reaction) may be employed to diagnose the variety of problem behaviors we are considering. DSM-II behavior disorders are defined in rather narrow terms. They provide very little flexibility for the diagnosis of disturbances which seem to be primarily symbolic manifestations of neurotic conflict or for classifying syndromes which arise from a state of neurotic family homeostasis. In some instances, particularly the runaway reaction of childhood or adolescence, the diagnostic parameters offered for the family and the youngster just don't seem to apply. This is true of a large number of youngsters whose primary symptom is running away from home.

If the behavior pattern is apparently of longer duration and relatively fixed, DSM-II provides a group of personality disorder categories. These include explosive personality (epileptoid personality), antisocial personality, and perhaps, paranoid personality. Many child psychiatrists are reluctant to utilize these diagnoses. They seem to imply a static and fixed condition, with a relatively poor prognosis. The fluidity of the developmental process and the potential for altering pathological family management techniques are encouraging realities. They mitigate against a narrowly phenomenological approach in this age group.

The GAP classification of psychopathological disorders in children is considerably more satisfactory in defining with some accuracy the continuum of disturbances which manifest through unexceptable patterns of behavior. The category of developmental deviations is extremely useful, especially in diagnosing the younger child. This category allows the clinician to stress the importance of constitutional factors, the family's response to these temperamental characteristics, and the influence of earlier unresolved reactive disturbances as they interact to produce the symptom picture. The reactive disorders are also more attuned to clinical reality than are the transient situational disturbances of DSM-II. Under the GAP classification, the focus is placed not so much on the degree of external stress as on the meaning of that stress to a specific youngster. Among the factors considered are the youngster's age, his level of psycho-social development, and any previous experiences which may sensitize him to specific events. At the same time, it is recognized that the immediate problem is primarily a response to a change in the youngster's living situation and his perception of that change.

Although the GAP classification also utilizes the category of personality disorder, it is with a clear recognition that the personality patterns described are part of a continuum ranging from relative normality to severe disability. In addition, the GAP classification recognizes that personality disorders are not static and may blend with the neuroses and psychoses under some circumstances such as increased environmental stress. The GAP classification also recognizes that youngsters who are predominantly neurotic and inhibited may resort to impulsive outbursts of antisocial behavior in severely threatening situations. Some of the flexibility in the GAP system accrues from the utilization of the symptom list. This allows the examiner to diagnose a youngster according to his overall developmental situation, and then to complete the phenomenological description by drawing the appropriate terms from the symptom List. Under this system, the common behavioral disturbances may be viewed as only one part of the clinical picture. It is then not necessary to confine the youngster to a narrow category which predicts his future adjustment. The personality disorders category is recommended only when the total personality configuration fits the degree of relative permanence and inflexibility of adaptive patterns implied in the diagnosis.

Within the personality disorders, the divisions seem closer to clinical reality as one encounters it in day-to-day practice. For example, the categories of overly dependent personality, oppositional personality, overly independent personality, and mistrustful personality describe broad patterns of attitude and defensive style which correlate well with commonly encountered clinical pictures. These diagnoses permit a focus on the larger patterns of behavior utilized by the child in his efforts to deal with temperamental quirks, family psychopathology, or early psychological trauma. They are categories which do not demand a phenomenological focus on isolated specific behaviors. Clinically, this is advantageous since it permits recognition of underlying sources of maladaptation and suggests ways of appropriate intervention. Again, the symptom list is utilized to specify important behavioral manifestations of the disorder, both for the sake of completeness and for the collection of data for statistical purposes.

For the large group of youngsters whose difficulties arise primarily from conflict with social norms, the GAP classification has suggested the category of tension-discharge disorders. This diagnosis includes youngsters previously included under such varying terms as antisocial personality, psychopathic personality, impulsive character, sociopathic personality, dyssocial personality, af-fectionless character, acting-out personality, neurotic character disorder, primary behavior disorder, and conduct disorder. Under the broad heading of tension discharge disorder, the GAP committee suggested two subcategories: (1) the impulse-ridden personality, and (2) the neurotic personality disorder. Although these two subgroups overlap, they do permit diagnostic differentiation between the group of youngsters who appear deficient in control and conscience development, and the group whose antisocial behavior seems to be a repetitive living out of neurotic conflict. The youngsters diagnosed as neurotic personality disorder typically show a tendency to repeat similar behaviors which have unconscious symbolic significance for them. They also show more evidence of guilt (although this may be demonstrated primarily through fairly transparent attempts to provoke punishment). In addition, they exhibit a capacity for object relation at a higher level than do those diagnosed as impulse-ridden personality. These relationships may be highly ambivalent. Nonetheless, the youngsters with neurotic personality disorder typically have not suffered the severe early deprivation with its resultant failure of emotional attachments which is seen in some impulse-ridden children.

Youngsters who would be diagnosed as group delinquent reaction under DSM-II are subsumed in the GAP classification under the category "sociosyntonic personality disorder." The GAP category is, however, considerably broader than group delinquent reaction. It is designed to include all youngsters whose behavior is primarily the result of compliance with social norms of the subculture, community, or family in which the youngster lives. The special factor here is that this same behavior might be unacceptable to the wider society. These youngsters have an adequate capacity for interpersonal relationships. They can conform to the code of behavior of their social setting. It is this code rather than the child that is at variance with the norms accepted by the remainder of society.

History

The history of professional interest in behavior disorders is a fascinating commentary on the difficulty the mental health field has encountered in its efforts to understand and treat problems of aggression. A variety of professional positions have appeared over the years. They seem clearly influenced by changing social attitudes toward the issue of youthful disobedience. Eissler[17] has suggested that much confusion results from the fact that alloplastic expressions of psychopathology share with normal behavior the utilization of action to alter reality. He also notes that while neurotic and psychotic patients clearly experience pain, the "delinquent" gives every evidence of enjoying his disability. Most modern psychiatrists accept the basic premise that severe disorders in social behavior result from psychopathology. In regard to this group of patients, however, their clinical practice still suggests a degree of unstated therapeutic nihilism. For example, Robin's[79] study of youngsters evaluated in a St. Louis child guidance clinic revealed that those with severe behavior problems were less likely to receive extensive treatment. This was true despite the fact (which her follow-up studies demonstrated) that this group of youngsters was at high risk for the development of psychiatric disorder in later life. This relative neglect of a significant group of disturbed youngsters has many roots. It is more difficult to engage these children and their families in meaningful therapeutic work, and they often respond to therapists in ways that are not calculated to enhance the professionals' sense of dignified competence. In addition, the bad behavior which characterizes these youngsters stirs strong and uncomfortable feelings in everyone, professional and nonprofessional alike. The temptation to respond to them with overt and covert punitiveness is certainly understandable.

This view, that the child is willfully bad and enjoying it at that, has a long and respectable history. In fact, it is only in recent years that problem youngsters have been viewed in any other way. Prior to the twentieth century, the antisocial child was regarded as willfully criminal, and his misbehavior was seen as a result of a conscious choice to be bad. Punishment was, of course, the proper response to such deliberate mischief, and the punishment tended to be harsh. For example, in the early nineteenth century, a ten-year-old child was hanged in England for stealing a letter from a mailbox. It is also possible that tendencies to deny the reality and seriousness of antisocial personality problems may be partially the result of reaction formation against such punitive attitudes. Certainly many workers in this field have tended to deny the presence of psychopathology in behaviorally disordered youngsters, preferring to view their behaviors as adaptive responses to social conditions. Although there is

a kind of cosmic truth to the idea that antisocial youngsters are victims of society, such a view tends to deny individual variation, predisposing family patterns, and the structuralization of typical patterns of dealing with other human beings. These disordered relationships usually persist even when social situations are drastically improved.

The difficulty in comprehending the real nature of antisocial behavior is demonstrated by the current attacks on the juvenile court system. Interestingly, the attacks are mounted with equal fervor by those who see the juvenile court as harshly punitive without the protection of due process,[77] and by those who accuse the juvenile court system of coddling vicious and hardened criminals who merely happen to be young chronologically.[53]

The juvenile court system has not always been regarded negatively. Near the turn of the century, the establishment of separate humanitarian courts for children in Chicago and the appearance a few years later of August Aichhorn's book *Wayward Youth*[2] promised a social and psychological breakthrough in the comprehension and management of problem youngsters.

Aichhorn[1] and the group of pioneering psychoanalysts, who followed his lead, had few illusions regarding the reality of internalized problems in their antisocial patients. They also clearly recognized the basically narcissistic structure of the delinquent personality and devised innovative methods of making contact with these youngsters. In spite of their clinical sophistication, the literature dealing with delinquency and behavior problems continues to report studies in which individual psychotherapy, utilizing traditional therapy techniques devised for neurotic youngsters, fails to produce positive results![15, 62, 71]

The implication of such studies is always that these youngsters cannot respond to dynamic psychotherapy and even suggests that this group of problems may be outside the legitimate area of psychiatric investigation. This attitude is reflected in the periodic appearance in the literature of diagnostic categories such as psychopathic personality, affectionless character, and primary behavioral disorder, which have tended to suggest a therapeutic nihilism in regard to some youngsters with antisocial tendencies.

In short, it may be that the intense emotional reactions occasioned by these disruptive youngsters have interfered with the orderly accumulation of data and experience. The result has been a disruption of historical progression toward deeper understanding and more effective treatment of this group of problems. Instead there is an erratic swing of opinion and a failure to build systematically on earlier insights and approaches of proven efficacy. Even landmark works such as Redl and Wineman's *Children Who Hate*[74] seem to be only isolated islands in a chaotic sea of speculation, superficial theorizing, and judgmental pronouncements.

Epidemiology

The occurrence and nature of specific patterns of disordered behavior is extremely variable. There is, to be sure, some tendency for particular geographic areas and historical periods to show rates of occurrence that are either very high or very low. This fact has led many sociologists to regard antisocial behavior as a purely sociological phenomenon. Their studies[57, 85, 93] demonstrated that certain urban areas were characterized by a high frequency of antisocial behavior, even though over the course of time, those areas of the city were populated by different ethnic, racial, and cultural subgroups. In addition, it seems true that the rate of antisocial behavior varies with conditions existing in the larger society. For example, any events that cause disorganization of community and family patterns result in an increased incidence of behavior disorders. Such events include war, natural disasters, and rapid social change resulting from advances in technology or the economy.

Other changes in society which are not completely understood also tend to produce alterations in the pattern of occurrence of disordered behavior. For example, currently there appears to be an increase in the number of girls involved in antisocial behavior as compared with past decades. The reasons for this are not immediately apparent, although they seem related to a decreasing tendency to protect and shelter adolescent girls. Of course, since all antisocial behavior is defined by the norms current in any given society, there is considerable variation between cultures and across time (within any given society) in the specific behaviors which are regarded as evidence of a personality disorder. For example, the sexual behavior of the average adolescent girl in the 1970s would have been regarded in America as clearly delinquent prior to World War I and would still be so viewed in much of Latin America.

In America the prevalence of antisocial behavior seems to have important socio-economic linkages. Conditions of poverty, lack of community cohesion, and the despair and anger toward the larger society which these conditions tend to engender explain the higher incidence of antisocial behavior in some low socioeconomic populations.[66] However, this is by no means a universal truth. In some communities, these conditions appear to result in a higher level of cooperative behavior than that observed in some affluent suburban settings where individualistic striving for achievement undermine proper concern for the young. Still, the poor family, which must struggle to meet basic survival needs, may have insufficient time or energy to provide appropriate parenting during young childhood. This emotional deprivation tends to produce a higher level of impulse-ridden, poorly socialized individuals. In addition, because of the lack of appropriate avenues for achievement, the antisocial gang tends to be more prevalent in poverty areas. The result is a higher rate of recorded delinquency, much of which falls into the category of the group delinquent reaction or the sociosyntonic personality disorder.

The occurrence of antisocial behavior often appears to be strongly related to age. The peak incidence of crimes against property, for example, is at age seventeen in America. In England the comparable age is fourteen. Certainly many people associate antisocial behavior with the adolescent age period. However, though with increasing age there may be an increase in the occurrence of some unacceptable behaviors, such as runaway, much of the apparent increase in delinquency is related to the fact that older children have a wider area of activity. As a result, their unacceptable behaviors are more likely to be noted and opposed by society. For example, many youngsters who are arrested for theft during adolescence reveal that they have stolen small items in the home and the nearby community for years without arousing significant concern. Other behaviors, such as lying, are normal for very young children and are often a source of concern in the adolescent only if they are associated with oppositional behavior or defiance of limits.

There is considerable controversy in the literature regarding the natural progression of the behavior disorders. For example, studies by Bovet[9] and McCord and McCord[57] showed that the majority of "juvenile delinquents" spontaneously outgrew their antisocial tendencies and had no further difficulty with the law during their twenties. On the other hand, Robin[79] and the Gluecks[34] reported a much more negative outcome. This confusion is probably the result of an unwarranted assumption that youngsters who misbehave represent a homogeneous population. These findings suggest again that the occurrence of specific behaviors cannot serve as a basis for deciding on the degree of psychopathology or the treatability of a given youngster. There is, in fact, wide variation along many axes among youngsters who demonstrate unacceptable behavior. This reinforces the need for careful diagnostic study; one must consider not only the character of the behavior, but the longitudinal history, general level of development, the quality of object relations, and the potential positive resources of the family and the community.

Clinical Course of the Behavioral and Antisocial Disorders

Because of their protean forms, it is impossible to describe any single typical clinical course for youngsters with behavioral and antisocial disorders. As previously mentioned, the group cuts across diagnostic categories in terms of both severity and basic personality structure. In addition, the child's explicit adjustment to society depends on the summation of multiple internal and external vectorial forces. These points, may have greater relevance when considered in reference to the following clinical vignettes which demonstrate the evolution over time of three "problem children."

MARILYN

At age thirteen, Marilyn was a beautiful young woman. She presented for her first psychiatric interview heavily made up, mini-skirted, and with her long blonde hair swept upward in sophisticated adult fashion. She could easily have passed as an eighteen year old. She was seductive, belligerent, profane, and completely uncooperative.

She had been sent to a residential treatment center because of explosive outbursts of unacceptable behaviors, including car theft, promiscuity, heavy use of alcohol, constant lying to her parents, and total defiance of their rules and expectations. Marilyn viewed her parents' reaction to her behavior as absurdly strict and unconscionably intrusive. She saw no reason why she should

change her pattern of behavior and insisted that for the first time in her life she was happy.

Marilyn's first few weeks at the residential school were a disaster. Not only did she personally defy every rule, but, with her beauty and charisma, she rapidly mobilized the entire patient population under her banner of hedonistic defiance. Her psychiatric interviews were torture for the therapist, who was constantly berated, manipulated, and challenged. She insisted that if he was any kind of man, he would recognize her right to dress as she chose and to engage in activities which gave her pleasure. But instead he was frightened of the school's staff and unwilling to stand and be counted in Marilyn's support. In short, in every manifest behavior and expressed attitude, Marilyn appeared totally committed to a colloused, hedonistic rebellion against all society's rules.

However, the past history revealed that Marilyn had been an overcompliant and somewhat excessively dependent youngster during her preschool and elementary school years. In fact, Marilyn's early attachment to her mother sounded extremely symbiotic. The mother told of several instances of she and Marilyn understanding one another without any verbal interchange, to a degree that was almost clairvoyant. In addition, Marilyn was always somewhat anxious regarding any separation from her mother. Even at age eleven, she was reluctant to spend the night at a friend's home. The father was curiously absent from the history; he was also functionally absent in the present. The mother stated that he was an extremely busy and successful businessman, whose frequent absences from the home were apparently accepted without comment by his wife and daughter.

Although the psychotherapy cannot be described in detail, it was possible to establish a therapeutic alliance with Marilyn. The psychotherapeutic work then focused on her ambivalent attitude toward males, especially her father. As therapy unfolded, she recalled her father's withdrawal from her at puberty and his obvious discomfort with her rapidly unfolding sexual maturity. She came to recognize that she regarded her sexual interests as wicked and inherently evil. As the surge of her sexual drives forced themselves into her awareness during adolescence, she concluded that this made it necessary for her to consider herself as a bad person. The problem was exacerbated by her precocious development which attracted the predatory interests of older boys. These posed an adaptive problem that she was too immature to manage.

As the therapeutic work progressed, her pro-vocative behavior diminished. She began to dress appropriately, found a renewed interest in her academic work, and became a constructive leader of the other patients. With the child-care staff, her posture became one of reasonable cooperative-ness and affection. After a few months of steady progress, she was able to return to her home where her acceptable adjustment continued.

Approximately a year after Marilyn returned home, her therapist received a phone call from Marilyn's father. He was in a state of near panic, because his wife had been arrested while shop-lifting from an exclusive department store in their home city. He wanted the name of a com-petent psychiatrist for his wife. It later developed that Marilyn's mother had been struggling with a variety of strong antisocial impulses for several years. The acts of thievery for which she was finally apprehended had been occurring regularly for the last six months. She was also involved in two emotionally superficial sexual affairs.

Although a complete history was never avail-able and the focus of Marilyn's therapy had cen-tered primarily on her relationship with her father, it seems likely that Marilyn's mother had utilized her daughter as a vicarious agent for disallowed antisocial strivings. The father's re-moteness from the family probably played an im-portant role in the etiology of both his wife's and his daughter's symptomatic behavior. It also seems probable that Marilyn's removal from the home and the successful treatment of her behavior dis-order tipped the balance toward the direct emer-gence of the mother's antisocial behavior.

Seven years later, Marilyn's therapist received a letter from Marilyn, who was then twenty years old. She indicated that she was engaged to marry a young man whom she described as "honest, decent, and fine." She was disturbed because the young man had no knowledge of her episodes of delinquency. She felt particularly guilty about her sexual escapades. She wrote that she spent a great deal of time struggling with painful memories of the degrading activities she had actively sought at age thirteen. She felt strongly that she should confess to her fiancé but was paralyzed by fear that he would find her unacceptable if he "knew the truth about me." She was particularly con-cerned that she would become a "phony hypocrite" like her mother by failing to disclose the truth about herself.

The therapist felt that Marilyn's anxiety was the result of a continuing inability to fully integrate her sexuality with a positive self-image. He spec-ulated that it was her present sexual interest in her fiancé, rather than her past misbehavior, which was the primary source of her current upset. In his reply to her letter he suggested that Marilyn recognize her emotional distress as an internal problem which required further psycho-therapy.

Several months later he received a brief note from Marilyn indicating that she had followed his advice to enter psychotherapy and that "the problem is now resolved."

CHARLES

Charles was admitted to the adolescent unit of a psychiatric hospital because of multiple and incessant behavioral problems. He was a tall, thin black boy of fifteen who would have been handsome except for the peculiarity of his facial expression and his mannerisms. He was fidgety and restless and his eyes bulged with a constant ex-pression of fear. He avoided direct eye contact and his jerky head movements directed his gaze around the room in a darting and furtive manner that marked him immediately as untrustworthy. His voice was high and plaintive and was usually raised in a whining demand to be understood. By this, Charles meant that everyone should validate his version of personal innocence in his unending war with authority. Charles was forever involved in such situations and was never in the wrong. If he was caught in the act and unable to lie or distort, he was always able to justify his behaviors as provoked by the various injustices which had been dealt him earlier, and was therefore the fault of others.

By age fifteen, Charles had compiled an as-tounding record of difficulties. He had been ex-pelled from seven different schools, had virtually demolished his own home during various rage outbursts in which he destroyed property indis-criminantly, and had been arrested three times for petty theft, vandalism, and trespassing. Away from adults, Charles did not engage in directly aggressive behavior. He had no friends of his own age in his neighborhood. In spite of the ambiva-lence and chaos which characterized their relation-ship, he seemed completely tied to his mother. Mother said that he had always been a difficult child, but his behavior had worsened over the past year since the death of his father. She blamed the father for Charles' difficulties. The father had made a considerable amount of money from varied activities of dubious legality. He had mar-ried Charles' mother fairly late in his life. She was several years his junior. When Charles was born, the father doted upon him and spent endless hours entertaining his young son. He gratified the boy's every whim and defended Charles against all efforts on the mother's part to establish limits or to control Charles' behavior. Upon further investigation it became clear that the mother had also played a significant role in Charles' misbehavior. She was herself quite impulsive and immature and was primarily envious of Charles because of his freedom from responsibility. Her efforts to control Charles were heavily tinged with poorly disguised hostility. This was based partly on infantile competitiveness and partly on her resentment of Charles' father. She had some reason to be angry. Her husband had squandered the large amounts of money he had handled through the years and had died almost penniless. Accustomed to luxury, she had been compelled to obtain employment to support Charles and herself.

In the hospital setting, Charles was initially a serious management problem. His strong proclivity to play practical jokes and to devise elaborate plots of stealthy revenge for assumed insults and mistreatment kept the unit in a constant state of uproar. It was difficult to prove that Charles was responsible for a variety of electrical malfunctions, instances of lost or stolen property, and one episode in which a staff member's automobile tires were slashed. At the same time, there was strong reason to believe that Charles was the guilty party in all of these events, especially since he was caught redhanded perpetrating several acts of vandalism.

In addition, even when he was not obviously breaking any rule, Charles had an uncanny capacity to irritate a variety of people at the hospital. His therapist was flooded with a stream of complaints about his young patient. When he confronted Charles with these accusations, Charles' voice would rise and his eyes would dart ever more swiftly around the room while he energetically asserted his innocence and retorted with criticism of the hospital staff and the other patients on the unit.

As Charles gradually learned that he would be held accountable for his behavior, he adapted to the unit's limits by giving up his provocative behavior and turning "informer." He devoted himself to uncovering the misdeeds of the other patients on the unit which he cheerfully reported to the staff. Naturally, this behavior made him extremely unpopular with his fellow patients. Charles denied that he cared about this and pointed out that his own behavior was now quite

acceptable. Although the staff attempted to define this as a new problem which required therapeutic work, neither Charles nor his mother were inclined to view his altered behavior in this way. Since he was now free of the behaviors which had concerned her, the mother grew increasingly insistent that Charles be discharged. The staff gave Charles frequent passes home, hoping that the unresolved issues would become apparent again so that mother would be willing to cooperate in further treatment. During these furloughs, Charles behaved in an exemplary manner. Finally, the staff was forced to discharge Charles, against their better judgment.

The mother did agree to allow Charles to remain in day hospital, psychotherapy, and the special education setting associated with the hospital. Under day care, Charles reverted fairly quickly to his previous pattern of behavior, although it seemed that his levels of hostility and mistrust were lower and that there was a greater quality of playfulness to his pranks and provocations. Nonetheless, his behavior was annoying enough to raise serious question about his ability to remain in the school setting without being rehospitalized.

During this period of treatment, about a year after his admission, Charles had shown an increasing interest in his therapist and a growing tendency to be more frank and open during his therapy sessions. This was a mixed blessing for the therapist, since Charles now revealed grandiose plans for his future. He was preoccupied with gaining a large sum of money and was not at all particular about the methods by which he might achieve this financial bonanza. For example, he was preoccupied with the Mafia for a time and considered seriously pursuing a career as a supercriminal. Other proposed projects included buying a gambling casino, becoming a financial wizard, and engaging in a variety of businesses, where he planned to use sharp and dishonest dealing to become rich quickly.

On the more positive side, Charles did seem to be showing greater interest in school and there was some evidence that his therapist's confrontations regarding the reality consequences of his behavior were having a slight impact. For example, Charles would occasionally admit now that he might have to work for a few years in order to save money and accummulate the capital that would allow him to initiate one of his get-rich-quick schemes. It gradually became clear that Charles needed money in order to bolster a severely deficient sense of self-worth. He intended to buy a Cadillac, a yacht, and an elegant home which he felt would impress everyone, especially girls. On the other hand, he stated that he had no desire for a close relationship with a girl, since all of them were out to get his money and he trusted none of them. Therapy during this time included multiple occasions when the therapist had to meet with Charles and his mother and hospital staff members, or teachers. The task in each instance was to clarify situations and reinforce appropriate limit-setting, while simultaneously trying to protect Charles from the excessive anger that his provocations tended to stir in several authorities.

As soon as some stability was achieved in this setting, the therapist recommended that Charles be enrolled in an ordinary private school. The only aspect of his treatment program that would continue was to be his individual psychotherapy. The mother was very dubious about the wisdom of this suggestion since, as mentioned previously Charles had already been expelled from seven schools. On the other hand, Charles was extremely enthusiastic about the proposal, though he frightened the therapist with dreams of straight A's and instant popularity in the new setting. In fact, Charles was closer to an accurate prediction of outcome than either the mother or the therapist. He adapted rather quickly to his new school, although he appeared for his therapy sessions in a state of total exhaustion which he ascribed to the horrendous academic workload in the school. Since he completely avoided any conflicts with school authorities, the exhaustion was more likely the result of the tremendous effort which he exerted to keep himself under control.

Charles began to report an entirely different view of authority. No longer did he attempt to enlist the therapist as an ally in an attempt to thwart the rules. Instead, he asked for help in controlling himself and for practical advice on how to improve his academic performance. During this time, Charles focused very little attention on his interaction with peers. His occasional comments suggested that he was both self-assured and brave, and less provocative in his interactions with other youngsters. Reports from the mother and the school confirmed this impression and described Charles as a boy who was well accepted by his peer group.

Toward the end of his first year in a normal school setting, Charles raised the question of termination. His social, athletic, and academic interests now seemed more attractive than the trips to the therapist's office. A thorough evaluation of his current situation suggested that termination was reasonable. During the course of the termination process, Charles showed appropriate sadness over leaving the therapist. Primarily, however, he was proud of his new capacity to conduct his own life in a constructive way. His comments about his course of treatment are interesting and perhaps instructive. Charles stated that inpatient treatment was "like putting a patch on." He explained that he recognized that the inpatient period of treatment did control his behavior by external means. He went on to say, "But when you leave the hospital that patch comes off and you have to see if you can do it yourself."

Charles felt the turning point in his therapy occurred when the therapist had sufficient faith in him to recommend placement in a school with normal peers. He seemed to have a clear awareness of the tolerance for pathology present in the therapeutic setting and an equally clear recognition that a similar tolerance would not exist in his new school. This recognition of reality led to his dogged determination to "make it." Although the effort cost him dearly in emotional energy for several months, its gratification in terms of academic and social success apparently convinced Charles that his previous notions regarding the road to self-satisfaction were inaccurate. It is interesting that as these attitudes changed, Charles' comments about his father grew less idealized and more realistic, and his evaluation of his mother turned from distrust and bitter hatred toward a moderately positive regard and a cooperative attitude.

MACK

Mack was a walking definition of the phrase "born loser." He was fifteen, sad, with ill-fitting clothes, and lank, uncombed hair. His posture, handshake, and personality were limp. He was referred for psychiatric evaluation by his probation officer because of multiple thefts, most usually of automobiles, in which he took his friends for "joy rides." He was undependable in his observation of family rules, especially when he was in the company of friends. He was also doing poorly in school. In the diagnostic interview and the treatment interviews that followed, Mack appeared consistently withdrawn and depressed, although in his own passive way, he was basically cooperative and friendly. He was unable to give any reason for his delinquent behavior and, in fact, did not seem at all interested in discussing his problems with the law. He did like to talk about cars and about his friends. The only animation he displayed occurred when he described an afternoon at the movies with his friends. The group had been so rowdy and boisterous that the manager finally asked them to leave.

Even this brief period of interest faded away quietly into the severe constriction of thought and affect that was characteristic of Mack. Mack seemed so intellectually impoverished that it was difficult to believe the psychological testing which showed average abilities.

Mack's parents were conventional middle-class people, who were embarrassed and shocked by Mack's repeated brushes with the law. They expressed a great deal of concern for Mack but had no idea why he should be having such difficulties. They described their marriage as tranquil and their other children as well adjusted and happy.

Shortly after beginning therapy Mack stole another car, thus revoking his probation. Through the intervention of his probation officer and his therapist, Mack was sent to a small work farm instead of the larger, more punitive reformatory for boys.

With Mack out of the family, the parents began to be more aware of marital discord and got in touch with the therapist for marital counseling. In counseling it was revealed that the mother carried the major responsibilities for child care in the family and resented it. She was also quite angry because she and her husband engaged in virtually no recreational activities together. Mack's father expressed his anger at his wife because of her sexual inhibition. He also talked in some detail of feelings of inadequacy as a father, particularly in regard to Mack. Gradually, he came to recognize his tendency to ignore and criticize Mack because of his belief that Mack was not as bright as his other children, an attitude that may have originated in Mack's apparently constitutional tendency to move slowly, cautiously, and timidly into new situations. The other children in the family had always been more aggressive, verbal, and outgoing.

Mack had an extremely positive experience at the youth farm. After his customary initial period of surveillance, he moved toward very warm relations with the male authorities at the correctional facility and became eager to please them. They recognized his need for status in the peer group and provided him with coaching and encouragement in developing his skills as a boxer. Mack had some minor success on the boxing team at the farm. He was much admired by the other boys, not so much because of his skill, but be-

cause of his dogged persistence and stoic indifference to pain. After a period of time, Mack was allowed to visit home. The family began to deal directly with the father's problems in setting firm behavior limits for Mack without becoming angry at him, rejecting him, or predicting antisocial behavior. The parents continued in counseling and the father's capacity to offer firm, friendly paternal guidance to Mack improved steadily.

At the time of Mack's release from the youth farm, the father again expressed doubt that Mack could adjust to the larger society. He was particularly reluctant to believe that Mack could do better academically. However, he was able to question these feelings and to consider the possibility that they originated within himself. He refrained from inflicting them on Mack. The youngster's adjustment was at first adequate and gradually improved. As his successes multiplied, he was able to attract a girlfriend for the first time and completely lost interest in the antisocial peer group that he had previously chosen as associates. For the first time, he began to maintain a "B" average at school and to talk of attending college.

At this point, the entire family was involved in family therapy sessions where Mack, in his quiet way, was often the one who put his finger on important emotional issues. He was of considerable help to a sister. At the time, she was having great difficulty with her feminine identification and experienced many neurotic concerns about her personal attractiveness. The father's respect for Mack grew steadily. Occasionally, Mack and his father would confer about important family decisions both at home and during therapy sessions.

At this point, some two years after Mack's initial psychiatric evaluation, the family was functioning well. Mack and his siblings dropped out of the family therapy since they did not appear to be experiencing adjustment difficulties. The father continued to be concerned about the marital sexual adjustment, and the parents continued in marital counseling. It became increasingly clear that most of the father's complaints related to personal sexual inhibitions which he projected on his wife, who was in fact adequately responsive. He desired a variety of somewhat exotic foreplay activities which he needed in order to become aroused; it was her rejection of these that led to his complaints. Gradually, he was able to accept responsibility for the difficulty and decided to enter analysis for treatment of his severe neurotic problems with masculinity.

The family therapy was terminated at that point, and the therapist did not hear from Mack again until his sophomore year of college. At that time, he called to request an interview. He told the therapist that he had done very well through high school and his freshman year of college, but that he had recently begun to experiment with marijuana at the insistence of a group of intelligent but somewhat bohemian friends that he had made at college. He stated that the second time he smoked marijuana, he experienced symptoms of depersonalization and anxiety that frightened him. Since that occurrence, he had become preoccupied with a belief that his steady girlfriend exercised excessive dominance over him.

He was bothered by a feeling that he was incapable of making his own decisions and that he was basically a "weak person." These feelings were threatening what had been a stable relationship with his girlfriend of over a year's standing. She resented his accusations that she was trying to run his life and tell him what to do. Mack knew intellectually that his girlfriend was not domineering and recognized that these feelings were extremely illogical. He stated that they had been involved with each other sexually for six months, that the sexual relationship was satisfactory, and that he hoped that the relationship would lead to marriage. He was now unsure that they could resolve their differences and achieve a harmonious relationship.

During the ensuing psychotherapy, it became clear that Mack had a neurotic disorder rather similar to his father's. However, it should be emphasized that during this entire course of individual therapy, Mack showed no tendency toward antisocial behavior. Even in fantasy, he demonstrated a strong element of superego control and gave no evidence of his previous delinquent adaptation. It is also interesting that his appearance was radically altered. In spite of his considerable overt anxiety, he now presented himself as an attractive well-groomed and basically self-assured young man, troubled by a fairly typical neurotic conflict which was highly egodystonic. He decided spontaneously to avoid drug use in the future and became symptom free during the course of a year's psychotherapy.

Discussion

These three cases illustrate a number of points. Most obvious is the tremendous diversity of dynamic patterns in the behaviorally disordered youngster. Although one could say that family psychopathology was present in each case, this would hardly do justice to the kaleidoscopic variety of influences which led Marilyn, Charles, and Mack into disruptive behavior. Marilyn was unconsciously but actively used by her mother to express, in a direct way, forbidden impulses that were pushing for overt expression. Mack, on the other hand, was not acting out his father's antisocial tendencies so much as he was attempting to compensate for an inadequate masculine model. He was also expressing his anger for being chronically scapegoated and rejected by parents who shared hidden feelings of inadequacy about their sexual roles.

Charles was simply living out the picture of the world that had been painted for him by his family. His father gratified his own hedonistic omnipotence directly and allowed Charles to share in the experience, while his mother reinforced the attractiveness of this style of life with her open envy and ineffectual and grudging adherence to the reality principle.

These examples were chosen for several reasons. First of all, each youngster turned out to be treatable, although initial presentation was not promising. Secondly, there was an opportunity to follow their future development and to observe some of the ways in which their vulnerabilities were manifested after their antisocial behavior was successfully contained. Finally, this longitudinal view permits a more convincing comparison of the variety of personality structures which can lead to serious behavior problems.

Marilyn, the most superficially defiant and unrepentant of our young offenders, was in many respects not only the healthiest of the three, but the one with the most solid superego formation. Mother had provided a corrupting influence, an initially subtle and later overt insult to the originally idealized source of Marilyn's values. In spite of this, Marilyn's subsequent reawakening of guilt feelings around sexuality suggests strong and even harsh conscience pressures. Perhaps the very strength of these prohibitions required Marilyn to attempt to deny all constraints and to affect an attitude of total derision toward all authority figures. The very intensity of her rebellion contained a counterphobic quality. Although the presenting picture was explosive and overwhelming, there were many clues that Marilyn's antisocial behavior was the product of an intense internal conflict. In her psychotherapy, it quickly became clear that her drive development was basically age-appropriate, with strong heterosexual interest, bisexual anxieties, and a fear of regression to a homosexual bond with her mother.

Charles, on the other hand, had a completely different personality structure. Superego development was minimal, since his identification with his asocial father was not counteracted by his relationship with an angry, rejecting mother. For her part, she demonstrated little concern for Charles' rights and seemed secretly to wish for a life free of reality problems. Charles' ego was poorly developed with little capacity for reality testing, binding of tension, or the elaboration of effective defenses against either impulse or anxiety. He lived in constant fear that he could not control himself or master the world around him which seemed overwhelming and excessively demanding. The result was a chronic state of restless agitation, only temporarily relieved by impulsive efforts to externalize this difficulty. Charles usually managed to maintain this world view through primitive defenses of denial, projection, and rationalization. Throughout his treatment, even during its relatively successful final stages, it was evident that Charles was fixated at several rather early pregenital libidinal positions. Oral greed, anal sadistic vengefulness, and infantile omnipotence dominated his fantasy life, and any capacity to see other human beings as more than an admiring audience was limited.

Mack's developmental configuration was different. He had some superego formation, but his values did not seem to arise from his basic personality structure. Instead, they were predominantly related to external models and were strongly dependent on the reinforcement of approval and praise coming from important others. He seemed able to transfer this orientation, first to a delinquent gang and then to the counselors and fellow students at the boys' farm who admired his toughness and courage in the boxing ring. Years later he showed no strong inherent antisocial tendencies when he returned for treatment of a neurotic disorder. On the other hand, he never mentioned feelings of conscious guilt in connection with his earlier delinquencies. In Mack's case, it is as though his conscience played a very insignificant role in his problem. His difficulties seemed much more related to an immature ego structure with an extremely poor self-image associated primarily with deficiencies in secondary narcissistic achievement. Mack provided little evidence of an observing ego or of a strong sense of personal direction. No internalized ego ideal acted to stabilize his personality. This personality feature seems very

possibly to have arisen from his constitutional passivity and his difficulty in dealing with novel situations while maintaining a sense of security. As a young adult, his neurotic symptomatology was precipitated when he utilized a drug which may have the effect of weakening ego boundaries and loosening the sense of personal identity. Many people find this sensation a pleasant release. Mack experienced it as a frightening loss of control over the direction of his life, a trauma sufficient to mobilize his underlying difficulty in assertive self-direction. With the return of the fear of passivity, he began to doubt his masculinity and to perceive his girlfriend as controlling and castrating. Fortunately, by this time, he had developed sufficient ego strength to recognize the internal origin of these anxieties and suspicions.

Though we will return later to the question of treatment in the behavior disorders, the tremendous differences in approach and method effective in these three cases should at least be noted in passing. It should also be recognized that the goals and effects of therapy, as viewed from a dynamic point of view, were quite different in the three cases. Marilyn benefited from a combination of limit setting (placement in a residential school) and fairly traditional dynamic psychotherapy, even though the content of the therapy was certainly incomplete and, to some extent, even wide of the mark in regard to the true dynamics.

Charles' treatment can barely be dignified with the name "psychotherapy." His therapist played a variety of roles including Dutch uncle, patient instructor, cheerleader, prophet, arbitrator and limit setter. The therapeutic posture was hardly objective, and the therapist was anything but a blank screen reflecting the emotional significance of his young patient's verbalizations. In short, Charles' therapist praised, scolded, preached, and persisted in a dogged effort to make himself personally important to Charles as an identification figure and a very active interpreter of the realistic ways in which Charles might gratify at least some portion of his limitless wishes.

In Mack's case, the therapist struck out after hardly coming to bat in the initial abortive attempt at outpatient therapy. Mack improved in response to a different living situation which was not formally therapeutic and in response to the changes produced in his management within the family through parent and family therapy.

The overall result also differed among these three youngsters. By circuitous paths, Marilyn and Mack achieved at least approximations of the combination of flexibility and conventional adaptation that passes for normality. On the other hand, at the end of therapy Charles remained a highly narcissistic and immature human being. Although these personality characteristics had come to be adapted to the demands of reality, Charles will probably remain a rather selfish and unscrupulous person. In all likelihood, this is not an unusual outcome in the therapy of antisocial youngsters. Needless to say, this raises interesting and troubling questions regarding the place of values and morality in psychotherapy and may pose potentially embarrassing questions to therapists who are both able and willing to "deceive the deceiver."[39]

The Specific Behaviors

The undesirable actions, which are the subject matter of this chapter, often occur in varying combinations in youngsters with serious behavior problems. However they do occasionally present as isolated points of concern. We shall now turn to a brief consideration of each form of misbehavior, its developmental origins and its natural and pathological course.

STEALING

The specific antisocial acts are closely related to a variety of social factors. Patterns of acting out change with alterations in cultural patterns. There may be a correlation between the high value placed on the possession of material goods in America and much of Western society, and the frequency of theft as a primary symptom of antisocial behavior. Until recent years, the social expectation that material goods should be accumulated by males was reflected in a higher incidence of stealing among boys as compared to girls. This gender distinction seems to be lessening, again perhaps in response to alterations in sex-linked social expectations.

Reported theft seems more common in lower socioeconomic class youngsters. Moreover, there is reason to believe that this is at least partially related to a variance in the reporting of petty theft. Affluent families have the capacity to protect their youngsters to a larger extent from formal legal action by making financial reparations and arranging private assistance. Certainly, in the course of psychotherapy of middle- and upper-class youngsters, one commonly encounters reports of

theft. These include shoplifting, bike stealing, motor theft, and other minor, as well as more serious, stealing. It is true, however, that certain kinds of theft seem to result from the juxtaposition of affluence and poverty. For example, when poverty-stricken, inner city youngsters have been placed in schools in well-to-do neighborhoods, there is a tendency for the poor youngsters to attempt to steal or extort money and other material possessions from their more well-to-do classmates.

Subcultural traditions also play a role in the incidence of stealing behavior in children. Those cultures and even subcultures within the capitalistic industrialized West, that have a more communal attitude toward private property, are clearly less troubled with thievery than are those countries and groups that attach status to the possession of goods. In all social groups, however, there appear to be some developmental and age-related patterns which are important in encouraging or preventing stealing.

Very young children appropriate any object which excites their interest and which is available to them. Of course, this acquisitive behavior cannot be regarded as stealing until the youngster is old enough to understand first of all the concept of the separateness of other individuals and eventually the idea of property rights. Both capacities tend to evolve during the period of separation-individuation as the recognition and awareness of himself and his mother as separate beings is gradually accomplished. The notion of property rights is learned first in an egocentric manner ("mine!"), and only later respected in regard to others. That is, the youngster first recognizes objects that are his and protests their removal before accepting a comparable privilege of other people to protect what is theirs. This lesson is learned at varying rates; the reluctance with which it is accepted is illustrated by the common saying "Finders keepers, losers weepers." In families where the youngsters' right to privacy and possession is not recognized, defended, and protected from the intrusions of both parents and siblings, the internalization of this aspect of morality is slow indeed. In these instances, the youngster's continued stealing results not so much from conflict or personality deviation as from a simple adaptation to a social system where property rights are not defined and mutually respected.

For a youngster to accept the inviolability of the property of others, he must also have a basic feeling that his needs will be adequately met according to the family's ability, in both the material and emotional spheres. For example, if other siblings are clearly favored with affection and gifts, it is understandable that the deprived youngster may devise his own system for equalizing the distribution of wealth. It is also commonly recognized that parents who are cold and emotionally withholding often become the targets for theft of material objects. In these instances, the stealing youngster appears to be utilizing the stolen object as a symbolic substitute for the withheld affection.

At least initially, stealing under these circumstances appears to be an effort to repair the ego damage occasioned by the rejection.[90] The youngster often appears initially to utilize the stolen object as part of an effort to maintain the fiction of a positive and loving relationship with the disappointing adult. Small children pretend and sometimes seem to believe that the frustrating parent has actually provided the stolen object as a loving gift. At times, the stolen object appears to represent a transitional object, an almost literal substitute for the parent. For example, the child may steal a valued possession of the parent which then appears to provide some comfort and psychological security to the child. In young children, there seems little awareness that the theft is hostile, and the intention does not as yet seem to be to inflict punishment on the parenting figures for their withholding attitude.

During latency, stealing is usually recognized as a forbidden act. However, it may continue as a symptom of an unsatisfactory parent-child relationship within the family. In addition, stealing is often utilized as a behavioral response to a variety of peer pressures. A youngster may steal from an enemy as an act of hostility or revenge. If the enemy is feared, the theft may be secretive, while, if the enemy is regarded as weak, the stealing may occur in a context of bullying or extortion. On other occasions, youngsters may steal from home or stores in order to obtain money or goods which can be distributed in an attempt to curry favor. Naturally, this ineffective method of making friends suggests a strong sense of personal inadequacy within the peer group and the probable existence of significant personal psychopathology, especially if it is a repetitive pattern.

Later in latency and during adolescence, stealing may be regarded as an act of bravado. Indeed, in some groups of youngsters, stealing may serve as an initiation ritual through which the youngster proves that he is one of the gang and not a "goody-goody." Some of this behavior seems more expressive of the widespread social uncertainty of the involved youngsters. They are struggling more

with what is proper moral conduct rather than expressing individual psychopathology. For example, many American adults would feel guilty if they stole from an individual. At the same time, they feel justified in cheating a large institution such as the federal government, an insurance company, or a large department store.

With appropriate parental management, most of these developmental variants of stealing behavior disappear spontaneously during maturation. Parents should be counseled to apply firm limits which include requiring the youngster to return the stolen object personally or to make other suitable reparation. When youngsters are too embarrassed or anxious to confront the victim alone, it may be necessary for the parent to accompany the youngster to give support while insisting that the youngster deal personally with the situation. The parents should be instructed to be sure that the youngster does not benefit from his theft under any circumstances. To permit such a gain from the activity may appear to the youngster to be condoning the behavior. The parents should also be encouraged to avoid moralizing, predicting future bad behavior, or in other ways implying that they now view their child as a thief. On the contrary, it should be made clear to the youngster that this behavior is totally out of character and unacceptable within the family tradition. When he has made appropriate atonement of the damage created by his act, the matter should be forgotten so that he can begin again with a "clean slate."

In addition to limit setting, the parents should be helped to comprehend any psychological factors in the family interaction which may have predisposed the youngster to stealing. The family must be made to understand that these factors merely explain the stealing and do not justify it. At the same time, they should of course be corrected if this is at all possible. Fortunately, this is often the case, since stealing may appear in response to transient family stresses in an otherwise basically functional family unit. For example, illness in a sibling may transiently result in relative neglect of other youngsters, who may in turn feel deprived and respond by stealing. In these cases, the stealing behavior should be suppressed in the way just described, but the young "thief's" need for greater attention and recognition as an important family member must be recognized and granted by the family.

Unfortunately, for many youngsters, if their stealing results from more serious impairments in emotional development, they do not respond to the management techniques described, and the thefts continue in spite of punishment and efforts to give them support within the family. These cases require careful evaluation of the individual and family dynamics so that effective therapy can be planned.

The Individual Psychodynamics of Persistent Stealing: As described, in most cases stealing begins as an effort to cope with a threat to a dependency relationship (stealing which appears later in development may have somewhat different dynamics, which will be described later). If the young child could describe his motivation for stealing, he might say "Since you refuse to give me what I need, I will have to take it."[19] If the frustration within the relationship becomes chronic, the stealing becomes more ingrained. The basic dynamics which support it then become altered in a way that tends to make the symptom more persistent. With advancing age, the element of hostility toward the frustrating adult becomes increasingly prominent. The desire to inflict pain upon him or on his symbolic equivalent adds another dimension to the need to steal. Many older youngsters will provide clues to this dynamics by admitting that one of the reasons they steal is to "get even" with their parents, whom they see as unfair. This admission does not do credit to the complexity of the internal dynamics.

The youngster may believe that if he were treated with more love and fairness, he would not steal. Clinically, this is not the case. In fact, therapists are often extremely upset when such a youngster steals from them. At this point in the development of stealing behavior, the youngster's structured internal dynamics might be paraphrased as follows: "I do not need or want you to give me anything. In fact, I hate you. I prefer to take whatever I want in order to please myself and to injure and humiliate you."

In other words, the stealing behavior has become to some degree a substitute for satisfying object relations. At this point, the youngster is extremely and understandably reluctant to trade the comfort of his defensive symptom structure for the uncertainty of an object relationship. After all, in his experience such bonds can be painful and unsatisfying. In the more extreme cases, many youngsters who steal are capable of only partial object relations and view people as "things" too.[82]

Where more mature object relations are retained, the youngster tends to project his own hostility onto others and often views people in general as exploitative, unreliable, and corrupt. This attitude toward other people and toward reality is maintained with characteristic defenses which both protect the youngster from internal guilt and also ensure a safe distance from other people. Because his basic unsatisfied needs are so great, he is regularly frustrated by even the most giving and understanding individuals he encounters. This is especially true if these individuals place expectations or demands upon him, as for example in the case of teachers. Denial is mobilized to avoid the acknowledgment of potential reality consequences, as well as to defend against recognition of the need for affection and respect. Displacement is widely used, and all adults are viewed as though they were the original frustrating parent figure. Any sense of guilt is suppressed and repressed with the aid of the aforementioned defenses. More than that, the youngster will often profess a sense of injured innocence. He is likely to develop a style of relating which predictably leads to rejection, thereby justifying his behavior. "Yeah, I steal, but they made me do it." The youngsters are often unaware that they must steal and prefer to believe that they have chosen a life of thievery because it is exciting, daring, and courageous, and justified as well.

Obviously this defensive posture has an erosive effect on the ego. Large elements of reality are ignored, especially those related to interpersonal interactions. Underlying depression and emptiness drive the youngster to increased theft, which in turn furthers the need for defensive operations to maintain a faltering homeostatis. A progression begins toward greater narcissism and greater recourse to infantile omnipotent fantasies. Gradually the alienation from others tends to increase. The only friends the committed thief can have are other thieves, and often he does not even pretend that there is honor between him and his comrades. They may admire each other, but they often recognize that, given the opportunity, their "friends" may well steal from them or use them shamelessly.

The secondary gain in stealing is so obvious as to obscure other dynamics of the behavior. The clear material benefits resulting from a successful theft often appear to the layman as a sufficient explanation for the motivation of the thief. The youngster who steals often is summed up angrily and briefly: "They take things because they want them and they don't want to work for them." Of course, this is one of the important reinforcers of stealing behavior and must be removed in the management of stealing as described previously. Still, it is rarely the most important motivation. Efforts to differentiate between cleptomania as a psychiatric symptom, and "purely" greedy theft, lead to a recognition of considerable overlap between the two views of this behavior.[27]

In addition to the acquisition of objects, many thieves find a secondary gain in the respect and adulation which they receive from other group members for an especially daring theft. Many of these youngsters do show a remarkable degree of ingenuity and cunning in devising their delinquencies and considerable skill and daring in their execution. Admiration for this kind of ability is not limited to delinquent gangs. It forms the basis for much of the plotting in popular TV and movie entertainment.

As mentioned briefly previously, not all stealing is predominantly pregenital. Compulsive stealing of a single specific item or a special group of objects which share similar qualities may represent an attempt to solve infantile sexual conflicts.[61, 82] For example, the theft of phallic objects by latency-age girls may represent a symbolic effort to obtain a penis. However, even in these instances, an underlying oral tendency toward passive or active receptiveness may play an important role in shaping the symptomatology. In a similar way, stealing by boys often appears to be motivated partially by an unconscious desire to obtain penis equivalents or to demonstrate through their daring and boastfulness their superiority to the father or father figures.[19] Car theft, particularly for "joy riding," may represent a substitute for sexual expression in some adolescents. According to Gibbens,[29] this is particularly common in middle-class males who have been excessively controlled in a matriarchal family. Some therapists have suggested a relationship between stealing and homosexuality and transvestism in some disturbed boys.[61] In these cases the stealing represents an identification with the depriving phallic mother and gratifies unconscious homosexual impulses toward the father. However, most authors agree that these higher level conflicts are strongly influenced by intense fixation at pregenital levels. To the extent that it substitutes for basic affection, stealing also represents an auto-erotic solution to conflicts at the sexual level. Thus, it is inevitably accompanied by a growing alienation from real objects. The result is an increase in self-abasement, narcissism, and impoverishment of the reality ego. This is reflected in a finding by Gibbens that delinquent boys reported a precocious beginning of sexual activity but a later "loss of interest" in girls.[30]

The deleterious effect on superego development is clear. This arises both from the psychopathological family structure and from the resort to stealing as a solution to the resulting sense of deprivation. The grudging attitude of the parent in early stages of development interferes with initial positive identification with external objects and thus disrupts the acquisition of a sense of basic trust. In later stages of development, bisexuality in the stealing youngster interferes with the conflict-free internalization of an idealized parent figure of the same sex.[61]

Some observers have suggested that youngsters who develop symptoms of stealing may be burdened by drives of unusual strength. Clinical observations have suggested to these observers that the youngsters are usually intolerant of frustration and deprivation. However, these observations are unsupported by a quantitative and systematic study of the relationship of temperament and the specific symptom of stealing.

Finally, in some youngsters, isolated episodes of theft may appear as a symptom of unconscious impulses which give rise to excessive guilt; the so-called "criminal out of a sense of guilt." In these cases, the stealing as such is relatively nonspecific. It derives primarily from the need to elicit punishment for unacceptable fantasies or guilt. Sometimes these arise from actual events; more often, perhaps, they are related to objectionable feelings or attitudes toward ambivalently loved objects. For example, a youngster may respond with episodes of stealing to the departure of a negatively regarded parent figure through divorce or to the loss of a sibling through serious illness or death. The stealing is intended to elicit punishment for his sense of hostile triumph.

Family and Interpersonal Dynamics in Persistent Stealing: The presence of obvious and severe family psychopathology is regularly noted in the literature dealing with youngsters who steal. Menaker[61] describes two typical family constellations. In the first, the mother is masculine and dominant and likely to assume a controlling and depriving attitude toward her son. The father in such a family is often weak, ineffectual, and somewhat effeminate. In the second family type, the mother is extremely narcissistic and self-centered, while the father is tyrannical and distant. In two cases of Menaker's small series, the youngsters came from single parent families. Menaker saw this circumstance as contributory to the failure of adequate resolution of the oedipal situation and the internalization of a functional superego. In the first two family patterns, the mother's inability to give adequate nurture was coupled with the father's unsuitability as an object of identification.

These combined to establish the personality patterns which often lead to compulsive stealing.

The importance of the presence of covert antisocial tendencies within the family has been noted by Johnson and Szurek.[43] In a surprising number of cases, however, the parents reveal an overt absence of socialization, particularly in the area of property rights. The youngster's stealing may be ignored or rationalized until it becomes impossible to maintain this posture; even then the importance of the symptom may be minimized. In other families, the child's stealing is condemned, even while the parents are engaged in unethical business practices, deceptive and unfair treatment of neighbors and acquaintances, or other activities which suggest to the child that other people should be regarded as targets for exploitation.

There is a group of families where the youngster is encouraged to steal in order to meet pathological parental emotional needs. Thus, there are families in which a youngster's stealing behavior is encouraged by one parent in order to discomfort the other parent or to prove the spouse's inadequacy in the parenting role. Here, the covert intention is to demonstrate that the spouse is either too strict or too lenient. In all these instances, there is a basic disturbance of the communicative process. They are, in fact, designed to obscure the true meaning of verbalizations and positions, rather than to convey accurate and useful feedback regarding reality and the child's relationship to it.

The general comments regarding family psychopathology in antisocial youngsters are applicable to the specific symptom of persistent theft.

Specific Therapy Methods for Youngsters Who Steal: The basic task in the therapy of the habitual thief is to reintroduce object relationships as a replacement for the auto-erotic and narcissistic conflict solution represented by stealing. In many ways, however, stealing is an exciting and gratifying activity. As a result, this goal is more easily stated than achieved. It is often necessary to expend considerable energy in establishing a relationship which will bring the youngster to view his symptomatology as ego-alien.[51, 82]

The basic format for therapy may be either group or individual. Due to the pregenital core of the problem in stealing, cure is usually effected only through the establishment of an intensive positive bond to a parent substitute. In some group therapy situations, this positive object tie may be divided between the group leader and admired peers within the group structure.[73] In either group or individual therapy, the young thief often disappoints the helping figure by continuing to steal, often even from the therapist himself.

The tendency to steal within the therapeutic setting appears to be multi-determined. It serves as a defense against the anxiety aroused by the beginning attachment to the therapist or other helping figures. The goal of the theft is to re-establish the safety and superiority that arose from coping with the original depriving object. The youngster is saying, "I do not need your affection. There is no need for me to fear that you will deprive me. On the contrary, I deprive you." The countertransference problems produced by a youngster with such an intense need to "bite the hand that feeds" are obvious but nonetheless difficult to resolve. However, instances of being stolen from do bring the symptom into the therapeutic situation directly. They thus provide an unusual opportunity to effect a therapeutic alliance with that part of the youngster's ego which disapproves of his behavior. Levy's charming description of her treatment of "Peter" illustrates this technique.[51] It serves as well to display an excellent method for achieving the "ego split" which permits the development of a therapeutic alliance with the young thief.

The appearance of stealing within the therapeutic relationship also provides a basis on which to assess the youngster's ego strengths and capacity for object relatedness. That is, stealing which is distinctly personal and related to an effort to possess the therapist has a better prognosis than more random theft which seems unrelated to the importance of a given relationship in the child's life. Information of this kind from the therapeutic context amplifies and supports the impressions derived from the history. The previous pattern of stealing may indicate a focus on important persons in the child's life. This would suggest a continuing effort to establish meaningful bonds with real objects. Again, the behavior may demonstrate a more auto-erotic pattern which betrays a severe detachment from the real world.

Therapy of the persistent thief is never easy. The youngster is strongly defended against the establishment of the kind of emotional bond which is requisite for effective psychotherapy. Follow-up studies show that stealing is the most common childhood symptom reported by adults who are subsequently diagnosed as antisocial personalities.[79] The virulence of the symptom is self-evident. Therapy requires patience, continual self-assessment, and a capacity to maintain both an objective, confronting, honesty and a nonjudgmental attitude toward a symptom which is socially repellant and personally insulting. No one likes to be "ripped off."

RUNNING AWAY

In recent years, running away from home has become one of the most common presenting symptoms of youngsters referred for psychiatric care during adolescent years. Moreover, it is clear that many other youngsters who leave their homes without parental permission prior to the generally accepted age of emancipation are never evaluated psychiatrically. A large number of centers have appeared in most metropolitan areas entirely for the purpose of dealing with this problem. The philosophy and aims of these centers vary widely. Some of them seem to function primarily as an alternative to returning home. Staff and policy clearly reflect a bias strongly in favor of the adolescent's view of his life situation. Others do not claim to be therapeutic but are humanitarian, offering food and shelter and some protection for the youngster adrift.

This extensive pattern of running has its roots in very early levels of psycho-social development. Eighteen-month-olds have been known to toddle off and disappear. Three- and four-year-olds tend to stray beyond the geographical boundaries established by their mothers. This is a part of the work of separation-individuation. Sometimes these children hide from their mothers and ignore frantic calls to return. Sometimes this is a response to maternal overprotection. Just at the point that the youngster's curiosity about the world is growing, he encounters excessive restriction of his freedom of movement. In these instances, the behavior may become chronic if the parents cannot moderate their expectations to a more age-appropriate level. However, reasonable management is no guarantee against the periodic occurrence of such forays. Most youngsters, especially those with outgoing and active temperamental styles, are simply unable to resist the call of the unknown and the sense of freedom and excitement which accompany it. Fortunately, they usually have some awareness of their limitations. This is especially true if the mother has been active in teaching the realistic dangers of the world and the techniques of avoiding them. As the youngster's opportunities for legitimate exploration increase, his need to "run away" diminishes.

Somewhat older children also "run away." The runaway behavior at this age is more likely to occur in a setting of family conflict. The late oedipal or early latency child may decide to leave his home because of a strong feeling that he is unloved, mistreated, or unappreciated. Often the child fantasizes finding a new home where his position will be more favorable. The intention is communicated to the parent and the child goes to the home of a grandparent or some other member of the extended family, or to the home of a friend. Most parents are understanding of this syndrome; they recall that they themselves went through it once upon a time. The entire episode is handled lightly and sympathetically, often with friendly consultation between the parents and the adults to whom the youngster is running. At the substitute home the youngster is greeted as a visitor, pampered briefly, allowed to ventilate his complaints, and then returned home in a happier state of mind to discuss his grievances with his parents. Sometimes parents have been taught that the appropriate response is to help the youngster pack, thus, calling his bluff and demonstrating their unwillingness to consider the legitimacy of his complaints. Since the youngster's attachment to his family at this age is very strong, most youngsters will give in, thus "proving" to the parents that their firm management was the appropriate response. Other parents may go to the opposite extreme. They are so frightened by the youngster's anger that they may change reasonable family rules and thus set the stage for further bribery and intimidation. Naturally, the appropriate response is one of insisting on the maintenance of reasonable rules, even if these are unpopular with the child, while simultaneously conveying affection and a strong hope that the youngster will be able to be happy within the family despite the fact that he does not like some of its restrictions and expectations.

All runaway behavior reflects the young child's effort to negotiate conflicts between attachment to the parent and the simultaneous fears of being shamed, engulfed, abandoned, or otherwise damaged by this dependency. Developmental pressures toward autonomy play a role in the child's periodic wish to leave home, but, in most cases, parental attitudes play a more important role. All children enjoy games of running and being chased. However, the parent may suffer from unresolved oral conflicts which cause him to reject the youngster's dependent approaches or to force unwanted closeness on the child in order to gratify personal neurotic needs. In such instances, the achievement of gradual emancipation accompanied by a continuing affectionate bond is disrupted. Both closeness and separation become imbued with anxiety. The youngster vacillates between clinging behavior and aggressive rejection of any bond to the parent. In older children, this behavior is often accompanied by a conscious repudiation of the parent or a denial of any dependency needs.[5, 76]

To the clinician, repetitive and prolonged runaways during these early stages of development should be a danger signal. They suggest either severe disturbance in the youngster resulting from mental retardation, brain damage, or extremely deviant constitutional patterns, or they indicate a pronounced impairment of the parent-child relationship. Often both factors are operative, and the situation requires vigorous intervention to avert a growth pattern that is chronically and seriously maladaptive. Usually such truancy from home is associated with many other symptoms of a developing behavior disorder.[67]

During the adolescent years, runaway behavior involves a more complex range of possibilities. Each case must be carefully surveyed to determine the underlying causes of the behavior. Although every situation is unique, there are several characteristic patterns. They overlap, but may, more or less, be recognized as fairly discrete behavior clusters. In reviewing these, the reader should keep in mind the individual dynamics of the runaway. These include the search for a totally good object, sexual adventuring, and the expression of forbidden unconscious drives and, according to Schmideberg, a self-imposed and self-destructive abandonment.[82]

The Adventurer: Many of the youngsters who run away from home for days to weeks during midadolescence are probably fairly healthy individuals. The running is their way of seeking an opportunity to prove their self-sufficiency and capacity to survive in the larger world.[41]

Many of these youngsters come from affluent suburban families where they have been sheltered and taught that the surrounding world is extremely dangerous. Their desire to venture forth into this "urban jungle" may represent little more than a counterphobic self-prescribed rite of passage designed to overcome fears of independence. Although many of them describe minor difficulties with their parents or with school authorities, these do not sound serious. Often these problems contain a predominant theme of being underestimated and overly directed. On direct psychiatric examination, these youngsters do not show evidence of severe psychopathology. Their families seem equally free of severe disturbance, and the social history does not reveal evidence of earlier trauma

or serious impairment of the developmental process.

Most of these youngsters do not show a repetitive runaway pattern. They return home feeling older and wiser and resume their previous pattern of adjustment, often maintaining that the runaway experience was a valuable and important part of their development.

The Hedonist: These are youngsters who may superficially resemble the "Adventurer" since they too run without any evidence of severe conflict with family members or other important adults. The frictions which have been present tend to center around issues of freedom and obedience to rules. Superficially, the conflicts sound similar to those of "normal" runaways. However, closer investigation reveals that these complaints have much less substance. Indeed, it turns out that the hedonist feels irritated and constricted by even the most reasonable restraints on his absolute freedom to do as he wishes. Though such youngsters may not appear calloused or angry, their affability depends on the adult's willingness to give them their way on all matters that affect their immediate pleasure.

Although the families in this category appear to have genuine affection for their youngsters, a careful history shows that their limit-setting has always been ineffective. The parents tend to fear the youngster's anger and displeasure and have a long history of indulging the child and entertaining him lavishly. This approach may appear to work satisfactorily in the earlier years of development. Once the youngster's appetites become more adult, however, the inevitable conflict ensues. The parents attempt to curb the youngster's pleasure-seeking for the first time, and he reacts violently.

These youngsters tend to run away to groups of other youngsters who share their philosophy of life.[40] They do not go to adult-organized refuges for the runaway. Their motive for running, after all, is not to find assistance in dealing with family problems, but to engage in activities which would be forbidden in the family and community atmosphere. In a psychiatric evaluation they do not seem to be severely disturbed. They often assert that they enjoy the freedoms they have found away from home. At times their basically infantile viewpoint leads them to the kinds of physical illness that arise from overindulgence in drugs, the uninterrupted and sleepless pursuit of pleasure, and sexual promiscuity. Although the negative effects of their pleasure-seeking may lead to superficial promises to behave differently, they are difficult to treat successfully in an outpatient setting, even if the parents are cooperative and involved. Having tasted the joys of unfettered license, they tend to run periodically unless they are confined and slowly led to accept the requirements of living within the constraints of reality.

The Loner: The next three categories follow closely Stierlin's[91] classification of runaway youngsters based on family psychopathological patterns. His categories are based on the conceptualization that there are three types of families which produce an adolescent who runs away. The first of these, he describes as the excessively binding family. These families tend to hold their youngsters too close, either through excessive gratification of dependency wishes or through a process of "mystification" which prevents the youngster from becoming aware of his own wishes and desires. As the youngster reaches adolescence, he finds that his emerging sexual and aggressive drives cannot be contained within the family and wants to emancipate himself.

However, his knowledge of the external world and his capacity to relate to peers are extremely deficient. As a result, his skills in adapting to the world outside the home are markedly impaired. If he does attempt to run away, the absence is brief, since he is unable to find, attract, or utilize alternative sources of gratification. His loneliness forces a quick return to the family, but the adjustment there is also unsatisfactory, so that sooner or later the wish to run again recurs.

In the author's experience, this situation is malignant and difficult to alter. It is also dangerous, since the youngster's inability to find satisfaction within or outside the family may lead to severe depression and even to suicidal behavior.

The Hood: This runaway youngster is produced by a family configuration diametrically opposed to the family which produces the lonely runaway. Stierlin describes this family as one with an expelling mode. This child is experienced by his parents as an unwanted encumbrance to their own desires and pleasures. He is rejected and neglected. At the earliest possible age, he is forced to fend for himself and to meet his own needs in any way that does not require the parents' time and attention.

Such a youngster runs away from home basically because there is nothing there for him. The long background of deprivation and emotional coldness have had their predictable result, and the child is calloused, predatory, and unscrupulous. He does not trust emotional ties of any kind and is well prepared to maintain himself and succeed among the criminal element on the street. In short, he is a successful runaway but a hazard to conventional society. Naturally, it is extremely difficult to interrupt this adjustment mode by means of any currently known psychotherapeutic approach.

The Emissary: Stierlin's third family type does not bind or expel the child but sends the youngster on a "mission." These youngsters are subtly encouraged to leave the home in order to engage in activities which indirectly benefit one or both of their parents. Often the children act out impulses which are present within the parents but which the parents' superegos forbid them to express directly. (This state of affairs was described by Johnson and Szurek[43, 92] in their classic papers on "superego lacunae.") Other missions may be more related to the vicarious testing of ego possibilities. For example, in one of Stierlin's cases, a father is described who was frightened of changing jobs and moving to a new community; he seemed to utilize his youngster's runaway as proof to himself that the change was not as dangerous as he feared.

In these cases, the youngster's runaway is marked by extensive involvement in the activity which the family mission requires. For example, the daughter who is being utilized to act out mother's inhibited sexuality will be sexually active during her absence from the home. Most of these youngsters maintain some contact with the home and often report on their behavior by telephone or on their return home. Often one is amazed to learn that the parents have rather complete knowledge of the youngster's location and activities throughout the runaway period. This information is especially surprising in view of the lack of parental activity toward retrieving the youngster.

Naturally, this pattern is unlikely to improve without extensive changes in the family dynamics. This can be approached by direct treatment of the parents or through family therapy.

VANDALISM

As is the case with many other antisocial actions, vandalism has its origins in the innocent anarchy of early childhood. The young child crayons mother's walls because they are attractive and available receptacles for his creative urge, not because of an angry desire to destroy valuable property. However, the mother's response to this early behavior may be crucial in determining the youngster's later attitude toward property destruction. In homes where there is no pride of possession and children are not taught to value this social expectation, the youngster cannot internalize respect for the possessions of others. On the other hand, in households where material possessions are prized more highly than children, the child may come to despise valued property and develop a proclivity for attacking it as a symbolic extension of unloving adults.

These two sources of the vandalistic urge continue to be important even in the older child. In rundown neighborhoods where there is an absence of community pride, vandalism is rampant and casual. On the other hand, the rapid escalation of vandalism in public schools may well represent a vindictive reaction to the impersonal and even hostile atmosphere which many youngsters subjectively experience in these institutions. The appearance of graffiti, for example, on school desks, walls, and other exposed surfaces may serve at once to personalize the institution, to gain some sense of possessing it, at least in part, and at the same time, to retaliate for real or imagined neglect.[54]

In addition to these factors, vandalism must also be considered a response to a sense of powerlessness. In observing the play of young children, one frequently notes their pleasure in destroying houses they have built with blocks, clay figures, and other objects which they clearly value. These actions are often symbolic aggressive acts, the living out of fantasies which involve angry feelings toward important figures in their environment. They are also dramatizations of the youngster's fantasies of possessing great strength and power. Frequently these sequences are played out with obvious glee and satisfaction. The childish fascination with storms and explosions derives from a similar origin. It is clear that these tendencies are to some extent universally human, based perhaps on the simple fact that it is easier to destroy in a spectacular way than it is to construct something which gives a comparable sense of personal impact on the environment.

The inscription of graffiti would appear to be a somewhat modified expression of a similar need to obtain a sense of mastery over the material environment. According to Lomas,[54] the individual who marks or writes on a wall is expressing aggressive and destructive wishes to befoul and simultaneously possess the involved structure at the owner's expense. Lomas feels that this desire to "leave one's mark" is the central dynamic even in the scatological graffiti observed in bathrooms, especially men's rooms. In his view, the increased frequency of graffiti in these areas is related primarily to privacy. There is an opportunity to

write on the walls without being detected. In addition, pregenital and homosexual impulses may be accentuated in such sexually segregated surroundings designed for the expression of pregenital instincts. In older youngsters and adolescents, property destruction frequently appears as a response to limit-setting. The destruction may be an impulsive expression of frustration, such as kicking a door, breaking a window, or smashing a lamp. In these instances it seems clear that the hostility is displaced from the frustrating human object and expressed indirectly by destroying property. Often in these cases, there is a suggestion of both homicidal and suicidal derivatives, since the destroyed object may be highly valued by the child himself and may be his own possession.

Not all destructiveness is impulsive. It may be much more calculated and planned. The motives may be similar to those that inspire impulsive destruction, but the act represents a planned attempt at interpersonal revenge rather than a loss of impulse control. Some youngsters clearly act this way in a conscious effort to control the supervisory adult by reassigning roles, and intimidating and frightening the authority figure. In these instances acts of vandalism become tools in a power struggle centered on questions of control. Obviously this variety of vandalism is a common problem in detention homes, residential treatment centers, and psychiatric hospitals, since youngsters confined in such institutions often feel powerless and may be threatened by their enforced passivity.

Vandalism can, of course, become a psychopathological phenomenon in its own right. Seriously antisocial youngsters often engage in repeated acts of major vandalism as part of their generally angry relationship to the world around them. Some of these acts probably do not originate as a wish to destroy but represent thwarted attempts at burglary. For example, youngsters may destroy articles in a building, because they are frustrated by locks or by the failure to find valuables to steal. Other destructive acts are merely part of a theft, as in the case of telephones or coin-operated devices which are demolished in the process of looting their contents.

Other acts of vandalism serve more as defiant expressions of the power and fearlessness of adolescent gangs who run through the streets breaking off car antennae and destroying other property primarily to prove their courage and daring.[35]

Another pattern of vandalism is more clearly vindictive. It arises within a community and tends to be directed toward a scapegoated individual or family. Often these adults have refused to let youngsters play on their property, have called the police to complain of noise, or have interfered in conflicts between their offspring and other youngsters in the neighborhood. These unpopular individuals become the targets for relatively harmless pranks, such as having their trees rolled or their houses egged. Unfortunately, depending on the intensity of the conflict and the nature of the neighborhood, these pranks may lead to more serious acts of vandalism involving destruction of property.

It does appear that acts of vandalism are on the rise. To some extent, this is a social phenomenon which cannot be accounted for entirely from a psychiatric viewpoint. Apparently many adults and children feel alienated and have a low or absent sense of community pride. Without the respect for property which views the community as to some extent a joint possession, vandalism is inevitable. Two examples may illustrate the point. The first concerns a community center placed in a poverty area by a well-meaning social agency. During the first year of its existence, it was virtually destroyed by multiple acts of vandalism. The center's directors recognized the basic mistake in the center's conceptualization and organized a community-wide drive to involve community members in planning programs, repairing the center, and determining its design and appearance. This community organization effort was successful and there was no further vandalism.

The second example concerns a therapeutic wilderness camp for boys. The camp sponsors provided a dining room and bath facilities for the youngsters. The boys themselves constructed their personal domiciles utilizing materials provided at the boys' request by the camp. The shower house and dining room were frequent targets of vandalism, while the structures which the boys erected were never damaged.

In short, from a social point of view, safety arises from the presence of a strong sense of community interest in protecting property. Such material goods are regarded as somehow the shared possession of community members. When such a feeling is lacking or loses its strength, vandalism follows. This may result from an individual's failure to achieve a sense of personal belongingness and value within the community, or from a generalized lack of cohesion and shared concern. The act itself may be angry and personal, a subgroup defiance of community values, or a sanctioned acting out of the whole community's anger at the wider society.

The individual psychodynamics of vandalism are those of the unsocialized aggressive behavior disorders in general. Impulsive destructiveness is basically an expression of intense, largely unmodified, aggressive urges, often expressed rather unselectively against the environment. The event is common enough so that when Morris and associates[67] wanted to describe a group of aggressively disturbed youngsters for purposes of long-term follow-up study, they included "wanton destruction" as one of seven defining characteristics. This destructive behavior represents primarily a failure in ego control. It arises in situations where environmental structure is insufficient to channel behavior constructively to provide gratification, to limit frustration, or to give control.

Youngsters who habitually engage in planned and secret acts of vandalism often resemble Charles (the case presented earlier). They experience simultaneously a strong sense of aggressiveness and an intense fear of counterattack, then turn to secret destruction of property as a compromise between these opposing emotions. They cannot express their anger and frustration directly because of their fears of retaliation, so their resentment takes the form of ingenious acts of revenge directed against the belongings of those they regard as their enemies and frustrators.

The youngsters who destroy objects while out of control often feel ashamed and guilty about their destructive behavior. They may not express this attitude verbally, but they find ways to communicate their concern over their inability to control and direct their own behavior. The usual form of expression this takes is visible in their obviously negative self-image and their efforts to elicit control from adults. If the authority figures are unable or unwilling to provide such external controls, the children feel more anxious. As their tension mounts and their internal disorganization increases, they become even more destructive.

On the other hand, the youngster who uses vandalism as a premeditated and planned method of dealing with his interpersonal difficulties is less likely to view his destructive behavior as ego dystonic. If he is able to "get away" with his destructiveness, he often experiences a sense of mastery, superiority, and personal victory. Unconsciously, however, somewhere within him, he knows he is doing wrong. Unfortunately, the need to deal with unrecognized guilt requires youngsters of this kind to project hostility onto the environment. They regard their own destructiveness as the fault of others, and often feel victimized, and potentially vulnerable. These fears generate and justify even more vandalism, and a vicious cycle ensues.[48, 75]

The family dynamics in youngsters who are prone to vandalism vary considerably. However, the most frequent pattern is well described by Rexford and van Amerongen.[76] The mothers of the acting-out children feared their youngsters' demands would be insatiable. As a result, they had tremendous difficulty in being adequately giving toward their children. This deprivation was, of course, extremely frustrating to the child. On the other hand, the mothers had difficulty in setting limits on aggressiveness and destructive behavior. In their view, all limit setting was total deprivation and rejection. The authors felt that these behaviors resulted from the mothers' unresolved oral conflicts. Many mothers with such problems implicitly or explicitly encourage their children to act out against persons outside of the family. They seek thus to avoid facing these impulses at home in direct personal interaction with their children. This observation is borne out by common clinical experience. Despite obvious and overwhelming evidence of guilt, as long as the destructive behavior occurs outside of the home, parents of vandalistic children often deny the youngsters' involvement.

The treatment of youngsters who vandalize is, in most respects, similar to the treatment of behavior disorders in general. Destructive behavior which results from loss of control is approached with the traditional techniques of gradually exploring the youngster's particular anxieties and areas of ego vulnerability. These are corrected by the provision of sensitive interpretation and judicious limit setting, coupled with appropriate support and affection. The goal is to assist the youngster in gradually gaining capacity for delay and in acquiring more appropriate skills with which to obtain necessary gratifications. In many respects, the process of psychotherapy with these youngsters involves as much patient teaching as it does insight and interpretation. Collaborative therapy with the parents is of obvious importance. Their struggle is to learn to meet their youngsters' needs without unnecessary frustration of legitimate dependency requirements while maintaining appropriate limits on destructive aggressiveness. It is at best a difficult assignment; when mastered it is truly a great achievement.

The treatment of youngsters who utilize vandalism as a conscious defense against internal conflict is somewhat more complex. While it is necessary for these youngsters to recognize and accept their own aggressiveness, premature efforts to confront them may elicit paranoid defensiveness and a sense that they are misunderstood by the therapist. It is often necessary to focus first on the defensive nature of their belligerent stance while recognizing sympathetically their sense of vulnerability. This can be technically difficult, since, within the transference, these youngsters can be extremely provocative. In spite of this, the therapist must often remain forgiving and understanding, commenting primarily on the patient's fear of retaliation instead of reacting to behavior which, in a nontherapeutic setting, would inevitably incite counter-aggression. In short, the therapist needs to assist the patient to see himself as less evil, dangerous, and vicious, so that the youngster will be less fearful and thereby less in need of the stance of defensive belligerence. If the youngster's basic desire for self-assertion and self-protection are accepted and supported within the therapeutic relationship, the youngster is more likely to find himself an acceptable member of the community of man and to feel less need to strike the first blow in a defensive war.

CRUELTY TO ANIMALS

The subject of the proper treatment of nonhuman animals seems to be heavily invested with emotion. Many adults, presumably emotionally normal, extend tremendous amounts of energy and money in systematic efforts to seek out and destroy wild animals. Another large group of adults, also presumably healthy, have organized themselves into a movement whose prime function is to prevent cruelty to animals. In America, enormous sums of money are spent feeding, grooming, and providing veterinary care for a variety of loved and cherished animals. At the same time, many animals are killed and neglected at public pounds. These social phenomena suggest that both wild and domesticated animals play an important role in the emotional life of humans. However, they also suggest that society's guidelines for the valuation and treatment of animals are far from clear.

The infant and young toddler often handle animals in a way that from an adult point of view, would be described as cruel. However, much of this mistreatment is simply the outcome of the child's desire to manipulate, tug, twist, and pound a variety of objects in the environment; it is based on a lack of full awareness that the pet experiences pain. Nonetheless, one often recognizes the presence of a punishment motif in this play with animals. The older toddler begins to be aware that he is giving his dog a "spanking" for some real or projected naughtiness. Other mistreatment seems related to the youngster's sense of object possession and his belief that the object exists entirely for meeting his personal needs. Thus, if he is in a kind and loving mood, his dog is petted, but, if the child is angry or frustrated, the animal is kicked, ignored, or otherwise abused.

These difficulties between younger children and their pets tend to be worked out reasonably quickly if the pet is old enough to defend itself and to protest its mismanagement with counter-aggression. This is the reality-learning aspect of the socialization of impulses toward cruelty. In addition, anal and oral sadistic impulses are curbed in response to the expectations of the parents and other valued love objects. The ego defenses, notably reaction formation and repression, are brought to bear on the forbidden impulses, and they are curbed or actually reversed into strong sympathies and protective attitudes toward pets. In many children, reaction formation may disguise hostility toward humans, while the cruel and destructive feelings are acted out on animals.[28]

In older children, some sex differentiation tends to appear in regard to the treatment of animals. Many oedipal and latency age boys engage in rather random acts of cruelty toward animals. However, these actions are not usually directed toward pets or other valued animals. The victims are likely to be stray cats, flies, frogs, and other animals which are seen as unwanted or unattractive. Often these actions are carried out in groups and seem to represent proofs of toughness, masculinity, and the total absence of "feminine" squeamishness. Boys of the same age enjoy "hunting" birds and other small animals with air rifles. Although these activities can become sadistic, the primary aim seems more one of phallic dominance rather than sadistic torture. However, van Ophuijsen[69] has suggested that enjoyment of inflicting pain is not the primary goal in sadistic behavior. He states the goal is to perform certain acts on an object that is, or can be viewed, as insensible. At any rate, predominance of this type of play, particularly if it is pursued individually by a youngster, suggests that development is not moving ahead smoothly. Acts of cruelty directed toward valued pets in this age group are an even stronger alarm signal. The symptom may reflect a strong fixation at pregenital sadistic phases, massive feelings of phallic inferiority for which the youngster is compensating, or a severely disturbed role in the family system. For example, many youngsters are forced into a scapegoat role within the family group. They then turn their hostility toward family pets because the animals are the only family members below them in a hostile pecking order.

In evaluating aggressiveness of any kind, it is imperative to remember Hartmann and Kris's statement[38] that extreme aggressiveness may originate either from a defensive need to deny fear and vulnerability or as the direct expression of sadistic impulses. Often one is confronted with a combination which includes both defensive and expressive elements. This is the common state of affairs because much fear actually results from the projection of hostile and sadistic impulses onto the environment. Some authors[50, 69] state that these destructive impulses derive from the oral biting stage of development and may even, at their deepest level, represent derivatives of cannibalistic urges for oral introjection of the object.

This attention to the impulse life of the youngster, however, should not detract the therapist from a careful investigation of family dynamics and the actual life experiences of the child. Many youngsters who are cruel to animals have in fact been treated quite cruelly themselves. Much of their behavior represents a protective identification with the aggressor[23] and is primarily defensive in its origin. Defense and desire become interconnected within such youngsters; they have often been subjected to considerable frustration with the result that their anger and aggressiveness are increased.

Treatment is important for these cases since the surging and largely hidden rage within these children, as well as their need to define some helpless creatures as appropriate recipients for their cruelty, results in a weakening of their capacity for reality testing and for ego growth. The resolution of ambivalence and the capacity for true intimacy are obviously blocked by this profound splitting within the personality.

In assessing the significance of cruelty to animals through the course of development, there has been some retrospective evidence that it may represent an ominous precursor of homicidal potential at a later age.[6, 16] This correlation is by no means proven. For example, a recent small but well-conducted study[84] did not find a higher incidence of history of cruelty to animals in a group of ten adolescent boys who had murdered than in ten adolescent boys who had threatened homicide and in ten controls who had no history of homicidal ideation or behavior. In addition, it seems clear that large numbers of youngsters engage in these behaviors without any evidence of severe psychopathology in later life and certainly with no apparent tendency toward homicide. As Anna Freud[22] has noted, symptomatic behavior by children is not even a reliable indicator of the severity of developmental problems, much less a predictor of adult behavior. The vicissitudes of instinctual development and the kaleidoscopic array of ego defenses make it extremely difficult to trace directly the path of any specific behavior to its outcome in adulthood.

SEXUAL ASSAULT

As a presenting symptom, sexual assault is extremely rare prior to adolescence. However, precocious sexual activity, which may be quite aggressive, is common in the history of many antisocial children. There is a strong tendency for the behavior to be repetitive, a state of affairs that does not seem to be materially affected by punishment or confinement. This is not surprising since the behavior is obsessional, serving both id and superego.[82]

Although there are many dynamic variations among sexually assaultive youngsters, one frequently encounters a tendency toward general emotional immaturity, poorly developed social skills, seclusiveness, suspiciousness to the point of near paranoia in most human relationships, and a tendency toward isolation with excessive and bizarre fantasy. Family psychopathology is striking, with extremely poor parent-child relationships and blatantly pathological marital and parenting patterns.

Treatment is difficult because of the emotional isolation and suspiciousness which characterize these patients. Still, the natural course of the illness is so malignant that despite the patient's vigorous resistance, the clinician is obligated to attempt treatment. The rejection of treatment often comes not only from the assaultive adolescent but also from the family.

Tim, an attractive, mild-mannered, but remote young man of fifteen, was referred for psychiatric evaluation after threatening an older woman with a knife in a rape attempt. He was diagnosed as borderline, and inpatient treatment was strongly recommended. Tim protested this recommendation mildly and was immediately supported in his resistance by his parents. The parents were able to convince the juvenile court that Tim should receive outpatient psychotherapy, although they told the judge privately that it was their opinion that Tim needed no treatment at all. Within two weeks, Tim successfully raped a woman using exactly the same approach. He was then confined in a reformatory for a prolonged period. Within days after his release, he assaulted a third woman.

The specific psychodynamics of sexual assault are rather poorly understood. This probably emerges from the difficulty of successfully treating these youngsters by means of an unmodified psychodynamic approach. The data arising from diagnostic studies, as well as from some cases that were successfully managed with insight therapy, suggest certain common patterns. Much of the difficulty appears related to an extremely distorted mother-child relationship which is at once erotized and inhibiting. There is a lack of counterbalancing strength from the boys' fathers. These men are typically both emotionally cold and relatively ineffective. As a result, they provide little in the way of an adequate identification figure. The mothers, on the other hand, are viewed with extreme ambivalence; they serve at once as strong and powerful sources of emotion and as serious threats to the boy's masculinity. The mother is likely to be prudish and yet fascinated with her son's sexual thoughts and behavior. In one case, for example, the mother was preoccupied with the possibility that the boy would get in trouble sexually. She guarded against this eventuality by spying on him in his room to see if he was masturbating and by searching his room for "pornographic" reading materials which he might have secreted there. Aside from the sexual area, the boy's relationship with his mother may be cordial and even warm. The mother may be somewhat seductive, at least to the extent that she prefers her son's companionship to that of her inadequate marital partner.

The effect of this family structure on the boy is to produce intense preoccupation with sexuality and marked inhibition in regard to appropriate channels of socialization and dating. Girls are often viewed as extremely attractive from a purely sexual point of view, but as frightening when viewed in the context of a real relationship. They are seen at once as potential sources of excessive demands and of rejection. The result is a great deal of secretive fantasy and of loveless, and often bizarre, sexual encounter in which the girl is utilized as a masturbatory object. At the same time, the mother's close, admiring attachment often leads to a core of grandiosity in the youngster with expectations that others will recognize his extraordinary value and worth. These fantasies are in turn threatened by recognition of his own social ineptitude, along with marked feelings of masculine inadequacy, in the real world.

The impact of these distortions on the developing ego is catastrophic. These boys are naive and show a marked tendency toward a polarized view of life and relationships. Positive ties are seen in a very idealized light and the smallest frustration at the hands of a "friend" is perceived as a vicious betrayal of trust. This touchiness makes the normal give and take of a close relationship almost impossible to tolerate, and the youngster is often preoccupied with his image, status, and methods of forcing others to respect and admire him. The desire for power reflects the youngster's belief that control and coercion of others is a more reliable source of narcissistic support than their affection. The result is an increasingly narcissistic adjustment which is highly precarious. The extreme variance between the youngster's image of himself and his actual functioning leads to repeated and severe narcissistic injury in the course of daily living. If these are occasioned by a real 'or imagined rejection at the hands of a desirable girl, this girl is all too likely to be the object of sexual assault. The assaultive boy may also characterize certain types of girls, especially those who are popular with boys, as the generalized source of his discomfort. He may, therefore, attack a girl that he does not even know personally.

The sexual attack clearly represents a wish to possess the girl. It expresses both the patient's rage toward women and his intense need for sexual acceptance.

A sixteen-year-old boy, in treatment two years after he had assaulted a female classmate, was talking about the fact that he had not seen the girl in the neighborhood for some time. The idea occurred to him that she might have died during the previous two years. This thought made him instantly sad, and he began to cry. When asked about his tears, he commented that this would have meant she had a very short life and that his behavior toward her had made it unhappy. When the therapist commented that he had wished very much to make her happy, he nodded and began to weep bitterly. The interaction was particularly fascinating in view of the fact that the boy had always justified his attack of the grounds that the girl had "made fun" of him and was a "bitch."

The internal mental life of these youngsters includes a fragmented collection of images as numerous and complicated as the characters in a Russian novel. The simplest behaviors require a complex balancing of psychic forces and the striking of compromises between a variety of conflicting motives. These elaborate transactions are particularly striking in regard to sexual behavior. For example, a sexually assaultive youngster was caught exhibiting himself through the window of his bedroom. This was reported to the therapist.

When it was approached in the therapy session, the youngster became furious that the therapist had knowledge of the event. Upon careful exploration, he was finally able to discuss the reasons for this dangerous and unwise expression of his sexuality. He explained that his anger at the therapist's involvement was related to intense fear. He had made a pact with his conscience that he could perform this sexual act so long as he denied it and refused to admit to anyone that it was the result of his own sexual excitement. It was the abridgment of this agreement that had generated the fear and the rage. When he had been apprehended by his mother, he had explained to her that he had exposed himself only because he was "bored."

This characteristic complicates the treatment of these youngsters. In effect, one is not always sure who is speaking during a given therapy session. Depending on which imago is in control of the ego, the youngster at one time presents himself as an unsocialized sexual gratification machine, at another time as a prudish and judgmental critic of human frailty in any form, and yet again as a reasonable and cooperative human being. The therapist must learn to recognize the nonverbal accompaniments of these various ego states in order to assist the youngster to become acquainted with the different facets of himself, so that integration eventually becomes possible.

The countertransference problems in the therapy of these youngsters are very serious. It is extraordinarily difficult to predict or prevent a reoccurrence of the dangerous behavior. In a sense, the direct assaultiveness is similar to a perversion. It is likely to occur whenever specific internal conditions coincide with opportunity and provocation in the environment. The youngster's capacity to hide the deviant sexual impulses from himself as well as from the therapist makes it extremely difficult to make rational decisions regarding the length of inpatient treatment and the time when therapy can be safely pursued on an outpatient basis.

It is clear that both the juvenile justice system and mental health professionals need more information and greater willingness to work collaboratively in order to treat these youngsters with any hope of effectiveness and to protect society from their dangerous behavior.

LYING

Anna Freud[22] has suggested that falsification by youngsters be divided into three types: innocent lying, fantasy lying, and delinquent lying. Innocent lying refers to the young child's inability to separate inner and outer reality and his failure to distinguish between primary and secondary process thinking. Because of his developmental level, he makes statements which are objectively untrue but which, from the subjective viewpoint of the child, are quite valid. Fantasy lying is a later development which arises because of reality frustrations and disappointments for which the child compensates by elaborating regressive wish-fulfilling versions of life events which are more satisfying. Delinquent lying refers to a deliberate distortion of fact in order to gain a direct advantage over reality issues, that is, to avoid punishment or to achieve some material or interpersonal gain.

It is obvious that these three forms of lying overlap to some extent. For example, in antisocial youngsters, one frequently encounters delinquent lying which is so strongly colored by wishful thinking that the youngster himself comes to believe his fabrications. On the other hand, not all fantasy lying is devoid of delinquent motivation.

Lying must be evaluated not only within a developmental framework but in comparison with the social norms extant in the child's family and social group. Almost all adults lie at least to the extent that tact and social propriety encourage this solution to sticky interpersonal situations. Few mothers will tell a friend that the color scheme of the friend's new living room is atrocious. However, the mother may later state this candid opinion in the hearing of her child who has previously heard her praise the room extravagantly. Apparently most children are able to understand these "white lies" and utilize them acceptably as they grow older, although their innocent candor at younger ages may lead to an occasional embarrassing situation for the parents.

Unfortunately, in many families, the pattern of lying is much more extensive. The youngster observes one parent make a purchase and then deny it later to the spouse. Often enough, the youngster may be asked to be an accomplice in the deception. More common still are families in which the honest expression of feelings is a rarity, and a veritable labyrinth of lies is utilized to avoid not only unpleasant confrontations but even necessary and difficult problem solving.

In addition, subcultures and specific community enclaves vary tremendously in their standards regarding objective truthfulness. In some schools, for example, cheating is accepted as a matter of course and lying is an unnoticed necessary adjunct

to that behavior. Often, the rules for truthfulness vary considerably depending on whom one is talking to. For example, lying to adults outside of the family may be accepted by some groups of youngsters, while lying to each other is explicitly forbidden. By the same token, it may be acceptable to lie to youngsters who are not members of one's clique while complete honesty is required within the "in group."

The primary psychodynamic of lying is obviously related to wish fulfillment.[11, 19, 82] Sigmund Freud suggested that children fabricate in retaliation for the lies they are told by grownups regarding sexual reality.[26] According to Fenichel lying may also be utilized to reinforce repression and denial of unpleasant realities by the formula, "If people believe the unreal things that I tell them, perhaps real things that bother me are also untrue." (p. 529)[19]

From the standpoint of object relations, lying is at a somewhat higher level than stealing or other direct action-oriented antisocial behaviors.[11, 82] Lying represents a progression in at least two ways. First of all, it is a cognitive movement from pure action to thought and words which are generally regarded as a higher level of mental activity. In addition, lying is less narcissistic than stealing, in that it at least requires the involvement of another human being. A child may steal in order to deny the need for objects and a relationship to them (he can nurture himself and needs no one else), but lying requires an audience and thereby involves another human being. From a therapeutic point of view, lying is more useful in view of the fact that it reveals unconscious motives and wishes, at the same time that it attempts to delude the therapist. Brill has noted the similarity between lies and "artificial dreams," since both may be analyzed as important psychic creations. Brunswick[12] has suggested that all lying begins in the denial of the anatomical differences between the sexes, but also feels that lying within the therapy situation has potential therapeutic value.

The presence of extensive lying always indicates a felt sense of personal weakness or personal inadequacy in older children and adolescents. Thus, it is obviously a compensatory mechanism, particularly when it is primarily fantasy lying. It represents fantasy which requires a corroborating listener.

The relationship between the liar and his audience is of special importance. Obviously, it is still quite narcissistic. Habitual liars experience a relative lack of discomfort when their untruthfulness is exposed. Often they begin again immediately with a new series of fabrications, cheerfully ignoring the other person's angry reaction to being deluded. This observation suggests that a primary motive in lying is to deceive the self; the listener is utilized only as a support to that internal operation. This is also corroborated by the extent to which liars come to believe their own fabrications. The severest form of lying is called pseudologia phantastica. There, indeed, the dividing line between psychotic delusions and simple untruth becomes somewhat hazy. The everyday liar generally seems to retain the capacity to recognize the unreality of his statements. But it is sometimes difficult to be sure that the appreciation of reality is strongly cathected in individuals who demonstrate pseudologia phantastica. That is, it seems to be emotionally unimportant that their statements are not factually true. However, unlike the psychotic, the individual with pseudologia often seems to go to considerable trouble to make his stories plausible, including obtaining facts and information which lend a surface veracity to his productions.[11, 20]

Obviously, a strong commitment to lying tends to produce other distortions of personality development. Jacobson[42] has pointed out that the extensive use of denial replaces structural conflict by instinctual conflict. This affects thought processes, interferes with logical thinking, and predisposes the youngster to acting out (through injury to the development of reality testing); the external impact of habitual lying on object relations is even more clear. Other people react to lying with resentment. They are angry with and tend to reject untruthful youngsters. This is particularly likely, since many children who are unable to express aggression directly, utilize lying as a method of creating conflict between other people for the purpose of achieving a measure of control or of gaining vicarious gratification. As noted, parents of lying youngsters often utilize deceitful and corrupt parenting practices and personal behavior. It is not unusual for these parents to recommend to their children that they lie to the therapist in order to protect the parent or to avoid revealing family secrets which the parent regards as shameful or guilt-ridden. Collaborative therapy with the parents or the utilization of a family therapy approach are often essential to success in these cases.

In summary, the clinical course of lying behavior depends on cognitive and developmental issues, the extent to which the child internalizes moral codes regarding truthfulness, and finally the nature of the attitude toward veracity which exists in the family and the wider society.

FIRESETTING

Most children are fascinated with fire. Its universal symbolic power is well recognized and is reflected in everyday language and in literature.[8] Yarnell[99] has noted that young firesetters seem to be preoccupied with Biblical images of good and evil, in which fire is seen as a destructive but purifying force which can convert bad to good. She also points out that these images are widespread in the mythology of the human race.

Since fire is a fascinating phenomenon which is not well understood by the younger child, inadvertent firesetting by such children is not unusual. Many of these occurrences do not represent symptomatic behavior, but result from the child's faulty reality sense combined with an environmental opportunity which may be accidental or related to parental carelessness and lack of supervision.

However, it is clear that there are a small but significant number of youngsters who are pathological firesetters. This behavior is repetitive and often dangerous to themselves and others. The basic dynamics of the problem seem related to frustration and aggression. It often arises in response to hostile and rejecting parents, especially in younger children. According to Yarnell, firesetters in the six to eight year age range set fires only when under stress in the home situation. In each instance, fire was intended as a hostile attack on a frustrating family member and was set in the home or nearby. The child seemed frightened of the fire and it was quickly extinguished. Left with matches in the hospital, these youngsters showed no interest in or desire to start fires.

Because of its dramatic nature, firesetting has led to considerable speculation in the literature. Unfortunately, perhaps because it is a relatively rare symptom, there are considerable discrepancies between the findings of various individuals who have studied these children. Sigmund Freud[26] was the first to suggest a close connection between ambition, homosexual competition, fire, and urethral erotism. Other analysts continued to emphasize the connection between water play, enuresis, and the symptom of firesetting, connecting these to the fixation of sexual drive development at the level of urethral-phallic impulses.[7, 37, 88] However, in Yarnell's large study[99, 52] she found a limited correlation between enuresis and firesetting and did not always discover the preoccupation with water play others had noted. Silverman[87] on the other hand, in the study of two late latency firesetters, did discover a strong preoccupation with water play, as well as a conscious pleasure in observing fires and all connected with them. In this respect his cases resemble the adolescent group in Yarnell's study. Recent papers such as those by Vandersall and Weiner[95] and Kaufman and associates[45] have emphasized the general ego weaknesses of firesetters rather than specific dynamics.

Yarnell's older age group was made up entirely of males who differed considerably from youngsters who had set fires at an earlier age. These adolescent boys gave the details of their firesetting behavior with no evidence of anxiety or remorse. They started fires away from home after careful planning and enjoyed staying to watch the conflagration. They did not seem to have any interest in putting out the fires and, on the contrary, experienced a sense of exhilaration and release when the fire began which they very much enjoyed. These boys frequently operated in pairs. Although there was no evidence of overt homosexual contact between them, the intensity of the attachment between the pair and the tendency to have an active and a passive member suggested an unconscious attachment of this kind. Both Silverman and Yarnell have observed disturbed motility in these youngsters, often accompanied by learning disability. They also recognized the presence of severe psychopathology, particularly in the younger children, with disorganization of thought processes to a point approaching psychosis. During these states of extreme tension, the children were confused, appeared dreamy and dissociated, were preoccupied with vivid fantasies regarding fire, and seemed to be extremely agitated. The adolescent firesetters often appeared to enter a similar tense state of dissociation which was relieved only by firesetting and its consequent sense of release and fulfillment.

The individual psychodynamics of the firesetter are not well understood. This is particularly true in regard to explaining the specific symptom choice. It is clear that youngsters have been subjected to unusual mistreatment and have every reason to be angry and aggressive toward their environment. However, it is not clear why they choose firesetting as the avenue for expressing their impulses. The best clue would seem to reside in the similarity of their fantasies. These are primitive in character and expressive of some universal belief in the magical power of fire. When this observation is coupled with their generally regressed psychological level, disordered motility, and poor cognitive development, it suggests that these youngsters resort to firesetting because of its efficiency. They have developed no other techniques for so grand a release of their extreme tension and the full expression of their intense frustration and anger.

The younger children may represent an entirely different psychological syndrome from that encountered in the adolescent firesetter. In this older group, firesetting appears to be a more contained activity which bears many resemblances to a sexual perversion. Since these older pyromaniacs show a poverty of imagination and fantasy life, it is difficult to obtain solid information regarding the dynamics of their behavior. This problem may be increased by the fact that their firesetting seems to occur in a state of altered consciousness. Thought processes during this state of near-dissociation may simply be unavailable to them for subsequent dynamic exploration.

The parental and family contribution to the symptom of firesetting seems obvious from all case reports. These families are unusually rejecting and frustrating in their relationships with the patients. Siegel[86] has reported the case of one thirteen-year-old boy who set several dozen small fires. The boy's mother strongly resisted residential treatment for the youngster and insisted that the fire marshalls had forced the child to confess in spite of his innocence. Later in treatment, when she became angry at the child's physician, she threatened to call the youngster and tell him to set fire to the hospital. In this case, at least, there appeared to be a clear destructive symbiotic bond between mother and child and an obvious unconscious and/or conscious collusion in his destructive behavior.

Macht and Mack[56] described four adolescent firesetters whose fathers were associated closely with fire through their work or avocations. The fathers were absent from the home. The authors suggested the youngsters may have started fires from an unconscious desire to be reunited with the absent father.

It is fortunate that this syndrome is relatively rare, since treatment of the older age group appears to be quite difficult. Outpatient approaches are hazardous in view of the child's threat to his home and community. The family cooperation may be difficult to achieve although family therapy may serve not only to remove the symptom but to alter some of the basic dynamic origins of the youngster's rage.[65]

Inpatient treatment may be difficult to arrange. Many residential treatment centers refuse to admit known firesetters because of understandable anxiety about their threat to property and to the safety of other patients. This is an unfortunate circumstance since persistent firesetting is often only one of several indications that these children are in serious emotional difficulty. It also seems to be an unnecessary conservatism especially in the case of younger children. This group of firesetters rarely pose a danger outside of their homes. Firesetting can, however, be a real risk in inpatient treatment. The perpetrators are usually responding to staff and institutional tensions and may not have a history of firesetting.[8]

PROVOCATIVE BEHAVIOR

To some extent, of course, provocation is in the eye of the beholder. Clinicians are occasionally asked to evaluate youngsters who are regarded by their parents as provocative. Sometimes the child is merely exhibiting the normal physical liveliness of the young or the developmentally normal negativism which is an invariant part of the individuation-separation phase. These behaviors usually disappear with further maturation, unless the parents persist in their unrealistic expectations or fail to respond with appropriate management techniques.

There are other youngsters for whom provocation becomes a way of life. Two general groups may be described as typical constellations. One of these is well delineated by the diagnostic category "oppositional personality" under the proposed GAP classification. These youngsters have been depicted by others as passive-aggressive. Their provocativeness consists of dawdling, delaying, failing to perform tasks they have been told to do, and other patterns of passive resistance to authority. Occasionally, the behavior spreads to more important tasks such as attending school or eating properly.

The dynamics of this behavior are perhaps best conveyed by the cliche "passive aggression is the silver lining of servitude." Often this is objectively true, and the youngster is responding to an extremely restrictive and demanding parental environment which he does not dare to defy openly. In other situations, the parents are not excessively strict from an objective point of view but demand too much of the specific youngster. Because of their temperament, minimum brain dysfunction, or mild mental retardation, these children are unable to meet average age-appropriate expectations.

They experience them as too exacting. In older children, the passive-aggressive pattern may camouflage an inability to perform. For example, the youngster with a specific learning disability can avoid repeated humiliations by neglecting his assigned work in school.

The second group of provocative youngsters demonstrate their provocations in a more direct manner and in response to different motives. For a variety of reasons, some parents tend to respond and interact with their children only in situations of behavioral crisis. These youngsters utilize motoric behavior to invite parental contact, ranging from spankings, to physical restraint, to physical fondling.[66] Often this behavioral pattern occurs in families that are relatively nonverbal and with parents who lack skills in conceptualizing and implementing consistent behavioral limits.

Schmideberg has suggested that the small child feels intense envy of his parents' moral superiority because of his own personal sense of guilt.[82] If the youngster can provoke the parents into behaving badly, he may escape considerable anxiety and guilt by projecting his badness onto them while concurrently justifying his own aggressiveness toward them. Thus unjust reproaches and provocations are projected self-denunciations. The provocation serves as a verbal substitute for further acts of direct aggression. Later aggressions may, however, be justified on the basis of the parents' mistreatment of the child.

This pattern of provocative interaction is described by Kaufman and associates.[46] It is typical of the mother-daughter interaction in some cases of delinquent adolescent girls which they designate as anal and bisexual in drive organization. A more subtle form of provocation may occur in which the youngster merely focuses on the frustrations which the parent really has afflicted on the child while denying and forgetting positive and pleasant family interactions. The parents of such children often describe them as ungrateful and may in fact be provoked into an extremely withholding attitude toward the youngster since "nothing pleases them anyway."

Finally, provocation may occur as a structured family disorder. This syndrome is characterized by a mutual complaint from parents and child that the other party is causing them to misbehave. That is, the youngster admits that he gets into a fair amount of difficulty and that there are constant fights in the family, but he subjectively feels that these are the result of his parents' treatment of him. On the other hand, the parents admit that they are frequently angry with the youngster, punish him too much, and dislike him, but relate these feelings entirely to the child's constant provocative behavior and inability to accept the demands of family life. The syndrome has been reported primarily in the behavioral modification literature.[32, 80] According to these authors, the behavioral pattern results from a family system which mutually reinforces the child's provocation and the parents' angry response to it. Considerable success has been achieved by treatment approaches which utilize the parents as behavior modification therapists according to a plan developed in collaboration with them to extinguish the provocative behavior.[96]

In brief, then, provocation, while annoying to parents and other adults who must deal with the youngster, does represent evidence of considerable psychological development. It implies a sense of guilt over wrongdoing and an admiration for adults. Potentially, these may be utilized in a constructive way. Therapy with these youngsters involves helping them become aware of their aggressive and destructive drives without inducing excessive guilt. The goal is to help them handle their aggression through fantasy and to direct it into appropriately sublimated channels as well as to give it more direct verbal expression. As they become able to do this, they have less need to utilize provocation as an interpersonal sleight of hand in order to maintain an illustory sense of total perfection and goodness. Parents must also be assisted in their efforts not to respond to the provocation. Their natural tendency is to attempt to defend themselves by proving that they are good and it is the child who is bad. This approach merely increases the youngster's sense of guilt and his need to provoke.

DEFIANCE AND DISOBEDIENCE

All clinicians are familiar with the developmental origins of overt defiance and disobedience during the separation-individuation phase. This observation has extensive clinical grounding based on developmental histories and direct child observation studies. Clinicians are also well aware that the fate of this pint-sized revolution is dependent on complex intrapsychic factors in the parents, especially in the mother, and equally complex family system issues. In other words, if the family is able to respond to the young child's negativism as a healthy sign of individuation without either crushing it or being intimidated by it, it becomes gradually organized in the personality as a healthy capacity for independent thought

and self-assertion. Unfortunately, these propitious family circumstances do not always exist.

Defiant and disobedient behavior by young children is often the direct result of parental failure to provide clear expectations regarding behavior and to offer sufficient affection to elicit a primary positive regard from the child.[76] Parental difficulties in this area may, of course, be accentuated by constitutional deviancy in the child, which makes it difficult for the youngster to accept limits or to be comforted and gratified by normal parental techniques. In any case, the impact on the child is to create a capricious and cruel initial conscience formation. This harsh internalized set of expectations is feared and the child makes every effort to avoid its unrealistic requirements and to escape from the oppressive sense of guilt and badness. If helpful objects are available to the youngster, this internal conflict tends to be lived out with them. The child varies between periods of clinging and anxiety with tremendous fear of social disapproval and rejection, and other periods where the limits of the adults' acceptance are tested through aggressive and belligerent defiance and disobedience. This interaction at times appears to be an almost stylized game of crime, punishment, atonement, and reconciliation. The pattern tends to be interminable since the youngster is personally convinced of his wickedness and feels that the adults could not possibly forgive him if they were in fact aware of the real intensity of his destructiveness, especially of the degree to which it is directed toward the loved object itself. As a result, any superficial efforts to reassure these youngsters that they are in fact good, lovable, and accepted by the adult are doomed to failure. Even if the youngster believes in the sincerity of the adult and in fact sees it demonstrated through multiple episodes of forgiveness and acceptance, he still cannot allow himself this affection. It is as if he says, "That's all very well, but if you really knew how bad I was you would not remain so loving." (p. 39)[82]

If no caring adults are available or if past experience has led to strong distrust of the possibility of help, the defiant and disobedient behavior is even more marked. The youngster has a pressing need to prove that he is uncontrolled and uncontrollable; he searches for occasions when he can defy adult authority. The internal conscience and external authority figures are feared, hated, and fought. Enforced obedience produces extreme anxiety with fears of engulfment and total control, where voluntary obedience is unthinkable since it only reminds the youngster of his basic depression and longing for dependency.

The clinical course of defiance and disobedience cannot be summarized briefly. Its manifestations are so protean that a full discussion would include consideration of all the topics in this chapter. Many of the general comments regarding treatment of behavioral and antisocial disorders bear directly on the management of this behavioral pattern.

OUTBURSTS OF RAGE AND VIOLENCE

Outbursts of volcanic emotion which can only be described as rage begin in infancy when the youngster is frustrated or uncomfortable. This rage is mitigated originally by the mother's sensitive ministrations which comfort the child. In older children, temper tantrums appear as an organized remnant of the original undifferentiated rage. Even in the older infant, the violence which accompanies the rage is randomly directed. If a person comes too close he may be kicked, but the youngster is equally likely to strike his own head against the wall or to break material objects. Tantrums also occur in settings of frustration. They are more common and frequent when illness, lack of sleep, new surroundings, or other factors tax the ego's control mechanisms. It has been noted that there is a strong tendency for tantrum behavior to decrease in frequency with the development of articulate speech and the improved capacity to express both needs and grievances in verbal form.

Among older children, outbursts of rage tend to appear in situations where the youngster feels threatened with the possibility of real or symbolic personal injury. In some boys, and to a lesser extent girls, controlled expressions of rage and violence appear as a readiness to engage in physical combat. This serves not only for physical self-protection but to avoid real or imagined slights, insults, or humiliations in the interpersonal sphere. In many settings, the young school-age boy is required to demonstrate a willingness to fight as a proof of his courage and as a requirement for acceptance by peers.

These developmental problems are rarely a source of serious concern and tend to become less problematic with advancing age. However, there are a fairly large number of youngsters who continue to have explosive outbursts of rage often accompanied by dangerously violent behavior. This reaches a degree which interferes markedly with their social, academic, and family adjustment. There is considerable evidence to indicate that a central nervous system disability is implicated in a large number of these youngsters.[97] In others, no evidence of EEG abnormality, developmental deviation, or neurological soft signs are evident. In these cases, the behavior appears to result from severe personal psychopathology, often augmented by a family tradition of violence[63] or to arise from living in a subcultural environment which accepts violence as a legitimate solution to social difficulties.

The clinical course of youngsters with repetitive outbursts of rage and violence varies considerably according to the basic etiology of the problem. Many youngsters with an organic component tend to improve with age. This may come about because maturation of the central nervous system allows for greater impulse control, while social learning permits the capacity for more acceptable self-assertion and defense. Where the violence seems to derive from social expectations, the youngsters relinquish it when they reach a certain age and "graduate" from their violent gangs.[81] Those with severe regressive psychopathology (the violent youngster who is borderline or psychotic) seem to do very poorly in the absence of vigorous and prolonged treatment.[14]

Habitual defiance and disobedience are means of expressing aggression toward adults who are seen as frustrating and condemning. At the same time, the behavior serves as a defensive effort to avoid loss of autonomy and injury to the sense of selfhood. From an interpersonal point of view, the youngster's extreme defiance and disobedience are aimed at eliciting protection from the external environment. This serves to offset the youngster's terror of a total loss of control over his impulses, which he regards as evil and destructive. This multiple meaning of defiant and disobedient behavior accounts in some degree for the variability with which the environment interprets these actions. To some extent, the youngster is hostile and aggressive, and does enjoy his periodic triumphs over the environment. Therefore, when adults regard these youngsters as self-centered, spoiled, and enjoying it all, they are, to some extent, correct. At the same time, since the youngster is in fact afraid of his own impulse life, those adults who recognize the plea for limits in his behavior are equally correct.

In older children and adolescents, defiant and disobedient behavior may merely represent a continuation of such an earlier pattern. In these cases their history reveals that the behavior has been a constant presence since early childhood. In other instances, particularly during adolescence, this earlier pattern may be reactivated as part of the regression in the service of growth so typical of that time of life.

One needs also to remember that episodic occurrences of defiant behavior may be primarily defensive, particularly during adolescence. For example, there are times when the youngster fears that obeying would cause him to be overwhelmed by his own passive wishes. He may respond to frightening dependency or homosexual yearnings by resisting all efforts at control. Defiance and disobedience may also be responsive to general states of anxiety. At these times, the youngster may derive some relief from his internal fear by a demonstration of his defiance of adult authority.[84]

MANIPULATIVE BEHAVIOR

The word "manipulate" has as one of its definitions, "to manage or influence by artful skill." This definition suggests one important fact of manipulative behavior. Evidently, the capacity to influence others toward positive and constructive activities is an important skill. It tends to be highly developed in many individuals with leadership ability. This is no less true in the world of the child. The natural leader in a kindergarten class is already skillfully interpreting the emotional needs and vulnerabilities of fellow classmates and utilizing this information to organize and direct the group at play.

The broad subject of manipulation and its place in human behavior is far beyond the scope of this chapter. We will consider only the youngster for whom manipulative behavior becomes an end in itself rather than one means of accomplishing individual and group goals.

This young "con artist" may begin to demonstrate the pattern even in preschool years. It is usually not recognized, however, until elementary or junior high school. At this point, the child may be referred for psychiatric attention for a variety of presenting complaints. If his manipulative behavior is blatant enough to interfere with orderly functioning in the classroom or in other group contexts, the complaint may originate with an offended adult. The parents may refer the manipulative child because of their concern with his disruptive effect on the family, his basic dishonesty, their inability to control him, or because of their recognition that the youngster has no true friendships. Often the referral is the result of a variety of concerns, and the parents frequently appear somewhat confused and unable to state a single clear reason for their anxiety about the child.

The youngsters perceive the psychiatric interview as another occasion for manipulation. Sometimes they are successful in convincing the examiner that they have no serious difficulties. More frequently, they offend and irritate the clinician with their obvious attempts to subvert the purpose of the examination. This has been known to lead to a diagnosis of sociopathy of psychopathy.

As in any other psychiatric syndrome, there are wide ranges of severity. Milder forms may improve with maturation as the child becomes more subtle in his manipulative skills and more mature in regard to the purposes for which he utilizes them. In more severe cases, the manipulation becomes a stereotyped pattern with its own rewards. Youngsters caught up in this adaptive mode tend to be highly narcissistic. They have a limited capacity for true empathy or for pleasure in honest, intimate relationships. The capacity to coerce, intimidate, or trick others into behaving in desired ways becomes more important than the practical results of the manipulation. At times, the manipulator seems willing literally to "cheat to lose" as long as he can "cheat" successfully. The glee and triumph which accompany these successful maneuvers may occasionally be tinged with some remorse, and with recognition that the other person has been "used." However, transient twinges of guilt rarely provide enough motivation for the youngster to undertake the difficult and, to him, mysterious task of learning to relate in a more honest way.

This behavioral pattern is a basic component of the personality structure of most persistently antisocial youngsters. It will be considered in more detail later. Once manipulation is established as the primary pattern in interpersonal relationships, it has a strong tendency to persist. This is true both because of its intrinsic emotional gratifications, its predictable material rewards, and because it blocks any opportunities for interpersonal contacts that might evolve naturally in more gratifying ways. The manipulator must regard the remainder of mankind with suspicion and distrust, both to justify his own machinations and to maintain the vigilance required to continue successful manipulations. Naturally, treatment is difficult. These are serious realistic problems in establishing a therapeutic relationship with such youths. More important still, however, is the enormous potential for negative countertransference feelings.

Etiology of Antisocial Behavior

ORGANIC FACTORS

The importance of temperament as an etiological factor in behavior disorders has been convincingly demonstrated by the anterospective study conducted by Thomas, Chess, and Birch.[94] They described temperamental style according to nine characteristics: activity, rhythmicity, adaptability, approach-withdrawal, threshold for stimulation, intensity of responsiveness, prevailing mood, distractibility, and persistence.

The study focused on the interaction between the child's temperament and his environment, especially parental management techniques. Behavior disorders developed in situations where there was a poor fit between temperament and environmental response. The presence of any particular temperamental combination did not assure a youngster of normal development nor condemn him to development of a behavior disorder. However, the investigators did define a cluster of traits which they called the "difficult child." This youngster was characterized by the temperamental attributes of irregularity in biological functioning, a predominance of withdrawal responses to new stimuli, slowness in adapting to changes in the environment, a high frequency of expression of negative mood, and a predominance of intense reactions. Such a child was at high risk for the development of behavior disorder. In fact, 70 percent of the temperamentally difficult children in the study population did develop behavior problems.

According to this study, behavior disorders are initially a direct expression of the poor fit between temperament and management. The area of function in which the disordered behavior develops seems to be almost entirely environmentally determined. That is, failures in function appear in those areas where the youngster's temperamental characteristics prevent him from meeting family expectations or in areas where the parents fail to recognize the youngster's need for special training or assistance. The ways in which the youngster expresses his behavioral problems are more directly related to his temperamental style. The low activity, "slow to warm up" child demonstrates passive withdrawal and avoidance, while the high activity, high intensity youngster reacts more explosively to stress situations of poor temperamental-environmental fit.

The authors trace the emergence of the symptom picture, demonstrating the effect of the consequences of original symptoms on the development of the clinical profile. They also trace the tendency for the original action symptoms to be converted into attitudinal sets, ego defenses, and self-image distortions as the child's psychological and cognitive abilities mature.

The study included clinical management of the research subjects who later developed behavior disorders. Of those who required treatment, 50 percent responded to parental guidance based on educating the parent to the temperamental style of the youngster and the provision of direct advice about management. This high percentage of success, in view of the brevity of the parent guidance contacts (an average of less than three sessions), has important practical implications for overcrowded child guidance clinics.

Other authors have implicated constitutional factors as important etiological agents in the development disorders and antisocial behavior. The high percentage of enuretics among delinquent youths has been regularly noted in the literature, and Michaels[64] has suggested that a basic constitutional deficiency in control mechanisms underlies both the enuresis and the impulsive behavior.

Many youngsters with known central nervous system damage demonstrate distractibility, hyperactivity, and poor impulse control, which may lead to the development of behavior disorder. However, Thomas, Chess, and Birch note that temperamental characteristics and parental management strongly affect the outcome of even demonstrable central nervous system damage. The finding of a high frequency of EEG abnormality in youngsters with behavior disorder is generally accepted, but the exact role which these dysrhythmias play in producing behavioral symptoms is not clear. A similar statement could be made regarding the importance of mental retardation and the specific learning disabilities in predisposing a youngster to antisocial behavior.

It does seem safe to say that a variety of constitutional and organic factors may serve to make a youngster more difficult to socialize. They interfere with the development of both the reality sense and warm object ties within the family. Some organic conditions (such as encephalitis) may produce severely disordered behavior patterns without any apparent environmental or temperamental contribution.

PSYCHODYNAMIC FACTORS

Organic or constitutional factors may play an important role in the etiology of many behavior problems. This should not obscure the fact that they are basically psychological problems. Many of these disorders are the direct result of individual and family psychological conflict. Moreover, regardless of the inception of the difficulty, all problems in adjustment to social reality eventually demand resolution in terms of intrapsychic dynamics. Treatment approaches to any established behavior disorder are unlikely to be successful in the absence of an understanding of the typical motivations, defensive maneuvers, and the styles of relating which characterize this group of youngsters.

PSYCHIC TRAUMA

Over the years there have been various attempts to link impulse disorders to specific traumatic events arising in the course of development. Most of the traumata which have been considered important in the etiology of these disorders have been ascribed to deprivations in parenting. For example, the early statistical studies of delinquent behavior had already noted the high incidence of "broken homes" in the delinquent's background. More recently, Bowlby[10] focused attention on early maternal deprivation as an important cause of antisocial character development. According to these authors, the absence of adequate maternal care in early infancy interfered with the capacity for the development of affectionate bonds to other humans. As a result, the socialization process was seriously impaired. Freud and Burlingham[24] described a similar high incidence of serious behavior problems in the World War II war orphans who were separated from their parents for long periods.

Although some of the finer points of these studies have been challenged in the recent literature, there does seem to be overwhelming clinical evidence that severe early deprivation is an important factor in producing impulse-ridden youngsters with strong tendencies toward antisocial behavior.

Greenacre[36] has implicated severe psychic traumatization at early stages of development as the crucial factor in the development of the "psychopathic personality. She refers to these youngsters as "impulsive depressive."

Finally, the traumatic impact of the loss of important identification figures at crucial stages of development is observed frequently in the social history of youngsters with behavior disorders. These losses seem particularly traumatic if they are associated with a major disillusionment with the loved person. This often occurs in a bitterly contested divorce, in the face of desertion, or when a family member is sent to prison. The clinical picture tends to be characterized by a conscious hatred of the lost and disappointing object, accompanied by identification with the negative aspects of the loved one's behavior.

Ralph was a handsome, innocent-looking youngster of sixteen who was referred for psychiatric evaluation after armed robbery of a supermarket. In an interview situation, he was tense and angry and apparently free of remorse. In the course of the interview, it came to light that Ralph's father had been killed six months previously in an automobile accident that resulted from driving while heavily intoxicated. As he discussed his father's death, Ralph first expressed anger and disgust at his father's alcoholism but burst into tears when the interviewer commented that Ralph's father sounded like a fine man who had begun to make some serious mistakes in his life.

Following this interview, Ralph was able to recall with considerable warmth his attachment for his father through his earlier development and his personal guilt because he did not take his father's drinking seriously for many years. Instead, he tended to side with his father when his mother nagged about the excessive drinking. In spite of being under age, Ralph had, in fact, often accompanied his father to neighborhood bars and drank with him.

Following the accident, Ralph described himself as "just mad all the time." He was extremely irritable and got into many fights because of his readiness to take offense at the slightest challenge or frustration. He admitted that he drank heavily and claimed that being drunk made him feel better. At the same time, he engaged in most of his serious antisocial behaviors including the robbery while intoxicated.

After passing through a prolonged period of depression and grieving over the loss of his father, Ralph formed an extremely warm and dependent relationship with the therapist. He became curious about the therapist's life style, values, and habits. His antisocial symptomatology gradually abated without any further serious incidence.

CHARACTERISTIC DEFENSES

The structural defects in the antisocial youngster are sometimes viewed as belonging primarily to the superego. Redl speaks, for example, of the "guilt-exempt fun" of the juvenile delinquent. He describes the ego as operating in the service of this corrupt superego and notes that in regard to specific aspects of reality this ego is highly developed.[73] Similar observations have been contributed by Aichorn.[1]

These authors have described an ego which is highly skilled in assessing opportunities for successful delinquency and in the capacity to defend against any sense of guilt. In his relationship with reality, the delinquent is described as being hyperalert, extremely observant, and capable of developing elaborate and well-conceived plans for engaging in disapproved behavior without detection and punishment.

These skills are not limited to the cognitive and material world but include a shrewd and cunning understanding of the motives of others which, as described earlier, allow artful manipulation of people. For the most part, these "well-adapted" delinquents would best be diagnosed as "group delinquent reaction" or "sociosyntonic personality disorder."

The youngsters who fall into the group of "tension-discharge disorders," however, are not so readily differentiated from this sociosyntonic category. Despite their poorer ego development, they present superficially as hedonistic individuals who deny that they are troubled. They utilize denial, projection, rationalization, and displacement to justify their behavior and, to a varying degree, have perfected the interpersonal skills that assist them to maintain this outlook. For example, they are skilled at provoking anger and mistreatment by others, so that they can justify their misbehavior and avoid guilt. Even youngsters with neurotic behavior disorders must deal with the interpersonal consequences of their acting out behavior. It is this necessity, inevitably produced by the alloplastic nature of the symptomatology, which creates the surface similarities between youngsters with behavior disorders.

Often it is difficult to penetrate this veneer in order to make an accurate assessment of the antisocial youngster, particularly in a brief diagnostic period. The youngster's need to deceive himself and others is further complicated by the countertransference reaction which the delinquent defensive style tends to elicit in the examiner. It is not pleasant to be fooled or to have one's trust abused. To avoid these unpleasant experiences, there is a protective tendency to become cynical and distrustful of the antisocial youngster. This can reach such an extent that honest communications may be dismissed as subtle efforts at manipulation and obfuscation. The need to avoid

being "outsmarted" can seriously interfere with empathy and emotional sensitivity. Perhaps, in working with antisocial youngsters, it is preferable to be a trusting sucker, who is willing to try again rather than to beat the delinquent at his own game of distrust and the denial of legitimate emotion.

EFFECT ON THE EGO

From an adaptive point of view, the ego of antisocial youngsters is seriously impaired. Some authors have emphasized the difficulty these youngsters experience in impulse control. However, it may be more useful to see the eruption of impulses as a final effort to compensate for other ego deficiencies. The adaptive capacities of impulsive youngsters are highly dependent on external agents for a variety of functions including management of stimulation levels, directing and maintaining attention, modulating affect, and a whole range of subtle operations related to the regulation of interpersonal relationships, particularly those that are emotionally important. Ultimately, these are the skills which enable one to master the environment and to maintain secondary narcissism and a sense of adequate selfhood.

It may be that deficiency in these skills is the core disorder in antisocial youngsters. Such defects can result from temperamental extremes, from constitutional or organic defects in the ego apparatus, or from deficient parenting. Clinical experience suggests that the difference between the impulse-ridden child and the neurotic behavior disorder is quantitive rather than qualitative. The neurotic child who expresses an internalized conflict through antisocial behavior is withal demonstrating a relative ego weakness. He is unable to internalize and contain his unrest within his own personality boundaries.

Naturally, there are efforts to compensate for this basic deficiency. Some of these compensatory mechanisms can be observed in the superego pathology of the youngster, in his efforts to alter reality, and perhaps in some aspects of his relationship with his family. Lacking a capacity for mastery, he must attempt to maintain a sense of omnipotence.[17] His efforts to do so will now be discussed in more detail.

It is obvious that there are superego defects in antisocial youngsters. Clinically, this is demonstrated by lack of remorse or conscious guilt over actions that are clearly harmful or unfair to other people. Often this nonchalance regarding the rights of others and the importance of social norms is organized into a verbalized philosophy of life which is selfish, callous, and amoral. In addition to these clinical observations, there is research evidence that delinquents show a lower capacity for self-critical guilt than do controls.[4] Many writers have considered these conscience defects the primary problem in asocial and antisocial behavior.

Actually, this formulation applies more accurately to the gang delinquent or sociosyntonic delinquent. Youngsters with tension-discharge disorders show many indirect evidences of operative, even harsh, superegos. The basically self-destructive quality of much of their behavior, the frequent tendency to invite external punishment, and the vulnerability to periods of self-hatred and depression strongly suggest that the youngster expends considerable energy attempting to avoid powerful feelings of guilt. Indeed, these youngsters will go to extreme lengths in order to maintain a sense of grievance against the world, a sense of abuse which justifies their hostile and destructive behavior. Redl has been particularly articulate in describing this adaptive mode.[36] He tells of the almost delusional quality that pervades the youngster's sense of unjust treatment. Such a child may encounter repeated demonstrations of trustworthiness, friendliness, and kindness. Nonetheless, he has an enormous reluctance to relinquish a hostile interpretation of the motives and actions of others.

This need to demonstrate the inescapable necessity of their unacceptable behavior is pervasive. Conceivably, it could be dismissed as an effort to cope with external criticism and disapproval. However, the intensity of the effort and the amount of energy and time expended are disproportionate. Presumably such a youth cares little for the opinions and expectations of others. The degree of defensiveness suggests that its origin is more likely a response to important internal pressures.

There is reason to believe that the primary problem in antisocial disorders does not lie in the absence of appropriate superego restrictions. This conclusion arises from clinical experience. When a therapist does obtain a positive relationship with one of these youngsters, he frequently drops his defensive façade and reveals clearly that he is not only quite familiar with social norms and expectations but that he very much desires to adhere to these norms. The typical antisocial youngster will admit in the abstract that many of his behaviors are "wrong," and he makes plans to avoid these behaviors in the future. In the face of temptation, frustration, or anger, however, these good intentions disappear and the unacceptable behavior recurs. The youngster is then often disappointed with himself and anticipates disappointment and disapproval from the therapist. He engages in a variety of defensive maneuvers which seem directed toward avoiding superego retaliation. Schmideberg states that at this point in treatment, the child may come to recognize the obsessive nature of his behavior and become more cooperative in the treatment effort. That is, he becomes capable of a therapeutic alliance.[82]

These comments are not meant to deny the presence or importance of superego pathology in acting out youngsters. These youngsters marshall numerous techniques of superego corruption and avoidance and much of the therapeutic effort must be directed toward countering these maneuvers. This is necessary in order to render the behavior consciously unacceptable and thus amenable to therapeutic intervention. It is merely suggested that much of the superego distortion observable in antisocial youngsters of the tension-discharge variety may have another origin. It may represent a necessary accommodation to a basic defect in coping skills rather than a proximate cause of misbehavior.

The limited adaptive skills of the behaviorally disordered youngster are also reflected in his attitude toward reality. Many observers have noted that these children are in many respects quite skillful and ingenious in their adaptation to reality demand. However, prolonged observation of their manipulative efforts shows a stereotyped, repetitive pattern which in fact lacks the subtlety as well as the breadth of the normal child's impact on his environment.

Superficially, antisocial youngsters are "savvy," clever, and shrewd in their endeavors to alter reality to gratify their wishes and requirements. They are undeniably more effective in the short run in forcing others to accommodate to them. Often they appear willful and controlling; determined to have things their own way. For example, the normal youngster is willing, perhaps after a bit of grumbling, to adjust to his teacher's assignment of a difficult project. The youngster with a behavior disorder, on the other hand, may expend considerable energy in order to avoid the task or to convince the teacher that her expectations are too high. Often enough, he is successful, he avoids the task, and he is then viewed as someone who gets away with things while other youngsters are "knuckling under." In fact, the healthier youngster's superior coping mechanisms allow him the luxury of accepting the teacher's demand while the behaviorally disordered youngster is forced to the point of desperation to persist in his efforts to avoid a task that he cannot master. The point is that in typically human fashion, the behaviorally disordered youngster would prefer to be viewed as defiant, cheeky, or even bad rather than inept and overwhelmed.

Delinquents have also been found to be more egocentric (in Piaget's terms) than normal controls. A treatment approach based on role playing has been described and seemed effective.[13]

Another characteristic of the antisocial youngster's relationship with reality is his preoccupation with "action," "kicks," and a hedonistic search for pleasure. Often it is clear that these gratifications are sought at the expense of other people. Indeed, part of the fun seems to be the sense of power and dominance associated with the disregard of limitations imposed by various authorities. Naturally, this characteristic arouses resentment (and perhaps some envy) in those individuals who accept a more orderly and disciplined style of life. It may be that this understandable response accounts for the tendency to interpret much antisocial behavior as though it were motivated primarily by "secondary gain."

On closer observation, it seems that much of this frenzied search for activity is motivated by an underlying sense of helplessness. Typically, the antisocial youngster feels that he has little or no control over his life. His subjective experience is a feeling of being controlled by external forces, viewed either as real authorities, a vague "they," or as the blind winds of fate. Frantic efforts to control individuals, events, and situations may be recognized primarily as strivings to gain some illusory sense of impact and personal importance in the face of these malignant and powerful influences. From a psychological point of view, the antisocial youngster's assessment of his place in the world is correct. In fact, he is not master of his fate because of the previously-described ego deficiencies. Although he misunderstands the reasons for his lack of self-direction, his compensatory efforts to prove he is running the show are as understandable as they are ineffective in improving his situation.

The relationship between the antisocial youngster and his parents is extremely complex. Some of the intricacies of that relationship will be discussed later. One aspect should be considered here, however, in connection with his characteristic ego deficiencies. The youngster with a behavior disorder commonly uses his parents as ancillary ego agents, all the while denying that

their interventions are desired or helpful. These youngsters are masters of means for eliciting unusual degrees of parental support, direction, and even intervention in interactions with the environment. At times, this help is requested or demanded openly. More commonly, the youngster provides an indirect invitation for assistance through his constant failures in adaptation and his apparent lack of concern for his own health, safety, and future.

This parental overinvolvement is regularly observed by the clinician but is often thought of as the cause of the problem rather than as one of the compensatory mechanisms for dealing with the basic defect. Of course, the parents have reasons of their own for encouraging this pattern of relating. Still, the clinician should recognize the youngster's need for protection and direction and his active role in maintaining a hostile dependent interaction. No matter "who started it," the behaviorally disordered child has a strong investment in perpetuating it.

SYMPTOM STRUCTURE

In the behaviorally disordered youngster[94] the choice of specific symptom patterns seems primarily related to two factors. The first of these is temperamental. The youngster's temperamental style seems to some extent to dictate the pattern of expression of the disordered behavior. That is, the intense, highly active youngster is likely to involve himself in visible and aggressive violations of expected behavioral norms, while the excessively passive youngster is more likely to show patterns of avoidance, withdrawal, and passive aggression. On the other hand, the particular area of maladjustment seems to depend a great deal on environmental factors. These begin in the family when expectations exceed the youngster's coping skills, and, in general, where particular behaviors are rigidly overemphasized by the family and, in general, where such areas tend to become the sites of combat with society. On the other hand, skills and behaviors which are ignored or inconsistently managed may fail to develop, particularly if the youngster's temperament is inclined against that kind of mastery. To illustrate the two situations, the family may strongly emphasize academic performance with a youngster whose temperament makes sustained attention and perseverance difficult. Presently they will report that their youngster's primary behavior problems occur around school work. On the other hand, a family may be loosely organized with few routines. The youngster with a temperamental leaning either toward biological arhythmicity or long persistence may presently find it extremely difficult to adapt to situations where he is expected to follow a timetable.

The wider environment also influences these specific patterns of antisocial behavior. Membership in a gang, for example, may channel the youngster's behavior into those areas which are designated by the group leader or by the tradition of the particular gang. The factor of chance, unusual temptations, and environmental opportunities also strongly influence the choice of symptoms. Schools that monitor attendance carefully may have a relatively low level of unexcused absenteeism but a higher level of direct conflict between students and teachers, while other schools with loose requirements for attendance have a great deal of "skipping" but a lower level of overt conflict in the classroom. This element of opportunism in the antisocial youngster is again related to the ego weakness described earlier, since this deficiency makes the youngster unusually susceptible to temptation, group pressure, contagion, and other environmental factors.

The role of pathological identification in symptom choice is less clear. It does seem important, however, at least in a general sense. For example, behavior disorders are more common in families which contain a socially deviant parent model.[57] The effect of modeling may relate more to overall socialization than to the selection of individual symptoms. In some cases, it does appear that the youngster's symptomatology is clearly shaped by the specific behavioral problems of important adults in his life. Such direct emulation seems to be especially frequent following the loss of an ambivalently loved deviant identification model.

SECONDARY GAIN

The role of secondary gain in establishing and maintaining the symptoms of behavior disorder is probably exaggerated both by the patient and by other people. As already described, the patient often insists that he enjoys being the way he is and, at times, seems quite gleeful in regard to some successful antisocial escapade. Often the outside observer can only agree with this assessment and views the antisocial youngster as someone who is getting away with forbidden pleasurable activities. A similar view is frequently held by family members (and family therapists) who correctly perceive that the antisocial youngster is receiving more than his fair share of parental attention.

They conclude from this that it is the excessive attention which motivates the deviant behavior. However, it may be more accurate to view these "triumphs" over the restraints of reality as basic defenses against feelings of weakness and powerlessness rather than as "secondary gain." In other words, the basic psychopathology in the behavior disorder requires the youngster to redefine and alter reality in order to maintain precarious self-esteem and a sense of ego integrity. This is not a minor or a peripheral reinforcer of the symptom. is the designated patient.

Family Influences in the Behavior Disorders

INTRODUCTION

Since the family is the primary instrument through which the child is socialized, disturbances in family functioning obviously play an important role in the development and expression of behavior disorders. The complex interaction between the behaviorally disordered youngster and his family is subtle and variable from one case to another. However, some common patterns can be identified and may provide useful guidelines for the clinician faced with the problems of sorting out the tangled web of significant influences in the cases he studies.

In the interest of clarity, an artificial separation will be made between dyadic parent-child interrelation and family system patterns. In real life, of course, these forces are inseparable. The effectiveness of the individual parent is strongly influenced by the nature of the marital relationship, the number of children and their temperamental characteristics, the socio-economic situation of the family, and many accidental factors such as illness, death, and externally imposed disruptions of family unity. This relative field dependence, however, does not diminish the importance of the personality characteristics of each parent, since these mirror the parents' own growth experience, the parenting they received, and the ways in which they resolved their own developmental crises.

THE INFLUENCE OF PARENTING BEHAVIOR

A baseline experience of adequate nurturing in early infancy which is sufficiently caring, sensitive, and dependable to permit positive attachment to the parenting individuals is prerequisite to socialization. Unfortunately many mothers and fathers are unable to provide this basic requirement of the socialization process. The failure may be the result of external factors, as in the case of extreme poverty or other unusual stresses which interfere with the mother's capacity to make herself available to her infant. Failure may be caused by psychopathology in the parent which results either in rejection of the parenting role or serious interference with the capacity for interpreting and appropriately meeting the needs of the newborn child. Often the failure in basic nature is a result of a combination of both internal and external factors.

At any rate, where this developmental step is successfully negotiated, the family must maintain this positive bond while educating the young child to the demands of social living within the family. These capacities are tested first during the negativism of the separation-individuation phase and again during the triangular manipulations of the oedipal period.

The skill with which the parents deal with these pressures is affected by the activation of their own unresolved conflicts, as the child progresses through these developmental stages. Parenthood is itself a developmental stage. It requires the parents to rework their own sources of unresolved anxieties in each psychosocial phase, in the process of assisting their child to master successive developmental crises.

One of the important clinical implications of this understanding of parenthood is to indicate the importance of assessing the parents' commitment to social behavior. Behavior problems are produced when the parent consciously or unconsciously rejects the necessity for socialization. If the parent is consciously asocial, he provides a pathological model for the youngster. More than that, he establishes a family atmosphere which virtually requires the youngster to adopt an antisocial pose for the sake of survival within his own family. Where the commitment to the gratification of antisocial impulses is unconscious, it leads to a more subtle parent-child interaction in which antisocial behavior is overtly condemned while it is covertly promoted.

Thomas, Chess, and Birch have described the induction of behavior problems by parents who are not antisocial but merely eccentric, especially when they rear a malleable, "easy child" in their unusual, socially aberrant lifestyle.[94]

In addition to emotional readiness and personal integrity, the parents must also possess a reasonable level of comprehension of the society in which they live. Extreme variance can exist between family patterns and the expectations of the wider society. This may produce a situation in which the youngster is severely torn between family expectations and the behavioral requirements encountered outside the home. This pattern is frequently observed in first generation immigrants, families that move from rural to urban settings, or in subcultural groups that are strongly alienated from the official institutions of acculturation.

The parents must have not only emotional rapport with their child and a cognitive grasp of the larger society, they must possess sufficient skill and flexibility in communication to adapt this comunication to the developmental level of the child and his capacity to understand. One has the impressionistic sense that it is difficult to come by this skill in the isolated nuclear family of mobile modern America. In the past, contact with an extended family and a variety of children of assorted ages allowed these techniques to be absorbed without conscious effort. Obviously, this skill is somewhat dependent on the verbal skills of the parent. Clinically, verbal facility does seem poorly developed in the parents of many behaviorally disordered youngsters. This deficiency in fluency may be generalized and result from a lack of training and experience. However, an equally serious problem may be observed in many educated, articulate parents who intellectualize excessively. Their ineptness in translating feeling states into words prevents them from assisting their child to learn how to describe and convey feelings verbally.

There is some evidence that many of the skills of parenthood come together in effective expression around the structure of parental discipline. Singer[89] has demonstrated that patterns of discipline correlate highly with the presence and type of psychopathology in the child. He considers discipline from three points of view: policies, policing, and punishment. The parents of antisocial youngsters utilize discipline which is characterized by rigid and exacting policies, negligent policing to determine the degree of compliance with policy, and lenient punishment when infractions of the stringent rules come to light.

It seems reasonable that this approach to socialization could result from latent antisocial tendencies in such parents. Their failure to fully master their own impulses would produce a felt need for a multiplicity of constrictive regulations; but their vicarious pleasure in the youngster's misbehavior would interfere with conscientious enforcement of their prohibitions.

Finally, any consideration of deficiencies in the parental management of behavior must carefully avoid judgmental evaluations in isolation. The specific youngster who is the object of socialization efforts is also an important variable. Socialization is an interactive process, highly dependent on a variety of feedback mechanisms. It is not at all unusual to encounter families in which only one of several siblings develops a behavioral disturbance. Often the reasons for the poor parent-child relationship with this individual are sought entirely in the dynamics of the parents or in historical events which affected the family about the time of his birth. The explanation for the isolated failure in socialization may just as well lie in the unique behavioral characteristics of the youngster himself. Parental effectiveness is a relative matter which depends more on the "fit" between the parent and the child than on any absolute standards of proper parental behavior.

THE INFLUENCE OF FAMILY STRUCTURE

Family structure must be considered from both static and dynamic perspectives. There is considerable evidence that for boys,[4, 33] paternal absence, hostility, or uninvolvement in child rearing is strongly related to the development of antisocial behavior. This definable structural characteristic of families has value from the statistical and diagnostic points of view. However, the reason for the father's lack of effectiveness must also be sought in the dynamic interplay of family relationships. It is possible that the father may simply be too immature or emotionally disturbed to function in the parenting role. However, one must also consider the possibility that other family members are actively colluding to exclude him from a position of influence.[65] A similar comment could be made regarding the impact of an intrusive and excessively dominating mother on the socialization of the daughter. Both individual and family factors may be active in shaping this maternal posture.

There are other patterns of family structure which are commonly encountered with behavior disordered youngsters. One of them is scapegoating. This is a homeostatic mechanism which allows the family to contain a variety of tensions by assigning all negative characteristics and family problems to a single youngster. This child becomes "the cause of all our difficulties."

Another family pattern commonly encountered in families of behavior disordered youngsters is the utilization of the child as a substitute spouse to compensate for inadequacies in the marital relationship. For example, one severely antisocial girl of fourteen always became the confidant and protector of her mother whenever the father entered one of his episodic rages.

The "problem child" may be utilized as a single stabilizing focus of mutual concern and cooperative action for couples who would otherwise be in serious personal conflict. A variant of this pattern employs the child as a disposable pawn who is utilized to demonstrate the inadequacies of each parent. A common framework for this dynamic is the family in which one parent is extremely permissive and forgiving while the other parent is harsh and punitive. The "loving" parent blames the youngster's behavior problems on his poor relationship with the "strict" parent, while the "strict" parent feels that all problems would be resolved if only the lax parent would enforce rules. It requires only a short period of contact with couples like this to grasp the fact that the child and his welfare are only a smokescreen behind which the parents can conduct their vicious marital warfare.

These and other distortions of family structure are commonplace findings in the families of behaviorally disordered children. Diffuse and shifting generational boundaries, excessive closeness with blurring of ego boundaries between individuals, the converse situation of extreme distancing with the absence of mutual concern, and bizarre and pathological alliances between subgroups within the family all are quite common. In some cases, the youngster's behavior problems may result predominantly from his conscription to play a deviant role necessary to the survival of the family group. However, one must also consider the individual vulnerability of the behaviorally disordered child. The following vignette illustrates both the importance of family dynamic influences and the role of the individual child who is the designated patient.

LARRY

Larry, a fifteen-year-old boy, was referred for psychiatric treatment because he was friendless, the source of much family friction, and seemingly restless and tense at all times.

Larry was the youngest of three siblings. His parents stated they had no difficulties with his eighteen-year-old brother, who was about to leave home for college, nor with his sixteen and one-half-year-old sister. They mentioned no problems between them, although the mother indicated that she sometimes felt her husband was unduly harsh with all of the youngsters. Both parents were eager to recite the long history of Larry's adjustment difficulties. These dated back to early childhood when he was viewed as an impulsive and unhappy preschooler,. As he grew, the difficulties continued in the form of a variety of learning problems, school conflicts, and a long history of inability to make friends. The parents admitted frankly that they both found Larry irritating and had very few positive feelings toward him. They stated that his brother and sister shared these feelings, although the sister, a "patient and long-suffering" girl, occasionally made efforts to be supportive and friendly toward Larry.

Only with great reluctance would they consent to discuss the marital relation, which they said was "fine now." With some prodding, they described a rather marked change in their relationship as the mother had gradually become a much more active and assertive individual over the course of the marriage. At the time of the referral, she had obtained a job and was experiencing considerable success in the business world. Her husband indicated that he was pleased with these changes and that he found his wife a more interesting person now. He did admit to occasional periods of annoyance when his wife's new found interests interfered with her responsibilities as spouse and mother.

Following an extended diagnostic evaluation, family therapy was recommended because of the scapegoated position Larry held in the family. It was reasoned that individual work with Larry would be doomed without concommitant improvement in the atmosphere he encountered in his daily life at home. The family was reluctant to accept the recommendation, but, after some delay, they agreed to cooperate.

Larry's behavior improved dramatically in response to the first three months of family therapy. As he left the scapegoated role, there was a brief effort to replace him with the older son. This young man, however, was able to resist the assignment. This was in part because his college plans had already resulted in considerable emotional emancipation from the family. Over the next two months the marital conflict became explicit and then intense. What emerged was a deep and embittered power struggle between the parents. This stemmed from the father feeling emasculated and depreciated by his wife's wish to achieve success outside the home, while she regarded him as a martinet whom she tolerated only because she still needed his financial support until her business grew more successful.

Open and violent arguments between the parents became commonplace in the family sessions and at home. In a family therapy meeting, the father asked Larry if there was a reason for his avoiding the family dinner table over recent weeks through a variety of excuses and scheduling conflicts. Larry candidly admitted that the avoidance was purposeful since the tension and open bickering between the parents made him extremely uncomfortable and he wished to avoid it whenever possible. He added, "in some ways it was better when everyone was yelling at me." Two days later, he provoked his father into a violent argument and ran away from home briefly, successfully focusing his parents' united concern on his problems once again.

It is obvious that all of Larry's difficulties were not created by the pathological family structure. At least in comparison with his brother and sister, he was temperamentally difficult and apparently suffered from mild minimal brain dysfunction with a concurrent learning disability. His individual ego weaknesses predisposed him for selection as the family scapegoat. However, the family did exert tremendous pressure to retain him in this position, and even Larry himself began to recognize vaguely that his problems served to protect the solidity of the marital relationship. Larry was not able to maintain his gains until his parents entered marital therapy which successfully resolved their neurotic interpersonal conflicts.

The Extended Family: Another aspect of family structure which deserves more careful study relates to the influence of grandparents and other members of the extended family. Both literature and clinical experience strongly suggest that these relationships may be important in the etiology of behavior disorders. Clinically, for example, it often appears that grandparents, particularly the mother's mother, are frequently involved in the creation of the youngster's behavior problems. There is insufficient data to clarify whether this observation results from a previously existing, excessive attachment. Perhaps it merely reflects the fact that mother's frustration in dealing with a temperamentally difficult youngster may lead her to seek support from her own mother. In any case, it does appear that this pattern can serve to undermine mother's confidence and her intuitive readiness to deal with a difficult youngster. However, without controlled studies of the variety of child rearing patterns in three generational relationships within the general population, it is impossible to determine the importance of this factor.

Some of these family findings have been utilized by learning theory advocates. They seek to explain all behavior disorders purely on the basis of operant conditioning. They point out that the family's response to the child actually reinforces unwanted responses. At the same time, the parents' preoccupation with the misbehavior results in a failure to reinforce desired behavioral patterns when they do appear.

From a theoretical point of view, such a simplistic rendering of learning theory ignores the constitutional and temperamental characteristics of the youngster and does not really explain the full range of observable phenomena. Learning theory also ignores other complexities. It gives too little attention to the processes of cognitive and emotional development and the accompanying internalization and structuralization of earlier interactions. In spite of these deficiencies, however, learning theory and its applications are important in understanding symptom selection and as one aspect of a comprehensive treatment approach.

Therapy of the Behavior Disorders

OUTPATIENT PSYCHOTHERAPY

According to Thomas, Chess, and Birch, the treatment of choice for the young child exhibiting a behavior disorder is parental guidance.[94] This counseling is based on a careful diagnostic evaluation which focuses primarily on a painstaking delineation of the youngster's temperamental style and a study of those aspects of parent management which are dissonant with the development needs of the specific child. This approach ignores motivational or neurotic factors in the parent. It builds on the assumption that the basic difficulty is caused by the parents' lack of understanding of both the youngster's temperamental style and the specific approaches which would be effective in the youngster's socialization. For the young child, this approach has much to recommend it. Many parents are able to alter their behavior in a constructive direction in response to a greater understanding of their child's needs and under the influence of the therapist's authority and status as

an expert. For somewhat older children and for those with more severe problems, the aforementioned authors often recommend individual therapy for the youngster in addition to parent guidance. They focus this therapy toward helping the child to become aware of his own temperamental style in order to elicit his cooperation in adapting temperament to the demands of reality.

Older children, particularly in late latency and in adolescence, often require a more intensive treatment approach. By this time, distortions of self-image, interpersonal conflicts, and the elaboration of neurotic defenses have created a self-perpetuating system which is extremely difficult to interrupt. It can rarely, if ever, be altered merely by parent guidance or other environmental manipulation.

Another variant of the parent guidance approach involves training parents to conduct behavior modification programs with their behaviorally disordered child.[44] A careful review of the results of this approach suggests it has merit. One interesting finding is that parents too must be reinforced for desired behaviors within the program. Curiously, improvement in the child's behavior does not seem to be the strong reinforcer that it was expected to be.[18] Some behaviorists also report that successful interventions in one setting do not necessarily generalize to other settings.[70] For example, the youngster may require a dual program at home and school for successful modification of unwanted behavior.

INDIVIDUAL PSYCHOTHERAPY

Outpatient individual psychotherapy of serious behavior disorders is extremely difficult. Some controlled studies have suggested that it is of no value, as mentioned earlier. However, these studies suffer both from the brevity and type of psychotherapy offered and the failure to distinguish diagnostically between impulse-ridden youngsters and those with neurotic behavior disorders.

Almost all clinicians have had surprisingly positive experiences with some youngsters who are severely antisocial. While there are no scientific guidelines which permit absolutely accurate selection of those cases which can be treated in individual psychotherapy, many clinicians have a good practical "feel" for their own skills and limitations. The factors involved in successful cases probably include a preponderance of neurotic motivation for the antisocial behavior, relatively low family compliance in the antisocial pattern, and some accidental or artful factors which determine the depth of mutual interest and liking which develop early in the therapeutic relationship.

Even in successful cases, the therapeutic techniques, utilized with behavior disorders, vary somewhat from those used with neurotic youngsters. As a rule, limit setting and the interpretation of reality are important aspects of the treatment experience. These are rarely effective if they take the form of lectures, recriminations, or moralizing. Effective interactions usually arise naturally in the ongoing process of treatment. The youngster invites the therapist to break a rule, possibly for the therapist's convenience, and is reminded matter-of-factly, even lightly, that the therapist has found that it's best in the long run to "play it straight." The young patient teases his therapist that he is a "pretty square dude" and receives the cheerful reply, "I guess I am for the most part and I kind of like it that way." The youngster attempts to cajole or intimidate the therapist into collusion in a deception of the child's parents or other authority figures and is rebuffed in the effort firmly but without anger. The examples are legion, and the youngster's continuing efforts to corrupt the therapist are as numerous as they are ingenious. Of course, these painless lessons in integrity are accompanied by the therapist's continuing interest in the youngster's well-being and an indefatigable and genuine curiosity regarding the youngster's true feelings, motivations, and attitudes toward life.

Often one is severely tested by the antisocial youngster's efforts to alter the very character of the treatment process itself. The wayward patient seems intent on forcing the therapist to play a role in a real life drama which not only is unrelated to the true purposes of therapy but may even be threatening to the therapist's professional and personal identity.[31] Although all of these maneuvers may be regarded as varieties of transference behavior, they differ not only quantitatively, but qualitatively as well, from the distortions of the therapeutic relationship commonly encountered with neurotic patients. Perhaps these differences are to be expected in view of the antisocial youngster's peculiar ego deficiencies and his desperate need to obscure them by redefining and reshaping the reality around him.

The specific needs of the antisocial youngster do not alter the basic requirement for a therapeutic alliance or working alliance as a prerequisite for meaningful therapy. This alliance is achievable with many antisocial youngsters. In spite of his need to distort reality, including the true nature

of interpersonal relationships, the patient may well consider some aspects of his problem as ego dystonic. As in the treatment of any other youngster, this core of cooperation can often be expanded to include many behaviors and problems that the patient originally considered acceptable, or even valuable and essential to his self-esteem.[60]

In view of the interactive and interpersonal nature of the symptomatic behavior of the behaviorally disordered youngster, it is rarely feasible to treat him in the absence of a fairly intense alliance with his parents. Often this can be achieved only through collaborative treatment of the parents or some regular and periodic contacts with the entire family. Some therapists are able to treat the parents and the child concurrently in separate sessions. Most therapists find this technically difficult and potentially disruptive to the therapeutic alliance with both the child and the parents.

In summary, the individual outpatient treatment of the antisocial youngster is difficult. Still, in those cases where it can be accomplished, it is often the most powerful and thoroughgoing agent of lasting change for these children. The opportunity for an intensely satisfying dyadic relationship which provides opportunity for ego strengthening, repair of self-esteem, and the internalization of a positive identification figure offers the chance to correct the core disabilities in the behaviorally disordered child. The classic paper by Schmideberg remains one of the best guides to this process. Unfortunately, probably only a minority of these patients can be engaged meaningfully in a treatment program of this kind, at least initially. Other treatment methods may be dictated by the youngster's approachability or by practical considerations such as the availability of resources or his potential danger to society.

GROUP THERAPY

The group approach is often important in the therapy of antisocial youngsters. Its value in the inpatient setting will be discussed later, but it is also useful as an outpatient approach. Two types of groups have been used in the treatment of youngsters with behavior disorders. Older youngsters with primarily neurotic behavior problems may be included in groups treated by means of dynamically-oriented, exploratory group psychotherapy. The presence of the behavior problems in the group must be balanced by the inclusion of other youngsters with stronger egos and a more reflective approach to problem-solving. However, the action-oriented, impulsive youngster can be a valuable addition. His eagerness to challenge authority and his readiness to verbalize forbidden impulses may enliven and catalyze a group interactive process.[49, 59]

Younger children with behavior problems seem to respond better to groups which are more actively oriented. This "activity group therapy" engages the youngster in a structured group play situation in which verbalizations play a secondary role. Ego growth is accomplished through the promotion of a positive identification with the group leader (usually of the same sex as the single sex group), the modeling of appropriate resolution of interpersonal disagreements between group members, and through success experiences in mastering group tasks. Properly conducted groups of this kind often provide the behaviorally disordered youngster with his first experience of positive peer interaction and may result in considerable strengthening of the ego.

Group psychotherapy has also proved of value to severely antisocial older youngsters.[21, 47] As a rule, these groups work on altering the symptomatic antisocial behavior through an inspirational and educational approach. Vocational training may be the primary focus. Groups of this kind are quite effective.[58] During the early phases of the youngster's membership, they may depend on some external authority to enforce attendance. They are usually open-ended. In fact, one of the primary group tasks is to assimilate and rehabilitate new members successfully. A dedicated and skilled therapist can often create a nucleus of youngsters who discover that there are more pleasant and productive ways to live than the constant battling and hollow victories of delinquency. These "old members" build a strong group ethic of honesty, self-direction, and interpersonal fairness. With the therapist's help, they are able to confront the new member with his self-destructiveness and his deceptive style of relating to other human beings. Often they do this with considerable accuracy and empathy, because they recognize their own previous style in the resistances, defenses, and evasions of the new antisocial member.

A similar approach is often employed by the "detached worker" who does not construct a group but accepts the neighborhood gang as his clientele. Through a variety of strategies, he endeavors to be accepted by the gang membership, particularly its leaders, and then to alter the value system of the gang in a more constructive direction.[83]

FAMILY THERAPY

Family therapy may be valuable as an adjunct to individual or group psychotherapy, as a useful modification of approach during specific periods in the treatment process, or as the primary therapeutic approach with antisocial youngsters. Offer and Vanderstoep[68] are probably correct in asserting that there is a large element of self-selection that determines which families will accept and utilize family therapy. In cases of antisocial youngsters, the problem is often with the parents. Many of these families utilize external and mutual blaming as primary defenses.[98] Scapegoating parents are threatened by the recommendation of a family approach, since the decision to utilize this method clearly implies that they have a role in the youngster's problem.[72]

In spite of the technical difficulties in beginning and conducting family therapy with this diagnostic group, the technique does have important advantages, both diagnostically and therapeutically. Observation of the entire family often permits recognition of the important pathological deviations in family structure which were described above. These aspects of the problem are not always evident from individual interviews with the family members. Even clinicians who are not interested in the family interview as a therapeutic technique might seriously consider including at least one interview with the entire family in the diagnostic evaluation.

From a therapeutic point of view, the family approach is particularly indicated in those cases where the child's current symptomatology seems to be deeply imbedded in a state of neurotic family homeostasis. This includes youngsters who are severely scapegoated, this superego lacunae patients described by Johnson and Szurek, and some cases where the antisocial behavior appears to represent a maladroit attempt at separation from a "binding" or symbiotic family entanglement.

THE INPATIENT TREATMENT OF
ANTISOCIAL YOUNGSTERS

When the antisocial youngster's symptoms are too disruptive or too dangerous to himself or others, inpatient treatment becomes necessary. Available facilities include psychiatric wards in general hospitals, adult psychiatric hospitals, psychiatric hospitals with special programs and units for adolescents and younger children, residential treatment centers, therapeutic boarding schools, runaway houses, and group homes with some degree of therapeutic programming. These facilities vary widely in treatment philosophy and methods. They differ as well in the level of their behavioral expectations and in the stringency with which they enforce behavior limits.

Some are designed to deal with youngsters who have motivation for change and the ability to take at least partial responsibility for regulating their own behavior. At the opposite extreme are locked units which regularly accept extremely belligerent and defiant youngsters who deny any need for treatment. Even with this diversity of population and treatment approach, all of these institutions face certain common problems in treating antisocial children and adolescents. These include behavioral control, development of a pro-therapy atmosphere, parental management, and the provision of suitable transitional and after-care experiences to enable the youngster to return to the larger society.

These tasks will be discussed from the viewpoint of program design and staff implementation. Naturally, in practice, these two factors intertwine and influence each other. That is, program design to some extent determines the kind of staff members who will be comfortable working in a system, while staff composition and attitudes will tend to mold programmatic practices both officially and unofficially.

Program Design: Control of serious acting out behavior is usually obtained by some combination of the following techniques: a system of rewards and punishments, the attempt to foster a value system among the patients which encourages acceptable social behavior, the effort to develop positive emotional bonds to staff members who both provide a constructive social model and direct assistance to the youngster in controlling his behavior, and careful structuring of activities to decrease both the incentive and the opportunity for loss of self-control. Psychoactive medications are also utilized in an effort to decrease the youngster's anxiety and aggression. Of course, this method is susceptible to abuse. In understaffed or poorly organized programs, drugs may be used excessively. Instead of their judicious application in specific situations, they are administered wholesale and in high dosage to all youngsters in the program. This will render them placid, but so obtunded that they can hardly function, much less learn new skills.

The structuring of rewards and punishments in inpatient settings has been strongly influenced by the development of more sophisticated behavioral modification techniques. The rewarding of appro-

priate and desired behavior has virtually replaced the punishment of unacceptable behavior in most modern inpatient treatment settings. The specific designs of these reward programs vary widely, but many include a status system which permits the youngster to "earn" privileges and other desired experiences by meeting an increasingly demanding schedule of expectations. Often the rewards of rising in status include a higher allowance and the opportunity for more extended passes away from the hospital.

Many centers have allowed the patients themselves considerable responsibility in administering the reward system. Strong patient input in the decision-making process strengthens the reward system by adding peer approval to any more objective award which is granted. Moreover, it is one of the methods of encouraging a protherapy atmosphere in the patient group. This tendency is furthered by a clear staff permission for the patients to assist one another and by appropriate recognition of constructive interaction among members of the patient community. The patient group as a whole is encouraged to assist individuals who are upset or troubled, and the troubled youngster is urged strongly to accept and utilize this peer support.

Many programs clearly convey their expectation of positive group functioning by holding the entire patient group responsible for serious individual crises or infractions. This includes such behaviors as runaways and suicide attempts. At first glance this practice seems unfair, but closer investigation usually reveals substantial group collusion in serious episodes of individual acting out. The basic motive may be either vicarious pleasure or an expression of group hostility toward an excluded and scapegoated patient.

The intricacies of appropriate sequencing of patient activities cannot be adequately discussed in a general text. The clinical needs of each age group, the diagnostic mix of the patient population, and the practical problems of availability of staff and facilities make each situation different. However, scheduling of activities is an important matter. For example, without a transitional "winding down" time,[73] younger children, especially severely disturbed ones, cannot shift readily from an active and stimulating activity to one that requires quiet concentration. Adolescents need opportunities for strenuous physical exertion, supervised social contacts with the opposite sex, and an opportunity for unstructured "rap sessions" with one another and with staff. All these situations have the potential for stirring up conflict or overtaxing ego resources. They may need to be followed by organized, controlled contacts with staff which encourage stabilization and focus on reality demands.

Many programs include individual or group psychotherapy. This naturally encourages the formation of positive attachments and working alliances between the patients and their therapists. These relationships, along with the therapeutic insight and growth which they promote, are important sources of behavioral control. However, the patient spends even more time with the child care workers and nursing personnel. These staff members play a crucial role in the success or failure of any treatment program. If they are intuitive, well trained, and sincerely interested in the patients, they have an almost uncanny ability to induce positive behavior in even highly disturbed youngsters. Some of the issues involved in assembling, training, and keeping staff members of this kind will be discussed.

Programming for parental involvement in inpatient treatment is a thorny problem for reasons that are both practical and emotional. As indicated previously, the parents of youngsters with severe behavior problems are often themselves quite disturbed and may even have a vested interest in maintaining the youngster's pathology. The child's removal from the home sets off a veritable conflagration of separation anxieties, guilts, shame, and disruptions of the family homeostasis. Thus, the parents are not only people with chronic problems; at the point of admission they have often regressed acutely in response to the trauma of separation from their child. They may respond to this regression by presenting themselves as helpless and dependent, or they may defend themselves by approaching the hospital staff with attitudes of hostility, arrogant demandingness, or aloof disinterest. These psychological factors make it difficult to enlist the parents in a collaborative treatment effort for the child. In addition, the parents' apparent ineptness and hostility increase the natural staff tendency to identify with the child patient. The competitive atmosphere which often exists between parents and inpatient treatment staff contains significant contributions from both.

In addition to these emotional obstacles, there are often practical issues of geographic distance, job demands, and the responsibility for siblings which may make it difficult for some parents to cooperate actively in the treatment program. Some treatment centers respond to these factors by involving the parents only peripherally, if at all. This seems unwise, since the vast majority of behaviorally disordered youngsters will eventually return home. Unless significant family changes occur, there is a strong likelihood that many treatment gains will evaporate rapidly after the child leaves the hospital. The only exception would be where the institution is assuming a full parental role until the child is self-sustaining.

Once the decision is made to involve the parents actively, there are still many alternative approaches. Perhaps the most common arrangement involves concurrent parental counseling or therapy, often conducted by individuals who are not directly involved in the treatment of the child. In the hands of skilled staff who collaborate actively, this traditional model is often quite effective. Some therapists feel that this separated therapy arrangement has advantages. Centers that use this approach often structure a prolonged period in the early phase of hospitalization where the parents do not even visit the child. It is felt that this enforced separation crystallizes the issues of symbiotic overinvolvement between parent and child and exposes them all to the therapeutic process.[78]

Other centers feel that the parents should remain actively involved with the youngster from the very beginning of hospitalization. From the outset, they permit frequent hospital visits and even passes home. This programmatic arrangement is usually accompanied by a philosophical commitment to a family treatment model. Formal family therapy is started as soon as possible. Usually the same therapists are involved in treating both the family and the youngster in the inpatient setting.

Some programs go even further in their efforts to involve parents. For example, the parents may serve as advisors to the patient government or be provided with other avenues through which they are encouraged and allowed to influence the treatment program. Basically these programs aim to open the hospital to the family and to encourage contact between the youngster and his family and community to the greatest possible extent.

The problems of successful transition from the inpatient setting back into society have provided the major impetus toward the development of the more open programs described. In the more closed systems, the youngster often becomes excessively dependent on the hospital staff and the protected environment of the treatment center. Important family and autonomy issues tend to be slighted during the treatment process, and discharge home is marked by extreme regression and the return of symptoms. This is especially true if inpatient treatment has been prolonged. Many inpatient treatment centers seem to be moving toward briefer inpatient admissions with the development of partial hospitalization programs to provide some structure for the youngster and his family in the transition back to the community. In any model, transition and aftercare are best provided by the same therapists who treated the youngster during the inpatient stay. Although there are many practical problems in arranging continuity of care, it is important enough to warrant the trouble.

An interesting alternative to inpatient therapy is provided by therapeutic camping programs. These were pioneered by Campbell Loughmiller at Salesmanship Camp[55] and have now become quite numerous. There is both anecdotal and statistical evidence to suggest that the approach appeals to the adventure-oriented, antisocial youngster and that treatment results are good.

Staff Issues: The selection, training, and supervision of the people who actually take care of the youngsters twenty-four hours a day is perhaps the most important part of any inpatient treatment program. There are few solid criteria to guide the selection process. Program directors must depend on their intuitive judgment in choosing people who will be able to work well with the irritating and largely ungrateful antisocial child. The goal is to choose people who are able to set reasonable limits while maintaining a primary interest in motivations. Unfortunately, many potential staff members present themselves in that way in an initial interview but are unable to function on the "firing line" without becoming angry and punitive or being corrupted into unwarranted leniency.

Even the best staff need continuing training and supervision. Often it is wiser not to separate these two activities. Staff are often bored and annoyed by formal and pedantic classroom teaching. They respond with much more interest to teaching which is conducted around the problems raised in their everyday work with the youngsters. Often a confluence of specific behavioral patterns or treatment difficulties will give rise to a spontaneous request for more formal instruction. They will then benefit from extended discussion focused on the topics that are currently absorbing their interest.

Perhaps even more important than this direct instruction regarding motivations and their impact on behavior are the emotional lessons the staff learn through their interaction with one another. Most staff members resent being treated as though they were patients, "always being analyzed." However, if the program director and other staff members in authority positions are willing to candidly admit their own errors and to explore freely the emotional dynamics which cause them, it is usually possible to create an atmosphere of openness and emotional honesty. If these frank interchanges are conducted within a framework that clearly recognizes each individual's ultimate responsibility to behave professionally in patient care contacts, they usually result in a relaxed and cohesive staff group. Under the circumstances, staff members are able to be free enough to utilize their own intuitive skills, since they know they can turn to other staff members for support and direction when their intimacy with the youngsters leads to uncomfortable countertransference reactions.

In a setting of intense emotionality, staff conflicts are inevitable. It is often fascinating to observe how these problems between staff members lead rapidly to disturbances in the patient group. Many puzzling crises in inpatient groups can be understood only by investigating the group process issues current in the staff.

REFERENCES

1. Aichhorn, A., *Delinquency and Child Guidance: Selected Papers*, Fleishmann, Kramer, and Ross (Eds.), International Universities Press, New York, 1964.

2. ———, *Wayward Youth*, Viking Press, New York, 1935.

3. Axberger, G., "Arson and Fiction: A Cross-Disciplinary Study," *Psychiatry, 36:*244, 1973.

4. Bandura, A., and Walters, R. H., *Adolescent Aggression*, Ronald Press, New York, 1959.

5. ———, "Dependency Conflicts in Aggressive Delinquents," *Journal of Social Issues, 143:*52–65, 1958.

6. Bender, L., "Children and Adolescents Who Have Killed," *American Journal of Psychiatry, 116:*510, 1959.

7. ———, "Firesetting in Children," in *Aggression, Hostility, and Anxiety in Children*, Charles C Thomas, Springfield, Ill., 1953.

8. Boling, L., and Brotman, C., "A Fire-Setting Epidemic in a State Mental Health Center," *American Journal of Psychiatry, 132:*946–950, 1975.

9. Bovet, L., *Psychiatric Aspects of Juvenile Delinquency*, World Health Organization Monograph, No. 1, 1951.

10. Bowlby, J., "Forty-four Juvenile Thieves," *International Journal of Psychoanalysis, 25:*1, 1944.

11. Brill, A. A., "Artificial Dreams and Lying," *Journal of Abnormal Psychology, 9:*321–332, 1914.

12. Brunswick, R. M., "The Accepted Lie," *Psychiatric Quarterly, 12:*458–464, 1943.

13. Chandler, M. J., "Egocentrism and Antisocial Behavior: The Assessment and Training of Social Perspective-Taking Skills," *Developmental Psychology 9(3):*326, 1973.

14. COPELAND, A. D., "Violent Black Gangs: Psycho- and Socio-dynamics," *Adolescent Psychiatry, 3:*340, 1974.

15. CRAIG, M. M., and FURST, P. W., "What Happens After Treatment?" *Social Service Review, 39:*165, 1965.

16. EASSON, W. M., and STEINHILBER, R. M., "Murderous Aggression by Children and Adolescents," *Archives of General Psychiatry, 4:*1, 1961.

17. EISSLER, K. R., "Some Problems of Delinquency," in Eissler, K. R. (Ed.), *Searchlights on Delinquency,* p. 9, International Universities Press, New York, 1959.

18. EYBERG, S. H., and JOHNSON, S. M., "Multiple Assessment of Behavior Modification with Families: Effects of Contingency Constructing and Order of Treated Problems," *Journal of Consulting and Clinical Psychology, 42:*594, 1974.

19. FENICHEL, O., *The Psychoanalytic Theory of Neurosis,* W. W. Norton, New York, 1945.

20. ———, "Zur Oekonomik der Pseudologia Phantastica," *Internationale Zeitschrift fuer Psychoanalyse, 24:*21–32, 1939.

21. FRANKLIN, G., and NOTTAGE, W., "Psychoanalytic Treatment of Severely Disturbed Juvenile Delinquents in a Therapy Group," *International Journal of Group Psychotherapy, 19(2):*165, 1969.

22. FREUD, A., *Normality and Pathology in Childhood,* p. 119, International Universities Press, New York, 1965.

23. ———, *The Ego and the Mechanisms of Defense,* Hogarth Press, London, 1937.

24. ———, and BURLINGHAM, D., *Infants Without Families,* International Universities Press, New York, 1944. tional Universities Press, New York, 1944.

25. FREUD, S., "The Acquisition and Control of Fire," in Strachey, J. (Ed. and Trans.), *The Standard Edition of the Complete Psychological Works of Sigmund Freud,* vol. 22, pp. 187–193, Hogarth Press, London, 1964.

26. ———, *The Interpretation of Dreams,* Macmillan, New York, 1913.

27. FRIEDEMANN, M., "Cleptomania: The Analytic and Forensic Aspects," *Psychological Review, 17,* 1930.

28. GELEERD, E. R., "The Beginnings of Aggressiveness in Children," *Child Study, 34(4):*3–7, 1957.

29. GIBBENS, T. C. N., "Car Thieves," *British Journal of Delinquency, 8:*257–265, 1958.

30. ———, "The Sexual Behavior of Young Criminals," *Journal of Mental Science* (now *British Journal of Psychiatry*), *103:*527–540, 1957.

31. GIOVACCHINI, P., "The Difficult Adolescent Patient: Countertransference Problems," *Adolescent Psychiatry, 3:* 271, 1974.

32. GLUCK, M. R., and WYLIE, H. L., "Provocation: A Common Family Syndrome," Read at 13th Annual Convention, Southwestern Psychological Association, 1966.

33. GLUECK, S., and GLUECK, E., *Unraveling Juvenile Delinquency,* Commonwealth Fund, New York, 1950.

34. ———, *Juvenile Delinquents Grown Up,* Commonwealth Fund, New York, 1940.

35. GOLOMEIER, H., "Vandalism: The Effects of Unmanageable Confrontations," *Adolescence, 9:*49, 1974.

36. GREENACRE, P., "Anatomical Structure and Superego Development," *American Journal of Orthopsychiatry, 8:*636, 1948.

37. GRINSTEIN, A., "Stages in the Development of Control Over Fire," *International Journal of Psychoanalysis, 33:*416–420, 1952.

38. HARTMANN, H., and KRIS, E., "The Genetic Approach in Psychoanalysis," in Eissler, R. S., et al. (Eds.), *The Psychoanalytic Study of the Child,* vol. 1, International Universities Press, New York, 1945.

39. HOFFER, W., "Deceiving the Deceiver," in Eissler, K. R. (Ed.), *Searchlights on Delinquency,* p. 150, International Universities Press, New York, 1949.

40. HOMER, L. E., "Community-Based Resource for Runaway Girls," *Social Casework, 54:*473, 1973.

41. HOWELL, M. D., EMMONS, E. G., and FRANK, D. A., "Reminiscences of Runaway Adolescents," *American Journal of Orthopsychiatry, 43:*840, 1973.

42. JACOBSON, E., "Denial and Repression," *Journal of the American Psychoanalytic Association, 5:*61–92, 1957.

43. JOHNSON, A. M., and SZUREK, S. A., "The Genesis of Antisocial Acting Out in Children and Adults," *Psychoanalytic Quarterly, 21:*323, 1952.

44. JOHNSON, C. A., and KATZ, R. C., "Using Parents as Change Agents for Their Children: A Review," *Journal of Child Psychology and Psychiatry, 14:*181, 1973.

45. KAUFMAN, I., HEIMS, L. W., and REISER, D. E., "A Re-Evaluation of the Psychodynamics of Firesetting," *American Journal of Orthopsychiatry, 31:*123–136, 1961.

46. KAUFMAN, I., MAKKAY, E. S., and ZILBACH, J., "The Impact of Adolescence on Girls with Delinquent Character Formation," *American Journal of Orthopsychiatry, 29:* 130–143, 1959.

47. KIMSEY, L., "Outpatient Group Therapy with Juvenile Delinquents," *Adolescence, 1:*2, 1969.

48. KNIGHT, R. P., "Intimidation of Others as a Defense Against Anxiety," *Bulletin of the Menninger Clinic, 6:*4–14, 1942.

49. KRAFT, I. A., "An Overview of Group Therapy with Adolescents," *International Journal of Group Psychotherapy, 18:*461–480, 1968.

50. LEHRMAN, P. R., "Some Unconscious Determinants in Homicide," *Psychiatric Quarterly, 13:*605–621, 1939.

51. LEVY, E., "Psychoanalytic Treatment of a Child with a Stealing Compulsion," *American Journal of Orthopsychiatry, 4:*1–23, 1934.

52. LEWIS, N. D. C., and YARNELL, H., *Pathological Firesetting (Pyromania),* Nervous and Mental Disease Monograph Series, No. 82, Williams & Wilkins, Baltimore, Md., 1951.

53. LOBLE, L. H., and WYLIE, M., *Delinquency Can Be Stopped,* McGraw-Hill, New York, 1967.

54. LOMAS, H. D., "Graffiti: Some Observations and Speculations," *Psychoanalytic Review, 60:*73–89, 1973.

55. LOUGHMILLER, C., *Wilderness Road,* Hogg Foundation, Austin, Texas, 1965.

56. MACHT, L. B., and MACK, J. E., "The Firesetter Syndrome," *American Journal of Orthopsychiatry, 31:* 277–288, 1960.

57. McCORD, W., McCORD, J., and ZOLA, I. K., *Origins of Crime,* Columbia University Press, New York, 1959.

58. MASSIMO, J., and SHORE, M., "The Effectiveness of a Comprehensive Vocationally Oriented Psychotherapeutic Program for Adolescent Delinquent Boys," *American Journal of Orthopsychiatry, 33:*634, 1963.

59. MEEKS, J., "Structuring the Early Phase of Group Psychotherapy with Adolescents," *International Journal of Child Psychotherapy, 2:*391, 1973.

60. ———, *The Fragile Alliance,* Williams & Wilkins, Baltimore, Md., 1971.

61. MENAKER, E., "A Contribution to the Study of the Neurotic Stealing Symptom," *American Journal of Orthopsychiatry, 9:*368–377, 1939.

62. MEYER, H. J., BARGATTA, E. F., and JONES, W. C., *Girls at Vocational High,* Russell Sage Foundation, New York, 1965.

63. MICHAELS, J. J., "The Relationship of Anti-Social Traits to the Electroencephalogram in Children with Behavior Disorders," *Psychosomatic Medicine, 7:*41, 1945.

64. ———, "Parallels Between Persistent Enuresis and Delinquency in the Psychopathic Personality," *American Journal of Orthopsychiatry, 11:*260, 1941.

65. MINUCHIN, S., *Families and Family Therapy,* Harvard University Press, Cambridge, Mass., 1974.

66. ———, et al., *Families of the Slums,* p. 352, Basic Books, New York, 1967.

67. MORRIS, H. H., JR., ESCOLL, P. J., and WEKLER, R., "Aggressive Behavior Disorders of Childhood: A Follow-Up Study," *American Journal of Psychiatry, 112:*991–997, 1956.

68. OFFER, D., and VANDERSTOEP, E., "Indications and

Contraindications for Family Therapy," in Sugar, M. (Ed.), *The Adolescent in Group and Family Therapy*, pp. 145–160, Brunner-Mazel, New York, 1975.

69. Ophuijsen, J. H. W. Van, "The Sexual Aim of Sadism as Manifested in Acts of Violence," *International Journal of Psychiatry, 10:*139–144, 1929.

70. Patterson, G. R., "Interventions for Boys with Conduct Problems: Multiple Settings, Treatments, and Criteria," *Journal of Consulting and Clinical Psychology, 42:*471, 1974.

71. Powers, E., and Witner, H., *Prevention of Delinquency: The Cambridge-Somerville Youth Study*, Columbia University Press, New York, 1951.

72. Rabiner, E. L., Molinsky, H., and Grabnick, A., "Conjoint Family Therapy in the Inpatient Setting," *American Journal of Psychotherapy, 16:*618–631, 1962.

73. Redl, F., *When We Deal with Children*, p. 155, Free Press, New York, 1966.

74. ———, and Wineman, D., *Children Who Hate*, Free Press, Glencoe, Ill., 1951.

75. Reik, T., "Aggression from Anxiety," *International Journal of Psychiatry, 22:*7–16, 1941.

76. Rexford, E. N., and van Amerongen, S. T., "The Influence of Unsolved Maternal Oral Conflicts Upon Impulsive Acting Out in Young Children," *American Journal of Orthopsychiatry, 27:*75–87, 1957.

77. Richette, L. A., *The Throwaway Children*, Lippincott, Philadelphia, Pa., 1969.

78. Rinsley, D. B., "Intensive Psychiatric Hospital Treatment of Adolescents: An Object-Relations View," *Psychiatric Quarterly, 39:*405, 1965.

79. Robin, L. N., *Deviant Children Grown Up*, Williams & Wilkins Co., Baltimore, Md., 1966.

80. Russo, S., "Adaptations in Behavioral Therapy with Children," *Behavior Research and Therapy, 2:*43, 1964.

81. Sargent, D., "Children Who Kill—A Family Conspiracy?" *Social Work, 7:*35, 1962.

82. Schmideberg, M., "The Psychoanalysis of Asocial Children and Adolescents," *International Journal of Psychiatry, 16:*22–48, (p. 25), 1935.

83. Schwitzgehel, R., *Streetcorner Research*, Harvard University Press, Cambridge, Mass., 1964.

84. Sendi, I. B., and Blombren, P. G., "A Comparative Study of Predictive Criteria in the Predisposition of Homicidal Adolescents," *American Journal of Psychiatry, 132(4):*423, 1975.

85. Shaw, R. C., and McKay, H. D., *Juvenile Delinquency and Urban Areas*, Chicago University Press, Chicago, 1942.

86. Siegel, L., "Case Study of a Thirteen-Year-Old Fire-Setter: A Catalyst in the Growing Pains of a Residential Treatment Unit," *American Journal of Orthopsychiatry, 27:*396–410, 1957.

87. Silverman, J. S., "Phenomenology and Thinking Disorder in Some Fire Setting Children," *Psychiatric Quarterly, 31(Supplement):*11–25, 1957.

88. Simmel, E., "Incendiarism," in Eissler, K. R. (Ed.), *Searchlights on Delinquency*, pp. 90–101, International Universities Press, New York, 1949.

89. Singer, M., "Family Structure, Disciplinary Configurations and Adolescent Psychopathology," *Adolescent Psychiatry, 3:*372, 1974.

90. Socarides, C. W., "Pathological Stealing as a Reparative Move of the Ego," *Psychoanalytic Review, 41:*246–252, 1954.

91. Stierlin, H., "A Family Perspective on Adolescent Runaways," *Archives of General Psychiatry, 29(1):*56, 1973.

92. Szurek, S. A., "Notes on the Genesis of Psychopathic Personality Traits," *Psychiatry, 5:*1, 1942.

93. Tannenbaum, F., *Crime and the Community*, Columbia University Press, New York, 1938.

94. Thomas, A., Chess, S., and Birch, H. G., *Temperament and Behavior Disorders in Children*, New York University Press, New York, 1968.

95. Vandersall, T. A., and Weiner, J. M., "Children Who Set Fires," *Archives of General Psychiatry, 22:*63–71, 1970.

96. Wahler, R. G., et al., "Mothers as Behavior Therapists for Their Own Children," *Behavior Research and Therapy, 5:*528, 1965.

97. Woods, S. M., "Adolescent Violence and Homicidal Ego Disruption and the 6 and 14 Dysrhythmia," *Archives of General Psychiatry, 5:*528, 1961.

98. Wynn, L. C., "Some Indications and Contraindications for Exploratory Family Therapy, in Boszormenyi-Nagi and Framo," in *Intensive Family Therapy*, Harper & Row, New York, 1965.

99. Yarnell, H., "Firesetting in Children," *American Journal of Orthopsychiatry, 10:*272–286, 1940.

26 / Atypical Sex-Role Behavior

Richard Green

Syndrome Name

The behavioral picture to be described is known as boyhood or childhood transsexualism, atypical sex-role development, sissiness or tomboyishness, and cross-gender-role behavior. While DSM-II did not have a specific diagnostic name or code number, in DSM-II it is tentatively labeled "Gender Identity or Role Disorder of Childhood" and coded 302.60.

Syndrome Description

The behavioral picture includes the preference by a child for the clothes, toys, activities, and companionship of the other sex, and statements of wanting to be of the other sex.

Literature Review

The behavioral picture of young boys with dramatically atypical gender-role behavior was described in 1960 by Green and Money[19] and elaborated upon with a discussion of clinical management by the same authors in 1961.[18] Concurrently, Bakwin[2] described similar cases. Green and Money[17] and Green[14] described additional cases and features, as did Francis[10] and Stoller.[36]

Reports of comparable childhood behaviors recalled by adults appeared in the transsexual literature during this same period.[4, 16, 36] These studies give accounts of adult males and females who requested sex-change surgery. These patients recalled their early lives as replete with cross-gender role behaviors. For males, the feeling was that "as far back as they could remember" they felt and behaved as girls. Converse behavior was recalled by adult females requesting sex-assignment to male status.

More recent research with adult male and female homosexuals also points to the significance of early life cross-gender behavior for adult sexuality. Two-thirds of eighty-nine male homosexuals studied by Saghir and Robins[32] recalled "girl-like" behavior during childhood. The majority of the female homosexuals recalled tomboyish behavior during childhood, which frequently continued into adolescence. Significantly fewer adult heterosexuals recalled such childhood behaviors.

Gender Ratio

The ratio of boys to girls with a significant degree of cross-gender identification is difficult to judge because our culture affords masculine behavior a higher status. Thus, it penalizes a male child who displays feminine behavior but does not stigmatize a girl who is masculine. For example, parents do not bring their "tomboy" daughter for professional consultation whereas they may become concerned over "sissiness" in their son. As a result, the sex ratio of children seen in counseling facilities favors males by a wide margin. Perhaps another result is that more adult women recall being "tomboys" as children than adult men recall being "sissies."

The more compelling question is *when* is cross-gender behavior significant with respect to adult sexual identity? The ratio of adult males requesting sex change is about three to one,[16] and there is data suggesting that about twice as many adult males as females may be homosexual.[24, 25] It would, therefore, appear that a smaller percentage of masculine-behaving girls than feminine-behaving boys become sexually atypical adults.

Age of Onset

Cross-gender-role behavior begins early and takes several forms. Consider first, cross-dressing. In a series of sixty males evaluated by Green, three-fourths began cross-dressing before the fourth birthday; 94 percent by the sixth. Doll play is another form. In this series, 50 percent began before the third birthday, 93 percent before the fifth. Other factors are statements of wanting to be a girl, and typically, role-playing as a female. These also begin in the pre-kindergarten years. In general, there is a considerable delay from the onset of such behaviors to when the children are brought for professional evaluation (if at all). In our series, at the time of initial evaluation the average child's age was seven. For a period of three to four years, the parents had dismissed the behavior as a "normal passing phase." Even at or past age seven, more fathers than mothers were reluctant to seek evaluation. Many parents never seek consultation; indeed, the majority of transsexuals seen as adults were not evaluated during childhood.[13]

Sibling Sequence and Twin Study

In this series, sibling sequence has been random. There was no remarkable distribution of younger or older brothers or sisters. Fifteen percent were only children.

One feminine boy was a monozygotic twin. His co-twin was masculine. The pre-feminine twin was considered prettier as an infant; the pre-masculine twin was given his father's name. The pre-feminine twin contracted a major illness at about three years which persisted for another three years. During this time, his mother was primarily responsible for managing his extensive series of hospital visits, chemotherapy, and surgery. Concurrently, the co-twin was involved with learning to play ball with his father. At six and one-half, when the previously ill twin was medically cured, the father made an effort to engage him in the same socialization experiences already experienced by the co-twin. The boy had difficulty adapting, other adults said that one couldn't expect him to "keep up," and soon the father disengaged. The boy then spent his nonschool time indoors with his mother.

When evaluated at age eight, one boy was feminine in mannerisms and role-played typically as a female. On a variety of psychological tests which discriminate boys and girls, he scored in the feminine range. The co-twin was normally masculine.[12]

This case highlights the manner in which researchers need to look at differences in mother-son and father-son relationships within families in the search for understanding how children develop masculine or feminine gender-role preferences. Indeed, in all cases of boyhood femininity in which there is at least one male sibling, there is never more than the one feminine boy. Indeed, there are only a handful of reports of adult transsexual siblings.[31]

Cross-Cultural Data

The phenomenon of extensive cross-gender role behavior is reported for many cultures. These accounts also point to the adoption of cross-gender behavior very early in life. Other cultures have typically been more accommodating to such behavior, with the individual taking on a respected societal role. An example is the North American Indian designation "berdache" for young males who adopted feminine behavior. These persons were accorded an important position within their society and were not objects of derision (for a compilation see Green[12]). Regrettably, these anthropological accounts give no descriptions of etiology.

Clinical Course

Boys begin to show an interest in culturally feminine articles by the end of the second or third year. This may involve wearing mother's shoes or improvising women's attire. The degree of this interest is greater than that shown by other male siblings in the family. Subsequently it becomes a preference. The child begins to role-play female characters. This may manifest itself in the course of playing house. The boy is typically mother or little sister. A doll may be the boy's favorite toy and the doll play is typically female (e.g., playing with a Barbie doll).

Two-thirds of the boys in the series have been observed by parents cross-dressing more than twenty times. Ninety-one percent had improvised feminine clothes, compared to 13 percent of a control group of masculine boys.

When playing house, more than half of the feminine boys typically role-play as a female while none of the masculine boys do so. Again, more feminine boys role-play as mother, whereas none of the masculine boys role-play as mother. The feminine boys are very much involved in play-acting.

Pictures drawn of identifiable people by feminine boys contain females and rarely, if ever, include a male. The boy may say he is a girl or that he wants to be a girl. Preferred playmates are female, the boy stating "boys play too rough" (see below). Characters from TV and movies imitated are female.

Cross-dressing continues, "as often as you let him," in the words of his mother. The boy is very attentive to feminine fashion and frequently comment's on his mother's clothes.

Feminine gestures and mannerisms may become apparent and are noticed by other children. As the boy begins grade school, he avoids rough-and-tumble play and associates primarily with girls.

Within the home, the boy is much closer emotionally to his mother. He is more interested in the things she does and has little interest in the activities of his father. He may have said on several occasions that he would like to grow up to be like his mother, and rarely, if ever, states he aspires to be like his father.

During preschool years the parents usually have considered the behavior either "cute" or "funny" (in a positive way) and have not considered it as a harbinger of future behaviors. They may state that "all children go through such a phase." The mother is usually more aware of the feminine behavior.

With the beginning of grade school, the atypical behavior causes conflict for both the child and the parents. The child is called "sissy" and is teased by age-mates, teachers point out the atypicality of the child's behavior to the parents, and neighbors comment that the boy always plays with dolls, or dresses up like a girl when playing with their child.

The parents are initially reluctant to seek professional advice. They may attempt to discourage the boy's cross-dressing or his role-playing as a female, but the boy persists. More often than not, it is the mother who seeks professional help; the father continues to insist "he'll outgrow it."

Due to the lack of significant social conflict experienced by masculine-behaving girls, the female counterpart of this clinical picture is rarely evaluated. When it is, there is generally an account of a girl who always role-plays as a male, refuses to wear dresses, never plays with dolls, and states that she wants to be a boy. When this insistent attitude continues for several years and has not waned during the later grade school years, the parents may become concerned that their daughter will grow up to be homosexual.

Post-Childhood Behavior

Little research exists which has longitudinally followed atypical gender-role children into adolescence and adulthood. Three follow-up reports have looked at adult or late adolescent behavior in previously evaluated and/or treated feminine boys. The total number in these reports is less than thirty, and a small majority are homosexual, transsexual, or transvestic.[12, 26, 40] The male children in the current series (N=60) are entering adolescence and as many as possible will be reevaluated.

Organic Etiologic Factors

Considerable speculation and some research data point to a physiological factor that contributes to the development of atypical gender-role behavior. Much of this interest stems from neuroendocrine animal research. The influence of androgen on the developing brain has been an area of keen interest. A pioneering study demonstrated that exposing a female rhesus monkey in utero to exogenously administered high levels of testosterone proportionate not only had an *anatomical* effect (virilized external genitalia) but a *behavioral* effect as well.[39] Earlier work had documented the gender dimorphic play behavior of juvenile rhesus monkeys.[30] Young males more often participate in rough-and-tumble play, chasing, and making social threats. Females whose prenatal hormonal milieu was manipulated so that they received extra androgen, behaved more like young males. They became "tomboys." That there is a critical period for this influence is demonstrated by the fact that postnatal exposure to equivalent levels of androgen does not have a comparable behavioral effect.

A human analogy exists for this "tomboy" monkey model. The andrenogenital syndrome is an inborn error of metabolism. In this condition, an enzymatic deficiency in the production of cortisol results in overproduction of other adrenal cortical hormones which are androgenic. This overproduction begins in utero. Human females with this syndrome are also more boyish. Studies by Ehrhardt and co-workers[8] show that when compared with their hormone-normal sisters or unrelated controls, they are more interested in rough-and-tumble play and sports, and less interested in doll play and newborn babies. They are more often called "tomboy."

Some data exist describing human males exposed in utero either to high levels of estrogen or to lower than usual levels of androgen. A few case reports have appeared of adult males with malfunctioning testes (typically with Klinefelter's [XXY] syndrome), who have requested sex-change surgery.[1, 27] These patients recall their childhood as similar to that of the feminine boys described previously. However, most males with the XXY chromosomal configuration are not as feminine as these case reports[22] and the concurrence of the extra X chromosome, low testosterone levels, and feminine identity may be coincidental, rather than causally related. A controversial prospective study is underway in which a more representative sample of children with an extra X chromosome is being observed longitudinally. The research strategy is that of karyotyping consecutively born newborn males.[37]

Another research strategy has been the study of males whose mothers received exogenous female sex steroids during pregnancy. We evaluated sixteen- and six-year-old males whose diabetic mothers had been treated with diethylstilbestrol and progesterone during pregnancy in an effort to avert the problems of gestation in the diabetic.

The contrast group did not contain as many diabetic mothers, so a valid comparison is difficult. However, the males prenatally exposed to exogenous female hormones were less rough-and-tumble and athletic. It is important to note that they were not feminine in the manner of the boys described earlier. This suggests the need to look for an interaction theory that would embrace neuroendocrine and socialization influences.

Nature-Nurture Synthesis

Rather than postulating an either/or thesis of a neuroendocrine versus socialization etiology of atypical gender-role behavior, it is possible to see the two in an interactional pattern. As noted, there is research support for the concept that androgen levels at some period(s) of central nervous system development influence postnatal behaviors. These latter include rough-and-tumble play, interest in newborns, and perhaps the role rehearsal for this interest: doll play. These behaviors have considerable social consequence within the cultural milieu which sex-types them. A male child with a lack of interest in rough-and-tumble play and an interest in doll play will have an early peer group experience different from that of a boy with converse interests. The male child with an aversion to rough-and-tumble play will also have a different relationship with his father. He will be regarded differently from a boy (perhaps his brother) who does show an interest in such activity (especially when this is also an activity preference of the father). Indeed, the feminine boys described previously complained that boys play too rough. They enjoyed doll play and were emotionally more distant from their fathers than the control group of masculine boys.

If the parents of a boy with feminine inclinations positively reinforce or do not interrupt the behavior during early developmental years, the boy may begin to follow an atypical developmental route. Later, when entering school, he is likely to be called sissy. This label will continue to stigmatize him and will further prevent him from identifying with his male peer group or adult male models. While this hypothesis is speculative, it does provide a way of theoretically linking the disciplines of neuroendocrinology, sociology, and psychology in the search for a better comprehension of the earliest roots of sexual identity.[11]

Psychodynamic Factors

Stoller[36] has proposed that certain unusual maternal characteristics and early mother-infant interactions can lead to a separation and individuation of the male child from its mother. In such contexts, a male child is likely to be held for unusually long periods of time by the mother, frequently with skin to skin contact. The mother has a high degree of masculine identification; symbolically she makes the male infant into her feminized phallus. The boy develops a female identity as an extension of his mother's body. His femininity is not defensive; it is a conflict-free ego development that emerges prior to the usually described patterns of castration fear and oedipal conflict. According to Newman and Stoller,[28] such oedipal dynamics as do evolve in such children are delayed. Often enough they come about as a by-product of psychotherapeutic intervention. In such families, the fathers exert little influence on these boys during the early years, and the mother and son co-exist in a blissful symbiotic universe.

For the atypical female, Stoller[35] sees the psychodynamics differently. The mothers of masculine girls tend to be tired, long-suffering and sad, left alone too much by their husbands. The little girl moves into the vacuum created by her mother's sadness. She feels protective toward her mother and has conscious thoughts of taking care of her as would a husband (these fantasies are generally nonsexual in character, at least on a conscious level). The child then receives positive reinforcement for her masculine behavior, typically from the father.

Children with atypical gender-role development do not manifest any classic childhood neurotic syndromes. They do experience social conflict, however, in consequence of being teased. This may engender depression, school phobia, or social withdrawal. It is an appropriate reaction to peer group pressure.

Psychological Testing

There are a number of psychological tests which are specially sensitive to gender issues. In the It-Scale for Children,[6] children select a series of sex-typed activity choices, drawn on cards, for "It" (a neuter stick figure). Typical grade-school age boys and girls score differently on this test. The feminine boys in our series scored similarly to the typical girl.[12]

The Draw-a-Person test requires a child to draw a person on a piece of paper. Children of school age (and individuals of all ages through adulthood) are more likely to draw someone of their own sex.[23] The feminine boys in our series more often drew a female first. The masculine contrast group did not.[12]

In a playroom stocked with sex-typed toys, the feminine boys select toys similar to those selected by girls and different from those selected by the control boys. The preferred toy of the feminine boys is a Barbie doll, that of the masculine boys is a truck.[12]

When completing picture sequences which depict a male child joining an adult male or female in a culturally typical masculine or feminine activity, feminine boys more often select the female and a feminine activity.[12]

When requested to compose a story utilizing doll figures representing grandparents, a boy, a girl, and an infant, feminine boys utilize the female figures more than the masculine boys and spend significantly more time with the infant doll. These reactions are similar to same-age girls.[15]

Familial Structure

The composition and interrelationships of the families of children with atypical gender-role behavior, either directly observed or retrospectively described, varies with samples studied and methodologies utilized. A psychoanalytic-treatment study of homosexually-oriented and heterosexually-oriented adult males found that a higher percentage of the homosexual males recalled their parent-self relationships in a special way. Their material could be interpreted by the therapist to give a picture of mothers and sons enmeshed in a close, binding, seductive, and intimate relationship, and fathers and sons in a distant, absentee, or passive relationship.[5] This intergroup finding, though nonspecific for the development of homosexuality (there was overlap between the groups) was replicated in one questionnaire study, utilizing a nonclinical population.[9] However, another study, utilizing questionnaires and several hundred nonpatient heterosexual and homosexual males, did not find comparable differences in the descriptions given of earlier parent-child relationships.[33] While the 307 male homosexuals described their fathers and mothers as more rejecting and

less loving than the 138 heterosexuals, and themselves as less close to their fathers, this difference disappeared when comparing subsamples who scored low on neuroticism test scales. This study stresses the non-specificity of certain configurations of early parenting and suggests the possibility that problems between child and parent may predispose to non-specific neurotic behavior. These early relationships are neither sufficient nor specific to the development of homosexuality.

A psychiatric interview study of heterosexual and homosexual males and females found childhood parental discord more common among the homosexual males—52 percent versus 17 percent.[32] Additionally, for the homosexual males, 84 percent described their fathers as indifferent and uninvolved in their childhood home versus 18 percent of the heterosexuals. The adult male homosexuals less often recalled their fathers as family decision maker (40 percent versus 71 percent). More homosexual males recalled possessive mothers (41 percent versus 23 percent). More of the homosexual males lost a parent by death or divorce before age ten (27 percent versus 9 percent).

More the homosexual females reported losing one or more parents by death or divorce prior to age ten (39 percent versus 5 percent). The mothers of the homosexual women were more often described as dominant (53 percent versus 27 percent). The adult homosexual women recalled their relationships with their mothers as poor, and those with their fathers as good.

In research concerned directly with feminine boys, plus a matched group of masculine boys, and their parents, other patterns have emerged. As is typical for most families the mothers spent considerably more time than the fathers with the boys. However, estimates of the time the boy was held during his first two years did not discriminate the groups. On the other hand, the fathers of the feminine boys reportedly spent significantly less time with their sons during the second year of life compared to the fathers of the masculine boys. In addition, more fathers were separated from their sons before the child's fifth birthday.

Marital role-division was also studied. Five sectors were examined: financial management, leisure-time planning, child disciplinarian, family argument winner, and, a global designation, "boss." Compared to the fathers of feminine boys, fathers of masculine boys more often saw themselves as being the financially responsible spouse. For leisure-time planning, however, fathers of the feminine boys saw themselves as more responsible (fathers of masculine boys saw both marital partners sharing in this responsibility). The fathers of masculine boys were more likely to be the family argument winners. Family "boss" was more often seen as co-equally husband and wife by the mothers of masculine boys, and more often as the husband by the fathers of masculine boys.

Both fathers and mothers see the feminine boys relating best to females. Thirty-one percent of the masculine boys are seen as relating best to older boys, 58 percent to same-age boys and 2 percent to girls. By contrast 27 percent of the feminine boys relate best to older boys, 14 percent to same-age boys, and 63 percent to girls.

The degree to which mothers and fathers of the feminine and masculine boys report feeling close to their sons does not discriminate the groups. However, the feminine boys clearly prefer their mothers. By contrast, masculine boys either prefer their fathers or feel equally close to both parents. More of the feminine boys state their wish to grow up like their mother, while more of the masculine boys state their wish to grow up to be like their father.

Societal Role Change

A frequently asked question is: What will be the effect of the continued blurring of sex-roles on the development of cross-gender behavior? First, it is necessary to point out that sex-role blurring, like all social evolutionary processes, moves slowly. Nor does it engage all segments of the population simultaneously. Perhaps more has been written about the diminishing sex-role dimorphism in our culture than has taken, or will take, place. The vast majority of Barbie dolls are still bought for girls and most girls want them. The vast majority of trucks and guns are still bought for boys and most boys want them. Parents of sons who attempt to restrict war toys may report that their children improvise guns from sticks and reenact violent television dramas with neighborhood children.

If movement continues in the direction of less stereotypic sex-oriented behavioral expectations for children, it may affect the development of children who do not feel contented with their gender-role and who are in conflict because they are unable to live up to societal expectations. There are boys and girls who envy the clothes, toys, games and role expectations of the other gender. There are boys who, for whatever rea-

son(s), like to play with Barbie-type dolls, cook, wear "pretty things," and, in the concrete thinking world of childhood, feel they must *be* a girl to do these things because "that's girls' stuff." There are girls who see that boys get more freedom, do not have to be as neat, get to play games considered too rough for girls, and have higher social status. With continued blurring of sex-roles, such children should be able to select the activities of their choice without those selections affecting their self-image of maleness or femaleness.

As societal (herein translated as parental) expectations change, there should also be fewer children (especially males) who do not meet the behavioral expectations of their fathers. The regard for athletic prowess, for example, would diminish, as would the ensuing alienation that comes from paternal disappointment.

However, in this connection it is essential to keep in mind the difference between behavior and identity. There may be a subsample of children, with what is currently called atypical gender-role behavior, who manifest the behaviors in consequence of some innate or early life (years one to two) postnatal experiences which result in a cross-sex identity. For these children, changes in culture have less impact on their basic conflict (feeling like a female, though anatomically male). What may happen in such instances is that these children will present clinically with the residual noncultural differences between male and female. Boys will want to have babies and a vagina rather than a penis, girls will want to have a penis and to father children.

The future of the children currently manifesting such atypical gender-role behavior will be influenced by the degree to which the culture accommodates atypical sex-typed behavior in the next decades. Hopefully, the atypical children of today will enter a different culture when they come into adolescence, one less marked by the rigid sex-role stereotypes of the past. Hopefully too, psychotherapeutic intervention will help them accommodate to their "outsider" role and abort the progression of their syndrome into the despair of full-blown adult transsexualism.

Therapeutic Methods

ETHICS OF TREATMENT

Treatment intervention into the lives of children with atypical gender-role behavior raises ethical issues of considerable magnitude. It has become the subject of increasing controversy.

One viewpoint on the need for treatment is that it is a fault of society that sexually-dimorphic behavioral demands are placed on children and that society should change; not the "deviant" child. The thesis is elaborated further: Treatment reinforces and perpetuates societal sexism. Furthermore, treatment may cause greater harm to the child, because the child is not permitted free expression (natural behavior is suppressed), and the outcome is psychological damage.

The opposing viewpoint is that the children are experiencing conflict over their behavior, are being stigmatized by their peer group, and have parents who want them to be treated. The argument is advanced further: Society is not evolving rapidly enough to accommodate this generation's atypical children, and the children will experience increasing conflict as they enter adolescence, a period in the life cycle when they will be less amenable to change.

TYPES OF TREATMENT

The types of treatment to undertake is also an issue. Advocates of behaviorist principles have applied positive and negative reinforcement, sometimes utilizing a token economy, to reward and punish selective sex "appropriate" and "inappropriate" behaviors. These strategies have drawn the most fire from critics, but are also those most elaborately documented as effecting behavioral change.[29] Others have utilized more eclectic approaches. For example, a male therapist may seek to involve a boy in sex "typical" activities which the boy finds enjoyable in the hope of promoting a more masculine identification. Concurrently, parents are advised of ways in which they have been covertly or overtly encouraging cross-gender role behavior. Another important approach is to seek to improve an alienated father-son relationship.[20]

Group treatment methods for boys have also been used and have been coupled with group treatment for the parents. Here, the boys form their initial male peer group and interact with a male therapist. As in other group therapy situations, the children project their own atypical behavior onto others. They identify with the aggressor and criticize the other children. Within their own group contexts the parents see more readily how other people encourage feminine behavior in their sons.[12]

OUTCOMES OF TREATMENT

Which of these treatments (if any) are effective? In what way? What will be the outcome for those children who are treated and those who are not?

The few clinical reports to date all describe behavioral change in the children treated. These include reports of treatment by psychoanalysts,[21, 34] by behavior therapists,[29] by eclectic approaches with children and parents,[20] and by group therapy either alone[12] or coupled with a token economy.[3] Additionally, our series of feminine boys includes those who have not been formally treated following clinical evaluation. Many of these boys also show behavioral change.

What is true for each of these interventions is that all the children manifest more masculine behavior. The common denominator may be that in every case the parents became concerned enough to seek professional consultation about the boy's feminine behavior. For years prior to evaluation, they had either reinforced the behavior or ignored it. However, they eventually became worried. Their attitude toward the boy's behavior underwent change: they began to view cross-dressing, doll play, and female peer group preference as possible harbingers of a serious problem.

Which behaviors are affected by treatment, by clinical evaluation, or by changing parental attitudes toward atypical sex-typed behavior? Sexual identity may be conceptualized as having three components: (1) core morphologic identity—the sense of being male or female; (2) gender-role behavior—culturally dimorphic activities which typify males and females; and (3) sexual partner preference—heterosexuality, homosexuality, or ambisexuality. These three behaviors are probably sequentially developed and interrelated. Core identity appears to evolve and be set during the first two to three years, gender-role behavior is quite dimorphic by the fifth year, sexual partner orientation begins to become manifest near the onset of adolescence. The components are usually interrelated. Most males behave in a masculine way during grade school and later become erotically attracted to females. The converse is true for females. However, the three components may vary independently.

When the child with the behavioral syndrome described here is initially seen he is about seven to eight years of age. He typically knows he is male but would like to be a girl and/or prefers the activities of girls. He has not yet developed romantic crushes. Changing parental attitudes, clinical evaluation, and formal treatment, if any, primarily engage the second component of sexual identity—gender-role behavior. An attempt is made to convert a feminine-behaving boy into a more conventionally masculine-behaving one. For those boys who wish to be girls, the anatomical distinctions between male and female are underscored, as well as the biologic impossibility of truly "changing sex." Not directly engaged, however, is the third component of sexual identity. That a relationship exists between the second and third is suggested by the observation that having a grade-school homosocial peer group is positively correlated with a later heterosexual life style. The converse is also true. In other words adult male homosexuals more often report that, in childhood, girls were their best friends. Since one of the treatment methods with feminine boys is their inclusion in a male peer group, this permits at least some speculation about the potential effect of treatment on sexual partner preference.

PRINCIPLES OF TREATMENT

Detailed principles of treatment with examples have been elaborated elsewhere.[12] Essentially, an attempt is made to find activities which are interesting to the boy but which do not stigmatize him. The goal is not to metamorphose him into a Little League Star, a rough-house boy, or a boy devoid of esthetic interests. He may find handicrafts, board and card games, and reading to his taste. His peer group associations may be widened to include males, so that some of these activities can be engaged in with other boys. Special effort may be required on the parents' part to find boys whose interests are sedentary, but who are not themselves stigmatized as "sissy." In addition, the father-son relationship should be enhanced. There are father-son activities which do not require athletic competence but which can be mutually enjoyable. The group father-son programs of Indian Guides, a YMCA sponsored program, can be of considerable help. Here, outdoor camping, cooking, and indoor handicrafts are given priority.

LONG-RANGE SIGNIFICANCE

The long-term outcome for the treatment of very feminine boys remains to be determined. These youngsters need to be reevaluated during adolescence, and again as adults. Such a project would have to include a thorough analysis of all the intervening variables, not just whether or not they were treated (and how). Intrafamily influences, socialization experiences, and fantasies, all need to be weighed. A no-treatment group must be similarly studied. A nonevaluation group of previously "feminine" boys is difficult to evaluate in a comparable way due to the lack of objective data on the earlier childhood behaviors.

Analysis of the effects of treatment on very masculine girls will be more difficult. To begin with, there are far fewer patients, and in any case, in the natural course of events, tomboyism appears, for the most part, to fade with the onset of adolescence.

Conclusion

The behavioral syndrome of atypical gender-role behavior is a relatively recently described constellation of behavioral features. It has taken on social significance in that it has an interface with issues of sexism, the changing cultural mores for "masculine" and "feminine" behavior, and the politically activist work of the homophile (gay liberation) movement. Somewhere in this morass is the intriguing research and philosophical question of how children develop sexual identity, and the major therapeutic burden of a population of troubled children and parents for whom sexual identity has become a significant obstacle to psychological comfort. The child psychiatrist cannot here avoid the triple responsibility of researcher, clinician, and social reformer.

REFERENCES

1. BAKER, H., and STOLLER, R., "Can a Biological Force Contribute to Gender Identity?" *American Journal of Psychiatry*, 124:1653–1658, 1968.
2. BAKWIN, H., "Transvestism in Children," *Journal of Pediatrics*, 56:294–298, 1960.
3. BATES, J., et al., "Intervention with Families of Gender-Disturbed Boys," *American Journal of Orthopsychiatry*, 45:150–157, 1975.

4. BENJAMIN, H., *The Transsexual Phenomenon*, Julian Press, New York, 1966.
5. BIEBER, I., et al., *Homosexuality*, Basic Books, New York, 1962.
6. BROWN, D., *Sex Role Preference in Young Children*, Psychological Monographs, 70, No. 14, (No. 421), 1956.
7. EHRHARDT, A., and BAKER, S., "Fetal Androgens, Human Central Nervous System Differentiation, and Be-

havior Differences," in Friedman, R., and Richart, R. (Eds.), *Sex Differences in Behavior*, John Wiley, New York, 1974.

8. ————, Epstein, R., and Money, J., "Fetal Androgens and Female Gender Identity in the Early Treated Adrenogenital Syndrome," *Johns Hopkins Medical Journal, 122:*160–167, 1968.

9. Evans, R., "Childhood Parental Relationships of Homosexual Men," *Journal of Consulting and Clinical Psychology, 33:*129–135, 1969.

10. Francis, J., "Passivity and Homosexual Predisposition in Latency Boys," *Bulletin of the Philadelphia Association of Psychoanalysis, 15:*160–174, 1965.

11. Green, R., "Sexual Identity: Research Strategies," *Archives of Sexual Behavior, 4:*337–349, 1975.

12. ————, *Sexual Identity Conflict in Children and Adults*, Basic Books, New York, 1974.

13. ————, "The Behaviorally Feminine Male Child: Pretranssexual? Pretransvestic? Prehomosexual? Preheterosexual?" in Friedman, R., and Richart, R. (Eds.), *Sex Differences in Behavior*, John Wiley, New York, 1974.

14. ————, "Childhood Cross-Gender Identification," *Journal of Nervous and Mental Disease, 147:*500–509, 1966.

15. ————, and Fuller, M., "Family Doll Play and Female Identity in Pre-Adolescent Males," *American Journal of Orthopsychiatry, 43:*123–127, 1973.

16. Green, R., and Money, J. (Eds.), *Transsexualism and Sex Reassignment*, Johns Hopkins Press, Baltimore, 1969.

17. ————, "Prepubertal, Morphologically Normal Boys Demonstrating Signs of Cross-Gender Identity," American Orthopsychiatric Association Annual Meeting, 1964.

18. ————, "Effeminacy in Prepubertal Males—Summary of Eleven Cases and Recommendations for Case Management," *Pediatrics, 27:*286–291, 1961.

19. ————, "Incongruous Gender Role Behavior. Nongenital Manifestations in Prepubertal Boys," *Journal of Nervous and Mental Disease, 131:*160–168, 1960.

20. ————, Newman, L., and Stoller, R., "The Treatment of Boyhood 'Transsexualism.' An Interim Report of Four Years' Experience," *Archives of General Psychiatry, 26:*213–217, 1972.

21. Greenson, R., "A Transvestite Boy and a Hypothesis," *International Journal of Psycho-Analysis, 47:* 396–403, 1966.

22. Hambert, H., *Males With Positive Sex Chromatin*, Scandinavian University Books, Goteborg, 1966.

23. Jolles, I., "A Study of the Validity of Some Hypotheses for the Qualitative Interpretation of the HTP," *Journal of Clinical Psychology, 8:*113–118, 1952.

24. Kinsey, A., Pomeroy, W., and Martin, C., *Sexual Behavior in the Human Male*, Saunders, Philadelphia, 1948.

25. ————, et al., *Sexual Behavior in the Human Female*, Saunders, Philadelphia, 1953.

26. Lebovitz, P., "Feminine Behavior in Boys. Aspects of Its Outcome," *American Journal of Psychiatry, 128:* 1283–1289, 1972.

27. Money, J., and Pollit, E., "Cytogenetic and Psychosexual Ambiguity," *Archives of General Psychiatry, 11:*589–595, 1964.

28. Newman, L., and Stoller, R., "Oedipal Situation in Male Transsexualism," *British Journal of Medical Psychology, 44:*295–303, 1971.

29. Reekers, G., and Lovaas, O., "Behavioral Treatment of Deviant Sex-Role Behaviors in a Male Child," *Journal of Applied Behavioral Analysis, 7:*173–190, 1974.

30. Rosenblum, L., "Sex Differences, Environmental Complexity, and Mother-Infant Relations," *Archives of Sexual Behavior, 3:*117–128, 1974.

31. Sabalis, R., et al., "The Three Sisters: Transsexual Male Siblings," *American Journal of Psychiatry, 131:* 907–909, 1974.

32. Saghir, M., and Robins, E., *Male and Female Homosexuality*, Williams and Wilkins, Baltimore, 1974.

33. Siegelman, M., "Parental Background of Male Homosexuals and Heterosexuals," *Archives of Sexual Behavior, 3:*3–18, 1974.

34. Sperling, M., "The Analysis of a Boy with Transvestite Tendencies," in Eissler, R. S., et al. (Eds.), *The Psychoanalytic Study of the Child*, vol. 19, pp. 470–493, International Universities Press, New York, 1964.

35. Stoller, R., "Etiological Factors in Female Transsexualism: A First Approximation," *Archives of Sexual Behavior, 2:*47–64, 1972.

36. ————, *Sex and Gender*, Science House, New York, 1968.

37. Walzer, S., and Gerald, P., "A Chromosome Survey of 13,751 Male Newborns," in Hook E., and Porter, I. (Eds.), *Population Cytogenetics*, Academic Press, New York, 1977.

38. Yalom, I., Green, R., and Fisk, N., "Prenatal Exposure to Female Hormones. Effect on Psychosexual Development in Boys," *Archives of General Psychiatry, 28:*554–561, 1974.

39. Young, W., Goy, R., and Phoenix, C., "Hormones and Sexual Behavior," *Science, 143:*212–218, 1964.

40. Zuger, B., "Effeminate Behavior Present in Boys From Early Childhood," *Journal of Pediatrics, 69:*1098–1107, 1966.

---

27 / Disorders of Masculinity and Femininity

Robert J. Stoller

I shall approach my topic in an autobiographical tone; that should bring greater accuracy than an orderly, scholarly presentation. Since the data that underlie these thoughts come especially from the peculiar intimacy of psychoanalyses, making my self invisible reduces the reader's chance to glimpse the uncertainties, biases, disturbances in logic, and faulty conclusions.

As another way to protect the reader, I must note that the research has continuously forced changes in my opinions; one position after another has been knocked down by data, so that little that seemed sure in the earliest years has held up. However, with the optimism that probably sustains other researchers who persist on one subject, I always feel that today's concepts, theories, data, and conclusions are solid and pretty accurate—a pleasant, persistent illusion that keeps one going.

It is evident that one's motivations are a crucial factor in the form one's findings take. So let me say a bit more on that. The prime reason I did not get interested earlier in the study of masculinity and femininity was that I could not discern any significant issues when confronted by patients with gender disorders. Whatever my contribution, conscious and unconscious, to that attitude, psychoanalytic training in the 1950s contributed its share. At that time, analysts were not raising questions about the origins or maintenance of masculinity and femininity; analytic theory seemed sophisticated enough to account for any clinical event, any observation, any data collected by any method. Indeed, the final defense against new ideas was the plausible, though too glibly used, argument that loose pieces could be accounted for by biology (that great immeasurable force taking the place of God in modern explanations).

Despite an ongoing research project by Worden and Marsh, in our department at UCLA, I still found no interest in the subject, even after they invited me to interview patients for their study (the first careful one ever done) on transsexualism. The one patient I recall seeing for them excited no interest in me either in the clinical condition, though bizarre enough, or in stirring the belief that there were unknowns worth pondering. This patient was a biologically normal man who liked to put on women's clothes and be enchained in order to become sexually excited; so he was no more than a pervert whose condition could be well enough explained by a consideration of vicissitudes of instincts, libidinal fixations, and oedipal traumas. In those days, all analysts, and candidates, could handle such data without batting an eye.

What threw me off with such patients was the grossness of the pathology; explaining it took no effort. This innocence died one day, literally from one moment to the next. Worden and Marsh were done with their project but had made an appointment with a patient whom they had not seen but who was categorized as a "transsexual woman," (a biological female who nonetheless considered herself a man). They asked me to see her to tell her the research was finished.

Shortly before the appointment hour, I was attending a committee meeting in a conference room with one glass wall, which allowed us to see people pass. I was gradually becoming stuporous. A man walked by; I scarcely noticed him. A moment later, a secretary announced my 11:00 o'clock patient. And to my astonishment, the patient was not a woman who, as I expected, would act masculine and in the process be a bit too much; instead it was a man, unremarkable, natural-appearing. Suddenly, contemporary psychoanalytic answers were inadequate; although they were finely tooled to account for bizarreness, they could not clarify naturalness. I was now into issues of self identity, identification, the relationship of culture and the historical past to the development of the individual, perhaps even the unexplored territory (notwithstanding Hartmann's theorizing) of conflict-free development. What, for instance, are the psychodynamic relationships between acting, imitation, impersonation, imposture, multiple personality, habituation, incorporation, introjection, identification, internalization?

None of these issues was manifest at that moment, but, in the almost twenty years since, I have discovered that they had been present in some form. The years have brought them to consciousness, which then let me ask the questions that have made up the greater part of this research. Due to the fortunate circumstance of my being an analyst set free in a congenial university, this study has roamed about the subject of masculinity and femininity without the discipline of a proper research plan or the dictates of granting agencies, but haphazardly, in accord with what interested me. At first—phase one of the research —with roots sunk in medicine but those in analysis still forming, I was especially occupied with biological issues—the relationships between demonstrable physical defects and gender behavior, and with diagnosis—discovering syndromes and the physiology and/or psychodynamics that underlay them.

Hundreds of patients and their family members were seen. As the years passed, separate conditions in which gender aberration was present have condensed out of the fog, forming a range of differential diagnoses. Although this might in time have practical use, pointing toward different treatments, it serves me mostly for studying the development and maintenance of "gender identity" (the phrase I coined as a label for the differing degrees of masculinity and femininity that can be found in a person).

For clarity, a short vocabulary exercise: Sex (maleness and femaleness) refers to a biological realm with these dimensions: chromosomes, external genitals, gonads, internal sexual apparatuses (e.g., uterus, prostate), hormonal state, secondary sex characteristics, and brain. Gender (gender-identity) is a psychologic state: masculinity and femininity. (One often finds the term "sex role" or "gender role" used; role refers to a part one takes; there is no reference to one's intensity, intent, or commitment to the behavior. "Identity," on the other hand, implies that one's very being is involved. One *plays* a role; one *is* one's identity.) Sex and gender are by no means necessarily related. In most instances in humans, postnatal experiences can overpower already present biologic tendencies.

Here, then, is a differential diagnosis for cross-gender behavior (for males; a discussion of females follows). It needs confirmation. The essential criterion measured is observable behavior that, in the society from which the subject comes, is considered natural for members of the opposite sex, i.e., cross-gender behavior.

True Transsexuals

These are males with no known biological (including anatomical) abnormality, who, whenever seen for evaluation (as a child, adolescent, or adult) are the most feminine of all males, have never had an episode—for moments or extended periods—of being able to appear like or live in the role of an ordinary masculine male, and who have been so since the beginning of anything that can be labeled gender behavior. As a result of this powerful sense of femininity, they nowadays, sooner or later, request that their sex be changed. They consider themselves heterosexual, asking that that be measured by one's sense of self rather than by one's anatomy, do not have social or sexual relationships with homosexual males, do not enjoy their male genitals, do not have sexual relations with women, and do not become sexually excited by cross-dressing (putting on clothes of the opposite sex). In time, no matter what barriers are placed in their path, these people get female hormones that change the appearance of their secondary sex characteristics to female, the removal of facial and body hair by electrolysis, and operations in which testes and penis are removed, and a vulva and vagina simulated. A complex constellation of family dynamics, not found in any of the other conditions in this differential, seems the basis of the behavior; the two main features of this are a mother-infant, blissful symbiosis that is prolonged for years, plus a passive, absent father. (I shall enlarge a bit on this later.)

Secondary Transsexuals

In this condition, also found in biologically normal males, the presenting manifestation is a request for sex change, but the clinical pictures and causative forces are different from those in true transsexualism. None of these people has been unswervingly feminine since earliest childhood, and few ever reach the point of the natural-appearing, persisting femininity pathognomonic for true transsexualism. They have all had periods of living unequivocally the role of boy or man, and residuals of that masculinity can be found at the time of psychiatric evaluation. So, for instance, there usually is a history of sexual relations with women, at least intermittent commitment to masculine professions, periods of dressing and appearing like ordinary boys or men, pleasure in their male genitals, and/or, often, either persistent periods of overtly homosexual behavior or of genital excitement caused by women's clothes. In none of these cases is the family constellation of the true transsexual found.

Transvestites

Although the term "transvestism" is used for any cross-dressing (in fact, such a vague clinical concept can seem precise only if one transforms it with the scientific-sounding Latin), I restrict it to those, again biologically normal, who put on clothes of the opposite sex because the clothes are sexually exciting. Although this fetishism can occur in childhood, usually it is first manifested at puberty or later in adolescence. It is almost always found in men who are overtly heterosexual, of masculine demeanor, in professions dominated by males; and it occurs only intermittently, most of the subject's life being spent in unremarkably masculine behavior and appearance. Such men usually marry and have children. As the years pass, for many the fetishism cools down (but does not disappear, and there is an increased need to dress and consider oneself momentarily a woman. Although a few such men in time have strong transsexual wishes (secondary transsexualism), for most transvestites the impulse for sex change is contained by the much more dominant masculinity. In no cases has the true transsexual family constellation been reported; rather, one frequently finds that in early childhood, the boy was cross-dressed by a girl or woman with the purpose of humiliating him. In time, the humiliation is converted, via the perversion, to a triumph, especially as manifested by the ability to get an erection and orgasm despite being in women's clothes.

Effeminate Homosexuals

These are boys and men, again biologically normal, who, knowing and accepting themselves as males, prefer males as their sexual objects. When these people cross-dress, they do it neither because they believe they are somehow females (as do transsexuals), nor because women's clothes sexually excite them (as is true for transvestites). One should note also the meaning of "effeminate"; it is not synonymous with "femininity," which implies natural appearance. "Effeminacy" rather, indicates that there is mimicry—hostility—mixed with the desire to be like a woman. Once again, the transsexual family constellation is not found. Typically reported is a mother, who, while overprotective, is also hostile and punishing; she attacks any behavior in her son that smacks of masculinity, accepting him—"overprotecting" him —only if he drives what she considers masculine behavior out of his manifest behavior. Although some of these men have occasional thoughts of sex change, they prefer their maleness.

Intersexuals

These are people with biological disorders of sex that influence their gender behavior. They suffer defects of the sex chromosomes (e.g., XXY—Klinefelter's syndrome); or of the genes, without gross chromosomal disorder (e.g., androgen insensitivity syndrome); or iatrogenic prenatal conditions (e.g., progesterone-induced androgenizing effects in girls whose mothers were given progesterones to prevent abortion). These states somehow influence brain function (either abnormal androgenization of the brain, as in adrenogenital syndrome in otherwise normal females, or failure to adrogenize the brain as in XO—Turner's syndrome).

Those with Hermaphroditic Identity

As with the previous category, these patients have a biologic defect, but in this instance, the condition (hermaphroditism) does not act directly on the brain to produce cross-gender behavior. Instead, the behavior is the result of aberrant sex assignment; when parents are unsure if their child is male or female, that uncertainty will be reflected in the child's gender identity. Such people feel freakish, as if they are neither male nor female or as if they were both at the same time.

Psychotics

Cross-gender impulses in psychotics have long been described. I break this category into two classes. The first, the familiar one, is made up of those psychotics (more frequently men than women) who suffer hallucinations and delusions in which, against their will, they feel their bodies are being transformed into the opposite sex or they suffer hallucinations (e.g., of being homosexual) with voices accusing them of being flawed in their sex. The second group are psychotics who wish sex change, the transsexual wish being independent of the psychosis; when not psychotic, they still want to change sex.

Casual Cross-Gender Behavior

Without strong intent, children may experiment by putting on clothes of the opposite sex. In addition, adults, especially in carnival situations, will also "for the fun of it" put on a display of cross-gender behavior.

A differential diagnosis for females is not quite the same as for males. The main differences are as follows.

In true transsexualism, the same sorts of criteria hold for the clinical picture—the most masculine of biologically normal females, with no periods of femininity, and starting as soon as any gender behavior can be distinguished—but the etiological factors (described in publications elsewhere) are not quite the same.

Transvestism (fetishistic cross-dressing) is essentially unknown in females.

"Butch" homosexuality differs from the effeminate homosexuality of males in that the masculine homosexuals do not typically have the element of caricature in their masculinity that is found in effeminacy.

In the differential diagnosis of cross-gender behavior in children, perhaps the most important factor for the child therapist is the question of severity and of prognosis. Roughly speaking, one worries about the prognosis if the intensity of the behavior is great. For instance, casual cross-dressing is ubiquitous in children, but true transsexuals wish to dress only in the clothes of the opposite sex, play only the games of the opposite sex and only with the members of the opposite sex, and they announce their desire to change sex. Or, in the rarely seen child fetishist, the desire to handle or put on females' clothes (the condition is not reported in girls) is accompanied by visible excitement, often erections.

A few words about gender aberrance in puberty are in order. Having studied far too few adolescents, I must settle for hunches. It seems to me, so far, that none of the conditions in the preceding differential diagnosis (except psychoses) start in puberty or later; in those that seem to, one can find the origins earlier. There is evidence (again, in order to be brief, I do not cite it) that gender identity is laid down and fixed in the first few years of life. I, therefore, expect gender disorders to have their roots in those first few years, but that is not to say that all *sexual* aberrance is the result of infantile and early childhood experiences. Thus, for example, one may see homosexual behavior that is primarily the result of adolescent experiences, but I would be surprised if gender-colored homosexuality was so easily produced.

I suspect that much erotic, aberrant or normative, behavior that starts in adolescence is, to a great degree, the product of a society's definitions. Peer pressure is terribly important, as we all know, and it often takes years after adolescence before one's underlying tendencies will break free of peer conformity. I doubt, however, if significant gender behavior is created *de novo* as late as puberty, in the absence of either brain disease or great and persistent external trauma.

Although feeling free to speculate on many aspects of sexual behavior, I am not expert on most. As familiar as anyone else with the clichés and sacred beliefs, I really have little idea of which people do what to whom or when; even Kinsey and co-workers only scratched the surface.

And so I find myself not only without solid data in regard to adolescence but equally so in regard to the overt practices of young adults, middle adults, and old people. It is easy enough to assume that most people stay within a pretty constant style of behavior, having gotten up momentum (and even wild fluctuations can be one's style). But we know less about those who persist steadfastly in one manner for years and then (due to hormonal changes? partner changes? brain changes?) move off in a new direction. I recall, for instance, a fascinating case in the analytic literature of a man who for years drilled himself, including his genitals, with nails in order to get excited and then lost the need to do so, apparently in the absence of marked biological or environmental pressures. Perhaps an occasional senile old man begins tickling girls for the first time, and apparently a fair number of middle-aged men and women, in despair, start swinging in the jacuzzi, but these seem atypical solutions for phase changes.

This differential might help in evaluating those requesting "sex change," a subject on which I have opinions at odds with many colleagues. For instance, those quote marks. Here is how I see that: the patients wish a change of sex (no quotes), but what in fact is done by physicians is "sex change." That is, sex was not changed; sex change was only simulated. I think this treatment is given too freely, the indications not well defined, and proper follow ups not yet reported. The present situation is no more than a fad and a rush of enthusiasm that discredits the medical profession. Although there are, I think, patients for whom no other treatment is suitable, the procedures are too often indiscriminately provided and endanger the patients. These techniques should be considered experimental, that is, not in the ordinary practice of medicine but instead restricted to those major medical centers able, not only to give the best possible care, but also to execute careful research into these disorders. At present, if one has enough money, one can get the hormones that produce changes in secondary sex characteristics and the genital surgery, with no more indication for treatment than the capacity to pay the high fees.

We have no dependable statistics: we do not know how many patients have been treated or what have been the outcomes; we do not know what kind or how many surgical and psychiatric complications have occurred. We do not know how many people want such treatment nor if there are certain classes of people who request the treatment more often than others. For instance, it is generally believed that more males than females are transsexuals, but the usual definitions of "transsexual" are so imprecise and vary so much from author to author that there is no foundation in definition on which to build statistical studies. It is generally believed (probably correctly) that more males than females request sex change, but we do not know if this is because more males than females want the treatment, or because males seek it out more vigorously, or because females know it is not possible to create a penis surgically.

This clinical psychiatric research required no special psychoanalytic viewpoint, theory, or skills. As time passed, however, I wanted to use analysis to study origins of gender behavior, not just manifestations and classification. For gratification, then, as much as for scientific reasons, I came to use analysis more and more in the second phase of the research. This stage began in the midst of the first but has increased so that now almost all my clinical work is done by analysis. This effort is weak, however, in that I cannot find patients with massive gender disorders who want analysis. They wish only to change the outer world—their anatomy, the people they know, society. Therefore, my recent analytic practice has been restricted, with few exceptions, to parents of children with gender disorders. While the child is seen by a colleague, and one of the parents also, I have analyzed the other parent, thus far, only mothers. (The nature of analysis, obviously, precludes one's seeing many patients, and so one has to be satisfied with the depth of the data; the breadth—numbers of people seen—is terribly inadequate.)

Along with others, I have come to believe that if one wishes to understand origins of character structure in childhood, one cannot settle for information gathered in the transference. Although the analysis of the transference is a marvelous source of data on how the patient experienced childhood, one should not confuse that with what actually happened. To get closer to the latter, we must also find what the parents did. To me, it seems that the greatest advance that might someday move psychoanalysis to be the science it already immodestly claims to be, is detailed and controlled observation of children. When one adds to this the analysis of the parents who are in the midst of the child's development, one gets a better picture, though still not complete, than one can by the analysis of adults alone. So I am strongly biased in favor of the research-treatment situation

in which the child and his parents are all seen in deep and extended treatment.

Therefore, in the past fifteen years, I have been involved in a psychoanalytic "experiment," in which I have slowly worked my way along a sequence of families, the focal case being a boy transsexual and his parents, the others being families with boys having another form of gender defect. In the "baseline" case, the analytic situation revealed the dynamics that I think cause this condition: boyhood, or true, transsexualism; with these in the open, I went on to see a total of fifteen families with such boys (some in treatment, though not analysis, some just for extended evaluation) to test the hypotheses that had developed in the first family's treatment. What was found (briefly; the present circumstances do not require a convincing description of the findings, which have been published elsewhere in more detail): a mother who in her childhood, because of a sense of hopelessness created by her frozen mother, powerfully wishes to change her sex. With the failure of this, announced by the female appearances developed after puberty, she renounces consciously her transsexual desires, especially that for a penis, and in time, without love or erotic desire, marries. The man she marries is passive and distant, driven out of the household so that he is scarcely a presence. When such a woman gives birth to a boy she considers beautiful and graceful—the ideal penis, grown from her own body—she finds therewith a cure for her lifelong sense of hopelessness and anatomical inadequacy. She holds the infant against her body day and night for years, wishing never to let him out of touch or sight, since he is the constant cure for her bad feelings. She tries for as blissful and intimate a contact with her son as possible. The result is that, by a year or so of age, he is already acting femininely; she encourages every such manifestation. The boy's father, who could have broken up this symbiosis and, in addition, have served as a model for masculinity, literally is not present in the house in order to mitigate the feminizing effects.

On confirming these findings in the subsequent families, I have come to feel that the degree to which such dynamics are present in any family will determine the degree of femininity in a boy. The next step in the experiment, then, was to find other boys with comparable but not identical conditions to see to what extent the aforementioned effects varied. And so I have also worked in analysis with the mother of another very feminine boy, but one who also had masculine qualities, to determine what was different in *that* family to produce a different form of femininity; with the mother of an adolescent transvestite (fetishist); and the mother of a then two and a half-year-old boy who became sexually excited when fondling his mother's pantyhose. These data will in time be published; suffice to say here that in each case, there were differences in the attitudes of the parents, the way they handled the child, and the relationships between mother and father that could adequately account for the differences in the gender disorders of the boys. Unfortunately, psychoanalyses with me takes many years, and so this "experiment" proceeds slowly. One who wishes to do analytic research that *uses* the practice of analysis must be patient and not subject to an urge to finish his research.

For safety's sake, in assigning therapists to the various family members, each boy has been treated by a masculine, male psychiatrist, with the hope that masculinity could be more easily learned from a male. The converse would also be true in treating very masculine girls. (In fact, both male and female psychiatrists treated our girls; the results have been the same: poor) However, this need not be an absolute rule; perhaps a woman could encourage masculinity in a boy and, without providing the model herself, guide him toward finding appropriate models.

Although the subject was always gender identity, and although the subliminal aim was to understand more about ordinary people, I was bound to work at times with perverse people. Especially as I came to understand better the origins of extreme femininity in boys, I began thinking that not all aberrations were perversions, in the usual sense that perversion is used in psychodynamic circles. We analysts tend to believe that aberrant behavior of any sort is, in the absence of a clear biological force, the product of attempts to resolve traumas, frustrations, intrapsychic conflicts. Thus were explained the perversions; and—without, it seems, adequate evidence—all aberrations were considered perversions. But I was seeing people whose behavior, though most unusual, was not, so far as I have been able to determine, always the result of trauma, frustration, or intrapsychic conflict. So—the third phase of this study—I gradually came to the following conclusions:

By *aberration* here I mean an erotic technique or constellation techniques that one uses as his complete sexual act and that differs from his culture's traditional, avowed definition of normality. Sexual aberrations can be divided into two classes: variants (deviations) and perversions.

By *variant* I mean an aberration that is not primarily the staging of forbidden fantasies, especially fantasies of harming others. Examples would be behavior set off only by abnormal brain activity, as with a tumor, experimental drug, or electrical impulse from an implanted electrode; or an aberrant act one is driven to *faute de mieux*; or sexual experiments one does from curiosity and finds not exciting enough to repeat.

Perversion, the erotic form of hatred, is a fantasy, usually acted out but occasionally restricted to a daydream (either self-produced or packaged by others, that is, pornography). It is a habitual, preferred aberration necessary for one's full satisfaction, primarily motivated by hostility. By "hostility" I mean a state in which one wishes to harm an object; that differentiates it from "aggression," which often implies only forcefulness. The hostility in perversion takes form in a fantasy of revenge hidden in the actions that make up the perversion and serves to convert childhood trauma to adult triumph. To create the greatest excitement, the perversion must also portray itself as an act of risk-taking. (pp. 3–4)[1]

These speculations on perversion had a consequence, the fourth and present phase of the research—sexual excitement. The descriptions of the dynamics of perversion led me to think about the pornography used by these perverse people, wherein are easily found those dynamics: the construction of a script, whose principal purpose is to undo childhood traumas and frustrations by converting these earlier painful experiences to present (fantasies) triumphs. On the route, while constructing these daydreams (of which pornography is only one style), the patients also made use of mystery, secrets, risk-running, revenge, dehumanizing (fetishizing) of one's objects, and, especially, hatred as a manifest or latent presence in the storylines. But having found these in perversions and their pornographies, I realized that the same dynamics were present in the pornographies of everyday life and in the sexual excitement of the patients (non perverse) I had treated for years. A quick glance at the literature confirmed that others could find the same dynamics in their patients. In other words, I found I was studying normative sexual excitement and, for most people, that which makes excitement out of boredom is the introduction of hostility into the fantasy.

In time, this could lead to a new phase, the search for the circumstances in which affection, tenderness, love (nonhostility) participate in, perhaps even dominate, sexual excitement. The difficulty will be in finding suitable people to study.

Transsexual boys are very rare; yet their infancy

gave glimpses of dynamics that, far less intense but qualitatively similar, illuminated for me the dynamics of masculinity and femininity at large, of perversion, and of sexual excitement. The original finding was this: if an infant male has too intimate a relationship with his mother (her body and psyche) and if she tries to maintain that intimacy indefinitely in an ambiance of trauma-less, frustration-less pleasure, he will fail (not be well motivated) to separate from her body and psyche in the manner boys usually do. As a result, from the start, he is feminine. The consequent hypothesis is that the less these factors are present, the less he will be feminine. In what is called normal masculinity, these factors should be minimal. (And if there is *no* intimacy between mother and infant, there are risks of "excessive" masculinity—the phallic character—something like what is seen in the development of female transsexuals or phallic warriors. (Coriolanus is a nice example.)

Generally, of course, there is a period of marked intimacy between mother and infant, necessary for healthy development. But I hypothesize that even this minimal period and milder degree of intimacy leaves behind a trace, a touch of uncertainty that one's masculinity (identity) is intact. (In females this will be an anlage for femininity, but that ought not be a problem.) This early, usually reparable, flaw suggests that masculinity in males may not be quite as absolute and stable a state as Freud indicated, and puts in doubt part of his theory of the development of masculinity and femininity. Freud maintained, and the classical position of analysis has since been, that maleness is the superior biological state and masculinity the superior psychological state. Women, Freud said, confronted with their inferior genital, are forever doomed to a second-rate solution to life, one in which they must come to terms with their conviction of being castrated males. A crucial piece in this logic was the argument that, since one's first and most profoundly desired love object was mother, a female, the boy starts life heterosexual, while the girl must overcome primary homosexuality and the profound trauma of being penis-less, needing to salvage from this rubble a capacity to turn from loving her mother to loving a member of the opposite sex—at first, father.

I read the situation differently. To me, it seems that the first stage for both boys and girls is the intimacy with mother in which one is so merged that one does not know where mother leaves off and he/she begins ("proto-identification"); gender identity for boys, therefore, does not start with heterosexuality, nor with the triumph of the penis. Instead, there is a special obstacle for boys (for some, a peril) that must be overcome but that, in girls, is an indifferent issue insofar as gender development is concerned. This primeval problem —separating one's identity from mother's—sets up an inherent weakness in masculinity that may begin to account for the fact that men are overtly perverse, far more than women, and are so sensitive to their manhood being threatened. These ideas, if confirmed, undercut Freud's antifemale and antifeminine declarations.

REFERENCES

1. STOLLER, R., *Perversion*, Pantheon, New York, 1975.

28 / Enuresis

Thomas F. Anders and Ellen D. Freeman

History

Enuresis has been a clinical problem in Western civilization for more than 200 years. The nature of treatment methods during the eighteenth and nineteenth centuries indicates some of the underlying etiologic assumptions. Burning the sacrum to cause blisters and generate heat was used to increase the efficiency of sacral nerves; conversely, forcing patients to lie prone was used to cool them.[13] Mattresses were devised with protruding metal spikes and frames for pelvic elevation. In order to strengthen faulty sphincters, boys were provided with penile ligatures or had their prepuces sealed with collodion. Enuretic girls had rubber bags inserted into their vaginas and inflated with air to compress the bladder neck and urethra. Hyponosis[10] and electrical stimulation of the bladder and rectal sphincters[24] were also attempted. Severe restriction of fluid to the point of dehydration and the avoidance of deep sleep enjoyed their historical heyday. Clearly, enuretic children evoked anger. The modern successors of these approaches, such as waking the child during the night, fluid limitation, or the administration of salt tablets at bedtime[9, 21, 23, 46] have all been equivocal in their success. Today, as 200 years ago, enuresis still persists to plague children and their families.

The Physiology of Micturition

Motor control of the urinary bladder is an autonomic nervous system function. In infants, it is completely reflex; only with training is it later brought under voluntary regulation.[15] The detrusor muscle of the bladder and the internal sphincter are composed of smooth muscle, innervated primarily by parasympathetic nerves originating in the sacrospinal cord. Motor innervation of the external sphincter, a voluntary muscle, is from the pudendal nerve, which also carries sensory fibers to the urethra, penis, and clitoris. Basically, as the bladder progressively fills, its walls stretch until the tension rises sufficiently to elicit the "micturition reflex." This is felt consciously as a desire to urinate. This reflex is an automatic cord response; it can be inhibited or facilitated by higher centers in the brain. It is these higher centers which maintain constant tonic contraction of the external sphincter while keeping the reflex partially inhibited. When the individual desires to urinate, the sacral centers initiate micturition, and the external sphincter is inhibited.

Definition and Incidence

Enuresis[10] generally refers to the wetting of one's clothes, or one's bed, past the age of three years. It is estimated that 15 percent of children wet past the age of three.[9, 44] In a study of more than 4,000 British school children, followed longitudinally for seven years, some 12 percent were enuretic at four, and 7 percent at seven years of age.[3] This incidence has been reported to be lower in upper social classes and agrarian cultures.[3] More common in males, enuresis is often familial and usually disappears at puberty.

Because elimination patterns and attitudes toward toileting are largely sociocultural in origin, the definition of enuresis varies. We feel that confusion in the literature and among clinicians regarding incidence and treatment outcomes stems, in large part, from an inadequate definition of the problem. Four areas of symptom history are frequently not specified: (1) the developmental stage and age at which the symptom is considered disturbing; (2) the relationship of the symptom to organic and/or functional pathology; (3) the assessment of whether the symptom has recurred following a significant period of dryness (2° enuresis), or whether the symptom has persisted unabated since birth (1° enuresis); and (4) whether the symptom occurs predominately at night (nocturnal enuresis), during the day (daytime enuresis), or both.

It is our contention that the symptom of enuresis is part of several separate and distinct syndromes. In this chapter, we propose a new classification of enuresis which provides clues to underlying etiology and suggests appropriate methods of treatment. Although this classificatory schema remains tentative, it represents a synthesis of our own clinical experience and a review of recent literature. Its validity awaits definitive research.

Etiologies of Enuresis

ORGANIC CAUSES

Excessive urination on an organic basis is not common. It is, however, the presenting symptom of a number of systemic illnesses, including diabetes mellitus, diabetes insipidus, and other biochemical and/or genetic disorders affecting urinary concentrating mechanisms. Urinary tract infections account for some cases of excessive urination. Most clinicians distinguish such forms of incontinence, urgency, or excessive urination from enuresis. Loss of urinary control has also been a presenting symptom of epileptic disorders, myelodysplasia, and congenital anomalies of the bladder.

Urologists generally subscribe to one or another of two hypotheses. Some data support the notion that bedwetting may result from decreased bladder capacity. In one study of 120 children ranging in age from two to seven years, the authors concluded that when individuals are able to retain 10–12 oz. (300–360 cc) of urine, they are not enuretic.[35] Forcing fluids during the day was felt to expand bladder capacity, and, in three-to six-month follow-up studies, these speculations were confirmed. Other studies have confirmed the efficacy of "bladder stretching."[17, 44, 45, 47] Yet some investigators wonder why individuals with a small bladder, an intact nervous system, and a desire to remain dry could not awaken and go to the toilet. Asking the child to retain urine "until it hurts" raises ethical issues.

The other hypothesis suggests that obstructive uropathy in the absence of urinary tract infection leads to enuresis. To one uncontrolled study of 223 enuretics over the age of six, intravenous pyelograms, cystourethrograms, and direct visualization of the bladder and urethra under general anesthesia revealed obstructions distal to the bladder neck in over 95 percent of the children.[27] Beyond the obstruction, dilatation of the urethra and hypertrophy of the detrusor muscle with associated myogenic irritability were thought to result in enuretic episodes. Surgical relief of the obstruction has been advocated. Unfortunately, long-term follow-up reports of these patients have not been published, and attempts to confirm the results by others have been unsuccessful. The concept of valvular obstruction of this kind remains highly controversial.

Broughton and Gastaut,[5] by polygraphic monitoring, have defined a sleep-related "enuretic episode," which generally occurs one to three hours after falling asleep, as the child is shifting from NREM Stage 4 sleep to the first REM sleep period. In enuretic children, this sleep state change is associated with a body movement, increased muscle tone, followed by tachycardia, tachypnea, erection in males, and decreased skin resistance. Micturition occurs one-half to four minutes after the start of the episode, in a moment of relative quiet. Immediately following micturition, children are difficult to awaken, and, when aroused, indicate that they have not dreamed. Amnesia for the event is present the following morning. Broughton[4] has suggested that the NREM slow-wave sleep state provides the appropriate central nervous system dissociative state for enuresis to occur.

Several factors single out this type of enuresis. Evidence has been obtained that individuals with sleep-related enuresis have higher intravesical pressures than controls, especially in NREM Stage 4 sleep. They have more frequent and intense spontaneous bladder contractions and have more secondary contractions in response to naturally and artificially occurring increases in pressure. In addition, children with sleep-related enuresis have a higher incidence of associated sleepwalking, sleeptalking, and pavor nocturnus, all considered NREM dyssomnias. Finally, their family history is positive for enuresis.

In adolescents and adults in whom enuresis persists, the enuretic episode shifts to a later part of the night and occurs more commonly in NREM Stages 1 and 2 sleep or REM sleep. In these individuals, psychological conflicts and other symptoms often are present in addition to the enuretic problem.

PSYCHODYNAMIC CAUSES

A surprising paucity of data pertaining to enuresis has been published by child analysts; anamnestic material from adult analyses is also sparse. Yet psychoanalytic and psychodynamic explanations are bountiful. Psychoanalysts have viewed enuresis as a symptom of neurosis, perversion, or impulse disorder and emphasized its symbolic, instinctual origins. It has been assumed that the enuretic episode occurs as part of a dream which, in its manifest or latent content, reveals the unconscious conflict. Freud[11] considered enuresis to be a form of "pollution" or masturbatory equivalent. Gerard[12] described the characteristics of a group of children referred to a child psychiatry clinic for wetting. A minority had organic etiologies. A substantial group were described as using the symptom in a directly aggressive or passive-aggressive way. The majority, however, demonstrated a similar set of personality traits, including nighttime fears and a strong identification with the parent of the opposite sex. Katan[22] and Sperling[42, 43] emphasize the importance of fantasies of genital damage. Sperling contends that the wetting may represent "punishment" meted out to the parents for inflicting the damage and emphasizes the importance of power struggles between the mother and child. Distortions of body image, castration fantasies, and conflicts related to sexual identification have all been elicited from patients manifesting enuretic symptomatology. Sexual overstimulation of the child has also been noted to be present. Michaels[31,32,33] compared a group of institutionalized patients with controls at a nearby summer camp. Enuresis past the age of ten was more common in hospitalized males with psychopathic traits, such as stealing, assault, or firesetting. He considered enuresis as another manifestation of poor impulse control. All of these theoretical explanations share in common the notion that the symptom of enuresis is psychologically determined.

Both psychoanalytic and learning theorists have focused on toilet training as the point of origin for enuretic symptomatology. Psychoanalysts have emphasized the "power struggle" between parent and child as individuation and autonomy proceed. The conflicts and associated anxieties over phallic mastery also have been held responsible for the development of symptomatology. Learning theorists, on the other hand, stress the operant contingencies which surround toilet training. Either too little or too much reinforcement is thought to be related to learned habit patterns that are maladaptive but attention-generating.

Current pediatric advice regarding toilet training, largely stemming from writings of behavioral pediatricians such as Benjamin Spock, M.D., centers around shifting toilet training out of the area of parent-child conflict. Pediatricians, by and large, recommend that toilet training not be attempted until the child is both physiologically (eighteen months to two and one-half years of age) and psychologically ready (two to four years of age). The latter is indicated by the child's desire for and ease with toileting activities. Positive reinforcement, using rewards of affection as well as rewards of material and edible goods, has been suggested. Excessively high expectations for performance and punitive retaliation for lack of performance are to be avoided. Unfortunately, comparison studies of various toilet training procedures have not been done; nor have success or failure in toilet training been followed prospectively to determine later character development or neurotic symptomatology.

Treatment

There have been as many treatment approaches to enuresis as there have been etiologic theories. Unfortunately, studies of most regimens have lacked adequate controls and been deficient in the classification of the enuretic subjects. It is not surprising that the results of various treatment programs have been inconclusive and often confusing.

PHARMACOLOGIC METHODS

Belladonna, in use for a century, was thought to be effective for the treatment of enuresis because of its anticholinergic effects on the bladder.[14] Recent reports, however, suggest that other anticholinergic agents are not beneficial.[19, 25] Tranquilizers, soporifics, stimulants, anticonvulsants, antidepressants, and posterior pituitary snuff have all been tried with equivocal results.*

Currently, interest focuses on antidepressant medications. A double-blind study by Poussaint and Ditman in 1965[38] evaluated the effect of imipramine on fifty-four five- to fifteen-year-old enuretics. Imipramine was shown to be better than placebo in 69 percent of the attempts, and of equal effect in 25 percent. In addition, these investigators noted anecdotally that a number of children awakened during the night to urinate. However, it was those children who had demonstrated irritability as a side effect of the drug who were more likely to show improvement. These results have been replicated by others.[20, 39] Imipramine seems to be the only drug that is clearly effective in the treatment of enuresis, although its mechanism of action remains speculative. It appears to decrease the frequency of enuretic episodes, particularly those occurring in the deeper stages of sleep.[39] Imipramine is also noted to have anticholinergic effects. One investigator[40] suggests that when enuresis reflects a depressive symptom, the mood-altering properties of the drug are effective in treating the symptom.

BEHAVIOR MODIFICATION METHODS

Without focusing on etiology, learning theory has contributed to the physician's therapeutic repertoire. Mowrer and Mowrer[34] devised an apparatus in 1938 consisting of an alarm buzzer which could be set off by the discharge of urine onto a detector circuit. They reported good results, as have others.[48, 49] Yates[48] reviewed the behaviorist literature and hypothesized that enuresis represents a failure to develop adequate cortical controls over contraction of the detrusor muscle, either because of "inappropriate conditioning" (learning not to micturate to certain

* See references 1, 6, 8, 14, 18, 23, 28, 29, 36, 49.

stimuli), or because of inadequate physiologic maturation. Silberstein[40] reported that 85 percent of his enuretic subjects responded to a modified Mowrer device. The majority of behaviorists, who report success in their endeavors, do not find symptom substitution. Unfortunately, many of the studies are poorly controlled, the types of enuresis are inadequately defined, and the length of follow up is insufficient.

PSYCHOTHERAPEUTIC METHODS

All forms of psychotherapy have been attempted in the treatment of enuresis, ranging from brief psychotherapy, to family therapy, to psychoanalysis. Generally, when psychotherapy is initiated, enuresis is not an isolated symptom. Again, well-controlled outcome studies are not available to assess the effectiveness of this treatment method.

SITUATIONAL MANIPULATION (HOME REMEDIES)

Family cures abound for the treatment of enuresis. These include waking the child during the course of the night, changing the sleep environment, restricting fluids before sleep, and avoiding certain kinds of spices and/or nutrients. Frequently, regimens for parents address their own anxiety, and this is sufficient to alter the course of a child's symptoms. Fortunately, the maturation of bladder mechanisms also plays an important role in all treatment attempts.

A Proposed Classification for the Diagnosis and Treatment of Enuresis

An underlying assumption in our proposed classification schema is that enuresis is a symptom and not a syndrome or single disease entity. The symptom may appear in isolated form or may be associated with a number of other symptoms. In addition to an etiologic assumption, the proposed classification takes into account the developmental stage of the patient, whether the symptom is limited to the nighttime, the daytime, or both; and whether the symptom is primary (the patient has never had a sustained period of being symptom-free) or secondary (symptom onset after successful toilet training). We make the basic assumption

that enuresis is not diagnosed before the age of three.

As a general statement, we feel that, except in the case of anatomic/metabolic enuresis, vigorous treatment should be used sparingly, especially before school age. In general, the family's anxiety should be allayed and the enuresis explained within a developmental context. Only when the symptom begins to interfere with school performance or peer relationships, or when the family's response becomes excessively disruptive, should more vigorous specific treatment approaches be attempted. In those cases, the treatment method selected should conform to the specific type of enuresis as summarized in Tables 28-1 and 28-2.

The Organic Enureses

ANATOMIC-METABOLIC ENURESES

This class of enureses includes patients with organic pathology whose symptoms may be associated with urologic obstructions; anatomic deformities such as spina bifida occulta; metabolic or neurophysiologic disturbances such as diabetes and epilepsy; and symptoms that are secondary to genitourinary infection. The anatomic-metabolic enureses may be primary or secondary and occur at all ages. The symptom may be limited to the nighttime but more often occurs during both the day and night. Appropriate medical and/or surgical intervention should be implemented as soon as the diagnosis is confirmed. As mentioned previously, many physicians refer to this symptomatology as incontinence, frequency, or urgency, rather than enuresis.

SLEEP-RELATED ENURESES

NREM Dyssomnia (Arousal) Enuresis: In this class of enuresis, there is a strong family history, especially in the fathers. In addition, children who suffer from this type of enuresis frequently manifest other sleep-related disorders such as sleepwalking or sleep talking. During NREM Stage 4 sleep, subjects have higher intravesical pressure than controls, have more frequent and intense spontaneous bladder contractions, and have more secondary contractions in response to naturally and artificially occurring increases in pressure.[4] This type of enuresis occurs predominantly in males between the ages of three and nine years.

TABLE 28–1

The Organic Enureses

		TYPE (SEE TEXT)	AGE/SEX	TIME OF OCCURRENCE	TREATMENT
A.	Anatomic/Metabolic Enureses	Primary or Secondary	Any Age and Sex	Daytime and Nighttime	Surgery and/or Specific Medication
B.	Sleep-Related Enureses				
	1. NREM Dyssomnia Enuresis	Primary	3–9 Males	Nighttime	Imipramine 40–100 mg
	2. Hypersomnia Enuresis	Secondary	10+	Nighttime	Treatment of Narcolepsy/ Sleep Apnea Syndrome
C.	Enuresis with Mental Retardation	Primary or Secondary	Any Age	Daytime and Nighttime	Behavior Modification and/or Supportive Psychotherapy

TABLE 28–2

The Functional Enureses

		TYPE (SEE TEXT)	AGE/SEX	TIME OF OCCURRENCE	TREATMENT
A.	Sociocultural Enuresis	Primary	3–12 Both sexes	Daytime Nighttime	Education and Support
B.	Separation-Individuation Enuresis	Primary	3–7 Males predominate	Nighttime predominates	Psychotherapy
C.	Regressive Enuresis	Secondary	3–10 Both sexes	Nighttime predominates	Crisis Intervention and Behavior Modification
D.	Enuresis with Depression	Secondary	3–12 Both sexes	Nighttime predominates	Treatment of Depression
E.	Adolescent Enuresis	Secondary	12–20 Both sexes	Nighttime predominates	Treatment of Underlying Disorder

It is limited to the nighttime and seems related to either immature transition mechanisms that shift sleep states from NREM Stage 4 slow-wave sleep to REM sleep, and/or immature bladder controls that may be dysfunctional at this point in the sleep cycle. Because slow-wave sleep is generally limited to the early part of the night (except under conditions of extreme fatigue), a good history leads to the diagnosis. Enuretic episodes which occur in the first two hours after going to sleep are likely to represent this kind of disturbance. In contrast to this, episodes of wetting that occur just prior to awakening, in the early morning hours, are unlikely to be related to this problem. Imipramine may be indicated for this type of enuretic symptom when the child's daytime social and/or academic function is affected.

Da, an eight-year-old boy, was referred by his pediatrician because of nocturnal enuretic episodes that occurred two to three times weekly. He was the eldest of three children, and the only one who wet the bed. Although dry during the day since age three, nighttime dryness had never been accomplished. A genitourinary workup, including an intravenous pyelogram and voiding cystourethrogram, had been negative. Family and past history were positive, in that Da—'s father had suffered from primary nighttime enuresis untile age eleven. Da—'s younger six-year-old brother was reported to "walk" occasionally during sleep, and Da— himself had had night terrors as a toddler. Da—'s mother was asked to keep nightly enuresis logs by checking his bed before she retired. Most enuretic episodes during the subsequent two-week period occurred within two hours of falling asleep. Without polygraphic study, a presumptive diagnosis of NREM dyssomnia enuresis was made. Since Da— was experiencing no other adjustment problems and the family accepted the explanation of "immature bladder mechanisms," no treatment was instituted. He was followed over the next six months, and the symptom gradually disappeared.*

Hypersomnia Enuresis: Recently, the "sleepy" child has become the focus of attention. Hypersomnia in children too often has been labeled as laziness or malingering. Several reports have described narcolepsy and the sleep apnea syndrome in children.[16, 37] Both present with symptoms of hypersomnia (excessive daytime sleepiness) which are generally not considered significant by a physician until severe impairment of learning and social interaction have occurred. Both have been associated with secondary nocturnal enuresis. The youngest children described have been ten years

of age. Treatment of the underlying disorder alleviates the enuretic symptoms.

Ca, a Caucasian female of fourteen had an uneventful childhood until the age of eight, when she began to complain of progressively worsening headaches, daytime sleepiness, and nocturnal enuresis. She had been toilet trained at two and one-half without subsequent difficulty. The sleepy spells generally occurred in the classroom or in monotonous situations, unrelated to the headaches. Hospitalization with a complete medical evaluation on a university neurology service revealed no significant pathology. Because the symptoms had their onset around the time of parental divorce, they were attributed to psychosocial causes. In the years that followed, deterioration in her school performance progressed. Her IQ dropped to the dull range. A variety of medications were attempted but were unsuccessful. Following extensive sleep laboratory procedures, Ca—was diagnosed as having sleep apnea syndrome.[16] A tracheostomy was performed. At one-year follow up, she now attends ballet classes and actively rides horses. Her daytime somnolence and nocturnal enuresis have totally disappeared. She requires no medication. Unfortunately, she is still behind her classmates academically. A longer follow up will be necessary to gauge the reversibility of her cognitive deficits.

Cl, was the third-born in a family of five. His past history revealed a normal birth after an uneventful term pregnancy. His development was normal until the age of three. At this time he was observed to sleep late in the morning and to persist in his need for an afternoon nap. This was welcomed by his mother, who cherished the free time while he slept. He was toilet trained without difficulty by three years of age. By six, he still slept late in the mornings but began to present behavioral disturbances in the midafternoon. He would become "grouchy," obviously drowsy but fighting sleep. At night, similarly, he would fight going to sleep, seemingly frightened by a "fear of monsters." For the next two years he would fall asleep only with someone next to him. Nighttime enuresis developed. At age nine, Cl—would often sleep during his first class and again during midafternoon classes. At the age of twelve, Cl—does not read or write. He falls asleep regularly twice a day. Recently, while playing, he broke into a fit of laughter, fell to the ground, and was unable to move for about three minutes. This sudden episode of paralysis led to referral to the Stanford Sleep Disorders Clinic. Cl—is a typical narcoleptic patient whose polygraphic record demonstrated REM sleep onset periods.[37]

ENURESIS WITH MENTAL RETARDATION

Children with mental retardation have a higher incidence of enuresis. In the more profoundly retarded, the symptom seems related to a cognitive inability to understand the nature of the training requirement. Bladder and micturition mechanisms are, for the most part, intact. However, environmental isolation and emotional deprivation may

* We would like to acknowledge gratefully Drs. C. Guilleminault and W. Dement, of the Stanford Sleep Disorders Clinic, for allowing us to use the clinical examples in this article.

also represent prominent factors in the development of the symptom. In the less severely retarded, psychological conflicts, as detailed in following paragraphs, seem to predominate. Both sexes are affected. In most cases, enuresis is more commonly primary and responds to behavior modification regimens, environmental manipulation, and empathic support.

The Functional Enureses

Although the term "functional" denotes the absence of demonstrable organic factors, a psychosomatic approach presupposes that it is impossible to delineate mind and body sharply. Not infrequently, organic events or psychological stresses precipitate one or the other type of enuresis.

SOCIOCULTURAL ENURESIS

In this class of enuresis, we include behaviors which represent differences in toileting patterns. Clearly, cultures and social classes differ in their approaches to toilet training. Differences may be evident on both sides of the continuum; namely, on the one hand, certain parents may desire premature control before the child is ready for such a level of mastery, and, on the other, there are parents who will be neglectful of accepted norms. Generally, children with sociocultural enuresis are referred by professionals outside the family, especially pediatricians and teachers. Children vary in age from three to twelve years. Both sexes are equally represented. The wetting occurs both during the day and at night. Since no period of prior dryness had developed, the symptom is primary. Encopresis is frequently present. Empathic concern and parental education are the treatments of choice.

S, a four-year-old girl, was referred by her pediatrician because of enuresis and encopresis. Her father, in his middle forties, was a recent immigrant from a village in the Middle East. He and his American born, but uneducated, wife operate a "Mom and Pop" delicatessen and work twelve to sixteen hours a day. S— was brought to the store or cared for by her eleven-year-old sister (who soiled until she was seven and wet until she was nine). Ill-kept and undisciplined, both children wandered around the apartment at night and usually could be found in the morning in their parents' bedroom. Clearly, the parents were overwhelmed by the pressures of urban life, financial responsibilities, and the demands of raising two children. Emotional support and mobilization of child-care resources led to rapid alleviation of the symptoms.

SEPARATION-INDIVIDUATION ENURESIS

Separation-individuation, as defined here, refers to primary enuresis in which the power struggles between the developing child and caregiver are the major source of the problem. This class of enuresis occurs in children of both sexes and may begin as early as two and one-half years of age. Occasionally, organic enureses—in particular, the sleep-related enureses—may precede and serve as a nidus for later separation-individuation enuresis. Sleep studies of these individuals show no abnormal transitions between slow-wave sleep and REM sleep. Rather, the enuretic episode occurs during early morning hours, before awakening. It may occur in either REM or NREM Sleep Stages 1 and 2. Separation-individuation enuresis does occur during the daytime but is more prevalent at night and may be associated with nightmares. It may persist into adulthood. Attempts at behavior modification are generally unsuccessful. We recommend traditional forms of individual or family psychotherapy which attempt to resolve the underlying conflict. In older children, the conflict may have become intrapsychic.

H, an eight-year-old boy brought for evaluation following expulsion from his third private school in four years. His parents thought him "cute" and the school "intolerant"; his classmates, repeatedly inconvenienced by H—'s pranks, were furious. His teacher said H—would do "anything to get attention." Although H—'s birth was planned, he was clearly a nuisance as an infant and toddler to his socialite parents, who left him with a succession of governesses so they could pursue other activities. H—was trained for the daytime at three but began to have increasingly frequent day and nighttime wetting at five. There was no history of somnambulism, somniloquy, pavor nocturnus, or family history of enuresis. He had never set fires. H—was referred to a therapeutic school and received a course of intensive psychotherapy. The wetting was clearly related to his anxiety level and his struggle with his mother. After he and his mother stopped fighting, the enuresis stopped. His other problems responded more slowly.

REGRESSIVE ENURESIS

By regressive enuresis, we refer to secondary enuresis, which develops following a stressful event. This symptom is akin to the traumatic neurosis of adulthood and generally follows a childhood trauma, such as birth of a sibling, the loss of a significant adult, a move to a new house, separation, or illness. It generally begins between three and ten years of age, but if the trauma is sufficiently severe, it can occur in adolescence and adulthood. If persistent, it resembles more the pattern of separation-individuaton enuresis. It is equally prevalent in boys and girls and may be associated with nightmares or other symptoms of behavioral pathology. We refer to it as regressive, because the symptom represents a return to an earlier form of behavioral functioning. Techniques of crisis intervention to stabilize the situation and provide ventilation of the conflict are frequently helpful. In addition, techniques of behavior modification have been used successfully.

C, an eight-year-old boy, was evaluated to determine whether he was a psychologically suitable candidate for plastic reconstructive surgery. Despite the defect, he had made a good adjustment, was outgoing, sociable, athletic, and successful academically. After having been completely bladder trained at age three, he began to wet at age six after the birth of his brother. He was described as a "sound sleeper" who would sleep through the enuretic episode until morning if his parents did not change the bedclothes. There was no somnambulism, somniloquy, pavor nocturnus, or family history of enuresis. The wetting diminished in frequency at six and one-half and stopped altogether at seven. Corrective surgery was recommended.

ENURESIS WITH DEPRESSION

Childhood depression has been an ill-defined entity, although it is currently receiving more attention.[7, 26, 30] Enuresis may be a feature of some childhood depressions.[41]

E, an eight-year-old boy, was brought for evaluation because of poor school performance and "hyperactivity" which had not responded to an adequate course of methylphenidate (Ritalin). Neurological examination was within normal limits. The last in a sibship of six, he was toilet trained at two for nighttime but continued to wet occasionally during the day "because he doesn't want to stop playing," according to his mother. E—had set some small fires; when questioned, he stated they made him "feel good." Affect was, in general, constricted, and E—maintained a compliant stance with adults. A six-month course of psychotherapy resulted in improvement of all symptoms.

ADOLESCENT ENURESIS

Enuresis, with impulse disorders and other kinds of nonspecific psychopathology, are encountered in adolescence. In addition, enuretic symptoms having their origins in childhood sleep-related disorders or conflict situations may persist and become complicated by the stresses of the adolescent identity crisis. These types of enureses have been most frequently reported in institutions, though this may reflect sample bias.[31, 32, 33, 46]

J, a sixteen-year-old girl, was admitted to a psychiatric hospital after a recurrent LSD psychosis. She had also abused amphetamines, barbiturates, alcohol, and cannabis, and had been sexually active with both boys and girls. J—still wet her bed and had never been dry for more than a few months. She enjoyed looking at fires, which often excited her sexually. An EEG obtained during hospitalization revealed "14 and 6 positive spikes." A course of diphenylhydantoin failed to improve J—'s enuresis or her impulsivity. Her hospital course was stormy; she was extremely manipulative, stole money, and attempted to start several homosexual affairs.

Conclusion

Enuresis, a common symptom of childhood and adolescence, has been a problem in most cultures for centuries. Psychological, social, and biological components appear to contribute to the problem in varying proportions. In an attempt to clarify the relationship between these, to define the symptom better, to further the cause of research in the area of enuresis, and to evaluate better the outcome of treatment, we have proposed a comprehensive classification scheme for the enuretic symptom. This scheme takes into account functional and organic components, the developmental age of appearance, whether the symptom occurs predominantly during the day or night, and whether it is primary or secondary in its onset. We hope that this scheme will be useful to clinicians, to investigators, and especially to children and their parents.

REFERENCES

1. ABRAMS, A. L., "Imipramine in Enuresis," *American Journal of Psychiatry, 120:*177, 1963.
2. BACHET, M., "The Concept of Criminogenic Encephalosis," *American Journal of Orthopsychiatry, 21:* 794–799, 1951.

3. BLOMFIELD, J., and DOUGLAS, J., "Bedwetting: Prevalence Among Children Aged 4–7 Years," *Lancet, 170:*850–852, 1956.
4. BROUGHTON, R. J., "Sleep Disorders: Disorders of Arousal?" *Science,* 159:1070–1077, 1968.

5. ——, and GASTAUT, H., "Polygraphic Sleep Studies in Enuresis Nocturna," *Electroencephalography and Clinical Neurophysiology, 16:*16–625, 1964.

6. CAMPBELL, E. W., JR., and YOUNG, J. D., JR., "Enuresis and Its Relationship to Encephalopathic Disturbances," *Journal of Urology, 96:*947, 1966.

7. CYTRYN, L., and MCKNEW, D. H., "Factors Influencing the Changing Clinical Expression of the Depressive Process in Children," *American Journal of Psychiatry, 131:*879–881, 1974.

8. EPSTEIN, S. J., and GUILFOYLE, P. M., "Imipramine in the Control of Enuresis," *American Journal of Diseases of Children, 109:*412–415, 1956.

9. FINCH, S., *Fundamentals of Child Psychiatry*, Norton, New York, 1960.

10. FREEDMAN, A., and KAPLAN, H., *Comprehensive Textbook of Psychiatry*, p. 1383, Williams & Wilkins, Baltimore, 1967.

11. FREUD, A., *Three Contributions to the Theory of Sexuality*, Hogarth, London, 1962.

12. GERARD, M., "Enuresis in Childhood," *American Journal of Orthopsychiatry, 9:*45–58, 1939.

13. GLICKLICH, M., "An Historical Account of Enuresis," *Pediatrics, 8:*259–269, 1951.

14. GOODMAN, H., and GILMAN, A., *The Pharmacological Basis of Therapeutics*, 4th ed., Macmillan, New York, 1970.

15. GUYTON, A. C., *Basic Human Physiology*, W. B. Saunders, Philadelphia, 1971.

16. GUILLEMINAULT, C., and ANDERS, T. F., "The Pathophysiology of Sleep Disorders in Pediatrics," *Advances in Pediatrics, 22:*151–174, 1976.

17. HALLMAN, N., "On the Ability of Enuretic Children to Hold Urine," *Acta Paediatrica, 39:*87–93, 1950.

18. HICKS, W. R., and BARNES, H., "A Double-Blind Study of the Effects of Imipramine in Enuresis in 100 Naval Recruits," *American Journal of Psychiatry, 120:*812, 1963.

19. HOLT, P. S., "Drug Treatment of Enuresis: Controlled Trials with Propantheline, Amphetamine, and Pituitary Snuff," *Lancet, 2:*1334, 1956.

20. KALES, A., et al., "Sleep Laboratory and Clinical Studies of the Effects of Tofranil, Valium, and Placebo on Sleep Stages and Enuresis," *Psychophysiology, 7:*348, 1970.

21. KANNER, L., *Child Psychiatry*, 4th ed., Charles C Thomas, Springfield, Ill., 1971.

22. KATAN, A., "Experiences with Enuretics," in Eissler, R. S., et al. (Eds.), *Psychoanalytic Study of the Child*, vol. 2, pp. 24–55, International Universities Press, New York, 1926.

23. KIM, H., "Enuresis: Literature Review," *Clinical Proceedings of the Children's Hospital of the District of Columbia, 15:*155, 1959.

24. KUZNETOSOVA, Z. P., "Electrical Activity of the Sphincters of the Bladder and Rectum in Enuresis and Its Dynamics Following Tonicization with Diadynamic Currents," *Urologiya i Nefrologiya* Eng. Abstr., *37:*43–45, 1972.

25. LEYS, D., "Value of Propantheline Bromide in the Treatment of Enuresis," *British Medical Journal, 1:*549, 1956.

26. MALMQUIST, C., "Depression in Childhood and Adolescence," *New England Journal of Medicine, 284:*887–893, 955–961, 1971.

27. MALONEY, D. T., "Studies of Enuresis. I. Incidence of Obstructive Lesions and Pathophysiology in Enuresis," *Journal of Urology, 106:*951–958, 1971.

28. MARGOLIS, L. H., "Tofranil—Better than Belladonna." *American Journal of Psychiatry, 118:*76, 1961.

29. MARIUS, J. M., and WALTERS, T. J., "Enuresis in Non-Psychotic Boys Treated With Imipramine," *American Journal of Psychiatry, 120:*597–599, 1963.

30. MCKNEW, D. H., and CYTRYN, L., "Historical Background in Children with Affective Disorders," *American Journal of Psychiatry, 130:*1278–1280, 1973.

31. MICHAELS, J. J., "The Need for a Theory of Delinquency," *Archives of General Psychiatry, 10:*13–36, 1964.

32. ——, "Enuresis in Murderous, Aggressive Children and Adolescents," *Archives of General Psychiatry, 10:*490–493, 1962.

33. ——, *Disorders of Character: Persistent Enuresis, Juvenile Delinquency and Psychopathic Character*, Charles C Thomas, Springfield, Ill., 1959.

34. MOWRER, C. H., and MOWRER, W. A., "Enuresis: A Method for Its Study and Treatment," *American Journal of Orthopsychiatry, 8:*436–447, 1958.

35. MUELLNER, S. R., "Development of Urinary Control in Children," *Journal of the American Medical Association, 172:*1256–1261, 1960.

36. MUNSTER, A. J., STANLEY, A. M., and SAUNDERS, J. C., "Imipramine (Tofranil) in the Therapy of Enuresis," *American Journal of Psychiatry, 118:*76, 1961.

37. NAVELET, Y., ANDERS, T. F., and GUILLEMINAULT, C., "Narcolepsy in Children," in Guilleminault, C., Dement, W. C., and Passouant, P. (Eds.), *Narcolepsy*, pp. 171–177, Spectrum Publications, New York, 1976.

38. POUSSAINT, A. F., and DITMAN, K. S., "A Controlled Study of Imipramine in the Treatment of Childhood Enuresis," *Journal of Pediatrics, 67:*283–289, 1965.

39. RITVO, E., et al., "Arousal and Non-Arousal Types of Enuresis," *American Journal of Psychiatry, 125:*77–84, 1969.

40. SILBERSTEIN, R. M., "Enuresis: A Controversial Problem in Child Psychiatry," *Child Welfare, 52:*367–374, 1973.

41. ——, and BLACKMAN, S., "Differential Diagnosis and Treatment of Enuresis," *American Journal of Psychiatry, 121:*1204, 1965.

42. SPERLING, M., *The Major Neuroses and Behavior Disorders in Children*, Jason Aronson, New York, 1974.

43. ——, "Dynamic Considerations and Treatment of Enuresis," *Journal of American Academy of Psychiatry, 4:*19–31, 1965.

44. STARFIELD, B., "Enuresis: Its Pathogenesis and Management," *Clinical Pediatrics, 11:*343–350, 1972.

45. ——, "Increase in Functional Bladder Capacity and Improvement in Enuresis," *Journal of Pediatrics, 72:*483–487, 1968.

46. TEICHER, J. D., "Enuresis: Critical Review of the Symptom," *California Medical Journal, 32:*198, 1955.

47. TROUP, C. W., and HODGSON, N. B., "Nocturnal Functional Bladder Capacity in Enuretic Children," *Wisconsin Medical Journal, 70:*171–173, 1971.

48. YATES, A., *Behavior Therapy*, John Wiley, New York, 1970.

49. YOUNG, G. S., and TURNER, R. D., "Central Nervous System Stimulant Drugs and Conditioning Treatment of Nocturnal Enuresis," *Behavioral Research and Therapy, 3:*93–101, 1965.

29 / Encopresis

Susan M. Fisher

Terminology

Name of the syndrome: encopresis
Alternative or historical name: soiling, bowel accidents
DSM-II name and number: encopresis 306.7
GAP terminology: Under Symptom Listing I. C. 5. encopresis, continuing or regressive

Description of the Syndrome

Encopresis denotes uncontrolled defecation of emotional origin. It involves repeated, involuntary evacuation of feces into clothing without gross organic cause after the age of four years, with or without constipation. Isolated incidents are not included. Uncontroled defecation of organic etiology is referred to as fecal soiling or fecal incontinence. Characteristically, the encopretic child refuses to use a pot or toilet or postpones such use. Usually, the consistency of the feces is normal. When retention of feces is present, a foul smelling liquid can be discharged while the hard fecal mass is retained, distending the rectum. The soiling may be daily or only occasionally. In some cases, an organic cause may have been present initially, with derivative emotional conflict serving to perpetuate the behavior.

Primary and secondary encopreses have been distinguished in several ways. The history of their redefinition parallels the elucidation of the syndrome.

The History of Its Identification

The term encopresis is credited to Weissenberg,[43] who suggested its usage as a parallel to enuresis in 1926. However, Pototsky[33] first used the term in 1925. Before 1925–1926, the condition was included under the term "incontinentia alvi." The syndrome was first described in 1881 by Henoch.[19] In 1882, Fowler[14] treated two cases by reducing the psychological pressures in the environment.

In their classic study differentiating encopresis from congenital megacolon, Richmond and associates[36] suggested that the term "idiopathic or psychogenic megacolon" be used, since, in many cases, the rectum and colon are functionally dilated. Since the intestine resumes normal width after proper evacuation, Browne advanced the alternative term "colonic inertia."[7] Berg and Jones called the disorder "functional incontinence."[5]

Anthony[1] distinguishes among: (1) continuous encopresis—never trained, an aggressive, overactive, shameless, disinhibited child from a lax, dirty, lower socio-economic class family; (2) discontinuous encopresis—once toilet trained but soils later in response to stress, a neurotic, inhibited, ashamed child from a rigid, compulsive, higher class family; and (3) retentive soilers. Both retentive and discontinuous types were subjected to coercive methods of toilet training.

Easson[10] labels Anthony's continuous type "primary infantile encopresis," the discontinuous type with retentive episodes "primary reactive encopresis," and the discontinuous type with retention "secondary reactive encopresis." The sharp distinctions drawn among these categories have been questioned in several studies (see following paragraphs). In general, primary or continuous encopresis refers to a child who has never achieved bowel control. Secondary or regressive or discontinuous encopresis refers to a child who loses previously achieved control in response to stress.

Frequency, Incidence, Prevalence, Distribution, Cross-cultural Characteristic

DISTRIBUTION ACCORDING TO GENDER

Bellman did the largest controlled study on record.[3] She reviewed the seven-year-old population of 9,591 first grade children in Stockholm and found 132 cases. Sex distribution was 3.4:1, or 102 boys : 30 girls. The incidence of encopresis was 1.5 percent. The incidence for boys was 2.3 percent and for girls 0.7 percent. Boys and girls were 1:1 in the studied population. The incidence of enuresis in the same group was 5.8 percent. Enuresis among boys was 7.1 percent and among girls 4.4 percent.

Bellman found thirty-eight out of seventy-five carefully studied encopretics to be primary in type, and thirty-seven to be secondary or discontinuous. Twenty-eight of the seventy-five were also enuretic. Thus, her large study reveals no significant differences in the two groups.

However, Wolters[45] found the secondary form to be more frequent than the primary, thirty-one cases out of fifty. Selander and Torold[37] identified 60 percent as secondary; Eller[12] and Anthony[1] also found primary encopresis to be much more rare. Primary enuresis, on the other hand, is much more common than secondary enuresis. Anthony found primary encopretics were more often enuretic. Olatawura[29] got very different results. Seventeen of twenty-four secondary encopretics were enuretic, whereas only two primary encopretics wet their beds.

SOCIO-ECONOMIC DATA

Bellman found an incidence of 1.5 percent in upper, middle, and lower socio-economic groups (in accord with the electoral statistics for 1962). Many studies carried out on smaller populations in hospital clinics suggest a greater incidence in lower classes. These figures probably reflect the reluctance of higher social-class families to acknowledge the symptom, and their tendency to bring the child to a private physician. Bellman's sampling of 9,591 school children is, therefore, far more reliable and suggests that encopresis cuts across class lines.

Anthony reported that discontinuous soilers came mostly from middle-class or skilled working-class homes, and that primary or continuous encopretics came from socially incompetent families. Olatawura,[29] Selander and Torold,[37] and Berg and Jones[5] found that discontinuous soilers, coming from disorganized families, were only mildly disturbed. They also found that the continuous group included children of good familial and emotional backgrounds; in these cases brief psychotherapy, rather than retraining, was sufficient to produce cure.

AGE OF ONSET, USUAL AGE WHEN SEEN, AGE OF SPONTANEOUS REMISSION, IF ANY, CROSS-CULTURAL ASPECTS

The age of onset of encopresis reflects the culture's expectations for self-controlled defecation. In the United States, a child is thought capable of self-control by age two.[2, 39] In Scandinavia, the usual limit is three years.[37] Some primitive cultures don't expect full bowel control until age six.[44] Bellman reports that bowel control in Sweden is not generally established until the fourth birthday. Thus, for the Swedish child before the age of four, it would be difficult to distinguish encopresis from incomplete bowel training.

By definition, then, children with encopresis will usually be seen after the age at which controlled defecation is expected by parents and by the school.

Anthony reported seventy-five encopretics, age four through fifteen. He found that most boys stopped soiling at the onset of puberty, and girls in conjunction with menarche. Bellman found a decline in incidence after the eighth birthday. In her study, none of the children continued to soil after age sixteen except for two instances with short-lived recurrences under stress.

DISTRIBUTION WITHIN FAMILY PATTERN

Both Bellman[3] and Wolters[45] found no rank order within the sibling pattern. However, Hoag and associates[21] noted eight out of ten intensively studied encopretics were first sons. Bellman noted an overrepresentation of encopretics in the families of encopretic children, with none in the control group. Fifteen percent of the biological fathers had been encopretic between seven and fourteen years.

Clinical Course of the Condition Along with Associated Clinical Experience

Bellman's study of the seven-year-olds demonstrates encopresis to be a relatively long-term illness. Half her cases had persisted since infancy (primary or continuous), and in the other half, the symptom had appeared after an interval of adequate self-control (secondary or discontinuous). In two-thirds of the secondary encopretics, the symptoms began in conjunction with a major separation from the mother: the circumstances included birth of a sibling, start of school, going to summer camp, impending divorce, playing outdoors. Bemporad and associates[4] described two cases of frequent soiling that were coincident with the birth of a sibling. These began at age two after six months of continence. In three cases at age three to four years, the onset was related to separation from mother. In his series, age six was the most frequent age of onset and it related to starting school. Paradoxically, however, he found that the encopresis was intensified by reunion with the mother and that it then improved only upon a subsequent separation from her.

Characteristically, before seeking help, the mothers tried a variety of remedies, everything from severe punishment to spending hours in the bathroom with the child. Extreme maternal response to the encopresis has been noted by almost all writers on this subject. This is especially visible in relation to the nature of the toilet training. Bemporad makes a perceptive additional observation: he comments that the mothers of his encopretics frequently ignored or seemed oblivious to other, even more serious symptomatology, such as severe language disorder, emotional withdrawal, and near psychotic behavior. In addition, in other behavioral areas, the encopretic child often shows evidence of excessive maternal control.

Bemporad described an "emergency" session demanded by the mother of a shy, withdrawn, encopretic boy. The emergency was that the mother wished to give him a birthday party and he strongly protested. The mother wanted the therapist to convince the boy to have the party and also to reassure him that he would have a good time. The boy vehemently expressed his feelings that he would be embarrased by the party and that other children would not want to come. In front of the child, the mother stated that the party would be for her own pleasure, and she looked forward to the other mothers coming to visit her. She seemed to disregard her son's feelings and to center completely on her own needs.

Encopresis varies in frequency, even within the same individual. There are often free intervals of several weeks. By age seven only a fecal lump or two is deposited in the clothes, rarely a full bowel movement. Among seventy-five encopretics (Bellman[3]) by age seven, ten defecated into their clothing one to three times daily, thirty-two soiled one to three times weekly, and thirty-three, one to three times monthly. At age four to five, most of these children had soiled more often. All the children used the toilet irregularly and ignored reminders to do so.

Nocturnal encopresis is very rare. During the day, it seldom occurs at school, but often happens on the way home from school. The behavior usually takes place indoors. The child will stop playing, become motionless, and tense the back and gluteal muscles. In some cases, the children postpone going to the toilet until it is too late. In others, they deny anticipatory awareness. Many children hide their soiled clothing near the toilet or under the bed.

Paul, a nine-year-old white male, normal on physical examination, had been encopretic for two years. At one year of age, he was tied to his potty-chair by his mother and physical punishment was used in an attempt to toilet train him. During this time period, his alcoholic father deserted the family. Mother was obsessed with cleanliness and overprotective of her only son, refusing to let him fight with other kids, get dirty, or walk to school alone. Paul was obedient, conforming, a straight-A student, the teacher's pet, and neat in all ways—except for the encopresis. He related poorly to his peers, craved affection, cried easily, and loved going to church, although he had been forced by his mother to join at age four. His three wishes were: "(1) to be a good boy for the rest of my life, (2) to be able to buy Bibles and pass them out to everyone, and (3) to be able to control my bowels." He was desperately ashamed of his encopresis and his underclothes.

Hoag and associates[21] found that in primary encopretics the frequency of soiling varied from once to several times daily, whereas the secondary soilers had episodes of two to three times weekly. Bemporad also noted a high proportion of soiling at home and in the proximity of the mother. He reported children soiling while sitting only a few feet from the bathroom watching television.

Most encopretics can give no reason for their symptom and seem indifferent to it.

Bellman noted how closely encopretics are tied to their mothers, how difficult the fathers were to interview, and how little contact the boys had with their father. Bemporad described a dramatic and unexpected finding: that all encopresis abated rapidly or stopped entirely when fathers returned home or were induced to spend time with their sons. This effect seemed in no way related to the therapy of the child.[3]

Food refusal was more common in encopretics than in controls, as were nail biting, pilfering, truancy, disturbed sleep, speech disturbances, negativism, and stomach aches.[3]

Bemporad[4] observed a "sneaky, sullen, lazy"

quality to the oppositional behavior of the children which correlates with Bellman's finding that significantly smaller numbers of encopretics displayed defiance between two and three years of age. These are tense, easily frightened children, very prone to anxiety reactions and with poor self-esteem. They are excessively controlled, with occasional violent outbursts. They have trouble sharing with friends and are often demanding and dependent with peers. Schools see most of them as immature, with poor peer relations. There is a smaller, aggressive group that the schools describe as highly disruptive.

Figure drawing analyses reveal marked passivity, difficulty in self-assertion, and disturbance in the children's relationship with their mothers. Projective testing reveals frequent themes of being fed with different types of food. This seems consonant with the history of food refusal. In addition, aggressive fantasies predominate along with themes of unexpressed hostility.

Many encopretics have very poor body images and their drawings depict grossly immature figures. In Bemporad's series, all the children had low verbal and performance scores on the WISC. This fits with the clinical impression of frequent severe language disorder and a history of late development of speech. This delay in language development is consistent with the quality of immaturity these children project. In effect, they display the syndrome of "maturational lag." In some measure, this may account for the choice of encopresis as a symptom. For the occasional child it may be the dominating etiologic factor.

In many series, the encopretic boys are said to present a similar physical appearance: they are pale, poorly coordinated children with a sickly, asthenic look. Withdrawn and stubborn, they watch television after school and spend little time with peers. Their dependence on their mothers is characteristic, and they seem content to let her speak for and dominate them. At the same time a spiteful, vindictive, mistrusting quality is often described as peeking through this benign, resigned façade. They often pick on children younger than themselves, and, when encouraged to let loose on a punching bag, they lose restraint easily and recover it only with difficulty. Some writers describe them as passive but with a shallowness and emptiness that diminishes with treatment. One observer noted that most of the encopretic children seemed tacitly to accept deprivation and depreciation without overt anger or resentment. The most common attitude toward the symptoms was shame plus denial.

The encopresis usually disappears at the end of an interval characterized by ever less frequent bouts of soiling. It almost always disappears by puberty.

An important clinical distinction that has drawn much attention is the presence or absence of constipation. Bellman found no more obstipation in her group of encopretics than among the controls.[3] Gavanski[16] suggested 25 percent of encopretics are retentive. Wolters[45] found a large number to suffer from obstipation, and some authors consider the obstipation to be primary.[42, 47]

It is highly likely that the encopresis seen by pediatricians in pediatric settings may be a transient, symptomatic response to sudden stress. This would stand in contrast to the chronic condition that characterizes the more deeply disturbed children referred to child guidance clinics and psychiatrists.[9, 20] Hence, a variety of professional settings are sorting out varying kinds of encopresis. These differ not only in terms of their assigned diagnostic categories, but also in the severity of their concomitant psychopathology.

Organic Etiologic Factors

ENDOGENOUS FACTORS

Genetic, Constitutional: Several researchers have noted a high rate of language disorder and a uniform presence of neurological immaturity in encopretic children. This led them to believe that organic factors are relevant to the development of the condition. A specific constitutional predisposition is unlikely, but some children display the characteristic findings of maturational lag: difficulty controlling bodily functions, difficulty channeling aggressive impulses, and problems in the use of verbal and symbolic behavior. In her series of encopretics, Taichert[42] also noted low frustration tolerance, distractibility, short attention span, variable hyperactivity, and learning problems. She suspects that these characteristics influence the child's response to toilet training and make for severe learning problems with failure to respond to rectal distension.

These constitutional factors may play a role in the case of *some* children. Other investigators (e.g., Bellman) find no evidence to support this position and consider the quality of the toilet training experience and the mother-child relationship to be paramount.

Neurological, Congenital: Bellman found no more frequent histories of brain disease or brain trauma among encopretics than among the control group. All EEG's on the tested encopretics were normal.

The literature varies widely on the subject of intelligence and encopresis. Niedermeyer and Parnitzke[28] felt intellectual ability is unrelated to encopresis. Bellman agrees. Taichert noted that even with neuro-developmental difficulties, the IQ's of her encopretics were normal. Olatawura's series indicated a lower range of intelligence, and Bellman noted a rise in the incidence with a fall in IQ. The assumption was made earlier in the century that the ability to retain feces is related to intelligence. This is unfounded.

Bellman observed that her incidence study, which showed no relationship between encopresis and intelligence, was based on a school population that included neither "imbecile children at residential schools" or institutional cases with an IQ below 50. She considers such children extremely special cases.

Physiologic: Easson (1960) notes that from the beginning of life infants differ in their responses to defecation. In the first week, some infants become anxious and agitated before a bowel movement and contract their gluteal muscles and cross their legs. Others concentrate intently, and upon completion, relax in great pleasure. He feels there is a great deal of difference in the constitutional strength of the instinct governing bowel function.

Encopretics were found by Niedermeyer and Parnitzke to be retarded with respect to height and weight. Bellman found absolutely no differences between encopretics and controls.

EXOGENOUS FACTORS

Infectious: This is a murky area. Children may become obstipated in conjunction with fever and the presence of an anal fissure[6] resulting in a "megacolon" with overflow soiling. These children adopt an extended position on the toilet, and Richmond[36] points out that the muscles used in the extended position actually oppose defecation. Squatting is the best position. Richmond notes too that the distension of colon and rectum in encopresis is the result of fecal retention due to "resistive behavior." According to Fenichel[13] dyspepsia, diarrhea, rectal fissures, and anal fissures

all contribute to making the intestine a favored site for the expression of psychic conflict.

In opposition to these views, however, are the many reports of no greater physical illnesses among encopretics than among controls. Bellman[3] and Wolters and Wauters[46] found that, except for more complaints of anal fissure, encopretics had no more gastrointestinal disease, obstipation, or bowel complaints than controls. On colonic x-rays, there were no differences either, except for the expected rectal dilatation in those children who retained feces.

As noted previously, some authors see encopresis as the result of chronic obstipation with resultant overflow soiling. Psychological problems may either trigger the obstipation,[47] or result therefrom. Studies of the presence of obstipation in encopresis have produced widely varying results. (Bellman,[3] six out of seventy-five cases; Wolters,[46] twenty-four out of fifty cases.) It is, therefore, worth noting the several causes of chronic obstipation. These are: abuse of laxatives, impaired gastro-colic reflex, insufficiency of abdominal and pelvic muscles (as in large abdominal tumors), fever and anal fissure, ion disturbances such as hypocalcemia and hypopotassemia, colonic "atony" of unknown etiology, congenital megacolon, postoperative rectal strictures, spinal cord injuries, and spasticity of the anal sphincter.

Pinkerton[32] matched a group of encopretics with chronic obstipation resulting in retention of feces and overflow soiling against a control group of cases of simple obstipation. Both groups exhibited negativism, and both had a history of early toilet training. However, the encopretics were the subjects of significantly greater degrees of strict toilet training before they were sufficiently mature. Moreover, the mothers of the encopretic children were very tense and overanxious about toilet training. The simple obstipation cases responded to routine medical treatment. The encopretic children with obstipation required psychotherapy.

In short, the figures on the presence or absence of obstipation vary widely. A child can certainly be chronically obstipated without being encopretic; more to the point, a child can be encopretic with or without obstipation.

Selander and Torold consider the etiology of encopresis to be heterogeneous. They assert that many cases are based on a disturbance in the psychology of learning. In these instances, obstipation, unpleasant toilet training, an unsatisfactory relationship to the familial environment, and, possibly, a maturational lag, all combine to produce this syndrome.

Psychodynamic Factors

INDIVIDUAL

Toilet training is at the heart of encopresis. In reviewing 213 cases of encopresis, Huschka[22] introduced the concept of coercive training to describe an excessively rigorous, aggressive approach to the child. She felt coercive training was a sufficient cause of encopresis.

Kanner[23] pointed out that inadequate training can also cause encopresis.

Silber[40] noted that many of his encopretics were toilet trained by grandmothers, whose experience had been accumulated in an area of very aggressive training.

Anthony writes eloquently about this:

The potting situation, like every other early coupling situation, is full of an unspoken language in which a system of minimal cues plays its part. The mother requires to learn the natural rhythms of her child, the rate at which food moves . . . in his visceral organs and the sensitivities of the thresholds concerned in giving signals that herald a need. The average mother learns this language without much difficulty . . . In the normal training situation, the mother's prompt response to the child's physiological ones and her own communications during the process gradually make the child aware of his own cues, so that he is able, eventually, to take over mother's role in the potting situation and thereby become autonomous. . . . In my sample there were two sorts of deviation from the normal. There were mothers who hopelessly muffed all the cues so that the child's learning of them appeared to become deficient. He was spoken of as passing his motions without being aware of it. Then there were mothers who anxiously misinterpreted every physiological cue of the child, responding to each and every crisis with the production of the pot. In time, the child appeared to become hypersensitive to this association and would run frequently to the toilet under the merest pretext. . . . In one case, every time his mother got cross with a small encopretic boy he automatically pulled down his trousers. (pp. 148–149)[1]

Huschka graded toilet training as follows: inadequate—neglectful or inconsistent; moderate—cooperation between mother and infant; and coercive. Coercive training involved the frequent and intense use of shame and punishment for failure; use of suppositories and rigid schedules; unduly frequent placement on the toilet; high love premium on perfect performance; laxatives and introduction of thermometers or soap into the anus; refusal to put child on toilet in response to nonverbal cues but waiting for speech; mechanical means such as strapping to the toilet; training the child before he had the ability to control his evacuation.

Bellman found no difference between encopretics and controls as to when toilet training was initiated by the mothers. Twenty-five percent of each group trained the children early. But according to Huschka's criteria, coercive methods were used by 31 percent of the mothers of encopretics and only by 5 percent of the control mothers. Eight percent of the encopretics were never trained at all. All the controls had been trained.

The mothers of encopretics expected their children to be fully trained at an earlier age than was true for the control mothers. The first period of bowel control occurred earlier in the group of encopretics who developed secondary encopresis. Also, the earlier the mothers of encopretics expected their children to be trained, the earlier they were trained.

A striking difference between the mothers of encopretics and the control mothers was that the control mothers could make allowances for the different reaction styles of the different children in their family, and the encopretic mothers could not.

Fear of the pot or toilet was found in 13 percent of encopretics and in none of the controls.

Anthony described periods of transition in the toilet training process in which accidents are likely to occur. In the face of such early accidents, Bellman found that 24 percent of encopretic mothers beat their children. Only 5 percent of controls did. The control mothers felt accidents were to be expected and reacted with equanimity to the child's own upset response. The encopretic mothers described extreme loathing and disgust at such accidents, sometimes being unable to deal with the soiled clothing.

Where a good relation exists between child and mother, the youngster can let mother know if he cannot meet her demands, and she can empathize. This is less likely to happen in the family of the encopretic. Although poor communication can arise as a result of the symptoms, in most instances pot training had already been stressful for children before the symptoms began. Moreover, these are children who displayed less defiance between ages two and three than did the controls. It would seem that the violent response of the mothers to accidents tended to fixate the symptoms. Thus, even though the child with secondary encopresis may have had a pseudo-mature period, he is subsequently prone to regression.

Bellman found that if a mother's relationship with her child is basically good, any mistakes she might make in the actual conduct of toilet training are inconsequential. The frightened, compliant child, who is constitutionally passive (relative to his mother's nature), or whose mother is excessively demanding, will achieve a premature, unstable, and fragile structure of bowel control. This makes defecation the target site of potential response to all kinds of subsequent conflicts.

Mothers who react violently to accidents often enough end up feeling remorseful, then they become overly indulgent, and thus provide the encopretic child with a clear possibility of secondary gain. Many discussions with the mothers of encopretics suggest a pattern of maternal management that is inconsistent, alternatively overprotective, and harsh. Some mothers have a strong need for excessive closeness with their sons, which itself tends to promote immaturity.

Anna Freud's[15] development line "from wetting and soiling to bladder and bowel control" is relevant here. The four stages she describes are as follows: (1) complete freedom to wet and soil; (2) a shift in cathexis from oral to anal zone so that anal productions are highly charged; (3) bowel and bladder control are accomplished through identification with the mother, and maintained because of a positive relation to her; and (4) autonomous control of function emerges and is maintained independently from object ties.

The encopretic symptom often reflects the child's rebellion against the mother's nagging and excessive preoccupation with his bowel function. Noncompliance is the only method of revolt the child has. Lehman[25] comments on Freud's equation of feces with gifts, babies, and penises. He feels that an emotional equation exists: the withholding child feels he does not receive love from his mother and in retaliation refuses to give. The encopretic child starts with a similar premise, but he transforms the refusal into its opposite: if I have to give, you'll get only excrement. Lehman feels that the child's ambivalent attitudes toward his feces (they are at once both precious and valueless), reflect the parental attitudes toward defecation.

Lehman describes Bertha, a seven and one-half-year-old child, unwanted even before birth, whose domineering, obsessively clean mother nagged her to go to the toilet, refused to give her foods eaten by the rest of the family, demanded unnatural quiet, and would scold and strike Bertha at any resistance or disobedience. From birth on, mother was preoccupied with the child's bowels and trained her between two and three years by placing her on the pot every half hour, even on the street. Obedience and cleanliness were demanded with threats of sending Bertha to an institution. Though constipation had been present for many years, encopresis was precipitated by starting schools, an event equated by the child with desertion by her mother and placement in an institution. "Bertha's resistance to her mother's command that she have stools persisted even after the passage of feces. The child still attempted to retain the stool by holding it between the buttocks, thereby producing perianal dermatitis. Another factor was Bertha's intense desire for a baby, which she manifested in play fantasies and by mothering three neighbors' infants (the small child commonly infers that birth occurs by ways of the anus). Therefore, one may assume that, although Bertha's obstipation was originally a reaction of revolt, it was later partly sustained by the unconscious thought "I will make a baby by holding my stools till I have a big belly like Mrs. A's, Mrs. B's, and Mrs. C's just before they had babies." When given this interpretation, the child replied that whenever she received enemas for an attack of obstipation, her sister remarked that Bertha was having a baby. Bertha also stated that an infant is born covered with "food."

Lehman emphasizes the anxiety in encopretics, the fears of being washed down the toilet, the identification with feces as a body part. He notes that encopresis can be generated by phobias unrelated to defecation.

Ada, age six, next to youngest of six children, was encopretic from birth with inadequate maternal care in the first year of life due to parental illness. Her mother openly preferred the younger sister and was aggressive and antagonistic to Ada, demanding strict responses to discipline and punishing her with blows and locking her in a cellar with threats of a "deeper cellar." In six visits the mother and daughter were in better communication, and warmth was shared openly between them, as the child had shared herself with other relatives and neighbors. The soiling ceased, as well as fears of shadows and ghosts.

An abrupt relapse occurred three months later and, through questioning, it was learned that the recurrence immediately followed upon witnessing parental coitus. Much therapeutic work was done about Ada's jealousy, her fantasies of intercourse, her wish to be grown-up—with little change in the returned encopresis. It was then discovered that Ada passed feces only when she heard air raid sirens or fire engines. Ada then reported an old dream, dating back one or two years, in which she was on a porch, watching a fire engine drive along the street. Lehman suspected that the porch was her crib with sides like a porch railing that she had occupied in her parents' bedroom until she was three years of age, and he thought the fire engine driving along the street symbolized her parents' coitus, which she already had witnessed from her crib before she reached the age of three. Because of the obvious symbolism and because the relapse occurred after observing parental intercourse, the interpretation was given that the siren and its sounds stood for the mother in coitus, and the fire engine was the father. Immediately after this interpretation was made, all soiling ceased, and, ten months later, the encopresis had not returned and the fear of air raid sirens and fire engines had entirely disappeared.

D. G. Prugh and associates describe the normal child passing through the anal phase as follows: the child

appears to overvalue the feces in a magical narcissistic fashion and at times marked anxiety over their loss "down the toilet" or in other ways may be manifest. His fantasies of omnipotence regarding this object, the stool, and its fantasied use in attacks upon others may lead to an animistic misunderstanding, related to fears or retaliation involving fantasied physical damage to his own anal region or the interior of his body.[35]

Anthony wisely points out that this description of the normal child applies better to the older encopretic child. He suggests that the mother's management of the child in the anal phase must combine with other factors to produce the syndrome. These factors may include the child's responsiveness to incidental traumata, his sensitization by previous illness, and the impact of disturbed family relationships.

In his series, Lehman notes the presence of not only sadistic but strong masochistic trends. In fact, encopretics bring all sorts of punishment upon themselves.

In the beginning, soiling may be a way of clinging to infantile habits. Where parental warmth is lacking, it may also provide a form of substitute satisfaction. This is especially true as excretory products are a source of pride and pleasure in the first three years. The anally fixated child, subjected to early and coercive training, will have missed out on a period of messy enjoyment. Now he is bent on revenge and supremacy. Such an encopretic must use intense denial.

To sort out the individual meaning of the symptom, one would have to study the individual child. It can mean many things: in stress-related secondary encopresis, the symptom of soiling can reflect regression, as well as fears of anal castration. It can be a control device to maintain contact with mother, a passive-aggressive reaction to a feared authority, or some combination of or all of these in specific cases.

Bemporad[4] described the only female in his study, a seven-year-old-girl who was atypical of the family constellation marking his series, and one of several cases which impressed upon him the need to see encopresis as a symptom, not a disease. She became encopretic a few days after starting school, soiled only at school, and was sent directly home after releasing a bowel movement. The mother was not upset by the encopresis and seemed to enjoy having the girl home. No effort was made to stop the encopresis, no attempt made to send her back to school. The girl was immature for her age, intellectually very bright, and her family situation was chaotic. One older sister was encopretic, and a brother had transvestite behavior. It was felt that the encopresis masked a school phobia and served to end the separation from the mother.

D.G. Prugh[34] emphasizes the regression from oedipal conflicts in encopresis. He also noted that fecal smearing is rare in latency except in psychotic children. He emphasized that pleasure in anal self-stimulation and in withholding feces remains unconsciously conflictual.

It is relevant to note here that fecal smearing, or fecal messing, is a normal part of development comparable to the delight an infant takes in messing with his food. This pleasure in touching and playing is part of the developing autonomy of the child. We observe less fecal play than food play, probably because the adult disgust reactions are quickly perceived by the toddler, and because diapers are changed rapidly by caretakers.

In the psychoanalysis of an encopretic boy, Lustman[26] noted a fragmentation of thinking due to impulse breakthrough. He also noted inadequate superego formation.

Shane[38] presented a lengthy analytic discussion of work with an encopretic patient. He described the treatment as beginning at stage two of the developmental line where anal products are erotically charged. The child's difficulty in impulse control stemmed from the first year of life. Deliberate frustration had occurred, which precipitated poor sleeping and excessive crying. As a result, the internalized need-gratifying maternal object representation was poorly differentiated and faulty. Shane speculated that infants with depressed mothers turn to their stools as replacements for lost objects.[41] Shane also noted severe separation anxiety, severe castration anxiety, and homosexual problems in the analytic material from his case.

FAMILIAL AND INTERPERSONAL DYNAMICS

Many encopretics come from unhappy, disrupted homes. Lehman[25] noted extremes of attitudes between the parents. He described the mothers as "feminine dictators who expected their children to respond with the alacrity of soldiers." These mothers nagged at and ordered their children about, damaging their capacity for initiative. He attributed this to the mother's own perfectionism and anxiety. He found the fathers to be weak, although an occasional father had very rigid educational attitudes.

Olatawura[29] found that 46.6 percent of the encopretics he studied came from broken or disrupted homes. In the nonencopretic population of the psychiatric clinic, 28 percent came from such homes.

Bellman[3] noted that a larger number of encopretics had experienced separation from their mothers before the age of four than was true of the control group, and that the mothers of encopretics were more anxious and unstable.

Bemporad[4] viewed encopresis as part of a hostile dependent mother-child relationship. Because of early and coercive training the child has neither internalized autonomous control over excretory functions nor been willing to accept parental attitudes toward bowel control. Frequently, the mothers of encopretics ignore the verbal requests of their children. They ignore other evidence of psychopathology and are rigidly controlling and detached in significant areas of their lives.

According to Bemporad's findings, the mothers of encopretics were anger-provoking and ungiving; they resented family demands. Frequently depressed, they swung from states of withdrawal to excessively organizing the lives of their families. The siblings of encopretics tended to react to the maternal over-control in the form of delinquent, acting-out behavior. The encopretic symptom on the other hand got the attention of the withdrawn depressed mother at the same time that it punished her and rebelled at her overcontrol.

The remarkable diminution of encopresis with the return of an absent father suggests several explanatory possibilities. Mother may be less depressed and more giving when father is home.

Or father may act as a buffer between the boy and his mother. It is likely that time spent with father improves the encopretic boy's self-esteem and offers a hopeful model for further identification.

In fourteen typical cases, Bemporad found eight families broken by divorce; in the remaining six, the fathers were either completely away from home or frequently absent because of job schedules.

The fathers were not involved in the life of the family; where there was a stepfather, he was rarely at home. These fathers were passive and distant; they were uniformly neglectful, either through physical absence or by psychological withdrawal. They were isolated and intimidated by their domineering wives. The occasional paternal temper outburst seemed to some observers more a product of desperation than an attempt at assertion. They handled their depression by extrafamilial escape and emotional detachment. Moreover, this withdrawal seemed to them an acceptable mode of adjustment. Children were seen as the wife's territory.

Most writers have commented on the difficulty of getting the fathers to participate in the therapy of encopretic children. Bellman[3] noted the 15 percent incidence of childhood encopresis in the history of the fathers. Hoag[21] added that the fathers often are bossy, critical, rigid, and sarcastic in manner.

The marital relationships are obviously unsatisfactory. The mothers are described as self-involved with a remarkable lack of empathy for other people. They have subservient, unsatisfying partners who do not fulfill them. They are domineering, overly involved in the lives of their children, and complain about them openly. In numerous reports from many different countries, one sees again and again, the same descriptions of maternal vacillation between overbearing intrusion and rejecting exclusion. Under the domineering façade, these are depressed women who wish to be cared for.

SOCIAL IMPLICATIONS FOR "LIFE STYLE"

Psychosomatic disease has increased in our century.[18] In the 1870s, infants were not presented with the demands for bowel training until well into the second or third year. Toddlers defecated at their own leisure and pleasure.

By the 1930s, with indoor water sanitation more generally available, a population ever more sensitive to diet and fecal smells, and far more abundant household furnishings, the earlier casualness was transformed and, perhaps, rationalized.

In general, great differences occur between different cultures. These are visible in the techniques used to enforce conformity, in the age at which it is demanded, and in the extent of the self-control expect.[44]

Woodmansey questions the need for toilet training altogether.

Clearly, then, we search in vain for evidence that bowels need training. . . . Clean habits do not depend on being able to pass a motion to order: indeed no one at any age can do this to please himself or anyone else, unless he has been deliberately withholding his stool for the purpose. A normal child in an ordinary home is eager to conform to the cultural patterns of his family as soon as he is able to do so and he will adopt their toilet habits when his sphincter control is physically mature enough and not impaired by interpersonal friction or inner conflicts . . . nature does not subscribe to fashionable aspirations for excessively early sphincter control, and parents should not be alarmed if children do not regularly use the pot . . . until well into the third or even fourth year . . . control developed at leisure is likely to be more reliable than after more hurried methods. . . . (pp. 220–221)[47]

LEARNING AND BEHAVIOR THEORY

Defecation is a spinal reflex, and it can be involuntarily inhibited for a variable period.

Distension of the rectum produces awareness of a desire to defecate. During the period of toilet training, the mother teaches the child to associate cues of a full rectum with what to do about it, by utilizing the gastro-colic reflex and offering positive and negative reinforcements. This is shaping behavior. Stress can arise, either because mother is anxious or punitive, or from the pain of a lesion; the presence of stress may make this shaping more difficult. It is possible that there is a critical period for this learning.

Neale[27] suggests that if the sensation of fullness produced by a fecal mass moving into the rectum doesn't lead to defecation, then the subject may adapt. This adaptation may involve a loss of awareness of the need to defecate when the full feeling comes again. In fact, the encopretic child fails to respond to rectal cues, and either hoards feces until they leak or releases them in an inappropriate place. Thus, by dissociation, such a child keeps stimuli with unpleasant associations out of awareness.

One can hypothesize that some children who resist being toilet trained still fall within normal limits. They are simply late in developing the previously described skills. They need more time to mature. If such children are trained prematurely, they develop fear and recalcitrance. If a mother notices and accepts that her child is such a late developer, the encopresis may not occur.

The encopretic children-to-be may also resist training because they need to prolong the pleasures of defecation longer, or because there is a constitutional need to assert aggression that makes them resist learning. The sometimes violent maternal response to toilet accidents by these children can also paralyze learning.

Specific Therapeutic Methods for this Syndrome

Before a diagnosis of encopresis is entertained, a careful history must be taken to rule out any organic basis for the fecal soiling. Physical examination should include inspection of the anal area and a digital rectal examination to check the normality of the anal reflex for anal lesions, and for presence or absence of fecal material in the rectum. An absence of symptoms in the first six months of life should rule out Hirschsprung's disease. Barium enema and a biopsy of the rectal mucosal should be avoided unless clear evidence of Hirschsprung's disease is present.

Encopretics find enemas alarming; this form of intervention is undesirable. Large doses of laxative for stool hoarding are not only psychologically disturbing, but are quite ineffective with these children. The same is true of the use of cleansing enemas as an attempt to prevent fecal impaction. Stool softeners, tasteless and given in food, are sometimes helpful. A mild laxative, like milk of magnesia, can produce an incentive to defecate.

The key pediatric approach is to advise the parents to ignore the incontinence, and so to reduce the pressure on the child, to avoid unnecessary discussion with the child, and to stop record keeping and tallying. Experienced pediatricians report that, with parents who are able to understand the implications of coercing the child and who can abandon the pressure, 10 percent of the children improve within a few weeks. Usually, parents are unable to give up coercion and enemas, and psychiatric consultation is necessary.

Psychotherapy with an encopretic child is based on establishing a good relationship with the child and his parents. Lehman[25] reports that play therapy with associative verbal expression will reveal the unconscious attitudes. The combination of good relationship and eventual interpretation of conflicts should relieve psychological stress. It is also necessary to relieve environmental pressure.

Gavanski[16] reports the successful treatment of nonretentive, secondary encopresis with a combination of imipramine and psychotherapy This group of reactive encopretics has had the least optimistic prognosis. The encopretic symptom has here been part of a major regression and prolonged treatment was required. The removal of the symptom is reported to prevent further loss of self-esteem and the stigma of being "untouchable." Gavanski uses a combination of imipramine (10 mg t.i.d.), play therapy, and work with the parents. Where the encopresis is retentive, however, he felt imipramine is contraindicated.

Connell[19] employs play therapy for the child, with an emphasis on expressing frustrated hostility and the desire to mess. She combines this with family interviews, attempts to reeducate parents and offers advice about diet and mild laxatives. She suggests stressing rewards and giving up charting. She also uses imipramine, on the basis that encopresis may well be a depressive equivalent. She prescribes between 30 and 75 mg daily.

Many authors have noted a striking improvement in interpersonal relations once the symptom has stopped. Unfortunately, it is very difficult to sort out cause from effect. With such a negating symptom, by the time a child reaches treatment, the disturbing behavior and its distressing effects are in a self-perpetuating feedback process.

Woodmansey divides his treatment recommendations according to age group. If a mother consults about incontinence in a child under the age of four, he feels she is unduly concerned to achieve early cleanliness and that her pressure will disturb the smooth working of the bowel. His suggestion is to work with parents in order to get them to stop training. Of seven encopretics under the age of four, all acquired normal bowel control with this method of convincing the parents to "lay off." Four of the seven encopretic toddlers became clean after one interview with the mother, the fifth after three interviews.

For children of school age who are encopretic, he suggests enabling the child to experience a situation with his parents or his therapist in which he loses fear of punishment in general and of defecation in particular. This is sought for through direct psychotherapy with the children or modification of parental attitudes.

Woodsmaney[47] questions the highly prevalent notion that failure to toilet train is the operative aspect of the behavior of the apparently uninvolved mothers, who are sometimes burdened with immense social problems. He suspects that these vague, seemingly unconcerned, mothers may also be very punitive but do not recall this when being interviewed.

Anthony[1] emphasizes the importance of achieving a moderate disgust reaction. When it is weak, the encopretic child can develop a passive personality; when it is exaggerated, as it often is in the secondary, discontinuous, child, it is paramount to shift this to a more moderate response. In such a case, the disappearance of an extreme disgust response is a hopeful therapeutic sign.

Behavior modification is profoundly effective in the treatment of encopresis. A variety of techniques has been applied. Reduction of soiling has occurred through the introduction, rearrangement, or withdrawal of reinforcement contingencies. Examples of such reinforcers are social,[8] material,[24] token,[30] and activity.[17] Reinforcers have been hugs, praise, attention, goodies to eat, pennies, stars in books, coupons, playing with toys in the bath, and freedom of movement in hospital. By careful temporal patterning of toileting after meals, at specific intervals, during situations correlated with high incidence of soiling, the desired behavior occurs and can be reinforced. Different consequences can be attached to releasing feces into the pants versus into the toilet, and the child can learn the chain of response. At first, he is physically and verbally prompted. This is gradually given up and discriminative control is transferred to exteroceptive stimuli (clocks, meals) and interoceptive (intestinal sensations). Some tactics involve punishment or avoidance programs.[11, 27, 31]

Young and Goldsmith[48] described behavioral extinction of encopresis in a nine-year-old boy after two years of psychotherapy and family work in which the child developed the capacity to make and to use good relationships with people. In the two years of psychotherapy, the child also built up a great deal of ego strength and self-esteem. Nevertheless, he retained his symptom. Their conclusion was that this firm psychotherapeutic groundwork made the symptom extinction possible by making the boy accessible to a joint attack on the undesired behavior. This suggests that the symptom of encopresis can function to some degree autonomously, after the underlying conflicts have been resolved.

Pedrini and Pedrini[30] reported a case of primary, continuous encopresis in a child with a stormy home life and school problems. The mother interrupted play therapy after four visits and a school psychologist instituted a program with cooperative teachers. For three weeks, the teachers recorded the number and class times of defecation. The psychologist spoke to the mother and she agreed to cooperate in planning reinforcers, which were coupons to buy books. Then the psychologist spoke to the boy and explained the plan, and the boy was assigned to record the time of receiving his coupons.

From the fourth week on there was no defecation and in the fifth week other children in school began to talk to him. In the following school year, he had only one accident, and, by this time, all reinforcement had been stopped. The control apparently had been internalized.

The wide range of therapeutic techniques reflect the different origins and meanings of the encopretic symptom, as well as the training and predilections of the varieties of therapists. One aims for the best match in order to achieve symptom loss and personality development. Whatever the modality selected, be it direct psychotherapy with parents and/or child, with or without imipramine, or behavior modification techniques, one always begins with an adequate physical examination, attempts to reduce parental pressures and coercions, and seeks to maintain good relationships with the child and the family.

REFERENCES

1. ANTHONY, E. J., "An Experimental Approach to the Psychopathology of Childhood: Encopressis," *British Journal of Medical Psychology, 30:*146–175, 1957.

2. BAKWIN, H., and BAKWIN, R., *Clinical Management of Behavior Disorder in Children*, 2nd ed., Saunders, Philadelphia, 1960.

3. BELLMAN, M., "Studies on Encopresis," *Acta Paediatrica Scandinavica, 170:*1–151, 1966.

4. BEMPORAD, J. R., et al., "Characteristics of Encopretic Patients and Their Families," *Journal of the American Academy of Child Psychiatry, 10:*272–292, 1971.

5. BERG, I., and JONES, K. V., "Functional Fecal Incontinence in Children," *Archives of Diseases of Childhood, 39:*465, 1964.

6. BODIAN, M., STEPHENS, F. D., and WARD, B. C. H., "Hirschsprung's Disease and Idiopathic Megacolon," *Lancet, 1:*6, 1949.

7. BROWNE, D., "Contribution to a Discussion on Megacolon and Megarectum," *Proceedings of the Royal Society of Medicine, 54:*1055, 1961.

8. CONGER, J. C., "The Treatment of Encopresis by the Management of Social Consequences," *Behavior Therapy, 1:*386–390, 1970.

9. CONNELL, H. M., "The Practical Management of Encopresis," *Australian Pediatric Journal, 8:*273–278, 1972.

10. EASSON, W. M., "Encopresis—Psychogenic Soiling," *Canadian Medical Association Journal, 82:*624, 1960.

11. EDELMAN, R. I., "Operant Conditioning Treatment of Encopresis," *Journal of Behavior Therapy and Experimental Psychiatry, 2:*71–76, 1971.

12. ELLER, H., "Über die Enkopresis im Kindesalter," *Monatsschrift fuer Kinderheilk unde, 108:*415, 1960.

13. FENICHEL, O., *The Psychoanalytic Theory of Neurosis*, W. W. Norton, New York, 1945.

14. FOWLER, G. B., "Incontinence of Faeces in Children," *American Journal of Obstetrical Diseases in Women and Children, 15:*984, 1882.

15. FREUD, A., "The Concept of Developmental Lines," in Eissler, R. S., et al. (Eds.), *The Psychoanalytic Study of the Child*, vol. 18, pp. 245–265, International Universities Press, New York, 1963.

16. GAVANSKI, M., "Treatment of Non-Retentive Secondary Encopresis With Imipramine and Psychotherapy," *Canadian Medical Association Journal, 104:*46–48, 1971.

17. GELBER, H., and MEYER, V., "Behavior Therapy and Encopresis: The Complexities Involved in Treatment," *Behavior Research and Therapy, 2:*227–231, 1965.

18. HALLIDAY, J. L., "Epidemiology and the Psychosomatic Affections. A Study in Social Medicine," *Lancet, 2:*185, 1946.

19. HENOCH, E., *Vorlesungen über Kinderkrankheiten. Ein Handbuch für Aerzte und Studirende*, 4th ed., Hirschwald, Berlin, 1889.

20. HILBUN, W. B., "Encopresis in Childhood," *The Journal of the Kentucky Medical Association, 66:*978–982, 1968.

21. HOAG, J. M., et al., "The Encopretic Child and His Family," *Journal of the American Academy of Child Psychiatry, 10:*242–256, 1971.

22. HUSCHKA, M., "The Child's Response to Coercive Bowel Training," *Psychosomatic Medicine, 4:*301–308, 1942.

23. KANNER, L., *Child Psychiatry*, 2nd ed., Charles C Thomas, Springfield, Ill., 1953.

24. KEEHN, J. D., "Brief Case-Report: Reinforcement Therapy of Incontinence," *Behavior Research and Therapy, 2:*239, 1965.

25. LEHMAN, E., "Psychogenic Incontinence of Feces (Encopresis) in Children," *American Journal of Diseases of Children, 68:*190–199, 1944.

26. LUSTMAN, S. L., "Impulse Control, Structure, and the Synthetic Function," in Loewenstein, R. M., et al. (Eds.), *Psychoanalysis—A General Psychology: Essays in Honor of Heinz Hartmann*, pp. 190–221, International Universities Press, New York, 1966.

27. NEALE, D. H., "Behavior Therapy and Encopresis in Children," *Behavior Research and Therapy, 1:*139–149, 1963.

28. NIEDERMEYER, K., and PARNITZKE, K. H., "Die Enkopresis. Beobachtungen somatischer, pneum- und elektrencephalographischer sowie psychischer Befunde," *Zeitschrift fuer Kinderheilkunde, 87:*404, 1963.

29. OLATAWURA, M. O., "Encopresis: A Review of 32 Cases," *Acta Paediatrica Scandinavica, 62:*358–364; 1973.

30. PEDRINI, B. C., and PEDRINI, D. T., "Reinforcement Procedures in the Control of Encopresis: A Case Study," *Psychological Reports, 28:*937–938, 1971.

31. PERZAN, R. S., BOULANGER, F., and FISCHER, D. G., "Complex Factors in Inhibition of Defecation: Review and

Case Study," *Journal of Behavior Therapy and Experimental Psychiatry*, *3:*129–133, 1972.

32. PINKERTON, P., "Psychogenic Megacolon in Children: The Implications of Bowel Negativism," *Archives of Diseases of Childhood, 33:*37, 1958.

33. POTOTSKY, C., "Die Enkopresis," in Schwartz, O. (Ed.), *Psychogenese und Psychotherapie körperlicher Symptome*, Springer, Berlin, 1925.

34. PRUGH, D. G., "Toward an Understanding of Psychosomatic Concepts in Relation to Illness in Children," in Solnit, A., and Province, S. (Eds.), *Modern Perspectives in Child Development*, pp. 246–367, International Universities Press, New York, 1963.

35. PRUGH, D. G., et al., "On the Significance of the Anal Phase in Pediatrics and Child Psychiatry," in Gardiner, G. E. (Ed.), *Case Studies in Childhood Emotional Disabilities*, vol. 2, pp. 98–140, American Orthopsychiatric Association, 1956.

36. RICHMOND, J., EDDY, E., and GARRARD, S., "The Syndrome of Fecal Soiling and Megacolon," *American Journal of Orthopsychiatry, 24:*391–401, 1954.

37. SELANDER, P., and TOROLD, A., "Enkopresis," *Nordisk Medicin, 72:*1110, 1964.

38. SHANE, M., "Encopresis in a Latency Boy: An Arrest Along a Developmental Line," in Eissler, R. S., et al. (Eds.), *The Psychoanalytic Study of the Child*, vol. 22, pp. 296–314, International Universities Press, New York, 1967.

39. SHIRLEY, H. F., "Encopresis in Children," *Journal of Pediatrics, 12:*367, 1938.

40. SILBER, D., "Encopresis: Discussion of Etiology and Management," *Clinical Pediatrics, 8(4):*225–231, 1969.

41. SPITZ, R. A., and WOLF, K. M., "Autoerotism: Some Empirical Findings and Hypotheses on Three of Its Manifestations in the First Year of Life," in Eissler, R. S., et al. (Eds.), *The Psychoanalytic Study of the Child*, vol. 3/4, pp. 85–120, International Universities Press, New York, 1949.

42. TAICHERT, L. C., "Childhood Encopresis: A Neurodevelopmental-Family Approach to Management," *California Medicine, 115:*11–18, 1971.

43. WEISSENBERG, S., "Über Enkopresis," *Zeitschrift fuer Kinderheilkunde, 40:*67, 1925–1926.

44. WHITING, J. W. M., and CHILD, I. L., *Child Training and Personality*, Yale University Press, New Haven, Conn., 1953.

45. WOLTERS, W. H. G., "A Comparative Study of Behavioral Aspects in Encopretic Children," *Psychotherapy and Psychosomatics, 24:*36–97, 1974.

46. ———, and WAUTERS, E. A. K., "A Study of Somatopsychic Vulnerability in Encopretic Children," *Psychotherapy and Psychosomatics, 26(1):*27–34, 1975.

47. WOODMANSEY, A. C., "Emotion and the Motions: An Inquiry Into the Causes and Prevention of Functional Disorder of Defecation," *British Journal of Pedical Psychology, 40:*207–223, 1967.

48. YOUNG, I. L., and GOLDSMITH, A. O., "Treatment of Encopresis in a Day Treatment Program," *Psychotherapy: Theory, Research, and Practice, 9(3):*231–235, 1972.

30 / The Primary Anorexia Nervosa Syndrome

John A. Sours

All great things are decided not by machines or gadgets, but by will power. Whoever has it will finally prevail.

WINSTON CHURCHILL

Although the preceding words were spoken by a man hardly anorexic, they pinpoint precisely the human potential for ultimate will and victory. In this respect, the anorexic patient is a caricature of that will which aims at ultimate control, not only of the body and spirit, but of the total world. The measure of an individual's power in sadistic love relationships is the degree of suffering with which she can punish those who love her. And no better display of this power is apparent than in the anorexic's iron will to control the body by mind over matter. Mr. Squeer's admonition in *Nicholas Nickelby*—"Subdue your appetites, my dears, and you've conquered human nature"—is understood by any anorexic girl.

Adults forget that the adolescent years are the most sensuous period of life. The teenage girl revels in sensuous enjoyment and delight, yet blushes easily if discovered and often seeks ascetic and aesthetic goals as a means for cleansing herself of sexual feelings. She wants a waist as tiny as Scarlett O'Hara's and a life at "Tara." The anorexic girl, however, panics over her sensuality and feminine wishes. She tries to escape into a narcissistic sexless existence and live eternally in her bony substance.

Anorexia nervosa is a peculiar disturbance which, although recognized in the last quarter of the nineteenth century, has been fully appreciated only in the last three decades. It is a disturbance which ranges from minimal manifestations, often fleeting and imperceptible to both the patient and her family and friends, to a relentless course leading to starvation, severe cachexia, and eventual death.

The Syndrome and Its Nomenclature

Primary anorexia nervosa was first called "nervous consumption." It was the English physician, Gull, who so named the syndrome anorexia nervosa because of its resemblance to tuberculous consumption.[20] The disorder is currently referred to as "feeding disorder of thin fat people," "feeding disorder," "nervous malnutrition," "disease of the young and beautiful," and "weight phobia." According to DSM-II of the American Psychiatric Association anorexia nervosa is a disturbance listed under 306.5, "feeding disturbances."[1] In the classification of the Group for the Advancement of Psychiatry (GAP), it is listed under "Symptom List, I. Disturbances Related to Bodily Functions, A. Eating."[19]

For decades, the disorder has stimulated speculation about an organic etiology and controversy about psychiatric nosology.[3, 12, 16, 33] From the psychological point of view, "hysteria" has been the most popular diagnosis because of the patient's indifference to her starvation and cachexia, as well as the secondary gain from the disorder.[29] In the last three decades, however, traditional neurotic and psychotic diagnostic criteria are recognized as less sharply divided. Consequently, anorexia nervosa is no longer viewed as an entity in itself, a specific neurosis or psychosis, but as a developmental syndrome appearing within a variety of psychopathologies.

The Phenomenology of the Syndrome and Its Descriptive Variants

Anorexia nervosa is a feeding disorder with primary and secondary clinical features, both types connected with a variety of psychopathologies.[46, 47, 48] It is often referred to as a psychosomatic disorder;[51] but, in this respect, the terminology is imprecise, for to be truly psychosomatic, the disturbance would require an organic compliance as in bronchial asthma and gastric ulcers.[37, 53]

The primary anorexia nervosa syndrome is best described and defined by a clinical vignette.

An attractive, physically mature fourteen-year-old girl "decided one day" while in a gymnastic class that she was chubby and pudgy. She resolved to limit her carbohydrate intake and restrict her eating entirely to protein health foods. After the first week of this diet, she felt that she was still eating too much, to the point that she then restricted her diet to under 600 calories a day. Concurrently, she exercised more, trying new feats of endurance in gymnastics and becoming much more daring on the trapeze and rings. She then began to jog around the reservoir in Central Park, first contented with a daily run of a mile and a half; but within a month, she increased the jogging to three miles a day. She felt ecstatic during her jogging as she watched the ground pass by her untiring feet. In the mornings, her parents noticed that she was doing the Royal Canadian Air Force exercises, something her father had abortively attempted a few years before.

When her parents first commented on her diet, her initial response was that she was trying to eliminate all "junk foods" from her diet. Later, when pressed by her parents, she claimed that her appetite had diminished because of her increased academic load. She now studied until 1:00 to 2:00 A.M. every night. The parents voiced some concern about her late studying and early rising in the morning to do her daily jogging.

It became apparent to everyone about her that she was pursuing thinness as a pleasure in itself and that this pleasure far exceeded any pleasure she derived from eating. The pleasure of exercising her body and seeing superficial fat layers disappear was exciting to her. She found that being able to control her body, especially her appetite for food, particularly ice cream and cashew nuts, made her feel very superior to everyone. Her friends teased her at school because of the way she picked at the school lunches. They were annoyed with her, because she would entice them into the local ice cream store and recount with pleasure the additions and substitutions made to the store's fifty-nine flavors. Then she would order ice sherbet. After several bites, she would either discard it or, as she did more frequently, feed it to a passing dog, preferably a poodle. In fact, her interest in feeding others soon extended to the home and family where she instructed the cook in the preparation of unusual gourmet foods. She took back issues of *Gourmet* out of the family library and, much to the cook's annoyance, chose complicated and exotic menus. She spent hours on weekends shopping in the upper East Side gourmet stores for obscure foods. Her younger brother was an athletic lad with an enormous appetite. He became piqued with her, because she kept insisting that he eat at least double portions. At dinner, she often encouraged the maid to serve second and third portions to the entire family, while she herself stubbornly refused to eat even half of her first serving.

Her hyperactivity and extraordinary energy were soon noted by her teachers who thought that she had suddenly realized the importance of education and achievement. Although just beginning ninth grade, she attempted to raise her grades to A+s with the view of going to Radcliffe, from which her mother had graduated. About the third month of her dieting, her menstrual periods ceased. Since her menarche at age eleven, she had had regular periods except for a two-month interval a year before when she was hiking in Colorado. At that time, she had felt very attracted to a college boy. They had corresponded in the fall, but she then stopped writing to him.

When the boy invited her to Boston on a weekend, she was quite upset to discover that her control over eating had suddenly failed her. Friends of the family had taken her to a harborside fish restaurant where she had consumed two appetizers and several entrees, along with a half dozen rolls, three salads, and a variety of vegetables. After this frenzied gluttony in Boston, she was tempted to vomit. She decided, however, to restrict her food intake even more the following week.

Within a few months, she began to show some of the secondary signs and symptoms of the primary anorexia nervosa syndrome. She increasingly manipulated her environment around food, to the point that the mother began having outbursts of rage against her. Her mother told her to stop talking to the cook, feeding the family, and shopping in the local gourmet stores. Later, when she was hospitalized because of severe weight loss, the staff at the university hospital recognized that they would have to control her manipulative behavior on the ward. From the very first hospital day, she attempted to feed all the children. She became increasingly distrustful; she felt that her world was now conspiring to feed her in order to make her fat. Nevertheless, her weight had dropped to sixty pounds. By the seventh month of the illness, her condition continued to go downhill, and she remained convinced that her legs were "heavy" and that within a few years she would have voluptuous breasts. At times her family and the hospital staff noted that she appeared sad. Yet she never manifested any tearfulness or remorse, and there were never any insomniac nights. When her sleep was disturbed, it was apparent that she was struggling to resist an eating sortie to the kitchen.

The following patient illustrates a more infantile variant of the primary anorexia nervosa syndrome.

A thirteen-year-old girl, a tenth-grader in a local high school was admitted several weeks after her parents' first vacation. During the parents' absence, the girl had developed "flu" at home and stopped eating. She expressed annoyance to her grandmother that she was not able to eat the special foods her mother had prepared for her. Her weight fell from 130 to 100 pounds, but her pediatrician felt that this was not serious and expected her to go back to school on her parents' return. When the parents came back from vacation, the girl did return to school but remained a poor eater. Her family situation then began to deteriorate. She not only continued to eat next to nothing, but she started to have temper tantrums over everything that defied her will. Within four weeks, her weight had fallen to 93 pounds, and her behavior had regressed to babyish talk and senseless temper tantrums. She wandered about the house. She constantly sought for her mother's attention, and she became increasingly demanding and manipulative. Her father found himself unable either to intervene between child and mother or to comfort the mother. Presently, the girl was admitted to a university hospital for treatment.

According to the family's account, the girl had always been a "perfect child" and had derived the best from her "protective family atmosphere." The mother was dismayed at her daughter's illness. Father generally agreed with mother, but occasionally he made fun of mother by referring to her as "Portnoy's mother."

The child was described as "a very good girl. . . . She always, as a child, wanted to be with us all the time." The mother remembers her own childhood much in the same way, emphasizing that she was unable to cross the street until she was eleven years old because of her own overprotective mother. The mother was unable to recall the early developmental years, except to say that she was certain that "everything had been just perfect." The father worked at two jobs in order to maintain the family style at the level that his wealthy father-in-law thought appropriate for them.

When the girl had first gone to nursery school, she had been quite frightened, and it was only after three weeks that she permitted the mother to leave. When an attempt was later made to send the child to sleep-away camp, her homesickness was "too severe." The mother had prepared her for menarche, but admitted quite openly that she felt sorry to see her daughter becoming a young lady. She remarked that the girl had objected to puberty. She feared "big breasts" and looking like her fat grandmother. The mother was proud that her daughter devoted herself to her studies and was not "boy-crazy."

On hospitalization, the child was completely uncooperative. For the first two days, she had temper tantrums, refused to leave her room, and displayed several instances of hostile aggression which required a "quiet room." There was a persistent refusal to eat. She was aloof from both her peers and the staff members. In her therapy sessions, she expressed a fear of losing her mother and complained of the depression which she had felt during her mother's vacation.

Early in treatment, she began to cling to the therapist, asking questions, and seeking reassurance. After a month of treatment, the patient suddenly handed the therapist a sign-out letter indicating that she was homesick and wanted to return to her parents in a distant part of the state. When she found she could not obtain immediate satisfaction, she screamed, yelled, and banged on the walls of her room, demanding to be taken home. Her parents, however, responded to her letter quite firmly, saying that she would have to stay in the hospital. The patient then became childish. She acted and talked like a three-year-old, and asked her mother when she could be with her and be allowed to be "a baby once again." Finally, she retracted her sign-out letter and adopted a stance of compliant behavior, weeping and sobbing during sessions and, on occasions, even speaking baby-talk.

Several months later, the therapist went on vacation. The patient produced a second sign-out letter, screaming and yelling that she wanted to see her parents immediately and, if necessary, her lawyer. Within several days, however, after her weight had fallen ten pounds, she retracted the letter. This time she was aware that her sign-out letter was related to her anger at her therapist for leaving her for vacation. The following day, for the first time, the patient acknowledged the connection between her behavior and her feelings. She gave past examples of behavior in which, instead of expressing her anger and concern over separation, she had refused to eat, had cried, and had temper tantrums. "I would do anything but express what I have inside."

Secondary anorexia nervosa is often confused with the primary syndrome. It is encountered in hysterical noneaters. In these cases, the food refusal is not related to the desire of achieving autonomy, effectiveness, and complete control over the body and its instinctual life. The hysterical noneater complains bitterly about her weight loss and thinness and does not attempt to deny hunger and asthenia. The eating disturbance is a symbolic expression of conflict. Only seldom does it lead to full-fledged episodes of bulimia.

Schizophrenic noneaters are similar to the hysterical youngsters in that they too are not attempting to achieve autonomy, effectiveness, and absolute control over themselves and their instinctual life. If not too withdrawn from human contact, they will acknowledge their hunger and weakness. Their body disturbances do not necessarily include those of weight and physical appearances. The eating behavior is usually ritualistic and bizarre, frequently manifesting fantasies of cannibalistic incorporation and mutilation. Such schizophrenic noneaters also seldom have episodes of bulimia.

There are physical states that frequently manifest themselves with an anorexia nervosa-like picture. Cerebral tumors of the frontal lobe, diencephalon, and fourth ventricle can present with anorexia. Bradycardia, low basal metabolic rate, and high serum cholesterol in a starving patient should raise the question of hypothyroidism. On the other hand, tremulousness, tachycardia, sweating, voracious eating, and a rapid, racing pulse may well suggest the diagnosis of hyperthyroidism in the bulimic patient. Panhypopituitarism must be differentiated from anorexia nervosa. Both disorders are associated with secondary amenorrhea and decreased libido. In addition, hypotension, as well as constipation, are likely to be present in both; however, chemically, they are quite different. Plasma growth hormone response to insulin is normal in anorexia nervosa, although in cases of prolonged anorexic starvation, there can be pituitary depletion which makes the chemical differentiation more difficult. There are also isolated reports of patients with granulomatous disease of the small bowel presenting as severe anorexia and weakness. Fever and constipation, however, tend to be prominent in this gastrointestinal disorder, and radiographic examination of the small and large intestine show a symmetric pattern of skipping and fistulization.

There are also cases of anorexia reported where there is an accompanying diarrhea. These patients vomit frequently and experience electrolyte imbalance and secondary hyperaldosteronism.

History of the Syndrome

Although the syndrome was first described by Morton in 1689[36] and characterized then as "nervous consumption," the disorder apparently existed in early times, often hidden in religious beliefs and magic.[49] Between 1868-1874, however, Gull defined the syndrome clinically, calling it a morbid mental state and suggesting a hysterical etiology.

The French school of psychiatry, notably Laségue[27] and Janet,[24] pursued the hysterical nosological position. In 1895, Freud wrote, in one of his many letters to Fliess, that anorexia nervosa was basically a melancholia which seemed to appear in sexually underdeveloped girls.[14] He later commented on anorexia as a symptom in the case of "Dora."[15]

Psychiatrists continued to be interested in the disorder after the turn of the century. In 1914, however, Simmonds[44] reported several cases which he had studied endocrinologically. He attributed the physical findings of anorexia nervosa to a pituitary deficiency. These endocrine reports unfortunately confused the medical community, shifting the emphasis in clinical thinking and research in the direction of a primary organic etiology. With the more sophisticated clinical approach and laboratory techniques available today, it is hard to imagine that anorexia nervosa and panhypopituitarism could have been confused for twenty years. Yet, in the world medical literature, there is still strong medical opinion, which attributes the etiology totally to pituitary and/or hypothalamic dysfunction. Indeed, in some respects, this tendency has increased in the last several years.

In 1936 the psychogenetic viewpoint was reestablished by Ryle's study of young women who had experienced psychosexual traumata.[41] A psychoendocrine concept was set forth by Reifenstein in 1946 when he described several cases of amenorrhea that were demonstrably due to psychophysiological disturbances.[47]

Frequence and Cultural Determinants

Anorexia nervosa is primarily a disturbance of adolescent girls.[55] Usually the onset is between the ages of eleven and fifteen; about one-fifth of the cases arise after mid-adolescence. Sylvester[50] reported a four-year-old case. This onset distribution is also true for male patients, but the frequency for males as compared to females is one in twenty cases. Onset under eleven and past eighteen years is atypical for both sexes; in such instances, if they are truly anorexia nervosa, the outcome is less optimistic.

It is almost certainly true that currently there is an increase in the incidence of anorexia nervosa in the United States, Great Britain, Japan, and in continental Europe. Although there is clinical agreement about this, there are, however, few statistical figures to support this contention. The only approaches that can be mentioned are those of Pflantz,[33] whose sociological studies put the risk at fifty to seventy-five per 100,000. It is dubious, however, whether any epidemiological study could produce accurate statistics for anorexia nervosa.

In Europe, the disorder is frequently confused with depression in adolescence and early adulthood. Bliss and Branch's criterion[3] of twenty-five

pound weight loss furthered the confusion in the United States. Then there are anorexics who secretly vomit after each meal but are able to take in enough food to maintain a normal weight. And there are many young adolescent girls like those presented in the clinical vignettes, who begin a diet, carry it to extremes, and are sent by the parents to the family physician. Sometimes this ends in a fatherly confrontation by an acceptable family doctor whose firm reassurance and direction allow the patient to stop her dieting. Such aborted cases would not be included in an epidemiological study. Then, too, one sees milder cases which do not progress beyond a missed menstrual period and a few pounds of weight loss. These young girls stop their dieting and their menses return. Such patients tend to be the healthier, teenage girls who, in the first flush of puberty, encounter the characteristic oedipal anxiety. They respond with a transient mild ego and id regression from which they are able to emerge without formal intervention.

One also encounters extremely thin girls and young women who follow vegetarian diets, and very slender ballet students and ballerinas, all of whom manifest anorexic behavior and attitudes but who do not usually lose control and require treatment. In quite a different age group are thin spinsters, in their fifth and sixth decades, who over the years have been eccentric in their fear of weight gain and in their dietary practices. They do not consult a physician unless medical problems arise from their anorexia nervosa. There are also thin individuals who conceal their anorexia behind an alleged malabsorption syndrome which they insist resists treatment.

The reasons for the increased incidence of anorexia nervosa are not clear. It has been suggested that greater availability of food over the last fifty years, and the associated overnutrition may well have been an important factor, especially when linked with the increasingly early onset of menarche in Western society. Children reared in this culture are also pushed more quickly into adulthood with little structure and control by their family and society. There is a body of opinion that feels that the developmental issues of autonomy and individuation have become more difficult to negotiate in our society.[4] Whatever the influences have been, it is clear that there is a psycho-social factor in Western culture that does favor the syndrome. This is evident in Japan, where Westernization has increased the incidence of anorexia nervosa.

It is also apparent that the condition is more

common in middle to upper classes, especially in Jewish and Italian subcultures where food, eating, and family solidarity are all important. Nevertheless, the disturbances are also seen in "WASPdom." One is far less likely to see a case of anorexia nervosa in a clinic population of the poor. In ghetto groups, one tends to see, instead, such syndromes as pica and drug addiction. The difference in food availability in the ghetto is probably only one factor in this difference.

In these cases, there is often a background of disturbed nutrition in the family. Parents may have had a history of anorexia nervosa in their own childhood. And it is not uncommon to find a history of obesity in relatives. Interesting family patterns of eating are often elicited. The father of an anorexic patient, whose mother was once anorexic, chose his wife out of guilt toward his younger anorexic sister who captured their parents' attention through her illness. Twin and adoption studies of anorexia nervosa patients fail to identify any chromosomal genetic pattern; it seems safe to say that psychogenetic family experiences are responsible for multiple cases within a family.[21, 22] Sibling rivalry is often an important factor[52] as is a combined passive-aggressive fight against parental control and suppression.

Clinical Course

The primary anorexia nervosa syndrome is characterized by the elective restriction of food, pursuit of thinness as a pleasure in itself, a frantic effort to establish control over the body and its function, food avoidance, and preoccupation with eating. About 10 percent of anorexic girls have never menstruated. All manifest hyperactivity, increased energy output, and secondary amenorrhea. Phobic avoidance of food leads to shame and alarm at trivial weight gain. In 30 percent of patients the hyperactivity and amenorrhea, either primary or secondary, are prodromal to the eating disturbance.

The secondary signs and symptoms involve manipulation of the environment around food and diet, along with a distrustful attitude toward the significant people who form the patient's human world. Sadness, guilt (without full-fledged clinical depression)[17] and occasional bulimia are seen.

There are several clinical varieties of anorexia nervosa.[2] The disturbance may be subclinical and disguise itself behind a food-fad or vegetarianism. No matter how it is manifested however, the diagnosis must agree with the phenomenological requirements of the syndrome in order to insure that the disturbance is indeed primary anorexia nervosa. The true anorexia nervosa patient is fixed on food refusal as part of her pursuit of thinness. Her ego-ideal is to achieve autonomy and effectiveness through bizarre control over her body and environment. The patient's overall psychopathology can fall into the neurotic, borderline, or psychotic realms.[32, 46] In the borderline case, one tends to see mainly cognitive and perceptual disturbances centering on the body and its nutrition. Depressive features, if present, are related to despair and frustration in not achieving victory of mind over matter. Defensively, the borderline or psychotic anorexic starves herself in an attempt to stop physical, sexual, and emotional maturation and development lest she be overwhelmed by anxiety over the possibility of object loss through separation and individuation. She rallies obsessive-compulsive mechanisms to substitute for individuative feelings, perceptions and thoughts, and, through the pleasure of control and mastery, she finds sources of motivation. Through starvation she can enjoy this substitutive pleasure as well as discharge the tension connected with her hostility toward the mother.

Bruch[5, 7] is quite adamant in insisting on a triadic disturbance for the diagnosis. She feels that a disturbance in body image and body concept of delusional proportions must be present in order to establish the diagnosis. The pathology, she believes, is best expressed in the patient's lack of concern over emaciation and cachexia. There is also a distortion in the accuracy of perceptual and cognitive interpretation of stimuli arising within the body. These patients display a failure in interpreting enteroceptive signals of hunger and discomfort. So great is their need to deny hunger that they seem unaware of hunger and appetite. During the course of the illness their hunger tends to be variable. They either direct their attention to feeding others or assuage their hunger by bulimia and vomiting. Furthermore, their pleasureless affective state diminishes hunger. In addition, their anxiety laden sexual feelings often distract them from their hunger. At some point in the illness these patients, especially the less borderline ones, may reveal oral impregnation fantasies. Nevertheless, anorexic patients will report intense hunger, particularly during the middle of the night. They show nutritional disorganization with bizarre food preferences and cravings and in their eating habits they often alternate between food refusal and bulimia. Their overactivity is a denial of hunger and fatigue. They tend not to recognize affects and emotional reactions. Frequently, their rationalization for self-starvation is tied up with religious-ethnic values that support a food ideology. And finally, as the third part of the triad, these patients experience a paralyzing sense of ineffectiveness. They fear that they act only in response to the demands of others. This compliance is usually camouflaged by negativism and stubborn defiance.

There are three main clinical courses the syndrome is likely to take.[46] In the first form, the disturbance may appear in a young adolescent girl who is fearful of her pubescent instinctual life. She feels that she is ungainly and heavy; she perceives her body as "too sexy." She decides to limit her food intake with the aim of shutting down the metabolic processes in an attempt to reduce libido.[25] She develops a fear of eating and pursues a Spartan diet along with a hyperactive life. These girls try to sidestep sexual feelings and fantasies. They move regressively to an oral-aggressive position where incorporative wishes give rise to a fear of merging with and destroying or of being annihilated by the infantile inner object. The incipient loss of ego boundaries forces ego modification and defensive shifts. Isolation, hyperactivity, and food refusal guard against closeness. The passive helplessness of the ego is neutralized by negativism and omnipotence—part of the functional ego regression which aims at control of oral aggression and prevention of merger with infantile inner objects. Anorexic patients in this first group are arrested in the late phase of separation-individuation (on the way to object constancy) or in the early phallic-oedipal phase. Self-object representations are more separate and whole, and less splitting into good and bad occur. Defense mechanisms tend to be more mature with repression, reaction formation, and sublimation. These patients tend to experience first oral pregnancy wishes and fears, pregnancy fantasies, and later, under increased pressure of regression, they fear engulfment and abandonment.

Many of these adolescent girls escape the attention of their parents and physicians and spontaneously remit after they have demonstrated to themselves their ability to control pleasure, appetite, and body functions. Some, however, pursue a relentless course which brings them eventually to hospitalization for refeeding. In these cases, treatment is difficult and protracted. Nevertheless, the prognosis for symptom removal in these cases tends to be much better than is true for the other groups of anorexic patients.

There are variants of the first group—girls who briefly manifest dieting behavior and mild, early ego regression. There are anorexics who develop food refusal in conjunction with their school peers to such an extent that a "near-epidemic" of anorexia suddenly sweeps through a school. Such an anorexic school group is commonly seen in the spring of the year when six to twelve girls in a class decide to go on a diet, lose five to fifteen pounds, become "sisters" to one another and shun boys.

The second group is made up, for the most part, of middle to late adolescent girls. Occasionally, some late latency girls may fall into this category. In addition to the primary anorexia nervosa signs and symptoms, this group displays defects in ego structure and organization along with pregenital instinctual fixation and infantile object dependency. These patients feel threatened by engulfment during ego and id regression. Fear of genital sexuality forces them toward ever more primitive object relations and pregenital drive discharge. They fear merger of self with an infantile inner object, and they turn to magical devices to save the self from merger. By falling back on the mother's magic, the anorexic masochistically falls victim to the mother's own falsification of reality. Disturbances of body image, false perceptual and cognitive interpretations of bodily stimuli, and overall sense of ineffectiveness are clearly demonstrated in this group of anorexics. This is a group that Bruch and Selvini have studied for many years.* These patients have a developmental arrest at the symbiotic or separation-individuation phase. They fear engulfment, abandonment, and loss of autonomy and function on the defensive level of splitting, projecting, acting out and denying, all part of a failure in development.[32]

Another group is that of the male anorexia nervosa patients. These patients are usually prepubertal or early adolescent chubby boys who fear oedipal-genital feelings toward the mother.[9, 13, 54] In the wake of their regressive shift, they experience a fear of maternal dependency and, in some cases, of merger with the inner object. They view their chubbiness as an indication of femininity, weakness, and homosexuality. A strongly negative oedipal history and feminine identification are usually apparent.

There are other variants of anorexia nervosa. More often seen in London, for some reason, is

* See references 5, 6, 7, 38, 42.

the late adolescent or young adult woman who diets vigorously like a fashion model and who delights in displaying her sleek pretty body. She shows no avoidance of sexuality and, in fact, tends to act in a hypersexual fashion (although without orgastic pleasure or sensual delight). Another variant is the mild to moderate chronic alcoholic, often a chain-smoker, who restricts food intake in order to continue drinking without gaining weight.

A less characteristic type is the young adult woman, socially active and professionally ambitious, who pursues an intense social and sexual life as a means of denying hunger, eating, and loss of impulse control.

From time to time, there are anorexic patients who continue their self-starvation beyond their twenties. This comes about either through inadequate treatment or because of the marked severity of their pathology. When they are seen in their late thirties, it is not unusual to find the patient locked into a close symbiotic relationship with a parent. An example of this is a father who ensconced his thirty-five-year old daughter in an apartment near the family home. Over the course of twenty years, she had seen a variety of therapists. No therapy had been pursued beyond a year, usually because the father would not permit it. By the time the patient was thirty-five, the syndrome appeared fixed, and her behavior suggested an early organic brain syndrome. Often incontinent and confused, she was unable to recall recent events, to do simple arithmetic, or, in general, to manage her life. She required custodial hospitalization, after her father died.

Organic Etiologic Factors

The physical findings in anorexia nervosa are the direct result of starvation and are corrected by refeeding.[10, 43, 47] They include hypothermia, hypotension, bradycardia, bradyprea, primary or secondary amenorrhea, and decreased libido. Body hair is reduced except for auxillary and pubic hair; downy lanugo appears on the arms and legs. Weight loss usually gives the patient a cadaverous appearance. She lacks subcutaneous fat and is angular and bony. Breast tissue, however, is preserved, and there is essentially no atrophy of the external and internal genitalia. The skin is blotchy, sallow, and often clammy, especially in the case of bulimic patients who vomit a good deal and de-

velop peripheral edema and abdominal pain. In such instances, the skin looks dehydrated, scaly, desquamated, and sometimes has a peculiar yellow-orange hue from carotenemia (a result of vitamin A deficiency). The anorexic is often hypoproteinemic; and blood studies reveal an anemia, either iron-deficient or megaloblastic, and a leukopenia with relative lymphocytosis.

There are no apparent generic factors, even among cases within the same family.[52, 54] There is no indication of a clear-cut genetic pattern. Crisp[9, 10] and Pilot[39] have reported monozygotic twins with anorexia nervosa which was the outcome of family experiential and dynamic factors. There is nothing to suggest a neurological lesion, although tumors of the third ventricle can clinically present a picture of anorexia. Biochemical factors had been sought for even before Simmonds' endocrine studies.[44] Crisp[10] reported a series of fourteen patients who had an abnormally sustained insulin response to intravenous injection of glucose. Delta-glucose values usually return to normal after refeeding as does glucose tolerance. For reasons not clear, insulin response may be sustained at an abnormal level even after feeding. Water balance also returns to normal after refeeding, although starvation edema may persist for several months. On the other hand, after a few years of starvation, metabolic disturbances may become profound with the appearance of symptomatic epilepsy, confusion, collapse, potassium depletion, and cardiac arrest. Cardiovascular collapse may also occur. Abnormal EEGs (14 and 6-per-second positive spike pattern) have been found in compulsive eaters. Green and Bau[18] believe that this finding indicates a "neurological dysregulation" correctable by anticonvulsant medications. They believe psychodynamic factors only determine the pathoplastic form of the compulsive eating; i.e., whether the patient is anorexic or obese.

The total estrogen output usually approaches normal after refeeding. In some instances, follicle stimulating hormone (FSH) secretion can be low. Pituitary gonadotropin levels show no consistent rise to normal after refeeding which has suggested to Russell[40] that there is a measure of pituitary involvement. He could not tell from the data when the depressed levels were related to continuing poor nutrition, weight loss, a disturbance in the responsiveness of the pituitary gland to hypothalamic releasing hormones, or a defect in the regulation and secretion of gonadotrophin-releasing hormones. Katz and Weiner[27] have reviewed the endocrine literature which they believe suggests a functional defect in the anterior hypothalamus and "in additional, as yet undefined, aberration in ovarian function or in responsiveness to the gonadotrophins." The nature and causal relation of such an anterior hypothalamic defect, however, remain ill-defined.[23, 26] Further research is needed, especially with that group of anorexics who do not recover well after a nutritional crisis. They may engage in prolonged psychotherapy but continue to remain thin, amenorrheic, sexually inhibited, and unassertive. Many anorexic women never overcome sexual fears and inhibitions. Psychoendocrine studies are needed to broaden our understanding of this dimension.[45]

If thyroid function is disturbed, it returns to normal after refeeding; pituitary-adrenal function is characteristically normal in these patients.

Exogenous factors do not include toxic or infectious elements. Traumatic elements may well contribute to the onset of anorexia nervosa syndrome. There are cases in which blatant seduction or rape occurred premorbidly. Often it is learned in treatment that the girl's father responded seductively to her on many occasions, forcing the girl into a regressive alliance with her mother.

Oral contraceptive treatment can precipitate anorexia in young women who then become amenorrheic. Hormonal changes may bring about increased sexual feelings too frightening to be enjoyed.

Developmental and Psychodynamic Factors

Interpersonal and intrapsychic factors are readily apparent in the delineation of the two main groups of the primary anorexia syndrome.

The young adolescent girls in the first group often have had an early onset of puberty and an accompanying reactivation of oedipal wishes which now take genital form and force. Such patients show less severe disturbances in separation and individuation. Early histories indicate that they are not consistently tied to their mother. As toddlers and preschool children they enjoy transitional objects and play with toys. They tend not to be blatantly negativistic and less oppositional behavior is present in early childhood. Ambivalence is expressed openly; these children are not

strikingly compliant, and they are willing to give vent to both physical and verbal aggression. Although they are not regarded as destructive, they are not considered "perfect children." In the oedipal years, they are attached to father and enjoy his attention well into latency. Their affective life is always much more manifest in adolescence. Their regressions do not lead them to an archaic inner object where self-object differentiation is lost. Throughout their childhood, they have shown instances of mastery. There are several attempts at identification during the latency years, and there are some peer relationships. As adolescents, the second individuation-separation phase is experienced more comfortably albeit with the accompanying anorexia nervosa disturbance.

The second group of patients become symptomatic in the middle and late adolescence. Puberty appears for them at a later date. They show a marked denial of its every aspect. They display structural ego defects of the borderline patient dating back to th toddler years. Throughout their childhood, a lack of separateness from the mother is apparent. As it turns out separation-individuation was most difficult for them. They are passive, submissive children who cling to infantile objects. Ambivalence is not manifested. Aggression is directed toward the self through an identification with the ambivalently loved object. Their denial of affect leads to an inability to feel separate and whole. They manifest delusions about the body and display fluid dedifferentiation and fusion with the primary infantile object. In latency, attempts at mastery are numerous but appear superficial, empty, and not sublimatory. Identifications are minimal during the latency years. There is no "hero" world, no family romance fantasy. Instead, their fantasies often take the form of wishes for a prolongation of the safety of childhood by way of depending on the magical world of nature and animals. Although they do good school work, they derive little pleasure from their achievement. In early adolescence, sexual fears abound, as well as a generalized fearfulness of the outer world. Adaptation is poor. And any event, such as parental divorce, death, or depression, threatens the child's tie to the maternal object and confronts her with separation anxiety and abandonment depression. Likewise, new adaptive and individuative challenges (camp, change of school, etc.) accentuate defense mechanisms and heighten vulnerability to separation anxiety.

The developmental histories of all anorexia nervosa patients regularly include mention of strong parental emphasis on delay and control of pleasure. Oral gratifications are tolerated and, at times, overindulged until the toddler stage, when the child is prematurely encouraged to conform to a parental model of compliance and socially acceptable behavior. The care of these children is basically adequate, except that the parents do not encourage separateness and autonomy, especially at the time when the first separation-individuation process is taking place. At that point, muscular exploratory behavior, oppositional attitudes and negativism are conspicuously absent. The child must suppress and deny her own separation and individuation to insure maternal supplies. Consequently, the child invests in the object, not the self, leading to fears of loss of the object and is left clinging and feeling helpless. The mothers often set a pleasureless and controlling tone to the family atmosphere and transactions,[48] and the patient's individual needs are subordinated to mother's strict moral codes and rigid, ambitious and narcissistic ego-ideals. The child resorts to negativism as an expression of rage at the mother's demand that the child's self be left tied to the mother lest libidinal supplies be withheld.

Because of conflict and anxiety around sexuality and dependency, the anorexic patient experiences both drive and ego regressions. Because of the developmental need to relinquish the self to the object in order to insure material supplies, the borderline anorexic is very sensitive to regression. Bulemic loss of control threatens the ego, and in the ensuing regression, the ego confronts its defenses. Concomitant to the drive regression is the functional regression of the ego that overshadows the oral mechanisms found in anorexia nervosa. The pressure of ego control and mastery which was learned during the anal-muscular stage is heightened in the regression. The ego turns against drive satisfaction. Ego pleasures now lie in the control and mastery of the body, its movements, its sensations, and all the perceptions of bodily and affective states. The highly analyzed ego functions are clearly discernible in the perceptual and cognitive areas. Magico-omnipotent thinking is prominent. Cognitive and perceptual control becomes the *leit motif* of these children. They develop a defective representational schema, a cognitive organization built around a diffuse personal identity inculcated by their parents who oppose individuation and perpetuated by their ego style of control and mastery. The ego pleasure of control outweighs oral drive gratification.

Many of the signs and symptoms of anorexia nervosa are best understood dynamically in this context. The conceptual and perceptual attainment of absolute power and control of body, self, parents, and other significant object relations is central to the syndrome. Thus, conceptual and perceptual discrimination is comprised through denial and suppression of individuative feelings and actions. The narcissistic pleasure of attaining supreme thinness blurs both the realistic ugliness of cachexia and the craving for food. The pleasure of control dissociates body and affective feelings from perceptual impressions and mental representations. The pleasure of limitless energy and activity nullifies the sense of ineffectiveness and denies fatigue. The pleasure of a perfect performance, of a perfect ego-ideal through control and mastery, challenges the exalted ego-ideal of the parents. Lest this challenge to the parents bring about a crisis of conscience, the masochistic delight of suffering attenuates the strain of superego conflict.

Neurotic and borderline anorexics vary considerably in regard to ego function and ego defect. What is common to the group, however, as well as to their families, is the exaggerated mode of ego function typical of the anal-muscular phase of development. During toddlerhood, these patients are taught to conform to parental models of behavior which emphasize joyless performance, achievement, physical fitness, strict morality, and perfect normality. At the approach of pubescence and renewed oedipal strivings, a drive regression and a parallel ego functional regression result in analization of behavioral modes. Cognitive and perceptual processes are then geared for control and mastery, which in turn become more pleasureable than drive gratification. This style of ego functional regression seems typical of patients with anorexia nervosa.

Family and developmental studies demonstrate the pathological mothering and difficulties in mutual cueing in the early toddler stage. The early histories suggest that anorexics project a primitive aggression onto the mother with the result that they form an unduly cruel superego. The aggression leads to harshness in the hostile component of their ambivalence and a fearfulness of its expression. Perhaps the marked preponderance of female anorexics is due to difficulties which toddler girls have in the rapproachement subphase of separation-individuation[30] and to their more ambivalent relationship with their mothers. Constitutional factors may well contribute to this gender preponderance. Fixation points, regression, the strength and vicissitudes of the drives, and the health of the object relations are all important in understanding the early development of these children.

Anamnesis is not sufficient to bring out these developmental factors. Since the mothers are unable to provide a history, it is only through analytic reconstruction that one can learn such developmental data. Normally there is an increase in aggression concomitant with muscular locomotive development. In these cases, however, the anamnestic data suggest a less than usual degree of aggression during the toddler period. This may well be related to a sex difference in aggression or to a special diminution of aggressive drives in those girls who later go on to have anorexia nervosa. We are reminded that the anorexic child is not encouraged to have motor separateness from the mother. This hypoaggressive behavior works against the achievement of psychological separateness. Later on, these children have difficulty in coping with aggression during early phallic, phallic-oedipal, and latency years. Pathologic defenses are multiple and include splitting of objects.[28, 31, 35]

Therapeutic Approaches

There are many treatment approaches to anorexia nervosa varying from psychoanalysis to psychosurgery—from education to behavioral modification. Most often the treatment recommended is determined by the extent of the clinician's experience and by his own theoretical orientation and personal convictions.

Some therapists take a predominately medical approach based on the belief either that anorexia nervosa is an anterior hypothalamic disturbance or that a cachexia of 25 percent total body weight loss warrants immediate medical intervention.

Leucotomy is still used in England, but now it is reserved mainly for chronic intractable patients who must be tube fed in order to live. ECT and tube feeding have been less frequently employed in the last fifteen years.

The most common medical regimen today is hospitalization with a program of chlorpromazine and/or modified insulin. These are accompanied by a controlled high carbohydrate-protein diet and, if indicated, intravenous tube feedings. The goals of treatment then are simply the stimulation of appetite, reduction of anxiety, and acceleration of positive metabolic processes. In this medical program, psychotherapy may range from suppor-

tive to analytic, with a variable emphasis on family therapy and/or behavioral modification along with some limited individual psychotherapy.

A second approach emphasizes out-patient or private office treatment. The proponents of this method view the hospital as contraindicated, even for the most severely cachetic patients. Within this program, the therapist dissociates himself totally from the feeding problem and the overall medical management.

Both programs are paradigms and ignore the particular needs of the individual patients. Clearly a treatment program must be based on a sound diagnostic, psychodynamic formulation with a careful assessment of the patient's medical and metabolic status. The most critical question the therapist must decide is whether hospitalization is indicated. Where the starvation is relentless, a rapid weight loss occurs to below 50 percent of total body weight, overt psychosis is present, and there is a persistent refusal by the parents to draw back from direct confrontation with the child; these together warrant immediate hospitalization. However, the patient should go only to a medical unit which has had experience with anorexic patients and understands that the therapist cannot take part in the medical management.

Behavioral modification is often an effective approach to a severely cachetic patient who has refused to eat during hospitalization. Operant conditioning techniques can be very effective for rapid weight restoration at the time of a nutritional crisis. However, they are inadequate for long term maintenance of eating habits and weight maintenance. The hospitalized patient is rewarded either by permission to engage in physical activity once a prescribed weight is reached, or by being allowed visitors if she continues to eat the hospital diet. During hospitalization, feedback techniques can be very effective in the treatment of this disorder. This is particularly true when they are combined with contingent positive and negative reinforcements. Reliance on this treatment, however, can be disastrous in that it allows the patient to eat her way out of the hospital to where she can then lapse once again into severe starvation and later death without returning to her physician and therapist.

The family therapy approach can initially be useful in delineating the disturbed interactions that usually occur in these families. Since the anorexic's family group is imbued with the idea of superhuman normality, they are loath to reveal any family disturbance. Only family meetings bring to the surface the basic intragroup pathology.

The mother's narcissistic use of the anorexic patient immediately becomes apparent as does the inability of all family members to verbalize their aggression. In cases where the anorexia nervosa disturbance is more neurotically based, one often can see the seductiveness of the hysterical father in the family sessions.

Minuchin[34] believes that early family intervention breaks up the family conspiracy to avoid all conflicts and teaches the family how to negotiate its conflicts. He has his best results with cases of anorexia nervosa of recent onset. In his view, it is only the anorexic in the family who has been able to bring the family conflicts into the open. A power-play then ensues with the result that the parents desperately turn on each other with accusations. He sees the anorexic's family as helpless to fight with the child who in turn cannot fight for her own rights. He tends to view the families as "loving families" who need assistance in their language and communications. He does not comment on the sado-masochistic character structures present.

Conjoint family therapy for the parents is advisable in all instances, but the results are variable. Its effectiveness is greatest in those cases where the anorexia nervosa is of recent onset and has a neurotic to borderline coloration. The prognosis is improved and the indication for conjoint therapy increased if the child is under eighteen and has had anorexia for only a few months. Prepubertal onset, duration beyond five years, and persistence through adolescence are grave prognostic indicators. Like enuresis, multiple tics (Giles de la Tourette syndrome), and obesity, long-standing anorexia nervosa is extremely difficult to treat, because the eating disturbance can become autonomous from the original conflicts.

The technical aspects of individual therapy remain controversial. There is one view that tradi-tional psychoanalysis—even for the neurotic group of anorexia nervosa patients—should never be used. It is felt to enhance negativism and mistrust in these patients and does not help them understand their bodily and perceptual disturbances. The other view is that the patient should be confronted with the abnormality of her dieting behavior by telling her that dieting is her metabolic device for reducing her frightening sexual feelings and increasing her attachment to her mother. The first view is best represented in the work of Hilde Bruch.[5] She believes that strengthening the ego under the guise of therapy, in fact, often enhances the patient's sense of ineffectiveness and helplessness. The second approach, on the other hand, confronts the ego and enhances resistance. Whatever the individual therapeutic approach, no interpretive activity can be effective until the fact of resistance is recognized by the patient. The main barriers to a therapeutic alliance are denial, negation, disavowal, and omnipotence. Before these defenses can be dealt with, the patient must experience and identify her warded-off affects. It is imperative that she recognize in herself abject feelings of helplessness and loneliness. Countertransference difficulties with the anorexia nervosa patient are compounded by the patient's feelings that she is misunderstood and controlled by the therapist.

Once the therapeutic alliance is achieved, for many of the more neurotic anorexia nervosa patients, analysis is in fact possible. If the disorder is recognized early, if the patient is not a fragile borderline case and does not intend to become severely cachectic and physically ill, if the parents are able to accept and remain in conjoint treatment, and if the patient is allowed to continue individual therapy after symptom-removal, then the prognosis is good for both symptom-removal and characterological change.

REFERENCES

1. AMERICAN PSYCHIATRIC ASSOCIATION, *Diagnostic and Statistical Manual of Mental Disorders*, (DSM-II), American Psychiatric Association, Washington, D.C., 1968.
2. BERLIN, I. N., et al., "Adolescent Alternation of Anorexia and Obesity," *American Journal of Orthopsychiatry, 21*:387–419, 1951.
3. BLISS, E. L., and BRANCH, C., *Anorexia Nervosa*, Hoeber, New York, 1960.
4. BLOS, P., "The Second Individuation Process of Adolescence," in Eissler, R. S., et al., (Eds.), *The Psychoanalytic Study of the Child*, vol. 22, pp. 162–186, International Universities Press, New York, 1967.

5. BRUCH, H., *Eating Disorders: Obesity, Anorexia and the Person Within*, Basic Books, New York, 1973.
6. ———, "Psychotherapy in Primary Anorexia Nervosa," *Journal of Nervous and Mental Disease, 150*: 51–67, 1970.
7. ———, "Anorexia Nervosa and Its Differential Diagnosis," *Journal of Nervous and Mental Disease, 141*: 555–564, 1966.
8. CRISP, A. H., "Primary Anorexia Nervosa or Adolescent Weight Phobia," *The Practitioner, 212*:525–535, 1974.
9. ———, "Primary Anorexia Nervosa or Weight

Phobia in the Male: Report of 13 Cases," *British Medical Journal, 1*:334–338, 1972.

10. ———, "Anorexia Nervosa: Feeding Disorder, 'Nervous Malnutrition' or 'Weight Phobia'?" *World Review of Nutrition and Dietetics, 12*:452–504, 1970.

11. ———, "Primary Anorexia Nervosa," *Gut, 9*:370–372, 1960.

12. EISSLER, K. R., "Some Psychiatric Aspects of Anorexia Nervosa Demonstrated by a Case Report," *Psychoanalytic Review, 30*:121–145, 1943.

13. FALSTEIN, E. I., FEINSTEIN, S. C., and JUDAS, I., "Anorexia Nervosa in the Male Child," *American Journal of Orthopsychiatry, 26*:751–772, 1956.

14. FREUD, S., *The Origins of Psychoanalysis. Letters of Wilhelm Fliess, Drafts, and Notes,* Hogarth Press, London, 1954.

15. ———, "Fragment of an Analysis of a Case of Hysteria," *The Standard Edition of the Complete Psychological Works of Sigmund Freud,* vol. 7, pp. 7–122, Hogarth Press, London, 1953.

16. GALDSTON, R., "Mind Over Matter: Observations on Fifty Patients Hospitalized for Anorexia Nervosa," *Journal of the American Academy of Child Psychiatry, 13*:246–263, 1974.

17. GERO, G., "An Equivalent of Depression: Anorexia," in Greenacre, P. (Ed.), *Affective Disorders,* International Universities Press, New York, 1953.

18. GREEN, R., and BAU, J. H., "Treatment of Compulsive Eating Disturbances With Anticonvulsant Medication," *American Journal of Psychiatry, 131*:428–431, 1974.

19. Group for the Advancement of Psychiatry (GAP), *Theoretical Considerations and a Proposed Classification, Psychopathological Disorders in Childhood,* vol. 6, Report No. 62, Group for the Advancement of Psychiatry, New York, 1966.

20. GULL, W. W., (1868), "The Address in Medicine," in Kaufman, M. R., and Heiman, M. (Eds.), *Evolution of Psychosomatic Concepts,* International Universities Press, New York, 1964.

21. HALMI, K. A., and BRODLAND, G., "Preliminary Communication: Monozygotic Twins Concordant and Discordant for Anorexia Nervosa," *Psychological Medicine, 3*:521–524, 1973.

22. HALMI, K. A., and DEBAULT, L. E., "Gonosomal Anenploidy in Anorexia Nervosa," *American Journal of Human Genetics, 26*:195–198, 1974.

23. HALMI, K. A., STRAUSS, A. L., and GOLDBERG, S. C., "Familial Hypothalamic Disorder in Anorexia Nervosa," (in press).

24. JANET, P., *Les Obsessions et la Psychasthenia,* Félix Alcan, Paris, 1903.

25. JESSNER, L., and ABSE, D. W., "Regressive Forces in Anorexia Nervosa," *British Journal of Medical Psychology, 33*:301–311, 1960.

26. KATZ, J. L., "Psychoendrocrine Considerations in Anorexia Nervosa," in Sachar, E. J. (Ed.), *Topics in Psychoendocrinology,* pp. 121–134, Grune & Stratton, New York, 1975.

27. ———, and WEINER, H., "Editorial: A Functional Anterior Hypothalamic Defect in Primary Anorexia Nervosa?" *Psychosomatic Medicine, 17*:103–105, 1974.

28. KERNBERG, O. F., "Early Ego Integration and Object Relations," *Annals of the New York Academy of Science, 193*:233–247, 1972.

29. LASÉGUE, E. C., "On Hysterical Anorexia," in Kaufman, M. R., and Heiman, M. (Eds.), *Evolution of Psychosomatic Concepts,* International Universities Press, New York, 1964.

30. MAHLER, M., "On the First Three Subphases of the Separation-Individuation Press," *International Journal of Psycho-Analysis, 53*:333–338, 1972.

31. ———, and FURER, M., *On Human Symbiosis and the Vicissitudes of Individuation,* International Universities Press, New York, 1968.

32. MASTERSON, J. F., "Primary Anorexia Nervosa in the Borderline Adolescent: An Object Relations View," Presented at the International Conference on Borderline Disorders, Topeka, Kan., March 1976.

33. MEYER, J. E., and FELDMANN, H., (Eds.), *Anorexia Nervosa,* Thieme, Stuttgart, 1965.

34. MINUCHIN, S., *Families and Family Therapy,* Harvard University Press, Cambridge, Mass., 1974.

35. MODELL, A. H., *Object Love and Reality,* International Universities Press, New York, 1968.

36. MORTON, R., *Phthisiologia seu exercitationum de phthisi,* Daniel Bartholomae, Ulmae, 1714.

37. MOULTON, R., "A Psychosomatic Study of Anorexia Nervosa including the Use of Vaginal Smears," in Kaufman, M. R., and Heiman, M. (Eds.), *Evolution of Psychosomatic Concepts,* International Universities Press, New York, 1964.

38. PALAZZOLI, M. S., *Self-Starvation,* Chancer, London, 1974.

39. ROWLAND, C. V. (Ed.), *Anorexia and Obesity,* Little, Brown, Boston, 1970.

40. RUSSELL, G. F. M., "Metabolic Aspects of Anorexia Nervosa," *Proceedings of the Royal Society of Medicine, 58*:811–814, 1965.

41. RYLE, J. A., "Anorexia Nervosa," *Lancet, 2*:893–899, 1936.

42. SELVINI, M. P., *L'Anoressia mentale,* Feltrinelli, Milan, 1963.

43. SILVERMAN, J. A., "Anorexia Nervosa—Clinical Observations in a Successful Treatment Plan," *Journal of Pediatrics, 84*:68–73, 1974.

44. SIMMONDS, M., "Über Hypophysisschwund mit todlichem Ausgang," *Deutsche Medizinische Wochenschrift, 40*:322–330, 1914.

45. SMITH, S. L., "Mood and the Menstrual Cycle," in Sachar, E. J. (Ed.), *Topics in Psychoendocrinology,* pp. 19–58, Grune & Stratton, New York, 1975.

46. SOURS, J. A., "The Anorexia Nervosa Syndrome," *International Journal of Psycho-Analysis, 55*:567–576, 1974.

47. ———, "Anorexia Nervosa: Nosology, Diagnosis Developmental Patterns and Power-Control Dynamics," in Caplan, G., and Levovici, S. (Eds.), *Adolescence: Psychosocial Perspectives,* Basic Books, New York, 1969a.

48. ———, "The Anorexia Nervosa Syndrome: Phenomenologic and Psychodynamic Components," *Psychiatric Quarterly, 45*:240–256, 1969b.

49. STONE, J., "Early History of Child Psychiatry," *International Journal of Child Psychotherapy, 2*:264–308, 1973.

50. SYLVESTER, E., "Analysis of Psychogenic Anorexia and Vomiting in a Four-Year-Old Child," in Eissler, R. S., et al. (Eds.), *The Psychoanalytic Study of the Child,* vol. 1, pp. 167–187, International Universities Press, New York, 1945.

51. THOMÄ, H., *Anorexia Nervosa,* International Universities Press, New York, 1967.

52. VANDERSALL, T., "Anorexia Nervosa in Siblings," (in press).

53. WALLER, J. V., KAUFMAN, M. R., and DEUTSCH, F., "Anorexia Nervosa: A Psychosomatic Entity," *Psychosomatic Medicine, 2*:3–16, 1940.

54. WEINER, J. M., "Identical Male Twins Discordant for Anorexia Nervosa," (in press).

55. ZIEGLER, R., and SOURS, J. A., "A Naturalistic Study of Patients with Anorexia Nervosa Admitted to a University Medical Center," *Comprehensive Psychiatry, 9*:644–651, 1968.

31 / Disorders of Early Parenthood: Neglect, Deprivation, Exploitation, and Abuse of Little Children

Richard Galdston

Introduction

This chapter is an attempt to elucidate the ways in which the normal parent-child relationship can become disordered during early parenthood. It includes descriptions of the resultant syndromes of deviant development among children whose parenting has become dysfunctional. The signs and symptoms with which the children suffer are grouped according to the prevailing pattern of parenting behavior in which they have been raised, together with an attempt to characterize the pathological processes which have led to the parents' inability to provide their child with a relationship that promotes optimal growth and development.

Parenthood is a state that is defined by a relationship. The word "relationship" comes from the Latin *relatus*, the past participle form of the verb *referre*, to give reference to. The parent-child relationship describes the state of being in reference to each other, a condition which is essential for the welfare of the child and which establishes the identity of the adult as parent. This unique and intimate arrangement normally subserves the function of procreation, providing for conception, pregnancy, birth, and upbringing. When the relationship becomes disordered so that the parties become estranged or disoriented in the ways by which they give reference to each other, then each participant suffers a derangement in development as a consequence.

Relationship, the state of being in reference to, is normally a dynamic condition in which each of the parties alters his practices and point-of-view according to his needs while maintaining constancy and accessibility toward the other. Among these families, the parents and their children are victims of an arrest in their ability to form relationships which allow them the freedom to maintain a dynamic attitude toward their patterns of interaction. The normal functions of parenting, to promote growth and development toward regeneration, are subordinated to patterns of parental behavior which are dictated by requirements resulting from flaws in the parents' own developmental history. These defects are made manifest through dysfunctions in the parenting process which can be diagnosed by the symptomatology of the child. The past is perpetuated into the future at the cost of the present.

The very stability of these patterns of interaction becomes pathogenic, because neither the parent nor the child can obtain what they require of the relationship. The dynamics of growth are frozen by mounting frustrations caused by chronic disappointment leading to an impasse of mutual dissatisfaction. The disorders of early parenthood epitomize the problem of dysfunctional relationships, the importance of which Bowlby has emphasized:

Nothing in child psychiatry has been more significant in recent years than the increasing recognition that the problems its practitioners are called upon to treat are not the problems confined to individuals but are usually problems arising from stable interactional patterns that have developed between two, and more often several, members of a family. (p. 349)[5]

The Normal Functions of Parenting

Adults, who have recently become parents, will usually answer a question about why they had their infant by citing some characteristic that they find to be especially lovable, adding that they just wanted to have a baby. It is rare that the mere desire to become a parent is given as a reason for having a child, yet there is evidence to suggest that the longing to attain the state of parenthood is a powerful force in motivating reproduction, quite aside from the particular child to be born. Couples forego a great deal of individual freedom and expend considerable effort, time, and money in order to form a relationship with a totally unknown entity who will establish them as parents. The initiation and maintenance of this relationship can become the cause of sacrifice of personal gratification willingly made because of the fulfillment that the relationship itself provides the parents.

The reproductive relationship, upon which the state of parenthood is ultimately founded, has a long and complex personal history, originating in early infancy in the experience of being a baby to other parents. The precursors can be traced through the several stages in individual maturation, evolving out of early relationships: of the little girl to her dolls and the little boy's efforts to make things. The relationships of the creator and the caretaker to their activities evolve through each stage of maturation, expressing the dominant developmental needs of the child's body and mind. Each of these activities makes its contribution to future ambitions. Out of this process, there accrues a body of experience in fact and fantasy which gives form to an ideal, expressive of the longing for a reproductive relationship. This ideal appears at adolescence in a form, romantic at first, which only gradually reveals its procreative purposes with the appearance in daydreams of a family of children drawn out in the child's mind to embody favored names and longed-for attributes. The adolescent girl may imagine, "I'll have two girls and one boy and he'll be called Andrew and will play on the football team." The whole of it is evanescent, intense, bearing scant recognition of the realities. It represents a rehearsal in the search for the reproductive relationship which alone can bestow the status of parenthood upon what otherwise remains adolescent dreams.

In the biologic dimension, human adulthood is characterized and distinguished by the act of procreation founded upon the reproductive relationship. The process of parenting a child and the state of parenthood require the establishment and maintenance of a reproductive relationship, a unique arrangement of one mother, one father, and one child, each devoting his energies toward a shared field of functions. The presence of the child transforms the relationship of husband and wife into that of father and mother and child, a relationship that normally functions to support regeneration. When the transformation of that relationship founders, one or another of the dysfunctions of parenting may ensue with a resultant deviation in the development of the child.

The maintenance of the reproductive relationship requires that the participants devote considerable attention to one another. Particular child-rearing practices, the vehicle through which parental attention is delivered, vary in accordance with cultural factors, but the stuff of which it consists is universal. The normal function of parenting depends upon the ability to watch over and give care to the child, to provide surveillance and response. When the parent is free to take care of the child's needs, the child will thrive and realize his biological potential through maturation.

Parental care has a sensory and a motor component. Normal functioning of the parenting process rests upon the formation of a reasonably realistic perception of the child's needs as determined by the parents' understanding of sensory data derived from observations of the child. The ability to act in response to that perception in a fashion appropriate to the child's needs closes the sequence of parental attention in its normal functioning. Whenever the sensory-motor sequence of parental care is disrupted, the child becomes vulnerable to one or another of the dysfunctions of parenting, depending upon where and when and for how long the disturbances occur. The disorders of early parenthood transform the child through a dysfunction of the parenting process made manifest by a disturbance in the quantity and/or quality of care. They represent miscarriages of parental love.

Dysfunctions of Parenting

The parenting process can be described as dysfunctional when the welfare of the child is sacrificed to the needs of the parent. The child suffers consequences which can be subsumed under four categories: neglect, deprivation, exploitation, and abuse. These are clinical entities, the signs and symptoms of which can be diagnosed in the child. Confirmation of the diagnosis rests upon obtaining a history of behavior and development from the parents. It should be emphasized that these dysfunctions in the parenting process are due to disordered relationships, and, therefore, are subject to changes, as are all things human. The terms are used to describe the prevailing pattern of relating in order to characterize the sensory-motor sequence of attention and response through which the parent and child relate to each other at the time.

NEGLECT

Definition: Child neglect can be defined as a disorder in the parent-child relationship characterized by a primary failure of the parents to endow the child with personal value. The child suffers from a lack of attention by the parents. There ensues a failure to perceive and acknowledge the child which is evidenced by scanty recognition of the child as belonging to, and depending upon, his parents.

Clinical Description: The neglected child reveals the consequences of physical and emotional starvation. Depending upon his age at diagnosis, the neglected child may present signs of malnutrition and lack of stimulation. Height and weight may be significantly retarded from the norms for age and sex. Psychomotor activity may be similarly behind the range of skills considered as the norm. Apathy is the predominant mental state with slowness to respond to stimuli which usually are the occasion for fright or withdrawal by the child. Neglect of physical care is often manifest by an accumulation of bodily filth, history of inadequate medical attention, and a paucity of objects for play. Dullness and listlessness characterize the mental status which is often within the range considered to be mentally defective, although the defect may be rapidly eliminated with the introduction of appropriate stimulation.

The essential feature of the clinical picture presented by the child is a primary relative retardation in development. When left to his own devices, the neglected child displays a poverty of spontaneous activity. The neglected infant, up to six months of age, shows slight interest in any part of his body. If thumb-sucking or other autoerotic activities are pursued, there is little evidence of pleasure on the part of the infant. Beyond the age of six months, the child shows a corresponding lack of interest in the environment beyond his body. There is little curiosity about his surroundings. The coming and going of other persons evoke neither interest nor fear. Preferred toys are rejected or meet with the most cursory of responses. The child appears not to know what to do with a toy and lacks the most elementary sense of play as a source of pleasure. Passive and joyless, the neglected child merely metabolizes as psychobiological preparation without evidence of having experienced emotion as a consequence of human intercourse. He functions essentially as an infantile vegetable.

Many children who had suffered from early neglect have subsequently been cared for by other persons who serve as parent surrogates. Depending upon the age at which this occurs, the clinical picture can be considerably ameliorated by the provision of more attention. However, such children give evidence of their earlier experience of neglect in their tendency to regress to a state of apathy whenever they are confronted with even minimal external stress. This liability to sudden and severe regression remains for many years despite the subsequent provision of adequate care. It appears likely that this vulnerability to profound regression in psychobiological functioning remains throughout adulthood as a liability to the formation of severe anaclitic depression.

Parents: Parents who neglect their child suffer from an inability to perceive, recognize, and acknowledge their child as belonging to them in a relationship devoted to the child's regeneration. This failure may be due to a restriction of available energies as in post-partum depression. It may be the consequence of immaturity as observed among adolescent mothers who see their infant as a doll to be played with rather than cared for. Parents afflicted with overwhelming grief due to bereavement from the death of a loved one, or those who have been afflicted with a sudden loss through illness or disaster, may neglect their infants or young child. In some instances the neglect may be viewed as situational and amenable to correction with the assistance of supportive persons within the context of the natural family or from agencies of society. Neglected children often develop a precocious capacity to fend for themselves and become capable of foraging for attention from others outside of their immediate family. Many children who have been neglected by their parents have managed to obtain care from grandparents, neighbors, or others, sufficient to attain a measure of maturation. Paradoxically, it is this very element of an absolute lack of attention by the parents which allows the young neglected child the freedom to fend for himself, if he can survive the early months of life. These children develop ingenuity at eliciting involvement with adults to whom they relate through active seduction. When placed in institutions or group placements, they often rise to positions of relative dominance manipulating others to assure their self-protection.

In other instances of severe and protracted neglect, the child can suffer from failure to thrive that is manifest by debility and cachexia which can be fatal if untreated. Adequate treatment of these children usually is dependent upon their removal to a medical facility where appropriate care can be provided. Such cases usually come from homes where the parents are quite willing to give the child up for placement or adoption. Review of the history with the parents often reveals that the advent of the child was denied during the prenatal period. The parents may have deferred obtaining prenatal care. The choice of a name for the child may have been postponed until several weeks after birth, and the selection of a name made by whim as an act of necessity. Other manifestations of a primary failure in attending to the advent of the child can be observed in a failure to assemble a layette or to make any of the usual preparations for childbirth which can be viewed as the human equivalent of nesting behavior.

The ultimate outcome of cases of child neglect depends to a significant degree upon the age and adequacy with which intervention is achieved. The very slackness of the attachment between the child and parents allows for their replacement by others to care for the child. If this is accomplished early in the child's life, within the first six months, and with appropriate attention, the child will probably recover from the early neglect with minimum evidence of enduring disturbance in development. However, if the neglect is not treated by the provision of adequate substitute care, the child will suffer from significant retardation in maturation, both physically and mentally.

Treatment requires early diagnosis and evaluation of the child and the parents with particular regard for the quality of the parents' interest in the child and their desire to attain the status of parenthood. Usually in cases of neglect, the parents are quite willing to give the child up for adoption if the intervention is early. Under such conditions, adoption is the treatment of choice for the child. The interruption of foster placements with its disturbance to the process of forming new attachments should be avoided if at all possible. The longer the neglect is allowed to go untreated, the greater the likelihood that the child will suffer retardation in development that will make subsequent adoption more difficult to implement. Such children appear much more likely to develop significant psychopathology of a delinquent or antisocial sort.

When the child is removed to a new situation, every effort should be made to provide him with relationships which are constant and accessible to him. Stimulation should be regulated in accordance with the child's development. When first exposed to new surroundings, many neglected children can only tolerate limited exposure to stimulation at a level that is considerably less than the normal range for their age.

For those children whose requirements for care bring them into a hospital setting, the usual therapeutic recommendation is for T.L.C., t.i.d., i.e., "tender loving care" three times a day. Such a recommendation is much easier to prescribe than to deliver, for many of these children are not particularly lovable at first because of the ravages that prolonged neglect have wrought upon their bodies and behavior. They do not afford their attendants the usual rewards for loving an infant or small child. There are no thanks, smiles, or chuckles of satisfaction likely to be forthcoming to please their caretakers. Their care requires a certain sort of person whose own needs for recognition will not interfere with the fact that having gone himself unrecognized, the neglected child has trouble recognizing others.

DEPRIVATION

Definition: Deprivation of the child can be defined as a disorder in the parent-child relationship characterized by the parents' valuation of the child as a nonhuman item. The child's humanity is denied, depriving him of human intercourse as a consequence.

Description: The deprived child has received a great deal, often an inordinate amount of attention from its parents, but that attention has been largely predicated on a major misperception, a delusion which renders a version of the child as a nonhuman object or an idea, often of an inanimate abstraction.

The child suffers from a combination of factors which depend to some degree upon the nature of the mistaken idea which the parents form about the child as a thing. Not only is the child likely to suffer from a lack of human attention, but he also is deprived of access to others who might intervene to proffer substitute recognition of his humanity. The deprived child is one who often has been raised in accordance with bizarre ideas such as toilet-training like a dog by rubbing his face in accidents; or fed in accordance with dietary ideology, such as the macrobiotic diet, as a source of supposed superior development. The limits of physical barriers may be completely removed to instill a sense of total freedom, or conversely, they may be rigidly imposed to develop superior discipline. Clothes may be used in a similar fashion to instill some desired attribute. Educational methods also may be implemented with a ruthless disregard for prevailing practices in favor of one or another bizarre ideology to which the parent sacrifices the child.

The early development of the deprived child may closely resemble that of the neglected child, but after six to nine months of age, the appearance of more bizarre forms of behavior distinguish the child who has been actively deprived of contact with other human beings. The appearance of self-induced vomiting and other forms of auto-erotic activity pursued to an extreme is illustrated by a three-year-old girl whose thumb-sucking was incessant until the terminal phalanx of her thumb fell off due to chronic maceration and secondary infection. Shortly after birth this child had been placed in a foster home with a number of children who were kept essentially for the money paid to their foster parent by the state. The child received the bare minimum of food and attention and was deprived of contact with any other adults. Such children develop bizarre and autistic practices which in some instances present as true cases of autistic development. In others, the appearance of autistic organization proves to be readily reversible with the introduction of supplementary association with other human beings.

In extreme cases of deprivation, the child may develop a failure to thrive syndrome which is so severe as to present the picture of marasmus. Often the parents will describe the child as having had a ravenous appetite and feeding voraciously, despite which the profound, unrecognized weight loss occurred When asked, they add a history of foul-smelling stools, suggestive of the possibility of a malabsorptive disease such as cystic fibrosis. Usually diagnostic evaluation of such children in the hospital fails to substantiate this condition. It appears more likely that their reported ravenous appetites and voracious feeding are due to misperceptions on the part of their parents. Usually they are very fussy and picky eaters who require a great deal of skillful and attentive nursing care before they can be restored to anything resembling normal food intake. On occasion the use of a central venous catheter for parenteral feeding is warranted by the extremity of the cachexia and the difficulty in establishing an adequate food intake by mouth.

Parents: Parents who deprive their child of human contact suffer from a primary misperception of their child. They do not recognize the child as being their biological issue but see him instead as a vehicle for an idea, an agency for a power or as an item to employ in a practice. These misperceptions are of a nonhuman order, and thus they are essentially psychotic in the degree to which they deviate from reality. These parents suffer from a psychotic distortion in their perceptions of their child although they may or may not show evidence of psychosis in other areas. Their denial of the child's humanity may be reflected in the choice of a bizarre name such as "Rover," or in the use of practices related to animals, such as keeping the child on a leash in the cellar. In some instances the parents are deeply involved in the promotion of some ideology, and they pursue their child-rearing practices in accordance with their preconception without any regard for the child's expression of his appetites. In some cases the parents are obsessed with a delusional preoccupation with the child's liability to death, and they take the child from clinic to clinic for treatment of numerous reported complaints. The hazards of overmedication become very real for such children.

The intensity and possessiveness of the parents' attention to the child is the diagnostic feature which distinguishes deprivation from neglect. The quality of the attention with which the child is raised is essentially psychotic in its lack of recognition of his human needs. The parents suffer from a segmental psychosis which has a profound effect in depriving the child of contact with other human beings or with themselves as mutual participants in the human condition.

The children whose parents have subjected them to this deprivation are the victims of a specific form of misuse. They are held prisoners in a form of solitary confinement. The stability of such an arrangement is not likely to endure for long, either because the child tends to deteriorate physically to the point of requiring medical attention for a failure to thrive syndrome, or the parents' ability to deny the child's humanity breaks down. Despite the inherent instability of the relationship, the parents who deprive their children are usually reluctant to give them up. Although they have little vested interest in themselves as parents, their need for the child to support their own psychic integrity is such that they usually bitterly oppose any efforts to remove the child from them. The urgency with which these parents guard custody of their child against all efforts to remove the child for proper care is of diagnostic import in differentiating deprivation from neglect. The quality of parental investment of attention in the deprived child differs from the relative uninterest which characterizes cases of neglect. These parents hold their child in great value, but the value lies in the capacity of the child to serve as a vehicle for the support of an item of belief essential to the maintenance of personal faith, no matter how deluded it might be. The fervor with which these beliefs are pursued rests upon the parents' need to deny some aspect of their own and their child's humanity. Deprivation is a disease

of denial; it tends to be categorical in its imperatives. The injunctions with which the parents
belabor the child are ill-suited to human growth
and development, and the deprived child tends to
founder and fail, with serious mental and physical
symptomatology, unless he receives effective
treatment by the age of five or six years.

Parents who deprive their children tend to be
the victims of major compulsive constraints on
their own behavior. These compulsions to restrict
their behavior in response to their own appetites
come to envelop the child, whose freedom to
fend for himself is severely limited by virtue of
his immaturity and dependence. The rigidity and
compulsiveness of his attitude toward himself and
his child distinguish the parent who deprives his
child from the parent who neglects his child. It
also serves to isolate the child from contact with
others and further deprives the child of the opportunity to form alternative relationships that
might subserve his human needs. The deprivation
from which these children suffer may or may not
include the physiological requirements for health,
adequate nutrition, clothing, and shelter. The
deprivation of sensory stimulation and the opportunity to obtain contact with human excitation
from surrogate sources appear to have the most
powerful effect in eroding the development of
these children.

With the advent of mobility, the deprived toddler becomes especially vulnerable to serious accidents, insofar as the parents may expose him to
hazards without physical barriers to his developing
motor competence. This is done often in a misguided effort to overcome obstacles to learning
without recognizing the child's humanity as the
basis for learning to take care of himself. These
children are exposed to the hazards of heights,
poisons, and other dangers in their surroundings
without the protection afforded by the cautionary
tales with which parents normally warn their
children. Conversely, some parents deprive their
toddler of any opportunity for physical contact
outside of an extremely restricted range, a cellar
or a garret, in order to protect him from contamination with outside influences or out of a profound
sense of shame about a child whom they perceive
to be evil incarnate.

EXPLOITATION

Definition: The exploited child is used by his
parents to service, or to defend against, the
unconscious demands of their own unmastered
appetites. The exploited child is used to perpetuate some part of the early symbiotic relationship
in order to subserve an obligatory parental claim
upon his energies for growth and development.
The exploited child develops specialized skills to
supplement defects in the parents' character structure. The exploited child is beloved by the parents
as human, but his value to them lies largely in
his usefulness in sparing the parents from the discomfort of unmastered intra-psychic conflict.

Description: The exploited child is distinguished
by the stigmata of precocious maturity. Early
specialization in the service of adult psychic requirements is made manifest by behavior which is
significantly premature and out of keeping with
other aspects of the child's being.

The mark of this condition is stamped on some
aspect of the child who appears to be a caricature
of an adult. By words, deeds, or posture, the exploited child demonstrates his efforts to function
in accordance with requirements for adulthood.
In the pursuit of this goal the child is obliged to
forego attitudes, practices, and values more appropriate to his chronological age. The functions
toward which the exploited child aims his development may be the gratification of, or prohibition
against, the adults' desires, or both. In any event,
the relationship is largely unconscious and goes
unrecognized by the parent. The child is often
quite fully aware of the exploitative relationship
but accepts it as natural, not having known any
other relationship to the parent.

Little children who have been exploited seldom
come to the attention of public social agencies,
because their parents neither neglect nor physically
abuse them. On the contrary, the exploited child
is usually held in intimate contact with the parents because of their need for the child to protect
them from their unmastered appetites. If the
little child does come to the attention of a public
agency, it is usually through some eccentricity
of his behavior. The three-year-old boy whose
mother made him wear a crash helmet to protect
him from falls off his tricycle when she pushed
him down a hill to inculcate toughness was clearly
serving needs other than his own. The four-year-
old girl who was posed for her birthday photograph with her hands outstretched so that she
couldn't be seen playing with herself was not
acting in response to prohibitions of her own. Unless there is a witness to the behavior, sufficiently
concerned to initiate intervention, most cases of
exploitation in early childhood go undiagnosed
and untreated. Instances of sexual exploitation
of little children by adults may go on for years
without detection, unless the child becomes suffi-

ciently conflicted about the behavior to develop symptoms that elicit medical attention. As long as the child is capable of behaving in accordance with the parents' requirements, the exploitative relationship has an innate stability which is extremely gratifying for both parties. The parents are spared from the anxiety inherent in conflicts about unmastered appetites and the child is secure in a sense of being highly valued. When, for whatever reason, the child is no longer able to subserve the parental requirements adequately, the exploitative basis for the relationship disintegrates leaving a void in which the child is likely to develop symptoms of a physiologic or behavioral breakdown in function. Thus the diagnosis of exploitation is most likely to be made at periods of rapid development and maturation when the traditional affiliations of child to parent are disrupted by biological and social requirements.

In the late preschool and early childhood periods, when separation from parental attachments is dictated by school attendance, the existence of intense, protecting functions by the parent may be revealed. The child has been employed by the parents as a transitional object furnishing the parent with a sense of comfort and protection against the ravages of unmastered issues of appetite regulation. Such children appear downright solicitous of their parents and apologetic about the requirement to separate, an act which they find less difficult than do their parents. The introduction of a preschool nursery experience proves to be intolerable for the parents who retrieve the child and keep him home. The parent is unable to travel out of the house unless the child accompanies her. In some instances the mother requires the child to be constantly in her sight day and night. These cases can be distinguished from cases of school phobia or separation anxiety on the part of the child by the observation that it is the parent who cannot bear to leave the child. Without the child's physical companionship the mother cannot bring herself to leave home or undertake any purposeful activity. In school phobia, on the other hand, it is the child who is primarily disturbed by the act of separation.

In other instances of exploitation, the child's physical health becomes a vehicle of parental anxiety and the child is utilized as the excuse for the solicitation of repeated reassurances from medical personnel. The parents and the little child travel from clinic to clinic in search of medical protection against items of unmastered intrapsychic conflict which the parents experience as a function of the child's body, a sort of extended hypochondriasis. No matter how many diagnostic tests are performed and despite repeated professional guarantees of health, the process recurs. Again and again the child's body is exploited in the parents' search for peace of mind.

With the advent of late latency and early puberty, the changes of adolescence reveal another order of symptomatology indicative of the presence of early childhood exploitation. The appearance of predelinquent, antisocial behavior in the child often uncovers a history of active parental promotion of physical violence throughout childhood in the expression of, and satisfaction for, unmastered parental aggression. Similar instances of parental exploitation of the adolescent's body for the vicarious gratification of unmastered sexual cravings can result in sexually promiscuous behavior among early adolescents. Often such behavior has been long present and only becomes identified when the social changes of adolescence render it more recognizable.

Conversely, there are children whose early childhood upbringing has been so freighted with moral strictures dictated in response to the parents' perceptions of their own appetites, that they are unable to seek fulfillment of their own desires. As they enter adolescence with its requirements of heightened responsibility for self care, these children are unable to do anything for themselves. They have been paralyzed by prolonged exposure to the moral constraints designed to contend with the threat of unmastered adult appetites. Some of these cases present with a renunciation of the desire to eat, as in cases of anorexia nervosa. Others abdicate any efforts to master heterosexuality and retreat into chronically asexual or homosexual adaptation. Still others develop chronically constrained conduct that allows them to act only in the service of the desires of another person, deriving only surrogate satisfactions.

Regardless of the particular parental appetite gratified or guarded against, exploitation during early childhood results in an intimate relationship between parent and child. There is an interaction between the intrusion of unconscious, unmastered parental desires and the child's accommodation through compliance in his motor responses. This interaction results in a functional fusion of the ego-operations of parent and child. This functional unit is vulnerable to profound disruption when maturation experiences involve separation. This vulnerability becomes manifest clinically at nodal points of development with the appearance of attitudes and practices often described as narcissistic in character. These phenomena can be understood as the residue of an early intense and hazardous sense of importance. Such a state accrues to a child whose early relationships have sent him forth upon the developmental mission of servicing his parents' intra-psychic requirements.

Parents: Parents who exploit their children to provide themselves with intra-psychic service are afflicted with defects in their own character structure. These flaws in development have left them vulnerable to a form of obligatory parasitism by means of which the child's development is skewed to service the parents' requirements. Since these needs are but dimly recognized, if at all, the child's function as a prosthetic device for the parents' psychic defects also goes unidentified. Neither parent nor child are conscious of their persistent fusion through function until some external event or internal development throws the relationship into turmoil at the threat of separation. The resulting symptoms vary but they tend to be in the form of a behavior disorder in which the parent and child act out their respective needs upon other persons, as they had previously served each other. This can be observed in the sudden eruption of sexual promiscuity in an adolescent child and the open marital discord of his parents which punctuates an incestuous arrangement.

The attachments between parents and child that result from the exchange of unconscious vows of intrusion and compliance persist despite a superficial picture of growth and development. The early signs of precocious pseudo-maturity are subsequently replaced by the appearance of an adolescent ego structure which is singularly deficient in the capacity to serve the child's own desires. Depending upon many earlier variables, the adolescent may thrash around in a series of self-destructive activities while searching for someone or something else to serve, or he may fall back upon himself in a variety of psychosomatic sufferings afflicting his own body. The parents of such children may either experience reciprocal symptoms in the form of mental suffering with depression, anxiety, or rage reactions, or they may turn to another child or adult to form another relationship based upon an exploitative pattern of attachment.

ABUSE

Definition: Child abuse can be defined as the physical assault upon a little child by an adult. It differs from corporal punishment in that the child is too immature for conscious knowledge of a misdeed.

Description: Child abuse typically presents with the signs and symptoms of the extreme ambivalence in the parent's attitude toward the child. A little child between the ages of six months to three or four years is discovered to have both fresh and old bruises and welts. There may be a history of old fractures of the long bones or skull. Recent and healed scars of burns may also be present.

In addition to indications of having been the victim of repeated physical violence, the abused child shows evidence of having received considerable physical care. The medical history may reveal repeated clinic visits at which the injuries were well cared for, if not accurately recognized as to etiology. The abused child has usually been well fed and dressed. His developmental milestones for height and weight are usually well within the range of normal and the level of psychomotor functioning which the abused child reveals is not readily apparent in an out-patient setting. The abused child is both beloved and hated by his parents, and his body bears the stigmata of the extreme ambivalence with which he has been perceived and cared for by them.

Little boys who have been physically abused tend to develop a proclivity to violent behavior as their prime mode of relating to others. In a group setting, they tend to violate the person and property of other children to a degree that far exceeds the norm for their age. It is not so much that they are more violent than other children but, rather, that violence remains their dominant mode of relating to others. They lack competence to express their wants or negotiate their emotions in alternative ways, without resorting to violence. Whether it be through the indiscriminate grabbing of that which belongs to others or the unprovoked assault upon others, the abused male child demonstrates the use of his major muscle mass as the dominant organ of his sensory and motor experience of interpersonal relations, as well as his own state of affective tension.

The little girl who has been physically abused tends to be inordinately dependent upon autoerotic activities as her source of comfort in the context of exposure to other children. She relies upon hair-twirling, thumb-sucking, and clinging behavior to a degree that exceeds the range for girls of her age. The desire to be held and the reliance upon sensory stimulation dominates her behavior and precludes participating in play or activities.

These patterns of behavior may be viewed as active and passive identification with the experience of violence as these children have come to know it at the hands of their parents. Unless these patterns of experience are revised through the addition of other ways of relating to adults, the patterns tend to become stabilized. The child's behavior is highly susceptible to change, depending upon his age and the vigor with which alternative experience with adults is introduced. The abused child readily integrates the addition of new relationships, often in a matter of days or weeks. This capacity to utilize new relationships with the elaboration of growth in ego skills can be viewed as a manifestation of the amount of love which has accompanied the abuse that the child has received. The abused child has been raised in the warmth of parental wrath which serves him better than neglect or deprivation by parents who are more indifferent to his humanity.

Parents: Parents who abuse their little child suffer from an inability to contain their ambivalence without resorting to the impulsive discharge of their emotions upon the child. Their perceptions of the child are exaggerated, often to the point of delusion. The child is seen alternatively as a saint or sinner, and their description of their child reflects their passionate attitude toward him. The term "monster" is frequently employed to express the fervor with which they experience the child. They vacillate between wildly inflated aspirations for the child and equally inappropriate disappointment and recriminations. The child is raised on a roller-coaster of parental expectations which creates a climate of highly charged emotions punctuated by outbursts of violence followed by periods of indulgence.

The abused child develops an intense attachment to his parents and they to him. This often confuses the problem of diagnosis because the child and parents display an interest in each other which appears to belie the likelihood of parental abuse. Further, the quality of the attachment compounds the problem of treatment because the abusing parent typically is strongly opposed to relinquishing the child and, when pressed, will resist any intervention that threatens to remove the child from his custody. If the child is hospitalized, the parents are exemplary in their devotion and eager to restore the child to their care. Once home, the likelihood of a recurrence of further abuse is great unless there is effective intervention. This fluctuation in attitude can be understood as an index of their ambivalence and their inability to contain the emotions which drive them. Absence makes their hearts grow fonder, but presence is more than they can bear.

Parents who abuse their child suffer from an inability to accept the fact of their parenthood. They look to the child to confirm the correctness, the validity, of their status as parents. The question of discipline assumes an obsessional importance to them, as if they relied upon the child's obedience to reassure them that they are, in fact, the parents they doubt themselves to be. This preoccupation can be understood as one of the sequelae to the rupture in the relationship with their own parents that abusing parents suffered as children. For example, a group of such families were studied in the Parents' Center Project for the Study and Prevention of Child Abuse. (This is a research service and training project staffed by members of Parents' and Children's Services of the Children's Mission: The author is Principal Investigator under support from the Grant Foundation, Inc.). Among these, none of the parents who abused their child were on reasonable terms with their own parents. Either they were totally estranged from their parents or they were locked to them in an intensely hostile, dependent basis.

This longing for, and inability to accept, the authenticity of their own parenthood, contributes to the impasse with which the abusing parent is afflicted. Often their choice of mate was impulsive with only the scantiest acquaintance before they committed themselves to parenthood. Nonetheless, the child conceived was born to a grand name chosen to reflect high hopes which were quickly dashed by the child's failure to realize the parental aspirations. Child abuse is an act that reflects the human capacity to entertain two intense and mutually contradictory emotions simultaneously. No other animal demonstrates this capacity to both care for and violate its offspring. There is an essential psychopathological core to the act of physical violence that distinguishes the syndrome. It consists precisely of this parental capacity to project distorted perceptions onto their young and to respond impulsively in accordance with their own delusions. Within the spectrum of human violence it lies somewhere between suicide and homicide.

Clinical Course: The natural history of these four syndromes varies greatly and allows for only the most general statements. Cases of neglect occurring in urban areas tend to be detected early through the intervention of public agencies or concerned individuals, or the child learns to fend for himself. Children who are actively deprived do not fare so well and early develop serious symptomatology.

Changes in the external circumstances and internal forces in the lives of the parents affect the prevailing pattern of relating to the child. The child who is neglected by an uninterested father while the mother works may be subjected to abuse when the mother is forced to assume care for the child when the husband gets employment. The child who is being exploited may be neglected when his services are replaced as result of the birth of another sibling or some other change in the composition of the family membership. The diagnosis of a syndrome of disordered early parenting describes the prevailing pattern of relating at the time of therapeutic intervention. It conveys an assessment of a dynamic state, subject to change in accordance with all of the factors that play upon the life of the family.

In general, patterns of deprivation and exploitation tend to be the most stable and, therefore, the most resistant to change. The pathological effects upon the children are the least amenable to early diagnosis and the most likely to result in serious disability. Neglect and abuse tend to be recognized earlier and are more responsive to therapeutic intervention.

Systematic prospective studies of the long-term consequences of these forms of parental dysfunction are lacking. Retrospective studies of individual cases indicate that early childhood neglect predisposes to a vulnerability to serious depression in the adult. Deprivation renders the child vulnerable to the development of an ego structure susceptible to subsequent psychotic disintegration. Parental exploitation disposes the child to deform his character structure toward the elaboration of a "false self" defined in accordance with the parental requirements. This contributes to maintaining a pattern of highly narcissistic motivations that persist into adulthood.

Prolonged exposure to physical abuse appears to shape an adult who relates to others primarily through the exchange of sado-masochistic intercourse.

All of these patterns of early development are liable to change, depending upon the quality of later relationships, but it appears that the experiences that prevail during the first five years of life go far to cast the die in which subsequent molding occurs.

Socio-Economic Factors

It is difficult to assess the importance of the role of socio-economic factors in the etiology of the disorders of early parenthood because of the great variation in the diagnostic process. The rearing of young children tends to be a private affair among all classes of society and is considered to be a personal matter. Under usual circumstances there is little occasion or opportunity for intervention by those outside of the immediate family. Preschool children have little access to professionals who might detect evidence of disordered early development. Among young children of the lower socio-economic classes who live in crowded urban areas, the occurrence of deprivation or abuse is more likely to be the occasion for attention from neighbors, clinics, or visiting nurses or social workers. On the other hand, exploitation and neglect often go undetected. Among middle and upper classes, deprivation and exploitation may be unrecognized for years, while neglect is more likely to be identified early.

Not only are the incidence and prevalence of these disorders difficult to establish, but the difference in the criteria for diagnosis according to socio-economic class compounds the problem. It is much easier to establish the diagnosis of neglect among lower-class urban poor than it is to diagnose deprivation among the well-to-do in the suburbs. The presence of supplementary hired caretakers for children, nurses, maids, or child psychiatrists, can serve to obscure the diagnosis of child neglect or deprivation.

The physical abuse of little children is perhaps the easiest diagnosis to establish, regardless of the socio-economic class. The reporting of such cases is mandatory in most states. This tends to facilitate recognition and intervention, although the requirements for effective therapy are probably less demanding than for cases of neglect or deprivation.

The lack of reliable figures on incidence and prevalence, either past or present, makes it a matter of conjecture as to whether these disorders are occurring with greater frequency among the population as a whole. Several social and economic factors can influence the incidence of these disorders.

Poverty: There is no doubt that poverty, wanting of adequate food and housing, is a cause of suffering for children as well as their parents. Nonetheless, there are many families who are afflicted by significant poverty without developing any of these disorders of early parenthood. Poor people have a lack of options in their child-rearing practices. They cannot hire substitute caretakers for their children. On the other hand, their residence, in housing projects or ghettos, makes it easier for them to find others to care for their children because of the proximity of friends or neighbors. Affluence tends to make it easier to hire socially acceptable surrogates to care for children, reducing the likelihood of case detection by public agencies.

Alcohol and Drugs: The use of alcohol and drugs to excess is associated, either as cause or effect, with a greater likelihood of impulsive behavior. Child abuse is usually an impulsive act, erupting out of circumstances in which there is a reduction in the controls of aggressive behavior, often associated with the use of drugs or alcohol by one or both of the parents. On the other hand, many parents who deprive or exploit a child do so in a context of strict moral or ideological constraints including the prohibition against the use of drugs or alcohol.

Religion: In general, regular attendance at church appears to protect against the likelihood of the disorders of early parenthood. It is not clear whether this is a coincidental or causal relationship. The ordering effect of extra-familial institutions appears to support families in their parenting functions.

On the other hand, the citation of quasi-religious doctrines of a moralistic nature is often encountered in the evaluation of parents whose deprivation, exploitation, or abuse of their child is justified by them as a matter of principle.

Race: The correlation of the disorders of early parenthood with racial or ethnic groups in the United States cannot be reliably isolated from the other variables in contemporary life. In general, those groups whose members live in some measure of continuity with their own traditions appear to be protected from these disorders. Family functions appear to be supported by membership in a body of interested persons whose attention serves to guard the parents against the vicissitudes of eccentricity. Those families who, for whatever reasons, are cut off from a sense of belonging to the traditions of an ethnic or racial identification, appear to be more vulnerable to the development of one or another form of disordered parental functioning. Physical and social mobility appears to increase the likelihood of this isolation.

Age of Parents and Size of Family: The younger parents of small families are more likely to be afflicted with dysfunctions in parenting than are the older parents of larger families. Whether it is a matter of learning or a function of self-selection, larger intact families with more than four children appear to be relatively free from these disorders, except for a form of exploitation in which the older children are left to care for the younger ones as parent surrogates.

Crime: The prevalence of criminal behavior appears to be correlated with the incidence of child abuse in that both are expressions of impulsive acts. Often abusing mothers have husbands with histories of criminal activity. The syndrome of maternal phobia, paternal antisocial acts, and child abuse appears to have a significant potential for the perpetuation of violence among the offspring, either as an active perpetrator or a passive victim.

Treatment

Systematic attempts to treat these disorders are too recent to allow for a reliable assessment of results. A wide variety of techniques is being employed. Traditionally, those cases which were brought to court relied upon the threat or actual removal of the child for foster placement. Recently, efforts have been made to strengthen family structure and function through a variety of techniques, with or without the reinforcement of legal injunction.

Most of these techniques depend upon the addition of one or more relationships to the lives of the parents in the hopes that the children will fare better as a consequence. The techniques can be subsumed under two general headings, those providing parent substitutes and those aimed at strengthening the parents in their own capacities to raise their children. Among the parent substitute approaches may be included the use of homemakers, visiting grandmother figures, daycare centers and foster care for infants and children, and the use of visiting nurses and paraprofessional mothers' helpers.

Among the techniques that aim primarily at strengthening parents in their own parenthood are the self-help groups such as Parents Anonymous, educational programs such as Parent Effectiveness Training, and the use of psychotherapeutic principles to promote greater parental responsibility. The Parents' Center Project for the Study and Prevention of Child Abuse is an effort to apply psychoanalytic concepts, through a variety of individual and group techniques, to the treatment of parents who are afflicted with these disorders. Concomitant treatment for their children in a therapeutic nursery is an integral part of the program.

Prognosis, Results of Treatment
and Prevention

The prognosis for untreated disorders of early parenthood is quite serious. It clearly warrants intensive search for more effective means of reaching disturbed families in time. Even if the parents, through their own maturation and learning, acquire an improved capacity to parent their children, it often comes only after significant damage has been done the child.

The evaluation of the relative therapeutic efficacy of the various techniques is difficult for many reasons. Since these disorders are due to disturbances in a relationship, and the treatment involves the introduction of another set of relationships, the variables become compounded and the construction of adequate controls taxes the ingenuity of research design. Furthermore, although the pathology derives from a disordered relationship, it is clear that it is not necessary for both parties to the relationship to change for improvement to occur in one. With the child's growth and development, critical periods of vulnerability will be passed, while the potential for change in the parents may be reduced with the passage of time.

Certain elements appear to be common among the approaches to these disorders that have had a measure of success. The introduction of a new relationship that offers a sense of constancy and accessibility appears to be essential to improvement. Whether that relationship be to a group, an individual therapist, or a movement of peers afflicted with the same problem, the sense of a supportive relationship in the search for competence as a parent appears to be essential. Agencies in which there is a rapid turnover in personnel or widely changing attitudes and practices cannot afford that sense. Neither can institutions that offer to take over the parents' job, for, by that very proposal, they give eloquent testimony to their belief that the parent is incapable of providing the child with a future.

Whatever the technique of treatment employed, ultimate success depends upon the parents' ability to grow in their capacity to raise their child. Such growth requires that the parents come to experience the child as their own true issue, to have and to hold in a reproductive relationship, the authenticity of which they can believe in as just and proper. How to best achieve that belief still remains a question to be answered.

REFERENCES

1. ARIES, P., *Centuries of Childhood*, Vintage Random House, New York, 1960.
2. BEAN, S. L., "The Parents' Center Project: A Multiservice Approach to the Prevention of Child Abuse," *Child Welfare, 50(5)*:277–282, 1971.
3. BISHOP, F. I., "Children at Risk," *Medical Journal of Australia, 1*:623–628, 1971.
4. BOWLBY, J., *Attachment and Loss: Separation*, vol. 2, Basic Books, New York, 1973.
5. ———, *Attachment and Loss: Attachment*, vol. 1, Basic Books, New York, 1969.
6. BRYANT, C., "Problems of Institutional Ineffectiveness," in Bryant, C. (Ed.), *Social Problems Today: Dilemmas and Dissensus*, pp. 167–340, Lippincott, Philadelphia, 1971.
7. CABANIS, D., and PHILLIP, E., "The Paedophile-Homosexual Incest in Court," *Deutsche Zeitschrift Für die Gesamte Gerichtliche Medizin* (Berlin), *66*:46–74, 1969.
8. ELMER, E., "Identification of Abused Children," *Children, 10(5)*:180–184, 1963.
9. GALDSTON, R., "Preventing the Abuse of Little Children," *American Journal of Orthopsychiatry, 45(3)*: 372–381, 1975.
10. ———, "The Burning and the Healing of Children," *Psychiatry, 35*:57–66, 1972.
11. ———, "Violence Begins at Home: The Parents' Center Project for the Study and Prevention of Child Abuse," *Journal of the American Academy of Child Psychiatry, 10(2)*:336–350, 1971.
12. ———, "Dysfunctions of Parenting: The Battered Child, The Neglected Child, The Exploited Child," in Howells, J. G. (Ed.), *Modern Perspectives of International Child Psychiatry*, Oliver and Boyd, Edinburgh, Scotland, 1968.
13. ———, "Observations on Children Who Have Been Physically Abused and Their Parents," *American Journal of Psychiatry, 122*:440, 1965.
14. GIL, D. G., "A Sociocultural Perspective on Physical Child Abuse," *Child Welfare, 50(7)*:389–395, 1971.
15. ———, "Physical Abuse of Children: Findings and Implications of a Nationwide Survey," *Pediatrics, 44 (Supplement)*:857–864, 1969.
16. GLASER, H. H., et al., "Physical and Psychological Development of Children with Early Failure to Thrive," *Journal of Pediatrics, 73*:690–698, 1968.
17. HELFER, R. E., and KEMPE, C. H. (Eds.), *The Battered Child*, University of Chicago Press, Chicago, 1968.
18. ISAACS, S., "Emotional Problems in Childhood and Adolescence: Neglect, Cruelty, and Battering," *British Medical Journal, 2*:756–757, 1972.
19. KEMPE, C. H., et al., "The Battered Child Syndrome," *Journal of the American Medical Association, 181*:17–24, 1962.
20. KOEL, B. S., "Failure to Thrive and Fatal Injury as a Continuum," *American Journal of Diseases of Children, 118(4)*:566–567, 1969.
21. MARTIN, H. L., "Antecedents of Burns and Scalds in Children," *British Journal of Medical Psychology, 43*: 39–47, 1970.
22. OLIVER, J. E., et al., "Five Generations of Ill-

treated Children in One Family Pedigree," *British Journal of Psychiatry, 119*:473–480, 1971.

23. PAVENSTEDT, E., and BERNARD, V. W. (Eds.), *Crises of Family Disorganization: Programs to Soften Their Impact on Children*, p. 103, Behavioral Publications, New York, 1971.

24. RESNICK, P. J., "Child Murder by Parents: A Psychiatric Review of Filicide," *American Journal of Psychiatry, 126*:325–334, 1969.

25. White House Conference on Youth, "Children in Trouble: Alternatives to Delinquency, Abuse, and Neglect," in *White House Conference on Youth, 1970*, Superintendent of Documents, U.S. Government Printing Office, Washington, D.C., 1970.

26. WIGHT, B. W., "The Control of Child-environment Interaction: A Conceptual Approach to Accident Occurrence," *Pediatrics, 44(Supplement)*:799–805, 1969.

---

32 / Failure to Thrive

John B. Reinhart

Failure to thrive is a syndrome more commonly diagnosed in pediatrics than in child psychiatry. The term is used to describe infants and children who demonstrate a failure of physical growth, malnutrition, and retardation of social and motor deveopment. Infants may present with a picture of marasmus (inadequate amino acid and calorie intake), with body wasting, or they may present with edema (Kwashiorkor syndrome) due to low protein, but adequate calorie intake. The term is most often used for infants in the first year of life who, after full term birth, have not grown at the expected rate in either height or weight. Although this syndrome of failure to thrive may be due to a variety of organic conditions, it is well recognized that perhaps 50 percent of children with this condition have their primary etiology in psycho-social factors,[16] and this is the focus of this section. After infancy, the syndrome of failure to thrive will disappear and blend into growth failure in the preschool years or later, which has been designated as "maternal deprivation" or "psycho-social dwarfism," a term which which implies that the parenting of these children is less than adequate to support growth in the physical as well as social, intellectual, and motor spheres.

But it has even been postulated, and needs to be investigated, whether or not delayed physical development in adolescence might not also be related to psychological and social factors.[29]

History

Modern psychiatric literature first recognized the association of growth failure and emotional deprivation in the description of infants and children living in institutions.[32, 34, 36] Other pediatricians at the same time reported similar findings and speculated that growth failure in children seen in pediatric clinics might also be due to psychological and social factors. Subsequently, the association of growth failure and emotional deprivation has been found to be a frequent finding among children who live in homes where there are disturbed family relationships. The problem has attracted the attention of both pediatricians and child psychiatrists, who are particularly interested in infants and young children.[2, 8, 15, 22]

In the first (1899) edition of his *Diseases in Infancy and Childhood* (under the heading, "Malnutrition in Infants (Marasmus)," Dr. L. Emmett Holt wrote:

The history in severe cases is strikingly uniform. The following is a story most frequently told. "At birth the baby was plump and well nourished and continued to thrive for a month or six weeks while the mother was nursing him; at the end of that period circumstances made weaning necessary. From that time on the child ceased to thrive. He began to lose weight and strength, at first slowly and then rapidly, in spite of the fact that every known infant food was tried." As a last resort, the child wasted to a skeleton, is brought to the hospital. (p. 661)[19]

In the tenth edition in 1933, under new editorship and authorship of L. Emmett Holt, Jr., and Ruston McIntosh, the same paragraph appeared; but later, under *Etiology* it ended with

Finally, it must be admitted that it is not always possible to find why certain infants *fail to thrive*. Such instances are regarded as due to some congenital weakness of constitution, a concept which is still far from satisfactory. A considerable number of premature infants fall into this group. (p. 661)[18]

This may have been the first use of the term, "failure to thrive," which has persisted in pediatric and child psychiatric literature since then.[32]

Incidence

Incidence of the syndrome of failure to thrive, or psycho-social dwarfism, will vary with the definition as well as the clinician's awareness. Just as in studies of incidence of child abuse, a related syndrome, all one can say is that this is one of the most common reasons for admission of infants to the hospital. It is more common among lower-economic groups, and "multi problem families." If thought of as a point in the continuum of abuse, sexual molestation and neglect, estimates are that one in every hundred children in America is so affected.

Criteria for Diagnosis

This diagnosis should meet the following criteria:
1. Weight should be below the third percentile at admission, and the infant should respond with significant gain after appropriate environmental stimulation and feeding are begun. Height may not be as severely affected, though this is probably a function of length of time of deprivation.
2. Usually these infants are retarded developmentally also and primary mental retardation may be suspected. Head size is normal and, as is the case with gain in weight, these children respond with increased motor and psycho-social development.
3. There is no evidence of any systemic organic abnormality. Renal, cardiac, central nervous system, or gastrointestinal and metabolic abnormalities must be considered, but, as stated before, 50 percent of children admitted will prove to be without organic disease.
4. History of child care should support the clinical diagnosis of neglect. Evidence of parent-child dysfunction should be expected, and a history of deprivation and ineffective parenting of the parents themselves is often found. Family stresses (financial, social, sexual, and otherwise) are usual, but are not necessary to explain parenting failure.

A syndrome that must be differentiated from failure to thrive secondary to psycho-social stress is the Diencephalic syndrome. This syndrome has its onset during the first year of life with a fatal termination, usually before two years of age. The Diencephalic syndrome results from neoplasms in the area of the hypothalamus and third ventricle. These infants have severe emaciation without depression of sensorium as a rule, and classically, the patient has the triad of marasmus, euphoria, and nystagmoid eye movements. Clinically these infants are quite different from the failure to thrive infants in that they seem to be alert, relate easily, and are not depressed.

There is general agreement[7] that the term "marasmus" be applied to children who are less than 60 percent expected weight for age and have no edema. The diagnosis of Marasmic Kwashiorkor would be applied to those who are less than 60 percent of expected weight but have edema; and that Kwashiorkor be applied to children who have edema and are between 60 percent and 80 percent of expected weight for age. Children who are 60 to 80 percent of expected weight for age without edema would be classified simply as underweight. Failure to thrive ("maternal deprivation syndrome") in infants is related to deprivation dwarfism, perhaps more aptly described as psycho-social short stature. This is a continuation of failure to thrive syndrome into an older age group of preschool or latency age children.

Mechanism of Growth Failure

Failure to thrive syndrome may be explained by undereating, secondary to dysfunction in the mother-child unit. And brain growth had been thought to be seriously affected on a permanent basis if growth failure is prolonged in the first year of life.

Animal studies have shown that emotional deprivation in early life can have detrimental effects on physical growth and intellectual and social functioning. However, infant monkeys,[20] totally isolated for a period of three to twelve months, did not reveal any abnormalities in body length or head circumference, and normal increases in weight occurred during the isolation. This was in spite of the fact that the animals demonstrated persistent behavioral abnormalities, which persisted after maturity with inadequate social and sexual adjustments. These animal experiments would seem to parallel the studies of human infants,[39, 40] in which, when food was offered, failure to thrive syndrome did not obtain.

Animal experiments suggest that there is a critical point in development when the size of an animal, arising from its previous plane of nutrition, determines its appetite thereafter, and hence, its rate of growth and dimension at maturity. At this critical time, no matter how liberal the diet, catchup growth does not occur. The ability of the animal to grow, after long periods of undernutrition, becomes progressively limited by the animal's chronological age when the catchup growth became possible. The earlier in the life of the animal the undernutrition is imposed, the more serious and permanent its effects will be. It is postulated that there is an organization of centers in the hypothalamus during the critical period and that, after that critical period, the responsibility of appetite, whether conscious or unconscious, is to insure that the intake of nutrients is only slightly more than enough to meet the current expenditures on growth and other activities of the body.[41]

The integration of the hypothalamus into the endocrine system makes possible a link between neural activity and feeling states, e.g., anger and sleep, and endocrine function. Secretion of human growth hormone during sleep is an example of this connection.

The exact mechanism of growth failure is not yet certain and the neuro-endocrine pathways are unclear. Hormones essential for normal growth are the pituitary growth hormones, thyroid hormone, insulin, and the gonadotrophic and sex hormones. Human growth hormone, produced in the pituitary, is controlled by a specific release hormone secreted by the cells of the hypothalamus. Growth hormone is required continuously through childhood and adolescence in order to attain normal adult stature. Deficiencies may simply be in the amount of growth hormone available or may extend to the release of other pituitary hormones as well. Hereditary isolated growth hormone deficiency occurs as both dominant and autosomal-recessive, but is rare in comparison to idiopathic hypopituitarism. Growth hormone itself does not act directly on growing cartilage, but causes the liver to secrete another hormone, somatomedin, which has to do with cartilage growth. Other factors such as growth hormone inhibiting hormone or somatostatin may be very important. Such hormones will be easier to synthesize than the human growth hormone itself, for they will be relatively small peptides (three to fourteen amino acids) compared to HGH which is a sequence of 190 amino acids.

Therefore, in addition to attention to diet and psychological and social environment, future treatment may involve the use of such hormones.

It is of interest, however, that cases have been reported where exogenous human growth hormone has failed to stimulate growth in children who, on change of environment, then began to grow satisfactorily.[14, 37]

Psychodynamics

Although psycho-social factors are considered to be primary in the etiology of this syndrome, the precise pathogenesis is not clear. Benedek[3] has described the importance of the symbiosis between the mother and her infant. Any breakdown in the communication system between mother and child can be seen contributing to the pathogenesis of the failure to thrive syndrome. If one considers the concept of congenital activity types,[5] it is easy to postulate on the infant's part, a failure to respond to the mother. Clinically this has been described to the degree that an infant has refused to suck and had to be gavaged or fed while sleeping, for the first eight months of life.[11, 12] Keen observers of mother-infant reactions have described infants as young as eight weeks becoming depressed upon the withdrawal of a mother's attention to them.[28] In one case, the baby had gained only nine ounces in a three-week period, after his mother weaned him so she could care for a four-year-old sib in the hospital. He was described as

extremely pale and listless, his fontanel was depressed, his skin inelastic and his expression lethargic. His conjunctival color was better than his general appearance would have suggested. He looked cold. I touched him again and made sure his skin was a normal temperature. (p. 507)[38]

A nurse described the treatment, which was to give the infant intense stimulation through many modalities by the mother, and the baby promptly responded. Speculation is that, had the child been placed in the hospital for observation and tests at this critical stage, the baby's condition could have deteriorated. This would seem to be a description of a child in the earliest stages of what has come to be described as failure to thrive syndrome.

In many studies, the frequency of prematurity has been noted, and this may be explained by the observations on maternal-infant attachments and the difficulty in "bonding" presented to the nursing couple by the occurrence of premature birth.[21]

595

The Infant

In the hospital, the infant with environmental failure to thrive has been distinguished as different from normal infants or those with organic failure to thrive by their more positive relations to objects and distant social approaches. Conversely, they do not respond as positively to close interpersonal interactions, such as holding and touching.[30]

Whether this is a behavior which precedes the development of the syndrome may be speculated.

The older child with a diagnosis of "psycho-social short stature" or "psycho-social dwarfism" or "deprivation dwarfism" may have obsessive-compulsive eating and drinking patterns[24] but also may not be so severely disturbed,[26] though retarded developmentally.

The Family

Studies of the families of the children who fail to thrive universally indicated that the mothers are in general, depressed, angry, helpless, and desperate and with poor self-esteem. As seems to be true in the syndromes of child abuse, these parents, too, have had poor nurturing themselves. Psychiatric studies of the parents are few, but one psychiatric study of twelve mothers[13] found ten of them suffering from character disorders, while only two were diagnosed as psycho-neurotic. This study made an extremely important point, that such a diagnosis will have a great deal to do with the strategy of intervention. Parents with character disorders have limited capacity to perceive and assess the environment, the needs of their children, and their adversive affective state. They also have limited capacity for relationship, to think literally and concretely, and are not good candidates for several problem-solving psychotherapy approaches. These parents are more likely to respond to action-intervention, need parenting themselves and an anaclitic relationship, and will need a treatment program which continues over a considerable period of time. In some cases, these parents will suffer from severe character disorders, so that attempts to relate to them will not be successful, and a change of the child's environment will be necessary.

In another study[10] three types of families were found. In the first group, young and immature mothers, relatively physically healthy and of good intelligence, were responding to object loss and were acutely depressed. They verbalized fears that the children would die or perceive them as retarded, and they were strained, constricted, or unsure in their behavior with their children. These families responded to intervention attempts and on follow up seem to be doing well.

A second group was seen as multi-problem families, with living conditions that were extremely deprived, crowded housing and scarce food. All children, including siblings, received poor physical care, and ten of fourteen were the last child in the family. The parents' behavior with their infants was much the same as in the first group, and the ability of professionals to intervene was limited because of the multiple, severe, and chronic problems the parents presented. On follow up, none of these children were doing well except those whose environment had been radically changed.

A third group of families was found in which the majority of the children received good physical care, but immunizations and well baby care were infrequent. Rehospitalization of these children was frequent. The most significant aspect was the mother's affect which was one of extreme anger and hostility. Their perception of the children was not in terms of illness or retardation but as "bad" or "out to get them." They handled their children in angry fashion, with frequent slapping and screaming. Without exception, they provoked anger in the nursing and medical staff involved with them, and on follow up, none of the children were doing well other than those who had been removed from their families. There was also strong evidence of abuse of those children who were still with their families.

In England, twenty years ago, it was found that the most important factors in the rehabilitation of families with failure to thrive infants were the steadiness of the husband and the good health and mental stability of the mother.[31] In a study of one hundred women, only thirty-nine were "outstandingly successful or progressing satisfactorily." There were twenty-five who were stated to be failures and thirty-six who were improved but still needed help. This was after a probation period of two years, with a "requirement to reside" in a training home for not less than four months for intensive residential training in mothering. As this syndrome is studied more, one can see that deprivation in infants has long-range serious consequence. For the children, mental retardation and emotional and learning disabilities are hazards. For some parents rehabilitation is not possible, even with intensive help, and termination of parental rights may be necessary.

The Treatment of Failure to Thrive

Infants who fail to thrive, providing laboratory studies and history are compatible with psycho-social reasons for the failure to thrive rather than organic causes, will require an assessment of the parents' ability to be involved in parenting of the specific child. It is possible for a mother or father to become involved with one child and not another. Observations of parent-child interaction will be of diagnostic import and continued observation has therapeutic value to the infant and the parent.

Initial therapy may require hospitalization, not only for protection of the infants but to treat the protein deficit, anemia, and vitamin deficiencies. There is an overlap of neglect and abuse, and this must be kept in mind. Hospitalization also serves to separate the infant from an anxious, if not hostile, environment and affords relief to the parents.

Depending on the assessment of the caretaking capacity of the parent, the infant, if feeding well and gaining weight, may be returned to the home environment from which it came; or it may need continued care in a foster home or other neutral environment while supportive and psychological therapy of the parents continue.

Important factors will have to do with the father-mother interaction, their interests in parenting, their abilities to receive support from others, family, friends, church, and other social institutions, their physicians and other health personnel. Because they are often "multi problem," "hard core," or "hard to reach" families, they may be neglected by the community. Traditional therapeutic methods such as psychotherapy which involves some degree of maturity often are not effective. "Aggressive casework," patience, and tolerance of their sometimes angry, defensive exterior is necessary to get at the unsure, unloved person beneath. In a sense these parents must be parented themselves in order to mature to the point where they can satisfactorily be nurturing parents to their children.

Treatment of the children will depend on the degree of deprivation they have suffered and the age and duration of that deprivation. This author[25] has seen a patient who had little physical growth in the first seven months of life, and who, on an alteration of the psycho-social environment, did respond, both in height and weight, as well as emotional and psychological development. Fifty years following the original observations, she was an adult who had advanced educational degrees and was in all respects normal. The amount of physical growth possible is remarkable, and the author has also seen a twenty-two-year-old young man who was the size of a four-year-old (forty-two and one-half inches) and had immature psycho-sexual development on admission to an institution. This young man, in a changed environment, and with only vitamin D given for rickets, grew some twelve and one-half inches in a period of thirty-six months (to the size of an average nine-year-old, fifty-five inches); and in the first year had sexual growth, in the sense that his genitalia grew from infantile size to full size adolescent male genitalia. However, intellectual gain, though it went from about nine months to approximately four years, did cease at that level, so that at the age of twenty-four he was still severely retarded.

In summary, treatment must be thought of in terms of the family. Parents are not born with the ability to parent; some do not learn and cannot be helped. Fortunately many families can be helped, but a wide range of supportive services will be needed.

The children will need proper feeding, and if the deprivation of nutrients has not been severe or prolonged, they will respond quickly. Usually these children have suffered stimulus deprivation and lack of emotional exchange with their parents. These deficits, if severe, are difficult to remedy and prolonged psychotherapeutic efforts, day care, group and individual therapy may be needed. Cognitive learning will improve to a much quicker degree than the defects in personality development.

If termination of parental rights is necessary, both those parents who will be forced to give up their children and those with whom the child will live will need help. And the child, too, will need appropriate attention, depending on its age and degree of disturbance.

Prognosis

Failure to thrive syndrome may be thought of as a continuum ranging from the relatively healthy family with a situational problem, depression, anorexia, and failure to thrive of a child, to the other end of the spectrum where the family's involvement with the infant is meager and perhaps even abusive. It would seem that a child may thrive but be subjected to parental dysfunction and abuse. Yet the failure to thrive infant has acute or often chronic difficulty in the parent-child relationship, which seems to lead to depression in the infant, with anorexia and failure to gain weight.

Prognosis seems to depend on the time of life during which the deprivation and failure to thrive syndrome exists and the degree of psychopathology of the child-environment interaction. Spitz's original follow up[32] on institutionalized children and Cravioto's[6] and Elmer's[9] studies showed severe psycho-social, as well as physical growth, retardation secondary to maternal deprivation and/or lack of adequate dietary intake. Recent studies suggest that undernutrition in infancy correlates with future lag in physical and mental development. It was noted that children seen in a hospital for undernutrition, which was corrected before four months of age, had developed normally three and one-half years later. Also, a pair of monozygotic twins varied quite differently, possibly because of the difference in their mother's feelings toward them. Investigators said "It seems impossible to separate undernutrition completely from associated environmental influences since they are part of the same entity."[4]

Reviews of the relationship of malnutrition and later mental development are not conclusive. In a study of boys of school age who had been hospitalized for severe malnutrition in infancy, results suggested the need to shift emphasis away from primary attention to malnutrition as a cause of functional impairment in later childhood to a broader concern for the ecology of child development.[27] Malnutrition is one of the array of variables that are hypothesized to influence the functional development of children. Though an attractive thesis, there is still not good scientific evidence that early malnutrition alone causes permanent mental impairment.

In the preceding study, the index boys had lower IQ's, did less well at school, showed less social ability at school, and were smaller physically than their comparisons.

These index boys lived in families that were more isolated socially, and they received less intellectual stimulation. Their caretakers had fewer human resources. More of them did not have a man around the house nor other people they could turn to for help, and they visited less often with relatives. They had fewer material resources, and it was suggested that the index caretakers were generally less capable than comparison caretakers and possibly less organized in a lesser intellectual ability.

Whereas the potential for catchup physical growth is great, particularly if the deprivation occurs after the period of rapid physical growth in the first six months of life, the prognosis for intellectual and emotional growth should be guarded. Early social deprivation may be modified if intervention is appropriate, and animal experiments have shown that isolated female monkeys who became mothers, if their infants persisted, "gave up the struggle against their own babies" and eventually achieved near normal contact.[19] Impregnated again, these same isolated females exhibited normal monkey maternal behavior toward subsequent offspring.

Also, similarly deprived and isolated infant monkeys, if exposed to "therapist monkeys" who provided a nonthreatening atmosphere, clinging rather than being aggressive, matured so that two years later their disturbance behaviors had disappeared.[35]

But in humans, more long-term follow up studies are needed of infants who fail to thrive. At this point, it would seem that Ainsworth's[1] statement is true, "that the effects on personality development of deprivation early in life, though not completely irreversible, are more resistant to complete reversibility in more cases than are intellectual functions."

REFERENCES

1. Ainsworth, M., "The Effects of Maternal Deprivation," *Public Health Paper 14*, World Health Organization, Geneva, 1962.

2. Barbero, G. J., and Shahein, E., "Environmental Failure to Thrive: A Clinical View," *Journal of Pediatrics, 71(5)*:639–644, 1967.

3. Benedek, T., "The Psychosomatic Implications of the Primary Unit: Mother-Child," *American Journal of Orthopsychiatry, 19*:642–654, 1949.

4. Chase, H. P., and Martin, H. P., "Undernutrition and Child Development," *New England Journal of Medicine, 282*:933–939, 1970.

5. Chess, S., "Individuality in Children, Its Importance to the Pediatrician," *Journal of Pediatrics, 69*:676–684, 1966.

6. Cravioto, J., and Delicardie, E., "Environmental Correlates of Severe Clinical Malnutrition and Language Development in Survivors from Kwashiorkor or Marasmus

Nutrition," *The Nervous System and Behavior*, p. 73–95, Scientific Publication, No. 251, Pan American Health Organization, 1972.

7. Editorial, *Lancet*, 2:302, 1970.

8. ELMER, E., "Failure to Thrive—The Role of the Mother," *Pediatrics*, 25:717–725, 1960.

9. ———, GREGG, G. S., and ELLISON, P., "Late Results of the 'Failure to Thrive' Syndrome," *Clinical Pediatrics*, 8:584–589, 1969.

10. EVANS, S. L., REINHART, J. B., and SUCCOP, R. A., "Failure to Thrive—A Study of 45 Children and Their Families," *Journal of American Academy of Child Psychiatry*, 11:440–457, 1972.

11. FELDSTEIN, G. J., "A Breast and Bottle Shy Infant at 21 Years of Age," *American Journal Diseases of Children*, 77:374–375, 1949.

12. ———, "A Breast and Bottle Shy Infant," *American Journal Diseases of Children*, 35:103–108, 1928.

13. FISCHHOFF, J., WHITTEN, C. F., and PETIT, M. G., "A Psychiatric Study of Mothers of Infants With Growth Failure Secondary to Maternal Deprivation," *Journal of Pediatrics*, 79(2):209–215, 1971.

14. FRASIER, S. D., and ROLLISON, M. L., "Growth Retardation and Emotional Deprivation: Relative Resistance to Treatment with Human Growth Hormone," *Journal of Pediatrics*, 80(4):603–609, 1972.

15. GLASER, H. H., et al., "Physical and Psychological Development of Children with Early Failure to Thrive," *Journal of Pediatrics*, 73(5):690–698, 1968.

16. HANNAWAY, P. J., "Failure to Thrive: A Study of 100 Infants and Children," *Clinical Pediatrics*, 9:96–99, 1970.

17. HARLOW, H. F., HARLOW, M. K., and DODSWORTH, D. O., "Maternal Behavior of Rhesus Monkeys Deprived of Mothering and Peer Associations in Infancy," *Proceedings of the American Philosophical Society*, 110:58–66, 1966.

18. HOLT, L. E., and McINTOSH, R., *Holt's Diseases of Infancy and Childhood*, 10th ed., Appleton-Century, New York, 1933. Quoted in Smith, C., and Berenberg, W., "The Concept of the Failure to Thrive," *Pediatrics*, 46(5):661–663, 1970.

19. HOLT, L. E., "Malnutrition in Infants (Marasmus)," in *Diseases in Infancy and Childhood*, Appleton, New York, 1889. Quoted in Smith, C., and Berenberg, W., "The Concept of the Failure to Thrive," *Pediatrics*, 46(5):661–663, 1970.

20. KERR, G. R., CHAMOVE, A. S., and HASLOW, H. F., "Environmental Deprivation: Its Effect on the Growth of Infant Monkeys," *Journal of Pediatrics*, 75(5):883–887, 1969.

21. KLAUS, M. H., and KENNELL, J. H., "Mothers Separated From Their Newborn Infants," *Pediatric Clinics of North America*, 17(4):1015–1037, 1970.

22. LEONARD, M. F., RHYNES, J. P., and SOLNIT, A. J., "Failure to Thrive in Infants," *American Journal Diseases of Children*, 3:60–612, 1966.

23. LIGHT, R. J., "Abused and Neglected Children in America: A Study of Alternative Policies," *Howard Educational Review*, 43(4):556–598, 1973.

24. POWELL, G. F., BRASEL, C. H., and BLIZZARD, R. M., "Emotional Deprivation and Growth Retardation Stimulating Idiopathic Hypopituitarism: I. Clinical Evaluation of the Syndrome," *New England Journal of Medicine, 276:* 1171–1283, 1967.

25. REINHART, J. B., "Failure to Thrive: A 50 Year Followup," *Journal of Pediatrics, 81(6)*:1218–1219, 1972.

26. ——— and DRASH, A. L., "Psycho-social Dwarfism: Environmentally Induced Recovery," *Psychosomatic Medicine, 31(2):*165–171, 1969.

27. RICHARDSON, S. A., "The Background Histories of School Children Severely Malnourished in Infancy," *Advances in Pediatrics, 21:*167–195, 1974.

28. ROBERTSON, J., "Mother-Infant Interaction From Birth to Twelve Months: 2 Case Studies," in Foss, B. M. (Ed.), *Determinants of Infant Behavior*, vol. 3, pp. 111–127, Methuen, London, 1965.

29. ROSENBAUM, M., "The Role of Psychological Factors in Delayed Growth in Adolescence: A Case Report," *American Journal of Orthopsychiatry, 29:*762–771, 1958.

30. ROSENN, D. W., STEIN, L., and JUES, M. D., "Differentiation of Environmental From Organic Failure to Thrive, Abstract from APS and SPR," *Pediatric Resident, 9(4):*262, 1975.

31. SHERIDAN, M. D., "The Intelligence of 100 Neglectful Mothers," *British Medical Journal*, p. 91, January 14, 1956.

32. SMITH, C. A., and BERENBERG, W., "The Concept of Failure to Thrive," *Pediatrics, 46:*661–662, 1970.

33. SPITZ, R. A., "Hospitalism: A Followup Report," *Psychoanalytic Study of Children, 2:*113–117, 1946.

34. ———, "Hospitalism—An Inquiry into the Genesis of Psychiatric Conditions in Early Childhood," *Psychoanalytic Study of Children, 1:*53–74, 1945.

35. SUOMI, S. J., HARLOW, H. F., and McKINNEY, W. T., "Monkey Psychiatrists," *American Journal of Psychiatry, 128(8):*927–932, 1972.

36. TALBOT, N. B., et al., "Dwarfism in Healthy Children: Its Possible Relation to Emotional, Nutritional and Endocrine Disturbances," *New England Journal of Medicine, 236:*783–793, 1947.

37. TANNER, J. M., et al., "Effect of Human Growth Hormone Treatment for 1 to 7 Years on Growth of 100 Children," *American Journal Diseases of Children, 46:* 745–782, 1971.

38. TAYLOR, R. W., "Depression and Recovery at Nine Weeks of Age: Introduction and Summary by Mollie S. Smart," *Journal of the American Academy of Child Psychiatry, 12(3):*506–509, 1973.

39. THOMPSON, R. G., and BLIZZARD, R. M., "Growth Failure, Deprivation and Undereating," *Journal of the American Medical Association, 211:*1379, 1970.

40. WHITTEN, C. F., PETTIT, M. G., and FISCHHOFF, J., "Evidence that Growth Failure From Maternal Deprivation is Secondary to Overeating," *Journal of the American Medical Association, 209:*1675–1682, 1969.

41. WIDDOWSON, E. A., and McCANCE, R. A., "A Review: New Thoughts on Growth," *Pediatric Research, 9:*154–156, 1975.

33 / Substance Abuse

Karl Frederick Nystrom, Adrian Lee Bal, and Viki Labrecque

Substance Abuse As a Syndrome

The abuse of any substance is not, in itself, diagnostic of a specific mental disorder, and the identifying label is dependent on the broader context of the abuse. That substance abuse should be considered as an entity and as a whole is a relatively recent concept; it unifies the often diverse thinking which arose out of the separate consideration of the abuse of one substance and another singly. Conceptually, a dynamic is established within which the pre-adolescent glue sniffer, the adolescent marijuana smoker, and the chronic alcoholic can be seen within the same frame of reference.

Within the classification of mental disorders in the DSM-II,[4] substance abuse might be associated with virtually any disorder. Situations in which the substance abuse exists as the causative element in the diagnosis are classified under a variety of categories listed as "psychosis associated with organic brain syndromes," "non-psychotic organic brain syndromes," "alcoholism," and "drug" dependence."

Individuals recognized to be prone to drug dependence or abuse are classified under "Personality Disorders and Certain Other Non-Psychotic Mental Disorders" as 301.89. This includes other personality disorders of specified types (immature personality, passive dependent personality, etc.).

Among children and adolescents, patterns of substance abuse might be found within the context of the following diagnostic categories:

Transient Situational Disturbances:

307.1 Adjustment reaction of childhood
307.2 Adjustment reaction of adolescence

Behavior Disorders of Childhood and Adolescence:

308.0 Hyperkinetic reaction of childhood
    (or adolescence)
308.1 Withdrawing reaction of childhood
    (or adolescence)
308.2 Overanxious reaction of childhood
    (or adolescence)
308.3 Runaway reaction of childhood
    (or adolescence)
308.4 Unsocialized aggressive reaction of childhood
    (or adolescence)
308.5 Group delinquent reaction of childhood
    (or adolescence)
308.6 Other reaction of childhood
    (or adolescence)

Conditions Without Manifest Psychiatric Disorder and Non-Specific Conditions:

316.1 Social maladjustment
316.3 Dyssocial behavior (classified in DSM-I as Sociopathic personality disorder, dyssocial type)[5]

The multiplicity of potential diagnostic categories among those who are also "substance abusers" underscores the fact that substance abuse is a symptom, however maladaptive, that might have virtually any diagnostic context. This jungle of appearances has served to conceal the essential unity of substance abuse. Instead, it has facilitated the focusing of individual attention and etiological consideration on each of these diagnostic categories. Within this chapter, an attempt will be made to establish the overall nature of substance abuse without overlooking the individual features of the separate agents.

Substance Abuse Described
As a Primary Entity

In his encounter with life and destiny, man has always striven to transcend his limitations. In keeping with this, the search for the perfect substance, which might alleviate all human woes and transcend all limitations, is deeply ingrained in mythology and in history. Man has searched for ambrosia, the food of the gods, the eating of which confers a godlike status. Soma, the long lost Vedantic substance which brought clarity, peace, and wisdom, has been sought intermittently for several millenia. The perfect anodyne has proved as elusive as the Holy Grail. Short of perfection, an endless number of lesser agents have been found and used for one purpose or another. The use of these imperfect substances has been accompanied by a multitude of pitfalls or hazards. In a primary sense, the abuse of a substance constitutes a failure to heed the hazards implicit in its use.

Hazards to be Considered in Psychoactive Substances

TOXICITY

Any substance ingested in excess is toxic. However, the general recognition that a drug is dangerous is rarely based on a recognition of its toxicity per se. Most often the reputation of a substance as either "safe" or "toxic" is relatively independent of its pharmacology. It is conferred by the culture as a whole on the basis of social practice and need. During the 1890s, arsenic was sometimes used in face powder to facilitate a fashionable pallor. Opium was a standard ingredient of most patent medicines. But cigarettes were widely reacted to with intense negativity as "coffin nails." The establishment of the Food and Drug Administration and the passage of Pure Food and Drug laws imposed a somewhat greater rationality on many such popular and misguided assessments of substances. None the less, a number of paradoxical attitudes about toxicity persist. Perhaps nowhere was this as evident as in the recent general relief felt in the United States when alcohol was re-espoused by the adolescent generation as its agent of choice.

POTENTIAL FOR CREATING ADDICTION

A substance is addicting if, once instituted, its continued use is necessary to prevent the occurrence of withdrawal symptoms. This implies the creation of a new physiological and biochemical homeostasis, one which supersedes the former equilibrium and includes the addicting substance. Within this new balance, a withdrawal of the substance leads to the biochemical and physiological readjustments associated with abstinence symptoms.

The concept of addiction is frequently expanded to include the related areas of tolerance and dependence, which are considered separately.

TOLERANCE

The development of tolerance to a substance describes a situation where an increasing amount of the substance is required to achieve a constant pharmacological effect, or, conversely, when continuing a constant amount is associated with a diminishing effect. This is caused by the development of more efficient metabolic pathways for breaking down the substance; these pathways form in response to its constant or recurrent presence. The phenomenon of tolerance varies both from drug to drug and from individual to individual.

In certain circumstances, tolerance becomes a key consideration. This is particularly true where it produces a desired pharmacological effect, but does not lessen a potentially lethal secondary action. Thus, with the opiates and the barbiturates, tolerance develops to the sedative properties but not to the respiratory depressant properties. This makes it possible for an individual to expire from anoxia secondary to respiratory depression while still awake.

DEPENDENCE

Dependence on a substance describes the emergence of an emotional reliance on its effect in order to continue to feel good. Dependence is the term most frequently used to describe relating to a substance in terms of a "need." However, it implies that the need is not based on a physical addiction and the avoidance of an abstinence syndrome, but rather on an emotional condition.

Western culture has placed a high value on self reliance and independence and has inculcated the concept that all people share these values to a great extent. In fact, each individual is highly dependent for the preservation of his emotional equilibrium on a large number of possessions and external circumstances, among them, a variety of substances. For the most part, these elements are not seen as dependencies at all, but as part of the fabric of life: home, land, family, work, friends, recreation, religion, food, sexual patterns, a hot breakfast, coffee, sugar for the coffee, tobacco, aspirin, antacid, a sedative. A barrage of advertisements invites everyone to cultivate new dependencies on new substances, which, once established, tend to perpetuate themselves by habit.

When a substance is not foreign to the culture, and when its use is not judged excessive, the concept of dependence is rarely invoked. Extension of this same process to a new or foreign substance, however, typically raises a popular fear of dependence or enslavement to the new substance. This concern transcends the limits of mere dependence itself and extends to include bondage to the substance, and regression.

REGRESSION CAUSED BY A SUBSTANCE

In itself, no substance has the power to create a life pattern of regression. There have been experiments in which the pleasure obtained from the stimulation of implanted electrodes was altogether compelling. Thus, when a rat or monkey was allowed the freedom to stimulate these pleasure centers, it engaged in this activity to the exclusion of attending to life-sustaining pursuits, and died. In mythology, Ulysses protected himself from a related situation by tying himself to the mast of his ship so that he could hear the siren's song without being free to yield to its overwhelming seductiveness and so led to his destruction. In fact, however, no drug has the power to divert an individual from the fulfillment of his higher aspirations. The myth that certain substances do have this power continues to be given credence by a short circuit of logic which is ancient in origin and persists to this day.

Culture and civilization perpetuate themselves by means of the "higher" accomplishments of their members. Whether or not Freud's classical assessment that civilization is built on repression is overly pessimistic, it is true that civilized man harbors many regressive longings. Typically, the culture defines and limits the extent to which regression is permissible, and ritualizes the form that it may take.

Parents usually hope that their offspring will grow up to be self-reliant. The unpleasant alternatives are death or dependence, often on the parents themselves. Consequently, as children discover their own capacity for sensual gratification, it is hoped that the overall context is one in which there is progress toward independence.

From era to era there have been differing behaviors that were popularly accepted as danger signals. Whenever they appeared, they aroused concern about the ultimate independence of the child. The pool hall, tobacco, masturbation, and alcohol have all had their day; each has been regarded as a primary sign of a wish to escape from the task of growing up. Each has meant that corrective measures were necessary.

When viewed as primary "evils," the elimination or suppression of the offending act or agent might seem necessary to assure optimal development. Within the context of the frequent power struggle

as to whether the future course of an adolescent is continued dependence or preparation for independence, these elements have often provided a focus for the battle; one generation has argued for their harmlessness, the other for their danger. In the course of these various debates, it is assumed that it is the presence or absence of some such element that determines whether or not an individal (or a generation) will achieve a fulfilling adulthood. This is an error in logic.

The question hinges, instead, on whether society will allow the individual to achieve an adult role. Sometimes a particular social arrangement makes it impossible for a given youth (or class of youth) to function within a context of justified hope for a productive future. This always creates a state of depression. It also gives rise to a series of compensatory pursuits, ranging from narcissistic regression to a predatory criminality. On the other hand, those who do become successful adults share a common experience. Somewhere during their growing years, they were regarded as potentially able; they understood that they could in time fill a position above their present capacity. Ordinarily young people are helped to grow in this way within a relationship of supportive optimism provided by an older, more accomplished adult. When an individual regresses to a position of overwhelming preoccupation with the pharmacological effects of drugs, he is likely to be seen as a misfit, a dropout, a parasite, handicapped, disabled, or psychiatrically ill. Individually, he may be ignored, eliminated, supported, rehabilitated or "treated," segregated or assimilated. Collectively, the number of these individuals provides a measure of the overall health of the society and constitutes a pressure for social and political change. It has been observed that the concern and most vigorous efforts at suppression of marijuana coincided with the time of the greatest opposition to the country's national policies on the part of the young. This led to the greatest development of a "counter culture" the United States has ever experienced. But this is not really unique. Other substance abusing subgroups exert their own pressure. The heavy drinking businessmen and the heroin using unemployed ghetto dweller share a profound sense of unfulfilment, albeit in different areas. They also make their presence felt.

ILLEGALITY, STIGMA, OR TABOO OF A SUBSTANCE

Each society and subgroup has always had its own list of permissible substances which may be used or abused, and forbidden substances which may not. The use of any of the latter constitutes a violation of propriety, taboo, or law and is categorized as abuse. Over the last several hundred years, there have been many additions to and deletions from the list of substances whose use is given general social approval. There is, however, a frequently repeated pattern which characterizes the first introduction of a foreign substance into a given culture.

Initially, the use of the new substance is dependent on the reputation and charisma of those who launch it. On its introduction into England by Sir Walter Raleigh, the smoking of tobacco was seen as exotic and startling. (There is a story of one gentleman being doused with water by his well-intentioned valet who apparently thought he was on fire.) It was also associated with the romance of England's enterprise and discovery in the new world; the act of smoking tended to confer on the smoker some of the glamor of these adventures. In Russia, Japan, and China, however, the merchants and seamen, who introduced tobacco, were associated with no such positive connotation, and the use of tobacco was outlawed on pain of death.

During such time as the substance is illegal or frowned upon, its users tend to be recruited from the disaffected or rebellious classes, who use it as an expression of defiance. The puritanical elements of society in seventeenth-century Holland disapproved of the use of coffee; at the time, its role as a stimulant had exciting and romantic connotations. Rebellious intent could then be signaled by publicly drinking a cup of coffee. This had as strong a symbolic value as the public drinking of whiskey, smoking of tobacco, wearing of perfume, or smoking of marijuana has had in other places and times.

The spread of the use of a new substance has rarely been influenced by laws aimed at its repression. Indeed, as time goes by, an initially disreputable substance may take on a more positive quality because its new users are among the upper classes. In Japan, when the use of tobacco had extended to the court, punitive legislation was repealed and artistically carved pipes were introduced.

Once the use of a substance becomes general, its romantic properties undergo rapid attrition unless it is used to symbolize a new conflict. For example, a "second wave" of reaction to tobacco occurred when women began to use it to express their equality with men. Otherwise, the symbolic value of the use of a substance must be artificially instilled through advertising and promotion.

Individual Dynamics of Purposeful Substance Abuse

When the topic of substance abuse is discussed, it usually goes without saying that this refers to purposeful abuse. The social matrix into which this abuse fits has been described in terms of ignorance, habit, and the culture. In individual terms, however, the following dynamics set identified substance abusers apart from these others.

The syndrome is characterized by a depressive base. The individual becomes preoccupied with the feeling brought about by the abused substance. In time, this leads to a self-destructive course. This pattern is described in the section on alcohol under "Personality Structured Family Dynamics of Alcohol Abusers." Within this pattern, the particular circumstances of the affected individuals vary. They are best studied along parameters which define the immediate gravity of the situation and the requirements which make for differing therapeutic approaches. The following considerations reflect the status of involvement within this syndrome:

Age of Onset: As the child's consciousness expands in the course of growth, again and again his experience amounts to the discovery and mastery of the unknown, the organization of confusion. From an early age, one boundary about which children are aware and curious is that between the "light of the common day" and the various altered states of consciousness with which they become familiar. The implications of dreaming and waking are sorted out within the limits of their experience. The child daydreams and there is an interest in the meaning of death. Rocking, breath holding, head banging, eye squeezing, spinning, and masturbation are among the common modes of exploring the shores of the uncharted ocean within. For many a child, there is an appreciation that these limits are closely allied with the magic and mystery of existence.

The normal context for such childhood discoveries is one in which the exploration and experience of the outside world is actively encouraged. Under optimal conditions, it is toward this dimension that the major thrust of life energy is directed. The inner experience, however, remains as an alternative interest, to be cultivated differently. In the absence of sufficient satisfaction in relating to the outside world, however, it is likely to be sought to a greater extent. The reality of this choice was the theme of a popular children's book,

The Water Babies, of several generations past. Currently, it is absent from the shelves of most libraries. Here is described an underwater world to which unhappy children may turn in the event of more trouble on earth than they can bear, and here they are lovingly nurtured by a kind Old Lady. The protagonist is an abused young chimney sweep who finally opts for the hopeful unknown at the bottom of the pond, in preference to the depressing known.

Any child may seek refuge within an experience of narcissistic regression by means of purposeful substance abuse. In general, the earlier the age at which this occurs, the more basic will be the impediments to his attaining a satisfactory relationship with the real world. The implications might be an inborn limitation of his ablity to connect to the world, a hypersensitivity to the frustration which accompanies all mastery and growth (frustrated omnipotence), or a deficit in the quality of the support available for his growth at that time. The younger the age at which an inward regression facilitated by substance abuse is sought, the more all inclusive the probable necessary remedies. The grammar school dropout glue-sniffer is likely to be more depressed than the high school dropout PCP (Angel Dust) user. The younger child requires far more help. The assistance needed to establish the basic prerequisites to further growth such as trust and initiative is much greater than that demanded by later, more advanced requirements. Although subsequent maturational difficulties, such as those surrounding the establishment of sexuality or a vocational choice, can reactivate the more basic themes of doubt or distrust, an older individual has had at least some experience in successful growth behind him; he has an experiential alternative. A younger child often does not.

In response to stressful factors which affect a predictable percentage of their age-mates, the vast majority of child and adolescent substance abusers retreat into their abuse in the company of a peer group. The social, familial, and individual dynamics in the life of the contemporary teenage abuser are likely to position him within a well-defined mainstream of abusers rather than to single him out as an individual with problems uniquely his own. In the case of a youngster poised on the brink of substance abuse, the essence of his situation is an absence of a constructive vision of his continuing life and life role, and a lack of appropriate support in the direction of fulfilling whatever vision he does have. As a rule, these circumstances exist where specific external determinants combine with important intrapsychic aberrations. The pattern will be described in the section on alcohol.

Social Context of the Substance Abuse: When a youth seeks a chemically influenced state in a group context, it is significantly different from the solitary pursuit of a similar state. Isolated abuse is likely to imply that the person feels uncomfortable even when alone. This suggests a more fundamental discomfort than behavior arising in the company of others.

The Degree of Pharmacological Effect (or Impairment) Sought: The substance taker who seeks a state within which he is "under the influence" represents a different magnitude of problem than one who seeks oblivion. Within this range, the greater the need to escape and the greater the impairment sought, the more serious the implication.

The Frequency of Abuse: The more frequently an individual places himself under the influence of a substance, the more likely that the abuse will complicate his life pattern and lead it in a regressive direction.

The Extent to Which the Abuse Interferes with the Continuity of the Pattern Within Which It Exists: It is self-evident that the gravity of a pattern of substance abuse is proportional to the extent to which the life pattern of the abuser is disrupted. This disruption might result from any of the hazards implicit in the substance's use.

The Availability of a Course Alternative to Immersion Within a Pattern of Substance Abuse: A fundamentally sound individual will possess a potential for a creative, positive solution to his life difficulties; a fundamentally healthy society will have a fulfilling position potentially available to whoever might aspire to a measure of productivity. The most complete obstacle to the establishment of a productive pattern is an ignorance of how to establish supportive social bonds, along with an unavailability of the external structures necessary to sustain an adequate level of growth.

The Essential Unity of Substance Abuse: The dynamics of abuse patterns of specific substances will be described under those sections. A focus on the individual drugs, however, should not obscure the overriding unity of substance abuse as an entity.

The specific agents abused are likely to vary with the times, the locale, the social situation, the availability, the cost, or the fashion. The adolescents of the 1970s are likely to be poly-abusers, with substances taken either sequentially or together. As a result, whatever diagnosis might be made with regard to their abuse of one substance or another would vary depending on the time they come to professional attention. The essential position of today's adolescent alcoholic, yesterday's "acid-head," and tomorrow's abuser of whatever else, is the same. Shifts in the style of chemical abuse are noteworthy but not ultimately meaningful, and the concentration of concern on the particular agent—heroin, marijuana, or alcohol—is misplaced.

The appropriate focus is the child whose development is blocked and whose future as a productive and fulfilled individual is jeopardized. The chief concern should lie in the sphere of primary prevention among the susceptible populations who are at high risk. Secondary treatment of established abusers is pathetically inefficient and generates only a modest success rate. There have been many attempts to attribute the problem of abuse to the pharmacological effects of a specific drug, and to hope either to control or to cure the problem through the suppression of the agent. These have been universally expensive, useless, and indicative only of an essential misunderstanding of the generic basis of the situation.

As the effects of the individual substances and their place in the scheme of things are considered, mention will be made of certain unique aspects of their roles as agents of abuse. Since alcohol is the substance whose use and abuse provide a model for the consideration of substance abuse generally, the section on alcohol will include the essence of the presentation of this syndrome.

The Depressants:
Alcohol, Barbiturates, Tranquilizers

ALCOHOL

Historical Notes: Alcohol has been history's number one drug. The vicissitudes of religious, cultural, and individual persuasion have resulted in a continuously evolving interaction between man and alcohol. Today, many of the traditional restraints to the abuse of alcohol seem to have lapsed. More than at any other time in history, the social effects of alcohol use are being determined by continuing unchecked abuse patterns within the vulnerable portions of the population. This continuing consumption and attendant abuse are effectively encouraged by vigorous advertis-

ing. The current ramifications of society's relationship to alcohol, and, by extension, to substance abuse generally, are vast and confused. The ensuing frustration and helplessness among the statesmen parallel the feelings of the adolescents about whom they are concerned: Washington, D.C. has the highest per capita alcohol consumption of any city in the country.

Concomitants and consequences have always existed to the abuse of alcohol (as well as to other substances). However, the additional possibility of estrangement from society in favor of living within a subculture of fellow-abusers is relatively new. For many years, opium haunts had existed in the Orient as a last way-station for the dissolute or for those whose lives had lost meaning. American "skid row" areas, however, did not become established until after the Civil War. At that time, many soldiers had fallen into alcoholism and could not readily return to the mainstream of society. They tended to frequent the same haunts, creating in the process a subculture of "Bowery bums." Currently, the largest influx of younger recruits to this life style has occurred since the depression of the 1930s. Significantly, the camaraderie among the drop-outs facilitates a lower suicide rate than among their alcoholic counterparts who remain in the larger community.

THE PHARMACOLOGY OF ALCOHOL

The frequent, ritual use of alcohol in social contexts acts as a potentiator of the prevailing mood. Birthdays, weddings, wakes, farewells, returns, coming of age, holidays, parties, etc., are all occasions where this use finds social approval. These are also situations in which children and adolescents are likely to experience a feeling of envy; they often feel excluded from the festive mood. The difference between the effects on one individual or another depends on the dosage, the personal meaning of the occasion, and the individual's personality, past drug experience and physiological status. The effect that is usually sought within these contexts is for the alcohol to create or enhance euphoria, enthusiasm, and a sense of excitement, and thus facilitate a more open, less anxious social interaction.

These anticipations correspond to the pharmacological effects of low levels of blood alcohol concentration (BAL). This is the most accurate reflection of dosage as it is experienced by the individual. The BAL depends on the food contents of the stomach and on the rate of absorption, detoxification, and excretion. The initial enhancement of excitation by alcohol is evident both in its effects on single nerve cells and on overall psychological function. As the BAL increases, however, the energizing effect is reversed; by the time the BAL is greater than .05 percent, verbal performance, learning, memory, and problem solving are all impaired.

As the BAL increases with more drinking, the onset of detrimental pharmacological effects is often masked by the anticipation of further enhancement. Anxiety is decreased after the ingestion of four to six ounces of alcohol, but by the time eight ounces have been consumed, it returns to the predrinking level.[92] As drunkenness is approached (at a BAL of .11 percent), the subjective feeling is that of being dizzy and delighted, exhilarated and stimulated. This is at variance with objective measurements. Personality changes typically occur in the direction of increased superficiality, impulsivity, and disorganization, qualities corresponding to specific impairments found in tests of sensory-motor and intellectual function.[89] Ego function changes in terms of decreased conventionality and there is loss of motivation which will continue on to relaxation and stupor as the BAL continues to rise. Personality shifts are likely to occur in the direction of more preoccupation with physical aggression and sex, coupled with decreased restraint.[69] Speech becomes thick, movement and coordination clumsy.

With increasing BAL, the prime effect is that of central nervous system depression, similar to what occurs with other anesthetics. With a BAL of .20 percent, the motor functions of the brain are grossly affected and the clinical state is "drunk and disorderly." At .30 percent, there is stupor, severe sensory impairment and dejection. At .40 percent, coma and anesthesia exist; the individual is "dead drunk." With BAL of .50 percent (or somewhat higher), the more primitive brain centers controlling breathing and heart beat are affected and death occurs.

The quality and course of the intoxication are also affected by the cogeners present in the drink. Cogeners are small molecule hydrocarbons which differ from one beverage to another and impart to each its characteristic flavor and aroma. Their concentration varies from a low in vodka (3.3 mg/ 100 ml) to a high in bourbon (2.85 mg/ml). More than 300 cogeners have been identified in wine. High cogener beverages show a greater risk than those with low cogeners.

The multiplicity of secondary pharmacologic effects from and sequelae to the use of alcohol are too extensive for full coverage here. The public

health ramifications of these elements however, are sufficiently widespread, inescapable and pathogenic, to warrant statement. They will serve as background to a consideration of the implications of alcohol abuse by children and adolescents, and the course of the alcoholism potential in such abuse.

SHORT TERM EFFECTS OF ALCOHOL
ON THE BODY

Nervous System: The role of alcohol as a CNS depressant is thought to be based on its effects on neurotransmitter release and biogenic amine metabolism. Specifically, at BALs greater than .30 percent,[89] a decrease occurs in MAO (mono-amine oxidase) and serotonin activity.[26]

Circulatory System: Alcohol impairs the mechanical performance of the heart, probably by depressing the efficiency of the myocardium.[58] Peripheral circulation is affected by a vasodilatation effect on the arterioles supplying the surface of the skin and by vasoconstriction of the arterioles within both the muscles and deeper skin.

Digestive System: In the stomach, alcohol increases the secretion of HCL and delays evacuation. At alcohol levels of 20 percent, hypersecretion of mucous occurs along with hemorrhages. Pancreatitis may follow, either as result of the blocking of the pancreatic duct from a spasm of the sphincter of Oddi, or by forcing HCL and bile up the duct as a result of vomiting.

Hepatic Function: The metabolism of both ethanol and its chief breakdown product, acetaldehyde, takes place in the liver. When this happens, there is an almost complete cessation of the metabolism of other substrates. With a constant alcohol consumption, the ethanol induced inhibition of the citric acid cycle causes a sharp decrease in fat oxidation which facilitates the accumulation of fat in the liver at a rate of up to 80 gm per day.[68]

LONGER TERM EFFECTS OF ALCOHOL
ON THE BODY

Diseases Attributed to Withdrawal:
1. Delirium tremens: Characterized by restlessness, irritability, hallocinosis, disorientation, a significant incidence of epileptiform seizures, and a 15 percent mortality.
2. Alcohol epilepsy: These are (rum fit) seizures which occur twelve to forty-eight hours after cessation of drinking. They are seen in individuals whose EEG, apart from this, is normal.

3. Abstinance or withdrawal syndrome ("the shakes"): The person is tremulous, overalert, easily startled, and sleepless.

Diseases Related to Nutritional Deficiencies:

1. Korsakoff's psychosis: This involves amnesia, disorientation, and confabulation. It is related to thiamine deficiency and is reversible with treatment.

2. Wernike's syndrome: This is manifested by tremor, ataxia, oculomotor palsies, memory loss, and confabulation. It is related to thiamine deficiency and is usually reversible.

3. Alcoholic deterioration: The affected person displays impulsivity, dementia, personality disintegration, and diffuse, irreversible cortical degeneration secondary to avitiminosis. It can be arrested with intervention.

4. Alcohol-vitamin deficiency polyneuritis: This includes parasthesia, weakness spreading from the legs to the trunk and arms; it can be reversed with treatment.

5. Alcoholic cerebellar degeneration: A condition of irreversible ataxia.

Diseases Resulting from the Effect of Alcohol on Premorbid Psychopathology:

1. Acute alcoholic hallocinosis: The patient suffers from terrifying hallucinations whose content is often accusing and homosexual.

2. Pathological intoxication: Hyperactivity, impulsivity, and amnesia occur superimposed on a hysterical substrate. Minimal alcoholic intake will precipitate such a reaction.

3. Alcoholic paranoia: This involves a delusional system and homosexual projections in a person with a premorbid paranoid personality.

Diseases Related to the Effect of Alcohol on the Gastrointestinal System:

1. Alcoholic gastritis: This includes inflammation and congestive hyperemia of the stomach; vomiting and incidental peptic ulcer are present.

2. Mallory-Weiss syndrome: Hematemesis related to vomiting is present along with retching. Lacerations of gastric mucosa occur.

3. Decrease of vitamin absorption from small intestine.

4. Pancreatic insufficiency and pancreatitis.

5. Fatty Liver: As much as 200 percent increase in the weight of this organ.

6. Alcoholic hepatitis: The systemic symptoms are fever, leukocytosis, and jaundice. It is a precursor of central sclerosing, hyaline necrosis, portal hypertension, and cirrhosis.

7. Laennec's cirrhosis: 10 percent of severe alcoholics develop this illness after ten to fifteen years. It involves portal hypertension, esophageal varices, and hemorrhage. These, along with hepatic failure, are the primary causes of mortality. The incidence of this condition is on the rise. Fifteen percent of those affected show an associated development of primary liver cell carcinoma.

Diseases Related to the Effect of Alcohol on the Circulatory System:

1. Alcoholic cardiomyopathy: Manifested by congestive heart failure, its dynamics are unknown.

Diseases Related to Effects on the Musculoskeletal System:

1. These include the acute, subclinical, and chronic myopathies. The patients experience cramps, weakness and muscle wasting. This is most common in the legs.

Endocrinological Disorder:

1. Silvestrini-Corda syndrome: This is a condition displaying the triad of Laennec's cirrhosis, testiculor atrophy, and breast enlargement.

Dermatologic Disorders Frequently Associated with Alcoholism:

1. Nummular eczema
2. Furunculosis
3. Rosacea
4. Seborrheic dermatitis
5. Secondary telangiectases

Cancers of Upper Digestive Tract, Respiratory Tract Related to Alcohol Use:

1. The nature of these associations is presently unknown.

THE DEVELOPMENT OF TOLERANCE
AND DEPENDENCE

Many people experience pleasurable effects and associations when they use alcohol. This carries with it a potential for the creation of psychological dependence. For different individuals, specific circumstances may impart to the intoxicated state a sense of being able to attain social adequacy, overcome depression, diminish anxiety, facilitate sexual gratification, and help establish intimacy. Any of these would tend to reinforce a drinking pattern quite early in a person's experience with alcohol.

Even with infrequent ingestion, tolerance to the pharmacologic effects of alcohol can ensue. The development of tolerance is thought to be physiologically related to the mechanisms which underlie physical dependence and withdrawal; the understanding of these relationships and dynamics is incomplete Hangover symptoms are in fact a mild withdrawal illness, but a full syndrome occurs only after prolonged and heavy drinking.

The circumstances of alcohol use in the United States are such that its potential for abuse is tremendous. Given its easy availability, social acceptability, its status as a sign of having come of age, and the broad lack of understanding of the associated problems, there is at present little to act as an effective restraint on its further use and abuse. Some investigators have felt that the incidence of adolescent alcohol users in the population has remained approximately constant over the last fifty years. However, most have felt that the incidence of young alcohol users has increased. Among these users, an approximately constant percentage will become abusers. These abusers display a wide variety of styles of abuse having to do with differences in class and subgroup. The essential sameness of the problem, however, renders these differences in style hardly worth mentioning; the corporation lawyer with his martinis at lunch, the truck driver with his six-pack during the ball game, the high school student with his pop-wine at the drive-in, and the matron with her champagne are all fit examples.

The various patterns of alcoholism and abuse (i.e., "long-term alcoholic," episodic intoxication, pathological drunkenness, etc.) do not contribute to an understanding of the roots, course, or solution of the problem. Hence, in this context, they will only be mentioned in passing. These matters of individual circumstance describe something of the complex interrelatons inherent in life. However, in considering substance abuse as a generic entity, they only provide a false focus.

There remain unanswered questions as to the preferential organic susceptibility of certain individuals and groups (i.e., Irish, American Indian, and Oriental). Some peoples have been said to acquire a pernicious pattern of alcohol use, affected by much less of it than is required to affect others. Essentially these are questions of individual threshold, a variable every individual should learn to respect with regard, not only to alcohol, but to everything.

The concept of "condition specific learning" has also been put forward as a possible basis for alcohol use. It is suggested that those who have learned under the influence of alcohol must get drunk again in order to use that learning. The existence of such a phenomenon may account for the fact that it does not seem possible to "retrain" alcohol abusers to be moderate social drinkers. The pattern seems to persist and can be re-triggered by even minimal drinking.

There is also a suspicion that infants born to drinking mothers may, as adults, have difficulty in assimilating alcohol in moderation. The question raised is whether the effect of an early metabolic familiarity with alcohol models the later handling of this substance as an adult.

EPIDEMIOLOGY OF ALCOHOL ABUSE

As of 1971, the U.S. Department of Health, Education, and Welfare estimated that there were 95 million users of alcohol in this country, 9 million of whom were abusers and 6 million alcoholics. This estimate was conservative at the time; as of 1975, it is calculated that there are 9 million problem drinkers and 9 million alcoholics, 18 million abusers in all. There are currently 5 billion gallons of liquor, wine, and beer sold annually for more than 23 billion dollars (up from 16.4 billion in 1969). Among alcohol users, there are significant differences in the likelihood of becoming abusers.[18] The distinguishing areas are these:

Sex Differences: Although among high-school-age youth, there are approximately an equal number of male and female drinkers, girls drink less than boys. In 1965, the Department of Health, Education, and Welfare estimated that 28 percent of male drinkers become heavy drinkers as opposed to only 8 percent of female drinkers, and there are at least five times as many male alcoholics as female (1 million women, 5 million men). Of those deemed heavy drinkers (12 percent of the general population), half are heavy-escape drinkers, whose excessive drinking is in the service of avoiding personal problems and social pressures (6 percent of the general population). A possible inference is that the level of mastery involved in achieving a satisfactory adjustment as a male is more difficult to attain and involves more frustration in this society than is necessary to fulfill a satisfactory female role.

Age Differences: Of the heavy drinkers, the highest proportion are found in men between the ages of thirty to thirty-four and forty-five to forty-nine (30 percent). Among the women, the highest proportion (10 percent) are between the ages twenty-one to twenty-four and forty-five to forty-nine. Among high school students, there has been a steady increase from 1968 to the present (1975) of those who drink. This includes those that drink at all, those that drink more than ten times yearly, and those whose drinking has caused problems. Presently, nearly 90 percent of male high school seniors drink alcohol, and 14 percent to the point of abuse.[39] Other estimates of the incidence of problem drinking in high school run as high as 50 percent.

Social Class Difference: Among all drinkers, the proportion of those who drink heavily tends to be higher in the lower socio-economic groups than in the higher. This observation is borne out by studies which show that 15 percent of semi-skilled and service workers who drink are, in fact, heavy drinkers.[18] More work per unit remuneration is apparently the curse of the drinking classes, but whatever the social class, frustrated competitive strivings are a common denominator.

City Size Differences: Residents of large urban areas show a consistently higher rate of heavy drinking than do residents of small towns.

Other Variables: Patterns of alcohol use and abuse are also unequally distributed according to ethnicity (fewer Jews, more Irish), religious practice (churchgoers less, unaffiliated more), and marital status (single and divorced more, married less). Of those children whose parents are alcoholic, 50 percent will presently become alcoholic themselves.

THE PHENOMENOLOGY AND SOCIAL
CONSEQUENCES OF SUBSTANCE ABUSE
(ALCOHOL)

The general assimilation of alcohol into American social life makes it the agent best suited for the covert expression of themes of frustration, depression, and destructiveness. If, in time, another substance is chosen, alcohol will then share this role with the new entrant.[54] Which substance comes to occupy this role varies with time, place, and fashion; in any case, alcohol has long been and remains the most popular means of developing destructive life styles. While no substance has a pharmacology which in itself can establish a commitment to destructiveness, the consequences and concomitants of alcohol abuse do in fact determine such a course. The associated phenomena are commonplace and widespread.

CONSEQUENCES WITHIN THE FAMILY

Within families where alcoholism flourishes, the children are both the victims of this pattern and the prime candidates for its perpetuation in the next generation.

They are prone to many forms of disturbance. These stem from the effects of parental deviance and social rejection. Within the home, the children are frustrated by the unpredictability and instability of the parents, who erratically punish

and praise, use the children against each other, and remain concerned totally with their own problems. During sober periods, the youngsters are often coddled and indulged; when the drinking occurs, however, they become subject to violent temper outbursts, inappropriate displays of nudity, abusive language, threats, and unprovoked punishment.[17, 48, 70] In their confusion, these children often blame themselves for their families' problems. Socially, these children are rejected on many counts. There is the stigma of their parents' alcoholism, their repertoire of socially disapproved behavior. They are further disadvantaged in terms of an increased incidence of school problems, educational failure, legal entanglements, and physical neglect.[19]

Both male and female children from such families have difficulty establishing appropriate adult sex roles. The male alcoholic's lack of self-discipline, dependence, irresponsibility, and sense of inadequacy are all at odds with an accepted masculine role and lead to identification problems in his children.[25] Sons are particularly affected; their essential male identification becomes dubious. If they identify with their father, they may later become problem drinkers; if they identify with their mother, there are immediate problems with heterosexual adjustment. Often enough, they remain mother-fixated behind a façade of macho toughness.[74, 90] Daughters tend to suffer severe neurotic problems and often seem unable to achieve a mature feminine sexual relationship as an adult. Half of the children from alcoholic homes, as compared to 10 percent of children generally,[79] are considered abnormal by their teachers. They show symptoms of emotional insufficiency, tension, depression, immaturity, and uneasiness. Their behavior is frequently deviant; it may include groundless fear, temper tantrums, opposition to authority, fighting with other children, school troubles which range from bad conduct to truancy, and isolated play.[9] The groundwork for the perpetuation of difficulties is laid early; of those who later develop an alcoholic pattern, 50 percent come from such a background.

In a family context of general stress and disagreement, with much arguing about who cares for whom and how, the dependency needs of the child are likely to be met in an erratic manner. Often there is major conflict about how these needs should be satisfied.[70] Within the child there is an exaggerated anxiety about revealing these needs; as a result they become intensified. As a defense against this inner pain, the child assumes an independent façade behind which the search for dependency-need satisfaction continues on a guarded but infantile level. Beset by doubts as to whether these needs will be met, the child does not develop a capacity to delay gratification. This low frustration tolerance often takes form as a tendency to impulsive action, argument, anger or withdrawal.[14]

A child with this developmental pattern retains the conflict about dependency as the covert but unmodified central issue in his personality structure. This fixation preserves a symbiotic, romanticized concept of how dependency needs might ideally be met, and the child attempts to ease the hurt to his injured self-esteem by seeking some approximation of gratification of these dependency strivings. In order to accomplish this, the child establishes a manipulative and self-centered style of connecting to others. Inevitably, this is associated with basic doubts as to self-worth and with feelings of inferiority, hostility, defensiveness, and guilt.

Ultimately, the child cannot work out issues of negative feelings, guilt, hostility, or, for that matter, of love and affection; there is simply insufficient maturity. This deficit is often hidden by the development of a superficial sociability and the avoidance of close personal relationships. In this way, an aura of adequacy, or even of superiority, may be developed without the risk of complications and anxiety. Issues of dependence, anger, and disappointment are avoided.[14] Underneath it all, the infantile ideals as to what might constitute a good relationship persist.

People who feel essentially inadequate because they are unable to elicit fulfillment of dependency needs consistently fear and try to avoid situations which test their adequacy. Intimate relations and work tasks are experienced[19] as threats to the preservation of their façade. As the pattern of avoidance continues, the child accumulates a backlog of nonaccomplishment and disconnectedness. This provides an external confirmation of inferiority feelings.

This sequence deepens the underlying depression. The associated anger can either be turned against others, or directed back at the self. The use of alcohol (or other substances) in this context is initially experienced as a respite from the stress of depression, a chemically induced euphoria. A person who is characterologically blocked from establishing an external basis for self-esteem and a state of good feeling about himself is immensely vulnerable. He becomes likely to turn to a chemically created good feeling and

is a good candidate for this to become an end in itself: a substance related "escapism."

The progression of this pattern, however, results in a general decline in the child's ability to create satisfaction in his external relationships. There is a decline as well in the ability of the substance to facilitate a compensatory euphoria. At the point where the choices are narrowed to chaos outside and depression inside, or oblivion through substance abuse, a slow suicide described by Menninger[72] ensues.

This capsule description of the intrapsychic development, difficulty, and destruction of a prototypical substance abuser defines the negative trends which assault him as he grows. Either these prevail, or they are prevailed against. The establishment of this pattern is reflected as well in his social patterns.

PERSONALITY STRUCTURE AND FAMILY DYNAMICS OF ALCOHOL ABUSERS

Alcohol abusers and other substance abusers tend to share certain personality traits. In their fully expressed form these traits lead to a life pattern of frustration and failure in interpersonal relationships. When this social difficulty is coupled with an extreme form of substance abuse, the result is a slow suicide with a myriad of associated problems. In their partially expressed form, these traits predispose to an erratic life course within which each resumption of substance abuse signifies the change to a destructive pattern ("falling off the wagon"). When this grouping of traits and associated life patterns is not present, the use of alcohol, or of any equivalent substance, is not likely to be linked to this set of overall destructiveness. In such instances, the substance abuse does not tend to progress.

In sum, the personality traits shared by potential and active substance abusers are dependency (often with an independent façade), low frustration tolerance, impulsivity, self-centeredness (narcissism), emotional isolation (often with a superficial sociability), feelings of inadequacy and depression. These traits signify characteristic ego defects; they develop within an individual on the basis of maturational experiences within a certain style of family. The pattern of this development is nowhere clearer than in the so-called "alcoholic family" in which similar personality and ego difficulties are predictably transmitted to 50 percent of the offspring. A description of this pattern follows:

DEVELOPMENT OF PATTERNS OF SUBSTANCE
ABUSE AMONG ADOLESCENTS

As adolescents grow up, there is a typical sequence in which the use of various substances are
introduced to their peer group.[38]

This sequence is as follows: (1) coffee and tea;
(2) beer and wine; (3) hard liquor; (4) tobacco;
(5) marijuana or hashish; (6) hallucinogens, stimulants, or depressants; (7) narcotics.[38, 54] These
substances are introduced with a wide time interval between each agent-grouping. This implies a
discrete decision making process with regard to
the use of the substance at each level. The available data tend to negate the hypothesis that it is
the use of one drug which leads to the use of
another. Instead, there seems to be a distinct subgroup of potential substance abusers who become
differentiated through their pattern of assimilating
these substances.

This subgroup of potential abusers share the
personality and developmental experiences just
described. Within a student population, they are
identifiable by virtue of specific characteristics.
They tend to ascend the hierarchy of drug use
rapidly and to use drugs for pleasure rather than
for curiosity. They are likely to be social and
gregarious and to date early; and more of their
time is spent with friends than in organized pursuits such as sports, homework, or religious activities. On the whole, they perceive themselves as
misunderstood by, and at odds with, parents,
teachers, and social institutions. They regard their
peer group interaction as more important than
intellectual preparation for a place in society as
a whole.[38] Their numbers include the overtly deviant, the delinquent, and the truant. In many
important ways they continue to be driven by
their internal needs as opposed to their need to
assimilate into the social order. Inevitably they
generate concern as to how they may be helped
to establish a constructive and integrated life for
themselves.

Although it may be too early to draw solid
conclusions on the matter, it is the prevailing impression that there is an absolute increase in the
incidence of both the use and abuse of alcohol
among adolescents. This increase does not seem to
exist among other age groups, and the longer
term implications of this possible trend are conjectural. If it is true, this increased abuse of
alcohol signals an increased allegiance to self-
absorbed and destructive life themes among the
youth of America.

Treatment and Therapeutic
Approaches to Substance Abuse

The essential change needed in the lives of substance abusers (or those vulnerable to the development of this syndrome) is to bring about
a fundamental alteration in their mode of connecting both to adults and to their peer group. Here,
success implies that they have been helped to
attain a positive self-concept. This must be based
on establishing connections in which their real
dependency needs can be met. Perhaps the essence
of the experience is to be able to share an optimistic and realistic vision of a fulfilling future with
an adult whom they respect.

Basic to this syndrome is a profound sense of
unfilled dependency needs along with self-defeating
attempts to attain compensatory gratification. This
intrapsychic state is expressed in terms of pseudo-
independence, low self-esteem, hypersensitivity to
the risks inherent in growth, anger, oppositionalism, delinquency, and depression. Direct attempts
to limit the destructiveness inherent in this attitude usually do not succeed. The only recourse
open to the youth is the establishment of a growth
promoting alliance with a mature person and
with his ideals. Through such a connection, a
positive growth oriented frame of reference may
supplant the negative assumptions connected with
the syndrome of abuse. Lacking such a connection and the accompanying inner change, the destructiveness in the internal state will find a host
of ways through which it can be expressed.

As any parent knows, humans are ambivalent
about growing up. At best, loss of infantile dependency is compensated for when creative autonomy is well rewarded; a more mature form of
mutually contributing dependencies is then established. At worst, as children grow, they find some
way to perpetuate their dependency on their parents. With increasing age, the symptoms of this
dependency-seeking continue to change. They are
accordingly responded to with differing qualities
of concern; thus, excessive thumb sucking, excessive masturbation, and excessive use of psychoactive substances elicit qualitatively different responses from parents and society as a whole.

THERAPEUTIC CONSIDERATIONS IN TREATING
SUBSTANCE ABUSE

Each facility for the treatment of alcohol
abusers attempts to alleviate alcohol related diffi-

culties in its own way; only the language and style differ. Thus: missions encourage repentance, prisons hope for "going straight," psychiatric institutions look for insight and "working through," social workers hope to "mobilize independence," and medical doctors warn that "the body can't take any more." For each approach, however, the rate of recidivism is within the range of 75 to 90 percent. And yet, as a result of the work of each of these modalities, there are some alcoholics who change their level of function.

Those who do abandon a pattern of abuse and take up a course with greater possibility of fulfillment are defined in the process as those for whom there is hope; for whom change is possible. Functionally, progress can be made toward a more basic "working through" of the core dependency of the abuse pattern. Some individuals shift out of an abuse pattern solely on the basis of some profound inner experience; it is far more usual, however, for such changes to take place within a facilitating interpersonal context. Either way, the abuser overcomes the emptiness which he has been attempting to fill with drugs or alcohol. A sense of significant identity or a commitment to an idea or mission supplants the feeling of hunger and need which underlies the abuse pattern.

Such a pivotal relationship may develop between an abuser and another person without regard for their categorical qualifications. Psychiatry describes the process in terms of identification, attachment, and working through. Whatever the terms, the process is similar, whether it involves a clergyman, probation officer, social worker, doctor, psychologist, group leader, nurse, teacher, friend, or anyone else. The pitfalls, too, are similar. The differing contexts within which these connections are made depend on the indefinable subtleties which cause some people to be attracted to each other, and others not. The possibilities are as limitless as life itself.

If there is to be any enduring change made in the life style of the abuser, a certain sequence must ensue. The initial phase of attachment gives the promise of improvement; but if that possibility is to be realized, however, it must be succeeded by "working through" to a solidly realized position of constructive functioning. Here again, the means by which this process is facilitated are varied and ultimately mysterious. It is not possible to quantify the exact preconditions necessary for the successful crystallization of a higher level of function. Whatever the specifics, they will include a dynamic balance of support and aloneness, love and anger, hope and despair, consolidation of gain and coping with loss, and growth of inner awareness or strength. Additionally, there will always be a sphere within which the newly acquired strengths can be exercised: in potential relationships for the isolated, in potential training for the unskilled, in potential work for the passive, in potential reward for the skeptical, and in potential help for the rough spots en route.

PITFALLS TO PROGRESS IN TREATMENT

Alcoholics and other substance abusers are known to most professional "helpers" as extremely difficult therapeutic challenges. Few therapists enjoy working with them because of the characteristics outlined previously. Once a pattern of failure and frustration has developed, the abuser is likely to repeat it over and over again. The same helper is then once more in a position of having to handle "the situation," each time with more and more negativity.

The usual pattern is this: on the heels of a crisis involving substance abuse, a potentially helpful relationship is established on both sides, with the hope that the establishment of this relationship heralds a change in the life pattern. All other things being equal in the total life picture, the abuser continues with the therapeutic relationship in high hopes that some facilitating magic will somehow ensue; that he will be rescued. In the course of time, of course, this magic change fails to materialize. Disappointment then leaves the substance abuser full of tension, anger, and longings, the usual solution to which is another excursion into abuse. The aftermath of such episodes is a re-grouping of the therapeutic alliance within a context of mutual disenchantment. The gradual crystallization of roles defines the relationship as that between a frustrated (or ineffectual) helper on the one hand, and a disappointed (or pessimistic) abuser on the other.

The essential failure of this process lies in the fact that it repeats within the transference the dependent expectations and disappointment of the child. Moreover, it does this without either working through the ambivalence or establishing viable peer relations within which both positive and negative feelings can be experienced. Where such a peer connection does take place, it provides an "other-oriented" reference as the basis for action. One experiences living in terms of being the proponent of a significant idea, of having a "mission" or purpose. In the absence of this basic shift, the experience of "reform" or abstinence is one of deprivation, and a return to the abuse pattern is assured.

THERAPEUTIC SUCCESS IN WORKING WITH SUBSTANCE ABUSERS

The essence of facilitating change among substance abusers, of helping them achieve productive life patterns, lies within the area of peer relatedness. As described, the typical course of a helping relationship recapitulates the development of the difficulties without opening any path toward a new realm of experience within the peer group. Whatever outward signs of improvement might have flourished during the "honeymoon period" with the therapist, peer relations are likely to have preserved a quality of being either an alliance of losers, frustrated competitiveness, or passive-aggressive submission.

The creation of peer bonds is a process which requires a very special social situation. This involves a consistent and supportive peer group, which possesses both appreciation of the difficulties and optimism for the ultimate accomplishment of the necessary changes. Although there will be group leaders, the group as a whole, rather than any individual, will be tacitly acknowledged to be the primary focus. The life patterns of most substance abusers have served to exclude them from such a supportive peer situation. Moreover, among many of the nonabusers deemed "successful," the same self-centered, competitive dynamics are present as among the abusers; the difference is that the successes are winners in the same game in which the abusers are the losers.

ALCOHOLICS ANONYMOUS

The healing professions have generated many proposals for providing substance abusers with therapeutic situations. When implemented, any such proposal will make a number of professionals available and establish a clientele. Presently there will be some rehabilitated program "graduates" who have established more productive life patterns. Within most programs, the drop-outs, recidivists, and perpetuators of the abuse pattern outnumber those who have made fundamental changes. The most notable exception to this generality is found within the structure of Alcoholics Anonymous, whose present membership is approximately 800,000. The elements contributing to this relative success will be discussed here.

The initial advantage of this program is based on its voluntary nature, those who are unwilling to make a commitment to change tend not to become involved. There is a familiar repertoire of promises that "it will not happen again" or a denial that any problem exists at all, which is frequently part of a continuing alcoholic pattern. Some cities have instituted programs in which drivers with multiple arrests for drunken driving have a choice of participating in an AA program or losing their drivers' licenses. It is not known whether the rate of success with these coerced members is as great as with others.

Once an alliance with AA has been made, the individual abuser becomes an equal-based participant. It is, however, implied that the group is the authority to which one relates about the problem. This process in itself dilutes the transference. This is a useful effect, because of the peer status of the helpers and because of the greater capacity of the group as a whole to work with the probable backsliding as the connection is tested. Participation implies that the narcissism which demands a mother-child type dyad in which to function has been held in abeyance by the structure of the group. Or, it may mean that the group has become the mother.

Another advantage of the AA approach is that participation provides a channel for both time and energy which might otherwise be searching for a theme, if not a bottle. A "Great Idea" is offered to which one may make a commitment: the idea of getting out of a terrible and destructive life pattern against all odds, and of helping others to get out as well. Cynics have identified the process as one in which there is an alternation between the roles of rescuer and rescued. In fact, unless a group is stagnant or inbred, this is not a flaw but a strength. Group participation is fostered from both the giving and receiving end. The process of both giving and receiving help, as well as congregating to share experiences, has much in common with the function of any group of close friends who have given and received help from one another over the years.

The great diversity of AA groups makes it likely that a group can be found where the majority of the individuals are truly peers. There are groups of mental patients, professional people, homosexuals, entertainers, teenagers, laborers, and those with special religious inclinations. Additionally, there are groups for teenagers whose parents are alcoholic, 50 percent of whom might themselves be (statistically) expected to develop alcoholic patterns.

The structure of the organization is such that the development of more constructive modes of peer relationship is implicit in the course of participation in an appropriate group. This group, moreover, is likely to be similar to an alternative peer group with which the abuser might otherwise be pursuing a destructive course; in any case, once he belongs, he is very far from living in isolation.

THERAPEUTIC TREATMENT SETTINGS

There are many elements which contribute to the relative success of the AA format. These are not the exclusive province of that organization; indeed, these factors are basic to the success of any group which attempts to work with substance abusers. Each city has organizations aimed at providing this kind of help, and each separate group has its own reputation, vicissitudes, supporters, detractors, successes and failures. Many of these organizations had originally aimed at abusers of specific agents; now they have expanded their scope to include poly-abusers or abusers of agents other than those they originally addressed.

As has been described, the family is the basic unit within which the potential abuser learns the flawed interactional and emotional patterning which provides the foundation for his difficulty. All treatment units function as family surrogates and hope to provide the participants with corrective modeling. At present, work is being done with alcoholics in which family members or close friends are included as "co-patients" during the final period of an eight-week, in-patient program. This approach, called "familization therapy," organizes a therapeutic family of about thirty people of both sexes and all ages. Within this group, interactional patterns are both lived out and examined. The goal of the work is to enable the abuser to establish more sustaining and supportive relationships; these, in turn, will act to minimize the frustrations which are the stimuli for escape into an episode of abuse.

Many cities have a number of live-in programs for adolescents and young adults that serve those whose flawed social patterning and substance abuse necessitate an all-inclusive surrogate family context. In such a setting, alternative living styles can be learned, while the old patterns are held in check. Such organizations as the Salvation Army's Manhattan Project, and Cri-Help are peer-group oriented programs which attempt to provide their participants with a fulfilling experience in living.

Other group homes serve primarily as foster placements for young people with juvenile court entanglements. They utilize psychodynamic approaches that are closely related to those described. Such homes frequently employ psychiatric consultants to assist in maintaining a therapeutic process and to help avoid the regressive enactment of the same patterns that led to the original difficulties.

CONTAINMENT SETTINGS, THERAPEUTIC AND OTHERWISE

For a great many victims of this syndrome, the patterns of destructiveness and substance abuse include an inability to participate voluntarily in an alternative process. Ultimately, they get themselves locked up in a setting which is designed to prevent harm to themselves or to others. It is quite often a matter of chance whether a given adolescent with a constellation of substance abuse and behavior problems will be dealt with by the juvenile court or by a psychiatric hospital. As a rule, however, depressive manifestations and bizarre destructive behavior are more evident among the hospitalized.

In any case, by far the larger number of these young abusers is handled by the juvenile court system, and the facilities employed are most often equivalent to a junior prison. At best, destructive behavior is limited during the duration of the confinement, and the ensuing probationary period may be one in which useful alliances are established either with a probation officer or a group home. While the outward manifestations of the problem pattern may be checked, the usual inner experience is one of sustained connection to the old ways. The interpersonal patterns tend to be either cold or brutalized. Survival is facilitated by an inner promise that the future holds more of the old comforts, including alcohol and drugs, but that next time incarceration will be avoided. Occasionally, counseling during this period proves to be helpful; it is often accepted under duress, however, and the destructive themes are minimized in homage to the fact that one is being "observed." Although this kind of forced compliance is not a mature position, it recapitulates the normal and common status of children who are unwillingly obliged to follow the directives of their parents "for their own good." Hopefully, in the course of this supervised period of dissembled virtue, constructive pursuits will supplant the process of covert resentment.

A minority of the adolescents haled into court are only on the verge of adopting the personality dynamics associated with substance abuse. Such youngsters will be sufficiently jolted by the experience of actually being incarcerated, or having therapy "threatened," to "clean up their act," i.e., cultivate alternative behavior. In essence, the "limit testing" aspect of their behavior has discovered that a firmly held limit does exist. If their parents failed to respond to destructive behavior with clear constraint, then society would do so.

The majority of those who appear in the juvenile courts, however, are on their way to becoming committed to a continuing pattern of recurrent trouble and destructive acting out. The punitive, limit-setting structure provided by the court becomes the senior party to a dialogue which too often continues into adulthood. This format is consciously resented. However, it is maintained because it fills powerful unconscious dependency needs. Indeed, it serves as an alternative to the destruction and chaos that would otherwise accompany the substance abuse. Although this form of abuse does not in itself cause a pattern of criminality, those juvenile offenders who are abusers often pursue a more serious course of delinquency than those who are not.[50]

The generality seems to be that the majority of those who become established in a pattern of alcoholism or substance abuse persist in that pattern to the point of their own dependence or destruction. The most common outcome is some mixture of alternating abuse, destructiveness, dependence, and reform, with an accompanying chronic depression and a shortened life span. Among young people, a picture of accelerating abuse serves notice that they are on the brink of despair, and that help is mandatory.

Even the better programs aimed at those who have become entrenched in an abuse pattern can claim only modest success. Most of the institutions established to contain the abusers or treat the consequences of abuse are simply futile. Given these facts, it follows that the most effective outreach to the potential and early abuser lies in preventative work in the social, political, economic, and cultural sphere. Many of the corrective instruments which must be brought to bear at the interface between the abuser and society have been described in connection with the workings of Alcoholics Anonymous. Further discussion of the necessary facilitators to resolve abuse patterns will be included in the final section on "Primary Prevention."

There are a number of treatment modalities available for older alcoholics which are seldom employed with adolescents. Private sanitariums, hospitals, alcoholic units, and the like rarely work with adolescents; their developmental status essentially excludes them from assimilation into such a milieu. Such programs tend to have a recurring clientele unless integrated into an overall corrective plan such as described with AA. Disulfiram (Antabuse), which renders an individual susceptible to becoming ill if alcohol is ingested, is a treatment adjunct rarely employed in adolescents, although it might conceivably be useful in certain instances.

An exploration was attempted to study the potential of LSD as an aid in the disruption of alcohol abuse patterns, but political realities interfered. In certain instances, the initial work gave promise of some success.[1] Implicit in this and in other methods that have fallen from favor is an essential element identical to that described and still employed: an alternative to alcoholism which provides a theme within which maladaptive patterning can be worked out.

Barbiturates

Among the depressants, known as "downers" to the abusing adolescents, barbiturates are the most frequently employed as agents of abuse. The pharmacology and the subjective effect of these agents is similar to alcohol, and seems to represent the preferred "high" sought by the majority of contemporary adolescent abusers. The pharmacologic effects involve a progression through states of sedation, hypnosis, and anesthesia, to coma, and to death.

MEDICAL USES

The discovery of the hypnotic properties of barbital in 1903 by Fischer and Von Baeyer marked the beginning of the rapid development of the barbiturates as medical agents. Phenobarbital, introduced in 1912, became the standard treatment for epilepsy and a commonly employed sedative. Varying substitutions on the basic barbituric acid nucleus facilitated the development of shorter acting compounds whose effects lasted six to eight, as opposed to eight to sixteen, hours. Amytal (1923) and Seconal (1930) were favored as hypnotics ("sleeping pills") whose effects would have worn off by morning. In the mid-1930s, sulphur-containing derivatives were synthesized and found to possess very brief durations of action (fifteen minutes to one hour) and were introduced as intravenous anesthetics. Thiopental (Pentothal, 1935) was the first of this group.

Further uses of the barbiturates include intravenous use of short-acting compounds for the control of acute convulsions, as a pre-anesthetic sedative which reduces the amount of anesthesia required for surgery, and as an adjunct to psychotherapy for the retrieval of suppressed material ("Truth serum").

PHARMACOLOGY

The usual hypnotic dose of the short acting barbiturates is 100 to 200 mg. When used as a sedative, one-fourth to one-third of this dose is prescribed. Anesthesia occurs with approximately 1 gm and coma with 3 gm. Death will ensue at about the same dosage as is necessary to induce coma. The longer acting agents require about 5 gm to achieve the corresponding effect. In order to prevent intentional overdosage, physicians are advised to prescribe these drugs in amounts insufficient to cause serious poisoning: no more than thirty 100 mg capsules of short-acting, and no more than 5 mg of long-acting.[7]

Barbiturates are absorbed rapidly through the stomach wall in the presence of the normal gastric acidity. Antacids and a basic stomach, however, cause the ionization of barbiturates and absorption is delayed. Similarly, a full stomach retards the rate of absorption so that a dose which might otherwise produce profound depressive effects may cause only mild sedation.

Elimination of long-acting barbiturates depends largely on their unchanged excretion by the kidneys. Short-acting barbiturates, however, are metabolized by the liver, and the rate is controlled by drug-metabolizing enzymes. Since the formation of these enzymes is accelerated following repeated exposure to barbiturates, a tolerance to short-acting barbiturates is quick to develop and figures significantly in the abuse characteristics of these compounds.

In combination with other drugs, other CNS depressants (tranquilizers, narcotics, and alcohol) augment the depressant effects of the barbiturates, while CNS stimulants (caffeine and the amphetamines) counteract this depressant effect. Thus, in many drug related deaths, a combination of alcohol and barbiturate has been found.

The toxicology of the barbiturates parallels that of alcohol. In amounts of three to five times the hypnotic dose, tremor, incoordination, visual difficulties, and thinking difficulties appear. These effects are evident in about one-half hour, last two hours, and disappear in four to five hours. The nervousness, tremor, and headache seen the next day are equivalent to a hangover. Five to ten times the usual hypnotic dose causes moderately

severe poisoning, and fifteen times the hypnotic dose is life-threatening.

Treatment of barbiturate poisoning consists of supporting blood pressure and respiration, while facilitating the urinary excretion of the drug through diuresis or by the use of the artificial kidney. There are no antagonists to barbiturates.

BARBITURATE ABUSE AND DEPENDENCE

The dependence liability of barbiturates was not recognized until the early 1950s, a full fifty years after their introduction. In 1950, Isbell and Fraser,[47] working at the United States Public Health Service Hospital at Lexington, described the pattern of chronic barbiturate intoxication and withdrawal. More recently, it has been recognized that the nonbarbiturate hyposedatives and the minor tranquilizers also create a barbiturate-like dependence.

The barbiturate-dependent state resulting from ingestion of larger than therapeutic doses over a period of time is similar to alcoholism but does not lead to the related disease states of malnutrition, mental deterioration, nerve damage, liver disease, and visual defects.[8] The dependent state, while under the influence of the drug, is characterized by symptoms similar to alcohol intoxication. There is a psychological dependence, a craving to continue to use the drug. Physiological dependence develops as well, and abstinence precipitates a withdrawal syndrome of delirium, convulsions, and fever. A tolerance to the effects of the drug develops so that increasing doses are required to produce indications of an overdose. There is also a mutual cross dependence with alcohol, other hypnosedatives, and minor tranquilizers.[7]

Tolerance to the effects of barbiturates develops largely on the basis of hepatic enzyme induction. As a result, the rate of metabolism of the drug is increased by the continued presence of the drug. Further tolerance results from a decrease in the sensitivity of the CNS to barbiturates and other depressants. Although individuals differ in terms of the maximum dose to which they develop tolerance, each person has a certain limit to which tolerance can develop. Beyond this point, additional barbiturates result in symptoms of acute intoxication. For short-acting barbiturates, tolerance is often complete at doses up to 500 mg/day. However, at doses greater than 800 mg/day, there are always some signs of intoxication. The acquisition of tolerance does not mean that it takes any more barbiturates to reach a lethal dose; it only implies that there is an increase in the amount required to cause clinical drunkenness.

All of the nonbarbiturate hypnosedatives and all of the minor tranquilizers share certain characteristics in common. They produce symptoms of intoxication, tolerance, dependence, and an abstinence syndrome similar to that seen with alcohol and the barbiturates. These agents include meprobamate (Miltown and Equanil), glutethimide (Doriden), methyprylon (Noludar), ethchlorvynol (Placidyl), methaqualone (Quaalude), chlordiazepoxide (Librium), and diazepam (Valium).

Drug dependence develops with the barbiturates and other depressants at dosages five to seven times the therapeutic dose taken on a daily basis. The exceptions to this generality are the minor tranquilizers, diazepam and chlordiazepoxide. These require a multiple of ten to thirty times the therapeutic dose to produce physical dependence. A daily dose of 600 to 800 mg of secobarbital or pentobarbital taken for a period of thirty-five to fifty-seven days is sufficient to produce withdrawal symptoms, serious enough to require medical attention.

Given a drug dependent state, an attempt at abstinence is followed by an asymptomatic period of from eight to sixteen hours. During this time, signs of intoxication diminish and the patient may be mistakenly assumed to be improving. The onset of the withdrawal reaction is then heralded by anxiety, agitation, confusion, insomnia, nausea, and vomiting. Coarse tremors of the face and hands appear along with increased deep tendon reflexes. Pulse and respiration rates increase, and there is a rise in blood pressure, with a tendency for postural hypotension accompanied by fainting. After twenty-four to thirty hours of abstinence, these "minor symptoms" intensify and are followed by the major symptoms of convulsions and delirium.[7] Although convulsions may occur between the second and eighth day of abstinence, they are most common at about thirty hours.[45] These seizures are sufficiently similar to typical grand mal epilepsy that the one may easily be mistaken for the other. In the course of a two or three day period of insomnia, a psychotic state similar to alcoholic delirium tremens gradually develops. Vivid and frightening auditory and visual hallucinations begin, often with a paranoid content and accompanied by exhausting agitation. This withdrawal psychosis may last anywhere from one or two days to several months; at length it terminates spontaneously with a prolonged sleep. It is thought that the hallucinosis may represent an attempt to make up for the loss of REM sleep

which accompanies barbiturate abuse.[28] An elevated temperature of somewhat above one hundred degrees occurs during the withdrawal psychosis. A continued rise in temperature is a life threatening sign.[29]

Medically supervised barbiturate withdrawal is accomplished by administering the short-acting barbiturates at the level of addiction and reduction of the dose by 100 mg. daily. The determination of the actual level of addiction cannot be made on the basis of patient reporting. The actual content of street barbiturates is both low and variable, and the reporting of these patients is usually grossly unreliable. The level of addiction is more reliably determined by response to test-challenge doses of short-acting barbiturates.

POTENTIAL FOR ABUSE

The barbiturates, the nonbarbiturate sedatives, and the minor tranquilizers possess similar pharmacologic and withdrawal characteristics. Nonetheless, compared to longer-acting phenobarbital, the dependence and abuse potential of the short-acting barbiturates is much greater. Nonbarbiturate hypnosedatives such as glutethimide and meprobamate possess an intermediate potential for abuse, and the minor tranquilizers diazapam and chlordiazepoxide are least likely to be used in this way. It turns out, however, that even these minor tranquilizers generate psychological dependence. This can be sufficiently intense so that it is often most difficult to achieve a voluntary abstinence from these agents after a period of use at a normal therapeutic level. There is little abuse of phenobarbital in spite of its liability for dependence. The reason seems to be that it does not have either an intense pharmacologic effect or a rapid onset. Similarly, the very short-acting barbiturates have not become agents of abuse; their duration of effect is too brief. In sum, the correlates of dependence and abuse potential are the quality, intensity, and duration of the drug effect,[30] parameters which make the short-acting barbiturates the inevitable favorites.[7]

EPIDEMIOLOGY

Since the abuse of hypnosedatives depends heavily on illicit production, it is virtually impossible to estimate with accuracy the extent to which these drugs are abused. In the late 1960s, it was estimated that a full half of the Lilly Company's production of Seconal was finding its way to the illicit market, nor were there any obvious ways this shunt could be controlled. Between 1966 and 1970, the volume of barbiturates legally produced rose at an annual rate of 18 percent. With half of the total production being short-acting barbiturates, as of 1962 this represented more than twelve doses of 100 mg for each person in the United States.[77]

Prior to 1970, there was no clear picture of increase in the abuse of hypnosedatives by nonmedical users and particularly by younger people. By 1971 secobarbital abuse was considered to have reached epidemic proportion in some locales, and secobarbital, particularly the illicit Mexican product, was thought to be replacing marijuana as the most popular illicit drug.[29] It is impossible, and finally unprofitable, to attempt to pin down overall trends with regard to hypnosedative abuse. As of 1975, in Los Angeles, the availability of street "reds" (Seconal) continued to be ubiquitous in the schools. But the number of instances of abuse and cases of withdrawal fell. Indeed, true dependence is something of a rarity among the adolescent population. This decrease may relate to a number of factors. There is greater sophistication among the using students; there is a higher incidence of patterns of multiple abuse which serves to reduce potential reliance on the barbiturates to "stay high"; and there may be a decrease in the content of the average "red," usually between 30 to 50 mg each as opposed to 100 mg in a pharmaceutical capsule. It is likely that at the most frequent level of usage, the majority of adolescent barbiturate abusers achieve a state of being "tranquilized" rather than intoxicated.

One recent, but logical phenomenon on the adolescent drug scene, has been the appearance of Valium as a street drug. Valium is the most widely prescribed drug in history; 15 percent of the population is taking it. At this rate, it finds a place in about 40 percent of the medicine cabinets of the country. Not surprisingly, it has become a drug widely pilfered by teenagers. Many parents, who have been careful to hide sleeping pills, have never considered Valium as requiring safekeeping; meanwhile, it is viewed by many adolescents as being about on a par with "reds."

The Opiates

HISTORY

Of all pharmaceutical agents, none generate more concern about their potential abuse than do the narcotic analgesics. The possibility of opiate addiction has been given conceptual precedence over the analgesic action of these drugs. This has been carried to the extent that in the United States, it is common medical practice for the terminally ill to be permitted to suffer needlessly so that the medical and nursing professions may avoid guilt about contributing to an ignominious deathbed addiction.

Opium eating, with a recognized dependence liability, had been common for centuries among Asian peasants; smoking opium followed the introduction of tobacco in the seventeenth century. A century later, opium eating had become fashionable among the upper and middle classes in England, particularly among artists, poets, and writers. Its use spread to the lower classes through an increasingly wide use of opium-containing patent medicines. Presently, it came to the United States from England, and from China by way of the influx of Chinese laborers to the West Coast.

In the mid-nineteenth century, the purification of morphine and the invention of the hypodermic syringe escalated the dependence liability of opiates. The first group to become addicted to intravenously injected narcotics was the great number of analgesic dependent wounded, caused by the Civil War. All of these circumstances combined to create a situation in which, by the late nineteenth century, an estimated 4 percent of the United States population was habituated to opiates.

The cures that were developed for opiate habituations invariably involved the substitution of one opiate for another. Heroin was introduced in 1898 as a new cure for morphine addiction with such encouraging results that the suspicion that it, too, was addicting did not occur for years.

Preliminary legislation aimed at the control of narcotic substances did little to ameliorate the problem. However, it did lead to increasingly strict control of these substances by the government. The Harrison Narcotics Act of 1914 eliminated the nonmedical availability of opiates, imposed a tax on opiates, and required the registration of persons involved in the distribution and manufacture of narcotics. Following these legislative actions and the increase in public concern and awareness, the number of habitual users dropped to one fourth of 1 percent of the United States population. Approximately the same holds true today.

The relative reduction in the use of opiates was probably also affected by a change in the prevailing attitude toward both agents and users. Initially, those who had become opiate dependent in the course of medical treatment were recognized as victims of unfortunate side effects associated with a useful agent, or dupes hooked on a patent concoction. Later, those continuing use of the opiates were seen as weak and as needing guidance. When the clinics set up to dispense opiates to official addicts were found to be providing some narcotics for unsanctioned use, they were closed, and increasingly stringent guidelines were established to separate the legitimate users of a problem drug from the narcotics abusers. Medically unsanctioned use of narcotics was forced underground, and users were increasingly viewed as scofflaws and criminals. The opiates themselves were seen as possessing a demonic hold on their users. The situation became a nightmare.

The process of criminalizing narcotics and those who use them culminated in the tragic conundrum of issues involving attempts to control the drugs and deal with the users that society faces today. At this point, bare mention will be made of the complex issues surrounding the Drug Enforcement Administration's fruitless attempts to choke off a supply of illegal opiates, and the frustration of "treating" committed addicts. In considering the vastly confused area of opiate abuse, a cardinal point to keep in mind is that any drug abuse is a phenomenon based on the presence and acceptability of the agent within the subculture. Further, the role played by the drug in the lives of the using population varies according to the overall life adjustment of the user. No drug can eliminate meaningful pursuits from the lives of its users. Those whose lives are lacking in rewarding life pursuits and commitments, however, are those who constitute the highest risk group for drug involvement.

That this is also true of involvement with the opiates is a recently recognized fact. It had long been an assumption of both professionals and the public that narcotics possess the power to take hold of a person's life, supplant the cultivation of alternative life themes, and lead to enslavement. Within the past decade, epidemiological studies of Viet Nam servicemen and adolescents who had become involved with heroin use have provided a different understanding of the interaction between the user and the agent:

1. Given a similarly stressed and homogeneous peer group, heroin use proceeds on the basis of peer to peer influence as opposed to the influence of a dealer or pusher on vulnerable individuals.

2. Ninety percent of heroin users are not addicted to the drug but are occasional users ("chippers"). Among those 10 percent who do become addicted, most withdraw themselves. At that point, they either desist or, after a period of time, become "chippers." Present estimates place the number of addicts nationwide at 400,000.[13]

3. There appears to be no reliable difference between the capacity of chippers and nonusers to fulfill their social obligations and pursue constructive life themes. However, habitual users show a poly-abuse pattern as a rule. The destructive themes in their lives are more often furthered through alcohol, depressants, or marijuana than through heroin itself.

4. In his involvement with the drug, the heroin addict has provided himself with a life pursuit: getting the drug, having the drug, etc. The fact is the addict perceives life as revolving around narcotics as a center. All the failure, the difficulty, and the pleasure in his life are attributed to the drug.

Currently there appears to be a rise in heroin use. The pattern of spread has shown an increase among middle-class whites in middle-sized cities as opposed to black and Latin American populations in large metropolitan areas. The phenomenon has aroused public concern, especially since it is evident that all of the attempts to affect the course of the use of heroin have been essentially ineffectual. This is only one aspect of the growing poly-abuse of multiple illegal substances. This practice is engaged in by large segments of the population who otherwise appear to be following a nondeviant course. Among other issues, there is the long-standing fear that these drugs will cause a breakdown in the structure of society.

The increase in the use of many drugs, including heroin, reflects the direction of social change. In a sense, it defines the direction of a new normative behavior. Similarly, the extent to which heroin and other agents are used is a reflection of the degree to which society affects its less integrated members. The problem of destructiveness is not a drug problem but a social problem. The solutions to such problems must then be social solutions, and cannot be achieved through the regulation of drugs. To imagine that the Department of Environmental Affairs or any regulatory agency might provide a meaningful change in the direction of the lives of the problem abusers is to fall into the error of the heroin addict himself. He sees all life in terms of the presence or absence of his drug.

PHARMACOLOGY

There are pharmacological generalities that apply to all of the narcotic analgesics. These include opium, its chief derivatives, morphine, codeine, the semisynthetic opiates, and the synthetic opiates.

None of the newer agents are clinically superior to morphine, nor do they lack the pitfalls of tolerance, physical dependence, and psychological dependence associated with its use.

Ten mgs of intramuscularly injected morphine, repeated every four hours, will provide analgesia sufficient to relieve severe pain. Moreover, it will accomplish this with relatively little sedation or respiratory depression. Although there may be individual variations, all of the opiates and synthetic opiates have about the same incidence of unwanted side effects. Morphine remains the standard of comparison. Less severe pain can be effectively relieved with orally administered codeine, meperidine, methadone, etc., particularly in combination with aspirin.

Narcotics produce sedation, tranquility, euphoria, and sleep. They are used for these reasons in situations where anxiety and dysphoris are associated with pain, as in terminal cancer and myocardial infarctions. Similarly, they are often used preoperatively.

Following the intravenous administration of an opiate, two distinct parts of the experience have been described. The instantaneous and brief "rush," representing the initial impact of the opiate on the brain, is overwhelmingly pleasant for most people. It has been likened to a huge, total body orgasm. Often there is a sense of increased psychomotor activity and energy called "drive," and an intense abdominal sensation with itching and flushing of the skin called a "thrill." The longer lasting "high" following the initial rush is one in which consciousness is dreamlike and pleasant. The person is shielded from the kinds of distress caused by emotions, cares, anxieties, and hedonistic drives. This "high" is accompanied by a religious-like turning inward of attention. There is a profound sense of well-being, and a tendency to go "on the nod," to drift suddenly into a brief sleep which is ended by a sudden awakening. This state has been likened to a regression to the tranquil, protected existence of the fetus, far removed from the drives and tensions of the real world.

OPIATE POISONING AND OVERDOSE

Each year, clinical, accidental, or suicidal overdose is believed to kill 1 percent of heroin dependent persons. The clinical presentation of an opiate overdose includes pinpoint pupils, depressed respiration, a state of stupor or coma, and subnormal temperature. There will be needle marks on the skin, and morphine will be present in the urine. The slowed respirations and irregular and often gasping, and are associated with hypoxia and cyanosis. This respiratory depression may lead to shock, cardiopulmonary arrest, and death. These symptoms are dramatically reversible with a narcotic antagonist.[21]

Another mechanism of opiate poisoning has been described as acute intravenous narcotism; it is responsible for many of the sudden deaths in heroin addicts. The clinical picture of opiate toxicity is accompanied by a severe exudative alveolar pulmonary edema. Often the presentation is that of frothy white edema fluid filling the trachea and oozing from the mouth and nostrils. Although the outcome is frequently death, in twenty-four to thirty-six hours a return to a normal status may occur either with or without treatment. If the patient survives the first critical hours, chances for recovery are good, although compromised pulmonary function persists for months. This syndrome was described by William Osler in 1880, but an adequate explanation of the mechanism remains obscure.[31] The syndrome is not fully responsive to the narcotic antagonists nor does it behave exactly as an idiosyncratic allergic reaction to heroin or an adulterant.

The toxic or lethal dose of morphine varies from one individual to another, but, generally, overdose is unlikely with 30 mg parenterally or 120 mg orally. Tolerance to the respiratory depressant effect occurs rapidly with repeated use, and no upward limit to the development of tolerance has been found.

MEDICAL PHARMACOLOGY

The analgesic action of the opiates can be predictably quantified. Ten mg of morphine (or the equivalent dose of another opiate) acts to increase the capacity of an individual to tolerate pain. At the same time, there is no loss in the ability to perceive the character and intensity of the painful sensation. The experience of anxiety, fear, panic, and suffering does not occur, and the narcotized person seems oblivious to his pain. The duration of this effect is four to six hours, with a peak at one hour. No other sensory modalities are affected by the opiates.

Deep sleep is the usual consequence of a 15 to 20 mg dose of intravenous morphine in a pain-free adult. Even at these levels, there is no significant motor incoordination, slurred speech, or convulsions. At dosages above 30 mg, serious toxicity may occur with progressive unconsciousness and insensibility leading to coma, respiratory arrest, and death.

Psychological effects tend to be much more subjective and variable according to the individual, group, and setting. The most commonly reported effects are drowsiness and mental clouding, along with feelings of heaviness, warmth, and an inability to concentrate. Physical activity is decreased and there is a lessening of the motivation to seek food and sexual gratification, or to express aggressivity. Others experience an increase in activity, energy, and strength.[52]

Mood changes are similarly variable. Most normal pain-free persons respond to a therapeutic dose of an opiate with feelings of anxiety, fear, discomfort, and often with nausea, vomiting, and dizziness. Having experienced this dysphoric response, these people actively avoid its repetition. Other individuals experience euphoria, an unrealistic sense of well-being, content, and peacefulness. For those who experience it, this euphoric effect is augmented by a higher dose.

OTHER MEDICAL USES

There are no more effective cough suppressants than the opiates. The antitussive dose can be administered orally and is generally lower than the analgesic dose. The dyspnea of pulmonary edema secondary to left ventricular failure is relieved by the opiates. This probably occurs because of reduced fear as well as peripheral vascular effects. Opiates are also the most effective antidiarrheal agents. Again, they are effective orally at lower doses than the analgesic dose.

PHYSIOLOGICAL CHANGES

The major actions of the opiates take place within the central nervous system, primarily the brain, and are both physiological and psychological. The pinpoint constriction of the pupils caused by the opiates is pathognomonic of toxic overdose. The major physiological effect of the narcotic analgesics on the central nervous system is respiratory depression; the critical chemoreceptors are desensitized to increases in carbon dioxide levels through a direct action on the respiratory centers in the brain stem. The extreme sensitivity of these centers facilitates a measurable respiratory depression at doses too low to alter the state of consciousness. This depression is dose related; in opiate overdoses, it proceeds to respiratory arrest and death.

Following intravenous administration, initial changes in the alpha-synchronization of the EEG pattern are compatible with relaxation, drowsiness, and euphoria. Within a half hour, decreases in the alpha and increases in the theta and delta activity are seen, a pattern resembling sleep. At toxic levels, meperidine and some other synthetic opiates are sometimes associated with CNS excitation evidenced by tremors, muscle twitches, and seizures.

NARCOTIC ACTIONS

Man is particularly sensitive to the narcotic actions of the opiates. These actions consist of analgesia, drowsiness, mood change, and a clouding of consciousness. Despite extensive study, the mechanism of action of these drugs within the CNS remains unknown.

TOLERANCE

Tolerance is said to exist when increasing amounts of the drug are necessary to produce the same pharmacologic effect. It occurs rapidly with all of the opiates and synthetic opiates. All of the effect of the opiates are subject to the development of tolerance, albeit at different rates. With increasing tolerance, analgesic, sedative, and emetic effects are totally diminished, whereas the pupillary and bowel actions are only minimally affected.

Another type of tolerance is developed toward the feelings of euphoria and well-being caused by morphine and heroin. With chronic administration, these feelings are diminished and replaced by lethargy, apathy, withdrawal, boredom, hypochondriasis, and an amotivational syndrome.

The development of tolerance is dependent on the pattern of use. When dosages on the therapeutic range are administered intermittently, the desired effects can be obtained indefinitely. Because tolerance to the respiratory depressant effect develops more rapidly than to the euphoric effect, there is a built-in safety factor in the process of addiction. A high degree of cross-tolerance exists from one opiate to another. The development of tolerance occurs most rapidly with morphine. Following the cessation of administration, tolerance is quickly lost to a great extent, although some degree of this tendency remains for as long as a year.

PHYSICAL AND PSYCHOLOGICAL DEPENDENCE

Physical dependence refers to the alteration of the physiology of the body in the presence of the drug so that the normalized steady state depends on the continued presence of the agent. It develops with all of the opiates and synthetic opiates. Discontinuance of the drug results in a characteristic abstinence-withdrawal syndrome which lasts until the body readapts to a drug-free state.

Dependence develops at a slightly slower rate than tolerance. The severity of the abstinence syndrome depends on the rate at which the drug is removed from its site of action. Thus, a cessation of the administration of morphine, following several weeks of twice daily usage, may create no recognizable symptoms. In contrast to this, however, only a few days of morphine given four times daily will produce a definite syndrome upon administration of a narcotic antagonist.

The severity of the withdrawal syndrome increases rapidly with a cessation of dosages in the lower and middle ranges; at the equivalent of 500 mg of morphine daily, it reaches a peak beyond which there is no further worsening. Cross dependence is the ability of one drug to maintain the dependent state of another and suppress the withdrawal syndrome. There is complete cross dependence between morphine and methadone, but only partial cross dependence between morphine and meperidine.

Psychological dependence can be said to have occurred when an individual considers the effects of the drug necessary to maintain an optimal state of well-being. With the opiates this may occur after repeated usage. There is a continuum of psychological dependence from a mild desire at one end of the spectrum to a craving or compulsion at the other. In its extreme form the need to be constantly under the influence of the drug is an all consuming preoccupation; it appears to be a chronic relapsing disease. The majority of normal individuals who have experienced the effects of the opiates have no difficulty avoiding repeated use.

There are recognized traits shared by most opiate addicts (depressed, schizoid, oral dependent, hostile, sexually immature, low frustration tolerance). However, there is no accounting for the development of an addiction on the basis of any individual characteristics or as a result of the capacity of the opiates to alleviate discomfort. The overall answer to the question of individual susceptibility must take a number of points into account. These include the complexities of the social matrix, the volitional status of the person, and the consequences of the drug use.

NARCOTIC WITHDRAWAL

At about the time when the next dose of the opiate might be expected, the addicted user will exhibit a variety of purposive symptoms aimed at getting more of the drug. Four to six hours after the last dose, complaints, pleas, manipulations, demands, etc., reflect the drug-craving of early narcotic withdrawal. The administration of a narcotic antagonist is associated with a short, very intense withdrawal developing in a few minutes and peaking in half an hour.

SOCIAL IMPACT OF THE OPIATES

The 6 billion dollars a year paid by the users of heroin to obtain their drug through illicit channels buys them the same amount of drug that could be bought for 20 million dollars through legal channels. ($11,000 per year per addict as compared to $40 per year per addict.) Of the total heroin distributed illegally, 45 percent is used by those involved in the distribution network. A great deal of criminality is spawned by the addict's pursuit of means to finance his habit and is unrelated to any drug effect. On the other hand, opiate users are in fact less likely to commit crimes of violence than are users of alcohol, amphetamines, or barbiturates.[43]

It appears that the majority of even heavy users of heroin function rather well in society, just as do many alcoholics. The concern and the cost generated by the malfunctioning and thieving heroin addict is a phenomenon only indirectly related to the opiates themselves; the social prerequisites for the contemporary American difficulties with heroin are unique to this time and place.

Under existing circumstances, the health hazards connected with the use of heroin are enormous. It is estimated that the death rate among heroin users is 1 percent per year. As a rule, the causes of death relate to factors such as contamination, serum hepatitis, and accidental overdose rather than to the pharmacology of the drug itself. The more recent epidemiology of heroin use has involved a shift to employed Caucasians living in smaller cities and away from large cities and unemployed nonwhites. At this point, it is not known whether this is associated with a lower mortality.

No attempt will be made here to review the tragic and complex history of recent attempts to deal with the difficulties of opiate abuse. Suffice it to say that among those associated with programs dealing with addicts, it is at present officially acknowledged that heroin addiction is a chronic, relapsing disease. Present goals do not extend to abstinence, but are increasingly limited to the establishment of intermittent heroin-free periods during which there is an alternative alliance to methadone. This limitation of goal can only be seen as a compromise and a defeat. (A source of the same kind of frustration was experienced by the missionaries when they provided the Polynesian women with shirts so that their breasts could be covered. The women modified the design by cutting holes in the front.) The establishment of either rationality or equanimity under such circumstances is most unlikely. Meanwhile, the shifts in pattern and vicissitudes of supply and demand of heroin function quite independently of the regulatory agencies, whose very nature seems wedded to frustration.

The Hallucinogens

There are three chemical classes of hallucinogens: (1) indoles; (2) phenethylamines; and (3) cannabinols. The indoles include LSD, psilocin, psilocybin, bofatenine, DET (diethyltryptam), DMT (dimethyltryptamine), yohimbine, and ibogaine. The phenethylamines include mescaline, peyote, MDA (3,4-methylenedioxyamphetamine), MMDA (4,5-methylenedioxy-3-methoxyamphetamine), and STP (DOM or 3-methyl-5-methoxyamphetamine). The cannabinols (Cannabis Sativa L.) as well as phencyclidine (PCP), both potent hallucinogens are discussed in their own sections. The anticholinergics also possess hallucinogenic properties and will be included in this section.

HISTORICAL NOTES

Hallucinogenic drugs have been used through the ages by many cultures. They have served as intoxicants, spices, and for recreation, as well as for rituals. For example, the peyote cactus (of which mescaline is the psycho-active agent) is traditionally used by the Yacqui Indians of Northern Mexico in their religious rites. The resulting altered state of consciousness is channelled trance-like into their sacred rituals and dances. In the United States today, this practice continues; the Native American Church has been exempted from many provisions of the Controlled Substance Act for the ceremonial use of mescaline.

In the tenth and twelfth centuries, two episodes of mass poisoning are recorded with more than 40,000 deaths. These were caused by LSD-like natural-occurring ergot alkaloids which contaminated wheat and rye tainted with the fungus *claviceps purpurea*. Naturally occurring belladonna alkaloids have been used for centuries for their hallucinogenic effect. Many adolescents today have experimented with the anticholinergic *datura stramonium* (jimson weed or stinkweed) and scopolamine. Unfortunately, the ignorance and trust with which they often ingest these potent agents result in frequent instances of serious toxicity.

The work of Moreau de Tours[75] began the modern scientific investigations of hallucinogenic drugs. His description of their effects influenced a generation of curious nineteenth century poets and philosophers; among them were Rimbaud, De Quincey, Baudelaire, Coleridge, and Keats. Although there were many earlier scientific reports, Lewin's systematic study of 1964 marked the beginning of modern scientific research.[64] His work proposed the notion that the mescaline influenced state could be studied as a model psychosis. He reasoned that this model could be used to provide insight into the nature of clinical psychoses. This hypothesis was first suggested by Thudichum's 1884 theory that toxic metabolite, a naturally occurring mescaline analog, might cause clinical psychoses.[87] A quantum jump in the study of the hallucinogens occurred in 1938 when Hofmann[42] in his Sandoz Research laboratory in Basel, Switzerland, was preparing a number of semisynthetic derivatives of the ergot alkaloids all based on the d-lysergic acid nucleus. He found that these new compounds caused uterine contractions in laboratory animals as well as serving as very strong stimulants. On April 16, 1943, Hofmann accidentally ingested a minute quantity of one of these compounds and became the first to experience the potent hallucinogenic properties of LSD-25. In 1947 the Swiss psychiatrist, still of the Psychiatric Clinic of Zurich University, started a full-scale study of the agent.

By the summer of 1966, the media had succeeded in capturing the public imagination with glowing and seductive accounts of the effects of LSD. There were claims that it could enhance creativity in art and music, lead the way to spiritual enlightenment, and help architects design better buildings; it was spoken of as a "wonder drug" able to help solve life problems, enhance pleasure, and treat mental illness. The nationwide backlash was that increasing numbers of youthful LSD intoxication casualties flooded psychiatric clinics and emergency rooms.

As the pitfalls of LSD became recognized, especially on the college campuses, the government intervened and federal laws were passed making possession, selling, or manufacturing LSD illegal. This law was called the "Drug Abuse Control Amendment of 1965." In May of 1966, all sponsored grants for research on the drug were cancelled, and Sandoz Laboratories stopped their production. The specific focus on LSD obscured the generality that the public health ramifications of substance abuse and toxicity among young people is a continuous—but ever changing story. Consequently a most interesting agent was relegated virtually exclusively to illicit use—and will remain so for a generation.

The hallucinogens are not a distinct class of drugs. A variety of centrally active agents cause hallucinations, delusions, illusions, mood changes, paranoid ideation, and psychotic-like states. These include the alcohols, bromides, analgesic antagonists (nalorphine), cocaine, insecticides (parathion), antimalarials, cholinesterase inhibitors (diisopropyl fluorophosphate), amphetamines, and corticosteroids. The distinguishing feature of the hallucinogens is their ability to alter the nature of consciousness, perceptions, thoughts, and feelings in a way usually experienced in dreams only.[86]

LSD

Also known as d-n, n-diethyl lysergamide, d-lysergic acid diethylamide, lysergsaure diathylamid, d-LSD-2S and lysergide or delysid, LSD is a naturally occurring alkaloid. Produced by several varieties of morning glory (convoluulus, ipomoea sidaefolia, and rivea corymbosa) and by claviceps purpurea, a fungus which parasitizes wheat and rye—the usual hallucinogenic doses range from 100 to 400 micrograms.[93] LSD is relatively simple to synthesize; it can be made either chemically from lysergic acid, one of the ergot alkaloids, or by a deep fermentation process. The synthesis of lysergic acid, however, is accomplished with great difficulty.

On the street, LSD is generically referred to as "acid"—varieties including white lightning, blue dots, yellow dots, purple wedges, wedges, green caps, blue caps, yellow caps, brown caps, paisley caps, blotter acid (piece of blotter), and "window pane" acid (thin gelatin segments). Street LSD varies considerably in price, dose, and contaminants: *caveat emptor.*[73]

The hallucinogens, psilocybin and psilocyn, occur in psilocybe mexicana, a mushroom indigenous to Mexico and used ceremonially by certain Indians there. The pharmacology of these agents is similar to that of mescaline, and an oral dose of 4 to 8 mg results in a "high" lasting about six hours.

Bufotenine is structurally related to serotonin. It is naturally derived from the dermal secretions of the toad L. bufo, and from the seed of the plant piptadenia peregrina. It is taken as snuff by certain South American Indians and can also be injected for its hallucinogenic effects.

DET and DMT (dimethyltryptamine and diethyltryptamine) are administered by injection or by smoking one of these chemicals with tobacco, marijuana, or other plant material. Their effects last for less than one hour but produce a strong hallucinogenic effect. DMT occurs in the seeds of certain plants in the West Indies and South America. The seeds have been used for snuff for centuries in Haiti where they are believed to facilitate communication with the gods.

Yohimbine and ibogaine produce hallucinogenic effects as well as aphrodisia and a cocaine-like euphoria. They are administered by injection.

Mescaline is the primary active ingredient of the peyote cactus (1. phophora Williamsii). The mescaline is concentrated in the "buttons" or buds of the plant. These are powdered and taken orally. A dose of 350 to 500 mg of mescaline will have an effect lasting five to twelve hours.

MDA (3,4-methylenedioxyamphetamine) and MMDA (4,5-methylenedioxy-3-methoxy amphetamine) are structurally related to the amphetamines and mescaline. On the street they are available as a powder, tablet, or liquid which can be taken orally, "bonged" (smoked in a bong pipe), snorted, or injected.

STP (DOM or 3-methoxy-4-methyl-5-methoxy amphetamine) like MDA or MMDA can be classed as a psychotomimetic amphetamine, being hallucinogenic in addition to having the stimulant effects of an amphetamine. STP, a name borrowed from the oil additive, referred to serenity, tranquility, and peace rather than to its chemical constituents. It is about one hundred times as potent as mescaline, and one thirtieth as potent as LSD.

The hallucinogenic anticholinergics are the belladonna alkaloids, scopolamine, and jimson weed leaf. As implied, these create atropine-like side effects. The natural alkaloids are found in the genus, solanaceae (nightshade family), most commonly from Datura stamonium (jimson weed or stinkweed) and Hyoscyamus niger (black henbane). The therapeutic dose ranges from 1.4 to 1.0 mg for scopolamine and jimson weed. The hallucinogenic dose is 10 mg or more. Many nonprescription sleeping aids (Nite Rest Capsules, Quiet World Tablets, Sedate Capsules, Sleep-Eze

Tablets, and Sominex) contain scopolamine, which causes sedation and amnesia at low dosage; but they are often abused both accidentally and purposely. Jimson weed can be taken orally as a tea from the cooked leaves or directly eaten as seeds or leaves. Overdose, with prolonged hallucinosis, is common among experimenting youth.

Clinical Applications: In the following discussions, LSD will provide a prototype for the hallucinogenic substances. The anticholinergic drugs will be considered where they differ from the generality.

Originally the LSD induced "model psychosis" was thought by several pioneer investigators to resemble schizophrenia. Later, however, it was found to differ substantially from that disorder in spite of a similar element of depersonalization. Today research with LSD is strictly limited and controlled by the Food and Drug Administration; it has in fact been minimal since the epidemic of abuse in the late 1960s.

In the early 1960s, there was research which explored the applicability and safety of this drug for the treatment of various physical and mental disorders. Its use in the treatment of alcoholism and as an antidepressant and facilitator of composure during terminal illness was promising.[56, 65] In evaluations of creativity under the influence of LSD,[24, 44] many persons felt that their capacity for creative thinking was enhanced. Further study indicated a promise of usefulness in autistic children[84] and sexual dysfunction—impotency, frigidity and homosexuality. The widespread public use of these drugs for mental exploration, excitement, pleasure, and religious experiences created many toxic psychoses, sometimes with conspicuous and tragic consequences. The initial positive charisma was reversed, and to this day negative reaction to any use of these agents continues to persist.

Psychological Effects: Following the ingestion of an average 150 mcg dose of LSD there is usually a latent period of thirty to forty-five minutes. The initial response experienced has been characterized as a feeling of depersonalization or of being "once removed" from the self. In inexperienced users, this sensation may trigger anxiety, setting the tone for a "bad trip." The nature of the drug experience is highly dependent on setting, expectation, and anxiety level. There is a great risk of serious upset when drug-naive subjects are given LSD without their knowledge (at one time, an all too frequent occurrence).

As the drug experience progresses, there are commonly time-space distortions, mood fluctuations, unusual or autistic associations, and perceptual alterations of the visual and auditory environment. An enhanced attentiveness and heightened perceptual acuity is frequent, often with psychodelic embellishment such as rainbow auras or a sense of seeing the molecular structure or movement of objects and living things. Occasionally subjects experience synesthesia, the translation of one modality of sensory experience into another —as, for example, music eliciting visual phenomena or colors bringing forth olfactory perceptions.

The total experience of LSD is frequently felt as profoundly spiritual and accompanied by a new sense of the meaning of life, love, commitment, or the nature of reality. For the enthusiasts of the drug in the later 1960s, it was a severe disappointment that a chemically induced millenium was not at hand.

The true hallucinatory experience (a visual or auditory perception without a basis in external reality) is rare with LSD. When present, it is usually more accurately described as a "pseudo-hallucination," since there is no loss of critical self-judgment during the experience.

A significant mood change is almost always present; the feeling tone may range from euphoria to dysphoria, anxiety, and tension. The resultant mood may remain constant during the drug experience, or a marked lability may ensue. Occasional individuals respond with confusion, disorganization, panic, and diminished capacity to deal with their surroundings. Some of the negative responses which occur with significant frequency include autistic or simplistic thinking, catatonic-like withdrawal, or excitement and perseveration. The question of why some subjects respond to the drug with a disintegration of their resources or a toxic psychotic state remains unanswered. It is however, not true that those who do experience psychotic reactions with LSD were somehow unstable to begin with or "riding for a fall" anyway.

Long after the pharmacological experience with LSD, there is a possibility of feeling once again as if one were under the negative influence of the drug. This has been dubbed a "flashback." The nature or even the existence of this phenomenon remains doubtful. When the adolescents become absorbed with the sensations of the drug state, there is an inevitable diminution in age appropriate growth and mastery. During the time when the charismatic LSD using counter-culture was at its height, it was feared that the drug itself could divert youth from maturation and independence. At present, psychodelic experience seems to have no special premium placed upon it by multiple substance abusing youth.

Anticholinergics possess both an hallucinogenic effect and an atropine-like side-effect. At a dose of 10 mg or more, there is restlessness, hyperactivity, or agitation—all followed by clouding of the sensorium, disorientation, and hallucinations. Delirium or coma may follow.

Mechanism of Action: It was observed early that LSD blocks the action of 5-hydroxytryptamine (serotonin) on the isolated rat uterus.[35] This led to Shaw's[95] later speculation that LSD's hallucinogenic effect arose from its antagonism to serotonin in the brain. Studies[32, 33] involving free and bound serotonin have been proposed to elucidate the basis of LSD's hallucinogenic effect. Other studies demonstrate no correlation between the antiserotonin activities and hallucinogenic potencies. Bradley[15] noted that LSD increases the responsiveness of the reticulum formation to sensory input without lowering the threshold to direct stimulation. Whatever LSD's mechanism of action, the pharmacodynamic action responsible for the hallucinogenic effect is associated with this increased stimulation.[11, 27, 76] Beyond this, the mysteries of neuro-chemistry persist.

Physiologic Effects: LSD has few physiological effects. It is absorbed from the intestine completely and readily, and there is no advantage to parenteral administration.

The subject often experiences a loss or increase of appetite, nausea, dizziness, headaches, palpitations, and periods of shivering with hot flushes. The pupils are dilated with consequent photophobia. There are moderate increases in heart rate, blood sugar, and blood pressure.

The drug is not addicting and there are no psysiological withdrawal symptoms. There can be an emotional dependence in those who experience the drug effect as euphoric. When labeled with C_{14}, LSD is found in highest concentration in the liver and kidneys. In the brain it is concentrated in the cerebral cortex, hippocampus, basal ganglia, and thalamic nuclei.[49] Most of the metabolites of LSD are excreted from the liver into the feces.[82] Behavioral changes are observed as the brain concentration slowly decreases.

Methylamphetamine crystals ("speed") interact with LSD to create a magnified awareness of the tachycardia, anxiety, and muscle tremor and a high likelihood of a "bad trip" or "bummer." Appel[6] found that if the catecholamines, for example, are depleted with reserpine,[12] the LSD effect is enhanced.

Tolerance: Tolerance to LSD develops in both normal subjects[46] and schizophrenics.[22] It occurs rapidly, and administration more than twice a week is associated with significantly diminished effect. There is no lethal dosage known in humans; but monkeys die after receiving 5 mg per kg of body weight.

TREATMENT OF LSD TOXICITY

A laboratory assay for blood LSD level does exist. Since, however, it is functional for only three hours post-ingestion, it is clinically useless.[2] The diagnosis of LSD toxicity is dependent on history. Phenothiazines block the action of LSD and are useful in controlling the acutely intoxicated state. A benzodiazapam (Valium) given IM may also be helpful.

Some steroids[12] and progesterone[59] are antagonistic to LSD. It has also been reported that niacin and serotonin[16, 80] are effective in reducing the effects of LSD.[3]

PCP: ANGEL DUST

Phencyclidine (PCP) was developed in the 1950s as an analgesic and anesthetic. It was also being investigated during that period for its potential in the treatment of and research into mental disorders. Clinical trial with humans showed that the drug produced too many unpleasant side effects for recommendation of its use, and such treatment with humans was discontinued in 1965. However, the drug was found to be an effective anesthetic for animals and is available for veterinary use.

PCP is easily manufactured and appears in many forms, such as crystalline powder, tablets, and capsules. It has been sold as THC or mescaline (or a number of other street drugs without PCP's reputation for being unpredictable). Reports of abdominal cramps, bloody vomiting, diarrhea, and coma following ingestion of PCP are attributed to one of the by-products of the synthetic process.

Phencyclidine appears to have markedly different effects at different dose levels, varying from mild euphoria, to acute psychotic states, to coma.

Meyers and associates[73] claimed that the sensory disturbances produced by PCP were similar to the effects of sensory deprivation. The resemblance of the acute psychotic state produced by PCP to schizophrenia has also been researched. This similarity was related to impaired ability to organize sensory input. PCP has also been found to aggravate existing psychotic states to a greater extent than LSD or mescaline.

Peripheral signs of PCP use include muscular incoordination, flushing, sweating, dizziness, and mild relaxation of the arteries. The adverse side effects make it of prime medical concern.

Pharmacologic Effects: Phencyclidine is a white, stable solid, soluble in water and alcohol and can be administered in a variety of ways. Studies of the toxicity of PCP revealed that the dose required to kill 50 percent of the animal population to which it was administered was approximately 180 mg per kg (oral).[20] Evidence on tolerance and withdrawal is incomplete.

Research suggests that the principal site of action is the sensory cortex, thalamus, and midbrain. The effects of PCP vary with the species, producing hyperactivity in mice and apparent depression of CNS activity in man. Large doses of PCP are associated with leukocytosis, hypertension, and tachycardia and may cause coma, convulsions, and death.

Epidemiology: Use of PCP was first found in the Haight-Ashbury district in San Francisco in 1967.[73] The drug was not popular, possibly because of the side effects, and was soon being marketed with another name (e.g., "Hog") or as another substance (e.g., THC or LSD). The LAC/USC Medical Center street drug identification program found PCP being marketed as hashish and THC, and some marijuana was found laced with PCP. Interestingly, of the eight or nine samples of supposed THC, all checked out to be PCP. In the month of March, 1976, the most frequently encountered drug was PCP and well over half of those samples were represented as THC.

PCP does not appear to be the agent of choice among the drug using population. Nonetheless, many are ingesting it in the belief that it is their preferred drug.

Subjective Effects: With low doses (1 to 5 mg), PCP has effects similar to those of many other psychoactive drugs. Euphoria has been described, occasionally combined with numbness. An increase in dosage generally leads to a state of confused, excited intoxication with changes in body image due, perhaps, to impaired proprioceptive feedback. Feelings of depersonalization, apathy, and estrangement are often reported. Increased doses are frequently associated with acute, psychotic-like episodes complete with auditory hallucinations, withdrawal, and paranoid ideation. The number of adolescents admitted with toxic psychosis based on PCP abuse has gone beyond that generated by any other agent. At present (1977) in Los Angeles, it is the most frequent cause of hospital admission with a psychotic presentation.

MARIJUANA

History: Marijuana (cannabis sativa) consists of the dried leaves and stems of the hemp plant; these can be smoked, chewed, or prepared as tea. A stronger preparation can be made by drying the resin of the marijuana plant; this preparation is called hashish. Both marijuana and hashish have been used by man for thousands of years.

The effects of marijuana were probably first studied scientifically by Moreau de Tours.[75] He believed that much about insanity could be elucidated through having normal subjects, including himself, experience transient psychotic states. He claimed to have achieved these psychotic-like states through the use of marijuana.

Articles on marijuana published between 1840 and 1900 were generally positive, finding marijuana useful for a variety of maladies and reporting no side effects. Scientific interest in the effects of marijuana on psychiatric disorders resulted in a series of articles both in the United States and in Britain. Lindemann and Malamud[66] tested marijuana on psychiatric patients and found that it produced withdrawal in schizophrenics, while neurotics reported apprehension and time sense disturbance.

The active ingredient, tetrahydrocanabinol (THC), was synthesized in 1940 under the name of Synhexyl. In 1947, Stockings[85] reported positive results using 60 to 90 mg of Synhexyl with depressed patients. Reported side effects were minimal with increased heart rate and apprehension occurring only at higher doses. These findings were not, however, replicated in subsequent studies, possibly because lower dosages were used.

The history of concern about marijuana use reportedly goes back to medieval Islam. The legal status of marijuana in the United States became an issue in the 1920s. General concern was aroused in the Southwest because of the widespread use of marijuana among Mexican laborers. In 1932, marijuana regulation was left to state option, but continued pressure led to the Marijuana Tax Act of 1937, whereupon marijuana use became a federal offense. Associated with these changes was an intensive public relations program warning against the use of this agent.

In the 1960s, marijuana again aroused public concern as the nation's youth made it the drug of choice. The use of marijuana was no longer confined to minority groups, but had spread to every social level via the disaffected young. The increased use stimulated considerable research on the physiological, psychological, and social effects of marijuana use. It also stimulated the passage of the Comprehensive Drug Abuse and Control Act (PL 91-513) in 1970. During 1970 and 1973 Congressional hearings and public debates dealt with the issues of decriminalizing or legalizing the use of marijuana.

Pharmacology: Tetrahydrocanabinol (THC) is the major psychoactive ingredient in this substance and one of its isomers, delta-9-tetrahydrocanabinol, appears to account for most of the psychological effects. The amounts of THC found in marijuana samples have varied widely, but are generally less than 1 percent. Other cannabinoids (specifically cannabidiol and cannabinal) appear either to augment the effects of delta-9-THC or to have psychological effects of their own.[55, 81]

The insolubility of the cannabinoids, along with concern for the stability of their preparations, has posed considerable problems for research. Many researchers have also been concerned about error factors in dosage. Even though research has shown that reasonable dosage control can be achieved using the smoking process, many researchers failed to control a larger source of variance, that is, butt length. New methods of administration, including parenteral administration, have permitted more closely controlled dosage in research on psychological and pharmacological effects of the cannabinoids. It would make sense that the most sensitive measure of dose would be the level of cannaboids and metabolites in body fluids and tissues.[36] Some evidence indicates that once a dose has been administered, a metabolite of delta-9-THC, called 11-hydroxydelta-9-THC, is primarily responsible for the psychological effects.[62]

There are obvious ethical aspects to the administering of high and frequent doses to humans. As a result, studies investigating tolerance to the effects of marijuana and cross tolerance to other drugs have primarily involved subhuman species. Tolerance to the behavioral effects of the cannabinoids has been shown in studies using pigeons as subjects.[71] Cross tolerance between cannabinoids[71] and between cannabinods and alcohol[78] has been reported.

Epidemiology: As has been mentioned, much of the interest in marijuana was generated by its association with the radical movements of the late 1960s. The issue was clouded because of the general public alarm at the attack on the established social order. Marijuana use was thought to be the basis for the suddenly rebellious and unorthodox behavior of the young. In this atmosphere, research has been directed toward elucidating the possible harmful, long-term effects of its ingestion; because of experimenter bias, however, the research findings have been controversial. This reflected itself many times in poorly designed studies. Epidemiological studies can answer many of the questions concerning long-term use of marijuana, and in the United States considerable data are becoming available. The Federal Bureau of Narcotics and Dangerous Drugs predicted in 1972 that by 1976, 50 million people will have experienced marijuana. The Shafer Commission survey[77] (1972) reported that 13 million people used marijuana regularly.

Marijuana use is not confined to the young. Arrest rates show that marijuana use continues into the late twenties and thirties, and that 14 percent of the users were in professional occupations. This would indicate that not only is there widespread use of marijuana, but that the users are to be found at all levels of the socio-economic structure.[96] Two studies carried out in Oregon and three others carried out across the country by the Washington Drug Abuse Council indicate that, as of 1974, more people were trying marijuana, but the number of regular users was decreasing (*Clinical Psychiatry News*, 1976). The final answers on marijuana use can come only from the data that are now becoming available from large numbers of regular users.

Subjective Effects: Experiences reported by marijuana users appear to depend on the psychological makeup of the user, and the amount ingested. Research generally confirms that marijuana can be distinguished from a placebo. Studies[44] have shown that as long as doses are above threshold, environmental conditions play little, if any, role in the way subject rate marijuana. With moderate doses, subjects generally report euphoria, and, with higher doses, there have been some reports of increased apprehension. Perceptual distortion is rarely reported, as are hallucinations and other evidence of the kind of space disorientation produced by stronger drugs. The feeling tone most often described is a sense of physical and emotional well being.

Tobacco: Nicotine

Smoking is so widespread that it is seldom recognized as the inhalation of the drug nicotine. Public awareness of the cardiovascular and pulmonary morbidity and mortality related to the smoking of tobacco has not deterred its use, except among the medical profession. In fact, the prevalence of cigarette smoking in America is increasing, a tribute to the power of advertising and to the addictive qualities of nicotine. Among youth, the smoking of cigarettes continues to have a significant role in proclaiming the coming of age and independence; the only conjoint sign that speaks both of oral dependence and adulthood.

BACKGROUND AND PHARMACOLOGY

Although nicotine has no therapeutic use, it has been extensively studied. In 1863, Traube found through his work with dogs, that nicotine causes bradycardia.[40] Later it was discovered that nicotine has a dual action, initially causing stimulation and later a blockage of the vagus, the mechanism for the cardiac slowing. It has been known since the work of Langley[60] that the autonomic ganglia are the site of action. Here, in the postsynaptic membrane, there is a receptor site where nicotine combines with acetylcholine, first stimulating and then causing blockage. The association of tobacco with pulmonary neoplasms, emphysema, and heart disease has assured continuing research on this drug, as it continues to increase its mortality in the population.

IDENTIFICATION

Nicotine is an alkaloid which comes from nicotiana tobacum and nicotina rustica. In the average cigarette, the nicotine content is approximately 2 percent, and in denicotinized cigarettes about 1 percent. It is a clear oily liquid which turns brown in light and, interestingly, is an effective insecticide in 40 percent solution.

PHARMACOLOGY

There is about 3 mg of nicotine absorbed into the body for every cigarette smoked. Three mgs. of nicotine inhaled have the same effect as 1 mg of nicotine injected IV. As with any drug, the effects and metabolism vary from one individual to another. Generally, there is an increase of parasympathetic activity in some organs (the gastrointestinal tract and salivary glands) and an increase in sympathetic activity in others (heart, pupils, and blood vessels).

Nicotine causes both stimulation and depression of the respiratory system. A 2 mg injection will cause a stimulation of respiration. In higher doses, a direct effect on the neuromuscular junction leads toward paralysis of the respiratory muscles. Heymans showed that the nicotine effects the carotid bodies.[41]

Nicotine from cigarette or pipe smoking results in an increase in heart rate ranging from several to fifty beats per minute. There may be a slight increase of blood pressure and cardiac output typical of sympathetic stimulation.[83] Nicotine can affect the cardiovascular system from a number of sites: autonomic ganglia, adrenal medula, chemoreceptors, the parasympathetic system, and the carotid bodies.[41] After smoking three cigarettes, there are significant EEG changes:[91] a fall in skin temperature due to vasoconstriction, antidiuresis (by inhibition of vasopressin secretions from the hypophysis), and finger tremor.

Inhalants (Volatile Organic Solvents)

Regardless of the attendant danger, the inhalation of volatile solvents as a means of getting intoxicated is very popular among children and adolescents. Among the easily obtained products so abused are glues, lighter fluid, paint thinners, and aerosols. Less readily available are the volatile anesthetics (i.e., ethers), hydrocarbons, carbontetrachloride, amyl nitrate, and other groups such as propyls and butyls. Brain damage, hepatic damage, and renal damage have all been associated with the inhalation of trichloroethane and trichloroethylene. Proteinuria, acute renal failure, and hepatic failure are associated with prolonged glue sniffing. These agents cause fatty degeneration of the liver, kidney, and heart. Abuse of these volatile substances has complicated the diagnosis for hepatitis, gastroenteritis, and acute renal failure. Post mortem examinations following sudden deaths in youths intoxicated with volatile substances suggest that arrythmias are the direct cause. Toluene, which is common in glue, can cause atrioventricular block in laboratory animals within two minutes; the mechanism of action involves a direct effect of the sinoatrial node and atrioventricular conduction system.

The most frequently abused volatile substances are the aliphatic hydrocarbons, which can be either fluorinated or chlorinated. A complication of the inhaling of commercial products is that they are often contaminated with more toxic ingredients than the pure solvent itself. These substances are classified as anesthetics along with the ether and alcohols.

THE ATTRACTIVENESS OF INHALANTS TO THE ADOLESCENT

Solvent abuse has little to recommend it except to the users who find it attractive: the hangover is very light (compared to alcohol and barbiturates), the gratification is immediate, and the duration is short. More than that the agents are easy to get and legal to carry, inexpensive, and readily available.

ADMINISTRATION

Inhalation can be accomplished directly from the fumes in a container, from a cloth or plastic bag, or from an aerosol sprayed directly into the nose or mouth (with possible freezing of the oral and pharyngeal tissues).

A survey of school children by Linder[67] indicated that in the elementary school, inhalants were second to alcohol abuse. By junior high, they had dropped to sixth place. Volatile substance abusers tend to be underprivileged boys (age range: seven to seventeen years). Solvent sniffing is rarely seen in adults with the exception of amyl nitrate inhalation by adult male homosexuals.

COMPLICATIONS

Toluene, acetone, hexane, and naphtha are all less toxic than gasoline, benzene, carbon tetrachloride, and zylene. While under the influence of the drug, people are accident prone. There is a longer term risk of danger to the bone marrow, heart, lungs, brain, kidneys, and liver. Death has been due to respiratory arrest, cardiac failure, or physical exertion. Aerosols can cause a block in the air passage at the larnyx by freezing the throat. Another danger is the possibility of suffocation from falling into the solvent filled rag or plastic bag.

TREATMENT

Since there are no special methods for managing the intoxicated sniffer, supportive therapy, with bed rest and monitoring of the urinary output is the best treatment.

The Amphetamines: Cocaine, Phenmetrazine (Preludin), Methylphenidate (Ritalin), and Premoline (Cylert)

INTRODUCTION

There has always been a use for substances which can relieve fatigue, increase alertness, improve the mood, and enhance a sense of well-being. In contemporary Western society, the stimulants nicotine and caffeine are a part of everyday life. The fact that the more potent agents have serious pitfalls—dependence, liability, abuse potential, physical and emotional sequelae—has typically been a painful discovery made some time after the initial enthusiastic discovery. At this point, publicity and warnings about the pitfalls of caffeine and nicotine fall on deaf ears.

The ease of establishing a dependence on these agents accounts for the frequent development of a pattern in which stimulants are employed to launch a lively, confident day, and depressants relied on at night to facilitate sleep. This pattern interferes with the body's natural biological rhythms and is presently associated with many difficulties. Stimulants are relied on to preserve wakefulness and to allow the person to function beyond the intrinsic capacity of his body. In time, this builds up to a "crash" period associated with depression and fatigue. Such an unpleasant state is all too easily regarded as a reason for ingesting more stimulants. Tolerance develops quickly, a circumstance which predisposes toward an attempt to maintain the effect with higher dosage. Excessive quantities or prolonged reliance on these agents to overcome natural tiredness and sleep is associated with physical exhaustion, delirium, and psychosis.

Early signs of toxicity include repetitive touching and picking of the body, self-centered preoccupation, paranoid ideation, and short temper. There is a diminished capacity for self-criticism and acceptance of feedback, and a god-like sense of being right. Higher dosages are associated with hallucinations, headache, chest pain, dizziness, tremor, agitation, panic and hostility, as well as flushed skin with sweating and abdominal cramps. Amphetamines increase the plasma concentration of fatty acid, and long-term use is associated with vascular degeneration, particularly in the brain. Death can occur from hyperpryexia, convulsions, cardiovascular or respiratory collapse, or suicide. Psychoses secondary to stimulant abuse may be clinically indistinguishable from paranoid schizophrenia; these conditions persist long after withdrawal.

Chronic high dosage users usually experience great difficulty in giving up their habit. Unpleasant withdrawal symptoms can last up to a week and include severe insomnia, impaired perception, with possible hallucinations, anxiety, depression, and suicidal ideation. The depressive symptomatology can persist for weeks and months; this provides a powerful motive to return to the use of the stimulant. Physical dependence per se, however, is not known.

Conspicuous abusers who favor these agents exclusively—the "speed freaks"—tend to be wild, unsocialized, violent, and deteriorated. There seems to be fewer of these individuals in evidence now than during the "drug cult" era of the late 1960s. Other amphetamine—abusing types include the depressed schizoid, the ambitious hypo-manic over-extender who burns the candle at both ends. Among adolescents, amphetamine abuse is rarely seen is isolation; it tends rather to be associated with a poly-abuse pattern.

CLINICAL USEFULNESS

Amphetamines are analeptics, reversing depression from the anesthetics, narcotics, and hypnotics. They are essential in the treatment of narcolepsy, and in this disorder they facilitate a normalization of wakefulness and attention span. They are useful in the treatment of hyperkinetic children for whom they paradoxically serve as a "tranquilizer," an effect which usually disappears during puberty. They are anorectic agents of some value in weight reduction, though less so than commonly believed. They have been used to provide an extra burst of endurance or energy; cocaine for the race horse and dextroamphetamine for the competitive athlete may make a winner,[61] but also cause a scandal. They serve to facilitate the absorption and retention of information, a particularly common practice among medical students. Their capacity to act as a "psychic energizer" is experienced as pleasurable; it potentiates verbal output but does not increase the capacity to listen to the same extent. Although equally true for grammar school children, the pitfalls of these agents were discovered before these agents were ever used with youngsters.

Amphetamines were introduced as a nonprescription drug in the form of benzedrine inhalers. It was many years before their abuse was recognized, initially among adolescents and prisoners. On further investigation it appeared that prior to its regulation, the most widespread amphetamine abuse was to be found among students and housewives. As with other agents with an abuse potential, following the establishment of regulation, the affected population shifted. Today it is largely confined to groups associated with sociopathy.

When dextroamphetamine and the analogs were employed as a central stimulant, the usual clinical dose was 5 mg, one to three times daily. Abuse has been reported at levels up to 1000 mg IV every two to three hours. Among heavy abusers, intravenous administration is accomplished by dissolving and injecting oral preparations. This is accompanied by a certain incidence of pathology from contamination of the water and equipment; this can take the form of thrombosis, strokes, and/or abscesses.

The treatment of clinical toxicity due to the CNS stimulants is symptomatic: bed rest, supportive care, and appropriate sedation (diazepam, chlorpromazine, or barbiturates).

COCAINE

Cocaine is an alkaloid obtained from the leaves of erythroxylon coca, the South American coca plant. (It can also be synthesized from ecgonine.) In these leaves, cocaine attains a concentration of 1 to 2 percent. Coca has been cultivated since prehistoric times, and its leaves are commonly chewed for refreshment and to relieve fatique.

Cocaine occurs chemically as a colorless crystal or as a white, crystalline powder. It was first isolated by Gaedcke in 1855. It is classified as a local anesthetic. The largest consumers of the leaves are the cola beverage manufacturers, who preserve the flavor after decocaining the leaves.

Although cocaine is still employed as a local anesthetic for ear, nose, and throat surgery, most of the cocaine in this country is of illegal origin for illegal use. It is usually sold on the street as a 5 to 50 percent white powder cut with other substances such as starch or lactose. It is usually taken by nasal inhalation ("sniffing" or "snorting"), with the aid of a straw or a "coke" spoon. Less often it is injected. Cocaine immediately produces a subtle euphoric state with a sense of heightened cognition and energy. Blood pressure, heart rate, and body temperature are increased. Appetite is reduced. Its social pretense has the positive charisma of conspicuous consumption, the effect of the pharmacology being slight for a usual street price of one hundred dollars per gram. Because cocaine is legally classed as a narcotic, the consequences of possession are disproportionate to the hazards.

Cocaine blocks nerve conduction. It stimulates the central nervous system, especially the cerebral cortex. Cocaine is absorbed from all sites of application. If taken orally, it is hydrolyzed in the gastrointestinal tract and inactivated. It is metabolized in the liver and excreted unchanged in the urine. A 20 mg dose is sufficient to cause toxic side effects; the fatal dose is approximately 1.2 gm.

OTHER AGENTS

The other CNS stimulants are essentially similar to the amphetamines with regard both to their pharmacology and abuse potential. The subjective quality of the stimulation may vary from agent to agent as does the equivalence per milligram as compared to dextroamphetamine. Methylphenidate (Ritalin) is most widely used for the treatment of hyperactive children and for the narcoleptic syndrome. Pemoline (Cylert) was introduced in 1975 as an agent for the treatment of the hyperkinetic syndrome. A variety of agents formulated specifically as anorectics include chlorphentermine (Pre-Sate), diethylpropion (Tenuate), fenfluramine (Pondimin), chlortermine (Voranil), mazindol (Sanorex), phendimetrazine (Plegine), phentermine (Wilpo), and benzphetamine (Didrex). A given individual may experience greater nervousness or more unpleasant jumpiness with one of these than with another. Basically, their effectiveness as an aid in weight reduction is limited to periods less than a month and to small amounts of weight.

Conclusion and Overall Treatment Guidelines

The medical treatment of any serious disease is fated to be accompanied by an inevitable incidence of failure. Drug abuse involves young people whose overriding need has been to maintain the experience of euphoria in their lives at the cost of their potential to establish creative, constructive, and loving pursuits; under such conditions the incidence of treatment failure is high.

The drug-dependent life style tends to perpetuate itself. It does so by force of habit and through the positive re-enforcement of the drug experience. It is not easy to achieve any lasting help for a life pattern incorporating the destructive use of substances. If change does occur, the essence of the experience is for the abuser to learn constructive ways to create emotionally relevant interactions in his life. In a life busied with its own destruction, even the most benign pharmacological agent can become a dominating force. There are many approaches which might serve as the basis for a program to assist substance abusers. The attainment of success, or the lack of it, however, depends on what is created within the patient's social and interpersonal sphere. This can only be alluded to implicitly; it exists between the lines of the printed material. A lasting cure of a pattern of substance abuse depends on having learned the high art of constructive living.

Each group or individual who works with substance abusers has a set of guidelines and a philosophy which constitute the inner structure of the program. The person as a whole and the actual function of the group are the embodiment and practice or expression of that philosophy. The test of the treatment is whether it gives rise to an emotionally sustaining and significant alternative to the pattern of abuse and its associated destructiveness. The potential availability of such a viable alternative is a prerequisite; the actual connection depends on the complex interplay of human togetherness and estrangement.

Those with established patterns of substance abuse always possess some means of forming intense interpersonal bonds, at least through some form of anger and negativity—and within their lives, this is an overworked option. They are frustrated by the experience of being themselves and are often competitively disadvantaged. In the face of this, they become skilled at perceiving possible censure and "put down." They anticipate it in silences, are most attentive to the negative connotations of others' behavior, and find ways to generate bursts of negative or angry engagement in those about them. Transforming the emotional economy of such an individual is sometimes as difficult and complex as the establishment of world peace; the apparatus of peace must be created, and its quality experienced while the war machine is being disengaged and moth-balled. In the case of the individual, the uncertainties and self-doubts implicit in civilian life must be tolerated and finally preferred to the stereotyped certainty and predictability of a hostile and defensive encounter. (The typical life experience and personality development of a substance abuser was described in the section on alcoholism.)

It has long been recognized that it is easier to fortify health than to cure the disequilibrium of disease. By the same token it is also easier to facilitate the development of a positive and abuse-resistant emotional economy than to transform a pre-existing, despair-compensating pattern of destructiveness. Indeed, where children have been offered the opportunity to experience themselves as negative entities, this reparative task has proved most difficult. Successes are rare.

THE ROLE OF THE SCHOOL

The schools are among the social institutions most often in a position to counter the establishment of destructive trends in the personality of children. Within the classroom, it is possible to provide the child with a positive experience of himself. By the same token it is equally possible for negative trends to be reinforced and furthered.

Where the families have not provided a context of growth and support, the school offers the children another arena for working out this essential issue. On the other hand, where the school joins the family and repeatedly frustrates and humiliates the child, it serves as a powerful confirmation of a negative identity. The end result is to invite withdrawal or delinquency.

If a child is to develop an attachment to the educational process, he has to have a positive and emotionally significant feedback experience in the classroom. Where this is absent, school and, indeed, any connections with an adult-directed social process are experienced as ordeals best avoided. Invitations, or pressures, to take part in some process which brings no anticipation of reward beyond the booby prize will be declined, passively or actively. When a youngster tries to compensate, to find his way, in a peer dominated social arena, the development of his educational skills is often bypassed. Instead he develops an apparently adult social life.

THE ESSENTIAL MISDIRECTION OF CURRENT CONCEPTS OF ABUSE PREVENTION

A discussion of educational methodology might seem far afield from a consideration of major obstacles in the prevention of drug abuse. In fact, this topic is close to where the problem lies. Any triumph over insects must see beyond flyswatters; all crucial advances probably began in error.

Meanwhile, the children of this generation are being molded to a significant degree within a classroom structure which can be summarized as "traditional"—a teacher, with desk and blackboard in front of rows of students. There is the smartest kid in the class and the dunce. Toward the end of the academic scale are those disadvantaged by nature, nurture, nutrition, and negativity. In the early grades, the more obviously handicapped may be provided with special educational opportunities. The more dramatic problems in the lives of these special children generally elicit more charity than will the later signs of trouble among older youth.

Any child who does not gain a sense of worth, support, and satisfaction from his school is already in trouble—and a later expression of the trouble may be substance abuse. If he is to learn and to grow, each child must be solidly rooted within a context in which he is valued. Typically, for that population at highest risk for substance abuse, the schools fall short of creating a positive emotional climate. As the grades advance, there is usually an increase in academic competitiveness. For some this leads to a greater sense of deficit, which, in turn, provides a basis for inferiority feelings. All too often, when attempts are made to help the disadvantaged, the focus falls on their academic difficulties. This leaves the emotional pre-conditions for failure unchanged. Minority students are especially apt to fail to establish a constructive relationship with school. For its part, the school is often impotent in its efforts to educate them. One way out has been the policy of social promotion. This means that, regardless of the level of scholastic accomplishment, in the absence of egregious behavior the youngster always moves on to the next grade. For these students, the moment of truth regarding their actual position in the world is delayed for a time. It comes to them at the point that they attempt to enter the job market or to go to a college, on a level beyond their actual abilities.

For a very few, individual and family counseling has been a pivotal experience. It is impossible to know how many of these high risk children might ideally have been helped. School is the interface between society and the young; as such it will either succeed or fail at this basic remedial emotional task. Once the youngster is out of school, the chance of effecting this change becomes increasingly slim.

Among the older youngsters, school is less important. For them, there is often no available context to act as an instrument of change. Neighborhood peer groups seldom help the individuals with problem behavior; the healthier youngsters disassociate themselves, and the troubled ones add to the problems. For the adolescent, it is impossible to generalize about the causes of change. There is no equation for the transformation of a destructive and drug-abusing life style to one which is constructive and associated with an appropriately autonomous status.

THE ROLE OF PSYCHIATRY

Psychiatry can study and strive to understand the phenomena associated with substance abuse: the pharmacology, the phenomenology, the historical antecedents, the psychodynamics, and the sociology. Psychiatrists will also be called upon to work with substance abusers and must assess what makes for change to a more constructive commitment. Hopefully there are many instances where the psychotherapeutic relationship will be crucial, and where emotional change allows for constructive development within the broader social context. To date, it can scarcely be said that psychiatry has done more to help deal with this problem than many other groups or concerned individuals who establish a relationship with a substance abuser.

Dr. Harden Branch, former president of the APA once stated that psychiatry must strive to retain a professional status within a world where there is an abundance of competition to provide psychological services. In order to do this, it must develop an understanding of the limits of its usefulness and applicability. In dealing with substance abuse, the overall role of psychiatry does not extend far into the area of treatment. As medical doctors with a special expertise in understanding human behavior, psychiatrists can aspire to deal effectively with the relatively few substance abusers who do present themselves to the profession. They can also seek to increase their knowledge of the influence of social institutions.

It is regrettable to have no advice to offer on the subject of eliminating substance abuse, nor any method for guaranteeing help for a particular individual. Although much has been learned about the agents of abuse, human self-knowledge remains entangled in error. The history of the regulation of these agents is ridden with irony and tragedy, an example of the sort of thinking which makes it seem logical to attack the automobile after an accident—or beat up the driver who prefers a wreck to a ride. The establishment of perspective in this area demands a rare attainment of knowledge, wisdom, patience, power, and humility. Most professionals who have worked with substance abusers can attest to the frustrating consequences of trying to help them with the usual imperfect attainment of these attributes. Hopefully the knowledge so far achieved will provide a means to avoid repeating or perpetuating past errors. Hopefully, too, it will point the way toward a wise development of human potentiality.

REFERENCES

1. ABRAMSON, H. A. (Ed.), *The Use of LSD in Psychotherapy and Alcoholism*, Bobbs Merrill, New York, 1967.
2. AGHAJANIAN, G. K., et al., "Persistence of Lysergic Acid Diethylamide in the Plasma of Human Subjects," *Clinical Pharmacology and Therapeutics, 5:*611–614, 1964.
3. AGNEW, N., and HOFFER, A., "Nicotinic Acid Modified Lysergic Acid Diethylamide Psychosis," *Journal of Mental Science, 101:*12–27, 1955.
4. American Psychiatric Association, Committee on Nomenclature and Statistics, *Diagnostic and Statistical Manual of Mental Disorders*, 2nd ed., (DSM-II), American Psychiatric Association, Washington, D.C., 1968.
5. American Psychiatric Association, Committee on Nomenclature and Statistics, *Diagnostic and Statistical Manual of Mental Disorders*, (DSM-I), American Psychiatric Association, Washington, D.C., 1952.
6. APPEL, J. B., et al., "Chemically-induced Alterations in the Behavioral Effects of LSD-25," *Biochemical Pharmacology, 13:*861–869, 1964.
7. ASTON, R., "Chemical, Pharmacological and Dependence Characteristics of Hypnosedatives and Minor Tranquilizers," in National Commission on Marihuana and Drug Abuse, *Drug Use In America: Problem in Per-*spective, U.S. Government Printing Office, Washington, D.C., 1973.
8. ———, "Characteristics of Drug Dependence to Barbiturates, Alcohol, and Tranquilizers," in Mule, S. J., and Brill, H. (Eds.), *Chemical and Biological Aspects of Drug Dependence*, Chemical Rubber Company Press, Cleveland, 1972.
9. BAILEY, M. B., HABERMAN, P. W., and SCHEINBERG, J., "Distinctive Characteristics of the Alcoholic Family," *Report of the Health Research Council of the City of New York*, August 30, 1965.
10. BARR, H. L., OTTENBERG, D. J., and ROSEN, A., "The Cross Use of Alcohol and Drugs by Addicts and Alcoholics—Patterns of Previous Abuse of Alcohol in a Group of Hospitalized Drug Addicts," *Proceedings of the Fifth National Conference on Methadone Treatment*, vol. 1, 1973.
11. BECK, R. A., GOLDSTEIN, L., and PFEIFFER, C. C., "Stimulant Effect of Psychotogenic Drugs Demonstrated by Quantitative EEG," *Pharmacologist, 5:*238, 1963.
12. BERGEN, J. R., KRUS, D. M., and PINCUS, G., "Suppression of LSD-25 Effects in Rats by Steroids," *Proceedings of the Society for Experimental Biology and Medicine, 105:*254–256, 1960.

13. BLAINE, J. D., BOZZETTI, L. P., and OHLSON, K. E., "The Narcotic Analgesics: The Opiates," in National Commission on Marihuana and Drug Abuse, *Drug Use In America: Problem in Perspective*, U.S. Government Printing Office, Washington, D.C., 1973.

14. BLANE, H., "The Personality of the Alcoholic," in Chafetz, M. E., et al. (Ed.), *Frontiers of Alcoholism*, Jason Aronson, New York, 1970.

15. BRADLEY, P. B., "The Effect of Amphetamine and D-lysergic Acid Diethylamide (LSD-25) on The Electrical Activity of the Brain of the Conscious Cat," *Journal of Physiology, 120:*13–15, 1953.

16. BRENGELMANN, J. C., et al., "Alleviation of the Psychological Effects of LSD in Man by 5-Hychoxytryptophan," *Journal of Mental Sciences, 104:*1237–1244, 1958.

17. BRODIE, H. K. H., "The Effects of Ethyl Alcohol in Man," in National Commission on Marihuana and Drug Abuse, *Drug Use in America: Problem in Perspective*, U.S. Government Printing Office, Washington, D.C., 1973.

18. CAHALAN, D., CISIN, I., and CROSSLEY, H., *American Drinking Practices*, Rutgers Center of Alcohol Studies, New Brunswick, N.J., 1969.

19. CHAFETZ, M. E., "The Alcoholic in Society," in Grunebaum (Ed.), *The Practice of Community Mental Health*, Little, Brown, Boston, 1970.

20. CHEN, G., et al., "The Pharmacology of 1-(1-phenylcylohexyl) piperdine-HCL," *Journal of Pharmacology and Experimental Therapeutics, 127:*241–250, 1959.

21. CHERUBIN, C. E., "The Medical Sequelae of Narcotic Addiction," *Annals of Internal Medicine, 67:*23–33, 1969.

22. CHESSICK, R. D., et al., "Tolerance to LSD-25 in Schizophrenic Subjects," *Archives of General Psychiatry, 10:*653–658, 1964.

23. CHWELOS, N., et al., "Use of LSD in the Treatment of Alcoholism," *Quarterly Journal of Studies on Alcohol, 20:*577–590, 1959.

24. COHEN, S., *The Beyond Within*, Atherton, New York, 1964.

25. CORK, M. R., "Alcoholism and the Family," paper presented at the annual course of Alcohol and Drug Addiction Research Foundation, University of Western Ontario Press, London, Ont., 1964.

26. DAVIS, V. E., and WALSH, M., "Effect of Ethanol on Neuroamine Metabolism," in Isreal, Y., and Mardones, J. (Eds.), *Biological Basis of Alcoholism*, pp. 73–102, Wiley-Interscience, New York, 1971.

27. ELDER, J. T., JR., and DILLE, J. M., "An Experimental Study of the Participation of the Sympathetic Nervous System in the LSD Reaction in Cats," *Journal of Pharmacology and Experimental Therapy, 136:*162–168, 1962.

28. EVANS, J. I., and LEWIS, S. A., "Drug Withdrawal State in EEG Sleep Study," *Archives of General Psychiatry, 19:*631–634, 1968.

29. FINKLE, B. S., "Ubiquitous Reds: A Local Perspective on Secobarbital Abuse," *Clinical Toxicology, 4(2):*253–264, 1971.

30. FRASER, H. F., et al., "Death Due to Withdrawal of Barbiturates," *Annals of Internal Medicine, 38(6):*1319–1325, 1953.

31. FRAUD, U. I., SHIM, C. S., and WILLIAMS, W. H., JR., "Heroin Induced Pulmonary Edema," *Annals of Internal Medicine, 77:*29–35, 1972.

32. FREEDMAN, D. X., "Psychotomimetic Drugs and Brain Biogenic Amines," *American Journal of Psychiatry, 119:*843–850, 1963.

33. ———, et al., "LSD-25 and the Status and Level of Brain Serotonin," *Annals of the New York Academy of Science, 96:*98–106, 1962.

34. FRIEDMAN, S. A., and HIRSCH, S. E., "Extreme Hyperthermia after LSD Ingestion," *Journal of the American Medical Association, 217(11):*1549–1550, 1971.

35. GADDUM, J. H., "Antagonism Between Lysergic Acid Diethylamide and 5-Hydroxytryptamine," *Journal of Physiology, 112:*15*ff*., 1953.

36. GALANTER, M., et al., "Effects on Humans of Delta-9-Tetrahydrocannabinol Administered by Smoking," *Science, 176:*934–936, 1972.

37. GERSHON, S., and LANG, W. J., "A Psycho-Pharmacological Study of Some Indole Alkaloids," *Archives Internationales de Pharmacodynamic et de Therapie, 135:*31–56, 1962.

38. HAMBURG, B. A., KRAEMER, H. C., and JAHNKE, W. A., "A Hierarchy of Drug Use In Adolescence: Behavioral and Attitudinal Correlates of Substantial Drug Use," *The American Journal of Psychiatry, 132(11):*1155–1163, 1975.

39. HARFORD, T. C., "Patterns of Alcohol Abuse Among Adolescents," *Psychiatric Opinion, 12(3)*, 1975.

40. HEUBNER, W., et al., "Historische Notiz Über Die Entdeckung der Synapsen in Autonomen Nervensystem Mit Holfe Des Nikotins," *Archiv fuer Experimentelle Pathologie und Pharmakologie, 204:*33–35, 1947.

41. HEYMANS, C., BROUCKAERT, J. J., and DAUTREBANDE, L., "Sinus Carotidins et Actions Stimulantes Respiratoires de la Nicotine et de la Lobeline," *Comptes Rendus Societede des Seances de la Biologie et des Sesfiliales, 106:*469–471, 1931.

42. HOFMANN, A., "Psychotomimetic Agents," in Burger, A. (Ed.), *Drugs Affecting the Central Nervous System*, Marcel Dekker, New York, 1968.

43. HOLAHAN, F. F., "The Economics of Heroin," in Wald, P. M., and Hutt, P. B. (Cochairmen), *Dealing With Drug Abuse: A Report to the Ford Foundation*, pp. 255–291, Praeger, New York, 1972.

44. HOLLISTER, L. E., "Marihuana in Man: Three Years Later," *Science, 172:*21–29, 1971.

45. ———, and HARTMAN, A. M., "Mescaline, LSD, and Psilocybin, Comparison of Clinical Syndromes, Effects on Color Perception and Biochemical Measures," *Comprehensive Psychiatry, 3:*235–241, 1962.

46. ISBELL, H., et al., "Tolerance to Diethylamide of LSD-25, *Federation Proceedings, 14:*354*ff*., 1955.

47. ———, and FRASER, H. F., "Addiction to Analgesics and Barbiturates," *Pharmacological Reviews, 2(2):*355–397, 1950.

48. JACKSON, J. K., "Alcoholism and the Family," *American Academy of Political and Social Science Annals, 315:*90–98, 1958.

49. JACOBSEN, E., "The Clinical Pharmacology of the Hallucinogens," *Clinical Pharmacology and Therapeutics, 4:*480–503, 1963.

50. JACOBI, J. E., et al., "Drug Use and Criminality in a Birth Cohort," in National Commission on Marijuana and Drug Abuse, *Drug Use in America: Problem in Perspective*, U.S. Government Printing Office, Washington, D.C., 1973.

51. JAFFE, J. H., "The Maintainance Option and the Special Action Office for Drug Abuse Prevention," *Psychiatric Annals, 5:*10*ff*., 1975.

52. JAFFE, J. M., "Report at American Medical Association Conference on Medical Complications of Drug Abuse," American Medical Association, Washington, D.C., 1972.

53. JONES, R. T., "Biological Effects of Cannabis: 1972 Literature," in National Commission on Marijuana and Drug Abuse, *Drug Abuse in America: Problem in Perspective*, U.S. Government Printing Office, Washington, D.C., 1973.

54. KANDEL, D., and FAUST, R., "Sequence and Stages in Patterns of Adolescent Drug Use," *Archives of General Psychiatry, 32(7):*923–932, 1975.

55. KARNIOL, I. G., and CARLINI, E. A., "The Content of Delta-9-Trans-Tetrahydrocannabinol (Delta-9-THC) Does Not Explain All Biological Activity of Some Brazilian Marihuana Samples," *Journal of Pharmacology and Pharmacy, 24:*833–835, 1972.

56. KAST, E., "Pain and LSD-25: A Theory of Attenua-

tion of Anticipation," in Solomon, D. (Ed.), *LSD, The Consciousness-Expanding Drug*, G. P. Putnam's Sons, New York, 1964.

57. Klepfisz, A., and Racy, J., "Homicide and LSD," *Journal of the American Medical Association, 223(4):* 429–430, 1973.

58. Knott, D. H., and Beard, J. D., "Changes in Cardiovascular Activity as a Function of Alcohol Intake," in Kissin, B., and Begleiter, H. (Eds.), *The Biology of Alcoholism. II Physiology and Behavior*, Plenum Press, New York, 1972.

59. Krus, D. M., et al., "The Influence of Progesterone on Behavioral Changes Induced by Lysergic Acid Diethylamide (LSD-25) in Normal Males," *Psychopharmacologia, 2:*177–184, 1961.

60. Langley, J. N., et al., "On the Local Paralysis of Peripheral Ganglia and on the Connection of Different Classes of Nerve Fibers with Them," *Proceedings of the Royal Society*, Series B., *46:*432–431, 1889.

61. Leak, C. D., *The Amphetamines, Their Actions and Uses*, Charles C Thomas, Springfield, Ill., 1958.

62. Lemberger, L., et al., "11-Hydroxy-Delta-9-Tetrahydrocannabinol: Pharmacology, Disposition and Metabolism of a Major Metabolite of Marihuana in Man," *Science, 177:*62–64, 1972.

63. Levick, L. J., and Levick, S. N., "Testicular Choriocarcinoma in LSD Users," *Journal of the American Medical Association, 217(4):*475–476, 1971.

64. Lewin, L., *Phantastica: Narcotic and Stimulating Drugs*, Dutton, New York, 1964.

65. Lewis, D. J., and Sloane, R. B., "Therapy with LSD," *Journal of Clinical and Experimental Psychopathology, 19:*19–31, 1958.

66. Lindemann, E., and Malamud, W., "Experimental Analysis of Psychopathological Effects of Intoxicating Drugs," *American Journal of Psychiatry, 13:*853–881, 1934.

67. Linder, R. L., Lerner, S. E., and Wesson, D. R., "Solvent Sniffing: A Continuing Problem Among Youth," *Proceedings of the Western Pharmacology Society, 18:* 371–374, 1975.

68. Lundquist, F., "The Metabolism of Ethanol," in Israel, Y., and Mardones, J. (Eds.), *Biological Basis of Alcoholism*, pp. 1–52, Wiley-Interscience, 1971.

69. McClelland, D., et al., *The Drinking Man: Alcohol and Human Motivation*, Free Press, New York, 1972.

70. McCord, W., and McCord, J., *Origins of Alcoholism*, Stanford Press, Stanford, Calif., 1960.

71. McMillan, D. E., et al., "Tolerance to Active Constituents of Marihuana," *Archives Internationales de Pharmacodynamie et de Therapie, 198:*132–144, 1972.

72. Menninger, K. A., *Man Against Himself*, Harcourt, Brace, New York, 1938.

73. Meyers, F. M., et al., "Incidents Involving the Haight-Ashbury Population and Some Uncommonly Used Drugs," *Psychedelic Drugs, 1:*139–146, 1967–1968.

74. Mik, G., "Sons of Alcoholic Fathers," *British Journal of Addiction, 65(4):*305–315, 1970.

75. Moreau de Tours, J. J., "Du Hachich et de L'Alienation Mentale," in *Etudes Psychologiques*, Masson, Paris, 1845.

76. Murphree, H. B., et al., "Quantitative ECG Analysis of the Effects of LSD and d-Amphetamine in Man," *Federation Proceedings, 21:*337ff., 1962.

77. National Commission on Marihuana and Drug Abuse, *Drug Use in America: Problem in Perspective*, U.S. Government Printing Office, Washington, D.C., 1973.

78. Newman, M. L., et al., "Delta-9-Tetrahydrocannabinol and Ethyl Alcohol: Evidence For Cross Tolerance in the Rat," *Science, 175:*1022–1023, 1972.

79. Nylander, I., "Children of Alcoholic Fathers," *Acta Paediatrica, 49:* Supplement 121, 1960.

80. Pare, C. M. B., and LaBrosse, E. H., "A Further Study on the Alleviation of LSD in Man by Pretreatment with 5-Hydroxytryptophan," *Journal of Psychiatric Research, 1:*271–277, 1963.

81. Paton, W. D. M., and Pertwee, R. G., "Effects of Cannabis and Certain of Its Constituents on Pentobarbitone Sleeping Time and Phenazone Metabolism," *British Journal of Pharmacology, 44:*250–261, 1972.

82. Rinkel, M., "Pharmacodynamics of LSD and Mescaline," *Journal of Nervous and Mental Disease, 125:* 424–427, 1957.

83. Roth, G. M., and Shick, R. M., "Effect of Smoking on the Cardiovascular System of Man," *Circulation, 17:*443–459, 1958.

84. Simmons, J. Q., et al., "Modification of Autistic Behavior with LSD," *American Journal of Psychiatry, 122:*1201–1211, 1966.

85. Stockings, G. T., "New Euphoriant for Depressive Mental States," *British Medical Journal, 1:*918–922, 1947.

86. Stoll, W. A., "Lysergsaurediathylamid, ein Phantastikum aus der Mutterkorngruppe," *Schweizer Archiv fuer Neurologie, Neurochirurgie und Psychiatrie, 60:*279–323, 1974.

87. Thudichum, J. W. L., *A Treatise on the Chemical Constitution of the Brain*, Balliere, London, 1884.

88. Vinar, O., "Analogien Zwishen Schizophrenon Erkrankungen und der LSD-Psychose," *Psychiatrie Neurologie und Medizinische Psychologie, 10:*162–166, 1958.

89. Wallgren, H., and Barry, H., *Actions of Alcohol: Biochemical, Physiological and Psychological Aspects*, vol. 1, Elsevier, New York, 1970.

90. Ward, R. F., and Faillace, L. A., "The Alcoholic and His Helpers: A Systems View," *Quarterly Journal of Studies on Alcohol, 31(3):*684–691, 1970.

91. Wechsler, R. L., "Effects of Cigarette Smoking and Intravenous Nicotine on the Human Brain," *Federation Proceedings, 17:*169ff., 1958.

92. Williams, A. F., "Social Drinking, Anxiety, and Depression," *Journal of Personality and Social Psychology, 3(6):*689–693, 1966.

93. Wilson, C. O., et al., *Textbook of Organic Medicinal and Pharmaceutical Chemistry*, 6th ed., Lippincott, Philadelphia, Pa., 1971.

94. Wolfgang, M. E., *Patterns in Criminal Homicide*, Patterson Smith, Montclair, N.J., 1975.

95. Woolley, D. W., et al., "Evidence for the Participation of Serotonin in Mental Processes," *Annals of the New York Academy of Science, 66:*649–665, 1957.

96. Zinberg, N. E., "Teenage Alcoholism and Drug Abuse," Letter to the *New England Journal of Medicine, 294(1):*561, 1976.

34 / Accident Proneness

Raymond Sobel

Introduction

Accidents are the major health problem of children and adolescents in the United States. They are responsible for more fatalities and disabling conditions than all diseases combined. Each year they account for 25,000 deaths plus the loss of a million years of life expectancy among American children and adolescents.[15] The annual cost to the nation has been estimated to be $47.1 billion. Accidents produce more misery, waste more lives, and end more careers than any other single cause. Children and adolescents account for a very large proportion of these injuries and fatalities. There has, however, been little basic investigation of the relationship of somatic and mental illness to this problem.

Definition and Description

Accidents are unplanned, unpredictable, and unexpected events which result in injury. The same event, e.g., falling down a flight of stairs, will be recorded medically as an accident if it results in injury, but will not be called an accident if the individual sustains no harm, i.e., has a "near miss." Psychiatrically, an accident may be considered to be a form of injury-producing behavior.

Accident Proneness

The term, accident proneness, has three different meanings, each of which has its own diagnostic, therapeutic, and preventive implications. It is important to distinguish among accident proneness, a classical psychoanalytic concept that describes a persistent self-destructive personality; accident liability, a statistical concept of increased risk of accident from multiple causes; and accident repetitiveness, a behavioral pattern of variable duration.

Accident proneness should be confined to that small minority of persons who persistently and repeatedly sustain unanticipated and undesired self-injury. In most cases, these accidents have little to do with the impulse for self-destruction. It is true that over certain intervals, these children and adults have more accidents than the population at large. Nonetheless, the theory that all accidents are the result of persistent self-destructive tendencies has little basis in fact. It has achieved a totally unwarranted legitimacy and reminds one of the words of H. L. Mencken: "For every human problem, there is a solution that is simple, neat, and wrong."

Description of the Syndrome

All children are accident prone by nature. Their increased tendency toward accidents is the resultant of the interactions of the child, the agent of harm, and the psychological, social, and physical environments. The interplay of these factors determines whether an accident will occur, how serious it will be, and whether or not there will be repetition.

The use of the term accident implies that the event is unanticipated, undesirable, unpredictable, and unintended. In this regard, an accident resembles Freudian parapraxes[5] which do not "just happen" by chance; instead they occur as the result of forces which are not immediately evident. In the case of children, accidents occur when there is a disturbance in the equilibrium between the self-preservative behavior of the child, the protective behavior of society, and the environmental hazard. Children are free from harm and behave safely when these factors, each with its own history and determinants, are at an optimal level. Behavior becomes unsafe and there is higher risk of accident when their interaction reaches a certain critical point, often triggered by chance.

History of the Concept of Accident Proneness

The concept of accident proneness was developed early in this century. It was noticed that within a given population (say a factory work force), a minority of persons had one, two, or even three accidents, whereas the majority of the work force had none at all.[7] It was then inferred that these persons were "accident prone." This conclusion was reached without further scientific or critical inquiry and was given a psychoanalytic interpretation by Dunbar in 1943.[3] She maintained that accidents in children and adults were the result of a specfic kind of psychopathology which involved a lingering and continuous drive toward self-destruction. This plausible theory was derived from a small number of accident repeaters; it was subsequently generalized to explain all accidents. It had a profound effect upon subsequent research by pediatricians and child psychiatrists; indeed, many efforts were made to identify and document those personality traits consonant with the theory. However, Dunbar[3] and Menninger[14] did not realize that the psychodynamics of accident repeaters, a deviant group of individuals, could not be extended to the population at large. They were also unaware of the "Poisson Distribution which states that on a purely chance basis[2, 6] in any given time span, it is only a minority of the population which will suffer most of the accidents.

In fact, if the same factory population is followed for another year, once again a minority would have incurred most of the accidents. This time, however, the group would not contain the same individuals who had had accidents during the previous years. Accident repetitiveness certainly does exist, but it is a transitory phenomenon. In fact, only very few children and adolescents continue to have accidents repeatedly over long periods of time.

So persuasive was Dunbar's concept that it was more than a decade before accidents were psychologically studied from any other viewpoint. With the notable exception of McFarland's work,[13] until 1970 behavioral studies suffered from inadequate data, simplistic conceptualization, and appalling methodology. McFarland introduced the ecological or systems approach to the study of accidents and examined the phenomenon as a host-agent-environment interaction. In the early 1960s, two symposia were conducted on the behavioral approaches to studies of accidents.[1, 23]

These, together with Haddon, Suchman, and Klein's landmark publication,[8] revolutionized approaches to understanding accidents of children and adults.

Thereafter, several studies of children with repeated accidents were published which attempted to delineate specific personality characteristics.[25] It appeared that the children who suffered accidents were energetic, aggressive, and impulsive, with strong tendencies to motor discharge of tension. Nonetheless, the studies produced little, if any, evidence that such traits were more common in accident-incurring children than in an accident-free control group. More recent studies have demonstrated that these aggressive and assertive traits alone do not account for accidents in children. They are better understood as the child's manifestations of a disturbance in a larger interpersonal field.[12, 20] Current concepts tend to explain repeated accidents on the part of the child as a symptom of disturbance within a family group which is experiencing acute or chronic stress. Accordingly, it suggested that the term "accident proneness," with its exclusively individual connotation, not only fails to explain adequately the cause of accidents, but also distracts from thinking about accidents as the end result of a disturbed social system.

Frequency, Incidence, Prevalence

The occurrence of accidents varies greatly as a result of the interactions mentioned previously.

Age: Accidents account for almost one-half of all deaths among children. In adolescents and young adults, accidents claim more lives than all other causes combined and are responsible for about four times more deaths than the next leading causes, suicide and homicide.

Sex: Males have more accidents than females at all ages, but the disparity is at its peak during adolescence when the male death rate is four times that of females.

Type of Agent: Table 34-1 illustrates the leading causes of accident deaths in children and adolescents by age and accident type.[15] Motor vehicles are by far the major cause, even though car accident deaths per 10,000 have been reduced drastically. This has occurred despite a six-fold increase since 1933 in the number of vehicles and the number of miles traveled.

The type of accident is closely related to the

TABLE 34-1

Leading Causes of All Deaths—1974

	UNDER 1 YEAR		1–14		5–14		15–24	
	# OF DEATHS	DEATH RATE*	# OF DEATHS	DEATH RATE*	# OF DEATHS	DEATH RATE*	# OF DEATHS	DEATH RATE*
Motor Vehicle	224	7	1,322	10	3,332	9	15,905	41
Drowning	—	—	850	6	1,320	3	2,390	6
Fires, burns	136	5	654	5	569	1	—	—
Ingestion of food, object	442	15	163	1	—	—	1,088	2
Firearms	—	—	—	—	—	—	832	—
Falls	87	3	159	1	—	—	—	10
Other	564†	18	734	6	1,816	5	3,985	3
Total Accidents	1,453	48	3,882	29	7,037	18	24,200	62

* Deaths per 100,000 in each age group.
† 50% due to suffocation.
NOTE: Reprinted by permission of the publisher from National Safety Council, *Accident Facts*, (Chicago: National Safety Council, 1976). © 1976 by The National Safety Council.

child's developmental level and social role. Pre-school children tend to have home accidents such as poisonings, burns, and falls, or to be injured as passengers in a car. With increasing autonomy, poisonings decrease, and high-risk behavior by children results in pedestrian accidents, falls, sport injuries, and the like. In adolescents, the major agent is the automobile as is well known to insurance underwriters and to the parents of teenage drivers.

Socio-Economic Factors: Urban surveys of burns and accidental poisoning have stressed the importance of such contributing factors as low socio-economic status, unemployment, overcrowding, and frequent changes of residence.[17]

Studies of the epidemiology of accidents have shown that, at least in rural areas, low socio-economic status or economic deprivation by itself does not necessarily result in a higher accident rate.[20, 21] Rather, it is the family stress associated with poverty and social deprivation which seems to be the causal factor.

Course of the Accident Phenomenon: It is virtually impossible to reach adulthood without having had a disabling injury, i.e., one which results in medical attention and which causes one full day or more of restricted activity (National Health Survey definition). The sequence of events leading up to an injury and following it has been described by Hirschfeld and Behan.[10] In their study of industrial accidents, they found that preceding the accident, there was inevitably a conflict

between a need to work for pay, status, companionship, pride, etc., and an inability to keep on doing so. They concluded that the accident, as well as the disability which might ensue, comprised a conflict solving device. A similar process has been noted in conflicts related to dependency; this has been observed in children and adolescents who have accidents during time of family stress.[20, 21] Such findings parallel the conclusions reached from investigations of the relationship between physical illness and life stress. These show that illness tends to occur at a characteristic point in an individual's life. Typically, there had been an increase in the number of life changes and degree of stress.[16] In individual cases, it appeared as though the illness served a useful purpose for the person by "solving" otherwise insoluble problems.

If one views the accident process in this fashion, the agent and the environment provide the arena in which the pre-existing conflict of the child or adult can be acted out. This may afford a partial explanation of why most children have few accidents. Injury may serve no purpose for them if it is not associated with primary or secondary gain. This may also explain why most accident repeaters cluster their injuries over relatively short periods of their lives. In their case, repetition of the sequence may be necessary to relieve the conflict. This can be achieved either through primary need gratification or by secondary removal from the life situation as the result of injury.

Etiology

For accidents, the epidemiologic model has proven to be the most useful explanatory construct. It states that accidents are not "accidental," i.e., due to chance alone, but are the end result, or the by-product, of the failure of the host-agent-environment system to maintain security. These general considerations apply to all accidents regardless of age or developmental level.

Genetic and Constitutional Factors: No genetic or constitutional predisposition to accidents has ever been documented. The slight correlation reported between the accidents of children and their parents may be attributed to many factors other than heredity.

Physical Factors: One would expect that bright-eyed, bushy-tailed, or hyperactive children would be more prone to accidents. Although this is true of children incurring injuries, it is not true of poisoning or automobile accidents. This is not surprising, since children who are superior in muscular coordination are more likely to be attracted to sports and games which expose them to higher risk, hence to injuries.

Intelligence: No studies have shown that intelligence plays a role in accidents. Although the brighter child may be more curious and intrusive, his greater risk may be canceled out by his awareness of the consequences of his behavior. There is no evidence that mentally retarded children sustain more accidents than children of normal intelligence. Whether this is due to learned cautiousness or to greater societal protection is not known. There is a dearth of studies of this aspect of the question.

Developmental Level: This factor, together with its accompanying variable, family interaction and stress, are important determinants of accidents. Illustrative paradigms of two developmental periods will be examined: poisoning in infancy and childhood, and traffic crashes in adolescence.

Infancy and Childhood: The characteristic relevant features of the child at this level of development are dependency, orality, magical and animistic thinking, and rudimentary concepts of time and causality. These factors, together with family disorganization, a lapse in maternal protectiveness, and the presence of toxic agents may result in accidental poisoning. In a study of accidental poisoning in 367 families living in a predominantly rural area, it was found that childhood poisoning is a function primarily of parental pyschopathology and family disturbance.[20] Contrary to what common sense would dictate, the frequency of poisoning was found to be unrelated to safety (accessibility of toxic substances), level of motor development, intelligence of the child, birth complications, and parental accident proneness. There was some suggestion that childhood emotional disorder and accidental poisoning are related, but the most significant correlations by far were those between poisoning and measures of maternal psychopathology. Significant relationships are also found between childhood poisoning and indices of family stress and strain, i.e., parental arguments, fights in the home, environmental stress, and a psychiatric finding of family pathology.

In the light of these findings, poisoning of infants and preschool children can be seen as one of the terminal links in a process which starts with a failure of mothering. This leads to the frustration of a number of the child's needs, specifically for dependency, autonomy, and security. Depending upon the nature of the mother's failure, the level of the child's development and the specific need frustrated, the resulting self-poisoning can be seen as an act of defiance, a bid for attention, a coercive attempt to achieve dependency, and/or an expression of anger deflected from the mother to the self. These findings have been replicated by Holdaway in New Zealand[11] and by Husband in Great Britain.[12]

Adolescence: The major characteristics of this developmental level include: psychological and biological lability, a resurgence of sexual impulses, a need for autonomy and disengagement from the family, experimentation with social roles, a shift of dependency from the family to the peer group, and the establishment of identity. In the highly mechanized American society, the car culture has become both literally and figuratively a major vehicle through which adolescents, directly or symbolically, work out their normal problems of growth and development. In the course of a single evening, the teenage male may use the car to act out a host of impulses and defenses—some quite conscious, others totally out of awareness. These might include: escape from family and parental pressures, rebellion against authority, assertion of his maleness, acceptance or refusal of the highway rights of others, experimentation with alcohol, enactment of a wish to be a racing driver, or derivation of status from peers by virtue of the car's prestige and power. His car may also provide him with a mobile and private place for love-making, hopefully far from the prying eyes of the adult. Studies of teenage traffic accidents and violations have established statistically significant correlations of traffic accidents with the impulsivity, rebelliousness, risk-taking, and thrill-seeking behavior of adolescent males.[18] For male drivers, these factors seem to be at least as important as driving skills, or the exposure to risk measured by the mileage driven.[9] Studies also demonstrate the significance of psycho-social variables in the causation of accidents in adolescence. Using path analysis, a somewhat more sophisticated mathematical model of the accident process,[4] it was possible to demonstrate that family and life stress increased the adolescent's vulnerability to accidents in two different ways: (1) directly, through the possible effects of anxiety and preoccupation with perceptual-motor driving skills; and (2) indirectly, through the effects of defensive coping styles such as "macho" behavior in boys, which expose the adolescent to higher risk. These relationships do not apply to females since the only correlate of girls' traffic accidents is the number of miles driven. This finding may provide an explanation for the significant difference between males and females in accidents of all types. Sex-role stereotyping tends to inhibit female aggression and self-assertion; females may, therefore, engage in less high-risk behavior in order to relieve stress and emotional conflict. In one example, girls from disturbed homes showed twice as much depression as boys from comparably pathological backgrounds. It is suggested that in response to social stress in adolescence, girls may tend to become depressed, whereas boys tend to act out. The outcome provides substantially different reasons for their traffic accidents. However, one should take note that using the most modern methods, measurement, and statistical analysis, the mutual interaction of the adolescent driver, his vehicle, the mileage driven, and the family and peer group accounts for and predicts only 17 percent of the causality or variance. These methods are useful for large cohorts; it is quite a different matter to seek to understand the genesis of a single accident. This is still best accomplished through the traditional retrospective methods of psychiatry in which the events leading to the accident are psychodynamically reconstructed.

The individual psychodynamics of the accident process are far more complicated and varied than the original hypothesis that attributed this to self-destructive "accident proneness." Nonetheless, such cases do in fact exist. In fatal accidents, conscious or unconscious suicidal motivation can often be demonstrated or inferred from the life events immediately preceding the accident.[19]

Waller[24] has demonstrated a close link between unintentional shootings, crashes, and acts of violence.

These two paradigms, childhood poisoning and adolescent traffic crashes, highlight the fact that accidents are not accidental and that, among their other causes, there are important psychiatric components. It is suggested that accidents are but one possible outcome of an individual's failure to cope adequately with the physical and psychosocial environment. It is only through detailed, individual, retrospective analysis of each case that one can understand why one child in a family is a poison repeater, another a bedwetter, and a third, an obsessive-compulsive neurotic. The data suggest that, in many instances, the close relation of alcohol abuse to traffic crashes in adolescence is probably not due to the direct interference of alcohol with driving skills. This may be a spurious correlation due to the fact that adolescents under pressure are likely both to drink and have accidents, as means of coping with stress. What is specially worthy of notice here is the failure of all investigators to identify any specific family or personal psychodynamic syndrome common to all accidents. It is more likely that the important causative factor is quantitative, i.e., the magnitude of social stress or family disorganization, rather than any qualitative variation. Only now is there a beginning understanding of why, in the same disturbed family, one member becomes alcoholic, another depressed, and still others have accidents.

When the clinician encounters an accident in the life of his child patient, it is best to consider this as symptomatic of a larger disorder in the child's life and social field. In these cases, it behooves the therapist or diagnostician to look carefully into the areas mentioned previously: the family structure, organization, and function, the family life style, the child's assigned role within the family, the models of identity, the approved means of coping with frustration, etc. In many cases, this will prove to be rewarding and may even have later preventive effects. This is especially true of those children who are evincing a pattern of accident repetition.

Prevention

Both the epidemiologist and the psychodynamic approach to accidents of childhood and adolescence have implicated a multifactorial etiology.

This involves disturbances in the relationship of the host, agent, physical environment, and psychosocial milieu; yet in recent years, the only headway which has been made in the actual prevention of accidents has been the result of passive restraints on the individual's risk-taking behavior. Typical examples are the mandates imposed by state and federal law, by the Office of Safety and Health Administration (OSHA), or, indirectly, by insurance companies as a condition of insurability. A brief list would include the use of motorcycle helmets, passive seatbelt restraints, collapsible steering columns in automobiles, nationwide safety packaging of drugs and toxic agents, lowering of the speed limit to 55 miles per hour, and the elimination of open railroad grade crossings. The often violent opposition of the public to these imposed restrictions tends to document the psychodynamic theories of accident genesis detailed previously, particularly those which suggest that, among males, the accident is often an unintended outcome of excessive risk-taking in demonstrating masculinity.

Attempts to prevent accidents through education of the child, the parent, and the community have been tried repeatedly. Although they have great appeal, unfortunately, they have failed miserably. It is evident that they have not recognized the inordinately complex causes of the accident phenomenon and have focused on the weakest link in the causal chain. Despite many prior years of costly poison prevention education, reductions in the accidental poisonings of infants and toddlers occurred only after the introduction of safety closures and packaging. Significant reduction of traffic fatalities in this country has been due to industry opposed and consumer neglected engineering improvements, not to driver education or safety campaigns. The first major drop in the motor vehicle death rate in over thirty years was not due to voluntary safe driving. It was the result of the oil embargo which led to the imposition and strict enforcement of a 55 mile per hour speed limit.

Conclusion

The family is the most important part of the child's environment, and family disorganization, the major cause of childhood accidents. Hence, the preservation or restoration of family integrity and well-being should be the primary method of accident prevention for children and adolescents. For the clinician, this implies an awareness of the accident as symptom of both individual and family disequilibrium. It requires a willingness on his part to go beyond education and simple elimination of hazard. A thorough family evaluation should be the first step. It should include a home visit and detailed examination of the family's life style. The family role of the child whose presenting symptom is an increased liability to accident should be explored. In those few cases where accident proneness is the result of self-destructive tendencies, individual and/or family therapy may be the treatment of choice.

REFERENCES

1. Association for the Aid of Crippled Children, *Behavioral Approaches to Accident Research*, Association for the Aid of Crippled Children, New York, 1961.
2. Ciba-Geigy Corporation, "Poison Distribution," in *Scientific Tables*, 6th ed., Documenta Geigy, p. 186, Ardsley, N.Y., 1962.
3. Dunbar, H., "Accident Habit," in Dunbar, H., *Psychosomatic Diagnosis*, Hoeber, New York, 1943.
4. Duncan, O. D., "Path Analysis: Sociological Examples," *American Journal of Sociology, 72:*2, 1966.
5. Freud, S., "The Psychopathology of Everyday Life," in Brill, A. A. (Trans.), *The Basic Writings of Sigmund Freud*, Modern Library, New York, 1938.
6. Froggat, P., and Smiley, J. A., "The Concept of Accident Proneness: A Review," *British Journal of Industrial Medicine, 21:*1, 1964.
7. Greenwood, M., and Woods, H. M., *Report of the Industrial Fatigue Research Board No. 4*, Medical Research Council and Department of Scientific and Industrial Research, Her Majesty's Stationery Office, London, 1919.
8. Haddon, W., Suchman, E. A., and Klein, D.,

Accident Research: Methods and Approaches, Harper, New York, 1964.
9. Harrington, D. M., *The Young Driver Follow-Up Study: An Evaluation of the Role of Human Factors in the First Four Years of Driving*, Department of Motor Vehicles, Sacramento, Calif., 1971.
10. Hirschfeld, A. H., and Behan, R. C., "The Accident Process," *Journal of the American Medical Association, 186(3):*193, 1963.
11. Holdaway, M. D., "Accidental Burns and Poisoning of Children in the Home," *New Zealand Medical Journal, 75:*280, 1975.
12. Husband, P., "The Accident-Prone Child," *The Practitioner, 211:*335, 1973.
13. McFarland, R. A., "Psychological and Behavioral Aspects of Automobile Accidents," *Traffic Safety Research Review, 12:*71, 1968.
14. Menninger, K., *Man Against Himself*, Harcourt Brace, New York, 1937.
15. National Safety Council, *Accident Facts*, National Safety Council, Chicago, 1976.
16. Rahe, R. H., et al., "Social Stress and Illness Onset," *Journal of Psychosomatic Research, 11:*213, 1964.

17. SAVAGE, J. P., and LEITCH, I. O. W., "Childhood Burns: A Sociological Survey and Inquiry into Causation," *The Medical Journal of Australia, 1*:1337, 1972.

18. SCHUMAN, S. H., et al., "Young Male Drivers: Impulse Expression, Accidents and Violations," *Journal of the American Medical Association, 200*:1026, 1967.

19. SELZER, M. L., and VINOKUR, A., "Life Events, Subjective Stress, and Traffic Accidents," *American Journal of Psychiatry, 131*:903, 1974.

20. SOBEL, R., "The Psychiatric Implications of Accidental Poisoning in Childhood," *Pediatric Clinics of North America, 17(3)*:653, 1970.

21. ———, and UNDERHILL, R., "Family Disorganization and Teenage Auto Accidents," *Journal of Safety Research, 8(1)*:8, 1976.

22. ———, "Psychosocial Antecedents of Automobile Accidents in Rural Adolescents," in *Proceedings, 18th Conference of the American Association for Automotive Medicine*, p. 417, Toronto, 1974.

23. SUCHMAN, E. A., and SCHERZER, A. L., *Current Research in Childhood Accidents*, Association for the Aid of Crippled Children, New York, 1960.

24. WALLER, J. A., "Unintentional Shootings, Highway Crashes, and Acts of Violence: A Behavior Paradigm," Paper presented at the 3rd Congress on Medical and Related Aspects of Motor Vehicle Accidents, New York, 1969.

25. WEHRLE, P. F., et al., "The Epidemiology of Accidental Poisoning in an Urban Population, II" *American Journal of Public Health, 50*:1925, 1960.

35 / Sleep Disorders

Steven Luria Ablon and John E. Mack

Introduction

Sleep disturbances in childhood are common. Their characteristics change at different ages and they vary from mild responses to inevitable developmental stresses, to severe disturbances, markedly altering the child and the family's life. Early attempts to explain childhood sleep disturbances usually attributed them to various bodily dysfunctions such as gastrointestinal distress. For example, in the latter half of the fifth century B.C. the Greek physician Hippocrates[14] wrote, "Then later when he sits down to dine, food is distasteful to him and he cannot eat his customary dinner. Instead, the food causes colic and rumblings and burns the stomache; he sleeps poorly and is disturbed by violent nightmares." This situation has changed greatly. At present, sleep disturbances are conceptualized in terms of a complex interplay of multiple factors. Sigmund Freud's *Interpretation of Dreams*[30] and Anna Freud's *Normality and Pathology in Childhood: Assessments of Development*[28] are important landmarks in the organization of psychological theories about sleep, dreaming, and child development. These two major works combined with the contributions of many other investigators clarified the impact of multiple determinants in sleep disturbances: (1) external factors that threaten the child's security; (2) traumatic memories; (3) developmental stresses such as attaining autonomy and independence; (4) instinctual forces; (5) the state of the ego in terms of reality testing and cognitive development; and (6) the regressive characteristics integral to the process of sleeping.

In addition, beginning in 1953, Aserinsky, Kleitman, and Dement,[5, 17] utilizing electrophysiologic recordings of sleeping infants and adults, recognized the presence of regular sleep cycles with accompanying periods of rapid eye movement. As the field of sleep physiology expanded, there was increasing clarification of the role of factors such as the phases of sleep, fever, and drugs in sleep disturbances. As a result, it has been possible to begin to relate psychological and physiological processes in understanding disorders of sleep. From this perspective, it is apparent that before discussing individual syndromes of sleep disturbance, it is important to review our present understanding of the physiology of sleep. Following this, the effect of psychological maturation on sleep disturbances in childhood will be reviewed. Sleep-connected problems such as bedtime rituals, fear of the dark or of sleeping alone, difficulty falling asleep, and recurrent awakening at night will be discussed. Since the nightmare embodies the conflicts of the child and reflects his development at different ages, it will be used as the prototype of a childhood sleep disorder. In this way the impact of developmental stresses at different ages as seen in the example of the nightmare can be applied to other sleep disturbances of childhood. The sleep disorders subsequently discussed in individual sections will include night terrors, somnambulism, enuresis, narcolepsy, and hypersomnias.

The Physiology of Sleep

The present understanding of the physiology of sleep has been clearly set forth in a number of review articles and books.* These studies are the result of sleep profiles obtained from subjects observed nightly by the use of electroencephalographic (EEG), electrooculographic (EOG), and electromyographic (EMG) recordings transmitted to polygraph machines. Electrodes are placed on the scalp to record brain activity, at the outer canthus of each eye to measure eye movements, and beneath the chin to monitor muscle tone. In special studies, parameters such as heart rate, respiratory rate, gastric secretions, and penile tumescence are also monitored. The massive amount of data that is accumulated can then be carefully analyzed.

Normal Sleep

Currently, normal sleep is conceptualized as a series of repeated cycles representing phases of brain and body activity. There are two major categories of sleep, rapid eye movement (REM) sleep, and nonrapid eye movement (NREM) sleep. NREM sleep is divided into four stages. Usually when a person falls asleep, Stage 1 sleep is recorded. It is characterized by a low amplitude, fast frequency electroencephalographic pattern, and an absence of REM. Sleep progresses into Stage 2 and then into the deeper sleep of Stages 3 and 4. Stage 2 is characterized by EEG patterns containing "spindles" of twelve to fourteen cycles per second and/or K-complexes, with continuing low amplitude fast frequency activity. K-complexes are defined as EEG tracings having a well defined negative sharp wave which is immediately followed by a positive component.[72] Stages 3 and 4 sleep show a generalized slowing of frequency and an increase in the amplitude of the electro-

* See references 1, 41, 42, 43, 44, and 51.

encephalographic waves. Progressively in Stages 3 and 4 sleep, high amplitude, low frequency waves dominate the recording. There is a return from Stage 4 to Stages 3 and 2 sleep until after approximately seventy to one hundred minutes of NREM sleep, the first REM period occurs. The cycle is repeated throughout the night, and the cycles are similar except that as sleep continues there is less Stage 3 and 4 sleep and longer REM periods. REM sleep is characterized by a low amplitude, fast frequency EEG pattern, bursts of eye movement, and a marked decrease in muscle tone. Depending on how long a person sleeps, there are about four to six REM periods a night. In the normal young adult, the approximate proportions of the various sleep stages are: REM, 20-25 percent; Stage 1, 5 percent; Stage 2, 50 percent; Stages 3 or 4, 20 percent.

There are differences in sleep patterns at different ages.[47, 81] Premature infants appear to have the largest amount of REM sleep. REM sleep comprises approximately 80 percent of total sleep in premature infants, and this decreases to about 30 percent by the second half of the first year of life. These figures are difficult to establish because physiological and behavioral parameters recorded in premature infants and newborns are not easily divided into clear REM and NREM periods. Sustained periods of the high amplitude, slow frequency pattern of Stage 4 sleep are not present until the end of the first year of life. The percentage of Stage 4 sleep is 20 percent to 25 percent in children, approximately 10 percent in young adults and then becomes minimal or absent in people over sixty-five years of age. In addition, in children the time from lights out to the onset of sleep is shorter than in adults; at the same time, the first REM period does not occur until after approximately two hours of sleep. This is because children have a greater percentage of Stage 3 and 4 sleep and because these stages are more prominent in the early hours of sleep.

REM Sleep

During REM sleep, neurophysiological and biochemical measures reflect increased activity. Rather than supporting the general idea that sleep is peaceful and quiet, levels of activity during REM sleep indicate a level similar to a waking state. Pulse, respiration, and blood pressure show wide variations during REM sleep and only slight changes during NREM periods. Penile erections occur predominantly during REM periods. There are increased levels of a number of hormones during REM sleep, such as anterior and posterior pituitary hormones, catecholamines, and 17-hydroxycorticosterone. Furthermore, dream recall occurs in about 70-80 percent of awakenings from REM sleep in contrast to approximately 10 percent from NREM periods.

The Newborn Period

As the newborn infant matures, a diurnal pattern of sleep and wakefulness develops. During the first three months there is a progressive physiological and psychological maturation that results in the establishment of a pattern of wakefulness during the day and sleep at night ("settling"). In their comprehensive study of night waking in early infancy, Moore and Ucko[61] report that by three months, about 70 percent of babies sleep from midnight to early morning, by six months 83 percent have settled, while 10 percent never sleep through the night in the first year of life. Among infants who have settled, about one-half of them have subsequent periods of night waking for more than four weeks duration. There is disagreement as to how soon day-night patterns become established, with some authors reporting such patterns as early as the first ten days of life.[76] The evolution of a sleeping pattern is similar to other early developmental accomplishments, such as the smiling response or purposeful motor activity. It is an early precursor of ego development. The emergence of a diurnal sleep pattern seems to be a product of innate biologic maturation and environmental stimulation, satisfaction and frustration.[31, 61, 63, 66] The reciprocal exchange between the mother and infant in areas such as feeding, activity, holding, and playing affects the child's level of tension and the development of a stable sleep pattern. How much the relationship between the child and his environment affects the unfolding of an innate biologic timetable is controversial. In their study, Moore and Ucko[61] suggest that early settling is independent of sex, birth weight, seasonal changes, sleeping arrangements, and transient illness. On the other hand, difficult birth circumstances, especially anoxia, seem to predispose an infant to delayed settling as well as to many other problems.

Three to Twelve Months

In contrast to the first three months of life, after the third month, the infant's sleeping pattern seems more influenced by environmental factors. Three months is not only the approximate age by which most infants have settled, but also the time when the sleep EEG becomes similar to that of an adult.[1, 81] After three months, the infant's sleep polygram shows sleep beginning with a sustained NREM period, and the sleep recordings can now be divided into REM sleep and the stages of NREM sleep. This is a period of rapid perceptual development. The infant receives increased sensory experience and stimulation from his environment. Hand-mouth co-ordination develops along with ocular fixation, and the recognition of familiar images and sound. Sleeping time gradually continues to decrease during the day, resulting in an eventual pattern of morning and afternoon naps along with a ten to twelve hour period of unbroken sleep at night.

During the first year, a number of environmental factors can be seen to play a progressively greater role in disturbances in sleep patterns. Among these are changes in the physical sleeping arrangements, separations from the mother, and prolonged and marked alterations in the mother's emotional state. Marital discord, a death in the family, or a new pregnancy may contribute to increasing maternal depression, anger, or ambivalence. This extends all too readily to the infant-mother relationship. For the most part, these disruptions are transient, although severe trauma may give rise to a persistent sleep disturbance. In the second half of the first year, parental anger or anxiety about sleep disturbances may compound the problem. Parents often report that a child waking at night enrages them. They feel inadequate as parents, or discouraged about parenthood. In the great majority of situations, these problems can be remedied by seeing to it that the bodily needs of the child are met in a gratifying and relatively consistent manner, and by an empathic appreciation of the parents' anxieties and stresses. Some changes in the environment can be helpful, such as moving the child from the parents' bedroom or avoiding overstimulation at bedtime. For example, the parents of a normal, developing seven month-old baby were distressed because, after sleeping through the night since four months, he had recently begun wailing and crying many times during the night. They were upset by the child's apparent discomfort and unhappiness and took turns rocking the baby and rubbing his back. Gradually the parents became fatigued and angry. They were advised to let the baby cry for a few nights and see what happened. After two nights of occasional, intermittent crying, the child again slept through the night. The parents were pleased, less tired, and less irritable. This supported the previously established, mutually gratifying relationship between the child and his parents.

The Second and Third Year of Life

Gesell and Ilg[34] considered sleep disturbances as developmental characteristics of the age group eighteen to thirty months. These disturbances include nightmares, pavor nocturnus, somnambulism, bedtime rituals, reluctance to go to sleep, and fear of sleep. In many instances, these disorders are a result of uneven development or the stress arising from shifts through the phases of normal development. Such developmental disturbances are more common than sleep disturbances arising from neurotic conflicts. As Anna Freud points out,[28] in the second year of life, falling asleep entails loosening the child's ties to the very people and outside world which have so recently become increasingly appreciated and valued. Albeit temporary, this loosening of attachment occurs at this point only with difficulty and tension.

Developmentally, the infant progresses from a stage of need satisfaction to one of object constancy. In the complex cognitive, emotional, and perceptual maturational process which occurs, the infant moves from total concern with satisfaction of its needs to a strong attachment to the need satisfying object. Finally, the object for its own sake, independent of gratification of the child's needs, becomes vitally important. However, in the period between eighteen and twenty-four months, the toddler is in an extremely vulnerable situation. Despite the child's intense involvement with the mother, object constancy has not been fully developed. When the mother is out of sight, the toddler cannot maintain a sufficiently stable internal image of her presence. In effect, his limited cognitive ability does not enable him to reassure himself of the mother's continued existence. This is elegantly observed and described by Mahler[59] in her formulation of the process of separation and individuation. In discussing the phases of separation and individuation, Mahler describes how the toddler will practice leaving and returning to the mother for emotional "refueling." At about sixteen to eighteen months of age, however, during the "rapprochement" phase, he can more fully recognize his separateness from the mother. The infant will now play separately, while periodically wanting to share with the mother his new skills and experiences.

Thus reluctance to go to sleep is a prevalent disturbance in toddlers. Procrastination at bedtime and the use of "transitional objects" such as a blanket or a teddy bear are attempts to manage the separation anxiety. Sometimes the parents indulge the child with lengthy bedtime rituals which may delay the child's development of his own capacity to master the separation process. However, if reasonable limits are established concerning the bedtime rituals and the child still has anxiety about bedtime, the problem should be explored further. As Kessler[49] points out, the use of the transitional object at bedtime as comfort and security in the face of separation should be left largely to the child's initiative. If the parents too actively direct the child toward the use of a comforting object, they endow it with their authority, and support the child's magical thinking. In the long run, this makes it difficult for the child to relinquish such an object of his own accord. During the second part of the second year, separation anxiety diminishes as object permanence becomes more established, and as the toddler's verbal skills develop. The child becomes increasingly able to use language to master the separation anxiety. At this age it is common to hear parents tell of a toddler who screams whenever he is left with the babysitter. However, as soon as the child can articulate the fact that the parents are away, even in the most rudimentary language such as "Mama, Dada, car," the anxiety diminishes.

In the toddler stage, sleep disturbances are frequently related to overstimulation or to frightening experiences that have occurred during the day. The resultant anxiety and tension continue into the night and may be expressed in nightmares. Injuries, operations, or prolonged separations are examples of the kind of anxiety-laden experiences the impact of which is revived during the ego regression of sleep. This is consistent with children's attempts at mastery through repetition. Freud[29] too spoke of this when he described dreams in traumatic neuroses as attempts to restore control over catastrophic experiences. In the course of the dream, the individual allows himself to feel the apprehensive affect that was absent in the original trauma. It is also possible that the REM period and its associated anxiety dreams can function as an adaptive mechanism. They can help the process of assimilating and mastering overwhelming stimuli in the safe environment of the motoric blockade accompanying REM sleep. In addition, during the regressive experience of sleep, Mack[57] delineates how, not only recent traumatic events, but a series of partly overwhelming past experiences can be revived in nightmares. Since the toddler cannot distinguish between nightmares and reality,[68] a fear of going to sleep may develop. Many authors have observed that in toddlers' nightmares their daytime fears are expressed in terms of being chased or attacked by animals, monsters, or witches. As the cognitive ability to distinguish dreams from reality develops, the difficulty in falling asleep because of fear of nightmares subsides.

For the toddler, the conflicts of the anal phase of psychosexual development play an important role in the genesis of sleep disturbances. Bornstein[9] and Fraiberg[26] provide excellent clinical descriptions and analyses of these conflicts. In addition to dangers in the outside world, the child experiences aggressive impulses within himself that cause anxiety. He comes to recognize that certain actions risk displeasure from his parents. This displeasure involves a loss of approval and even the loss of the parent. The toddler's struggle with aggressive impulses is apparent in toilet training where, for the sake of his parents' approbation, the child is asked to submit to their requirements. Psychoanalytic exploration of the nightmares of toddlers frequently reveals anxiety and conflict over loss of control. This centers particularly around soiling and wetting, but it relates as well to other forbidden instinctual wishes that derive from the anal, as well as the oral developmental levels. This type of sleep disturbance frequently improves if the parents reduce the pressure on the child to accomplish toilet training. In addition, the toddler is comforted by the physical presence of the parents, their calm and their affection. This reassures him that his aggressive wishes have not magically harmed them, that his parents are not angry at him, and that they will continue to help his shaky ego protect him from temptations and trouble. Although the parents' physical presence reassures the child, it is too stimulating for the child to sleep in the parents' bedroom. Such a practice may arouse new anxieties that disrupt sleep. Furthermore, after a few nights in the parents' bedroom, the child experiences the return to his own bedroom as a deprivation. In effect, it is a new separation with increased anxiety and difficulty sleeping. A common and effective way of helping the toddler with these problems is to leave the bedroom door partially open so the child feels less isolated and recognizes familiar surroundings.

The Three to Six Year Old

Melitta Sperling[78] states that during the oedipal period (age three to six), mild and transient sleep disturbances are typical in our culture. More severe disturbances, however, with acute exacerbations and persisting sleeplessness, are indicative of an emotional disorder. On the basis of his experience at the Hampstead Clinic, Nagera[63] confirms this impression. In his experience with preschool children, it was rare to find any who did not experience some difficulty in sleeping, such as waking at night, nightmares, fears of ghosts or wild animals, and reluctance to sleep alone. At this age, in addition to attempting to master unresolved earlier developmental issues, every child struggles with the emotional frustration of aggressive and sexual wishes which gradually become repressed. These conflicts and anxieties are more complex than at earlier stages. Aggressive and competitive wishes focus not just on parents but also on siblings and friends. In addition to fears about wetting and soiling, anxiety about masturbation is prominent. The case of a four-year-old girl, who was seen because of anxieties concerning her father's death a year earlier, exemplifies a number of these issues. She had a period of nightmares, during which she screamed for her mother and said she dreamed of monsters and gorillas chasing her. In her psychotherapy, the gorilla was revealed as representing her own aggressive feelings toward her mother, her father, and her therapist. In addition, she played a game of pretending to be asleep. When everyone's eyes were closed, she would pretend that a bat would come, tickle and wake her. The bat was represented in the play by a paper glued to a popsickle stick, and the tickling gradually focused on the pubic area. As this material unfolded, the anxiety about masturbation became apparent. She described how the tickling was exciting but it scared and worried her. At another point in the treatment, the child told of waking from a bad dream in which she was at school.

She dreamed that she and a boy in her class went to the bathroom to make wee-wee. When they got undressed, she became scared and woke up.

Nightmares reflecting oedipal conflicts are frequently noticed in this age group. A five-year-old girl was seen in treatment because of her fears and her active avoidance of competition and aggression. This was most marked in relation to her sister, a year and a half younger, who constantly bossed her around. The patient described a recurrent nightmare in which a scary, mean witch, dressed all in black, chased her and tried to kill her. As the dream was explored, the child described how she preferred to spend time with her father, and her annoyance with her mother and younger sister because they always joined them. She also recounted how the nightmare reminded her of the witch in her favorite daydream. This daydream was a mixture of fairy stories, which described how a brave, young prince scaled a castle wall, fought a man "queen-witch," and rescued the young princess, subsequently carrying her away with him. These dreams portray typical oedipal concerns such as competition with the parent of the same sex for the attentions of the parent of the opposite sex, fear of retaliation for aggressive and sexual wishes, and interest in romantic family stories. The content of the child's nightmare is presented in abbreviated form. In fact, in the preschool age, as Anna Freud[27] noted, children's dreams often have many of the complex characteristics of adults' dreams, such as complicated symbolization, condensations, reversals, and distortions.

Another difficulty in the preschool period is the child's fear of falling asleep lest he die and never awaken. Sometimes this is related to children's difficulties in understanding the concepts of death and time. Parents' explanations that being dead is like sleeping forever are confusing for the child. By this age, children may have known someone who died and are trying to understand this. Furthermore, children personalize what they hear and this account of death serves to demonstrate to them their own vulnerability. Nor is it unusual for a child to fear that his own aggressive wishes will be discovered, and that death will be the punishment. These aggressive wishes are often externalized, and, as a result, the child may become afraid of ghosts, wild animals, and the dark —and is reluctant to go to sleep. Or, the child may develop elaborate bedtime rituals. A common occurrence during the oedipal period is for the child to find a reason to come to his parents'

bedroom in the middle of the night. He may say the faucet is dripping or a fly is buzzing and waking him. These problems often provide a pretext for the child who is trying to satisfy his curiosity about what happens at night in his parents' bedroom.

There are a number of criteria for attempting to decide how or whether to intervene in sleep disturbances in the preschool age. Transient, mild sleep disturbances are common and generally subside as the child normally masters the developmental conflicts of this age. However, when the interference with sleep is acute or prolonged, or when it results in a degree of fatigue or anxiety that compromises the child's relationships with parents and friends and diminishes attention in school, psychiatric evaluation is definitely warranted. Usually the sleep problem itself responds fairly rapidly to psychotherapeutic intervention and parental guidance. However, the underlying conflicts often require considerably more time to resolve. Sometimes the child's sleep disturbance is related to the parents' own conflicts over unresolved childhood fears and conflicts. They may have longstanding difficulties, for example, with separation anxiety, depression, loneliness, and warded off hostility, or problems of coping with their own persisting oedipal struggles. In such circumstances, extended, intensive work with the parents can be rewarding. A six-year-old boy who was sleepy and unable to attend to the work in class often talked about his conflicts concerning sleeping in his mother's bed. Interviews with the mother revealed that since her separation from her husband, she had kept the child awake to watch television with her for "company." In addition, she believed he had feelings and needs very similar to hers. She took him to bed with her ostensibly to offer him the extra reassurance and comfort she felt he needed since his father had left. In actuality, she was also meeting needs of her own.

Latency or Primary School Period

(Ages Six Through Eleven)

Around the age of six, to some extent, the child will have mastered and repressed the sexual and aggressive drives of the oedipal period and begun to develop an independent conscience. He or she then moves into the latency period. To some degree the child has to contend less with pressure from drives. The maturing ego is better able to cope with conflicts and anxieties, especially if there has been a relatively successful resolution of the conflicts of the oedipal period. For this reason, there is a decrease in the frequency of nightmares and other sleep disturbances. Latency age children are less interested in learning about what happens in the parents' bedroom and in having the parents' company at night. As such children are progressively permitted to establish their own patterns at bedtime, their conflicts and anxieties become focused on activities before sleep such as reading, listening to a radio, or playing games. Sometimes the requirements for reading at bedtime become compulsive and complex; they seem to be attempts to ward off erotic fantasies, and/or masturbatory temptations and activities. Also, latency age children experience occasional insomnia or trouble falling asleep, which is largely related to the persistence into the evening of the excitement surrounding the activities of the day.

Analyses of children with sleep disturbances in latency[57, 63] reveal that when they are persistent and disruptive, the child is struggling with unresolved conflicts. These often derive from earlier stages of psychosexual development as well as from the oedipal period. The child is thus contending with internalized conflicts of the oral and anal periods rather than with the vicissitudes, the stresses, and the strains of normal development. In latency age children, then, the nightmare often reflects developmental struggles from earlier periods. These dreams are increasingly complex and elaborate. The apparent attempts the child makes at a logical presentation of their content parallels his investment in organizing and mastering information in his waking life. In addition, the harsh superego of the first half of latency is reflected in nightmares. It is seen in the punitive potentialities of events and in the menacing characteristics of human or quasi-human creatures that populate these dreams. Rather than depicting the parents or their displacements directly in the form of dangerous animals, the latency child's more sophisticated dreaming ego frequently attributes to teachers and peers internal concerns about criticism, standards, and requirements. Furthermore, cognitive development is more advanced at this age. It is a stage where, once awake, the child can clearly distinguish dreaming from reality. Latency age children report a sense of an observing self even while dreaming: something seems to help wake them if the dream is too frightening. By ages eight to eleven, the ego has developed to the extent that recurrent nightmares are unusual. Their appearance at this point indicates that some form of pathology must be considered.

Adolescence

With the onset of puberty, there is an intensification of the drives. Variable amounts of ego regression appear as part of the reworking of earlier conflicts and anxieties. Blos[8] refers to this aspect of adolescence as the second individuation phase. Nightmares and other sleep disturbances in adolescence parallel the re-emergence and reworking of previous conflicts and anxieties. In adolescence, cognitive development expands dramatically. There is a marked increase in intellectual abilities, including an increased capacity for abstraction. This adds richness and complexity to nightmares. The organization of an ego ideal with the progression from narcissistic homosexual to more mature object-related heterosexual attachments gives new dimensions to the adolescent's dreams. At this point in growth, nightmares often derive from a family disturbance in which separation of the child from the primary objects is highly charged and conflicted for both parents and child. Many adolescents are caught up in an intense struggle to remove themselves from their parents emotionally and physically. As a result, they are reluctant to turn to an adult for help, especially for such sleep disturbances as nightmares. Other youngsters perceive nightmares as an important symptom, or recognize that their life is seriously compromised or endangered in other ways and seek help.

It is beyond the scope of this chapter to review in detail the developmental tasks of adolescence and the expression of this maturation in nightmares and other sleep disturbances. Nevertheless, a brief description of the nightmares of one sixteen-year-old girl may be useful. It illustrates how a youth standing at a relatively advanced and tumultuous developmental stage goes about reworking earlier conflicts.

This bright, young high school student was referred after the divorce of her parents. She sought help for recurrent nightmares which had become intolerable. She was the older of two children in a Catholic, middle-class family. The following excerpts are characteristic of the nightmares and other troubling dreams which led her to request treatment: She dreamed that she was following a car which ran over a pedestrian crossing the road. When she drove up to the body lying in a puddle of blood, she realized in horror that it was her mother. As she got out of her own car, her mother's body grew bigger and bigger until it reached an immense size and began to crush her.

On another occasion, she dreamt that when she came home from school her father met her with the news that her mother had died. During the dream itself, she was aware that she experienced no sadness at her mother's death. As the dream progressed, her father told her that her mother was actually alive. He explained that her mother's pretending to be dead had to do with her sister's confirmation. The parents did not want the patient to be jealous and felt that if the mother appeared to be dead, her sister's confirmation would become unimportant. In other dreams, there was a recurrent theme of the appearance of a terrifying devil. Her anxiety was so great that she was unable to describe the devil except that he was of a bright yellow color. She always awakened from these nightmares with an intense feeling of panic and had to go into her mother's room repeatedly to be comforted and to reassure herself that her mother was alive. On many occasions she felt she had to spend the rest of the night in her mother's bedroom.

An examination of these dreams in the context of the ongoing issues of this youngster's psychotherapy revealed many elements which represented the reworking of earlier developmental issues, as well as attempts at trying to resolve present conflicts. The parents' divorce had upset her deeply and left her with many unrecognized angry feelings toward both of them. The feelings were especially strong toward her mother, whom she held responsible for not being able to keep her father's interest. The divorce also left the patient feeling vulnerable. In addition, she had very ambivalent feelings about the plan that had been developed to send her away to boarding school in the near future. These feelings were clearly expressed in her nightmares which also contained elements of earlier separation issues. Along with the problems of separation, residual conflicts from various developmental stages were elaborated in themes of sibling rivalry, sadism, and sexual attraction to the father.

Nightmares

Nightmares have been described in the medical literature at least since the time of Hippocrates in ancient Greece.[14] Over the years, descriptions have varied, stressing different aspects of the syndrome. In his pioneering study of nightmares in adults, Ernest Jones[40] emphasized the aspects of dread, a sense of oppression or weight on the chest interfering with respiration, and a feeling of helplessness and paralysis. In children, as Mack[58] points out, there is certainly marked anxiety, but paralysis and respiratory difficulty are not commonly experienced. By popular usage, a general description of nightmares in children has emerged. It includes the occurrence of a dream arousing sufficient anxiety and fear to awaken the child at least partially. Recent physiological studies have confirmed early clinical impressions[35, 40, 78] that such a general definition is too imprecise. In the field of nightmares, one might say that different breeds and strains can be distinguished. Recent studies by Broughton[10] and Gastaut,[32] subsequently confirmed by many other investigators, indicated that nightmares occur during two different stages of the sleep cycle. The phenomena associated with the terms anxiety dreams or nightmares most closely resemble the sleep disturbances occurring during REM periods. On the other hand, pavor nocturnus, or night terrors, are associated with what is understood as an arousal reaction from slow wave sleep (predominantly Stage 4, sometimes in cases with less severe anxiety with arousal from Stage 2). This distinction seems useful, not only physiologically, but also psychologically, and for that reason, nightmares will be used to refer to REM anxiety dreams and pavor nocturnus to slow wave arousal phenomena.

The REM nightmare usually is related to a prolonged dream. There is rarely screaming or talking, and the anxiety is of moderate to severe character rather than of desperate quality. In these nightmares, during the minutes before waking, the autonomic response is also relatively mild. In addition to an increase in respiratory rate, the heart rate may increase by 25 to 40 percent. Fisher and associates[21] describes this in terms of a "desomatization" that diminishes anxiety. It may perhaps be related to the fact that the REM period is already physiologically activated as if in preparation for danger.

It is probable that the occurrence of REM nightmares some time during childhood is universal. Estimates of the frequency and distribution of these dreams is limited and difficult to interpret because of the lack of clarity previously noted in the definition of the various types of anxiety dreams. A number of authors report the incidence of nightmares in various and overlapping age ranges.[2, 25, 55] In general, nightmares seem to be most common in the preschool years and decrease after about age six. Mack[57] states that children's dreams and nightmares can be evaluated most fruitfully within a developmental context. In his case illustrations, he elucidates how nightmares express the current anxieties and conflicts in the child's life in relation to earlier developmental issues that are revived and recapitulated during the regressive process of sleep. Kessler points out that nightmares are intimately related to other sleep disturbances such as difficulty falling asleep, bedtime rituals, or sleep phobias.[49] In the latter situations, conflict and anxiety overwhelm the ego's defenses prior to, rather than during, sleep.

Night Terrors

Night terrors, or pavor nocturnus, are characterized by intense anxiety, piercing screams, and greatly increased manifestations of autonomic disturbance. They are often associated with sleepwalking and retrograde amnesia for the entire episode. The importance of distinguishing night terrors from the more common night mares or anxiety dreams has been emphasized by numerous investigators.* In the past ten years, confirmation and clarification of these differences has depended on electroencephalographic observations in the sleep laboratory. That is, as previously outlined, night terrors occur during arousal from slow wave Stage 4 sleep, while nightmares or anxiety dreams occur during REM periods. These recent findings make previous estimations of the frequency of night terrors less dependable. Nevertheless in the general population, such estimates as we have of the incidence of night terrors suggests that they occur in approximately 3 percent of all children.[47, 53, 77] They are perhaps slightly more frequent in boys than girls. They occur throughout childhood, but are most common between ages five and seven; by puberty they have become distinctly unusual. Hällström,[37] in a study of night terrors in three generations, suggests a genetic origin transmitted as an autosomal, dominant trait, but clearly this area requires further investigation.

The phenomenology of night terrors can be divided into pre-arousal and post-arousal periods. In the pre-arousal period, Fisher[21] has suggested that on a given night the greater the amount of Stage 4 sleep, the greater the intensity and frequency of the night terrors. Although Fisher's studies[20, 21, 23] included predominantly adult subjects, his findings seemed to extend to his child subjects and to children in general. Most Stage 4 activity is present in the first few hours of sleep. This is consistent with the finding that most episodes of night terrors occur early in sleep, about two-thirds of them during the first non-REM period. In addition, in contrast to REM nightmares, where there is a relatively mild autonomic discharge, in night terrors there is an explosive autonomic discharge with a marked increase in cardio-respiratory activity.

Arousal in the night terror begins with loud, terrified screams, usually associated with cries for help, along with gasping and garbled entreaties or moans. The child will often sit up in bed and stare wide-eyed, as if pursued and tormented by some ineffable terror. He is oblivious to his parents' worried faces, soothing words or embraces. The child may stumble out of bed and wander about in a desperate way. Occasionally the child will hurt himself and may be violent. He is dissociated, relatively unresponsive to the environment, and may be delusional or hallucinating. During this period, the autonomic activity is extreme in contrast to the mild autonomic discharge during a REM nightmare. During a night terror, within a half a minute the heart rate may triple to 180 beats per minute and respiratory rate shows a moderate increase. There is no evidence of seizure activity and the EEG is similar to a waking pattern. Within minutes, the elevated levels of autonomic activity subside, and the child can be helped to return to bed and sleep. A child may have multiple night terrors in a single night. In the morning, characteristically, there is no memory of the events of the previous night.

In contrast to the complex and elaborate dream content obtained from dreams during the REM periods, the paucity of content obtained during Stage 4 sleep and during the night terrors has resulted in the impression that night terrors arise out of a "psychological void." Night terrors have been viewed as an expression of delayed central nervous system maturation consistent with the

* See references 1, 10, 20, 21, 23, 32, 43, and 48.

finding that most children outgrow these episodes. Studies[8] have indicated that in subjects prone to night terrors and nightmares sounding a buzzer during Stage 4 sleep produces night terrors. The same buzzer stimulus during REM periods does not have this effect. When content is obtained from a Stage 4 night terror, it is usually not complex or elaborate, but rather a single vivid image related to physical experiences such as being crushed, falling, or choking. Nevertheless, often the brief but vivid vision can be seen to have some identifiable content or psychodynamic organization. Fisher and associates[22] report that when subjects are awakened during night terrors, in 58 percent of the episodes some mental content such as a frightening feeling can be recalled. In occasional instances, an elaborate dream is remembered.

The onset of night terrors can frequently be related to a recent event such as a hospitalization, a mother's prolonged absence from the home, conflict between the parents, or the death of a family member or close friend. For example, a six-year-old boy had a night terror after a number of disturbing events had occurred in his life. During the preceding year, the family had moved three times because of the father's occupational reassignments. The moves entailed living in two foreign countries where English was not spoken, two changes of school for the boy, and lengthy absences by the father who was away on trips. Two months before the first night terror, the child and friends were playing in the ruins of an old house. An older boy started a fire which quickly got out of control. The children barely escaped from the fire, which was difficult to extinguish and almost spread to nearby buildings. The child was questioned by the police and fire department, and the parents feared a lawsuit. The night terrors began one week later and occurred one-half hour after the onset of sleep. The child screamed, "Help, Mommy!", sat bolt upright in bed, and stared wide-eyed about his room. He was gasping and his whole body trembled with fear. His parents tried to talk to him and restrain him as he got out of bed and stumbled out of his room, but he seemed totally unaware of them. Minutes later he went to bed and back to sleep. In the morning he could not remember the incident. Over the next year, the child had about six episodes of night terrors. Except for anxieties about the moves and school changes which were well within what might be expected, he adjusted well. The night terrors subsided without psychiatric intervention. By age eight and one-half, the boy

and his family had moved back to the western United States and his growth and development continued to be good. He had no further night terrors.

In night terrors, the relative contributions of psychodynamic and biologic factors are difficult to determine and may vary greatly from one child to the next. Heuristically, however, the concept of ego regression during sleep is useful. During Stage 4 sleep, sleep descends to its greatest depth. Perhaps it is this that facilitates the loss of reality testing, weakening of psychological defenses (especially of repression), and the emergence of primary process thinking. At this time, a massive eruption of anxiety emerges around traumatic events or around the reopening of previously unsettled, developmental issues. In contrast, during REM nightmares there is a relatively high level of central nervous system activation. In conjunction with this, the anxiety is more controlled and perhaps even organized and mastered to a degree. In night terrors, the anxiety seems uncontrolled and unintegrated. In attempting to determine what, if any, intervention is indicated, a number of factors should be reviewed. The overall ego capacities and developmental progress[28] of the child, the child's mastery of present and past developmental issues, and the character of recent traumatic events and environmental stresses all need to be weighed. It is only from such a wholistic perspective, that a determination can be made as to whether the night terrors are related to a conflict that is interfering with the child's development, or whether they are likely to be mastered by the child's own ego capacities. In the former situation, referral for a comprehensive evaluation of the child and family is necessary to formulate a program for therapeutic intervention.

Pharmacologic management of night terrors has not been extensively studied. Diazepam, which suppresses Stage 4 sleep, has been reported[24] to decrease the frequency of night terrors in adults. Imipramine has also been reported to be effective.[24] However, since night terrors occur infrequently and children tend to outgrow them, and because many medications have undesirable side effects for children, pharmacologic treatment is rarely indicated or advisable.

Somnambulism

It is estimated that somewhere between 1 and 15 percent of children walk in their sleep at some time.[45, 51, 53] Sleepwalking may be slightly more common in boys and is often associated with night terrors and enuresis. Monozygotic twins have been reported to be concordant for somnambulism six times as frequently as dizygotic twins.[6]

A typical episode of sleepwalking includes a regular sequence of events. The child abruptly sits up in bed. His eyes open but have a distinctly glassy, unseeing character. There is considerable disagreement as to the dexterity and complexity of the actions performed by the sleepwalker. In general, the child leaves his bed and, although his movements are clumsy, he rarely falls or collides with objects or furniture. The length of the episodes may vary from less than a minute, with the activity confined to sitting up in bed, to half-an-hour or more, during which the child opens drawers and doors or even leaves the house. The episode generally ends with the child returning to bed. During the sleepwalking, the child may mumble a few words spontaneously or in response to questions. These are often difficult to understand, however, or to put into a useful context. When the child awakens, there is amnesia for the entire episode.

A child may sleepwalk several times a week. Episodes of sleepwalking occur in the first hours of the night. Studies in sleep laboratories have shown that somnambulism occurs during arousal from slow wave sleep Stages 3 and 4. Sleep walking can be induced in somnambulists, but not in normal children, by lifting them to their feet during Stage 4 sleep.[46] In addition, Kales and associates[46] reported that the sleepwalking episodes began with a paroxysmal burst of high voltage, slow frequency EEG activity. These investigators proposed that such activity suggests an immaturity of the central nervous system. They base this on the fact that this activity is common in children and decreases as they grow older. Moreover, in older children who are sleepwalkers, it occurs to a much greater extent than would be expected in normal children of that age.

Janet described sleep walking as an hysterical dissociative symptom.[39] It is commonly supposed that sleepwalking is the acting out of a dream. This is not readily reconcilable with the discovery that sleepwalking occurs during NREM sleep. Numerous studies[62] have attempted to relate sleepwalking to various degrees and types of psychopathology, and to certain personality patterns. In children, even more than in adults, such efforts are inconclusive. Nevertheless, episodes of somnambulism often do seem related to tensions in the child's life. Therefore, as with night terrors

and nightmares, a child with somnambulism should be evaluated in terms of recent and past developmental difficulties, family problems, recent traumatic events, and environmental stresses. A decision about what, if any, intervention is necessary depends on the extent of the stresses in the child's life and on his ego's ability to master them on its own. As with night terrors, possible interventions include environmental changes, individual and/or family psychotherapy, and pharmacotherapy. Despite their ability to suppress Stage 3 and 4 sleep, diazepam and flurazepam, both benzodiazepines, have not been effective in a clear-cut way in reducing the frequency of somnambulistic episodes. Imipramine has been reported to reduce the frequency of sleepwalking episodes.[67] However, since imipramine did not seem to alter Stage 4 sleep significantly in the children treated, its mechanism of action remains unclear. Because of potential adverse effects of these medications, and because sleepwalking in children usually subsides within several years, conservative management is advisable. In order to protect the child prone to sleepwalking from injury, it is essential to remove dangerous objects and secure doors and windows.

Enuresis

Enuresis, or bedwetting, is a common disturbance of sleep. The prevalence of enuresis is difficult to determine because investigators differ as to the age at which they consider bedwetting to be pathologic. Moreover, statistics vary depending on whether studies are done in psychiatric clinics or in general populations of school children. Approximately 10 to 15 percent of children in the four- to five-year-age range still wet the bed.[64] Children outgrow enuresis (with one study[65] reporting 90 percent of the children "dry" by age seven, and 97 percent by age twelve). Approximately 1 percent of military recruits are found to be enuretic.[56] Enuresis is more common in males.

It is important to distinguish primary from secondary enuresis. Children who have never developed full bladder control are said to have primary enuresis, while secondary enuresis refers to the establishment of an extended dry period followed by subsequent loss of bladder control. As with night terrors and somnambulism, primary enuresis seems to have a familial pattern.[36] In primary enuresis, the possibility of organic problems such as lesions of the genitourinary system or of the spinal cord should be considered. Secondary enuresis is often the result of psychologic factors, although organic problems such as diabetes mellitus, diabetes insipidus, or cystitis are possible etiologic factors. The relationship of enuresis to developmental and neurotic conflicts is a large and important issue which is discussed in Chapter 28 of this volume. This section focuses on the relationship of enuresis to the sleep cycle.

Episodes of enuresis occur predominantly during NREM periods. As with night terrors and somnambulism, bedwetting occurs during arousal from Stage 4 sleep. Broughton and Gastaut[11] have defined characteristics of bedwetting episodes. They note that enuresis usually occurs during the first few hours after falling asleep when the child is moving from Stage 4 sleep prior to entering the first REM period. At this time, there are general body movements, increased muscle tone, tachycardia, tachypnea, and penile tumescence in males. Within several minutes following the burst of activity just described, during the period of relative motor and autonomic quiet, the enuresis occurs. After the bedwetting, it is difficult to wake the child, and dreams are rarely reported.[70] If the child is left wet for the remainder of the night, dreams of being wet may be recovered. In the past, this led to the belief that micturition occurred while the child dreamed of being wet. However, the dreams of being wet, rather than occurring at the time of micturition, seem to be the incorporation in subsequent REM periods of the child's awareness of being wet. In additional studies,[12, 33] Broughton and Gastaut have found that during Stage 3 and 4 sleep, enuretic children have higher intravesicular pressure than controls. These children also have stronger and more frequent spontaneous bladder contractions.

There are several approaches to the treatment of enuresis. First it must be established whether the child has primary or secondary enuresis. If the bedwetting is secondary and prolonged, a predominance of emotional factors is most likely. Psychiatric evaluation with subsequent psychotherapy are indicated. In younger children with primary enuresis, and in cases with a family history of enuresis, the syndrome may represent some degree of immaturity of the nervous system which the child will outgrow. Whether this is the case, or whether concomitant emotional factors suggest psychological problems requiring psychotherapy, are issues that must be assessed on an individual basis.

The question of urologic studies to exclude organic causes is problematic. Such procedures can be psychologically traumatic in their own right and should be instigated only if information from the child's history or from routine physical examination and laboratory studies suggests the possibility of a repairable defect. An important concern is the parent's reaction to and management of the bedwetting. Parents should be helped to be understanding and not punitive, in order to avoid contributing to the child's guilt and anxiety. A number of investigators have found that imipramine is an effective treatment for enuresis.[45, 60, 70] Imipramine is said to reduce intravesicular pressure by its anticholinergic properties and to reduce REM and Stage 4 periods of sleep. Nevertheless, although Kales and associates[45] found imipramine to be effective in reducing the frequency of enuresis, this effect was apparently independent of sleep stage alterations. Problems with the use of imipramine for enuresis include a tendency for the children to relapse after the drug is discontinued and lack of experience and information concerning possible adverse effects of long-term use of tricyclic medications in children.

Narcolepsy

Narcolepsy is a syndrome whose expression takes the form of irresistible episodes of sleep. These characteristically last about fifteen minutes. Yoss and Daly[85,88] have described a narcoleptic tetrad consisting of sleep attacks, cataplexy, sleep paralysis, and hypnagogic hallucinations. A full tetrad occurs in about 10 percent of cases; sleep attacks and cataplexy in about 70 percent; sleep attacks, cataplexy, and hypnagogic hallucinations in about 25 percent; sleep attacks and sleep paralysis in less than 5 percent.[89] In 1877 Westphal[80] described a case of narcolepsy in a thirty-six-year-old bookbinder. Subsequently, narcolepsy received little attention except for psychodynamic formulations of its being a defense against unacceptable sexual or aggressive affects. In the 1960s, a major new dimension in the understanding of narcolepsy developed when sleep EEG studies became prominent and were used to investigate the disorder.

The incidence or prevalence of narcolepsy is unknown. The majority of cases begin between the ages of ten and twenty. Approximately 5 percent of the cases are said to begin before the age of ten,[89] although childhood symptoms of recurrent drowsiness may not have been recognized as narcolepsy until later years. The onset of narcolepsy is fairly common in young adults, with 25 percent occurring after age twenty, 18 percent after age thirty and new cases rarely being reported after age forty.[80] Case reports of narcolepsy include more males than females and suggest a familial pattern with a possible single, dominant mode of inheritance.[16, 52] Cataplectic attacks may first begin a number of years after the onset of sleepiness.[86] The sleep attacks are said to occur after meals, during monotonous or boring situations, and during times of stress. They sometimes can be delayed and a person can be awakened during the sleep attack. Although the period of sleep can last several hours, a period of about fifteen minutes is more common. After a sleep attack, another episode is not likely to occur for one to several hours. The sleep attack can be dangerous, as when driving an automobile, especially since sometimes there seems to be no sense of drowsiness or other warning signals before sleep. Cataplexy, a sudden complete or partial loss of muscle tone, can also result in serious injuries, largely as a result of falls. A cataplectic attack can last from a few seconds to as long as thirty minutes and is frequently initiated by an outburst of emotion such as anger or laughter. Sleep paralysis usually occurs when falling asleep, but also may occur upon waking. It is characterized by flaccidity lasting only a few seconds. However, the conscious awareness of the inability to move is usually terrifying. The paralysis can often be interrupted by shaking or calling to the child. Hypnagogic hallucinations are dream-like, sometimes terrifying, auditory and visual perceptions. They tend to occur at the same time as the sleep paralysis, though sometimes they take place independently.

Studies in the sleep laboratories reveal that daytime episodes of narcolepsy are frequently episodes of REM sleep. The cataplexy and sleep paralysis are consistent with the motor blockade characteristic of the REM period, and the hypnagogic hallucinations are not unlike terrifying REM dreams. In these subjects, night sleep began with an REM period rather than the usual period of approximately seventy minutes of NREM sleep preceding the first REM period.[71, 73] Roth and associates[74] proposed that narcolepsy without accessory symptoms is due to a disturbance of the NREM sleep system. They explain that in narcolepsy with cataplexy, sleep paralysis, or hypnagogic hallucinations, there is always a disorder of REM sleep which is associated in most instances with a disturbance of the NREM sleep system. The nature of the disorder of the NREM sleep system requires further elucidation. Narcolepsy, especially in the presence of accessory symptoms, seems to be primarily a disorder of REM sleep. However, conditions of narcolepsy with cataplexy have been reported in subjects with only NREM attacks.[74] In addition, Zarcone[82] points out that, along with the primary idiopathic narcolepsy of REM and NREM types, there are secondary forms of narcolepsy on a postencephalitic, posttraumatic, or drug-dependency basis.

The symptoms of narcolepsy are often attributed to laziness, emotional difficulties, or lack of a sense of responsibility. This makes establishing the proper diagnosis crucial. A careful study of the history of the episodes can be very useful in suggesting a diagnosis of narcolepsy. For example, a fourteen-year-old girl was referred to a local family health clinic because she fell asleep in class, especially around 10:00 A.M. and 2:00 P.M. almost every day. She described sensing an overpowering need to sleep that she could not delay. If she was standing up or even sitting down at these times, her knees felt weak. No history of sleep paralysis or hypnagogic hallucinations could be elicited. She did report that from the time these episodes began, she did not sleep well at night. During the day, she would sleep for twenty to thirty minutes and would wake feeling alert and refreshed. There was no family history of similar symptoms. The girl had had a mild case of mononucleosis several months before the onset of her symptoms. Otherwise, she was and had been in good health. She was an excellent student, outgoing and popular, but had become increasingly anxious, embarrassed, and humiliated by these episodes. She often missed or tried to schedule her classes so that she could nap in privacy at these times. Although narcoleptic episodes have been reported to be associated with increased emotional tension, this could not be documented in this girl prior to the onset of the episode.

If a child has a history suggestive of narcolepsy, evaluation in the sleep laboratory should be undertaken if possible. Such an evaluation may show the presence of sleep onset REM periods, which is essentially pathognomic of narcolepsy. When sleep onset REM periods are not documented, the presence of primary idiopathic narcolepsy of the NREM type cannot be excluded. Furthermore, the differential diagnosis of narcolepsy[89] includes Klein-Levin syndrome, Pickwickian syndrome, sleep apnea, hypersomnia, hypothyroidism, hypoglycemia, and epilepsy. Other conditions that should be considered are myasthenia gravis, multiple sclerosis, intracranial space occupying lesions, anemia, uremia, sleep deprivation, adrenal insufficiency, schizophrenia, dissociative reactions, and other psychoneurotic states.[89]

Once the diagnosis of narcolepsy has been established, a treatment or management program should be undertaken because the syndrome is not known to resolve spontaneously. Analeptic drugs such as methamphetamine and methylphenidate hydrochloride (Ritalin) have been found to be effective.[83, 84, 87, 88] These drugs are known to suppress REM sleep, but whether it is this factor or their general stimulant action which accounts for their effectiveness is unclear. A constant potential danger with amphetamines is drug abuse. The patient becomes tolerant to the dose level, takes more medication, and may experience depression without the drug. This leads to a vicious cycle in which the amount of amphetamine is increased to avoid both the sleep attacks and the depression. Imipramine has been reported to be effective in treating cataplexy,[3, 38] but not the sleep attacks. The combined use of amphetamines and imipramine is potentially dangerous because a combination of a release of catecholamines at the neuronal synapse (amphetamines) and blockade of the re-uptake of catecholamines (imipramine) may cause a hypertensive attack. Nevertheless, Zarcone[89] reports excellent experience with this combination. Finally, the monoamine oxidase inhibitor, phenelzine, has been used successfully in subjects with intractable narcolepsy.[82] However, monoamine oxidase inhibitors should be used only with the utmost caution until their effectiveness, long-range risks, and side effects in children have been thoroughly evaluated. In addition, it should be mentioned that in mild cases of narcolepsy, arranging the day to provide a nap period, or to avoid dangerous activity such as driving, may be a satisfactory solution. When there are unrelated or related concurrent emotional problems, psychiatric evaluation and treatment are clearly indicated.

Hypersomnias

Hypersomnia is a syndrome characterized by excessive amounts of sleep. The episodes of sleep are not irresistible as in narcolepsy, and cataplexy or hypnagogic hallucinations are not usually reported. In approximately one-third of the cases, a condition, which Roth[75] terms "sleep drunkenness," is present. This includes extreme difficulty in waking completely, especially from nocturnal sleep. Along with this, the patient experiences confusion, disorientation, poor motor coordination, and a tendency to return to sleep.[75] The episodes of sleep may last from hours to days. Usually the etiology of hypersomnia is unknown. Occasionally it is secondary to organic brain disturbances such as encephalitis, cardiovascular disease, or head trauma.

There are several special forms of hypersomnia. The Klein-Levin syndrome is associated with bulimia. It is a rare syndrome occurring preponderantly, if not entirely, in adolescent males. It is characterized by the onset of periods of extreme somnolence interrupted by episodes of ravenous eating. These occur several times a year and last from several days to several weeks.[50, 55] Critchley[15] adds the observations that the syndrome eventually disappears spontaneously and that the megaphagia is possibly more in the nature of compulsive eating than a true bulimia. The Pickwickian syndrome is associated with extreme obesity, respiratory insufficiency, and drowsiness.[13]

The general incidence and frequency of hypersomnia is unknown. Idiopathic hypersomnia often begins in early childhood, but may also become manifest in the second and third decades, and, less often, later.[75] There seems to be a familial tendency in this condition, with perhaps a higher incidence in males, but this is unclear.[75] The hypersomnias appear to have a relatively unchanging stationary course in the subject's life. Studies of hypersomnia in sleep laboratories generally suggest that, in these cases, the sleep stages and patterns are similar to normal patterns.[71, 75]

In subjects with hypersomnia, periods of sleep apnea (absence of breathing) ranging up to thirty to sixty seconds occur.[89] Sleep apnea is a universal occurrence in infants between ages one and three months. It seems to follow a familial pattern and may be related to the sudden infant death syndrome.[43, 79] In infants, sleep apnea occurs most often during REM periods, while in hypersomnia and also in narcolepsy sleep apnea occurs during both REM and NREM periods.[43]

In evaluating children with hypersomnia, a thorough investigation to elucidate possible organic (especially neurologic) and psychologic causes must be undertaken. Hypersomnia, as Hartmann points out,[7] may be related to attempts to avoid emotional tension as occurs in depressive, phobic, anxiety, or even psychotic states. Although amphetamines have been effective in treating hypersomnia in adults,[3] this course of treatment at the present time cannot be recommended for children except in very special circumstances.

Discussion

In this review of the nature of sleep disturbances in childhood, the complex interplay between psychological and central nervous system development has been apparent. Although development in the psychological apparatus and in the central nervous system are intimately related, some sleep disorders appear more the result of immaturity in one system. For example, night terrors, primary enuresis (when not caused by an anatomical or physiological disorder), and somnambulism all occur during arousal from the deepest stage of sleep. This stage comprises 20 to 25 percent of sleep in children, and decreases to 10 percent in young adults, while being only minimally present, or even absent, in people over sixty-five years of age.[47] These facts are consistent with the importance of central nervous system maturation in these disorders. Also supporting the role of central nervous system immaturity as at least one important factor in these conditions is the observation that they become progressively less prevalent in older children and young adults. Numerous reports have recognized the familial nature of these disorders. This can be understood in terms of a genetic predisposition to delayed or divergent central nervous system maturation.

In the newborn, the diurnal pattern of sleep and wakefulness is based on the innate rhythms of the immature central nervous system. In both physiological and psychological development, this diurnal rhythm gives way progressively to more complex relationships among the central nervous system, internal psychic and external environmental factors in the determination of sleep—waking patterns. Until approximately age three months, the pattern of sleep and wakefulness appears to be predominantly the result of innate biologic maturation. At that point, about 70 percent of infants sleep from midnight to early morning.[61] After that, age environmental factors such as stimulation, need satisfaction, frustration, activity, and feeding play a gradually larger role in determining patterns of sleep and wakefulness. As his psychological maturation proceeds, the child struggles to cope with an increasingly complex awareness of environmental and internal stimuli. His psychological development includes such goals as the attainment of object constancy (belief in the care taking person's continued existence when he or she is not in the child's field of vision), mastery of the phases of separation and individuation, as well as the tolerance and mastery of aggressive and sexual impulses and various anxiety states. Erickson's[18] terms such as basic trust, autonomy, industry, initiative, and identity also describe some of the important developmental accomplishments in childhood. It is these, as well as many other vicissitudes of psychological development, that seem to play the predominant roles in the development of several sleep disturbances. These include the REM nightmare, bedtime rituals, fear of the dark or of sleeping alone, difficulty falling asleep, and recurrent awakening at night. These symptoms are all properly classified as disturbances of sleep. They can also be seen as reflecting the child's attempts to master stage specific developmental anxieties and conflicts within the domain of sleep behavior.

The application of a conceptual framework that weighs the relative importance of both central nervous system and psychological development is useful in understanding the causation of some of the sleep disturbances in childhood. In other disorders such as narcolepsy and hypersomnia, however, such a developmental point of view is less useful. Both conditions become apparent after the early years of childhood, and the symptoms do not disappear during later childhood and adulthood. Rather than a maturational or developmental delay, both narcolepsy and hypersomnia seem to represent an ongoing disturbance. Roth[74] views their presence without auxiliary symptoms as disturbances of the NREM sleep system. In fact, there is clearly a disturbance of REM sleep when narcolepsy is accompanied by cataplexy, sleep paralysis, or hypnagogic hallucinations. Nonetheless, in the majority of cases, there still is a disturbance of the NREM sleep system. At the same time, to view narcolepsy and hypersomnia as disturbances of NREM sleep does not exclude the role of psychological factors in how the child experiences and adapts to these disorders.

In fact, in all of the disturbances of sleep in childhood, the difficulty in distinguishing psychological and somatic elements is similar to the issue posed by other "psychosomatic" problems. This is well illustrated in the case of night terrors. Gastaut and Broughton[32] view night terrors as a disorder of arousal. They state that individuals who suffer from night terrors seem to undergo physiologic changes that precipitate these attacks. They do not specify how the changes may be accentuated on certain nights so as to produce night terrors. Fisher[21] points out that a central problem is whether psychological activity precedes and generates each attack, or whether psychological factors have initially produced physiological changes that predispose to night terrors during arousal. Fisher takes the approach that certain night terrors have a psychogenic origin and are triggered by specific repressed mental content. Other episodes of night terrors, such as those precipitated by sounding a buzzer, are related to physio-

logic conditions such as relative amounts of Stage 4 sleep. That is, in most individuals the amount of Stage 4 sleep correlates directly with the frequency and intensity of night terrors. From such a vantage point it seems possible that electrophysiologic techniques for monitoring sleep provide a valuable methodology for expanding our knowledge about the relationships between central nervous system and psychological development. In this way, investigators in the field of sleep disorders of childhood may help in the elucidation of the mysteries of all psychosomatic processes.

REFERENCES

1. ANDERS, T. F., and WEINSTEIN, P., "Sleep and Its Disorders in Infants and Children: A Review," *Pediatrics, 50(2)*:312, 1972.

2. ANTHONY, J., "An Experimental Approach to the Psychopathology of Childhood Sleep Disturbances," *British Journal of Medical Psychology, 32*:19–37, 1959.

3. AKIMOTO, H., HONDA, Y., and TAKAHASHI, Y., "Pharmacotherapy in Narcolepsy," *Diseases of the Nervous System, 21*:704, 1960.

4. ASERINSKY, E., and KLEITMAN, N., "A Motility Cycle in Sleeping Infants as Manifested by Ocular and Gross Bodily Activity," *Journal of Applied Physiology, 8*:11–18, 1955.

5. ———, "Regularly Occurring Periods of Eye Motility and Concomitant Phenomena During Sleep," *Science, 118*:273, 1953.

6. BAKWIN, H., "Sleep Walking in Twins," *Lancet, 2*:446, 1970.

7. BAEKELAND, F., and HARTMANN, E., "Sleep Requirements and the Characteristics of Some Sleepers," in Hartmann, E. (Ed.), *Sleep and Dreaming*, Little, Brown, Boston; also in *International Psychiatry Clinics, 7*:37, 1970.

8. BLOS, P., "The Second Individuation Process of Adolescence," in Eissler, R. S., et al. (Eds.), *The Psychoanalytic Study of the Child*, vol. 22, p. 162, International Universities Press, New York, 1967.

9. BORNSTEIN, B., "Phobia in a Two-and-a-Half Year Old Child," *Psychoanalytic Quarterly, 4*:93–119, 1935.

10. BROUGHTON, R., "Sleep Disorders: Disorders of Arousal?" *Science, 159*:1070, 1968.

11. ———, and GASTAUT, H., "Polygraphic Sleep Studies of Enuresis Nocturna," *Electroencephalography and Clinical Neurophysiology, 16*:625, 1964.

12. ———, "Further Polygraphic Sleep Studies of Enuresis Nocturnus (Intravesicular pressures)," *Electroencephalography and Clinical Neurophysiology, 16*:626, 1964.

13. BURWELL, C. S., et al., "Extreme Obesity Associated with Alveolar Hypoventilation, A Pickwickian Syndrome," *American Journal of Medicine, 21*:811, 1956.

14. CHADWICK, J., and MANN, W. N. (Eds.), *The Medical Works of Hippocrates*, p. 18, Blackwell Scientific Publications, Oxford, 1950.

15. CRITCHLEY, M., "Periodic Hypersomnia and Megaphagia in Adolescent Males," *Brain, 85*:627, 1962.

16. DALY, D. D., and YOSS, R. E., "A Family with Narcolepsy," *Mayo Clinic Proceedings, 34*:313, 1959.

17. DEMENT, W. C., and KLEITMAN, N., "Cyclic Varia-

tions in EEG During Sleep and Their Relation to Eye Movements, Body Motility and Dreaming," *Electroencephalography and Clinical Neurophysiology, 9*:673–690, 1957.

18. ERIKSON, E. H., *Identity and the Life Cycle*, Psychological Issues, Monograph No. 1, International Universities Press, New York, 1967.

19. ———, *Childhood and Society*, W. W. Norton, New York, 1959.

20. FISHER, C., et al., "A Psychophysiological Study of Nightmares," *Journal of American Psychoanalytic Society, 18*:747, 1970.

21. ———, et al., "A Psychophysiological Study of Nightmares and Night Terrors. 1. Physiological Aspects of the Stage 4 Night Terror," *Psychoanalysis and Contemporary Science, 3*:317, 1974.

22. ———, "A Psychophysiological Study of Nightmares and Night Terrors. III Mental Content of Stage 4 Night Terrors," *Journal of Nervous and Mental Disease, 158*:174, 1974.

23. ———, "A Psychophysiological Study of Nightmares and Night Terrors, 1. Physiological Aspects of the Stage 4 Night Terror," *Journal of Nervous and Mental Disease, 157*:75, 1973.

24. ———, "A Psychophysiological Study of Nightmares and Night Terrors: The Suppression of Stage 4 Night Terrors with Diazepam," *Archives of General Psychiatry, 28*:252, 1973.

25. FOSTER, J. C., and ANDERSON, J. E., "Unpleasant Dreams in Childhood," *Child Development, 7*:77, 1936.

26. FRAIBERG, S., "Sleep Disturbances of Childhood," in Eissler, R. S., et al. (Eds.), *The Psychoanalytic Study of the Child*, vol. 5, p. 285, International Universities Press, New York, 1950.

27. FREUD, A., "Four Lectures on Child Analysis," *The Writings of Anna Freud*, pp. 19–36, International Universities Press, New York, 1974.

28. ———, "Normality and Pathology in Childhood: Assessments of Development," *The Writings of Anna Freud*, International Universities Press, New York, 1965.

29. FREUD, S., "Beyond the Pleasure Principle," *The Standard Edition of the Complete Psychological Works of Sigmund Freud* (hereafter: *The Standard Edition*), p. 32, Hogarth Press, London, 1955.

30. ———, "The Interpretations of Dreams," *The Standard Edition*, vols. 4 and 5, Hogarth Press, London, 1953.

31. GAENSBAUER, T. J., and EMDE, R. N., "Wakefulness

and Feedings in Human Newborns," *Archives of General Psychiatry, 28:*894, 1973.

32. GASTAUT, H., and BROUGHTON, R., "A Clinical and Polygraphic Study of Episodic Phenomena During Sleep," *Recent Advances in Biologic Psychiatry*, vol. 8, p. 197, Plenum Press, New York, 1965.

33. ———, "Conclusions Concerning the Mechanisms of Enuresis Nocturna," *Electroencephalography and Clinical Neurophysiology, 16:*626, 1964.

34. GESELL, A., and ILG, F. L., *Infant and Child in the Culture of Today*, p. 146, Harper & Brothers, New York, 1943.

35. HALL, J. W., "The Analysis of a Case of Night Terror," in Eissler, R. S., et al. (Eds.), *The Psychoanalytic Study of the Child*, vol. 2, p. 189, International Universities Press, New York, 1946.

36. HALLGREN, B., "Enuresis: A Clinical and Genetic Study," *Acta Psychiatrica et Neurologica Scandinavica, 32(Supplement 114):*1–159, 1957.

37. HÄLLSTRÖM, J., "Night Terror in Adults Through Three Generations," *Acta Psychiatrica Scandinavica, 48:* 350, 1972.

38. HISHIKAWA, Y., et al., "Treatment of Narcolepsy with Imipramine (Tofranil) and Desmethylimipramine (Pertofran)," *Journal of the Neurological Sciences, 3:*453, 1966.

39. JANET, P., *The Major Symptoms of Hysteria*, pp. 22–43, Macmillan, New York, 1929.

40. JONES, E., *On the Nightmare*, p. 20, Liveright, New York, 1951.

41. KALES, A., "Treating Sleep Disorders," *American Family Physician, 8(5):*158, 1973.

42. ———, *Sleep: Physiology and Pathology*, Lippincott, Philadelphia, 1969.

43. ———, and KALES, J., "Recent Findings in the Diagnosis and Treatment of Disturbed Sleep," *New England Journal of Medicine, 290:*487, 1974.

44. ———, "Evaluation, Diagnosis and Treatment of Clinical Conditions Related to Sleep," *Journal of the American Medical Association, 213(13):*2229, 1970.

45. KALES, A., et al., "Sleep Laboratory and Clinical Studies of the Effects of Tofranil, Valium and Placebo on Sleep Stages and Enuresis," *Psychophysiology, 7:*348, 1970.

46. KALES, A., et al., "Somnambulism: Psychophysiological Correlates. I All-night EEG Studies," *Archives of General Psychiatry, 14:*586, 1960.

47. KALES, J. D., JACOBSON, A., and KALES, A., "Sleep Disorders in Children," in Abt, L. E., and Reiss, B. F. (Eds.), *Progress in Clinical Psychology*, p. 63, Grune & Stratton, New York, 1968.

48. KEITH, P., "Night Terrors, A Review of the Psychology, Neurophysiology and Therapy," *Journal of the American Academy of Child Psychiatry, 14:*477, 1975.

49. KESSLER, J. W., *Psychopathology of Childhood*, p. 231, Prentice-Hall, Englewood Cliffs, N.J., 1966.

50. KLEINE, W., "Periodische Schlafsucht," *Monatsschrift fuer Psychiatrie und Neurologie, 57:*285, 1925.

51. KLEITMAN, N., *Sleep and Wakefulness*, University of Chicago Press, Chicago, 1963.

52. KRABBE, F., and MAGNUSSEN, G., "On Narcolepsy: I Familial Narcolepsy," *Acta Psychiatrica et Neurologica Scandinavica, 17:*149, 1942.

53. KURTH, V. E., GÖHLER, I., and KNAAPE, H. H., "Untersuchungen über den Pavor Nocturnus bei Kindern," *Psychiatrie, Neurologie, und Medizinische Psychologie, 17:*1–7, 1965.

54. LAPOUSE, R., and MONK, M., "Fears and Worries in a Representative Sample of Children," *American Journal of Orthopsychiatry, 29:*803, 1959.

55. LEVIN, M., "Periodic Somnolence and Morbid Hunger: A New Syndrome," *Brain, 59:*494, 1936.

56. LEVINE, A., "Enuresis in the Navy," *American Journal of Psychiatry, 100:*320, 1943.

57. MACK, J. E., *Nightmares and Human Conflict*, Houghton-Mifflin, Boston, 1974.

58. ———, "Nightmares, Conflict and Ego Development in Childhood," *International Journal of Psycho-Analysis, 46(4):*403, 1965.

59. MAHLER, M., "Symbiosis and Individuation: The Psychological Birth of the Human Infant," in Eissler, R. S., et al. (Eds.), *The Psychoanalytic Study of the Child*, vol. 29, p. 89, International Universities Press, New York, 1974.

60. MILLER, P. R., CHAMPELLI, J. W., and DINELLO, F. A., "Imipramine in the Treatment of Enuretic School Children: A Double Blind Study," *American Journal of Diseases of Children, 115:*17, 1968.

61. MOORE, T., and UCKO, L., "Night Waking in Early Infancy Part I," *Archives of Diseases in Childhood, 32:* 333–342, 1957.

62. MURRAY, E. J., *Sleep, Dreams and Arousal*, pp. 275–277, Appleton-Century-Crofts, New York, 1965.

63. NAGERA, H., "Sleep and Its Disturbances," in Eissler, R. S., et al. (Eds.), *The Psychoanalytic Study of the Child*, vol. 21, p. 393, International Universities Press, New York, 1966.

64. NESBIT, R., "Urethrovesical Malfunctions and Urinary Incontinence in Female Children and Adolescents," *Pediatric Clinics of North America, 19:*705, 1972.

65. OPPEL, W. C., HARPER, P. A., and RIDER, R. V., "The Age of Attaining Bladder Control," *Pediatrics, 42:* 614, 1968.

66. PARMELEE, A. H., SCHULTZ, H. R., and DISBROW, M. A., "Sleep Patterns of the Newborn," *Journal of Pediatrics, 58:*241–250, 1961.

67. PESIKOFF, R., and DAVIS, P. C., "Treatment of Pavor Nocturnus and Somnambulism in Children," *American Journal of Psychiatry, 128:*778, 1971.

68. PIAGET, J., *Play, Dreams and Imitation in Childhood*, p. 245, W. W. Norton, New York, 1962.

69. PIERCE, C., et al., "Enuresis and Dreaming," *Archives of General Psychiatry, 4:*166, 1961.

70. POUSSAINT, A. F., and DITMAN, K. S., "A Controlled Study of Imipramine (Tofranil) in the Treatment of Childhood Enuresis," *Journal of Pediatrics, 67:*283, 1965.

71. RECHTSCHAFFEN, A., and DEMENT, W., "Narcolepsy and Hypersomnia," in Kales, A. (Ed.), *Sleep: Physiology and Pathology*, pp. 119–130, J. B. Lippincott, Philadelphia, 1969.

72. ———, and KALES, A. (Eds.), *A Manual of Standardized Terminology, Techniques and Scoring System for Sleep Stages of Human Subjects*, National Institute of Health, Bethesda, Md., 1968.

73. RECHTSCHAFFEN, A., et al., "Nocturnal Sleep of Narcoleptics," *Electroencephalography and Clinical Neurophysiology, 15:*599, 1963.

74. ROTH, B., BRUHOVÁ, S., and LEHOVSKÝ, M., "REM Sleep and NREM Sleep in Narcolepsy and Hypersomnia," *Electroencephalography and Clinical Neurophysiology, 26:* 176, 1969.

75. ROTH, B., NEVGIMALOVA, S., and RECHTSCHAFFEN, A., "Hypersomma with "Sleep Drunknness," *Archives of General Psychiatry, 26:*456, 1972.

76. SANDER, L., et al., "Early Mother-Infant Interaction: A 24 Hour Pattern of Activity and Sleep," *Journal of the American Academy of Child Psychiatry, 9:*103, 1970.

77. SHIRLEY, H. F., and KAHN, J. P., "Sleep Disturbances in Children," *Pediatric Clinics of North America, 5:*629, 1958.

78. SPERLING, M., "Etiology and Treatment of Sleep Disturbances in Children," *Psychoanalytic Quarterly, 24:* 358, 1955.

79. STEINSCHNEIDER, A., "Prolonged Apnea and the Sudden Infant Death Syndrome: Clinical and Laboratory Observations," *Pediatrics, 50:*646, 1972.

80. WESTPHAL, C., "Eisenthümliche mit Einschlafen Verbundene Anfälle," *Archiv fuer Psychiatrie, 7:*631, 1877.

81. WILLIAMS, R. L., KARACAN, I., and HURSCH, C. J.,

Electroencephalography (EEG) of Human Sleep: Clinical Applications, John Wiley, New York, 1974.

82. Wyatt, R. T., et al., "Treatment of Intractable Narcolepsy with a Monoamine Oxidase Inhibitor," *New England Journal of Medicine, 285:*987, 1971.

83. Yoss, R. E., "Treatment of Narcolepsy," *Modern Treatment, 6:*1263, 1969.

84. ———, and Daly, D. D., "On the Treatment of Narcolepsy," *Medical Clinics of North America, 52:*781, 1968.

85. ———, "Narcolepsy," *Archives of Internal Medicine, 106:*168, 1960.

86. ———, "Narcolepsy in Children," *Pediatrics, 25:* 1025, 1960.

87. ———, "Treatment of Narcolepsy with Ritalin," *Neurology, 9:*171, 1959.

88. ———, "Criteria for the Diagnosis of the Narcoleptic Syndrome," *Mayo Clinic Proceedings, 32:*320, 1957.

89. Zarcone, V., "Narcolepsy," *New England Journal of Medicine, 288:*1156, 1973.

36 / Pica

Frances K. Millican, Christina C. Dublin, and Reginald S. Lourie

Name and Number

In current official terminology, pica is properly designated as: DSM-II (306.5) Feeding disturbance, (306.9) Other special symptom: pica.[1] According to the GAP classification it is listed as: GAP (H.17) Symptom disturbances related to bodily functions. A. Habit pattern; 17. Pica.[7]

Description

Children normally explore the environment by mouthing until at least twelve months of age. Occasionally some substances are swallowed. Some children are very persistent in their ingestion of nonedible substances, even preferring them to food, and continue in the habit beyond the age when such ingestion might be considered as incidental to normal oral interests. These children have the symptom of pica. Substances ingested include laundry starch, plaster, paint, paper, wood, crayons, cigarette ashes and butts, clothing, strings, pencils, and talcum powder.

Pica may be engaged in as an accepted cultural practice (eating clay or laundry starch); it may be a consequence of constitutional factors (such as organic brain damage); or it may be an expression of underlying emotional disturbances.

History

The symptom of pica is described as the craving for substances unfit for food. It acquired its name from the Latin word for the magpie, a scavenger bird. Pica has been known since antiquity and occurs on every continent.[2, 3, 14] Geophagy (earth-eating) has been described by physicians and ethnologists for nearly two hundred years. The phenomenon has been classified under four main headings: (1) cases in which the clay is regarded as a delicacy; (2) cases where clay is consumed as a substitute for food (usually during famine or because of poverty); (3) cases where clay or earth is eaten in connection with a religious or civic rite, as in the swearing of an oath; and (4) cases where it is supposed to have medical benefits, such as a cure for diarrhea, or to assure easy delivery of a baby, or, as in Java, to function as a slimming agent by creating a false sense of repletion. Diseases actually caused by earth-eating are well documented:[5, 18] they include constipation, anemia, and emaciation (cachexia africana).

Geophagy was known among the Indians of North America, but clay-eating among the blacks and poor whites, especially in the southern states, is of particular interest. The early cultural roots of pica in the blacks are found in the magical meanings and rituals of dirt eating in Africa. Pica was so frequent among black slaves, that sometimes mouthlocks were used to prevent suicide by ingestion of excessive quantities. Currently, laundry starch and clay are frequently ingested by black women, particularly during pregnancy.[15] Many mothers accept pica in their children, also: "all children eat dirt."

In the United States at present, pica occurs most frequently among the low-income black and white populations and in some Indian tribes; it is much less frequent in the more affluent white population. Nutritional lacks have long been ascribed etiologic significance,[3, 13] but controlled studies by Gutelius and associates[8, 9] did not demonstrate that any nutritional deficiency was etiologically related to pica. The psychiatric aspects of pica have been discussed by Van der Sar and Waszink,[24] Kanner,[11] Mellins and Jenkins,[10, 17] Wortis and associates[25] and the research team at Children's Hospital of the District of Columbia, Millican and associates,[20] Lourie and associates,[16] Layman and associates,[15] Millican and associates.[21] It was also discussed in a later follow-up study of the research population ten to twenty years later by Millican, 1975.[19] In early publications, Kanner[11] mentioned the relationship between pica and organic brain damage, and all authors have discussed the significance of the early mother-child relationship in the etiology. Much of the following discussion of pica is drawn from the findings of the studies conducted from 1950 to 1973 by a research team at Children's Hospital of the District of Columbia. This includes the last study, a demonstration service project designed to assist the families of children whose pica had resulted in lead poisoning to deal with the associated medical, environmental, and psychodynamic problems.

Frequency

GENDER

Among young children, there is no difference in prevalence between boys and girls. In older children and adolescents, the habit occurs more frequently in girls than in boys. In a recent follow-up study[19] of sixty children who had pica when young, twelve of the subjects (now ranging from twelve to twenty-five years) still had pica. Only two of the twelve were boys. It is rare among adult males.

SOCIO-ECONOMIC

A survey[22] of the prevalence of pica in three groups of children aged one to six years revealed

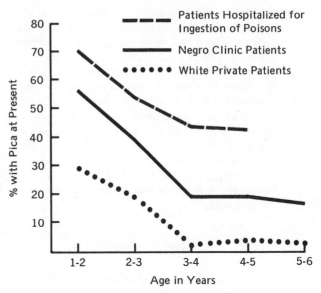

FIGURE 36–1

The Prevalence of Pica

NOTE: Reprinted by permission of the publisher from F. K. Millican, et al., "The Prevalence of Ingestion and Mouthing of Non-edible Substances by Children," *Clinical Proceedings of the Children's Hospital of the District of Columbia, 18:207–214, 1962.* © 1962 by *Clinical Proceedings of the Children's Hospital of the District of Columbia.*

that in the black low-income group, pica occurred in 32 percent; as compared with 10 percent in children from the white middle- and upper-income population. However, in a group of children hospitalized for accidental poisonings other than lead, the incidence was the highest, 55 percent. The prevalence of pica dropped sharply in both the black low-income and white middle- and upper-income groups after the age of three years. However, it was consistently higher in the black children at all age levels (Figure 36-1). Small samples suggested that children in the white low-income group and the black middle-income group had pica to a degree comparable to that occurring in the black low-income population. The greater incidence of pica in the black low-income group is at least partially due to the cultural acceptance of pica.

As previously indicated, ingestion of nonfoods may begin as early as the middle of the first year of life but usually declines with the normal developmental decrease in hand to mouth activity. There is a marked drop by the age of three years. When pica is present after the age of three, the possibility of organic brain damage or psychopathology must be considered.

Among patients with pica who had siblings old

enough to have possibly developed pica, the incidence was 27 percent among siblings of white subjects with pica and/or lead poisoning. Among blacks it was 54 percent, with an increase to 63 percent where lead poisoning was present.[21] In the study by Gutelius, and associates,[9] 58 percent of twenty-four children with pica had siblings with pica. In another study[8] 87 percent of children with pica had either mothers and/or siblings with pica. Mothers of children with pica had a high incidence of pica themselves (63 percent).[21] Pregnancy was frequently the condition under which the ingestion of laundry starch or dirt occurred.

Clinical Course

Where a combination of developmental stage, a high level of oral interest, and cultural acceptance co-exist, pica may occur in young children. A mother who has pica will often see no reason to discourage pica in her child. Indeed, rather than supplying controls, she may permit or encourage the habit.

As part of their play, children may ingest substances that are not food. However, as is noted by Anna Freud, "the neurotic element in any play activity is unmistakable when it becomes repetitive, monotonous and when it interferes with all other kinds of activities."[4] It is the repetitive, unrelenting nature of the activity that defines the symptom of pica, particularly after the age of eighteen months.

All the children studied showed a remarkable persistence in their pica. If holes in plaster were patched, they would dig new holes. One child searched for laundry starch when candy was available, others cried for newspapers to chew when food or popsicles were offered, or would leave any activity to engage in pica. Most were selective, preferring certain substances and going to considerable trouble to obtain them. Some children, especially the brain damaged, showed no discrimination and would ingest anything available.

In older children, the symptom of pica is more pathognomonic of either underlying organic brain damage or psychopathologic conditions.

Organic Etiologic Factors

Constitutionally, children differ in the intensity of their normal oral drives and also in their willingness to relinquish oral activities. More attention and external control may be required from parents of both the brain-damaged child and the child with an innately high degree of oral activity in order to help the child to forgo these activities in favor of the next stage of development. Chronic or intractable pica, which may be extremely difficult to modify, is often due to organic brain damage. This may be of any origin.

Exogenous factors—the issue of toxicity as it relates to the symptom of pica is not etiologic, i.e., in general, toxic factors are not involved in producing the symptom. At the same time, however, the symptom of pica is still the primary etiologic factor in lead poisoning of young children. The organic brain damage resulting from lead poisoning may produce irreversible pica. Failure to correct the symptom of pica earlier than, or concurrently with, lead poisoning before brain damage occurs, may result in cyclical pica. The pica leads to lead poisoning; the brain injured child engages in pica which exacerbates the lead poisoning, and so on.

Children who ingest lead-containing substances, particularly paint and plaster from old housing, carry an increased body burden of lead. In such instances, when infections alter the acid-base balance of the body, this may result in clinical symptoms of lead poisoning. The incidence of clinically symptomatic lead poisoning is seasonal, with more cases appearing in the sunny summer season.

Various writers have ascribed etiologic significance for pica to iron deficiency.[3, 13] Other nutrients have also been considered suspect. Pica has been resorted to for assuaging hunger pains when food was available.[2, 3, 14] Occasional children with pica are found to be grossly malnourished, and some are anemic. However, a controlled nutritional study at Children's Hospital of the District of Columbia[8, 9] compared children with pica to a normal control group. Anthropometric evaluation and clinical examination both showed the pica children to be normal. They did have somewhat less adequate diets, showed lower levels of ascorbic acid in the plasma, had slightly lower hemoglobin concentrations, more reported respiratory illnesses, and more recorded days of hospitalization than the control children without pica.

In contrast to these findings, two double-blind experiments failed to demonstrate that iron given intramuscularly or that a multivitamin and mineral preparation given daily were any more effective than were placebos in ameliorating or eliminating the habit of pica. In brief, pica was not caused by a deficiency of any of the nutrients studied. Poor economic conditions and inadequacies of child care are contributory both to the symptom of pica and to less than optimal nutrition of the child.[8, 9]

Psychodynamic Factors

In any given case, pica is the resultant of complex interacting etiologic factors (constitutional, organic brain damage, socio-economic, and emotional); as a symptom, it may be the expression of various underlying psychopathologic entities.

In very young children, still in the oral phase of development, persistent ingestion of nonedible substances is a distortion of normal oral interests. If it has about it a quality of driven intensity and it continues well beyond the first year, it can be considered to be evidence of oral fixation and early psychopathology. Children with previous pica, who have given it up, may regress to the symptom under stress. This may come about in the face of the birth of a sibling, loss of a parent, beginning school, or, later in life, during pregnancy.

In many cases, pica is a distorted form of instinctual seeking of satisfaction. It is engaged in impulsively as a defense against the loss of security caused by lack of parental availability and nurture. Psychic trauma due to separation from one or both parents occurs with significant frequency. Such separation may be in the form of physical separation but may also be related to employment of the mother, with replacement by inadequate or rapidly changing caretakers. Emotional difficulties in the mother, such as psychosis, depression, personality disorders, (especially the passive-aggressive, schizoid, or paranoid types), and alcohol or drug abuse may render her particularly unavailable for nurturing the young child.

One important contribution to the symptom on the part of many mothers is the encouragement of oral gratification. A pacifier is thrust forward, in response to the child's expression of anxiety, to serve as a substitute for a satisfactory personal relationship. As one mother said, "Whenever he fusses, I give him about an ounce of milk in a bottle." Some mothers are unable, or too overburdened, to listen or respond to the child's feelings. They find it more comfortable to shunt the child to oral satisfaction as a way of dealing with anxiety. Encouragement of orality also occurs in the form of late weaning (i.e., after two years) or vacillating weaning, or by the use of pacifiers well beyond infancy. Cases where excessive frustration of the oral drive contributes to the development of pica are found much less frequently.

The psychopathology of children with pica studied at Children's Hospital of the District of Columbia[22] covered a broad spectrum. The older children tended to have more severe disturbances. The diagnoses of children aged one and one-half to thirteen years is given in Table 36-1.[21] Of the twelve adolescents whose pica persisted to the time of follow-up,[19] half were either clinically depressed, or had manifested suicidal thoughts, gestures, or attempts. Viewed diagnostically, six of them were neurotic, four had personality disorders (primarily of the passive-dependent type), and two were borderline.

Depending on the defensive structure and psychopathology manifest by individual children, pica serves variously as incorporation, introjection, or identification. The other most frequently employed defense mechanisms, corresponding to those characteristic for each of the psychopathologic organizations, were repression, denial, avoidance, reaction formation, restriction of ego function, acting out, rationalization, and displacement.

The young children with pica showed a high degree of other oral activities, including mouthing of inedible objects, thumb-sucking, nail-biting, and feeding problems. As a group, they were somewhat retarded in their use of speech, and some even withheld speech. They showed conflicts about their dependency needs and around handling of aggressive feelings. They displayed considerable negativism. Sometimes children threatened their parents with "If you don't do ————, I will eat some paint."

In the follow-up study of sixty pica children, oral activities had persisted into adolescence in the form of pica itself (twelve), chewing on substances, thumbsucking (four), nail-biting, chewing gum, aberrant food habits (forty-five), and the use of alcohol (three), drugs (ten), and tobacco (fifteen). Three-fourths of the subjects were nailbiters. One-half had begun the habit at the time of original study, and 80 percent of all who were biting their nails originally persisted to the present. Two subjects bit their toenails, as well. A total orality score was devised for each patient and consisted of all the oral habits just described, weighed according to intensity. The seven who had the highest total orality scores showed severe difficulties in adjustment and serious psychopathology, with poor ego strength.

TABLE 36–1

Diagnoses of Children with Pica

| MAJOR DIAGNOSIS | ALL DIAGNOSES | | |
| | 6 YEARS AND OVER (N = 9) | 5 YEARS (N = 8) | 4 YEARS (N = 13) |
TOTAL GROUP (N = 95)			
None	2			
Brain Damage	14			
Severe		2	4	5
Suggestive		3	3	1
Mental Deficiency	1			
Severe		2	3	2
Mild		4	1	1
Psychosis	9	3	2	3
Psychophysiological	0			
Neurosis	8	2		2
Personality Disorder	28		6	6
Schizoid		3		
Other		1		
Transient Personality Disorder	33			

NOTE: Reprinted by permission of the publisher from F. K. Millican, et al., "Study of Oral Fixation; Pica," *Journal of the American Academy of Child Psychiatry*, 7:79, 1968. © 1968 by *Journal of the American Academy of Child Psychiatry*.

It was hypothesized that children with pica would be prone to addictive behavior and to depressions later in their lives.[21] Pica occurs in young children where the ego is still immature. The later evidence of the oral fixation did occur particularly in those subjects with poor ego strength. Kohut states that it is the lack of ego structure for soothing the self which leads to addictive behavior.[12]

Half of the sixty subjects who had childhood pica evidenced some degree of depression in adolescence. Even among the 55 percent who were seemingly making an adequate adjustment, underlying depression was present in certain subjects. Seven had made suicidal gestures or serious attempts. Only five were considered relatively free of neurotic, personality or behavior disorders. Six were borderline or psychotic.

In United States studies[15, 21, 22] children with pica are found more frequently in low-income families, and among black families where a matriarchal family structure and family instability are present. Relationship of the incidence of pica to ordinal position in the family or to the number of children present under the age of six is not of significance. However, the percentage of pica cases whose siblings have the condition, often learned from an older sibling, is over 50 percent in blacks and over 25 percent in whites.

Identification of the child with the mother is reflected in the 63 percent of children with pica whose mothers also indulged in the habit. Where a strong father figure was present, his meeting of the mother's dependency needs, his interest in the child, or his disapproval of the symptom appeared to act as a deterrent in the development or retention of the pica. In a solitary case, where pica was practiced by the father, in the form of starch eating, the female child, like the mother, did not have pica, whereas the four male siblings, identifying with the father, did.

Controlled study[8, 9, 21] revealed a marked difference in family coping styles, between normal and pica cases. Frequent changes of residence, poor housing, irregular employment, major emotional problems, and domestic disorganization characterize the pica families, despite the fact that the income level in both groups was equivalent. The relationship of a working mother as a contributing factor to the development of pica in the child pointed to the more subtle aspects of the quality of child care and family life styles. In cases where the mother's employment did not lead to the development of pica, the child care was frequently assisted by a grandmother, aunt, or close relative, with the mother remaining the "major caretaker." However, in cases in which the child developed pica, the employment of the mother frequently led to the pattern of care by rapidly shifting baby-sitters, often nonrelatives, or by farming the child out from the home to be cared for, first by one person, then another.

As has been discussed under the sections on "History" and "Frequency," cultural, socio-economic, and racial factors are all contributors both to the development of pica and to its recurrence.

Direct teaching or reinforcement of pica occurs in cases where mothers share their own favorite pica substances, such as laundry starch or dirt, with their children. In other cases, it is the defense that is learned; i.e., some form of oral activity as a defense against anxiety of various origins. Since the anxiety is frequently related to separation, it is useful to recommend that the parent attempt to discover what the child's anxiety is about, and spend time and give attention to that. It can also be suggested that rather than reinforce orality, the parent share other more developmentally useful activities with the child. This may be difficult for parents who tend themselves to utilize oral defenses. They do this in the form of pica itself, alcoholism, overeating, or drug abuse. With guidance, however, many parents are able to change their methods of handling their children.

Since pica children already manifest many other forms of orality such as nail-biting and thumb-sucking, it is not recommended that oral substitutions such as food snacks, chewing gum, or pacifiers be proffered to divert the child from the ingestion of nonfood substances. Such substitutions would reinforce orality, whereas age-appropriate play materials or activities with parents would strengthen trends toward normal development.

Although severe threats or punishment may be counter-productive, it is not advisable to remove pica substances from the child's mouth with too affectionate handling, lest this reinforce the behavior as a way of eliciting a warm parental response.[23]

Specific Therapeutic Methods

The therapeutic approach must be multidisciplinary in order to deal with the multiple etiologic factors, and with the interrelation between pica and lead poisoning. All medical histories of young children should include questions about pica. Every case of pica must be considered a presumptive case of lead poisoning until proved otherwise. These children are at risk not only for the serious sequelae of poisoning, from lead and other accidental ingestions, but also for later psychiatric disorders resulting from early environmental and psychic traumata.

Experience has shown that the best care for this condition is by a special clinic devoted to pica and lead poisoning, rather than by approaches that are either purely pediatric or psychiatric. Within a hospital setting, such a clinic is well accepted by parents and can handle both the medical and socio-psychiatric aspects of the children's illness.

The pica clinic team is headed by a pediatrician who is responsible for screening for lead poisoning. He maintains regularly scheduled follow up until the blood lead level is normal, the pica ceases, and the environment is lead-free. The other members of the team are the visiting nurse, social worker, psychologist, and psychiatrist. Since many of the families are hard to reach, they require home visits from the nurse or social worker. Knowledge of home conditions is necessary, and these team members can serve as skilled observers and offer guidance about handling problems in child development, health, and the symptom of pica. They can recommend temporary measures to protect the child from areas where lead is accessible until full de-leading is accomplished.

Social case work includes assistance in dealing with economic problems, liason with housing agencies to expedite de-leading or relocation, advise on handling problems in the family and/or mother-child relationship, aid in nursery or day care placement, and aid in securing protective convalescent care when necessary.

The psychologist or psychiatrist evaluates the emotional climate in the home, assesses the child's development, and looks for evidence of organic brain damage. They may recommend approaches for the social or emotional difficulties in the family, or direct adapted behavior modification techniques.

Experience underscores the importance, not only of a team approach, but of the desirability of minimizing fragmentation of services which is so frequently encountered by these families, who themselves are often struggling against disorganization. To this end, it is helpful for one team member to be the primary contact with the family and to serve as liason with other members of the team as needed.

The combined team approach involves an emphasis on education about the problem of pica and attendant medical hazards, improvement of child care, and the extension of supporting services to the family. This will prove sufficient in the case of many of the younger children whose personalities are still flexible. In those cases where pica is refractory, or where more fixed and severe psychopathology is present, as is often the case in white children, or older children or adolescents, psychotherapy should be instituted. Psychotherapeutic methods will depend upon the form of the psychopathology.

ACKNOWLEDGMENT

These studies were supported by Public Health Service Grants M-1445 RMH, RG-5923 R1, and R01MH15443.

REFERENCES

1. American Psychiatric Association, Committee on Nomenclature and Statistics, *Diagnostic and Statistical Manual of Mental Disorders*, 2nd ed. (DSM-II), American Psychiatric Association, Washington, D.C., 1968.

2. ANNEL, B., and LAGERCRANTZ, S., *Geophagical Customs*, Amquist and Wiksell, Upsalla, Sweden, 1958.

3. COOPER, M., *Pica*, Charles C Thomas, Springfield, Ill., 1957.

4. FREUD, A., *The Psychoanalytic Treatment of Children*, pp. 79–83, International Universities Press, New York, 1955.

5. GARDNER, J. E., and TEVETOGLU, F., "The Roentgenographic Diagnosis of Geophagia (Dirt-Eating) in Children," *Journal of Pediatrics, 51:*667, 1957.

6. GESELL, A., and AMATRUDA, C. S., *Developmental Diagnosis: Normal and Abnormal Child Development*, Paul B. Hoeber, New York, 1941.

7. Group for the Advancement of Psychiatry, Committee on Child Psychiatry, Psychopathological Disorders in Childhood: Theoretical Considerations and a Proposed Classification, vol. 6, Report No. 62, Group for the Advancement of Psychiatry, New York, 1966.

8. GUTELIUS, M. F., et al., "Nutritional Studies of Children with Pica," *Pediatrics*, 29:1012–1023, 1962.

9. ———, et al., "Treatment of Pica with a Vitamin and Mineral Supplement," *American Journal of Clinical Nutrition, 12:*388, 1963.

10. JENKINS, C. D., and MELLINS, R. B., "Lead Poisoning in Children; A Study of Forty-six Cases," *Archives of Neurology and Psychiatry, 77(1):*70–78, 1957.

11. KANNER, L., *Child Psychiatry*, 3rd ed., Charles C Thomas, Springfield, Ill., 1957.

12. KOHUT, H., "Introspection, Empathy and Psychoanalysis," *Journal of the American Psychoanalytic Association, 7:*451–473, 1959.

13. LANZKOWSKY, P., "Investigation into the Aetiology and Treatment of Pica, *Archives of Diseases in Childhood, 34:*140, 1959.

14. LAUFER, B., *Geophagy*, Field Museum of Natural History, Anthropological Series, 18, No. 2, Chicago, Ill., 1930.

15. LAYMAN, E. M., et al., "Cultural Influences and Symptom Choice: Clay-Eating Customs in Relation to the Etiology of Pica," *Psychological Record, 13:*249, 1963.

16. LOURIE, R. S., et al., "A Study of the Etiology of Pica in Young Children, An Early Pattern of Addiction," in Hoch, P. H., and Zubin, J. (Eds.), *Problems of Addiction and Habituation*, Grune & Stratton, New York, 1958.

17. MELLINS, R. G., and JENKINS, C. D., "Epidemiological and Psychological Study of Lead Poisoning in Children," *Journal of the American Medical Association, 158:*15, 1955.

18. MENGEL, C. E., et al., "Geophagia with Iron Deficiency and Hypokalemia—Cachexia Africana," *Archives of Internal Medicine, 114:*470, 1964.

19. MILLICAN, F. K., LOURIE, R. S., and DUBLIN, C. C., "Oral Autoerotic, Auto-Aggressive Behavior and Oral fixation," in Marcus, I. M., and Francis, J. J. (Eds.), *Masturbation*, International Universities Press, New York, 1975.

20. MILLICAN, F. K., LOURIE, R. S., and LAYMAN, E. M., "Emotional Factors in the Etiology and Treatment of Lead Poisoning," *American Journal of Diseases of Children. 91:*144, 1956.

21. ———, et al., "Study of an Oral Fixation; Pica," *Journal of the American Academy of Child Psychiatry, 7:*79, 1968.

22. ———, et al., "The Prevalence of Ingestion and Mouthing of Nonedible substances by Children," *Clinical Proceedings of the Children's Hospital of the District of Columbia, 18:*207–214, 1962.

23. SHERER, L., Personal communication.

24. VAN DER SAR, A., and WASZINK, H. M., "Pica (Report on a Case)," *Documenta de Medicina Geographica et Tropica, 4:*29–32, 1952.

25. WORTIS, H., et al., "Children Who Eat Noxious Substances," *Journal of the American Academy of Child Psychiatry, 1:*536, 1962.

37 / Tic: Gilles de la Tourette's Syndrome

Alexander R. Lucas

Terminology and Classification

The origin of the word *tic* is obscure. Its sound suggests the action it describes, and its onomatopoeic source is suggested by the similarity of terms in Western languages. *Tique, ticq, tiquet,* and *tic* were in common use in France for centuries. *Tug* and *tick* were early English equivalents. *Zucken, ziehen, zugen, tucken, ticken,* and *tick* were the German terms; *ticchio,* the Italian and *tico,* the Spanish. The word *tique* is said to have first been used to describe an affection of horses in seventeenth century France. Later the term was applied to humans.

Eighteenth century French physicians identified it with diverse conditions: André used the term *tic douloureux* in 1756 to designate painful trigeminal neuralgia, while in 1785 Pujol described simple painless convulsive *tic* which spread from the face to the arms, and the body as a whole.[58] In 1830, Sir Charles Bell,[7] in his classic study *The Nervous System of the Human Body,* described "spasmodic twitching" of the respiratory muscles, "spasmodic contortions" of the head and neck and "ludicrous jerking" of other muscles. "Muscular tic" was introduced in the English medical literature in 1852 by Marshall Hall.[37] He described patients with facial tics and contortions of other parts of the body. In contradistinction to the views of most other writers, he identified the movements as voluntary.

Tic is an involuntary, repetitive movement of a muscle or group of muscles. In child psychiatric literature, the term frequently is used interchangeably with habit spasm. Definitions often characterize tic as a spasmodic movement. It has variously been identified as a prototype of nervous habit in children, or as the motor manifestation of an abnormal neurologic discharge in the central nervous system. Much controversy still surrounds the understanding of its origin, its pathophysiology, and its psychologic meaning; so much so that some writers accept the presence of tics as incontrovertible evidence for emotional disturbance, while others consider them signs of organic brain pathology. The truth probably lies somewhere between these extreme positions. It is likely that tic can have a multiplicity of causes, influenced in varying degree by the organic substrate of the individual's central nervous system and by his intrapsychic, interpersonal, and social environment.

The monograph of Meige and Feindel, written at the turn of the century, still stands as the most comprehensive account of the phenomenology of tic. These writers differentiated between spasm and tic, defining spasm as the motor reaction resulting from a pathological irritation of any point in a reflex spinal or bulbo-spinal arc. A tic requires cortical involvement and is a coordinated and systematized motor action.[58]

Many, if not all, individuals have experienced an occasional tic. Tics may be isolated and limited to a single muscle or circumscribed muscle group, or they may be widespread, involving any and all

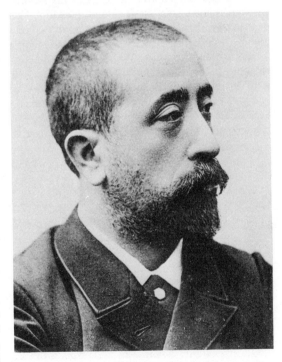

Georges Gilles de la Tourette

Courtesy of Dr. Howard P. Rome

parts of the body. They may occur at any age but are more common during certain developmental phases of childhood than during others. They may be fleeting and transitory in occurrence, episodic, or may become chronically fixed. They may represent the reaction to physical irritation, or to psychic stress. They may be manifestations of severe tic disease, known as Gilles de la Tourette's Disease or tic syndrome. Tic syndrome is a strikingly unusual condition manifested by a triad of symptoms: multiple tics, vocal tics of inarticulate noises, and coprolalia. Its eponym was given the disease by the students of Charcot to honor their colleague who reported the first series of patients.

Samuel Johnson (1709–1784), the great English critic and lexicographer, who died 100 years before Gilles de la Tourette published his treatise, very probably had the disorder. As a young man he was denied a position as headmaster in a boys' school because it was thought his facial contortions would affect the boys under his control. His convulsive starts and curious gesticulations suggested to a visitor in his home that he was mentally defective. He was said sometimes to seem to be a victim of St. Vitus' dance, his legs and arms jerking convulsively as if at the mercy of a nerve. He made singular ruminative noises with his mouth: chewing, clucking, sibilating, and blowing. The painter Joshua Reynolds declared that his odd gestures were apparent only when he was reading a book or lost in reverie. While his attention was engaged in conversation, his vocal mannerisms were silenced and his limbs stilled.[65]

Psychiatric classification becomes problematic because tic can represent a normal developmental phenomenon, a temporary tension state, a reactive disorder, a symptom occurring in many psychiatric disorders, or the major psychopathology in severe tic syndrome or tic disease. Both the DSM-II classification and the GAP classification include tic in their special symptom list. Thus, the term may be appended to any other primary diagnosis. When tic is the sole manifestation of psychopathology the DSM-II classification, "Tic," (306.2) may be used.[4] For multiple tic syndrome the "Psychophysiologic Musculoskeletal Disorder" category (305.1) is suitable. In the GAP classification, the most appropriate diagnosis is: "Psychophysiologic disorder, musculoskeletal, tic."[34] It is desirable, for explicitness, to describe the body part affected. Commonly the designation tic syndrome or its eponym, Gilles de la Tourette's disease, is included in the diagnostic description. When tic is symptomatic of another psychiatric condition, the primary diagnosis should be indicated, the term tic appended to indicate that it is a prominent symptom (Table 37–1).

Tics may occur in children with neurotic disorders, in psychotic children, in children with acute or chronic brain disorders, and in children with personality disorders. Notwithstanding Kanner's statement that no happy, secure child ever develops tics,[41] they may even occur in children without major psychopathology.

Description and Variants

TIC AS A PRIMARY SYMPTOM

Clinical Types: Willard Olson[63] made direct observations on tics in 700 school children. Based

TABLE 37–1

Examples of Classification of Tics

DSM-II CLASSIFICATION	GAP CLASSIFICATION
306.2 Tic of the eyelids	Psychophysiologic Disorder, musculoskeletal, tic of the eyelids
305.1 Psychophysiologic musculoskeletal disorder, tic syndrome (Gilles de la Tourette's Disease)	Psychophysiologic Disorder, musculoskeletal, tic syndrome (Gilles de la Tourette's Disease)
309.0 Non-psychotic Organic Brain Syndrome with intracranial infection, with tics of the face, neck, and left shoulder	Chronic Brain Syndrome, postencephalitic, with tics of the face, neck and left shoulder
285.8 Schizophrenia, childhood type, with body tics, echolalia and coprolalia	Psychotic Disorder of Childhood, with body tics, echolalia and coprolalia
300.13 Hysterical neurosis, conversion type, with tic of right arm	Psychoneurotic Disorder, Conversion Type, with tic of right arm

SOURCES: American Psychiatric Association, Committee on Nomenclature and Statistics, *Diagnostic and Statistical Manual of Mental Disorders*, 2nd ed., (DSM-II), American Psychiatric Association, Washington, D.C., 1968; and Group for the Advancement of Psychiatry, Committee on Child Psychiatry, *Psychopathological Disorders in Childhood: Theoretical Considerations and a Proposed Classification*, vol. 6, Report No. 62, Group for the Advancement of Psychiatry, New York, 1966.

TABLE 37–2

Inventory of Tics

A. FACE AND HEAD

Twisting hair
Grimacing
Puckering forehead
Raising eyebrows
Blinking eyelids
Winking
Wrinkling nose
Trembling nostrils
Twitching mouth
Displaying teeth
Biting lips and other parts
Extruding tongue
Protracting lower jaw
Fingering ear
Picking nose
Sucking thumb or fingers
Biting nails
Nodding, jerking, shaking head
Twisting neck, looking sideways
Head rolling
Head banging

B. ARMS AND HANDS

Jerking hands
Jerking arms; swinging arms
Plucking fingers, writhing fingers
Clenching fists
Striking head or body
Scratching
Manipulating genitalia

C. BODY AND LOWER EXTREMITIES

Shrugging shoulders
Shaking shoulders
Shaking foot, knee, or toe
Peculiarities of gait
Body rocking
Body writhing
Jumping

D. RESPIRATORY AND ALIMENTARY

Hiccoughing
Coughing
Hysterical laughing
Grunting
Barking
Sobbing
Sighing
Yawning
Snuffing
Blowing through nostrils
Whistling inspiration
Exaggerated breathing
Belching
Sucking or smacking sounds
Vomiting, regurgitating
Swallowing
Spitting and salivation
Clearing throat

E. MISCELLANEOUS

Repeating words, tunes, etc.
  (echolalia)
Repeating actions seen
  (echokinesis)
Uttering obscene words
  (coprolalia)

NOTE: Reprinted by permission of the publisher from W. C. Olson, *The Measurement of Nervous Habits in Normal Children*, (Minneapolis, University of Minnesota Press, 1929. © 1929 by The University of Minnesota Press.

upon a review of the literature, he first made a comprehensive inventory of tics (Table 37–2). Utilizing this inventory, he constructed a condensed list upon which actual classroom observations of children from kindergarten through eighth grade were based. This list included:

1. Oral (sucking thumb, sucking fingers, biting nails, protruding tongue)
2. Nasal (picking nose, scratching nose, wrinkling nose)
3. Manual (picking fingers, writhing hands, clenching fists)
4. Hirsutal (pulling and twisting hair, scratching head)
5. Aural (pulling ear, picking ear)
6. Irritational (scratching body)
7. Ocular (rubbing eyes, blinking eyelids, winking)
8. Genital (manipulating genitalia, thigh rubbing)
9. Facial (grimacing, twitching muscles)

Olson found no relationship between the number of these "nervous habits" and ages, but found the incidence to be higher in girls than in boys. He considered the habits to be relatively normal characteristics of all children. Olson recorded the frequency of each habit and accepted the broadest definition of tic. Many of the nervous habits he included are not considered tics by most writers. The study of Macfarlane, Allen and Honzik of 252 normal children between twenty-one months and fourteen years of age did not identify habits such as nailbiting or thumbsucking as tics.[53] The age incidence of these habits contrasts with that of tics. Nailbiting, in the Macfarlane study increased in frequency with age, while thumbsucking declined with age. Tics increased in frequency to age six and seven, and then declined.

Phenomenology: Meige and Feindel required a tic to meet certain criteria. They stipulated that a tic is a coordinated movement and that it is a purposive act. It is not an incoordinated movement as is chorea; the tiqueur does not strike his face when lifting a fork to the mouth or trip over his feet as does an ataxic person. The movement was first initiated by an external cause or by an idea. Through repetition it has become habitual and finally involuntary, having lost its original purpose. Its form, intensity, and frequency are exaggerated so as to assume the character of a convulsive movement, inopportune and excessive. Its execution is often preceded by an irresistible impulse and its suppression with malaise. Distraction and volitional effort diminishes its activity; it disappears in sleep. Meige and Feindel believed that it occurs in predisposed individuals who show other indications of mental instability. The prevailing mental defect, they felt, is impairment of volition (this could be equated to cerebral disinhibition). Thus, Meige and Feindel, in their masterful treatise, chronicled the origin and development of tic.[58]

Kinnier Wilson offered Cruchet's definition: "Tic consists in the execution—short, abrupt, sudden, irresistible, involuntary, inapposite, and repeated at irregular but frequent intervals—of a simple isolated or complex movement which represents objectively an act intended for a particular purpose."[88]

Margaret Mahler[54] defined tic as an involuntary motor automatism. She noted that it is difficult to draw the line between transient auto-erotic habits, repetitive manneristic movements, and true motor automatisms. In children who are fidgety and restless, their constant nervous movements may develop into tics. More often the transitory, tic-like habit movements frequently found in young children disappear without residue at school age. Mahler characterized symptomatic tic as consisting of distinctly patterned and more or less localized involuntary twitching. Such isolated tics as blinking or sniffing may, she felt, represent transient tension phenomena or they may represent a true psychoneurotic symptom as the symbolic expression of an unconscious conflict. Psychoneurotic tic she differentiated from tic syndrome which she considered to be an organ neurosis of the neuro-muscular apparatus (a psychosomatic disease). She emphasized the necessity of distinguishing between those tics which are a sign or symptom of various psychopathological conditions and the tics which in themselves represent the central disturbance.

The line between excessive activity and the normal restless motor behavior of preadolescent children is difficult to draw. This is also true for the line between hyperactivity and tics. The expectations and tolerance of the observer influence this demarcation. Redl[68] noted that normal preadolescents are characteristically extremely restless. Odd gestures, facial tics, and jerky movements are commonplace. The epidemiologic studies of Macfarlane and associates[53] and of Lapouse and Monk[43] have shown that mothers describe a very large proportion of their young children as "overactive."

TIC AS A SECONDARY SYMPTOM

Symptomatic tic, which Mahler[54] also called "passagère tic" when transient, was illustrated by the case of a four-and one-half-year-old girl who contracted her eye muscles in tic-like fashion, as if to see into the distance, when thinking intensely. Anna Freud and Burlingham[29] similarly described the condensation of motor actions and gestures into symbolic expressions as occurring when circumstances prohibit children from playing out the underlying conflicts.

Children described by Margaret Gerard[31] had symptomatic tic and constituted a homogeneous group of ten boys and three girls referred for psychiatric treatment. In this group, the occurrence of tic followed experiences arousing fear of being injured and represented a defensive response in aggression-inhibited children.

Mahler described tics as neurotic symptoms representing, in some cases, conversion symptoms and, in other cases, compulsions in an obsessive-compulsive neurosis.[54]

Tics as manifestations of bizarre motor actions in schizophrenic children were described by Lucas, Kauffman, and Morris.[52] The differentiation of schizophrenic children from those with severe tic syndrome was emphasized.

In contradistinction to children with symptomatic tic, Mahler[54] identified children whose multiple tics were part of an impulse or character neurosis as having tic syndrome.

OUTCOME OF TIC SYMPTOM

Two large-scale follow-up studies of children with tics seen in pediatric and psychiatric clinics have been reported. Torup[82] reported on 237 children seen at a general hospital. Two hundred twenty (93 percent) were followed up after periods varying between two and sixteen years. In 50 percent, the tics had disappeared; in 44 percent, there was improvement; and in 6 percent, they were unchanged. Corbett and co-workers[18] identified 171 child tiqueurs seen at psychiatric clinics. Eighty-nine, who presented with tics as the primary complaint, were selected for follow up. Data on seventy-three (82 percent) were obtained after periods varying between one and eighteen years. Forty percent had completely recovered from their tics, 53 percent were improved, and 6 percent were unchanged. These findings suggest that roughly half the children will outgrow their tics. What causes tics to persist in others is not clear.

History of Identification
of the Syndrome

According to Gilles de la Tourette,[33] in his 1818 "Treatise on Chorea,"[9] Bouteille had classified diseases characterized by spasms, convulsions, hysteria, and nervous origin as false chorea. Nonetheless, confusion about this class of disorders continued. Although the first case description was actually made by Itard[40] in 1825, Gilles de la Tourette credited Trousseau[83] as being the first to describe the disease succinctly. Itard's celebrated case was that of the Marquise de Dampierre, then twenty-six years old. Her symptoms began at the age of seven with jerking of the arms which spread to other parts of her body. Eventually vocalizations, and finally, obscene epithets became a prominent part of her affliction. Several reports on her progress by various observers appeared in the literature, and she was included among the nine cases reported by Georges Gilles de la Tourette in 1885[33] under the title of "Study of a Nervous Affliction Characterized by Motor Incoordination Accompanied by Echolalia and Coprolalia." Gilles de la Tourette stated that the Marquise had been seen at an advanced age by Charcot and continued to manifest her disorder. Obscene expressions, particular, "merde" and "foutu cochon," were included in her repertoire.

A multiplicity of case reports, often of a single or a few cases, appeared following the first description. No less than fifteen synonyms have been given for tic syndrome in the French, English, and German literature (Table 37–3).

Surveying the literature before 1968, Lucas[47] found 182 case reports. In recent years, the cumulative experience of many workers, some large-scale studies, and follow-up data have permitted the pooling of data and the statistical analysis of larger numbers of cases. This has been facilitated by several national and international workshops and panel discussions; by the formation of an organization (The Gilles de la Tourette Syndrome Association, Inc., Box 3519, Grand Central Station, New York 10017) devoted to the dissemination of information and the encouragement of research; and by the formation of an International Registry. Abuzzahab and Anderson,[3] largely responsible for establishing the registry, were able, in 1973, to report data on 485 cases.

TABLE 37–3

Alternate Historical Names for Tic Syndrome
(Gilles de la Tourette's Disease)

Maladie des tics convulsifs	Guinon, 1886[36]
Myospasia impulsiva	Guinon, 1886[36]
Tics convulsifs	Guinon, 1887[35]
Convulsive tic	Hammond, 1892[38]
Maladie des tics	Chabbert, 1893[14]
Mimische Krampfneurose	Bresler, 1896[10]
Maladies des tics	Wille, 1898[87]
Koordinierte Erinnerungskrämpfe	Köster, 1899[42]
Multiform tic	Prince, 1906[67]
Generalisierte Tic-Krankheit	Clauss and Balthasar, 1954[17]
Maladie des tics dégénérés	Kanner, 1957[41]
Psychosomatic tic	Daugela, 1961[22]
Tic de Gilles de la Tourette	Tobin and Reinhart, 1961[81]
Tourette's Syndrome	Challas and Brauer, 1963[15]
Multiple tic syndrome	Moldofsky, Tullis, and Lamon, 1974[60]

Gilles de la Tourette, in his monograph of 1885, described the syndrome as follows: The muscular disturbances often begin in the face or the upper limbs and are noted first by the teacher or the parent. Alternate flexing and extending of the fingers, and lifting of the shoulders may be noted. Eye blinking, drawing upward of the corners of the mouth, contraction of the masseters, thrusting of the tongue, and alternate flexion and extension of the neck muscles are noted. The movements then spread to affect the lower limbs, causing kicking and bending. Characteristically, there is a tendency to jump. Periods of remission and exacerbation were noted. Gilles de la Tourette noted that the mental status of the patient remains perfectly normal. He stated that the patient's life span is not shortened, but that the patient will probably always have the symptoms. He noted that Itard's patient had a persistence of her disease until she died. He described three distinctive phases in the development of the symptomatology. First, the patient has convulsive muscular jerking which may be confused with chorea; during the second phase, the convulsive movements are accompanied by inarticulate cries; and finally, coprolalia and echolalia are added to the other symptoms.

Mahler and Rangell succinctly summarized the symptomatology:

The classical syndrome . . . consists first in the appearance, usually at an early age, of a series of abnormal, uncontrollable involuntary movements, of gradually increasing intensity and frequency. These usually begin in the upper part of the body, in an upper extremity, shoulder or face, and spread in the course of time to involve the head and neck, trunk, and finally the lower extremities, so that eventually there may be widespread involuntary movements of the entire body, including kicking and jumping, twisting of the head and neck, quick movements of all the extremities, blinking of the eyes, grinding of the teeth, and projection of the tongue. There then appears the involuntary utterance of an inarticulate cry. This in turn is followed by the onset of echolalia and echokinesia, and finally a feature, which, when it appears, is pathognomonic for this disease syndrome, namely, the symptom of coprolalia. (p. 579)[56]

Frequency, Incidence, Prevalence, Distribution, and Cross-cultural Information

Tics occur more commonly in children than in adults. Their frequency increases until age six or seven and then the frequency declines. The musculature of the face, head, and neck is most often affected. Kanner[41] cited Boncour's 1910 study in which 23 percent of 1759 children between two and thirteen years of age were tiqueurs. In 1954 Macfarlane, Allen, and Honzik,[53] in a sample of 252 normal children between twenty-one months and fourteen years of age, found that tics and mannerisms reached their peak in girls at six years (10 percent) and in boys at seven years (11 percent). The incidence at ages above and below these peaks declined sharply and reached zero at age ten in girls and at age twelve in boys. One-quarter of each group had a record of this behavior at some age, a figure remarkably similar to that of Boncour. Lapouse and Monk, in an epidemiologic study of 482 children aged six to twelve, found unusual movements, twitching or jerking (tics) in only 12 percent.[43] Incidence at particular ages was not given.

The incidence of cases reported from children's psychiatric clinics varies from one case in 1,000 outpatients[52] to one case in 12,500 outpatients.[5] Abuzzahab and Anderson collected 430 published case reports plus fifty-five case reports in the International Registry. Seventy-one percent were males. This gender distribution of slightly more than twice the number of males as females is not unlike the gender distribution in children that come for treatment with other tics.[90]

Age at onset of symptoms was tabulated for 485 cases (Figure 37–2). The age of onset in 90 percent was between three and sixteen years, with more than three-fourths of the cases beginning between ages five and twelve years. Less than 4 percent were older than twenty years when symptoms began.

TABLE 37–4

Frequency of Symptoms

MOTOR SYMPTOMS:	
Facial tics	92%
Arm tics	78%
Leg tics	54%
Neck tics	53%
Eye tics	31%
VOCAL SYMPTOMS:	
Inarticulations	65%
Coprolalia	58%
Echolalia	23%

NOTE: Reproduced by permission of the publisher from F. E. Abuzzahab and F. O. Anderson, "Gilles de la Tourette's Syndrome: International Registry," *Minnesota Medicine*, 56: 492–496, 1973. © 1973 by *Minnesota Medicine*.

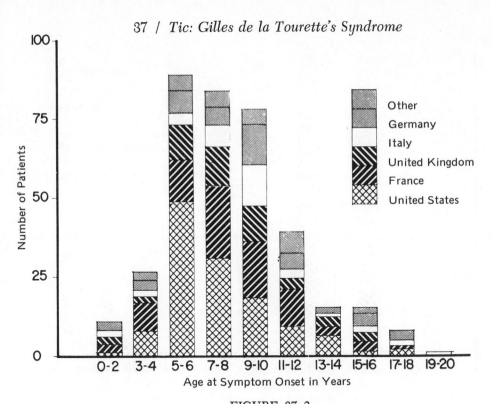

FIGURE 37–2

Age at Onset of Symptoms

NOTE: Reproduced by permission of the publisher from F. E. Abuzzahab and F. O. Anderson, "Gilles de la Tourette's Syndrome: International Registry," *Minnesota Medicine*, 56:492–496, 1973. © 1973 by *Minnesota Medicine*.

Frequency of symptoms as recorded by Abuzzahab and Anderson are tabulated in Table 37–4. Intellectual assessment with the Wechsler Intelligence Scale for Children, ascertained in forty-five cases, revealed an almost normal distribution except for a preponderance of scores in the bright normal range (Figure 37–3). In 106 other case reports less detailed psychometric information was given, with sixty-six cases described as being of "average intelligence," twenty-six "above average" and fourteen "below average."[3]

Cross-cultural analysis (Table 37–5) revealed a great preponderance of case reports from the United States and Western Europe. The American cases were younger at age of onset, had more tics of the neck and more coprolalia. Patients reported from France had fewer tics of the neck and eyes, and more echokinesis. The United Kingdom group showed fewer echophenomena, and the Italian patients demonstrated more eye tics. The German group was not significantly different from the group as a whole.[3]

TABLE 37–5

Cross-Cultural Distribution

NO. CASES	COUNTRY
174	United States
107	France
57	Germany
53	United Kingdom
46	Italy
48	Other:
	Eastern Europe, 25
	Scandinavia, 9
	India, 5
	Japan, 2

NOTE: Reproduced by permission of the publisher from F. E. Abuzzahab and F. O. Anderson, "Gilles de la Tourette's Syndrome: International Registry," *Minnesota Medicine*, 56: 492–496, 1973. © 1973 by *Minnesota Medicine*.

Clinical Course of the Condition

Typically, the first signs of the disorder are seen between the ages of four and ten and resemble the common transient tics of latency. Within several years, vocal noises develop which first resemble throat clearing, coughs or grunts, and later, loud barking sounds. Finally, usually near the time of

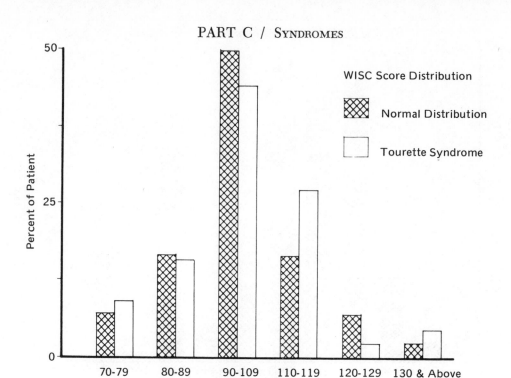

FIGURE 37–3

Intellectual Functioning

NOTE: Reproduced by permission of the publisher from F. E. Abuzzahab and F. O. Anderson, "Gilles de la Tourette's Syndrome: International Registry," *Minnesota Medicine*, 56:492–496, 1973. © 1973 by *Minnesota Medicine*.

puberty, coprolalia, the sudden outburst of obscenities, occurs. Echolalia and echopraxia are less common features of the disorder, although careful observation frequently reveals some evidence of mimicry and echophenomena.

True tics of the diaphragm frequently occur associated with violent expiratory noises. The diaphragmatic contractions associated with contractions of the abdominal musculature not infrequently result in abdominal pain. Tics of the trunk and lower extremities can become so severe as to propel a seated patient from a chair and to cause violent flexion of the trunk and limbs. So violent can such convulsive episodes become as to leave the patient totally exhausted.

Arthur Shapiro and co-workers[73] recorded the symptoms of thirty-four patients. They classified the tic movements as simple or complicated. Ninety-four percent of patients had facial tics, 91 percent had tics of the head, neck, and shoulders, 77 percent had tics of the upper limbs, 56 percent of the lower limbs, and 53 percent of the torso. Complicated movements occurred in 56 percent and included jumping, squatting, skipping, hitting, kicking, repetitive touching movements, startle reactions, esophageal spasm, and echopraxia (see Tables 37–6 and 37–7). Involuntary vocalizations occurred in all of Shapiro's thirty-four patients. Most frequently these assumed the form of grunts, barks, throat clearing, shrieks or yelps, high pitched squeal, odd accentuation of words, snorts, and coughs. Sniffing, lip smacking, echolalia, stammering, unintelligible sounds, guttural sounds, humming, and spitting occurred with lesser frequency. Coprolalia, not considered a necessary symptom by Shapiro, occurred in 53 percent. Great relief of tension and temporary decrease in other symptoms was reported when coprolalia could be expressed. Conscious supression of coprolalia markedly aggravated tics and other noises.

The course of the disorder is characterized by remissions and exacerbations of varying duration, a feature which makes the evaluation of treatment efficacy difficult. Although Gilles de la Tourette noted that mental deterioration did not occur, many of the early writers implied that there occurs progressive degeneracy and neurological deterioration, notions which have been incorrectly perpetuated by some neurological and psychiatric textbooks. Nor is the final outcome psychosis as was suggested by some writers. At the onset of adolescence, there is frequently an efflorescence of the symptomatology, and it is at this time that

TABLE 37–6

*Simple Movements in 34 Patients
with Tic Syndrome*

SYMPTOM	PERCENTAGE
Face	
Eyes	85.3
Nose	20.6
Lips	14.7
Mouth	5.9
Tongue	26.5
Forehead	14.7
Grimace	41.2
Total	94.1
Head, neck, shoulders	
Head	76.5
Neck	32.4
Shoulders	55.9
Total	91.2
Upper limbs	
Upper arm	11.8
Whole arm	52.9
Hands	26.5
Total	76.5
Lower limbs	
Upper leg	11.8
Lower leg	5.9
Whole leg	38.3
Feet	14.7
Total	55.9
Torso	
Thorax	17.7
Abdomen	5.9
Thorax and abdomen	38.3
Total	52.9

SOURCE: A. K. Shapiro, et al., "The Symptomatology and Diagnosis of Gilles de la Tourette's Syndrome," Journal of the American Academy of Child Psychiatry, *12*:702–723, 1973.

TABLE 37–7

*Complicated Movements in 34 Patients
with Tic Syndrome*

SYMPTOM	PERCENTAGE
Complicated movements	
Jumping	20.6
Squatting	2.9
Skipping	2.9
Hitting	11.8
Kicking	8.8
Total	35.3
Repetitive movements—touching	
Touch floor	2.9
Hesitate picking up things as if hot and touch things	2.9
Fingers touch chin, lips, tongue, throat	2.9
Right arm touch left ear, bull-like prancing, closed fist touch chest	2.9
Adjust belt, rub lips until chapped	2.9
Touch and kiss things, hold hand up	2.9
Dance-like movement, kicking	2.9
Touch people	2.9
Clutch throat and chest	2.9
Total	26.5
Other	
Startle reactions	8.8
Esophageal spasm	2.9
Echopraxia	11.8
Total	17.7
Total with complicated movements	55.9

SOURCE: A. K. Shapiro, et al., "The Symptomatology and Diagnosis of Gilles de la Tourette's Syndrome," Journal of the American Academy of Child Psychiatry, *12*:702–723, 1973.

coprolalia becomes most prominent. Often there is a gradual abatement of symptoms in late adolescence and through early adulthood. However, the symptoms may persist into adulthood. The usual patient learns gradually to camouflage some of his symptoms by performing motor acts which are less obtrusive than the symptoms or by pretending to clear his throat when an uncontrolled vocalization occurs.

Latent forms have been described by Mahler[54] and by Lucas[47] in children in whom tic symptoms are minor and remain arrested in *forme fruste.*

OUTCOME

Follow-up studies and accumulating data from the world literature suggest that patients do not, as a rule, follow a deteriorating course. Reports of psychotic decompensation exist, and fatal neurological degeneration has been known to occur in a patient who presented with multiple progressive tics. The rarity of such occurrences suggests that initially the wrong diagnosis was made. Mahler and Luke[55] reported on the outcome of ten children with severe tic syndrome. Follow-up duration was up to eleven years after dismissal from the hospital. They found no direct correlation between recovery from the tic syndrome and length or method of psychotherapy. In six patients, the tics had disappeared or were almost absent; one of these patients who had received the longest and "deepest" psychotherapy became schizophrenic; the other five were making a good social and personal adjustment. In four patients, the tics remained the same or progressed in severity; all but one of these four were making a poor social and personal adjustment.

Lucas and co-workers[52] followed fifteen patients who had received comprehensive long-term psychiatric treatment including residential treatment. Six of the patients were treated before pheno-thiazine or butyrophenone drugs became available. Follow up after a period of up to fifteen years in some cases showed that in six patients tics were absent or almost absent, in six the tics were improved, and in three the tics persisted. None had worsened. Two of the cases in whom the tics persisted had been followed up for only two and three years when the study was reported. The tics of these patients had improved three years later. The one remaining patient whose tics were unimproved had the briefest treatment—only two months of outpatient therapy.

In 1970, Lucas[48] reported further on the outcome of tic syndrome based on continuing observations of these patients and of others. He noted that treatment had a beneficial effect upon outcome. The nature of the family dynamics and the presence or absence of encephalopathy appeared to have no relationship to the fate of the tics as such. Social and personality adjustment continued to be poor in a number of the patients during late adolescence and early adulthood. Those patients with signs of encephalopathy and severe learning deficits in childhood continued to have the greatest adjustment problems. Good intelligence, absence of signs of brain damage, and good academic performance were the best indicators of eventual favorable adjustment, regardless of the family dynamics. In early adulthood, two clinical prototypes emerged: (1) the children who had demonstrated signs of brain damage and severe learning deficits tended to become isolated, socially inept young adults prone to impulsive acts and frequent temper outbursts. While the tics had improved and may have been almost absent, the life-long experience of social ostracism, together with repeated frustration and failure in school, appeared to have left permanent personality scars. Their job histories were erratic with frequent job changes. They had difficulty persevering, they reacted poorly to stress, and they found it hard to accept authority and supervision. (2) Those children who showed no signs of encephalopathy and who were academically competent were able to continue school, graduate from high school, join the military service, and sometimes go on to college. They were better able to compensate for their earlier frustrating experiences and had made an adequate social and personal adjustment. Interpersonal relations continued to be difficult, however, although some did marry. They tended to be more introspective and to require more external support than the average individual.

Organic Etiologic Factors

ENDOGENOUS FACTORS

Hereditary: Many authors have suspected and implicated a hereditary influence on the disorder and have alluded to family members who were tiqueurs. Trousseau said that the tics are often hereditary. Many isolated cases of tic occur, however, and until recently no documentation of the occurrence of the full-blown tic syndrome in more than one member of a family had been reported.

In 1973, three such reports were published independently. A mother-son pair was reported by Lucas.[46, 51] The mother, age thirty-one suffered severe tic syndrome beginning at age eight, for which she received psychiatric treatment at age ten. Symptoms diminished in late adolescence. She was married at age twenty and became almost completely free of tics in subsequent years. Her five-year-old boy developed jerking of the head and twitching of the shoulders and arms at age four and one-half. Skipping and dancing mannerisms occurred, followed by involuntary vocalizations, increased body tics and vocal tics. Sanders[69] reported two cases of Gilles de la Tourette's syndrome occurring in a man and his son. The father, seen at age fifty-four, had onset of tics at age seven, progressing in adolescence to involuntary vocalizations and coprolalia during his mid twenties. The son was seen at age twenty-three because of uncontrollable generalized body jerks and twitches, associated with explosive grunts, barks, and squeals of many years' duration. He began having facial twitching and grimacing at age eight. At that point his father thought the son was taunting and mimicking him. Friel[30] described two sisters, the sixth and fifth siblings, respectively, in a family of four boys and two girls. One, a twenty-eight-year-old woman, began having symptoms involving the face and neck at age eleven, followed by widespread tics and vocal grunts at age sixteen. Later, profanities occurred. Her sister, a thirty-four-year-old woman, also had the onset of symptoms at age eleven beginning with vocal tics. She had multiple motor tics, repetitive sniffing, and uttered inarticulate guttural sounds. The twenty-eight-year-old sister's eleven-year-old son had, since age ten, developed motor tics and then vocal grunts. The sisters had a total of six children; four of the six had definite and obvious multiple motor tics, but only one had the pathognomonic vocal component.

Moldofsky and co-workers[60] have suggested the

hypothesis that some patients with Gilles de la Tourette's syndrome have a genetically determined metabolic disorder. The preceding case reports give support to the hypothesis. They noted better response to haloperidol by patients who have a family history of tics. In their study of fifteen patients, they discovered that nine had at least one first-degree relative with tics. Other studies which reported family history of tics found lesser incidence. Shapiro and co-workers[75] reported that 12 precent of thirty-three patients had a family member with tics, and Fernando,[27] in a review of sixty-five patients from the literature, found 11 percent to have a family history of tics. Many case reports have not provided a careful review of family history.

Neurologic: While Mahler's work on tics is perhaps best known for its elucidation of psychodynamic mechanisms operating in children with tics, Mahler and Rangell[56] emphasized the presence of an organic substratum. They theorized, on the basis of the clinical manifestations, that there is an underlying defect in the striopallidal connections of the basal ganglia. While many writers have speculated about possible organic etiologic factors, little hard evidence has emerged from the many scattered case reports.

Report of autopsy in a patient with Gilles de la Tourette's disease by DeWulf and van Bogaert[23] revealed an entirely normal anatomic nervous system. In another autopsy report,[6, 7] an immature ratio of small to large neurocytes was found in the corpus striatum. The significance of this is uncertain. While neither of these reports has resolved the question of whether or not there are neuroanatomic changes, they confirm that tic syndrome may occur in the absence of major anatomic changes. Lucas and co-workers[52] reported that 60 percent of fifteen children showed psychological test evidence for encephalopathy and had significant learning difficulties resembling those of children with organic brain defects.

Shapiro and his co-workers at the Payne Whitney Clinic, New York Hospital-Cornell University Medical Center, have carried out extensive studies in the largest series of patients followed at one center. Detailed demographic, birth, developmental, and family history studies[76] of thirty-four patients, who received careful psychological and psychiatric evaluation, revealed evidence for organic impairment of the nervous system in 77 percent by psychologic tests, in 54 percent by neurologic evaluation, and in 50 percent on the basis of the psychiatric evaluation. The finding by Shapiro and co-workers,[75] of 35 percent incidence

of left-handedness, much higher than expected in the general population, lends additional weight to the possibility of cerebral damage in some of the patients. Childhood developmental abnormalities were reported in the histories of 52 percent of the patients.[75]

Biochemical: The predilection by the phenothiazine and particularly the butyrophenone drugs for the basal ganglia gives further support for the belief that this may be the site of a metabolic disturbance in the syndrome. Snyder and his associates[79] proposed the intriguing hypothesis that there is a hyperactivity of dopaminergic systems in the corpora striata of patients with Gilles de la Tourette's disease. This hypothesis was based on the knowledge that haloperidol, unique in its great potency for blocking dopamine receptors, is the most effective drug in treating the disease. Conversely, the drug L-dopa, whose action is attributed to the dopamine it forms, can produce stereotyped tic-like movements of the face and limbs. Moreover, d-amphetamine, which also produces hyperstimulation of dopamine receptors in the corpus striatum, has been demonstrated to cause tic-like motor movements in animals and can do so in man. Snyder and co-workers noted that their hypothesis has not been proved by the demonstration of a biochemical abnormality, but suggested its value for the rational development of pharmacotherapy for the condition. If haloperidol relieves the symptoms of Gilles de la Tourette's disease by blocking dopamine receptors in the corpus striatum, they cautioned, this does not establish that excess dopamine activity is the cause of the condition. Symptoms could be unrelated to dopaminergic neurons, yet antagonized by blocking dopaminergic activity. Another mechanism of increasing dopamine concentration in the corpus striatum, namely through impairment of γ-hydroxybutyrate (GHB) metabolism, was suggested by Moldofsky and co-workers.[60]

The striking clinical similarities of tic syndrome to Lesch-Nyhan syndrome was pointed out by Moldofsky and co-workers.[60] Lesch-Nyhan syndrome is an X-linked recessive disorder of uric acid metabolism beginning in early childhood and showing the features of gout. It is associated with intellectual impairment. Additionally these patients exhibit uncontrollable violent jerking and choreiform movements. Vocal components—explosive grunts, cries, and obscenities—are characteristic. Inordinate aggressiveness, and biting self-mutilation of the digits and lips has been observed. Deficiency of the enzyme hypoxanthine guanine phosphoribosyltransferase (HGPRT) has been demonstrated.[62] It is of interest that HGPRT is normally highly concentrated in the basal ganglia. Although Pfeiffer and co-workers[66] observed a tendency toward elevated serum uric acid in three cases of Gilles de la Tourette's disease, Moldofsky and his associates[60] investigated uric acid metabolism in eight cases of tic syndrome and could not find an abnormality.

The interesting occurrence of tic syndrome in four self-abusive children has been reported by Smith.[78]

Endocrine: There are no reports of endocrine changes or influences in tic syndrome. The role of putative neurotransmitter substances in the brain has already been reviewed.

Neurophysiologic: Electroencephalographic studies have not revealed a specific abnormality to elucidate the underlying brain pathology. However, a variety of abnormal findings are reported in individual patients. Field and associates[28] noted bilateral rolandic sharp waves in the recordings from six of seven patients. Lucas[47] reviewed fifty-eight reported electroencephalographic studies and noted that thirty showed evidence of abnormalities suggestive of cerebral dysfunction while twenty-eight had normal records. Lucas and Rodin[51] demonstrated a variety of abnormal electroencephalographic findings in eight of eighteen patients, ranging from mild nonspecific dysrhythmia grade I to severely abnormal, dysrhythmia grade III. No temporal relationship between abnormal electrical brain activity and the occurrence of tics could be demonstrated. No consistent relationship was found between electroencephalographic diagnosis and clinical evidence for encephalopathy. Wayne and co-workers[85] studied thirty-two of Shapiro's patients electroencephalographically. Of these, 50 percent had abnormal recordings, nonspecific in type. The absence of consistent findings on surface electroencephalography in these studies is not surprising, but does not negate the possibility of altered electrical activity in the depth of the brain. It suggests that tic syndrome occurs in patients with varying degrees of neurophysiologic dysfunction, some with diffuse abnormality of cerebral function.

EXOGENOUS FACTORS

Mechanical: Mechanical irritation has often been implicated in the initiation of tics. Hoppe[39] wrote that tic can develop as a result of an external irritation, or on the basis of an idea or both combined. As an example, he mentioned conjunctival irritation as a cause for eye-blinking. The habit may become established and persist even after the cause of the irritation is removed. Willard Olson[63] performed an experiment, in which rats were subjected to a cutaneous irritant. Tic-like movements developed and persisted after the disappearance of the irritation.

Movement restraint has also been implicated in the causation of tic. Often cited as evidence are the observations by David Levy[45] of head-shaking tics in hens confined for long periods in small egg-laying cages and the "weaving tics" of horses confined to stalls. He noted head-rolling and other stereotyped movements in infants whose movements were restrained by confinement to cribs. While Levy considered these movements analogous to the tics of hens and horses, he did not observe discrete tics in these infants. He found that other forms of mechanical restraint which prevented freedom of locomotion resulted in hyperactivity in children. Thesi Bergmann,[8] observing children immobolized by casts or frames on an orthopedic ward, did not find that this form of motor restriction resulted in tics. Nor did Corbett and co-workers[18] find movement restraint an important antecedent in their study of 171 tiqueurs. Nonetheless, Moldofsky and co-workers[60] noted that their patients with tic syndrome poorly tolerated motor or territorial restraint. Lesch-Nyhan patients, on the other hand, seemed relieved when they were physically restrained from self-mutilating behavior.

Toxic: Uncontrollable impulsive behavior, including compulsive laughing and crying, and other bizarre behavior is characteristic of the early stages of manganese poisoning.[61] Corbin and co-workers[19] pointed to its similarities to tic syndrome in speculating about an organic cause. They noted that similar phenomena are observed in patients who have suffered from encephalitis and identified the anatomic locus of such abnormal movements as strio-pallido-thalamic. No direct implication of toxic causation in cases with tic syndrome could be found in the literature.

Infectious: Selling[71] and Brown[11] suggested that respiratory infections such as sinusitis played a role in the etiology of tics. Corbett and co-workers[18] found no association of physical illness and the onset of tics. Creak and Guttman[20] suggested a relationship between chorea and multiple tics. However, there was no definite evidence of rheumatic infection in these patients. One of the cases described by Lucas and co-workers[52] documented rheumatic fever without associated chorea two years before the onset of tics. More often the diagnosis of Sydenham's chorea is suspected or incorrectly made at some time in the case histories of patients with tic syndrome. It has been suggested that some forms of chorea become chronic and resemble cases of tic syndrome.

Postencephalitic tics have been described. Gerstmann and Schilder[32] stated that, although tics following epidemic encephalitis are not rare, detailed reports are almost nonexistent. Wilder and Silbermann[86] reviewed such cases. Multiple tics may well be the sequel of CNS infection in some children. Another of the patients in the series of Lucas and co-workers[52] had the onset of tics a year after an illness which was probably encephalitis.

Traumatic: Mahler, Luke, and Daltroff[57] found that 33 percent of their cases had a history of abnormal childbirth. Pasamanick and Kawi[64] found 33 percent pregnancy complications in the mothers of fifty-one children who developed tics, as compared to 18 percent complications in a control group. Corbett and co-workers[18] did not consider toxemia of pregnancy, prematurity, and other birth abnormalities significant determinants of the disorder. Shapiro, Shapiro, and Wayne[75] did not find the history of perinatal distress in their patients to differ from that found in the population at large. Moldofsky and co-workers[60] postulated that nonresponders to haloperidol are inclined to perinatal abnormalities (based on three of four patients with history of perinatal distress who were haloperidol nonresponders).

Nutritional: Olson[63] focused on nutritional status as one of the determinants of tics and concluded from his observations that underweight children have more nervous habits than the normal at all ages. He noted that fatigue during the school day tends to aggravate the manifestation of nervous habits.

Psychodynamic Factors

INDIVIDUAL

From the time of the earliest descriptions of the syndrome, observers have noted the influence of environmental factors and personality characteristics in tiqueurs. Meige and Feindel steadfastly ascribed tic pathogenesis to a mental process. Alluding to a psychic predisposition they stated "not all who would may tic."[58] Wilson also noted a "psychical predisposition" behind all tic phenomena.[88] Although a neurologist, he was influenced by Freudian theory and made the psychodynamic interpretation that

grafted on a constitutional basis, tic makes its appearance in some cases (possibly in the majority) as the expression or outward manifestation of an *unconscious desire*—or better, as I am fully convinced, of a desire that is often but half-hidden from consciousness . . . experience leads me to emphasize the feature of *seeking a pleasurable sensation* in the genesis of enumerable tics. (p. 94)

Kanner[41] stated that, without exception, all tiqueurs have additional personal difficulties including restlessness, self-consciousness, sensitiveness, spoiled child reaction, overambitiousness, and overconscientiousness. Some are shy, seclusive, and readily embarrassed. He believed that "no happy, secure child ever develops tics" and noted there is always a close correlation between the intensity of the movements and the severity of the emotional strain to which the patient is subjected.

Ferenczi[26] regarded tics as a form of autoeroticism in which certain body parts had been genitalized. He referred to tics as "muscular memory traces" which are "abreacted" in the tic. Abraham[2] characterized the tic personality as a "pregenital conversion" and noted two important factors in the mental life of tic patients: (1) their well-defined anal character, and (2) their marked narcissistic makeup. In severe multiple tics (maladie des tics), all these characteristics are even more prominent than in patients with isolated and individual tic movements.

Fenichel, accepting Abraham's formulations, also characterized psychogenic tics as pregenital conversion reactions.[25] He described tic patients as showing archaic features of a regressed personality with a compulsive character and narcissistic orientation. He noted that some forms of tic have more connection with compulsions, as compulsive motor patterns may become automatic. Psychogenetically, he traced the development of tics thus: they are movements originating in past situations. The whole action, of which the movements form a part, has been repressed, and the repressed motor impulses return against the will of the ego. The repressed situations, whose motor intentions return in tic, are highly emotional ones representing either instinctual temptations or punishments for warded-off impulses.

The psychodynamics in a group of thirteen children with simple tics were described by Margaret Gerard.[31] Uniformity of intrapsychic and family dynamics was found in these tiqueurs. The tic, in each instance, followed a traumatic experience which aroused the fear of being injured. The tic became a defensive response of the small muscles which was appropriate at the moment of the trauma, but became inappropriate as it was further used in response to different fears. The children were aggression-inhibited youngsters. Margaret Mahler[54] characterized tic as an example of neurotic symptom formation with an underlying conflict. The original, instinctual impulse, censored by the superego, finds its outlet in motility through an unrecognized, condensed ego function, a quick, more or less involuntary, repetitious gesture or movement. The movement contains elements of discharge gratification and punishment. By Mahler's definition, the tic syndrome belongs to an essentially different psychopathological category from the psychoneurotic tic. She classified it an organ neurosis of the neuromuscular apparatus following the genetic and dynamic rules described by Alexander and Fenichel for psychosomatic disease. The personality of this type of tiqueur, according to Mahler, has constant and typical traits. It is characterized by a peculiar mixture of high intellectual endowment, emotional immaturity, and proneness to intermittent affectomotor outbursts (temper tantrums).

It must be remembered that psychiatric studies of psychosomatic disorders tend to have a built-in bias because of the selection of children referred for psychiatric evaluation and treatment. The larger the groups studied and the more heterogeneous the subjects, the greater the diversity of personality and psychopathologic features that will be found. Epidemiologic surveys reflect more accurately than do select groups the diversity of characteristics to be found in subjects with a particular symptom. Arthur Shapiro and co-workers,[77] in their study of thirty-four patients who had careful psychiatric and psychologic evaluations, found no confirmation for the major psychopathological factors reported in the literature as being etiologic. Although many of the patients exhibited some of these traits, the traits appeared to be psychological responses to the illness rather than factors in the etiology. Psychopathological states commonly believed to characterize patients with the syndrome included schizophrenia, underlying psychosis, obsessive-compulsiveness, inhibition of hostility, hysteria, somatization, higher IQ, and deterioration of intellectual and psychological functioning. Shapiro and co-workers concluded that common psychopathological factors do not characterize patients with Gilles de la Tourette's syndrome.

FAMILIAL AND INTERPERSONAL DYNAMICS

Margaret Gerard[31] found the mothers, and in some cases both parents, of her tic patients to be ambitious for the child in the realms of intellectual achievement and of conformance to nonaggressive behavior. The mothers were affectionate, but firm and controlling in their behavior toward the child, efficient and ambitious in work. The children were shy but had winning manners toward adults and conformed to adult authority.

Bruch and Thum[12] described psychosis in the mother of a boy with tic syndrome. She had made control of his aggression the goal of her life, rearing him with extreme psychic restraint.

Study of the family dynamics by Lucas and co-workers[52] revealed a diversity of psychodynamic interaction. In fifteen families, five showed signs of severe intrafamilial psychopathology with diffuse expression of intense aggression in the home. Eight families placed excessive emphasis on the inhibition of aggression similar to the dynamics described by Gerard. In this group, there were high expectations not only for academic achievement but also for behavioral conformity in general. A covertly seductive or sometimes overtly highly sexualized relationship between the patient and the parent of the opposite sex was common. Two of the families studied were well adjusted and demonstrated no discernible psychopathology. In the normal families, the children with tic syndrome had histories strongly suggestive of organic etiology: one with birth complications, and one with probable encephalitis.

The cumulative evidence of reports from the entire literature gives increasing weight to the impression that no uniform pattern of family dynamics is present in all families with tiqueurs. It seems plausible that an underlying neurophysiologic dysfunction is requisite to the development of tic syndrome. If the dysfunction is mild and the environment benign, the symptoms of tic may be minor and remain arrested in a *forme fruste*. Thus, with favorable environmental circumstances, understanding parents, good intelligence, and adequate learning opportunities, tics will probably not progress when the underlying predisposition is mild. In children exposed to punitive, threatening, and restrictive surroundings, however, with parents who lack tolerance and empathy and who are poor models for impulse control, the tics progress and develop into the classic symptoms of Gilles de la Tourette's syndrome. When the neurologic predisposition is overwhelming, the tic syndrome will develop in any child despite environmental influences.

SOCIAL IMPLICATIONS FOR "LIFE STYLE"

Children with tic syndrome are at high risk, not only from the standpoint of their physical handicaps but from the standpoint of developing serious personality, social, and learning complications. Early in the course of the illness, medical misdiagnosis is common. The variable symptomatology may all too easily puzzle those attempting to evaluate the child. Even when the bizarre behavior has advanced sufficiently to clarify the diagnosis, adequate treatment is usually difficult to find. Until quite recently, no effective medication was available. Poorly understood by their acquaintances and by professionals alike, and perplexed by their strangely disturbing uncontrollable symptoms, children with tic syndrome often view themselves as unique freaks of nature. Ostracized by their families and their peers in school, they are relegated to do their schoolwork in the hall, become social outcasts, and are often excluded from school altogether. Constant reproach and their own unacceptance of their behavior causes them to become introspective, guilt-ridden, and mournfully sad.

Early diagnosis, symptom alleviation, and supportive management, discussed in the section on treatment, should prevent or diminish the secondary emotional complications.

Learning and Behavior Theory

The proposition derived from learning theory is that tics are conditioned avoidance responses, evoked initially by stress and reinforced by the seeking for reduction of anxiety.[18] Corbett and coworkers[18] demonstrated that tiqueurs were superior to control subjects in reaction time and cited the study of Crown[21] which suggested that an exaggerated motor response to stress is characteristic of tiqueurs. The application of learning theory to the treatment of tics was described by Yates.[89] Other reports of treatment with behavioral techniques have been made by Walton,[84] Abi Rafi,[1] Miller,[59] and Thomas, Abrams and Johnson.[80]

Specific Treatment Methods

A great multiplicity of treatment modalities has been advocated in the treatment of tic and tic syndrome. Meige and Feindel[58] enumerated among the medicinal formulations in vogue at one time or another to cure tics: bromides, chloral, opium, zinc valerianate and gelsemium, quinine, cannabis, and arsenic. They concluded that all had proved equally inefficacious. Nonetheless, they conceded that transient improvement sometimes resulted with injections of morphia, atropine, and curare, and with inhalation of chloroform or ether. When a sedative was needed, Meige and Feindel preferred valerian as its unpleasant odor would discourage abuse of the drug. Counter-irritants such as mustard plasters, and cautery to the vertebral column; cold, hot, and tepid douches; baths; rhythmic traction of the tongue; thoracic compression; and electrotherapy have also been used without consistent benefit. Stimulants such as kola, coca, and caffeine are contraindicated.

Meige and Feindel anticipated principles of behavior therapy in the treatment they favored for tics. They believed that tics could be unlearned and described their approach as "treatment by reeducation." Graduated exercises of forced immobility, requiring the patient to remain perfectly still by exerting self-control were described. Beginning with a few seconds, the periods of immobility would gradually be lengthened.

It was the contention of Meige and Feindel that children should be corrected when tics are still "bad habits." They thought little of the idea that calling attention to them would aggravate them. Most physicians today would counsel parents to ignore mild tics, but this question is by no means resolved. It is probable that there are individual differences among children in their tolerance for such correction, and the wise physician would individualize his advice. Meige and Feindel did not countenance threats and penalties, however. They advocated structuring of the daily routine, keeping the child occupied in his leisure time, and the establishment of "good habits." They also recommended training of antagonistic muscles by practicing the opposite movement at the moment a tic impended. Meige and Feindel, however, cautioned prudence lest the tic be replaced by another one! In addition, they emphasized the implementation of what are basically sound principles of supportive psychotherapy.

Abuzzahab and Anderson[3] have tabulated the most frequently used modes of treatment in an analysis of 430 cases gleaned from the literature (Table 37–8). Almost 600 therapeutic trials were reported, with many patients given more than one type of treatment. The list has particular value in comparing the efficacy of drug treatment, but it should be remembered that treatment using a drug alone may be ineffective. Encouraging treatment results with phenothiazine drugs[50] and with halo-

TABLE 37–8

*Results of Various Treatments
in Gilles de la Tourette's Syndrome*

TREATMENT	NO. OF PATIENT TRIALS	TOTAL IMPROVED %
Psychotherapy	117	45
Hypnotherapy	27	15
Hydrotherapy	25	12
Isolation	19	26
Sleep therapy	13	54
Behavior therapy	12	25
Bed rest	6	33
Shock therapy	25	20
CO_2 Inhalation	11	18
Physical therapy	9	56
Thalamotomy	3	33
Lobotomy-leucotomy	2	50
Sedatives[1]	98	19
Haloperidol	63	89
Other Antipsychotic Tranquilizers[2]	81	48
Antidepressants[3]	17	24
CNS stimulants[4]	17	18
Anticonvulsants[5]	16	19
Antiparkinsonians[6]	7	29
Spontaneous Remissions	14	(3.3% of patients)

[1] Sedatives: ethanol, chloral hydrate, ethchlorvynol, bromides, barbiturates, meprobamate, chlordiazepoxide, diazepam, oxazepam, hydroxyzine, methaqualone, arsenic, paraldehyde.
[2] Antipsychotic tranquilizers: reserpine, rauwolfia alkaloids, chlorpromazine, promazine, triflupromazine, thioridazine, prochlorperazine, trifluoperazine, chlorprothixene, fluphenazine, perphenazine, thiothixene, piperacetazine, promethazine.
[3] Antidepressants: imipramine, amitriptyline, nortriptyline, doxepin, protriptyline, isocarboxazid, phenelzine, iproniazid.
[4] CNS stimulants: amphetamine, d-amphetamine methamphetamine, methylphenidate.
[5] Anticonvulsants: diphenylhydantoin, primidone, trimethadione, ethosuximide, paramethadione.
[6] Anti-parkinsonisms: belladonna alkaloids, trihexyphenidyl, benztropine mesylate, orphenadrine, diphenhydramine, L-dopa, amantadine.
SOURCE: F. E. Abuzzahab and F. O. Anderson, "Gilles de la Tourette's Syndrome: International Registry," *Minnesota Medicine,* 56:492–496, 1973.

peridol established the latter drug as the most effective specific treatment method. Haloperidol is a butyrophenone drug with potent action in blocking dopaminergic pathways in the brain. Favorable results were first noted by Seignot in France,[70] by Caprini and Melotti in Italy,[13] and by Challas and Brauer in the United States.[15] Accumulating experience[16, 49, 72, 74] has confirmed

the selectivity of haloperidol in markedly reducing or alleviating the tics. Vocal noises are sometimes more easily controlled than generalized body tics. Most children will respond to daily doses in the range of 2 to 6 mg when environmental stress is mitigated or when the children are removed from stressful environmental influences. Treatment should be initiated with 0.5 mg initially and daily increments of 0.5 mg used until the desired clinical effect is obtained. Administration is twice daily because of the drug's long duration of action. Daily doses of up to 180 mg have been reported.[74] However, great caution should be exercised if the daily dose exceeds 16 mg. High doses are generally not necessary and can produce disturbing and hazardous side effects. Haloperidol can be remarkably effective in reducing the singularly disturbing, incapacitating symptoms of Gilles de la Tourette's syndrome and in aiding the child to maintain his usual academic and social pursuits. However, excessive sedation can also interfere with school performance. It is not known whether haloperidol or other drugs favorably influence the natural course of the illness. The answer must await the results of long-term follow-up studies. Nonetheless, the diminution of incapacitating symptoms can immeasurably help the patient's life adjustment. In particular, early treatment can prevent the secondary social isolation, personality decompensation and school failure.

Once the diagnosis of tic syndrome is established, treatment should be multifaceted, aimed not only at diminishing the tic symptoms themselves but the secondary symptoms of poor self-esteem, social isolation, school failure, and depression which may supervene. After careful individual assessment of the child and of the family, treatment should be directed to all those aspects of the child's functioning in family, school and social environment which perpetuate and aggravate the disorder. Treatment may thus include special remedial education, individual supportive psychotherapy, direct work with the family, and possibly residential treatment for the child. Before effective drugs were available, Eisenberg, Ascher, and Kanner[24] had emphasized that the clinical manifestations are responsive to the social environment. They noted that capably administered psychotherapy is of assistance to the child and family in dealing with the social consequences of the illness, and modifying intrapsychic tensions that aggravate the symptoms.

REFERENCES

1. ABI RAFI, A., "Learning Theory and the Treatment of Tics," *Journal of Psychosomatic Research, 6:*71–76, 1962.

2. ABRAHAM, K., *Selected Papers on Psychoanalysis,* Basic Books, New York, 1953.

3. ABUZZAHAB, F. E., and ANDERSON, F. O., "Gilles de la Tourette's Syndrome: International Registry," *Minnesota Medicine, 56:*492–496, 1973.

4. American Psychiatric Association, Committee on Nomenclature and Statistics, *Diagnostic and Statistical Manual of Mental Disorders,* 2nd ed., (DSM-II), American Psychiatric Association, Washington, D.C., 1968.

5. ASCHER, E., "Psychodynamic Considerations in Gilles de la Tourette's Disease (Maladie des Tics)," *American Journal of Psychiatry, 105:*267–276, 1948.

6. BALTHASAR, K., "Über das Anatomische Substrat der Generalisierten Tic-Krankheit (Maladie des Tics, Gilles de la Tourette)," *Archiv für Psychiatrie und Zeitschrift Neurologie, 195:*531–549, 1957.

7. BELL, C., *The Nervous System of the Human Body,* pp. 137–153, Longman, Rees, Orme, Brown, and Green, London, 1830.

8. BERGMANN, T., "Observation of Children's Reactions to Motor Restraint," *Nervous Child, 4:*318–328, 1945.

9. BOUTEILLE, E. M., *Traité de chorée,* Vincard, Paris, 1818.

10. BRESLER, J., "Beitrag zur Lehre von der Maladie des Tics Convulsifs (Mimische Krampfneurose)," *Neurologisches Zentralblatt, 15:*965–972, 1896.

11. BROWN, E. E., "Tics (Habit Spasms) Secondary to Chronic Sinusitis," *Archives of Paediatrics, 74:*39–46, 1957.

12. BRUCH, H., and THUM, L. C., "Maladie des Tics and Maternal Psychosis," *Journal of Nervous and Mental Disease, 146:*446–456, 1968.

13. CAPRINI, G., and MELOTTI, V., "Una Grava Sindrome Ticcosa Guarita con Haloperidol," *Rivista Sperimentale di Freniatria, 85:*1–6, 1961.

14. CHABBERT, L., "De la Maladie des Tics," *Archives de Neurologie, 24:*10–41, 1893.

15. CHALLAS, G., and BRAUER, W., "Tourette's Disease: Relief of Symptoms with R 1625," *American Journal of Psychiatry, 120:*283–284, 1963.

16. CHALLAS, G., CHAPEL, J. L., and JENKINS, R. L., "Tourette's Disease: Control of Symptoms and Its Clinical Course," *International Journal of Neuropsychiatry, 3 (Suppl. 1):*95–109, 1967.

17. CLAUSS, J. L., and BALTHASAR, K., "Zur Kenntnis der Generalisierten Tic-Krankheit (maladie des tics, Gilles de la Tourette'sche Krankheit)," *Archives of Psychiatry, 191:*398–418, 1954.

18. CORBETT, J. A., et al., "Tics and Gilles de la Tourette's Syndrome: A Follow-up Study and Critical Review," *British Journal of Psychiatry, 115:*1229–1241, 1969.

19. CORBIN, K. B., et al., "Further Observations on Tourette's Syndrome," *Asian Ocean Congress of Neurology, 2:*447–453, 1967.

20. CREAK, M., and GUTTMAN, E., "Chorea, Tics and Compulsive Utterances," *Journal of Mental Science, 81:*834–839, 1935.

21. CROWN, S., "An Experimental Enquiry into Some Aspects of the Motor Behavior and Personality of Tiqueurs," *Journal of Mental Science, 99:*84–91, 1953.

22. DAUGELA, M. Z., "Psychosomatic Tic: A Case Report with Discussion," *Clinical Proceedings of Children's Hospital* (Washington), *17:*235–240, 1961.

23. DEWULF, A., and VAN BOGAERT, L., "Etudes Anatomo-Cliniques de Syndromes Hypercinétiques Complexes: III. Une Observation Anatomo-Clinique de Maladie des Tics (Gilles de la Tourette)," *Monatschrift für Psychiatrie und Neurologie, 104:*53–61, 1941.

24. EISENBERG, L., ASCHER, E., and KANNER, L., "A Clinical Study of Gilles de la Tourette's Disease (Maladie des Tics) in Children," *American Journal of Psychiatry, 115:*715–723, 1959.

25. FENICHEL, O., *The Psychoanalytic Theory of Neurosis,* pp. 317–321, W. W. Norton, New York, 1945.

26. FERENCZI, S., "Psycho-Analytical Observations on Tic," *International Journal of Psycho-Analysis, 2:*1–30, 1921.

27. FERNANDO, S. J. M., "Gilles de la Tourette's Syndrome: A Report on Four Cases and a Review of Published Case Reports," *British Journal of Psychiatry, 113:*607–617, 1967.

28. FIELD, J. R., "Gilles de la Tourette's Syndrome," *Neurology, 16:*453, 1966.

29. FREUD, A., and BURLINGHAM, D. T., *War and Children,* International Universities Press, New York, 1943.

30. FRIEL, P. B., "Familial Incidence of Gilles de la Tourette's Disease, with Observations on Aetiology and Treatment," *British Journal of Psychiatry, 122:*655–658, 1973.

31. GERARD, M. W., "The Psychogenic Tic in Ego Development," in Eissler, R. S., et al. (Eds.), *The Psychoanalytic Study of the Child,* vol. 2, pp. 133–162, International Universities Press, New York, 1946.

32. GERSTMANN, J., and SCHILDER, P., "Über Organisch Bedingte Tics," *Medizinische Klinik, 19:*896–899, 1923.

33. GILLES DE LA TOURETTE, G., "Étude sur une Affection Nerveuse Caractérisée par de l'Incoordination Motorice Accompagnée d'Écholalie et de Coprolalie (Jumping, Latah, Myriachit)," *Archives de Neurologie, 9:*19–42, 158–200, 1885.

34. Group for the Advancement of Psychiatry, Committee on Child Psychiatry, *Psychopathological Disorders in Childhood: Theoretical Considerations and a Proposed Classification,* vol. 6, Report No. 62, Group for the Advancement of Psychiatry, New York, 1966.

35. GUINON, G., "Tics Convulsifs et Hysterie," *Revue de Médicine, 7:*509–519, 1887.

36. ———, "Sur la Maladie des Tics Convulsifs," *Revue de Médicine, 6:*50–80, 1886.

37. HALL, M., "On Muscular Tic," *Lancet, 2:*510, 1852.

38. HAMMOND, G. M., "Convulsive Tic: Its Nature and Treatment," *Medical Record, 41:*236–239, 1892.

39. HOPPE, H. H., "The Treatment of Spasmodic Disorders," in White, W. A., and Jelliffee, S. E. (Eds.), *The Modern Treatment of Nervous and Mental Diseases,* vol. 2, Lea and Febiger, New York, 1913.

40. ITARD, J. M. G., "Mémoire sur Quelques Fonctions Involontaires des Appareils de la Locomotion, de la Préhension et de la Voix," *Archives Générale de Médicine, 8:*385–407, 1825.

41. KANNER, L., *Child Psychiatry,* 3rd ed., Charles C Thomas, Springfield, Ill., 1957.

42. KÖSTER, G., "Ueber die Maladie des Tics Impulsifs (Mimische Krampfneurose)," *Deutsche Zeitschrift für Nervenheilkunde, 15:*147–158, 1899.

43. LAPOUSE, R., and MONK, M. A., "An Epidemiologic Study of Behavior Characteristics in Children," in Quay, H. (Ed.), *Children's Behavior Disorders,* pp. 3–21, Van Nostrand, Princeton, N.J., 1968.

44. ———, "Fears and Worries in a Representative Sample of Children," *American Journal of Orthopsychiatry, 29:*803–818, 1959.

45. LEVY, D., "On the Problem of Movement Restraint: Tics, Stereotyped Movements, Hyperactivity," *American Journal of Orthopsychiatry, 14:*644–671, 1944.

46. LUCAS, A. R., "Report of Gilles de la Tourette's Disease in Two Succeeding Generations," *Child Psychiatry and Human Development, 3:*231–233, 1973.

47. ———, "Gilles de la Tourette's Disease: An Over-

view," *New York State Journal of Medicine,* 70:2197–2200, 1970.

48. ———, "Follow-up of Tic Syndrome, in Gilles de la Tourette's Syndrome," vol. 1, Abuzzahab, F. S., and Anderson, F. O. (Eds.), *International Registry,* pp. 13–17, Mason Publishing, St. Paul, Minn., 1970.

49. ———, "Gilles de la Tourette's Disease in Children: Treatment with Haloperidol," *American Journal of Psychiatry,* 124:243–245, 1967.

50. ———, "Gilles de la Tourette's Disease in Children: Treatment with Phenothiazine Drugs," *American Journal of Psychiatry,* 121:606–608, 1964.

51. ———, and Rodin, E. A., "Electroencephalogram in Gilles de la Tourette's Disease," *Diseases of the Nervous System,* 34:85–89, 1973.

52. Lucas, A. R., Kaufman, P. E., and Morris, E. M., "Gilles de la Tourette's Disease: A Clinical Study of Fifteen Cases," *Journal of the American Academy of Child Psychiatry,* 6:700–722, 1967.

53. Macfarlane, J. W., Allen, L., and Honzik, M. P., *A Developmental Study of Behavior Problems of Normal Children Between Twenty-One Months and Fourteen Years,* University of California Press, Berkeley, Calif., 1954.

54. Mahler, M. S., "A Psychoanalytic Evaluation of Tic in Psychopathology of Children," in Eissler, R. S., et al. (Eds.), *The Psychoanalytic Study of the Child,* vols. 3/4, pp. 279–310, International Universities Press, New York, 1949.

55. ———, and Luke, J. A., "Outcome of the Tic Syndrome," *Journal of Nervous and Mental Disease,* 103: 433–445, 1946.

56. Mahler, M. S., and Rangell, L., "A Psychosomatic Study of Maladie des Tics (Gilles de la Tourette's Disease)," *Psychiatric Quarterly,* 17:579–603, 1943.

57. Mahler, M. S., Luke, J. A., and Daltroff, W., "Clinical and Follow-up Study of the Tic Syndrome in Children," *American Journal of Orthopsychiatry,* 15:631–647, 1945.

58. Meige, H., and Feindel, E., *Tics and Their Treatment,* Wilson, S. A. K. (Trans. and Ed.), Sidney Appleton, London, 1907.

59. Miller, A. L., "Treatment of a Child with Gilles de la Tourette's Syndrome Using Behavior Modification Techniques," *Journal of Behavior Therapy and Experimental Psychiatry,* 1:319–321, 1970.

60. Moldofsky, H., Tullis, C., and Lamon, R., "Multiple Tic Syndrome (Gilles de la Tourette's Syndrome)," *Journal of Nervous and Mental Disease,* 159: 282–292, 1974.

61. Naby, S. A. E., and Hassahein, M., "Neuropsychiatric Manifestations of Chronic Manganese Poisoning," *Journal of Neurology, Neurosurgery and Psychiatry,* 28: 282–288, 1965.

62. Nyhan, W. L., "Clinical Features of the Lesch-Nyhan Syndrome," *Archives of Internal Medicine,* 130: 186–192, 1972.

63. Olson, W. C., *The Measurement of Nervous Habits in Normal Children,* University of Minnesota Press, Minneapolis, 1929.

64. Pasamanick, B., and Kawi, A., "A Study of the Association of Prenatal and Paranatal Factors with the Development of Tics in Children," *Journal of Paediatrics,* 48:596–601, 1956.

65. Pearson, H., *Johnson and Boswell: The Story of Their Lives,* Harper and Brothers, New York, 1958.

66. Pfeiffer, C. C., et al., "The Serum Urate Level Reflects Degree of Stress," *Journal of Clinical Pharmacology and New Drugs,* 9:384–392, 1969.

67. Prince, M., "Case of Multiform Tic, Including Automatic Speech and Purposive Movements," *Journal of Nervous and Mental Disease,* 33:29–34, 1906.

68. Redl, F., "Pre-adolescents: What Makes Them Tic?"

in Redl, F., and Wineman, D., *When We Deal With Children,* pp. 395–409, Free Press, New York, 1966.

69. Sanders, D. G., "Familial Occurrence of Gilles de la Tourette Syndrome," *Archives of General Psychiatry,* 28:326–328, 1973.

70. Seignot, J. N., "Un Cas de Maladie des Tics de Gilles de la Tourette Guéri par le R. 1625," *Annales Societe Medico-Psychologique,* 119:578–579, 1961.

71. Selling, L., "The Role of Infection in the Aetiology of Tics," *Archives of Neurology and Psychiatry,* 22: 1163–1171, 1929.

72. Shapiro, A. K., and Shapiro, E., "Treatment of Gilles de la Tourette's Syndrome with Haloperidol," *British Journal of Psychiatry,* 114:345–350, 1968.

73. ———, and Wayne, H. L., "The Symptomatology and Diagnosis of Gilles de la Tourette's Syndrome," *Journal of the American Academy of Child Psychiatry,* 12:702–723, 1973.

74. ———, "Treatment of Tourette's Syndrome with Haloperidol, Review of 34 Cases," *Archives of General Psychiatry,* 28:92–97, 1973.

75. ———, "Birth, Developmental, and Family Histories and Demographic Information in Tourette's Syndrome," *Journal of Nervous and Mental Disease,* 155:335–344, 1972.

76. ———, et al., "Tourette's Syndrome: Summary Data on 34 Patients," *Psychosomatic Medicine,* 35:419–435, 1973.

77. ———, et al., "The Psychopathology of Gilles de la Tourette's Syndrome," *American Journal of Psychiatry,* 129:427–434, 1972.

78. Smith, R. H., *Gilles de la Tourette's Syndrome in Self-Abusive Children* (unpublished manuscript), 1973.

79. Snyder, S. H., et al., "The Role of Brain Dopamine in Behavioral Regulation and the Actions of Psychotropic Drugs," *American Journal of Psychiatry,* 127:199–207, 1970.

80. Thomas, E. J., Abrams, K. S., and Johnson, J. B., "Self-monitoring and Reciprocal Inhibition in the Modification of Multiple Tics in Gilles de la Tourette's Syndrome," *Journal of Behavior Therapy and Experimental Psychiatry,* 2:159–171, 1971.

81. Tobin, W. G., and Reinhart, J. B., "Tic de Gilles de la Tourette," *American Journal of Diseases in Children,* 101:778–783, 1961.

82. Torup, E., "A Follow-up Study of Children with Tics," *Acta Paediatrica,* 51:261–268, 1962.

83. Trousseau, A., *Clinique Médicale de l'Hotel-Dieu de Paris,* vol. 2, pp. 198–212, J.-B. Ballière et Fils, Paris, 1865.

84. Walton, D., "Experimental Psychology and the Treatment of a Tiqueur," *Journal of Child Psychology,* 2:148–155, 1961.

85. Wayne, H. L., Shapiro, A. K., and Shapiro, E., "Gilles de la Tourette's Syndrome: Electroencephalographic Investigation and Clinical Correlation," *Clinical Electroencephalography,* 3:160–168, 1972.

86. Wilder, J., and Silbermann, J., "Beiträge zum Ticproblem," *Abhandlungen aus der Neurologie, Psychiatrie, Psychologie und Ihren Grenzgebieten,* 43:1–100, 1927.

87. Wille, H., "Ueber einen Fall von Maladie des Tics Impulsifs (Gilles de la Tourette'sche Krankheit)," *Monatschrift für Psychiatrie und Neurologie,* 4:210–226, 1898.

88. Wilson, S. A. K., "The Tics and Allied Conditions," *Journal of Neurology and Psychopathology,* 8: 93–109, 1927.

89. Yates, A. J., "The Application of Learning Theory to the Treatment of Tics," *Journal of Abnormal Social Psychology,* 56:175–182, 1958.

90. Zausmer, D. M., "The Treatment of Tics in Childhood," *Archives of Disease in Childhood,* 29:537–542, 1954.

38 / Suicide and Suicide Attempts

Joseph D. Teicher

Introduction

An important step in the study of suicidal behaviors is definition and classification. The literature generally reveals semantic confusion, unclear definition, and inconsistent, contradictory use of terms. The development and validation of methods for categorizing and measuring such behaviors are progressing, especially measurment of suicidal intent and risk. Current studies are increasingly provocative but far from definitive. Research is needed to further understand suicidal ideation and gesture. The meaning of single and multiple attempts with varied populations is an additional area of study. There is also a need to evaluate the person's biography, family constellation, and culture. Suicidal behavior is at the very least a deviation from normative social adaptation. It is apparent that the etiology of suicidal behavior involves a multitude of causes; this probably accounts for the relatively slow progress in understanding and classification.

This author's research was basically descriptive in character. Combined with various etiological models, i.e., ecological (Durkheim), developmental, learning theory, genetic, biological, and neurophysiological, it offers a comprehensive approach to the problems. Difficulties abound. In animals the "cry for help" is often considered innate. In man it is probably cultural. Certainly few suicide attempters use the available suicide prevention centers. Indeed, the frequent inability of the attempter to assume a patient role and request help is frustrating to most studies.

Scope of Problem

There is a high prevalence of suicide attempts among adolescents. This is severely underrepresented in the actual reported rates. Suicide is the second cause of death among adolescents and youth in the United States. It is estimated that about 4,000 young people between ages fifteen and twenty-four kill themselves each year. Con-

jectures about the number of attempted suicides place them at about 400,000 per year. Rates for teenagers of both sexes, fourteen to nineteen years, have gone up 200 times.[5] Under fifteen, suicides are infrequent, but the fifteen- to nineteen-year-old group has an overall rate of 5.7 per 100,000 population.[41, 42] White male adolescents have the highest annual rate, 9.0 which is more than three times the rate for white females. Nonwhite males have a rate of 5.8 and nonwhite females, 3.2. No one tabulates standardized, official data on suicide attempts; accordingly these have to be estimated. The estimates are that eight to ten times as many youngsters attempt suicide as complete it, an annual rate of 45.6 per 100,000.[6] The rate of completed and attempted suicide is, conservatively, 51.3. Automobile accidents are the most frequent cause of deaths in the fifteen- to nineteen-year-old group, yet few are classified as suicides. There is little doubt that, for some youths who survived, these were in fact suicide attempts.

Suicide and suicide attempt increase is a phenomenon throughout the Western world.[22] In Canada, too, the suicide rate for males has risen sharply; in Japan the rate declined sharply. In Great Britain, both suicide attempts and suicides have been referred to as a major epidemic.

If clinical experience is an indicator, the rise is evidenced in major medical centers. The degree of conflict among figures from different sources does not inspire confidence, except to make it all too clear that the trend is upward. Currently, the best estimate is that 12 percent of all the suicide attempts in the nation are made by adolescents, and 90 percent of these by adolescent girls.[43] Without many exceptions, suicide attempters tend to be young. The majority fall between the ages twenty to thirty years, with the peak years between twenty and twenty-four. Moreover, in recent years the average age of the attempters has decreased. Almost universally, in all countries, there is a preponderance of female over male attempters. However, the sex differential of two or three females to one male may be lessening. All reports state that ingestion of medicines is the most common method chosen. Barbiturates have the dubious distinction of heading the list. Psychotropic drugs, tranquilizers, and drugs combined with alcohol are common. The multiple drug use among the young, as well as the lack of information about the potential lethality of these drugs, has serious medical effects.[11]

Nonwhite Suicide Attempters

Meaningful social class comparisons cannot be made. Assessments of social class are not standardized even within the same country. It has been noted that there are fewer attempts in rural areas; that among Indians, those with nontraditional backgrounds are more likely to be suicide attempters; and that there are substantial differences between white and nonwhite attempters. Few studies have undertaken to compare the various psychosocial aspects of communities in different countries in order to account for differing suicide rates. One study, for example, found a lower rate in Edinburgh than in Seattle. This was attributed to Edinburgh's cultural tradition of less violence, its less socially mobile society, its smaller percentage of racial minorities, and its lower incidence of alcoholism. In most cities in which behavior was studied, the common problems were alcoholism, serious illness, and loss of loved ones.[26]

The differences between white and nonwhite implies that suicides are higher among blacks. In New York City, suicide rates for nonwhites of both sexes between ages twenty to thirty-five have exceeded white suicide rates for over fifty years. In Los Angeles, the suicide rate for young people has risen in the twenty- to twenty-nine-year-old group. Forty percent of all black suicides and 30 percent of all Chicano suicides occur within that group.[32] Compared with whites, relatively few nonwhites may be treated for suicide attempts. Nonetheless, studies of attempters seen in emergency services of general hospitals suggest that rates of suicide attempts in the nonwhite population are in fact much higher. Emergency services are overrepresented among the lower socio-economic levels; they may spuriously present the suicide attempt rate as higher for lower classes. The rise in nonwhite suicide rates may be associated with urbanization and the exposure of families to new, unfamiliar stresses, such as joblessness and father absent households.

Periodically a great deal is written about the alarming number of suicide attempts and the high suicide rate at Indian reservations. Careful demographic studies have not been done. But studies of the biographies of adolescent suicides and suicide attempters have been initiated. Some investigators found that during their developing years, 70 percent of those in the suicide group were cared for much of the time by more than one person. Forty percent of the primary caretakers had five or more arrests; 50 percent had two or more losses by desertion or divorce. Eighty percent had one or more arrests in the year preceding death. For the Indian youth, those arrested at an early age and those with a large number of arrests in a twelve-month period were high suicide risks.[8] The authors concluded that those who committed suicide experienced far more disruption in their early years and far more early losses. Even though a nuclear family may be relatively intact, these critical times were often chaotic and unstable, i.e., grandmother taking over care of child because of the arrival of another child.[8]

The Suicide Attempt

It is not enough to dismiss a suicide attempt as an impulsive act. All too often it is treated as a crisis situation resulting from a temporary upset, with each episode regarded as an independent event. Nor is it accurate to consider it merely an insincere gesture (death is not intended), or an act for which the individual is not responsible. Nor need the suicide attempt result from a restricted view of alternatives stemming from a depression.

In the great majority of cases, the suicide attempt is a considered act, planned in advance, and, from the perspective of the adolescent suicide attempter, weighed rationally against other alternatives and selected over them. The more "conventional" techniques of solving a series of longstanding problems have been tried and have failed, e.g., rebelling, withdrawal, running away from home, physical violence, psychosomatic complaints, etc. At this point, suicide (where death is intended but does not result), or the suicide attempt (where only an attention-getting device is intended) is perceived by the attempter as the only possible solution to his problems. More often than not, those who adopt the drastic measure of an attempt as an attention-getting device find that this too fails to open an avenue to a solution to their problems. In fact, it generally makes matters worse. Without relief, the adolescent is then convinced, or soon becomes convinced, that death is the only solution to what appears to him as the chronic problem of living. Such a view does not necessarily constitute an arbitrary or irrational conclusion on the part of the adolescent. It is based on the adolescent's very real experiences with life and a recent history characterized by progressive social isolation from meaningful personal relationships. Such an exclusionary process not only constitutes the adolescent's problem, but serves simultaneously to exclude him from the resources necessary to solve it.[39]

Suicidal Feelings

The author studied over one hundred college freshman as to suicidal ideation. Some 70 percent had had a recent suicidal thought or thoughts. A survey of suicidal feelings in a general population was also revealing: 8.9 percent of 720 adult subjects interviewed reported suicidal feelings in the past year. In 3.5 percent, the feeling prevailed that life was not worthwhile; 2.8 percent wished for death; 1 percent thought of actual suicide; and 0.6 percent had in fact made a suicidal attempt. Coincident with suicidal feelings, the subjects reported depression and had experienced recent stressful events and somatic illness, and felt they were socially isolated. They were more likely to be female.[23]

Pertinent Literature

Moodiness, sadness, and depression are readily observable as part of the emotional experience of adolescence. Indeed, when these feelings are not exhibited, one may wonder about the individual's emotional health. However, when the adolescent actually attempts to act on his morbid fantasies, one does not ascribe this behavior to normal developmental processes.[17] Anna Freud[12] points out the paucity of understanding of many adolescent processes. She ascribes this to the fact that the two usual analytic investigative methods, re-

construction and analysis, prove to be less productive when applied to adolescents than when applied to either children or adults. In adolescence, libido is tied up fully with real, present, or recently lost objects. This presents difficulties in psychoanalysis, similar to those found during love affairs and mourning. Suicidal wishes may occur during adolescence stemming from the reversal of the affect of love to hate toward parents, with displacement to the self.

Sigmund Freud[13] discussed the suicidal attempt of an eighteen-year-old girl who jumped onto a railroad track. Besides the conscious motivation of despair over the loss of the love object, Freud emphasized the oedipal disappointment suffered by the patient with her father when she was fourteen and mother had borne a son. The suicidal attempt was both the fulfillment of self-punishment and the attainment of the very wish which, when frustrated, had driven her into homosexuality. This was the wish to have a child by her father for now she "fell" through her father's fault. (p. 162).

Zilboorg[44] noted a sharp rise in the rate of suicide at the age of fifteen and sixteen. He emphasized that, in children, suicide resulted from oral spite or oral aggression, whereas during puberty it is the primitive and semi-ceremonial outcome of frustrated genital wishes (rather than a product of oral aggression) (p. 29). However, he states that the problems in females probably had more to do with oral strivings and spite, and in males, were more concerned with loss of love functioning as castration for an oedipal wish (p. 30). In Eissler's view,[9] adolescence may end in suicide if the resistances to, and the fear of, impulses and fantasies concerning heterosexual or substitute gratifications are so strong that the ego cannot cope with these new demands (p. 224). Erikson[10] considers adolescent suicide to be the outcome of an attempt at an identity based on a negative identity choice. Such an identity would be based on all those identifications and roles which, at critical states of development, had been presented to the individual as most undesirable or dangerous, and yet, real (p. 87).

In an early publication, Schneer and coworkers[30] pointed out that events and ideation leading to youthful suicidal behavior are not specific. Instead they may emerge from any one of the many overwhelming crises that arise at this time of life in the areas of sexual development and/or control of aggressive urges. Reactions to previous traumatic experiences determine the behavior. In their series, among the events considered significant were separation from parents or important others, discovery of forbidden activity, defiance, parental restrictions, criticism, discovery of adoption, school expulsion, and bodily attack. Thoughts about punishment, separation, being unloved and unwanted, hurting or killing parents and siblings were common. In common with others, these authors emphasize that the most significant finding was the factor of parental loss or separation. The father was usually absent, and the mother, while present, or in contact, was likely to be detached. The crisis of identity (in the sense of fulfilled identification as male or as female) was particularly significant for the increase of suicidal behavior among adolescents. For them, this action provided the infantile solution of fusion with the mother.

Schneer and Kay[29] studied a series of eighty-four cases. They concluded that these youngsters experienced a great deal of anxiety or exaggerated guilt and aggression. More specifically, however, the additional loss of, or separation from, one or both parents, in varying degrees, at crucial periods in libidinal and ego development (the preoedipal, oedipal, and revived oedipal conflict at puberty) was a major force that predisposed the adolescent to suicide. This appears to the authors to be:

omnipotent, regressively infantile behavior in coping with an explosive oedipal conflict involving loss (destruction) of the sadomasochistic attitude in the child. Then, at adolescence, after a profound sense of rejection was experienced (through death, prolonged departure, illness, etc.) separation, whether provoked by the adolescent in the independence bid for an identity or whether initiated by the parents, constitutes too severe a narcissistic mortification for the emerging adolescent ego. The suicide, in promoting "sleep" (surcease from restless, emotionally labile adolescence) enables fusion with the object (mother). (p. 181)

One investigator[31] emphasized the disturbed relationship between the parents, especially mother and child. He emphasized that basic parental feeling toward the child was that the child was a burden. This feeling was evidenced from infancy and was conveyed to the child unconsciously. Moreover, the self-destructive acts are partial fulfillment of the mother's unspoken demand that the child be nonexistent. Another author[27] discusses the hypothesis that a significant number of suicidal patients receive suicidogenic messages from the family members or other people that are significant to them. One clinician[28] presented interesting data which led to the conclusion that the suicide attempter is the expendable child.

Separation

Note the frequent insistence that separation during critical periods of development from either parent, and identity formation based upon the identification with a sado-masochistic, rejecting mother are major determining factors in suicidal attempts. The research by the author and his co-workers essentially confirms this.

In evaluating a large number of suicides and suicide attempts in adults, there is considerable evidence of an association between childhood deprivation and the development of depressive syndromes. The group of investigators associated with the author believed that the death of a parent during the oedipal period or puberty led to a morbid identification with the dead person and a predisposition to suicide in later life. They hypothesized that unresolved object loss in childhood resulted in an inability to sustain object losses in later life. This in turn led to depressive reactions culminating in suicidal behavior. For the suicides, the death of a parent was the more prominent factor. For the attempted suicide, a loss by desertion or divorce was more common.[7] At Kings County Psychiatric Hospital, Brooklyn, New York, 330 patients with suicide attempts were studied. The authors concluded that to create a vulnerability to suicide attempts, multiple rather than single separations are of primary importance.[34]

On the other hand, separation during critical periods occurs in many lives without subsequent suicidal attempts. The frequency of both separations and parental loss has been noted repeatedly as part of the development of the attempters. The loss of love object is an important aspect of the developmental process, but it is not only an issue because of its presence or absence. It must be viewed as part of a process, with particular attention paid to when it occurred and/or recurred. Furthermore, it may be that it is not the loss of a love object per se that is so distressing but the loss of love, i.e., the reciprocal intimacy, spontaneity, and closeness that one experiences in a primary relationship. Both suicide attempters and the control adolescents had high rates of parental loss in early childhood. One group attempted suicide; the other did not. Is it parental loss in early childhood per se that predisposes to depression and suicide in later life? Or is it rather that the loss is an important aspect of a process viewed within the total context of the person's life?[15, 16]

The Three-Stage Progression in Suicide Attempts

Studies by this author and his co-workers at the Los Angeles County-University of Southern California Medical Center since 1963 show that 75 percent of adolescent suicide attempters between ages thirteen to eighteen are girls with the average age being sixteen. The usual means employed was the ingestion of pills which were readily available. The studies show that the five years prior to the attempt are marked by many personal, medical, social, and family difficulties. The case histories were built on information received in an interview with the adolescent, conducted within forty-eight hours of the attempt, and on another interview with at least one parent, usually the mother. Each interview was guided by a structured schedule covering five basic areas of inquiry: the suicide attempt, family relations, peer relations, attitudes toward and performance in school, career aspirations.[35]

The case history comprised two separate stories: the adolescent's autobiography and his biography as constructed by the parent. Additional data from transcribed recordings of therapy sessions, suicide notes, and later information received from significant others were also incorporated when available. The accumulted data comprised the adolescent's biography. Discrepancies in perception between the adolescent and parent were systematically analyzed. The study focused on how these discrepancies acted to escalate the total family conflict, especially since the onset of adolescence. What emerged was the picture of a three-stage process leading to the suicide attempt.

Ultimately, the three-stage process leads to social isolation and this in turn culminates in a suicide attempt. The three stages are: (1) a long-standing history of problems, from childhood to early adolescence; (2) a period of escalation, during which new problems associated with adolescence are introduced; (3) a final stage, the weeks and days immediately preceding an attempt, characterized by a chain reaction breakdown of the adolescent's few remaining primary associations.

LONG-STANDING HISTORY OF PROBLEMS

The following is a partial listing of long-standing problems, with approximate percentages, which characterize the biographies of adolescent suicide attempters:

1. 20 percent have a parent who attempted suicide.
2. 40 percent have a parent, relative, or close friend who attempted suicide.
3. 72 percent have one or both natural parents absent from the home (divorced, separated, or deceased).
4. 84 percent of those with stepparents felt they were contending with an unwanted stepparent.
5. 58 percent have a parent who was married more than once.
6. 62 percent have both parents working (or, when there was only one parent present, that parent worked).
7. The average number of serious, problem-making environmental changes experienced by the adolescent suicide attempter is 10.42 (examples: parents remarrying, family members in hospital, death in family, changing schools, siblings leaving home, foster home placement, being in juvenile hall, etc.).
8. 16 percent have serious problems with a parent due to that parent's alcoholism.
9. Large numbers live with persons other than parents (foster home placement, left with relatives for prolonged periods).
10. Families show marked residential mobility. An unusual number of school changes, and siblings leaving the home are common findings.

Suicide attempters experienced 53 percent more environmental changes than did the control group. The suicidal adolescent had been subject to one and three-fourths times more residential mobility and about twice as many school changes, and had lived with persons other than parents twice as often. Parents of suicide attempters had left, died, or remarried in three times as many instances as had parents of the control adolescents. The sum of these findings strongly suggests that the suicidal adolescent is far more subject to unexpected separations from meaningful social relationships in earlier life than are the controls.

ESCALATION OF PROBLEMS

Most of the problems associated with this second stage seem to revolve about a parent's trying to contend with a new, unfamiliar stage of development, namely, adolescence. Often, what is viewed as a "behavioral problem" by the parent is regarded by the teenager as conventional adolescent behavior. The parent feels, "He always used to be a nice boy, but lately (the last few years) I don't know how to handle him." At the same time, the adolescent feels that his parents don't understand him and punish him inappropriately. He responds with rebellion or withdrawal as "adaptive techniques" of self-defense. Withdrawal behavior usually occurs in the later stages of this process. The escalation stage is generally characterized by an uneasy resignation to the problem, and both parents and adolescent "stop trying."

Several areas representative of the escalation stage are depicted separately in the following paragraphs.

Behavior Problems: Adolescent suicide attempters reported that 89 percent of all "behavioral problems" they had ever exhibited began within the past five years.[35] Actions such as rebellion (sassiness, defiance, rebelliousness), withdrawal into self (with symptoms characterized by gloominess and ranging from minor reluctance to emotional withdrawal), lying, and physical withdrawal (running away from home) are viewed by parents as behavioral problems. The adolescent, however, while he recognizes them as behavioral problems, also views these as adaptive techniques. He knows they constitute difficulties to the parent; but to him, they are a means of dealing with a stressful situation within the family. The adolescent is hopeful that the parents will share his dual perspective and will regard his acts, not just as misbehavior, but also as an indication that a problem exists. He hopes further that his parents will recognize in his behavior a serious attempt to bring the problem to their attention through the only means available to him.

Time after time, the teenager attempts new ways of telling his parents about his troubles. He tries all of these "adaptive" techniques and finds, to his continued frustration, that his parents persist in viewing each new act as an additional bit of misbehavior. The parents are unable to grasp the adolescent's definition of the situation. As coping techniques are expended fruitlessly, the available options may narrow down to a suicide attempt as an attention-getting device. That failing, suicide may remain the only remaining way out.

Illness in the Family: A significant situation that contributes to the escalation of problems for the suicide attempter is physical or mental illness within the family (not necessarily an illness that afflicts the attempter himself). In 48 percent of all cases, either the adolescent, parent, or sibling was treated for mental illness or serious physical complaint within five years prior to a suicide attempt. Fifty-four percent of adolescent suicide attempters had been treated for some physical complaint or mental disturbance (including previous suicide attempts) within the past five years. Thirty-two percent had some serious physical complaint, 16 percent had some emotional disturbance, and 6 percent suffered both physical and mental disturbances. Thirty-six percent of the parents of adolescent suicide attempters had been treated for either a serious physical complaint or mental disturbance within the past five years (including, in four cases, suicide attempts made by the parents). In 14 percent of all cases, suicide attempters had a sibling or close relative other than a parent living with them who had been treated for a serious physical complaint or mental disturbance within the past five years.[35]

Intrafamily illnesses and hospitalizations serve to disrupt seriously the usual composition and interaction of the family and add considerably to the problems faced by the adolescent; e.g., they may result in: (1) his dropping out of school; (2) losing a parent from the household, often for the first time and for an extended period; (3) possibly losing a parent through death; or (4) the adolescent's assuming a parental role in caring for the sick or for younger siblings and taking care of the household or family business.

School: In 36 percent of all cases, the adolescent suicide attempter was not enrolled in school at the time of the attempt; only rarely, however, was poor scholarship the reason for dropping out. In 89 percent of these cases, the reasons given for nonattendance in school also contributed to the suicide attempt. One-third of those adolescents out of school at the time of their suicide attempts were absent for medical or related reasons: illness, pregnancy, prior suicide attempts (44 percent of all attempters had one or more previous attempts). Another 28 percent were out of school due to "behavioral problems" (acting up in class, "mental instability," fighting). Eleven percent were not attending school due to their being in juvenile hall. An additional 17 percent were out of school because of lack of interest, or due to dislike for the particular school they had been forced to attend. Forty-nine percent of suicide attempters (only 13 percent of control adolescents) stated they had begun truancy within the past five years. Another factor which placed a strain on the adolescent and his ability to remain in school is illustrated by the common statement, "I don't feel I can wait until later to begin earning money." The data about school are presented because it is one area where prevention is neglected, and where it ought to begin.[35]

Peer Relations: During the interviews, suicide attempters (and control adolescents) frequently expressed their liking for school, not primarily for academic reasons, but for the social life that school provides. To be excluded from school was considered by these adolescents tantamount to exclusion from one of the key potential resources for establishing meaningful social relationships. This is even truer for the suicide attempter who has already been excluded from many of the resources ordinarily open to the average teenager. One must wonder whether programs designed to increase and extend adolescents' interrelationships with peers and teachers would reduce the potential for suicide attempts.

It is not surprising to find that 23 percent of suicide attempters (zero percent of the control group) either agreed or strongly agreed to a statement: "There is no one to turn to when I need to talk to someone." During the interview, 18 percent of the suicide attempters admitted that they had no good friends to turn to in times of troubles. Only 3 percent of control group adolescents found themselves in a similar situation. Thus, pathetically, 46 percent of the suicide attempters (to 20 percent of the control group) either agreed or strongly agreed: "One of the worst things about my troubles is that they always seem to be without a solution when I have them."[35]

Incidentally, failure to achieve adequate peer group relatedness is an important finding in the assessment of suicide potential. In the adolescent task of loosening the parental ties, peers provide a major defense against the ensuing feelings of isolation. The potential attempter's dependent needs are so intense that his peers are often threatened and they reject and sequester him. The last defense is the romance.

THE FINAL STAGE: THE ROMANCE

By the end of the escalation period, the parents have been totally alienated. The adolescent yearns to reestablish the spontaneity, openness and intimacy that he feels characterized the earlier relationship with his parents. Granted that these ideal relationships were realized imperfectly at best by the suicide attempter during his childhood, they have by this time deteriorated to a state of nonexistence.

One of the few remaining possible relationships which could re-establish the needed conditions is a teenage romance. The adolescent whose biography is characterized by effects of the first two stages will pursue intensely what appears to be his last chance to establish a primary relationship. In this pursuit, he may expend all his time and energy and have little left for casual friendships, even for a good friend of his own sex (21 percent of female suicide attempters compared to

5 percent of control females considered their closest friends to be boys).[35] As a result, previous friends, close or casual, are usually alienated during the courtship. When this romance fails, the adolescent is left with no one. The last defense is gone, and he is left alone feeling abandoned and isolated.

Of those 36 percent of all suicide attempters who engaged in a serious romance, all were in the terminal stages of the romance. Earlier in the study, it was noted that 22 percent of all girls attempting suicide, compared to zero percent of control girls, were either pregnant or believed themselves to be pregnant as a result of their romance.[35] In such cases, pregnancy further alienates the adolescent from society. Rejected by the boyfriend or his family, abandoned by her parents when their help is most needed, subject to rejection and verbal abuse by her peers and, more often than not, with school a minor consideration, the youngster's isolation appears to be complete. There seems to be no way out. Living is a chronic problem; to end it, death appears to be the only solution.

Special View of Male Attempters

These youths experienced maternal deprivation during their first year of life. Characteristically, there was also an intensely ambivalent relationship with a male during their early years. This person functioned as the elder male in the home. In eight of thirteen male adolescents, who were studied intensively, the onset of suicidal behavior occurred concurrently with serious suicide preoccupations by their mothers or mother surrogates. All these boys professed love for their nagging, ambivalent mothers who they often felt did not love them. Because of the infantile dependence of such youths, the mother's depression, anger, rejection, withdrawal, and disapproval have a devastating effect. The mothers make demands on the boys to be maternal husbands, care for them, and relieve them of responsibility. The youths, struggling against being narcissistic extensions of their mothers, are conflicted because of their own dependency and their identifications with these powerful female presences.

When the relationship with the mother, girlfriend, or maternal surrogate is seriously threatened, e.g., through the appearance of a new rival or by an incident of rejection, enormous anxiety is generated. The suicide attempt expresses the response to this catastrophic affect. Suicidal preoccupations on the part of the mother were consistently present. The adolescents avoided separation from their mothers by identifying with their mother's depressed suicidal state. This was a hostile identification. At the same time it was a frantic, "useful" attempt to hold on to the "good object" since the teenagers had no other. They were never able to free themselves in a meaningful way from infantile dependent and ambivalent relationships with their mothers. The actual suicide attempt is in fact a striving to avoid separation from the mother and to continue identification with her.[20]

Role of the Physician and the Problem of Prediction

In light of problems typically revealed by the suicide attempter's biography, the importance of the adolescent's contact with his physician during the weeks and months preceding an attempt cannot be overestimated. Most of the patients studied had kept their suicide attempts secret. They were accordingly not seen by physicians following these earlier attempts. It was only through physician contacts in the wake of more recent suicidal attempts that these earlier ones were ever discovered.

The physician's interest in the adolescent and the aid he offers for dealing with his problems (beyond the usual attention directed to any specific physical complaint) may mean the difference between life and death for such a patient. The suicide attempt itself results from a complete breakdown of meaningful social relationships. Uncovering adolescent attitudes, either through lengthy interviews or by questionnaire, is certain to be time consuming. However, without the insight which emerges from considerable contact with suicidal persons over a prolonged period, the suicidal person is not readily distinguished from the "normal" member of society. It is for this reason that these procedures are undertaken.

Without exception, a first suicide attempt comes as a great surprise to both the parents and peers of the adolescent attempter. The physicians of such adolescents are, similarly, usually caught off guard. There is no indication in any of the cases studied at Los Angeles County-USC Medical Center that referring private physicians were given advance warning. This is not surprising, since there exists no convenient means for anticipating a suicide attempt. To detect an impending suicide attempt, a good deal must be known in advance about the individual involved; and the routine contacts of everyday life do not normally yield such information. In the comparisons made between a control group of adolescent suicide attempters, one point upon which both experimental and control groups agreed is that secrets are an essential part of life particularly during adolescence. In this respect, the adolescent suicide attempter finds himself in a disadvantaged position, since effective therapy often is dependent on his divulging many of his secrets.

By the time the adolescent makes an attempt, he usually has pretty well convinced himself that "talking about his problem gets him nowhere." His past experience strongly supports this view. Insofar as he is concerned, such an attitude does not represent a spontaneous or arbitrary opinion. The suicidal youth is not easily distinguished from others because his biography is not common knowledge. Those rewards which give the normal adolescent sufficient reason to live have, in the course of time, been taken from the suicidal youth. If the physician is to treat him effectively, he must invest the time and effort needed to uncover more information than that necessary for a medical evaluation. Our studies reveal that a high percentage of illness for which the suicide attempter sought a physician's aid fell into the category of "functional physical complaints not given to specific diagnosis."

The adolescent contemplating suicide often seeks out the physician. As a patient, the youth believes there is hope for him here, a potential for help. The doctor's position is somewhat unusual in providing the suicide attempter ready access to a last possibility of rescue when all others have failed. Furthermore, the doctor is one of the few people in whom the adolescent may feel free to confide and to confess. This is a function of the objectivity, impartiality, confidentiality, and anonymity assured in the doctor-patient relationship.

No less important to those seeking help is the presumption that the doctor holds "office" in one of the most powerful existing agencies of help: science. The doctor has a moral obligation to use this privileged position to the best advantage of those seeking his services. Bearing in mind the availability of information which he alone is in a position to elicit, and being cognizant of experiences and attitudes held by the adolescent suicide attempter, it may be prudent for the physician to compile thumbnail biographical sketches of his adolescent patients, covering the following three stages:

1. Is there a long-standing history of problems preceding adolescence?
2. Is there an escalation of problems during adolescence? (Typical problems are described previously).
3. Is the stage set for a finale characterized by a chain reaction dissolution of what remains of the adolescent's meaningful social relationships?

Most adults do not wish to recapture the emotional turmoil of their adolescent period. This is reflected in the remarkable blindness many physicians demonstrate in dealing with troubled adolescents—even those who have attempted suicide. Where the relationship with the physician may literally be the adolescent's lifeline, the means by which the attempter seeks to escape ultimate alienation, doctors too often "get rid of" the suicide attempter as soon as the medical or surgical problem is eased. The anxiety the disturbed adolescent provides in the doctor fosters blind spots and a singular unawareness totally uncharacteristic of his other doctor-patient relationships. The attempter is so hungry for relationships that his life is literally maintained through a firm connection with an interested human. This applies with unusual force to the doctor, whose skills have special significance. In the face of this, it behooves all physicians to ask themselves hard questions about blind spots.[40]

Treatment

Whether the suicide attempter is seen in the hospital, at home, or in the office, the moment the therapist engages with the young person, his effort should be directed toward becoming the "lifeline" for the adolescent.[38] Clinically, the adolescent is anxious, depressed, insecure, guilty, and apprehensive because of the parental reaction of anger and hurt. Often enough he is clinging and always feels dreadfully alone and vulnerable. The loneliness or alienation is more painful than the depression or anxiety. There may be active, continued suicidal ideation. The parents, usually the mother, are angry, concerned, occasionally guilty, but soon hostile. They defend themselves with massive denial. Father, usually stepfather, considers it all quite a bother and exhibits a relative unconcern. Both the parents and the physician (who may have known the youth) are surprised by the attempt; it is unexpected. Despite the long history of problems recounted with mothers, after their suicide attempt, the girls, surprisingly, uniformly described their mothers in glowing, idealized terms with denial of any flaws.

The suicide attempt is an overdetermined symptom. Whether it is primarily attention-getting or is, in fact, a real attempt to die, it is always to be regarded as serious. If possible, the young patient should be hospitalized, even if only briefly. This serves many functions. Further acting on suicidal ideation is prevented; anxiety is often diminished. The "mothering" atmosphere of the ward, (preferable to a private room for a young person), plus the support of the other patients, offers a caring, protective, and safe milieu. One may have difficulty discharging these patients from the hospital. They tend to cling to the staff and to other patients.

From the initial contact, the psychiatrist offers himself as an attentive, empathic person who can always be reached and is available when needed. The aim is to establish rapport, a beginning trust, an image of a stable, caring, supportive, significant person in the life of the alienated adolescent. Contact—the lifeline—isn't necessarily personal; a telephone call is a tie too. One patient's attempt was aborted when she was able to locate her therapist across the continent. In view of the many problem areas, as noted previously, one attempts some resolution of the most critical issues, usually the broken romance and the parental reactions. It is important to enlist the parents' cooperation, passive or active, in the treatment plan before the patient's discharge. One deals with the parents' anger, guilt, concern, and, in our hospital cases, with reality problems such as arrangements for treatment for the young person, school problems, etc. In any case, the attempt is made to point up parents' involvement in the attempter's problems and to encourage them to participate in the treatment program.

Inevitably, the young person focuses on the precipitating event which is fully discussed. Despite the denials that appear soon after recovery from the attempt, there is direct work to be done with the feelings of depression and suicidal ideation. Ideally, prior to discharge from the hospital, the patient should have some understanding of the forces and factors behind the suicide attempt. Nonetheless, the bond determinedly established between the "always available" therapist and the patient may well be sufficiently firm to prevent further suicidal actions and to permit a therapeutic engagement.

As noted, the commonest precipitating factor is a rejection by a boyfriend or girlfriend. This reactivates feelings of an earlier loss of love and support from a parental figure. When there had been early positive experiences, the young person has something to fall back on; he can absorb the broken romance as an unhappy event rather than as the culmination of a process of progressive social isolation. The adolescent's task of detaching from parental authority is especially painful for the suicide attempter with impaired object relations. The detachment is experienced as an abandonment, the separation anxiety is great, and the feeling of aloneness is frightening and adds to the pain. Feeling alone, empty, and helpless, there is resentment toward forcibly abandoning the past. The normal adolescent ego feels forced to relinquish old attachments and to form new ones, and does so.

The suicide attempter's ego is weak, able to make attachments only feebly, and unable to detach. After the escalation period, unable to express overt aggression, the traumatized adolescent's ego is overwhelmed by feelings of helplessness. Bibring[4] pointed out that any condition which forces a feeling of helplessness upon the infantile ego predisposes to depression. This is clearly seen in the depressed adolescent. To note again, the male adolescent's identification with the suicidal mother appears increasingly crucial in those who clearly had difficulty resolving the symbiotic tie and the associated separation-individuation conflicts. The threat of object loss, the narcissistic shifts, and the identity struggles are indeed acute. Caught up in such attachment to mother, the oedipal complex is distorted.

Lorand[19] revived the concept of the ego ideal, as postulated by Sigmund Freud, as a useful theoretical concept and guide to the treatment of the depressed, suicidal adolescent. In the "lifeline" approach this is of particular importance. The precipitate of the old picture of the parents, the expressions of admiration for the perfection which the child attributed to them, is the ego ideal. The root pathology of one form of depression lies in not being able to live up to the aspirations of the ego ideal.

The earliest difficulties of ego ideal development and identification disturbances that occur at the beginning of ego development help to form the basic structure from which later pathology emerges. This leaves its mark on the later growth and structure of the personality. Our case studies give strong support to this thesis. In our cases, the precipitate of the old picture of parents from the earliest period of development was inadequate and unsatisfactory. Mother was described as cold, unperceptive, providing little warmth or encouragement even though the basic physical necessities of cleaning, feeding, etc. were cared for.

Capacities for experiencing understanding, permissiveness, and love will be achieved through identification with a new, albeit transient ego ideal. The therapist takes this role. He is the focal point around which the patient's early conflicts are reviewed. One is constantly aware of the suicide attempter's insatiable need for love. In therapy, the adolescent experiences and tests in reality a new kind of relationship with an object, one that affords a dependable attachment, a model, in fact, an ego ideal. Despite the marked inner, repressed rebellion against authority, the adolescent's evident need makes for a therapeutic alliance. Direct support is essential to help the young person cope with daily conflicts and current difficulties which involve parents, school, peer and sibling relationships, and goal commitment.

The accumulation of repressed rebellion against and hatred toward the external world (superego) makes for self-accusation and reproaches. These become so violent that strong self-destructive tendencies arise. Threats, ideas, and fantasies about suicide are frequently expressed. The adolescent may seek out challenging and dangerous situations, such as reckless driving or motorcycling. In this way, he tries to defend himself against feelings of helplessness. Acting out tendencies may be used as a defense or to prevent loss of identity. Acting out tendencies of a self-destructive nature have to be considered as a reaction to a stress situation and as a bid for the environment to provide love and care for the patient in his hopeless and helpless misery. Psychosomatic symptoms are a frequent source of refuge.

Lorand emphasizes the classical psychoanalytic view. Self-destructive tendencies, plans or attempts serve the need for self-punishment and, at the same time, punish the frustrating, abandoning object. The aggression felt toward the frustrating object is turned against the self. Other unconscious guilt feelings emerge with renewed vigor and join with the current aggression. Collectively, these evoke a strong need for self-punishment which in turn leads to self-castigation and remorse.

The adolescents with suicidal tendencies are preoccupied with violent hatred and ideas of revenge. The therapeutic aim is to encourage an awareness of the good qualities of the superego and to enable the patient to consider re-establishing a new type of ego ideal and superego. Always, suicidal ideation and depressed feelings must be analyzed before tension reaches a high degree and the still weak ego is overstressed. Under favorable circumstances, the infantile conception of the frustrating objects will change to a new kind of appreciation.

Prediction of Suicidal Potential

Since so much is unknown about the development of adolescent suicide attempters, prediction is difficult. It is known that those who make an attempt are at a much higher risk for future acts of this kind. Also, those who leave suicide notes are at a higher risk; the note is a significant warning. Obviously, the preceding statements have prognostic significance. High risk persons probably can be identified. Many professionals have attempted to develop suicide prediction scales. At best, however, the level of prediction is still too low to warrant individual application. Biological studies, too, are far from definitive. Investigations of catecholamines, as well as other neurotransmitters, in critical brain areas may eventually elucidate the biological mechanisms that underlie suicidal and other deviant behaviors.

The belief that suicidal behaviors are predictable is valid as a belief in principle, but not in fact. Even elaborate statistical methods will not solve the problem of prediction until our understanding of the causes deepens. This will happen when investigators come to grips with the data collected. Only then will they be able to recognize where data are not adequate or not thoroughly analyzed.[3, 36]

Diagnosis

There is much variability in diagnostic criteria, particularly with adolescents. Moreover, medical records are variable and yield inaccurate data. The largest number of adolescent suicide attempters are not psychotic. Regardless of the label placed on them, the overwhelming clinical, observable fact is that, at the time of the attempt, they are depressed.

Prevention

Primary prevention lies in strong family life and re-establishment of standards which at one time served to integrate the person within a social group. Presently, they do not appear to be effective resources for a young person. Nor are schools effective resources today. All too often, the peer support and teacher or counselor support is lacking, since truancy or dropping out eventually closes the school to the youth. Yet, if school counselors and nurses could become more aware of the high risk adolescent, they would be an invaluable resource.

Secondary prevention is focused on those who have made an attempt. Here, treatment for the adolescent and his family is essential, difficult, often frustrating, and anxiety producing. The role of the family physician and importance of milieu have been discussed previously.

Suicide prevention centers are valuable in helping to meet the challenge. Some 200 suicide prevention centers began operating in communities during the 1960s, utilizing valuable manpower and considerable funds. Unfortunately, high risk adolescents do not contact prevention centers, and there is little evidence to demonstrate that these centers are effective. In one study,[18] suicide rates for the cities studied had risen significantly from 1960 to 1969. Neither the presence nor absence of a center was found to affect the suicide rate. Although these agencies may not prevent suicide, they may be useful as crises intervention centers or to coordinate services for the local mental health agencies.

Pre-adolescent Children Who Attempt Suicide

Suicide attempts in children are not common if one judges only by hospitalized patients. Children have limited access to lethal weapons, but there are always pills and opportunities for dangerous behavior. However, there are no accurate figures on the incidence of attempted suicide in children. Here too, families and physicians often conceal such attempts.

At the Los Angeles County-University of Southern California Medical Center, increasing numbers of children under twelve are admitted for "accidental overdose." It is common knowledge that children have a high rate of accidents, and it should not be surprising that many are sub-intentioned suicide attempts. In preschool children, accidental injuries are the most frequent cause of death, with motor vehicle fatalities dominating, followed by drowning, fire, and suffocation. In view of the fact most accidents are preventable, it would be difficult even to speculate whether any of these in fact are suicidal, and whether the child was "expendable." One to 5 percent of all children under ten years of age admitted to child psychiatric facilities have a history of a threat or an attempt to kill themselves.[1]

In general, childhood suicide attempts appear to be impulsive acts, usually motivated by feeling badly treated and by the desire to punish those who would grieve at their death. Running in front of cars, jumping from roofs, attempted hanging, placing one's head in a plastic bag, and the ingestion of pills are the common modes. The relative frequency of suicidal attempts is so much greater in the teenage period that far more attention is paid to this age group. In general, the child who threatens to kill himself is expressing his rage toward his parents, usually his mother. But to the young child's mind death is not permanent. To him, it often means a way to a better life, or somewhat like the phoenix myth, a wish to re-unite with the all giving, good mother. However, recent work indicates that children are more concerned with death than was previously recognized. Observers have noted that death is explored frequently in a variety of sober play activities.[2, 37] Those who do seriously attempt to kill themselves are usually very disturbed, with very pathological family situations and, as a rule, with a very sick mother.

In one study, one-half of all children with suicidal behavior came from intact families. Abundant evidence existed of long-standing individual and family psychopathology. More than 75 percent of a total of 170 had a history of emotional disorders of more than one year duration. Prior to the attempt, 40 percent had displayed signs of depression in the form of social withdrawal, loss of initiative, changing scholastic performance, sadness, crying spells, and sleep disturbance. Unfortunately, as is true in a number of studies about children, adolescents are included and muddy any conclusions. Nonetheless, a significant environmental factor that emerges is again the element of loss by death, desertion, or separation.

Some observers have noted that suicidal children often are those who do not take part in school activities outside the classroom. They are socially isolated, have no close friends, and may show reading or learning difficulties. Such learning problems are a frequent symptom of family pathology. The child also may feel he can no longer tolerate the pain of living and that his adaptive attempts to fulfill his needs have come to nothing. Regardless of his concept of death, he views it as a solution to his difficulties. Children suffer depression with behavioral and somatic symptoms as the outward manifestation. In a number of children seen, deviant behavior may be the only, or at least an effective, means of arousing maternal concern, however punitive. It is preferable to a total absence of concern. A reasonable conclusion, based on clinical experience, is that the suicidal child wishes to alter an intolerable living situation that is beyond his capacity to change and to punish significant persons in his life.

There is no careful, well-controlled study of attempted suicide in children that sheds more light on this area.

REFERENCES

1. ACKERLY, W. C., "Latency Age Children Who Threaten or Attempt to Kill Themselves," *Journal of the American Academy of Child Psychiatry*, 6:242–261, 1967.

2. ANTHONY, S., *Discovery of Death in Childhood and After*, Basic Books, New York, 1972.

3. BECK, A. T., RESNICK, H. L. P., and LETTIERI, D. J. (Eds), *Prediction of Suicide*, Charles Press, Bowie, Md, 1974.

4. BIBRING, E., "The Mechanism of Depression," in Greenacre, P. (Ed.), *Affective Disorders*, International Universities Press, New York, 1953.

5. CANTOR, P. C., *Personality and Status Characteristics of the Female Youthful Suicide Attempter*, unpublished doctoral dissertation, Columbia University, 1972.

6. CHORON, J., *Suicide*, Charles Scribner, New York, 1972.

7. DARPAT, T. L., JACKSON, J. K., and RIPLEY, H. S., "Broken Homes and Attempted and Completed Suicides," *Archives of General Psychiatry*, 12(21):213–216, 1965.

8. DIZMANG, L. H., et al., "Adolescent Suicide at an Indian Reservation," *American Journal of Orthopsychiatry*, 44(1):43–49, 1974.

9. EISSLER, K. R., "Notes on Problems of Techniques in the Psychoanalytic Treatment of Adolescents," in Eissler, R. S., et al. (Eds.), *The Psychoanalytic Study of the Child*, vol. 13, pp. 223–254, International Universities Press, New York, 1958.

10. ERIKSON, E. H., "The Problem of Ego Identity," *Journal of the American Psychoanalytical Association*, 4:56–121, 1956.

11. FOX, K., and WEISSMAN, M. M., "Suicide Attempts

and Drugs," Paper presented to the American Orthopsychiatric Association, New York, 1973.

12. FREUD, A., "Adolescence," in Eissler, R. S., et al. (Eds.), *The Psychoanalytic Study of the Child*, vol. 13, pp. 255–278, International Universities Press, New York, 1958.

13. FREUD, S., "The Psychogenesis of a Case of Homosexuality in a Woman," in *The Standard Edition of the Complete Psychological Works of Sigmund Freud*, vol. 18, pp. 147–172, Hogarth Press, London, 1955.

14. GOULD, R. E., "Suicide Problems in Children and Adolescents," *American Journal of Psychotherapy, 19:* 228–246, 1965.

15. JACOBS, J., *Adolescent Suicide*, Wiley-Interscience, New York, 1971.

16. ——, and TEICHER, J. D., "Broken Homes Viewed as a Process," *International Journal of Social Psychiatry, 13:*139–149, 1966.

17. JACOBSON, E., "Adolescent Moods and the Remodeling of Psychic Structure in Adolescence," in Eissler, R. S., et al. (Eds.), *The Psychoanalytic Study of the Child*, vol. 16, pp. 164–183, International Universities Press, New York, 1961.

18. LESTER, D., "Effect of Suicide Prevention Centers on Suicide Rates in U.S.," *Health Service Reports, 89:* 37–39, 1974.

19. LORAND, S., "Adolescent Depression," *International Journal of Psychoanalysis, 48:*53–68, 1967.

20. MARGOLIN, N. L., and TEICHER, J. D., "Thirteen Adolescent Male Suicide Attempts," *Journal of the American Academy of Child Psychiatry, 8:*272–285, 1968.

21. MATTSSON, A., "Suicidal Behavior as a Child Psychiatric Emergency," *Archives of General Psychiatry, 20(1):*100–109, 1969.

22. Metropolitan Life, "Suicide—International Comparisons," *Statistical Bulletin, 53:*2–5, 1972.

23. PAYKEL, E. S., et al., "Suicidal Feelings in the General Population," *British Journal of Psychiatry, 124(5):* 460–469, 1974.

24. PEDERSON, A. M., AWAD, M. D., and KINDLER, A. R., "Epidemiological Differences Between White and Non-White Suicide Attempters," *American Journal of Psychiatry, 130(10):*1071–1076, 1973.

25. PERLIN, S., *A Handbook for the Study of Suicide*, Oxford University Press, New York, 1974.

26. RIPLEY, H. S., "Suicidal Behavior in Edinburgh and Seattle," *American Journal of Psychiatry, 130(9):* 995–1001, 1973.

27. ROSENBAUM, M., "Suicide: Role of Hostility and Death Wishes From Family and Society," Paper presented to the Southern California Psychiatric Society, September, 1972.

28. SABBATH, J. D., "The Suicidal Adolescent—The Expendable Child," *Journal of the American Academy of Child Psychiatry, 8:*272–285, 1969.

29. SCHNEER, H. I., and KAY, P., "The Suicidal Adolescent," in Lorand, S., and Scheer, H. (Eds.), *Adolescents*, pp. 180–201, Hoeber, New York, 1962.

30. ——, and BROZOVSKY, M., "Events and Conscious Ideation Leading to Suicidal Behavior in Adolescence," *Psychiatric Quarterly, 35(7):*507–515, 1961.

31. SCHRUT, A., "Suicidal Adolescents and Children," *Journal of the American Medical Association, 188:*1103–1107, 1964.

32. SEIDEN, R. H., "Why are Suicides of Young Blacks Increasing?" *HSMA Health Reports, 87(1):*3–8, 1972.

33. SHNEIDMAN, E., and FARBEROW, N., *Clues to Suicide*, McGraw-Hill, New York, 1957.

34. STEIN, M., GLASBERG, H. M., and LEVY, M., "Childhood Separation Experiences and Suicidal Attempts," Paper presented to the American Orthopsychiatric Association, New York, 1973.

35. TEICHER, J. D., "A Solution to the Chronic Problem of Living: Adolescent Attempted Suicide," in Schoolar, J. C. (Ed.), *Current Issues in Adolescent Psychiatry*, pp. 129–147, Brunner-Mazel, New York, 1973.

36. ——, "The Enigma of Predicting Adolescent Suicide Attempts," *Feelings*, vol. 4, no. 4, Ross Laboratories, Columbus, Ohio, 1972.

37. ——, "Children and Adolescents Who Attempt Suicide," *Pediatric Clinics of North America, 17(3):*687–696, 1970.

38. ——, "Treatment of the Suicidal Adolescent—The Life Line Approach," *Excerpta Medica, International Congress Series, 1(15):*747–751, Excerpta Medica Foundation, Amsterdam, The Netherlands, 1967.

39. ——, and JACOBS, J., "Adolescents Who Attempt Suicide," *American Journal of Psychiatry, 122:*1248–1257, 1966.

40. ——, "The Physician and the Adolescent Suicide Attempter," *Journal of School Health, 36:*406–415, 1966.

41. United States Department of Commerce, Bureau of Census, *Statistical Abstracts of the United States*, Government Printing Office, Washington, D.C., 1974.

42. United States Department of Health, Education, and Welfare, *Teenagers: Marriages, Divorces, Parenthood and Mortality*, Statistical Series 21, No. 23, Department of Health, Education, and Welfare, Washington, D.C., August 1973.

43. WEISSMAN, M., "Epidemiology of Suicide Attempts, 1960–1971," *Archives of General Psychiatry, 30(6):*737–746, 1974.

44. ZILBOORG, G., "Considerations on Suicide with Particular Reference to That of the Young," *American Journal of Orthopsychiatry, 7:*15–30, 1937.

39 / Habit Disorders

Carolyn B. Robinowitz

The habit disorders, such as thumb sucking, nail biting, head banging, rhythmic movements, hair pulling, and tics had occupied a central position in the early literature of child psychiatry. Currently, however, they are not considered to be specific disease entities and are not so designated in the present systems of classification and nomenclature. By and large, these auto-erotic activities are related to stages of development. Amount of activity, as well as persistence, has an impact on the degree of psychopathology.

DSM-II refers to disorders of habit and training as "Special Symptoms" (306), further specifying tics (306.2) and other psychomotor disorders (306.3) as well as other nonspecific symptoms (306.9).[1] They describe the occasional patient whose psychopathology is limited to a single specific symptom. By and large, however, these disorders do not appear in isolation. They are the result of underlying disturbances, which can range in severity from normal healthy response (GAP)[20] to psychosis or mental retardation. In view of this, classification systems need to take the underlying psychopathology into account. Thus, the habit disorders are commonly seen in reactive disorders. These appear in the DSM manual as situational reactions (307), neurosis (300), behavior disorders of childhood and adolescence (308), (the Psychoneurotic disorders and personality disorders of the GAP classification[20]), psychosis, and organic brain syndrome, as well as part of a normal response (q.v.).[1]

It is clear that the habits described do not themselves allude to the history or etiology of the particular adaptational pattern. Although each disorder will be discussed in specific detail, it is important to note that the important areas of investigation must always be the conflicts and disturbances which the habit (symptom) may represent.

Thumb Sucking

DESCRIPTION

Thumb sucking is the earliest form of habitual manipulation of the body. It is extremely common during the first two years of life. At this age, it is likely to be regarded as a problem only by overzealous parents who have been warned of its potential ill effects. In general, however, it becomes a cause for concern only if it persists into school age. Thumb sucking per se is rarely sufficient reason for psychologic referral; it tends to appear as one of a constellation of behaviors or feelings which in aggregate present problems.

HISTORY

Babies have always sucked their thumbs. In early Renaissance paintings, infants were often pictured with thumbs in their mouths, appearing serene and tranquil. Only in the nineteenth century was the act regarded as harmful or pathologic. Dentists reported on the certainty (later studies[50] dispute this) of dental malocclusion in thumb suckers; twentieth century physicians, in their concern about germs, warned of the dangers of fingers in the mouth. Psychologists condemned thumb sucking as "unsocial" and stated that use of a dummy or pacifier to quiet babies was near criminal because it would damage the developing child's personality. Kanner (p. 548)[23] described in some detail the varied and ingenious devices designed to prevent the hands from being brought to the mouth, noting that the reason for stopping thumb sucking was to develop the child's moral character.

FREQUENCY AND INCIDENCE

Thumb sucking usually begins during the first months of life, often during the teething period, if not earlier. Estimates of its frequency range from 15 to 60 percent of all children. Observation of sixty-five infants aged three to twelve months at a well-baby clinic documented some finger or thumb sucking in forty-four, or two-thirds, although only thirty-one engaged in this activity for an extended period.[34] There is no difference in incidence according to sex, nor according to performance on Bayley or Denver scales. The behavior usually disappears by latency. In retarded school age youngsters, however, finger and thumb sucking, as well as other habitual body manipulations, are rather common. Thumb sucking is quite rare in adolescence.

Accessory movements are often seen. They include such behaviors as pulling on the body, especially the hair or ears, and twisting or rubbing blankets or toys. In older children, especially, manipulations of the genital area are likely to accompany thumb sucking.

Cultures which are less restrictive about sucking in general allow longer use of pacifiers and tolerate thumb sucking at a later age. Cross cultural data suggest that the Spanish-American, and Afro-American cultures do not regard the habit as deviant until much later in latency.[46]

Thumb sucking is particularly common when the child is lonely, sad, or depressed. It is likely to appear at bed time or at other times of separation. Hunger, shame, excitement, anxiety, and even boredom have also been implicated.

In spite of historical warnings, there are few physical effects directly attributable to thumb sucking. There is no evidence that thumb or finger sucking causes gastro-intestinal dysfunction. Temporary dental malocclusions may be spontaneously reversed if the habit does not persist after age six or seven, and there is disagreement as to the effect of thumb sucking on permanent teeth. Some authorities state that dental abnormalities are rare even in chronic cases.[50] There are infants and children who suck so vigorously that ulcerations of the thumb or lips are formed; these are also reversible.

ETIOLOGY

Developmental: For infants, sucking is a gratifying reflex action designed to ensure survival. It is the means by which an infant receives food. Sucking on nipples, pacifiers, or thumbs is soothing to infants, many of whom fall asleep in the course of this activity.

Although finger or thumb sucking may begin as a reflex, it is found to be pleasurable and soothing in its own right. Gesell[16] observed that it was associated with hunger during the first few weeks of life, and that later it was connected with teething. Levy[34] implicated inadequate or insufficient sucking during feeding, an experience which left the infant unsatisfied and in need of further gratification of this kind. Other studies, however, have failed to support the hypothesis that deprivation forms the etiology of thumb sucking.[43] In studying children who had been fed with the cup from birth or early infancy, Sears and Wise[49] could not demonstrate any relationship between sucking deprivation and thumb or finger sucking.

Davis, Sears, and Miller[10] did demonstrate that there were differences in the sucking responses of babies fed with cup, bottle, or breast during the first ten days of life. They attributed these differences to the association of sucking with gratification of hunger and thirst.

PSYCHODYNAMIC FACTORS

In his "Three Contributions to the Theory of Sex,"[15] Freud described thumb sucking as an infantile sexual manifestation in which the erogenous significance of the lip zone is maintained through deprivation or overstimulation. This oral fixation was correlated with adult behavior in which drinking, smoking, and eating disturbances, including choking and globus hystericus, as well as emphasis on sexual lip activities such as kissing were all related to thumb sucking in infancy. It has been suggested[12] that parents make an unconscious connection between thumb sucking and masturbatory activity. Their own early conflicts and concerns about masturbation are reactivated when they observe their children, and thus they overrespond to their children's thumb sucking.

Youngsters who thumb suck may report fantasies of being suckled at the mother's breast, as well as devouring or fellatio. Thumb sucking can be related to loss or separation, in which the child symbolically tries to overcome his pain and anxiety by attaining the remembered infantile sensation of being full and satiated. The thumb may serve as a replacement for the "other;" in particular, when accompanied by a blanket or toy, it may represent a transitional object. In older children, the thumb may serve the function of imaginary companion to ward off feelings of loneliness. Turning to thumb sucking in times of stress may represent a withdrawal from a situation which is too frightening or overwhelming to face except through regression to a younger age, an age at which one is cared for (and the child, by virtue of the thumb, provides his own care).

There is no specific family psychopathology associated with the symptom. However, the concern exhibited by parents, as they attempt to stop the habit, may cause further stress in the parent-child relationship, worsening, rather than ameliorating the habit.

TREATMENT

In infants and young children, no treatment is needed. Efforts should be made to see that a variety of adequate gratifications are available, and that, wherever possible, excessive environmental stress is reduced. Parental awareness of the principles of child development should be explored, and there should be ample opportunities for the child to suck, chew (as able), be held and cuddled, play, and rest.

Mechanical restraints or noxious substances are rarely effective in removing the symptom. In fact, they may cause additional tension and stress. Nagging, too, may serve to reinforce the thumb sucking and increase parent-child discord. In mild cases, distraction to other activities may be useful. Removing the thumb from the mouth of the sleeping infant or toddler may also serve to interrupt the pattern.

In older children, and especially those of school age, thumb sucking suggests that the child is striving to cope with an intrapsychic or interpersonal burden that is beyond his resources. In keeping with this, a careful evaluation of the child, including intrapsychic, interpersonal, and environmental factors, should be made. Counseling and/or psychotherapy to deal with the causes may also relieve the symptom, particularly if treatment is coupled with remediation in social relationships or scholastic settings.

When thumb sucking itself becomes a major battleground between parent and child, symptom removal by use of behavior modification techniques may be indicated. The goal is to improve the parent-child relationship and foster the child's pride in his/her ability to discard an ill-regarded activity. Use of rewards, punishments, and support by teachers have been helpful in developing successful behavioral programs. With symptom removal, there has been notable improvement of parent-child relationship and in the child's socialization and school performances; nor have any immediate ill effects or spread of the problems to other areas been observed.

Nail Biting

DESCRIPTION

Nail biting is one of the most common habits of childhood and adult life. Parents rarely seek medical help for nail biting that is unaccompanied by other habits or problem behaviors, and its presence is usually noted as an incidental finding, if it is noted at all. Nail biting may be associated with picking at the nails or cuticle or with picking or biting the toe nails. It can become so intense and extreme that infection or even destruction of the nail may result.

HISTORY

Historically, nail biting was regarded as a severe symptom of considerable magnitude (earlier descriptions of habit disorders tended to focus on this as a special and unique form of psychopathology). Kanner cites both Cramer (p. 552),[23] who regarded nail biting as "an exquisitely psychopathic symptom," and Berillon (p. 553),[23] who spoke of it as a sign of "degeneration." More recent literature refers to it as an example of motor discharge of tension.

FREQUENCY INCIDENCE

Nail biting usually begins about age three and increases in incidence until age six. Its incidence levels off for three years and then increases again at age nine, reaching a peak from ages thirteen

to fifteen. At the peak, some 40 to 45 percent of children are said to be nail biters. Approximately one-half cease between age sixteen to eighteen. A small, persistent minority continue to bite their nails through adulthood. Nail biting has been associated with motor restlessness, restless sleep, tics, and other forms of body manipulation including thumb sucking and nose picking.

There is no significant difference in the gender of nail biters, although reports indicate that males persist longer in biting nails than do females. There is no correlation between intelligence and nail biting, nor is there any significant relation between this habit and delinquency or enuresis, both of which, the early literature cited as related. Nail biting is somewhat more common in children who stutter (although some authorities feel this may be related more to a general state of tension than to the specific symptom and syndrome). Twice as many children reared in an institutional setting bit their nails as compared to children raised in foster homes.

In spite of frequent historical assertions that nail biting causes malocclusions, there is no evidence in orthodontic studies to support this theory. There is also lack of evidence to support the likelihood that nail biting causes dental trauma or gingivitis. Sucking habits are frequently said to cause malocclusion, if engaged in strongly between six and twelve years of age. But sucking involves the labial and lingual muscles in quite a different way from nail biting, and it is this stress on the muscular balance which has been implicated in maldevelopment of the teeth and bite.

It has been suggested that nail biting is an extension of thumb sucking, in that at about age three, thumb sucking tends to disappear and nail biting tends to come into view. Nail biting tends to be given up during later or mid-adolescence in response to disapproval from peers and is replaced by other habits or bodily manipulations, such as gum chewing, cigarette smoking, doodling, nose picking, or hair twirling.

In contrast to the more calm or placid thumb suckers, nail biters at any age are described as hyperactive or fidgety. Most persons bite their nails in moments of fear or stress, such as when they fear disapproval, read an especially sad, scary, or exciting story; take a test; face a battle; etc.

PSYCHODYNAMIC FACTORS

Nail biting seems most related to tension states associated with real or imagined danger or excitement. Viets[56] found that there was a greater frequency of tense home situations among nail biters and commented on the presence of broken homes and alcoholic parents. Often the parent of a nail biter has been, or continues to be, a nail biter himself, and overprotection is not uncommon.

Many authors feel that finger and thumb sucking serve a definite need for oral gratification in the infant, with nail biting serving a similar purpose in the older child. Since nail biting often begins during the phallic period, it may be an unconscious and displaced form of masturbatory activity. However, in contrast to thumb sucking, it is an intrinsically destructive activity. Thus, it may also serve a self-destructive purpose. In effect, it involves injury to the child and may function as a possible self-punishment for destructive and unacceptable thoughts and fantasies. The mechanism of turning against the self may here be paramount.

Nail biting may also be seen as the response of a generally compliant child to the myriad rules, regulations, and demands placed on him or her, particularly if the child is not very flexible, does not receive positive support and feedback, or attain success. Disappointment and anger are then expressed by nail biting. This is both an indirect form of hostility which is provocative to adults (who regard it as "disgusting") and the payment for this act (the hostility is also turned inward in retaliation).

It is clear, however, that nail biting itself is not indicative of any psychopathology, nor is there any particular family constellation or personality type which is a *sine qua non* for nail biting.

TREATMENT

The most efficacious treatment is directed at removal of the causes of tension responsible for nail biting. Treatment per se is usually not indicated in mild cases, as the nail biting will generally be replaced by some more acceptable activity at a later age. Nail biting is said to be lessened when there is opportunity for more vigorous muscular or athletic activity, as well as more protection from the avoidable forms of excitement or stress. It has been suggested that obtaining the child's cooperation through the use of star charts (a form of positive reinforcement), or the purchase of a manicure set (which may enlist the child's pride or vanity), may be helpful in diminishing the symptom. For younger children, occupation with distracting toys, activities, or hobbies may lessen tension and diminish opportunities for nail biting.

For more severe nail biting, treatment should be directed toward eliciting and dealing with the responsible intrapsychic and environmental factors, thus responding not to the symptom but to its cause. Although the literature is full of descriptions of devices and restraints designed to prevent the hand from reaching the mouth, as well as noxious tasting substances, which make biting or chewing of nails or fingers unpleasant, taken in aggregate, these seem to have little effect. In fact, these approaches may well become punitive and thus worsen an already stressful situation. In addition, they are likely to complicate the parent-child relationship and provide another area in which parent and child can battle. Indeed, the amount and intensity of attention paid to the nail biting may in itself serve as a reinforcer.

In older children, aversive conditioning has been used (with the consent and co-operation of the child), as has positive reinforcement. This is particularly likely to be invoked when the symptom persists after the more basic tension generating conflict has been dealt with. As in all such approaches, attention must be given to the underlying problems which may remain after alleviation of the symptom.

Rhythmic Body Movements

Rhythmic motor habits such as rocking and head-banging are quite common in infants and toddlers. Rocking may be seen during sleep or the waking state. The baby gets up on hands and knees and rocks back and forth, often so violently as to move or break the crib or play-pen, or even to hurt himself. Head-banging is a rhythmic motor habit in which the child repeatedly strikes his head against a solid object, often the head of the crib. It is often accompanied by rocking.

In infancy, these generally represent benign, self-limited conditions which are associated with normal development, and which terminate around the second birthday. In older children, these may be part of more serious disorders, such as organic brain syndromes, mental retardation, or autism. In such cases, these habits are components of the specific cluster of self-destructive or bizarre symptoms which define the illness. Head-banging, and occasional rocking, can also be seen in blind children who are otherwise normal.

HISTORY

These rhythmic motor habits are well known in the pediatric and psychiatric literature.[36] Spitz[52] noted a high incidence of body rocking, but no head-banging, in institutionalized children and attributed this to a disturbed mother-child relationship. Anna Freud[14] reported head-banging by institutionalized children, relating it to institutional life, while Kravitz and associates[27] emphasized the response to auditory and tactile stimulation, which was a distinguishing characteristic of head-banging as opposed to body rocking.

FREQUENCY AND INCIDENCE

In his 1949 report, Lourie[36] noted the presence of rhythmic motor habits in 15 to 20 percent of a pediatric clinic population. He observed that incidence was only half as frequent in private pediatric practice. Both rocking and head-banging first appear in the latter half of the first year of life, and most commonly when the infant is moving from one developmental stage to another. Thus, rocking may begin, or become more pronounced, when the child is about to go from sitting to standing, or from crawling to walking. Head-banging is often accompanied by rocking. In about 50 percent of cases, the rocking appears first and may continue after the head-banging stops. As a rule, these habits cease by the second birthday, but in about 5 percent they may persist for months or even years. A small but significant number of children maintain these behaviors until age ten. On a more limited level, rocking has been seen briefly as normal in early adolescence. These habits are at least twice as common in boys as in girls.

Rhythmic movements are more common in the first child in the family, less so in the second, and increasing less so therafter. Head-banging occurs in other children in the family only 20 percent of the time. Very few of these children are thumb suckers (about 10 percent as opposed to the usual reported incidence of 30 to 50 percent of a normal pediatric clinic population). Few have associated temper tantrums (but many were not yet of the age at which such behaviors were more likely to occur).

ETIOLOGY

There is no specific etiology known. The age of onset tends to support the theory that the rhythmic movements serve initially as tension relieving phenomena and as a means of satisfying maturational instinctual needs as well. It has been noted that the age of onset corresponds to the average age of eruption of the lateral and central incisors, with exacerbation of the habit at the time of eruption of a new group of teeth. The absence of crying with rocking and head-banging suggests that pain, if present, may be neutralized by the kinesthetic, auditory, and rhythmic motor sensations or pleasures. Rhythmic motor movements are also seen when a child's or infant's movements are retricted, for example, during confinement to bed or to a cast, thus supporting the concept of tension release. Development is normal as reflected in the EEG and neurological examination.

PSYCHODYNAMICS

In the presence of such incomprehensible and dramatic motoric behavior, parents often fear that such intense movements represent a psychological disorder. In fact, however, disturbing emotional factors in the environment do not usually seem to be present. In two-thirds of the youngsters evaluated by Kravitz and associates,[27] the mother-child relationship was judged to be good. In about one-fourth of the cases, there was separation of mother and child by death, divorce, hospitalization, institutionalization, or mother working. No specific psychopathology was noted.

The rhythmic body movements have been described as a purposeful response to inner or external sources of tension, which the infant then brings under his own control. There is a giving up of interest in other people at this time in a somewhat "autistic" manner. Freud felt that the head-banging of institutionalized children represented self-directed aggression against the child's own body and was related to separation and institutional life. Infants who engage in these activities are felt to have considerable energy but to be slow to engage in new activities or approach people. There is no correlation with the development of later personality disturbance in children whose only "abnormality" consists of rhythmic body habits.

Children become aware of the anxiety of their parents and may maintain the habit in order to obtain their parents' attention. Secondary gain can thus cause a habit to persist beyond the usual age of disappearance, especially in a disordered parent-child relationship. When the habits are associated with severe underlying conditions such as mental deficiency or psychosis, their significance must be evaluated in the context of the total symptomatology.

TREATMENT

In most youngsters with rhythmic motor habits, the activities will cease spontaneously and no specific treatment is necessary. However, some of the movements can become violent enough to injure the child or damage the surroundings, as well as create noise or disturbance. This raises the possibility of putting stress on the parent-child relationship, a stress that flows from the habits themselves. Therapy may, therefore, be useful in reducing the activity. The replacement of the rhythmic movement with a rhythmic auditory stimulus, such as a metronome or hand tapping to synchronize with the rhythmic movement of the child was suggested by Lourie.[36] Outlets for more purposeful and acceptable rhythmic motor activities such as dancing, swinging, etc. should be encouraged. Chronic head-bangers should have a complete physical and neurological evaluation, as well as psychological investigation. In particularly violent, disturbing, and tenacious cases, sedatives and tranquilizers in small amounts may be helpful in breaking the cycle. In severe cases, a helmet may be needed to protect the head. In situations where the movements are manifestations of an underlying physical and/or psychological disorder, treatment should be directed at the primary condition.

Trichotillomania

DESCRIPTION

Hair pulling leading to alopecia, with or without trichophagia, represents one end of a continuum of activities involving the hair. The associated disorders include fingering, stroking, and twirling, as well as the intensified brushing, patting, and hair arranging of adolescence. The hair may be pulled out in patches and then eaten, caressed, or discarded.

HISTORY

According to Greenberg and Sarner (p. 482)[19] the term "trichotillomania" was first used by Halopeau in 1889 to describe "an irresistible urge to pull one's hair." In spite of its common occurrence, especially in its milder forms, little is found in the psychiatric literature about the syndrome. Clinically, it is more amply described by the dermatologists to whose attention it primarily comes.

Barahal[5] reported on a large series primarily taken from an older and institutionalized population. Kanner[23] described two mentally retarded children whose hair pulling was one of several patterns of physical manipulation. Buxbaum[9] gave a detailed account of the treatment of two young girls whose hair pulling seemed a kind of fetishism.

FREQUENCY AND INCIDENCE

Females with this complaint far outnumber males. Case reports cover the age span from toddlerhood through adulthood. The paucity of case reports or reviews prevents the determination of more specific age groupings. Clinicians agree, however, that the hair pulling, which may represent increased body manipulation (like thumb sucking or nail biting), is an extension of normal behavior. It is increased again during adolescence. A small number have a family history of alopecia, but other siblings rarely have the same symptom.

CLINICAL COURSE

The majority of youngsters who pull their hair in childhood probably do not come to the attention of a psychiatrist. Greenberg and Sarner[19] reported that in more than 50 percent of their cases, there was some other symptom present that lead to seeking psychiatric help. Most patients saw a general physician, pediatrician, or internist before psychiatric referral, and again, more than 50 percent of all their patients were treated with salves, steroids, or ultraviolet irradiation for a variety of skin conditions. Over half were worked up for thyroid dysfunction, although the youngsters studied were euthyroid. Few had significant dermatologic disease per se, although many complained of itching or burning of the scalp at some time or another. One could then question whether the condition could be precipitated by a dermatologic disorder of the scalp, causing increased awareness of scalp sensation, followed by a secondary irritation related to the initial rubbing, scratching, and manipulating.

PSYCHODYNAMIC FEATURES

Greenberg and Sarner[19] emphasized the high proportion of antecedent actual or threatened significant object loss prior to the onset of hair pulling. Moves, birth of a sibling, death of a sibling, and illness of a parent were present in the histories. Two-thirds of their patients reported moderate to severe depressive episodes which usually began before hair pulling was manifest. These depressive trends were defended against, as was the hair pulling itself, by denial and rumination. The pervasive guilt and anxiety, as well as the hypochondriacal concern with body image, seemed to be related to the intense efforts of the affected youngsters and their parents to find a "physical" cause or cure for their hair loss.

The psychology of the symptom appears to be multi-determined. Symbolically, hair represents beauty, attractiveness, and virility. Sexual conflicts can be displaced onto the hair which may be cut without pain and which will grow back easily. The expression "tearing one's hair" represents despair and grief. Saving or eating hair can represent oral regression with incorporation of and identification with mother. The more common auto-erotic stroking and pulling of hair during childhood, thus, is also a sign of the incomplete separation from mother's body; the children use part of their own bodies as transitional objects. This is accompanied by a high frequency of preoccupation with eating and overeating, and the findings of depression and real or threatened loss through death or separation.

Hair pulling can be aggression turned against the self, or punishment to avoid the retaliation of a sadistic parent, as well as symbolic death or castration for unacceptable sexual or destructive wishes. It may also represent a self-referred depressive equivalent of the rage directed towards the object. Then again, it can be a more acceptable form of masturbation in which the child is reminded of his or her own existence by the feeling that hair pulling elicits.

In girls, hair pulling, leading to alopecia, may represent the denial of femininity, and the girl may thus attempt to resolve the oedipal conflict, identifying with father, while wishing to be close to mother (Greenberg and Sarner[19] reported two patients whose alopecia was in the distribution of their father's baldness). For the male child, the self-inflicted castration emphasizes that he is not in competition with father for mother, but is rather like him in his baldness.

Hairlessness is often seen to be innocent childishness. As genital hair develops in puberty (along with active sexual fantasies and longings), there is an increase in hair pulling. In one case of a fourteen-year-old girl with anorexia nervosa and trichotillomania, as the condition progressed, along with the loss of hair, there was also a loss of her breast contours and menstrual periods. Collectively these represented a regression to childhood innocence.

FAMILIAL AND INTERPERSONAL DYNAMICS

Although nonspecific for hair pulling per se, as an expression of parent-child conflict, the histories and families of many of these patients are pathologic. Apparently, parental concern or preoccupation with hair is communicated to the child, as is demonstrated by the upsurge of anxiety in the mothers of adolescents whose hair begins to grow back. Apparently, these parents have difficulty allowing the increasing adolescent desires for autonomy and mastery to go unchallenged.

The mothers of youngsters with trichotillomania have been described as ambivalent, competitive, double binding, alternatively infantilizing and parentifying, and critical of hostile or aggressive behavior by their children. During their own development, the mothers themselves have experienced feelings of unmet dependency needs and regarded their parents with resentment and disgust.

The fathers tended to be helpless, passive, and ineffectual men who were dominated, manipulated, and overwhelmed by their wives, and given to expressing their aggression more covertly. Weak and aloof at home, many were more successful in their work or social experiences outside the family.

The mother-daughter relationships tend to be ambivalent. They are characterized by hostile dependency and mutual fears of separation. The intense love-hate relationship tends to exclude the father as well as the other siblings, and, for the youngsters themselves, it spreads to anyone outside of the family relationships. The daughters become the ambivalent recipients of their mothers' own unfulfilled ambitions and are often given the burden of obtaining the longed for fulfillment. The mothers can then respond with anxiety to their daughters' strivings, causing the youngsters to fear their own competitiveness or desires for autonomy. Within this context, the hair pulling is regarded as deliberate. An immense power struggle ensues as to which person is in charge of the hair (or of the wig used to cover the bald areas).

In families where sons have this condition, there does not tend to be this degree of ambivalent or symbiotic conflict between the boys and their mothers. With their sons, the mothers are more often overprotective or seductive, while the boys learn to defend against their own aggression.

SPECIFIC THERAPEUTIC METHODS

By and large, the therapy should be directed at the cause, the child's developmental struggles and the disturbed parent-child relationships, rather than at the symptom itself. Depending on age and specific dynamics, individual child therapy, with collaborative treatment of parents, would deal with all the issues involved in the disorderd functioning. Family therapy or group therapy has been quite successful with adolescents and their families. In the situation where the child is retarded, or where development is otherwise normal and the family picture is less pathologic, behavioral therapy, to remove the symptom, has been successful. In the wake of such treatment re-occurrence has been rare, nor has the development of other symptoms been noted.

Masturbation

INTRODUCTION

Masturbation is a normal auto-erotic activity which appears at certain development stages. Its inclusion in a section on "habit disorders" stems from the historical definition of masturbation as a pathological activity. At the present time, masturbation must be viewed in the context of physical and psychic growth and development, as well as from the outlook of the socio-cultural setting within which it occurs. Even in sexually permissive western society, most adults continue to have some conscious or unconscious anxiety, shame, or guilt about masturbatory fantasy or activity.

DESCRIPTION

In 1967, the American Psychoanalytic Association defined masturbation as a "volitional genitally-directed rhythmic self-stimulation which produces sexual pleasure." In general, males are more apt to engage in manual manipulation. Females may use thigh rubbing and pressure, or rubbing with objects (e.g., toys), as well as using fingers to manipulate the clitoris and genital area.

In infancy, masturbation begins with the baby's discovery and exploration of body orifices and sensations. Kinsey described rhythmic body movements (pelvic thrusts) with tension and release in infant males as early as five months. Except for the absence of ejaculation, this seemed to correspond to orgasm.[25] In general, however, manual masturbation requires some control of smaller muscles. Hence, earlier in development, other autoerotic activities such as rocking tend to occur.

During the first years of life, masturbatory activity is ubiquitous and may be viewed by parents with varying degrees of tolerance. As the child develops sphincter control and becomes more socialized, parental concern over persistent or noticeable masturbation increases. The timing of a request for outside intervention is based on a number of factors, including the child's behavior and the parents' background, concerns and conflicts about masturbation.

HISTORY

Masturbation has been described as "harmful," "sinful" and responsible for a number of diseases including schizophrenia, general paresis of the insane, "early insanity," and a host of abnormal mental and physical behaviors. The Biblical injunction against withdrawal (onanism) as a means of contraception has also been considered an injunction against masturbation. The earlier pediatric and psychiatric literature contained many warnings about masturbation and often described management in judgmental or moral terms.

FREQUENCY AND INCIDENCE

Masturbatory activity begins in the first year of life; at one time or another it is seen in almost all children. Spitz[52] noted that in the absence of good interaction between mother and child there was an absence of genital play. He postulated that routine care of the child stimulates a variety of pleasurable sensations which the child then attempts to reproduce. Similarly, deprived children were more likely to engage in auto-erotic movements such as rocking or head-banging.

By the third year of life, the exploratory behavior becomes modified and is seen as more definitive masturbatory activity. These patterns diminish in frequency and intensity as the child reaches school age. This shift is related to superego development and resolution of the Oedipus complex, as well as to an increased focus on skill development (cognition, socialization). Retarded children may continue to engage in obvious masturbatory activity, much to the distress of parents and teachers. This activity is related to ego deficits and delayed development.

In latency, with maturation, defenses work more effectively and adequately. Sublimation and repression occur, and masturbation is far less frequent (although it may still persist). In latency, both the activity and the fantasies are repressed, allowing for the development of sublimated derivatives in the form of intellectual skills, game play, and creativity.

With the onset of puberty, all auto-erotic activities increase. Genital masturbation occurs in response to sexual tensions. The anxiety associated with masturbation may be related to shame and guilt, and the associated fantasies contain themes of death or loss of control. It is these fantasies in particular rather than the action or the sensation as such that evoke the untoward reactions. Francis and Marcus[13] have noted that it is in adolescence that the degree of indulgence or prohibition of masturbation becomes most problematic. Masturbation may also be in the service of growth and development, foster object relatedness, and assist in the delineation of inner and outer reality. The bizarre or perverse fantasies accompanying masturbation may be regressions in the service of the ego. Genital masturbation, especially in the boy, may serve as an anchor to genital levels of development. Basically it can subserve many functions. It can be a direct expression of a yearning for pleasure; it can be a source of self-comforting in the face of external frustration; it provides a site for sexual experimentation through fantasy, and a compensation for failure when sexual activity with others does not work out.

ETIOLOGY

Since masturbation per se is not an indication of pathology, its presence and persistence take on different meanings at different times of life. Arlow[2] observed that symptom formation insulated blocking of tension discharge through masturbation. Excessive masturbation may be linked to castration anxiety, incestuous fantasies, and conflicts about aggressive urges. Malone[37] studied children in lower socio-economic families in which there was much aggressive acting out by adults in the environment. He noted that among such children there was less overt auto-erotic activity. Meers[41] analyzed ghetto children with inhibitions, character disturbances, and premature sexualization of activities. He noted that overt masturbatory activity persisted in spite of parental prohibition and punishment.

In adolescence, many youngsters masturbate excessively as a way of avoiding even small amounts of tension. The practice may interfere with maturation and the development of frustration tolerance. Many nonsexual activities, such as reckless driving and accident proneness, may be masturbatory equivalents or substitutes.

Inadequate suppression of masturbation may inhibit relations with peers (particularly of the opposite sex) and delay the beginning of heterosexual activities. In lonely, isolated young people such turning to the self for solace and gratification can become habitual. This usually brings with it intense conflicts involving guilt, shame, and self-devaluation.

The absence or inhibition of masturbation may also be problematic and significant of difficulties in early separation and individuation, autistic or anaclitic withdrawal, depression, inhibitions, etc. Once again, the activity per se must be considered in concert with historical and developmental information, as well as the presence of other signs or symptoms.

The role of the parents is an important one. It is their anxiety, conflicts, and concerns which define what is, and what is not, "excessive." Their response to these manipulations may precipitate or add to difficult parent-child relationships. The role of parental responses in etiology and management should be thoroughly explored.

TREATMENT

The prime factor in initiating treatment is determining the cause of the symptom. Occasionally, masturbation exists in isolation, and the meaning of this behavior must then be explored in detail. More likely, it is part of a constellation of symptoms and problems representing developmental lag, deviation or disturbance; it may be associated with neurotic conflicts or with more severe pathology. Treatment is primarily psychological and should be aimed at understanding or resolving conflicts. When masturbation is part of a more complicated problem, its treatment should be part of the total treatment plan. As the child improves, this will be reflected, among other ways, in a diminution of masturbatory activity. In the case of the inhibited or deprived child, of course, the reverse will be true; improvement may be signalled by the appearance of "normal/developmental" masturbatory activity.

In the case of excessive masturbation, help and encouragement can be given a child to promote socialization and lessen the obvious activity. However, parents, physicians, and teachers should avoid too strong prohibitions which can lead to increased shame, guilt, and anxiety. The numerous approaches and devices developed to minimize accessibility of the genitals (e.g., restraints) should be avoided. This approach only increases the likelihood of symptom substitution; more than that, it increases the evocation of shame or guilt, without understanding and devoting attention to the etiology of the problem.

Behavioral therapy may be useful in treating retarded children as part of socialization activity and general strengthening of ego functions and can be considered as part of a total treatment plan.

REFERENCES

1. American Psychiatric Association, Committee on Nomenclature and Statistics, *Diagnostic and Statistical Manual of Mental Disorders*, 2nd ed. (DSM-II), American Psychiatric Association, Washington, D.C., 1968.

2. ARLOW, J., "Masturbation and Symptom Formation," *Journal of the American Psychoanalytic Association, 1:* 45–58, 1953.

3. BAKWIN, H., "Erotic Feelings in Infants and Young Children," *American Journal of Diseases of Children, 126(1):*52–54, 1973.

4. ———, and BAKWIN, R. M., *Clinical Management of Behavior Disorders in Children*, pp. 427–438, W. B. Saunders, Philadelphia, 1966.

5. BARAHAL, H., "Psychopathology of Hair Plucking (Trichotillomania)," *Psychoanalytic Review, 27:*291–310, 1940.

6. BENTLER, P. M., "A Note on the Treatment of Adolescent Sex Problems," *Journal of Child Psychology and Psychiatry, 9(2):*125–129, 1968.

7. BERNSTEIN, A., *Some Relations Between Techniques of Feeding and Training During Infancy and Certain Behavior in Childhood*, Genetic Psychological Monographs, vol. 51, pp. 3–44, 1955.

8. BORNSTEIN, B., "Masturbation in the Latency Child," in Eissler, R. S., et al. (Eds.), *The Psychoanalytic Study of the Child*, vol. 8, pp. 65–78, International Universities Press, New York, 1953.

9. BUXBAUM, E., "Hair Pulling and Fetishism," in Eissler, R. S., et al. (Eds.), *The Psychoanalytic Study of the Child*, vol. 15, pp. 243–260, International Universities Press, New York, 1960.

10. DAVIS, H., et al., "Effects of Cup, Bottle, and Breast Feeding on Oral Activities of Newborn Infants," *Pediatrics, 2:*549–558, 1948.

11. EIDELBERG, L., "A Contribution to the Study of the Masturbation Fantasy," *International Journal of Psychoanalysis, 26:*127–137, 1945.

12. ENGLISH, O., and PEARSON, G., *Common Neuroses of Children and Adults*, p. 96, Norton, New York, 1937.

13. FRANCIS, J. J., and MARCUS, I. M., "Masturbation: A Developmental View," in Marcus, I. M., and Francis, J. J. (Eds.), *Masturbation from Infancy to Senescence*, International Universities Press, New York, 1975.

14. FREUD, A. J., and BURLINGHAM, D., *Infants without Families*, International Universities Press, New York, 1944.

15. FREUD, S., "Three Essays on the Theory of Sexuality," in *The Standard Edition of the Complete Psychological Works of Sigmund Freud*, vol. 7, Hogarth Press, London, 1953.

16. GESELL, A., and ILG, F., *Feeding Behavior of Infants*, Lippincott, Philadelphia, 1937.

17. GIBNEY, H. A., "Masturbation: An Invitation for an Interpersonal Relationship," *Perspectives in Psychiatric Care, 19(3):*128–134, 1972.

18. GLENN, J., "Testicular and Scrotal Masturbation," *International Journal of Psychoanalysis, 50(3):*353–362, 1969.

19. GREENBERG, H., and SARNER, C., "Trichotillomania, Symptom and Syndrome," *Archives of General Psychiatry, 12:*482–489, 1965.

20. Group for the Advancement of Psychiatry, Committee on Child Psychiatry, *Psychopathological Disorders of Childhood: Theoretical Considerations and a Proposed Classification*, vol. 6, Report No. 62, Group for the Advancement of Psychiatry, New York, 1966.

21. HAMMERMAN, S., "Masturbation and Character," *Journal of the American Psychoanalytic Association, 9:* 287–311, 1961.

22. HARLEY, M., "Masturbation Contacts," in Lorand, S., and Schneer, H. I., *Adolescents*, Harper, New York, 1961.

23. KANNER, L., *Child Psychiatry*, 3rd ed., Charles C Thomas, Springfield, Ill., 1957.

24. KESTENBERG, J. S., "A Developmental Approach to Disturbances of Sex-Specific Identity," *International Journal of Psychoanalysis, 52(1):*99–102, 1971.

25. KINSEY, A. C., et al., *Sexual Behavior in the Human Male*, W. B. Saunders, Philadelphia, 1948.

26. KLEEMAN, J. A., "Genital Self-Discovery During a Boy's Second Year: A Follow-Up," in Eissler, R. S., et al. (Eds.), *The Psychoanalytic Study of the Child*, vol. 21, pp. 358–392, International Universities Press, New York, 1966.

27. KRAVITZ, H., et al., "A Study of Head Banging in Infants and Children," *Diseases of the Nervous System, 21:*203–208, 1960.

28. KRIS, E., "Some Comments and Observations on Early Autoerotic Activities," in Eissler, R. S., et al. (Eds.), *The Psychoanalytic Study of the Child*, vol. 6, pp. 95–116, International Universities Press, New York, 1951.

29. LAMPL-DE GROOT, J., "On Masturbation and Its Influence on General Development," in Eissler, R. S., et al. (Eds.), *The Psychoanalytic Study of the Child*, vol. 5, pp. 153–174, International Universities Press, New York, 1950.

30. LANGFORD, W., "Disturbance in Mother-Infant Relationship Leading to Apathy, Extra-Nutritional Sucking and Hairball," in Caplan, G. (Ed.), *Emotional Problems of Early Childhood*, pp. 59–76, Basic Books, New York, 1957.

31. LAUFER, M., "The Body Image, the Function of Masturbation, and Adolescence," in Eissler, R. S., et al. (Eds.), *The Psychoanalytic Study of the Child*, vol. 23, pp. 114–137, International Universities Press, New York, 1968.

32. LEVINE, M. I., "Pediatric Observations on Masturbation in Children," in Eissler, R. S., et al. (Eds.), *The Psychoanalytic Study of the Child*, vol. 6, pp. 117–126, International Universities Press, New York, 1961.

33. LEVY, D., "On the Problem of Movement Restraint," *American Journal of Orthopsychiatry, 14:*644–646, 1944.

34. ———, "Finger Sucking and Accessory Movements in Early Infancy; Etiologic Study," *American Journal of Psychiatry, 7:*881–918, 1928.

35. LEWIS, M., "Psychosexual Development and Sexual Behavior in Children," *Connecticut Medicine, 32(6):*437–443, 1968.

36. LOURIE, R., "The Role of Rhythmic Patterns in Childhood," *American Journal of Psychiatry, 105:*653–660, 1949.

37. MALONE, A., and MASSLER, M., "Index of Nail Biting in Children," *Journal of Abnormal and Social Psychology, 47:*193–202, 1952.

38. MARCUS, I. M., and FRANCIS, J. J. (Eds.), *Masturba-*

tion from Infancy to Senescence, International Universities Press, New York, 1975.

39. MASSLER, M., and MALONE, A., "Nailbiting—A Review," Journal of Pediatrics, 36:523–531, 1950.

40. MAZER, D. B., and MAHRER, A. R., "Developmental Factors in Masturbation: Family Background, Antecedents and Later Personality Patterns," Journal of Psychology, 79(1):21–27, 1971.

41. MEERS, D. R., "Contributions of a Ghetto Culture to Symptom Formation: Psychoanalytic Studies of Ego Anomalies in Childhood," in Eissler, R. S., et al. (Eds.), The Psychoanalytic Study of the Child, vol. 25, pp. 209–230, International Universities Press, New York, 1970.

42. MONROE, J. T., JR., and ABSE, D., "Psychopathology of Trichotillomania and Trichophagy," Psychiatry, 26:95–103, 1963.

43. ORLANSKY, H., "Infant Care and Personality," Psychological Bulletin, 46:1–48, 1949.

44. Panel, "Masturbation," Francis, J. J. (reporter), Journal of the American Psychoanalytic Association, 16(1):95–112, 1968.

45. Panel, "Masturbation," Marcus, I. M. (reporter), Journal of the American Psychoanalytic Association, 10:91–101, 1962.

46. ROBINOWITZ, C., "Cross Cultural Observations of Child Rearing Practices," Unpublished data collected at University of Miami, pp. 22–37, 1972.

47. RUTTER, M., "Normal Psychosexual Development," Journal of Child Psychology and Psychiatry, 11(4):259–283, 1971.

48. SCHWARTZMAN, J., "Onychophagy," Archives of Pediatrics, 56:599–604, 1939.

49. SEARS, R., and WISE, G., "Relation of Cup Feeding in Infancy to Thumb Sucking and the Oral Drive," American Journal of Orthopsychiatry, 20:123–133, 1950.

50. SILLMAN, J., "Finger Sucking Serial Dental Study From Birth to Five Years," New York State Journal of Medicine, 42:2024–2028, 1942.

51. SPIEGEL, N. T., "An Infantile Fetish and Its Persistence Into Young Womanhood, Maturational Stages of a Fetish," in Eissler, R. S., et al. (Eds.), The Psychoanalytic Study of the Child, vol. 22, pp. 315–328, International Universities Press, New York, 1967.

52. SPITZ, R., and WOLF, K., "Autoeroticism, Some Empirical Findings and Hypotheses on Three of Its Manifestations in the First Year of Life," in Eissler, R. S., et al. (Eds.), The Psychoanalytic Study of the Child, Vol. 3/4, pp. 85–120, International Universities Press, New York, 1949.

53. STERLING, M., "Use of Hair as Bi-Sexual Symbol," Psychoanalytic Review, 42:363–364, 1954.

54. TAUSK, V., "On Masturbation," in Eissler, R. S., et al. (Eds.), The Psychoanalytic Study of the Child, vol. 6, pp. 61–79, International Universities Press, New York, 1951.

55. TOOLEY, K., "A Developmental Problem of Late Adolescence: Case Report," Psychiatry, 31(1):69–83, 1968.

56. VIETS, L., "An Inquiry into the Significance of Nail Biting," Smith College Studies of Social Work, 2:128–145, 1931–1932.

---

40 / Psychoses of Adolescence

Sherman C. Feinstein and Derek Miller

No comprehensive overview of the incidence of emotional mental health exists at the high school level, but it has been conservatively estimated that 10 to 15 percent of the adolescent population, at some point in their development, will manifest a reaction requiring diagnostic evaluation or treatment.[14] The examination of statistical reports of inpatient programs indicates that approximately 10 percent of admissions are labeled as psychotic reactions, and a further 10 percent are diagnosed as adolescent schizophrenia.

The use of the term psychosis has led to much confusion and requires careful definition, particularly in the disorders of adolescence. Menninger[38] warns that the use of the term may imply a specific disease rather than a description of various forms of the "penultimate stage of organismic disequilibration and disorganization." In this chapter, the authors are attempting to make a clear distinction between psychosis (which mani-

fests itself as an altered state of consciousness with marked regression, fragmentation, and dissolution and is variously called schizophrenic psychosis, overt schizophrenia, as well as a transitional state) and schizophrenia proper (in which these symptoms may be present along with a pattern of isolation, apathy, poor object relationships, internal disorganization and incompetence and are accompanied by a disorder of thinking and feeling).

Within the developmental frame of reference, it is generally true that the earlier and more severe the impairment of the mother-child relationship, the more severe the developmental deficits. When a disruptive process is present in childhood, the achievement of self-structures and interpersonal relationships is impeded. Later stages of growth are likely to manifest a failure of integration of the personality, disturbances in social relationships, failure to form a sense of identity, and may result in the development of a thought disorder.

The classification of psychopathological disorders proposed by the Group for the Advancement of Psychiatry[25] states that during adolescence, psychotic reactions result in behavior which deviates from age appropriate responses. Psychotic disorder may be revealed by various behavioral clusters: impairment of emotional relationships manifested in aloofness or preoccupation and exaggeration of peer relationships; disturbances in sensory perception; bizarre behavior and motility patterns; resistance to change; outbursts of intense anxiety and panic; impairment of a sense of identity; and interferences with intellectual development.

The DSM-II classification[2] is incomplete concerning psychotic reactions of adolescence. Acute schizophrenic episode (295.4) is described as an acute onset of schizophrenic symptoms associated with confusion, perplexity, ideas of reference, emotional turmoil, dissociation, excitement, depression, and fear. Patients usually recover within weeks but disorganization may become progressive. Schizophrenia, childhood type (295.8), is reserved for those cases in which schizophrenic symptoms appear before puberty. Transient situational disturbances (307) and behavior disorders of adolescence (308) do not apply to the psychotic reactions of adolescence.

The DSM-III[1] classification will attempt to provide a broader approach to clinical diagnosis, making use of a multi-axial system that considers developmental disorders in children and adolescents (Axis II) in addition to the clinical psychiatric syndromes (Axis I), severity of psycho-social stresses (Axis IV), and the highest level of adaptive function in the previous year (Axis V). In the section listing conditions manifesting themselves exclusively in adolescence, psychosis is not listed as a clinical entity. In those adolescents with chronic handicaps (organic brain syndromes, mental retardation, or severe emotional impairment), the social and physiological pressures of adolescence may result in the development of a psychotic state which is secondary to the primary medical diagnosis (Axis III).

The following special categories of psychotic reactions are characteristic of adolescence and are predicated upon developmental considerations: (1) acute confusional state; (2) schizophrenic disorder, adult type; and (3) other psychoses of adolescence—regressive pictures of psychotic degree, transient catatonic states, and marked dissociative states with hysterical features.

The Psychotic Syndrome

A psychosis has been defined as "a complicated structure which may manifest itself in different ways, not only from one patient to another, but in the same patient at different times. Manifestations were formerly taken for the diseases themselves, and even yet it is of practical value to emphasize them as pictures of morbid states and as syndromes."[6] This concept presupposes different etiologies for different clusters of psychotic disorganization. Any of these syndromes can be understood as the result of an individual's aberrant response to stress, a reaction which involves both organic and emotional components.

Psychotic symptoms are designed to restore homeostasis. They may include: pervasive feelings of sadness, bizarre or excessive overactivity, autistic regression, extreme self-absorption, delusional preoccupation, hallucinations, and the acute discharge of sexual and aggressive impulses in an inappropriate manner. These reactions occur because the perceived stress causes the individual to experience actual or potentially intolerable experiences of helpless disintegration. The ensuing behaviors are, in addition, reconstitutive and represent an attempt at coping.

An individual's ability to cope with stress depends upon the vulnerability of the personality in in the face of the intensity of perceived stress. Perception is modified by neuro-physiological processes as well as by ego defenses. Psychoses, therefore, may occur because of aberrant neuro-endocrinological responses produced by genetic abnormality, drug toxicity with mind distorting drugs, physical illness including brain tumor, developmental stresses occuring in psychologically vulnerable individuals, and conflictual life situations. Psychosis can be understood as an extreme state of personality disorganization with organic and emotional components in which the individual's ability to interpret reality and behave appropriately is impaired. The altered state of consciousness may last a variable period of time, and sometimes its expression may be consciously controlled.

Recent research in the study of psychotic states emphasizes the structural aspects of the process.[7] Psychotic experiences are described as having form (heightened awareness, broadening of the experiential field, alterations in the sense of self, and perceptual and cognitive changes), and content (idiosyncratic memories, conflicts, and wishes), and their occurrence is related to areas of individual vulnerability to conflict. An individual possessing fragile character defenses or neuro-endocrinological vulnerability responds to the configuration of forces which overwhelms these defenses. This results in an impasse which leads to an altered state of consciousness; in childhood and adolescence, this severely impedes developmental progress.

Hecker in 1871 first termed a psychical disorder occurring during puberty "hebephrenia" (or Jugendirresein).[26] Kraepelin[34] denied a causal relationship between a subgroup of "dementia praecox" and puberty, stating that a large number of such outcomes occur in later adolescence. On the other hand, he observed that many psychotic reactions in adolescents had a favorable outcome, and this led him to conclude that adolescence could be a pathogenic factor.[45] This same conclusion was recently reiterated by Holzman and Grinker[28] in their studies of adolescent schizophrenia. Their data support the idea that serious psychopathology occurs, not only where there is social, intellectual, and physical incompetence, but also where stressful demands from societal expectations serve to potentiate disorganization.

Psychosis as a reaction and adolescence as a developmental phase have much in common. This may help explain the extreme vulnerability of adolescents to a wide variety of psychotic states. Adolescence is generally considered to be characterized by a loosening of ego structures derived from pressures from both emotional and physiological sources. These find expression in the form of aggressive and libidinal drives. The essential tasks of adolescence in the move to adulthood are directed toward achieving a modification of the unconscious idealizations of parents, the assumption of moral standards, the completion of sexual role identification, and the selection of an educational or career choice.[19] The establishment of a firm sense of self along with reformation of the ego-ideal, leads to a final consolidation of the superego and an adult identity.[21]

The manner in which adolescent tasks are accomplished is of great interest. Many authors have described the "second chance" available to the adolescent ego for revising earlier unresolved developmental conflicts. This is carried out by the dissolution of some ego structures during which regressive features are certain to appear. Anna Freud[17] wrote that intolerable anxiety produced by potentially close and threatening object relations may produce a defensive regression to the ego state of primary identification. Here the adolescent is dealing with the intense demands of object relationships along with certain heightened physiological processes resulting in a state of continuous alertness and vigilance and an increased sensitivity to stimuli.[20] The mechanism of partial regression to the phase of undifferentiated object relations is thus an essential step in eventually furthering ego development. During this process, the ego may show spurts in development accompanied by increased growth and mastery of intellectual pursuits and a general widening of interest in human endeavors.[14]

Similarly, research in the study of psychotic states has also emphasized the structural aspects of the process.[7] If comparisons between psychotic regression and normal adolescent process have validity, then our understanding of the psychotic process as a psychophysiological attempt to master overwhelming emotional and organic stress has important implications for theoretical and therapeutic explorations. The psychobiology of the altered state of conscioiusness, the psychic conflict, and the growth impasses all need further clarification; ultimately these may serve as an important breakthrough in the rapidly developing field of neuropsychophysiology.

Epidemiology

The importance of the epidemiological approach to mental illness has been emphasized by Henderson, Krupeinski, and Stoller.[27] Adolescence lends itself well to an epidemiological approach because this discrete age group, accessible to study while at school, is characterized by considerable physical, emotional, and social change which results in numerous pattern alterations condensed into a short time span. Many authors, however, believe normal adolescence is characterized by severe discomfort and turmoil. As a result, the difficulties in clarifying the diagnosis of psychotic reaction of adolescence make epidemiological study uncertain.

Holzman and Grinker[28] state that seventeen years is the high-risk age for the onset of the adult form of schizophrenic psychosis, with little variation across national boundaries. Mayer-Gross, Slater, and Roth[37] report that their study of first admissions to mental hospitals indicates that a marked increase in psychotic reactions occurs in the middle and late adolescent years. More adolescent males than females enter hospitals with schizophrenic psychosis and only in the adult years after age thirty-five does the ratio shift to a predominance of females.

Major methodological studies in the families of schizophrenic patients have attempted to evaluate the environmental, social, and genetic factors present. Studies of intrafamilial communication patterns, parental roles, and sexual attitudes suggest that an underlying factor or possibly a predisposition to schizophrenia exists in some families.[40]

Clinical Course of Adolescent Psychotic States

The early symptoms of psychotic reaction include heightened awareness, an intensification of sensory experiences, a broadening of the sense of the social field in which the individual lives, and alterations in the sense of self. Often there is externalization of conflicts with an increasing distortion of cognitive and perceptual experiences, and gradual development of a delusional system.

The content of the distorted thought processes is both idiosyncratic for the individual adolescent's experiential world and dependent on social system norms. The length of time the psychotic process lasts depends on the intensity of the stress, the strength of the adolescent's emotional resources, and the response of the environment to the process. Thus the psychotic experience is a defense against conflict, but it is also a form of communication about the individual's conflicts.

Initially there are early disturbances and fluctuations in perception and cognition. These distortions lead to attempts by the ego to cope and defend against the decompensation. If this fails, there results a pervasive experience of helplessness. Acute psychic pain then appears along with fear of loss of control, and finally an acute breakdown in reality testing which may be accompanied by panic dysphoria.

If there is successful resolution, a quiescent or chronic stage of psychosis occurs. Concept formation becomes aberrant and is associated with autistic preoccupation and interpretation of stimuli. The content of many of the delusions may indicate in advance the eventual mechanism of recovery.[16]

The phases of decompensation frequently seen are:

Stage 1. Conflict and impasse: a concatenation of developmental dilemmas frequently marks the onset of severe conflict; oscillations in mood may become overt.

Stage 2. A heightened awareness of the self: this ensues with a sense of urgency, a decreased need for sleep and a belief that something is about to happen; often there is an increase in visual and auditory acuity. Thoughts and perceptions begin to flood consciousness; emotions, particularly sexual feelings, increase in intensity.

Stage 3. Ideas of reference and influence become predominant. There is an increase in anxiety with progressive distortion of ideation and perception. Contamination of ideas and perceptions result in reality distortions which are frequently induced by religious, political, and philosophical conflicts.

Stage 4. Delusion formation is the final attempt to resolve the rapid disintegration of ego functions that is taking place. The delusions are usually understandable and based on the underlying distorted perceptions of the conflicted individual.

With the breaking down of control and the alteration of the experience of the self in the world, the patient may experience a certain relief. Perceptions can now be explored in their distorted form.

Reintegration is a variable process; its speed depends on the state of psychotic disintegration that has occurred. Often an admission to a hospital may produce immediate reintegration. On the other hand, on occasion, this can produce further decompensation. It is as if, for some individuals, hospitalization gives permission to regress and disintegrate. This response is not always clinically predictable. Supportive therapy which aims at clarifying reality may be helpful.

Acute Confusional Type

This type of psychotic reaction is often associated with confusion, complexity, ideas of reference, emotional turmoil, dreamlike dissociation, excitement, depression, or fear. It is considered in DSM-II (295.4) an acute schizophrenic episode. However, acute schizophrenia has a different clinical course and may require different specific therapeutic interventions. If acute confusional states, occurring during adolescence or post-adolescence, are treated as if they were schizophrenia, the prognosis may be worsened. For example, in an acute confusional state related to the developmental problems of the age period, too early treatment with phenothiazines is contraindicated, and hospitalization without appropriate support systems may produce an iatrogenic illness.

Acute confusional states are characterized by having an abrupt onset, often with intense anxiety, depression, confusion, depersonalization, and interference with the sense of identity. However, a true thought disorder or marked breakdown in reality testing is usually not seen. Any violence which may occur is usually directed against things rather than people and often occurs when an adolescent feels acutely overwhelmed by a perception of parent figures as being intrusive and powerful.

The acute confusional state which is associated with drug abuse has a different clinical course. The onset of such a state may be quite insidious. There are slowly developing changes in perception and behavior. Sometimes these may appear as an apparently explosive reaction to an overwhelming stress and may mimic the acute confusional state of identity confusion.

When adolescents suffering from acute confusional states are admitted to hospitals, it is advised to wait for some twenty-four to forty-eight hours before the use of phenothiazines is begun. In adolescents suffering from acute identity confusion, phenothiazines may worsen the situation because of the muscle splinting action of the medication. Adolescents who use physical activity to relieve tension may have this outlet interrupted, thus enhancing their confusion.

Hysterical-like features may occur in adolescents suffering from acute identity confusion. Jackson and Watzlawick[29] describe a situation in which young people feel trapped in a social nexus which limits their growth. At the same time, they find themselves in a stress situation from which there appears to be no escape. Among the other meanings, the psychotic episode is also an attempt to gain help and may assist the adolescent in influencing the surroundings to obtain such attention.

Sixty percent of patients who experience acute psychotic decompensation appear to experience manifest depressive symptoms; guilt, remorse, and perhaps suicidal thoughts.[10] These depressive symptoms are associated with ideas of being overwhelmed and helpless, and with the hopeless feeling that no one can possibly be satisfied.

Schizophrenic Disorder, Adult Type

The differentiation of adolescent schizophrenia into the classic subtypes; simple, paranoid, catatonic, and hebephrenic does not appear justified. The clinical descriptions of these syndromes were based on individuals who were hospitalized in inadequate therapeutic systems or who were untreated in an equally disturbed society at large.[39] However, no adequate therapy of psychiatric illness is possible without a working grasp of the psychological mechanisms of the disorder, its usual clinical course, and the age when it is likely to appear. The interrelationship of stress and support in family and society needs to be understood, along with the genetic, social, and psychological orgins of the personality which help explain the individual's perception of the world.

There is considerable argument over the clinical course of the schizophrenic syndrome. There are, however, two observations that can be offered. One is that schizophrenia is a reflection of the development over the years of increasingly inadequate ways of living with oneself and others. The second is that for a variety of reasons the individual perceives the environment as stressful and becomes overwhelmed with anxiety. This produces a stage of acute psychic pain which may eventually develop into panic. In its initial stage, this panic may or may not be apparent to an observer. This state of acute anxiety, which results in significant neuro-endocrine distortion, produces in time a psychological situation in which recent experiences are not used effectively and perception is distorted. The adolescent makes frantic and poorly co-ordinated efforts to resolve the experience of psychic disintegration caused by the acute schizophrenic experience. The psychotic resolution with its alteration of consciousness resolves the conflict in a spontaneous fashion. Under these circumstances, the diagnosis is likely to be confused with that of an acute confusional state. A possible hypothesis is that an emotionally supportive and highly reassuring human contact has been accidentally discovered. Alternatively, the patient may be reassured by an idiosyncratic perception of people or events.

Should acute tension not be allayed in this way, a variety of psychological responses are possible. These depend on the individual's previous life experience and current phenomenological situations. There may be further psychological dissociation with ever increasing anxiety in human contacts. Omnipotent solutions are sought in order to obtain a perception of control of the world and thus to obtain a measure of reassurance. Highly abstract symbolization of reality, magical transfers of blame, or the grandiosity of a paranoid solution may appear.

The theory of stress as a producer of the schizophrenic syndromes fits known psychological theories about the origin of schizophrenia. Furthermore, it does not contradict the concept of possible genetic or biochemical vulnerability as etiologically significant.[18] It also explains why schizophrenia was traditionally described as a deteriorating illness.

Although the reaction varies with age, social class, and the cultural setting of the individual, perceptual disorder produces an idiosyncratic series of social and psychological responses to the communications of others. In their turn, others in contact with the troubled youth respond to the effects of communications which result from his misperception. Thus a feed-back mechanism is produced. For the patient, perceptual distortion produces a reality response which may validate the distortion and/or increase the perception of stress; further distortion may then occur. Thus the concept of process schizophrenia or nuclear schizophrenia can be understood as the result of increasing stress as part of a feedback mechanism. It may well be that adolescents, who were schizophrenic children, have very little competent ego functioning available. The turbulence of puberty then becomes an overwhelming internal stress, and schizophrenia is the resultant adaptation.

Acute schizophrenia may become chronic schizophrenia as a result of inadequate therapeutic intervention. The individual may find himself in an environment which is so sociologically aberrant as to be incomprehensible; the iatrogenic response which then occurs results in chronicity.[43]

A clear differentiation must be drawn between two conditions. On the one hand is the general category of psychosis, which should be looked upon as an alternate state of consciousness characterized by marked regression, fragmentation, and dissolution and capable of rapid reintegration. On the other hand is the specific syndrome of schizophrenia, which should be reserved for those patients, both acute and chronic, where there is evidence of more serious thought disorder. That this differentiation is difficult is confirmed by Masterson's[36] study of adolescent diagnostic problems in which only a third of the patients with acute psychotic confusion presented clear findings of the characteristic syndrome seen in schizophrenic young adults.[28] This consists of thought

disorder, anhedonia, characterological dependency, impairment of competence, and a vulnerable sense of self-regard. Two-thirds initially presented clinical pictures of severe adjustment reactions of psychotic proportions or severe personality disorders. Although at times, a clear differentiation between severe characterological disorder, borderline psychosis, and schizophrenia may be inordinately difficult, further study eventually demonstrated the underlying pathological process.

The age of onset of adolescent schizophrenia appears to confirm the hypothesis that a significant etiological factor is an aberrant series of biochemical responses to stress. Traditionally "dementia praecox" appeared in early adolescence. In the late nineteenth century, this was a time of emotional turmoil, possibly even more intense than now, since pubertal changes were very rapidly followed by a societal demand for adult responsibility. Schizophrenia now typically appears in vulnerable adolescents either towards the end of a high school career, or in the middle stage of adolescence when social and psychological pressures are on the young to begin to behave in an adult fashion through resolution of adolescent tasks.

The clinical course of schizophrenic disorder in adolescents may begin with an acute onset over very few days, or may emerge slowly over a period of weeks or months. The exact nature of the disorder may only slowly be revealed. Masterson[36] reported that only 25 percent of cases in which the eventual diagnosis of schizophrenia was made could be properly labeled at the time of onset.

While psychopathological conditions usually pre-exist in these adolescents, certain events usually precede the precipitation of the psychotic reaction. In some cases, the onset of adult demands, the death of a significant person, or the stress of a heterosexual relationship may precipitate the illness. In some students, it does not appear until the end of a college career.

The onset of labile affective reactions, bizarre behavior, auditory or visual hallucinations, and evidence of thought disorder with suspiciousness, negativism, and persecutory delusions are common first signs of this illness. Psychosomatic complaints of a fixed nature and, at times, frank sexual seductiveness are other manifestations of a growing alteration of consciousness. Schizophrenia may also present with compulsive, delinquent behavior, or as an atypical anorectic pattern.

The disorganization may be of varying degrees of severity. The individual may show very appropriate contact with reality, but severe disorganization with almost complete disregard of reality awareness is not uncommon. This tends to make the diagnostic picture confusing. Disorganized states which immobolize the adolescent in social situations frequently interfere with purposeful action. Feelings of thought scattering, fears of social blundering, and emotional confusion are quite usual. A careful exploration may reveal that such disorganization has been present for several years. Many adolescents are terrified of the implications of the experience of growing alteration of consciousness, particularly while they retain an observing ego. Thus, they may present massive denial of their difficulties to concerned adults and psychiatrists. While the clinical course of adolescent schizophrenia is variable, there is a remarkably homogeneous pattern that tends to be in three phases: acute disorganization, integration, and a less well recognized, but equally important, phase of postpsychotic regression.[9]

ACUTE DISORGANIZATION

The phase of acute disorganization is characterized in many instances by manifestly chaotic behavior, combativeness, agitation, and withdrawal. There is evidence of the use of primitive defenses, particularly splitting. The world appears split and often the bad is characterized as belonging to sinister forces; devils or hallucinatory accusers. Often significant individuals in the life of the adolescent take on the qualities of evil. This may be a reason why acutely schizophrenic adolescents occasionally make impulsive attacks. Some patients temporarily manifest delusions of grandeur or ascribe omnipotence to their therapists or other staff members. The whole world, therefore, becomes a narcissistic extension of the patient. This may result in the reduction of anxiety with increasing emotional investment in the therapeutic milieu.

This increased emotional investment in the environment may eventually lead to an increasing vulnerability with the recognition that the grandiose expectations cannot be met. At this point intense depression and suicidal ideation may appear. The individual characteristically shows feelings of abandonment and vulnerability. In the acute schizophrenic process, as in a more chronic situation, the individual is unable to tolerate separation. Object loss leads to anxiety, depression, and a massive introjection of a sense of guilt.

INTEGRATION

With the reduction of anxiety, there comes an increased ability to receive support from the environment and slow integration occurs. The symptoms begin to disappear in the reverse order of their development. The speed of integration is increased by an appropriate social system, the use of neuroleptics and supportive psychotherapy. The therapy essentially helps clarify reality for the disordered patient.

THE POSTPSYCHOTIC PHASE

This most crucial phase of the illness is not commonly recognized and is thus not properly treated. It consists of a continuation of the regression, but with ongoing, gradual integration, leading eventually to remission. The postpsychotic phase may continue for a period of from three to as long as twelve to eighteen months. This is a period of great vulnerability. Further disorganization may occur if the adolescent is discharged abruptly from the therapeutic situation. In particular, the patient continues to be unable to tolerate separation. This is another common cause for the apparent appearance of a chronic schizophrenic process; this may then be understood as a societal, as well as a medically induced illness.

In the early period of the postpsychotic phase of schizophrenia cognitive and affective distortion may continue, often accompanied by feelings of confusion. Some adolescents commonly talk about feeling "spaced out." Adolescents who have abused drugs often continue to use them. By reproducing the feelings of confusion, they may get some sense of mastery over their own destiny. Adolescents in the postpsychotic phase frequently complain of insomnia, depression, neurasthenia, and show regressive behavior. Affective flattening may still be present. Psychophysiological disturbances are common in this period, in particular nausea, vomiting, diarrhea, headaches, amenorrhea, and various bodily aches and pains. In addition, it should be noted that there may be an increased sensitivity in females to side effects of various medication.

During this period, supportive psychotherapy is crucial. In addition, it is necessary for the adolescent patient to know that the support of a caring network is available, and they may come back into the hospital where they were originally treated for a brief period of time. When this need occurs, the same therapist should be assigned if possible.

The postpsychotic phase is particularly important because of the educational difficulties the adolescent may experience. There are serious problems of attention, and if school systems are not aware of this dilemma, the adolescent may suffer undue stress with resulting rapid regression. Comprehension may be difficult. Concrete thinking seems to predominate, and there are frequent reports of being unable to work or conceptualize. The adolescent frequently withdraws from others and may be found staring into space, apparently daydreaming or hallucinating; when asked about this, the adolescent frequently reports that he feels nothing. A diminished frequency of blinking has been described and, at times, a widening of the palpebral fissures.

The middle period of the postpsychotic phase shows gradual stabilization with the disappearance of insomnia. The adolescent becomes more concerned with appearance, there is an increased ability to concentrate and a clearing of memory. The capacity to discuss the previous acute disorganized state becomes available, and the adolescent now feels safe enough to talk about what has happened. Socialization improves and the adolescent becomes interested in group and heterosexual activities. At this time, adolescents may talk more freely about anxiety, potency, and separation, but many attempt to deny progress and are quite unable to consider the future.

After recovery from the postpsychotic phase, intermittent depression may continue for as long as a year, along with the resumption of premorbid functioning. Developmental turmoil may appear at this time and therapeutic assistance for the patient's family may be required because the patient may now undergo the growth which was not possible in earlier years.

Other Psychoses of Adolescence

Some borderline personality disorders show short psychotic episodes from which reintegration is rapid after removal of the immediate stress. However, some adolescents, who are diagnosed as borderline illness, really suffer from schizophrenia. Such adolescents may experience symptomatic remission of their schizophrenic symptoms and then, when stressed, become acutely schizophrenic again. These patients do well when given neuroleptic medication. Those borderline adolescents, who are not schizophrenic, may have a short

psychotic episode and do not need medication. The differential diagnosis is made on the basis of a repetition of similar psychotic reactions, whatever the stress, and the presence of a thought disorder in the schizophrenics.[32]

Adolescents with borderline illness may have a particular type of transient psychotic episode. Grinker and associates[24] identified a group of borderline patients who do not possess a sense of their own identity and have difficulty in relating to others. The authors found the development of object relationships impaired, and the patients, lonely, depressed, and enraged. While their rage may appear in many behavioral outlets, these are not sufficient to protect them from transient psychotic reactions which are superimposed on inappropriate, nonadaptive, and negative behavior. Masterson[36] describes a long-term study of adolescents who show a wide range of adolescent psychopathology, including transient psychotic episodes under developmental stress. These adolescents have a history of early loss and thus cannot cope with the developmental tasks of the age period.

Adolescents who suffer from chronic handicaps, either organic, intellectual, or emotional, may become psychotic under stress. In particular, when they face developmental tasks which their handicap makes insuperable, the result may take the form of massive regression accompanied by a brief psychotic episode. This psychotic state usually resolves with the reduction of stress. On the other hand, while the psychotic ideation associated with acute identity diffusion may be resolved, the adolescent still needs assistance to develop a cohesive sense of self.

A brief psychotic reaction may also be an early manifestation of affective illness, particularly of the bipolar type. The history of familial affective disorder, absence of thought disorder, and an early history of affective mood swings helps clarify the diagnosis.[13]

Organic Etiologic Factors

Endogenous factors in schizophrenia have been considered extensively in the literature, from the search by early neuropathologists for specific cellular changes to theories of psychotoxins, endocrine aplasias, faulty metabolic breakdowns, aberrant electrical discharges, auto-immune reactions, and lately defects in chemical, genetic, and corticothalamic physiology.[23] Kety[33] has criticized these trends toward explaining schizophrenia in reductionist terms as being highly subjective and experimentally incompletely controlled. These authors, in reviewing current organic theories of schizophrenia, conclude that none explained the disease completely and that psychodynamic factors must still be considered as playing a critical role. Bowers[7] also believes that the alteration of consciousness is owed either to neuro-chemical vulnerability or developmental failures related to prior experiences individually or in the family, or to a combination of these two factors. Lidz[35] explains that in the development of a psychotic process, egocentric cognitive regression occurs and consequently the filtering function of categorical thinking is greatly diminished. These psychological effects are the consequence of the psychoendocrinology of ego disintegration where corticosteroid and epinephrine levels are greatly elevated as part of the response to danger and high catecholamine production and filtration capacities of the reticular activating system are impaired.

Exogenous factors have been extensively studied in a search for neuro-chemical similarities between drug-induced psychodelic states and schizophrenic psychoses. However, as Freedman[15] points out, "History records our increasing urge to cope with dreary reality or dread with the aid of magic, drugs, drama, festival rites, and (with biological regularity) through dreams." Similarly in Erikson's[12] discussions of student problems, he mentions that, while characteristic disturbances occur at each stage of life, these reactions are essentially determined by the life tasks of that stage.

The psychotic reaction induced by toxic infections, trauma, and nutritional stresses may be highly idiosyncratic. Freedman's studies conclude that these exogenous stresses alter brain serotonin metabolism and increase the utilization of norepinephrine. On the other hand, the authors' experiences with adolescents undergoing psychotic episodes from ostensible exogenous causes lead them to conclude that in many cases a definite vulnerability exists which is only emphasized by the immediacy of the stimulation. This multidetermined causal complex should be considered, because the therapeutic approaches to psychotic reactions associated with exogenous stresses must include careful consideration of emotional, as well as mechanical, factors.

Psychodynamic Factors in Adolescent Psychosis

INDIVIDUAL DYNAMICS

Adolescence is a psycho-social process of adaptation during which identity firmly develops and separation-individuation is finally completed. It is not just a transitional period which reworks the conflicts of childhood; it is a significant developmental stage in and of itself. It can be understood both in terms of its internal dynamics, from the viewpoint of ego functions, and also from the viewpoint of psycho-social development.

The dynamic processes normally associated with adolescence are characterized by a loosening of ego structures as a result of pressure from emotional and physiological sources. The goal is to learn to deal with aggressive and libidinal drives. Thus the main task of adolescence is the synthesis of a cohesive ego containing a firm sense of self and capacity to deal comfortably with object relations. By the end of this period the healthy individual knows what and who he or she would like to be. Apart from the resolution of infantile object attachments, the development of a firm sense of self is impossible unless a phenomenological modeling takes place, built on the perception both of other human beings and of the interaction between them. For healthy adolescent development to occur, the presence of parent figures, a peer group, and extra-parental adults of meaningful emotional significance in the life of the young person are all required.

Psychotic adolescents, during the regressive period, may experience any process of identification as involving helpless dependence or humiliating submission to a sadistic, intrusive, controlling figure. Ultimately, the patient may perceive himself as engaged in a futile struggle with an overpowering individual who resembles the image of an attacking, persecutory parent. The adolescent's perceptual distortion of the other person means that the perceived identification models are unsatisfactory whatever they are really like. In addition, the psychotic is so helpless and overwhelmed by the regression that his or her behavior appears unrelated to anything others can do. As a result, the reality responses of others are distorted, and potential identification models become intensely persecutory. The individual perceived by the psychotic adolescent as a hostile attacker may eventually become a persecutor in reality. This reinforces the internalization of persecutory external objects.

This type of interruption of the process of identification helps explain why the adolescent psychotic, who is inadequately treated, has such a grave prognosis. Identification models change their attitudes toward the patient. The interactions between people which are also incorporated into the adolescent personality structure are likely to become pathological as well, resulting in distorted personality development.

FAMILIAL AND INTERPERSONAL

As an outgrowth of studies of communication phenomena, there has been a great deal of interest in the interpersonal and family aspects of schizophrenia. Sullivan[44] saw schizophrenia as related to malignant anxiety which developed as a consequence of disturbed communications early in the life cycle. Further contributors are Artiss[3] who saw schizophrenia as a special communication system, and Beck[5] who wrote that schizophrenia was less a disease than the idiomatic use of a special language to communicate in a grossly disturbed situation.

Within the family unit itself, Bateson and his co-workers[4] have described the "double-bind" form of disturbed communication as a characteristic of schizophrenic families. Wynne[47] worked therapeutically with the parents and siblings of schizophrenics in order to understand the active and actual input from the parents. He found that the family life of schizophrenics operated as a multi-person social system. This system was characterized by pervasive features demonstrating pseudomutuality, stereotyped roles, transactional thought disorders, a trading of dissociations, and shared focal attention. He and Singer[41] found that measures of communication deviances in parents consistently differentiated families with schizophrenic offspring from those with normal, neurotic, or borderline patients. In reviewing the literature on schizophrenia, Grinker[23] concluded that family patterns can be linked to the personality organization of its offspring, and that these patterns are interadaptive along with the social cultural matrix.

Therapeutic Approaches

GENERAL CONSIDERATIONS

Any treatment approach to the psychotic disorders of adolescence depends on various generic factors which influence the process and course of the illness. The prepsychotic personality with its developmental experiences and deficits, both emotional and neurobiological, demands a frame of reference related to the idiosyncrasies of the adolescent and his family. Adolescence creates certain specific stresses and requires particular therapeutic approaches appropriate to the individual, familial, peer, and educational needs of the age. Pubescence, separation, sexual experimentation, and loss experiences, all contribute to the onset of the illness. Separately or together, they serve as the precipitating circumstances for the psychotic reaction and may require enormous modifications in intrapersonal and interpersonal operations. Finally the altered state of consciousness brings with it a degree of destructuring. A typical clinical pattern of central nervous system malfunction follows which requires supportive and pharmacological care related to the protection of the individual's psychic and physical function.

When schizophrenia does appear during puberty, there are specific therapeutic problems. One of these is an aberrant response to tranquilizers. Puberty produces significant endocrinological and biochemical changes which are at their maximum for a period of some three years. During this interval, adolescents do not appear to react, as do adults, to a variety of psycho-pharmacotherapeutic agents, in particular to phenothiazines, amphetamines, and antidepressants.

For example, over a two-year period, a fifteen-year-old schizophrenic girl, who was also diabetic, was treated in the same clinical setting on three separate occasions with adult-adequate doses of phenothiazine. The first two attempts at treatment produced no remission of her psychosis. The first course was given when she was age thirteen, the next one year later, and the final course, nine months later. The last dosage schedule, started when it was apparent that she was approaching physiological maturity, resulted in remission six weeks later.

Psychiatric patients are usually hospitalized because of social problems observed or deduced by others. Most adolescent patients enter hospitals because of difficulties in personal relationships, behavior, or social performance at home, school, or in the community. Some are hospitalized because of behavior actually or potentially dangerous to the self or others, or because of conflicts with the law relating to acting out or drug abuse. Young people, at times, may directly request help from psychiatrists because of the psychic pain involved in disintegrative aspects of the adolescent process.

Compared to the usual practices in the community at large, many psychiatric hospitals have therapeutic social systems which are highly idiosyncratic in their way of life. This may make patients temporarily lose further touch with the reality of their existence. Initially most adolescents perceive hospitalization as sociologically and psychologically threatening. If such a placement is to be therapeutic, it has to take into account all of the special development needs of this age period and of the social and cultural setting from which the patient comes.

Psychotic adolescents experience an acute sense of helplessness which may be overwhelming. In order to deal with their alteration of consciousness, they try to conform to the implicit demands of the environment, which are consistent, rather than to explicit expectations which may be quite variable. Thus it is not unusual for acutely psychotic adolescents to take on a highly conflicted way of life. All adolescents carry on an intense struggle over an unconscious wish to regress. For the schizophrenic, however, a regressive solution is particularly appealing, and hospitalization may enhance its likelihood.

There are two indications for hospital placement of adolescents suffering from acute psychotic reactions: a pathological intra-familial home environment which inhibits all potentiality for growth and emotional support, or unusually serious problems created by the disturbed behavior of the adolescent—dangerousness to the self or others. The duration of hospitalization depends upon its quality; whether the program can meet the treatment needs of the patient; and on the intensity of the personality distortion created in the adolescent by the illness. The therapeutic approach to acute psychotic reactions then demands a proper integration of a sophisticated social system approach to the individual which meets both specific and nonspecific needs, the efficient use of neuroleptics, and adequate psychotherapy.

Adequate treatment of the psychotic syndrome consists of: (1) reducing stress, (2) altering perception of stress by providing emotional support so that the stress, although still perceived, is not felt to be as persecutory, and (3) providing a biochemical dampener to the stress response. Furthermore, since the symptomatic responses of the patient evoke more stress-producing environmental reactions, interruption of this feedback mechanism becomes necessary as the resulting emotional surrender may leave the patient totally helpless.

PSYCHOTHERAPY

Studies of good outcomes of psychotic reactions of adolescence clearly indicate that a positive therapeutic relationship is an important factor in achieving a favorable result. In addition, such a relationship can aid in the formation of a more favorable convalescent environment. These two factors are crucial in long-term recovery, since, beyond the remission of the acute psychotic process, there must be a resolution of the postpsychotic regressive state which occurs in a social context.[31]

In the early stages of the psychotic process, the therapeutic management may allow only for sensitive management of the milieu and the development and preservation of a trusting, supportive relationship. More formal insight-oriented psychotherapy is not usually possible until the psychotic state is in remission, and the regressive phase has been terminated.[30]

While it remains pertinent to inquire whether individual psychotherapy is efficacious and what type of psychotherapy is indicated, Dyrud and Holzman[11] conclude that a plurality of treatment techniques are called for. These may range from behavioral approaches which reduce the ambiguity of the environment to individual psychotherapeutic efforts which put additional stress on the patient and may be employed simultaneously or sequentially.

Certain therapeutic attitudes are particularly helpful in the treatment program. Severely disturbed adolescents need to know that, as far as possible, their therapist will be available to them as long as needed. If hospitalization is indicated, continuity of care should be available both as an inpatient and later as an outpatient. Kayton's study showed that a well-treated schizophrenic episode permitted the patient to continue individuation even after the termination of psychotherapy. Therapy, however, should continue for at least a year following a breakdown and remission.

Separation is a major stress for all individuals. It becomes a destructive one for those who suffer from a psychotic reaction, as they find it almost impossible to work through object loss. While psychotic adolescents also find it difficult to make object attachments, it is possible to dilute the intensity of primitive involvement with others by supplying a network of relationships in which many people provide a supportive, accepting environment. This promotes a feeling of safety without interfering with the individuality of the patient and maximizes the opportunity for influencing outcome.[31] It is all too easy for programs to encourage continued helplessness and not to discourage passivity and withdrawal. Overtly or covertly, such arrangements reject the adolescent, increase the sense of isolation, and help to produce poor results.

A fifteen-year-old girl was admitted to a hospital because of behavior dangerous to herself. She impulsively took an overdose of aspirin, was acutely delusional, and believed that all boys could influence her to become pregnant. In the initial stage of hospitalization, it was established that she had functioned reasonably well at school until the last few weeks of the summer semester when she became increasingly withdrawn. An excellent student, she was particularly interested in dance and music. The suicidal attempt occurred just before the start of the fall semester.

With phenothiazines, the psychotic reaction rapidly remitted, and she began to show an increasing ability to tolerate psychic tension. She started attending the hospital school. An evaluation of her living situation established that with adequate case work the family unit, which had been grossly overprotective, could promote emotional growth and support. While hospitalized, arrangements were made for her to continue to receive lessons from her teachers. Her friends were encouraged to visit her. She attended some classes in the hospital school and some in the local high school. The total duration of hospitalization was eight weeks.

In individual psychotherapy, it became evident that her disturbed behavior, perceptual distortion, and thinking disorder were in response to separation anxiety and attempts to cope with it. The stance of the therapist was to look at the existential cause of her pain rather than to discuss with her the nature of her symptoms or the possible cause of her breakdown. Her therapist's role was to help her in her contact with reality, and she was assured that he would be available to her for a prolonged period if she should require it. Initially, the frequency and duration of the therapist's contact with her depended on her attention span, her apparent inability to carry with her a memory trace (an introject) of her previous contact with him, and the degree of emotional support she seemed to need to help her maintain contact with the real world.

Toward the end of her hospital stay, the therapist saw her twice weekly for extended sessions. In addition, he saw her for a few minutes on other days. At discharge, he arranged to see her twice weekly as an outpatient, and six weeks later, the therapy sessions were reduced to once weekly. Drug treatment was discontinued after four weeks of hospitalization and was not needed thereafter. The content of the discussion with the therapist was designed to soften her self-punitive attitude toward her developing sexuality, to help her feel less guilty about her creative and affective impulses, and help her feel more separate while accepting reasonable support from her family. She was seen in all for a total of three months after she left the hospital. Again, at this time her rather pervasive depression and feeling of not being competent had disappeared.

It does not generally help to offer schizophrenic patients an infinite amount of love. This usually arouses rage. Interpretations may then be met with blank denial, and reality confrontation is likely to produce paranoid ideation. More appropriately, the patient's perception of the self is accepted and understood. An attempt is made to understand the schizophrenic experience as part of a current phenomenological stress. To some extent the patient's harsh self-criticism is taken over by the therapist and modified, but not denied.

This technique takes into account the narcissistic regression of the patient and the extreme omnipotence of his grandiosity. Fearful of closeness, schizophrenic adolescents tend to have poor discrimination between thought and action; they are self-engulfed. The stance which communicates to the patient, "I accept your hallucinatory or confused experience, and I agree with some of the concepts you express, but I will discuss with you what causes you, here and now, to have these experiences," basically reassures the patient that the therapist will not be overwhelmed by the patient's aggression.

A severely regressed, angry, postpubertal fourteen-year-old schizophrenic girl, overwhelmed with primitive sexuality and heavily abusing drugs, was admitted to an inpatient adolescent service. Since infancy, her relationship with her disturbed mother had been of a symbiotic character. For many months her therapist attempted to work with her in an interpretive fashion. She was given adequate doses of phenothiazines with little or no effect. During this phase of her treatment, she saw her parents frequently. Because it was believed that continuous contact with her parents encouraged regression and helped maintain the psychotic defense, her therapist decided to limit her parents' visits and for two months refused to let her see them. Throughout this time, she continued to be grossly psychotic. She was then told she could see her mother for very short periods providing she controlled her expression of angry feelings, attended school, and organized herself. The patient began to improve dramatically, ceased her disorganized psychotic verbalizations and began to integrate. The eventual remission of her psychosis can be understood as a result of her perception of her therapist as unafraid of her rage after she had projected her sense of omnipotence onto him. Once the symptoms remitted, the therapist was seen as a powerful sustaining figure, helping her deal more adequately with separation and individuation. The long-term treatment program envisaged that her hospitalization would not be an encapsulated experience.

Countertransference problems in work with psychotic adolescents are legion; the patients have a need to be cared for and seductively encourage the therapist to look upon them as infants. A therapist can easily incorporate the patient's anxiety, become threatened by the adolescent's aggression, and react in an angry fashion when the patient appears to refuse to get better. Attempts at the onset to engage in intensive psychoanalytic psychotherapy with a psychotic adolescent may be inappropriate. It is recommended that short, supportive sessions be held until adequate remission and resolution of the postpsychotic regression allow more intrusive explorations to occur.

Family and group approaches to the psychotherapeutic treatment of psychotic reactions and schizophrenia are valuable ancillary supports. Characteristic disturbances of communication are found, which are adaptive responses to the presence of a highly pathological individual in the group or family. These double-bind communications result in pseudo-mutual family structures which keep the pathological defense systems operating. Group and family therapeutic approaches should be considered as part of the overall effort to deal with these serious disorders of adolescence.

Psychopharmacological Approaches

Treatment of psychotic disorders has been revolutionized by the introduction of psychotropic drugs. While the discovery of the effectiveness of chlorpromazine led to the development of an entirely new approach, with extensive scientific expansion of psychopharmacology, unrealistic hopes for the cure of serious mental illness have not been realized.[46] However, as part of a total approach to the treatment of psychotic reactions of adolescence, the use of neurotropic drugs is essential.

Because of the lack of scientific studies, there is no evidence that the use of psychotropic drugs is more effective in schizophrenic children and adolescents than other types of approaches, singly or combined.[8] In addition, the rapidly changing physiology and emotional states during puberty and adolescence make the effects of particular pharmacologic agents highly unreliable. At best, powerful neuroleptics result in various side effects which are tolerated in order to achieve maximal results. The adolescent, however, may not always cooperate because of feelings of being externally controlled. Moreover, the frequent side effects may cause intolerable anxiety. For example, the muscle splinting action of the phenothiazines may lead the adolescent to feel restrained, or males on piperazines may experience impotence and

failure to ejaculate. Such identity and body image crises contribute to the difficulties in using neurotropic drugs in adolescents.

In spite of these difficulties, during the acute phase of the altered state of consciousness and the postpsychotic stages, drug treatment is indicated in the overall treatment plan. The following medications have been useful in adolescents.[42]

PHENOTHIAZINES

Phenothiazines are the most common drugs used in the treatment of schizophrenia. They include:

Aliphatics (chlorpromazine, promazine, triflupromazine); and piperidines (thioridazine, piperacetazine, mesoridazine): Chlorpromazine (Thorazine) was the first drug used in the treatment of schizophrenia in adolescents, and reports of its use have appeared in the literature for over twenty-five years. Outside of the United States, it remains one of the most common drugs used in this age group.

The piperadines, in particular thioridazine (Mellaril), are particularly effective for agitation, hallucinations, and delusions. They also are useful in treating those adolescents who show obvious signs of depression in association with the schizophrenic process.

Side effects with the phenothiazines are common. With chlorpromazine and thioridazine, drowsiness, apathy, lethargy, or somnolence are frequent, even with low doses. Individuals should be warned about the possible side effects as well as the possibility of allergic reactions which are not uncommon. Occasionally lens-stippling has occurred in patients whose chlorpromazine intake was relatively moderate. Benign side effects include fatigue and dry mouth. More serious side effects include leucopenia, jaundice, and dystonia. There is, however, a lack of information about the appearance of side effects, as to how much is a result of dose, age, and sex. In general, it would appear that the side effects are not related to dosage or age. The dosage must be carefully regulated so that learning processes are not inhibited but, at the same time, a therapeutic result is achieved. Daily interviews to determine the dosage effect, answer questions, and allay anxiety are particularly necessary in treatment of the teenager.

Piperazines (fluphenazine, perphenazine, trifluoperazine, acetophenazine, proclorperazine, carphenazine, butaperazine): The most commonly used piperazine in adolescents is trifluoperazine

(Stelazine). This drug seldom produces drowsiness or motor inhibition and only in isolated instances has it been reported to induce seizures. However, although dystonic reactions are rare even with high doses, extrapyramidal symptoms are noted; these include oculogyric crisis, akathisia, and head and neck dystonias. These quickly respond to anti-parkinsonism drugs (benztropine). These agents should not be continued indefinitely, but the dosage of tranquilizer should be reduced.[22]

BUTYROPHENONES

Haloperidol and triperidol are among the butyrophenones most commonly used. Haloperidol (Haldol) is a potent antipsychotic agent with a low incidence of side effects (dystonia). It is particularly useful in the treatment of adolescent psychoses, especially in those young people who show excessive hyperactivity. There are some reports that haloperidol is better than chlorpromazine in reducing impulsiveness, hostility, and aggressiveness. It is said not to produce the drowsiness and lethargy which interfere with learning, but high doses may result in side effects such as drowsiness, dystonic reactions, and muscle spasm.

OTHER AGENTS

Thioxanthenes (chlorprothixene, thiothixene): These two drugs, chlorprothixene (Taractan) and thiothixene (Navane) are reported to be useful in treatment of those adolescents who show signs of psychomotor retardation by providing stimulation along with antipsychotic properties. They are less likely to produce hematopoetic, liver damage, or photosensitivity reactions.[8]

Dihydroindolones (Molindone): Molindone (Moban) is a psychotropic with some characteristics of an antidepressant. Campbell[8] reports that with the exception of extra-pyramidal side effects, it has fewer untoward reactions than aliphatic and piperidine phenothiazines.

REFERENCES

1. American Psychiatric Association, Committee on Nomenclature and Statistics, Unpublished Draft, *Diagnostic and Statistical Manual of Mental Disorders*, 3rd ed., (DSM-III), American Psychiatric Association, Washington, D.C., 1978.
2. American Psychiatric Association, Committee on Nomenclature and Statistics, *Diagnostic and Statistical Manual of Mental Disorders*, 2nd ed., (DSM-II), American Psychiatric Association, Washington, D.C., 1968.
3. ARTISS, K. L., *The Symptom as Communication in Schizophrenia*, Grune & Stratton, New York, 1959.
4. BATESON, G., et al., "Toward a Theory of Schizophrenia," *Behavioral Science*, 1:251–264, 1956.
5. BECK, S. J., *Psychological Processes in the Schizophrenic Adaptation*, Grune & Stratton, New York, 1965.
6. BLEULER, E., *Dementia Praecox or the Group of Schizophrenias*, International Universities Press, New York, 1950.
7. BOWERS, B. B., *Retreat from Sanity*, Human Sciences Press, New York, 1974.
8. CAMPBELL, M., "Treatment of Childhood and Adolescent Schizophrenia," in Wiener, J. M. (Ed.), *Psychopharmacology in Childhood and Adolescence*, Basic Books, New York, 1977.
9. DONLON, P. T., and BLACKER, K. H., "Stages of Schizophrenic Decompensation and Reintegration," *Journal of Nervous and Mental Diseases*, 157:200–209, 1973.
10. DONLON, P. T., RADA, R. T., and ARORA, K. K., "Depression and the Reintegration Phase of Acute Schizophrenia," *American Journal of Psychiatry*, 133(11):1265–1268, 1976.
11. DYRUD, J. E., and HOLZMAN, P. S., "The Psychotherapy of Schizophrenia: Does It Work?" *American Journal of Psychiatry*, 130(6):670–673, 1973.
12. ERIKSON, E., *Identity: Youth and Crisis*, W. W. Norton, New York, 1968.
13. FEINSTEIN, S. C., "Diagnostic and Therapeutic Aspects of Manic-Depressive Illness in Early Childhood," *Early Child Development and Care*, 3:1–12, 1973.

14. ———, "Adjustment Reaction of Adolescence," in Freedman, A. M., Kaplan, H. I., and Sadock, B. J. (Eds.), *Comprehensive Textbook of Psychiatry II*. Williams & Wilkins, Baltimore, 1975.
15. FREEDMAN, D. X., "On the Use and Abuse of LSD," in Feinstein, S., Giovacchini, P., and Miller, A. (Eds.), *Adolescent Psychiatry*, Basic Books, New York, 1971.
16. FRENCH, T. M., and KASANIN, J., "A Psychodynamic Study of the Recovery of Two Schizophrenic Cases," *Psychoanalytic Quarterly*, 10:1–22, 1941.
17. FREUD, A., "Adolescence," in Eissler, R. S., et al. (Eds.), *Psychoanalytic Study of the Child*, vol. 13, pp. 255–278, International Universities Press, New York, 1958.
18. FROHMAN, C. E., BECKETT, P. G. S., and GRISELL, J. L., "Biologic Responsiveness to Environmental Stimuli in Schizophrenia," *Comprehensive Psychiatry*, 7(6):494–500, 1966.
19. GARDNER, G. E., "Psychiatric Problems of Adolescence," in Arieti, S. (Ed.), *American Handbook of Psychiatry*, Basic Books, New York, 1959.
20. GELEERD, E. R., "Some Aspects of Ego Vicissitudes in Adolescence," *Journal of the American Psychoanalytic Association*, 9:934–405, 1961.
21. GITELSON, M., "Character Synthesis: Psychotherapeutic Problems of Adolescence," *Journal of the American Orthopsychiatric Association*, 14:422, 1948.
22. GOODMAN, L. S., and GILMAN, A., *The Pharmacological Basis of Therapeutics*, Macmillan, New York, 1970.
23. GRINKER, R. R., SR., "An Essay on Schizophrenia and Science," *Archives of General Psychiatry*, 20:1–24, 1969.
24. ———, WERBLE, B., and DRYE, R. C., *The Borderline Syndrome*, Basic Books, New York, 1968.
25. Group for the Advancement of Psychiatry, Committee on Child Psychiatry, *Psychopathological Disorders in Childhood: Theoretical Considerations and a Proposed Classification*, Jason Aronson, New York, 1974.

26. HECKER, E., "Die Hebephrenie," *Virchows' Archives of Pathological Anatomy, 52:*394–429, 1871.

27. HENDERSON, A. S., KRUPENSKI, J., and STOLLER, A., "Epidemiological Aspects of Adolescent Psychiatry," in Howells, J. C. (Ed.), *Modern Perspectives in Adolescent Psychiatry*, Brunner-Mazel, New York, 1971.

28. HOLZMAN, P., and GRINKER, R. R., SR., "Schizophrenia in Adolescence," in Feinstein, S. C., and Giovacchini, P. L. (Eds.), *Adolescent Psychiatry*, Jason Aronson, New York, 1977.

29. JACKSON, D. D., and WATZLAWICK, P., "The Acute Psychosis as a Manifestation of Growth Experience," in Mendel, W. M., and Epstein, L. J. (Eds.), *Acute Psychotic Reaction*, Psychiatric Research Reports, American Psychiatric Association, Washington, D.C., 1963.

30. KAYTON, L., "Good Outcome in Young Adult Schizophrenia," *Archives of General Psychiatry, 29:*103–110, 1973.

31. ———, BECK, J., and KOH, S. D., "Postpsychotic State, Convalescent Environment, and Therapeutic Relationship in Schizophrenic Outcome," *American Journal of Psychiatry, 133(11):*1269–1274, 1976.

32. KERNBERG, O., "The Diagnosis of Borderline Conditions in Adolescence," in Feinstein, S., and Giovacchini, P. (Eds.), *Adolescent Psychiatry*, University of Chicago Press, Chicago, 1978.

33. KETY, S. S., "Biochemical Theories of Schizophrenia," *International Journal of Psychiatry, 1:*179–200, 1967.

34. KRAEPELIN, E., (1904), *Lectures on Clinical Psychiatry*, Hafner, New York, 1968.

35. LIDZ, T., "Foreword," in Bowers, M. B., Jr. (Ed.), *Retreat from Sanity*, Human Sciences Press, New York, 1974.

36. MASTERSON, J. F., JR., *The Psychiatric Dilemma of Adolescence*, Little, Brown, Boston, 1967.

37. MAYER-GROSS, W., SLATER, E., and ROTH, M., *Clinical Psychiatry*, 3rd ed., Williams & Wilkins, Baltimore, 1969.

38. MENNINGER, K., *The Vital Balance*, Viking Press, New York, 1963.

39. MILLER, D., "An Approach to the Social Rehabilitation of Chronic Psychotic Patients," *Psychiatry, 17:*347–358, 1954.

40. MOSHER, L. R., and FEINSILVER, D., *Special Report on Schizophrenia*, United States Department of Health, Education, and Welfare, Washington, D.C., 1970.

41. SINGER, M. T., "Family Transactions and Schizophrenia: 1. Recent Research Findings," *Excerpta Medica International, 151:*147–164, 1967.

42. SOLOW, R. A., "Child and Adolescent Psychopharmacology in the Mid-Seventies," *Psychiatry Digest*, October: 15–38, 1976..

43. STAINBROOK, E., "Toward a Theoretical Model of the Determinants of Acute Schizophrenic Behavior," in Mandel, W., and Epstein, L. J. (Eds.), *Acute Psychotic Reaction*, Psychiatric Research Reports, American Psychiatric Association, Washington, D.C., 1963.

44. SULLIVAN, H. S., *Schizophrenia as a Human Process*, W. W. Norton, New York, 1962.

45. VAN KREVELEN, D. A., "Psychoses in Adolescence," in Howells, J. G. (Ed.), *Modern Perspectives in Adolescent Psychiatry*, pp. 381–403, Brunner-Mazel, New York, 1971.

46. World Health Organization, "Psychotropic Drugs and Mental Illness," *WHO Chronicle, 30:*420–424, 1976.

47. WYNNE, L. C., "Family Transactions and Schizophrenia, II Conceptual Considerations for a Research Strategy," *Excerpta Medica International, 151:*165–178, 1967.

NAME INDEX

SUBJECT INDEX

Abandonment, 208

Abdominal pain, 365

Aberration, definition of, 545

Abortion, 368; habitual, 366

Abstract thought, 186

Abstraction, 419

Abused children, 21, 78, 588–590; failure to thrive syndrome among, 594, 596

Academic retardation, 52; *see also* Learning disorders

Accident proneness, 637–642; definition and description of, 637; developmental level and, 640–641; frequency, incidence and prevalence of, 638–639; genetic and constitutional factors in, 640; history of concept of, 638; intelligence and, 640; prevention of, 641–642

Acetophenazine, 720

Acne, 353

Acting out: in anorexia nervosa, 574; depression masked by, 327; in pica, 663; *see also* Behavior disorders

Action orientation, regional trait of, 89

Activity group therapy, 230

Actual neurosis, 197; hypochondriacal, 200–201

Acute brain syndromes, 382–384

Acute confusional state, 136, 138, 711–712

Acute depressive reaction, 327–329, 331, 333

Acute identity diffusion, 15

Acute illness, reactive disorders provoked by, 182

Acute school phobia, 215

Adaptation, 25–26; behavioral disorders of, 106; principles of, 7–14

Addiction, 601

Addictive behavior: pica and, 664; *see also* Substance abuse

Adjustment disorders, classification of, 131

Adjustment reaction, distinction between reactive disorders and, 174

Adolescent asceticism, 11

Adolescent disorders, classification of, 120

Adolescent enuresis, 554

Adolescent psychosis, 708–721; acute confusion type, 711–712; borderline syndrome and, 715;

clinical course of, 711; epidemiology of, 710–711; organic etiologic factors in, 715–716; psychodynamic factors in, 716–717; psychopharmacological approaches to, 720–721; schizophrenic type, 712–715; therapeutic approaches to, 717–720

Adoption: of neglected children, 583; family romance and, 25; identity formation and, 14; object loss and, 16

Adoption studies: of anorexia nervosa, 573; of hyperkinesis, 445; of minimal brain dysfunction syndrome, 429

Adrenal insufficiency, 656

Affect, integration of thought and, 161

Affect-meaning zone, 102, 105

Affective development, 104; deviations in, 186, 188, 190

Affective disorders: classification of, 117; hyperkinesis and, 445; in psychosis, 255; *see also* Depression

Affective tone, familial, 74–75

Aggression: alienation and, 14; anatomic basis of, in organic brain syndrome, 398; in anorexia nervosa, 576, 578; anxiety and, 201; in behavior disorders, 483; in borderline syndrome, 306, 309, 310, 313, 317; in cruelty to animals, 504; depression and, 205, 327; in encopresis, 559; in enuresis, 548; of epileptics, 389; in firesetting, 508; gender differences in, 35; Gilles de la Tourette's syndrome and, 680; in Klinefelter's syndrome, 397; masturbation and, 706; in oppositional personality, 243–244; in overly inhibited personality, 245; pica and, 663; precocious, 20–21; in psychophysiologic respiratory disorders, 357; in schizophrenia, 282; school phobia and, 454; sleep disorders and, 647–648; sound production and, 469, 471; sublimation of, 13; suicide and, 687; in theories of neurosis, 221; turned against self, 12; in vandalism, 502, 503

Aggressor, identification with, 13, 19; emotional deprivation and, 16

Agnosia, 151

Agoraphobia, 456

Akathisia, 385

Akinesia, 385

Alcohol abuse, 605–615; Alcoholics Anonymous for treatment of, 613, 614; anorexia nervosa and, 575; diseases resulting from, 606–607; epidemiology of, 608–609; family and, 609–610; heroin abuse associated with, 619; historical notes on, 605; incarceration and, 614–615; parenting dysfunction and, 591; among parents of hyperkinetic children, 56; pharmacological effects in, 605–606; phenomenology of, 609; pitfalls to progress in treatment of, 612; potential for, 608; residential treatment for, 614; short term physiological effects of, 606; social consequences of, 609; therapeutic considerations in treatment of, 611–612; tolerance and dependence in, 607

Alcoholics Anonymous, 613–614

Alexander's disease, 396

Alienation, 14; humanistic socialist concept of, 221

Aliphatics, 720

Allergic rhinitis, 356

Allergies: in asthma, 357; hyperkinesis caused by, 447; minimal brain dysfunction syndrome and, 435

Alloplastic behavior, 236

Alopecia, 353

Alper's disease, 396

Altered consciousness: in conversion hysteria, 202; in dissociative hysteria, 204; drug-induced, *see* Hallucinogens

Amaurotic family idiocies, 396

Ambivalent coexistence, 208

Amblyopia, 372, 373

Amenorrhea, 366–368; in anorexia nervosa, 570, 573, 576; in pseudocyesis, 370

American Group Psychotherapy Association, 230

American Psychiatric Association: Diagnostic and Statistical Manual of, *see* Diagnostic and Statistical Manual; referendum on homosexuality in, 166

American Psychoanalytic Association, 705

Epileptic delirium, 382–383, 388
Epileptic insanity, 207
Epinephrine, 348
Episodic behavior disorders, 138
Epistaxis, 360
Equanil, 617
Erections, frequent, 366
Ergot alkaloids, 623
Erotogenic zones, psychological significance of, 10
Erythromelalgia, 360
Essential hypertension, 361
Ethchlorvynol, 617
Ethological concepts of attachment, 324
Ethosuccinimide, adverse neurological reaction to, 384
Euphoria, 186; drug-induced, 610, 620, 621, 625, 627, 631
Excessive urination, organic causes of, 547
Exhibitionism, 11; precocity and, 20–21
Existentialists, 22
Expelling, transactional mode of, 223
Experimental child psychology, 101
Experimental method in learning theory, 100
Experimental neuroses, 198
Exploitation, 586–588
Explosive speech, 151
Extended family: behavior disorders and, 522–523; school phobia and, 461
Externalization, in school phobia, 454, 458
Externalizers, 212–213
Externalizing-internalizing behavior, 210–211
"Externalizing" symptoms, 150
Extinction, 102, 103
Extrafamilial relationships, development of, 67, 70
Eye contact, avoidance of, in psychosis, 254
Eye injury, 372

Factitious disorders, classification of, 117
Factor analysis in diagnosis, 113; of neurosis, 210
Fading, 103
Failure to thrive syndrome, 9–10, 78, 364, 593–598; criteria for diagnosis of, 594; deprivation and, 585; developmental approach to, 159, 162; familial factors in, 596–597; history of, 593; identification of, 593; incidence of, 594; mechanisms of growth failure in, 594–595; neglect resulting in, 583; prognosis in, 597–598; psychodynamic factors in, 595; treatment of, 597

Familial dysautonomia, 345–346
Familial psychodynamic factors: in adolescent psychosis, 717; in asthma, 358–360; in behavior disorders, 518–523; brain damage and, 50–51; cerebral palsy and, 391–392; in compulsive personality, 238; in conversion hysteria, 203; in cross-gender-role behavior, 535–536; cruelty to animals and, 504; defiance and disobedience and, 511; in depression, 323, 333–335; in developmental deviation, 192–193; diagnostic categories and, 113; in eating disorders, 82–83; in elective mutism, 478, 480; in encopresis, 564; in failure to thrive syndrome, 596–597; firesetting and, 508, 509; in Gilles de la Tourette's syndrome, 680; hyperkinesis and, 441, 447–448, 450–451; in hypochondriasis, 200; in hysterical personality, 240; lying and, 507; mental retardation and, 406–408; minimal brain dysfunction and, 424–426; neuroses and, 223–224; in obsessional neurosis, 205; in overly independent personality, 245–246; in overly inhibited personality, 244–245; in pica, 664; provocative behavior and, 510; in psychophysiologic disorders, 351–352; in psychosis, 274; in schizophrenia, 278–280; in school phobias, 216, 460–461; sexual assault and, 505; stealing and, 493–494, 496–497; in transsexualism, 541, 544; in trichotillomania, 704; vandalism and, 503; see also Mother-child relationship; Parenting disorders
Familial retardation, 408
Familism, 90; pathogenesis related to, 92–93; stabilizing influence of, 95–96
Familization therapy, 614
Family, 62–84; affective tone of, 74–75; basic functions of, 64–68; consequences of alcoholism in, 609–610; definition of, 64; delinquent, 80–81; disturbances in separation processes of, 76; finances-employment function of, 65–66; health function of, 66; homeostasis of, 76; identity and myth in, 76–77; incestuous, 80–82; in Jungian therapy, 228; life cycle of, 64, 68–74; motor activity level of, 74; multi-problem, 82; psychopathological disturbances in functioning of, 78–84; see also Parenting disorders; of runaways, 500; with schizophrenic member, 79–80; shelter-housing function of, 65; sociali-

zation and enculturation functions of, 67–68; studies of, 166; supplies-food function of, 65; treatment implications for disturbances in, 83–84, see also Family therapy; Familial psychodynamic factors
Family romance, 25
Family secrets, 25
Family therapy, 230; for anorexia nervosa, 578–579; for behavior disorders, 525; for school phobia, 463
Fantasy: in anorexia nervosa, 573, 574, 576; in borderline syndrome, 306, 309, 310, 314–315, 318–319; constitutional sensitivity to, 5–6; in depression, 330–332; disturbances of parenting and, 16, 18; in encopresis, 559, 563; in enuresis, 548; in family romance, 25; in firesetting, 509; in isolated personality, 246; in masturbation, 705–706; in neurosis, 214; object loss and, 16; in perversion, 545; in psychosis, 254; in school phobia, 458; sexual assault and, 505; stealing and, 496; in thumb sucking, 699; suicide and, 687
Fantasy lying, 507
Farber's disease, 396
Fastidiousness, levels of, behavior disorders and, 39, 41
Fatalism, regional trait of, 89
Fatty-acids, 294
Fatty liver, 607
Febry's disease, 396
Federal Bureau of Narcotics and Dangerous Drugs, 628
Feeding disorders, see Eating disorders
Feeling-orientation, regional, 96
Femininity, disorders of, see Gender disorders
Fenfluramine, 632
Fernald School, 404
Fever: delirium in, 382; recurrent, 370
Fetishism, 541
Fetus: cardiovascular functioning in, 360; nourishment of, 374
"Fight or flight" reaction, 345
Figure drawing analysis of encopretics, 559
Finances-employment function of family, 65–66, 68, 69
Fine motor disability, 420
Firesetting, 508–510
First Week Evaluation Scale (FES), 37
Fixation, 10–11; grief and, 22; in school phobia, 458; resulting from seduction, 23; see also Anal fixation; Oedipal fixation; Oral fixation
Flooding, 17, 226–227